Core Concepts in Pharmacology

FIFTH EDITION

Leland Norman Holland, Jr., PhD
Professor
Hillsborough Community College, Brandon, Florida, and
Polk State College,
Lakeland, Florida

Michael Patrick Adams, PhD, RT(R)
Adjunct Professor of Biological Sciences
Hillsborough Community College and
Pasco-Hernando State College, Florida
Formerly Dean, Health Professions
Pasco-Hernando State College

Jeanine Lynn Brice, RN, MSN
Adjunct Professor of Biological Sciences/Health Sciences
Saint Petersburg College and Hillsborough Community College, Florida
Former Professor of Nursing
Pasco-Hernando Community College,
New Port Richey, Florida

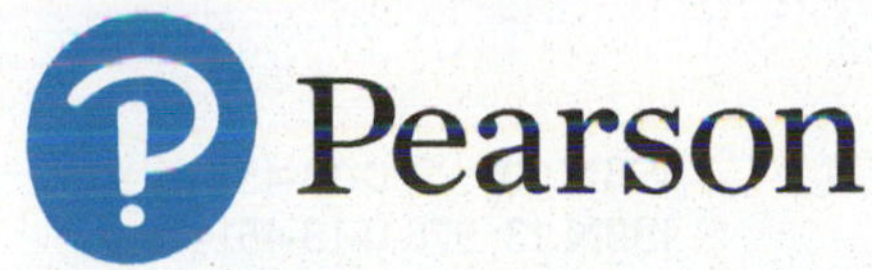
Pearson

330 Hudson Street, New York, NY 10030

Publisher: Julie Levin Alexander
Portfolio Manager: Pamela Fuller
Editorial Assistant: Erin Sullivan
Managing Content Producer: Melissa Bashe
Content Producer: Michael Giacobbe
Development Editor: Teri Zak
Cover and Interior Designer: Mary Siener
Vice President of Sales and Marketing: David Gesell
Vice President, Director of Marketing: Margaret Waples
Senior Product Marketing Manager: Phoenix Harvey
Director, Digital Studio: Amy Peltier
Full Service Vendor: iEnergizer Aptara®, Ltd.
Full-Service Project Management: Joy Deori, iEnergizer Aptara®, Ltd.
Cover Printer: Phoenix Color/Hagerstown
Printer/Binder: LSC Communications

Notice: The authors and the publisher of this volume have taken care to make certain that the doses of drugs and schedules of treatment are correct and compatible with the standards generally accepted at the time of publication. Nevertheless, as new information becomes available, changes in treatment and in the use of drugs become necessary. The reader is advised to carefully consult the instruction and information material included in the package insert of each drug or therapeutic agent before administration. This advice is especially important when using, administering, or recommending new and infrequently used drugs. The authors and publisher disclaim all responsibility for any liability, loss, injury, or damage incurred as a consequence, directly or indirectly, of the use and application of any of the contents of this volume.

A Note About Nursing Diagnoses: Nursing diagnoses in this text are taken from Herdman, T.H. & Kamitsuru, S. (Eds.), *Nursing Diagnoses: Definitions & Classification* 2015–2017. Copyright © 2014, 1994–2014 NANDA International. Used by arrangement by John Wiley & Sons, Inc. Companion website: www.wiley.com/go/nursingdiagnoses.

In order to make safe and effective judgments using NANDA-I nursing diagnoses it is essential that nurses refer to the definitions and defining characteristics of the diagnoses listed in this work.

Library of Congress Cataloging-in-Publication Data
Holland, Leland Norman.
Core concepts in pharmacology / Leland Norman Holland, Jr., Michael Patrick Adams, Jeanine Brice. — Fifth edition.
p. ; cm.
Includes bibliographical references and index.
ISBN-13: 978-0-13-451416-1
ISBN-10: 0-13-451416-5
I. Adams, Michael, (date) author. II. Brice, Jeanine, author. III. Title.
[DNLM: 1. Pharmacological Phenomena. 2. Drug Therapy. QV 37]
RM301.14
615′.1—dc23

2013042150

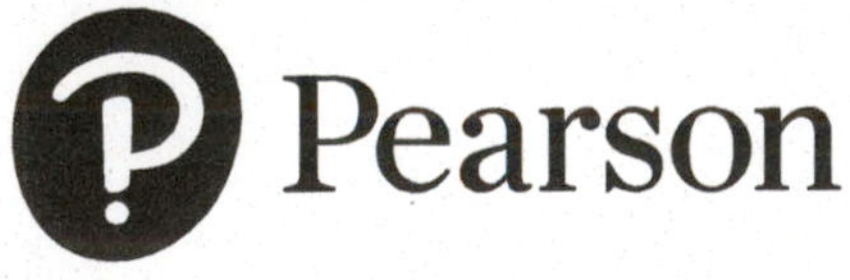

ISBN 10: 0-13-451416-5
ISBN 13: 978-0-13-451416-1

30 2021

Preface

Pharmacology is one of the most challenging subjects for those embarking on careers in the health sciences. By its very nature, pharmacology is an interdisciplinary subject, borrowing concepts from a wide variety of the natural and applied sciences. Prediction of drug action, the ultimate goal in the study of pharmacology, requires a thorough knowledge of anatomy, physiology, chemistry, and pathology as well as of the social sciences of psychology and sociology. It is the interdisciplinary nature of pharmacology that makes the subject difficult to learn, but fascinating to study.

This text presents pharmacology from an interdisciplinary perspective. The text draws upon core concepts of anatomy, physiology, and pathology to make drug therapy understandable. The text does not assume that the student comes to the course with a strong background in the natural or applied sciences. Instead, the prerequisite science knowledge necessary for understanding drug therapy is reviewed in each chapter that presents the core concepts in pharmacology.

Organization

The authors use numbered core concepts, a concise means of communicating to the student the most important pharmacologic information. These core concepts are stated at the beginning of each chapter, so that the student can get an overview of what is to be learned. They are repeated at the end of the chapter, with a brief summary of each important concept.

Disease and Body System Approach

Core Concepts in Pharmacology is organized according to body systems and diseases. The framework places the drugs in the context of how they are used therapeutically. This makes it easy for the student to locate all relevant anatomy, physiology, pathology, and pharmacology in the same chapter in which the drugs are discussed.

Prototype Approach to Drug Therapy

The vast number of drugs taught in a pharmacology course is staggering. To facilitate learning, this text highlights one or two most representative drugs in each classification as prototypes and introduces them in detail. **Prototype Drug** boxes showcase these important medications.

Focused Nursing Content

This text provides focused nursing content, allowing students quick access to essential content for safe, effective drug therapy. **Nursing Process Focus** charts provide a succinct, easy-to-read view of the most commonly prescribed drug classes. Need-to-know nursing actions are presented in a format that reflects the "flow" of the nursing process: nursing assessment, potential nursing diagnoses, planning, interventions (including patient education and discharge planning), and evaluation. Rationales for interventions are included in parentheses. The Nursing Process Focus charts clearly identify what nursing actions are most important.

New to this Edition

- **NEW CHAPTER!** *Preventing Medication Errors* recognizes the critical role of healthcare providers in contributing to safe medication practices.
- **NEW FEATURE!** *Drug Focus* boxes cover new and emerging drugs.
- **NEW FEATURE!** *Lifespan and Diversity* margin features address variations in nursing care based on patient age and disease or disorder.
- **UPDATED AND REVISED!** All drugs have been updated and prototypes adjusted to reflect modern drug usage.
- **UPDATED AND REVISED!** *Safety Alert* features throughout the text call attention to medication errors and The Joint Commission safety guidelines.
- **UPDATED AND REVISED!** End-of-chapter **NCLEX-PN®-style questions completely revised**. Complete rationales and NCLEX tagging are provided in an appendix.
- **UPDATED!** *Glossary* provided with definitions of all key terms.
- **COMPLETELY REVISED!** The *Nursing Process Focus* charts reflect current nursing practice.

DESIGN AND FEATURES

Focus on Core Information

The numbered **Core Concepts** identify ideas and provide an overview of the chapter.

Chapter 22

Drugs for Shock and Anaphylaxis

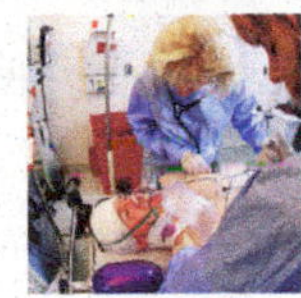

"Where am I? What happened? I really hurt."
Mr. Joshua Hanks

Core Concepts

22.1 Shock is a syndrome characterized by the collapse of the circulatory system.
22.2 The initial treatment of shock includes basic life support and identification of the underlying cause.
22.3 Intravenous fluid replacement drugs are given to replace fluids lost during shock.
22.4 Vasoconstrictors are administered during shock to raise and maintain blood pressure.
22.5 Inotropic drugs are useful in reversing the decreased cardiac output that occurs during shock.
22.6 Anaphylaxis is a type of shock caused by a hyper-response of body defense mechanisms.

Drug Snapshot

The following drugs are discussed in this chapter:

Drug Classes	Prototype Drugs
Fluid replacement drugs	Pr normal serum albumin (Albuminar, Plasbumin, others)
Vasoconstrictors	Pr norepinephrine (Levophed)
Inotropic drugs	Pr dopamine (Intropin)
Drug for anaphylaxis	Pr epinephrine (Adrenalin)

The **Drug Snapshot** provides an at-a-glance list of the drug classes and related prototype drugs covered in each chapter.

Key Terms

anaphylactic (ann-ah-fuh-LAK-tick) shock
antigen (ANN-tuh-jen)
cardiogenic shock (kar-dee-oh-JEN-ik)
colloids (KO-loyds)
crystalloids (KRIS-tuh-loyds)
hypovolemic shock (high-poh voh-LEEM-ik)
inotropic drug (eye-noh-TROW-pik)
neurogenic shock (nyoor-oh-JEN-ik)
septic shock (SEP-tik)
shock

Key Terms help students review important vocabulary terms.

Concept Reviews are questions placed strategically throughout the chapter to stimulate student comprehension and retention as they read.

CONCEPT REVIEW 22.2

- How can inotropic drugs reduce the symptoms of shock without causing vasoconstriction?

Prototype Approach

The prototype approach introduces the one or two most representative drugs in each classification in detail. **Prototype Drug** boxes highlight these important drugs.

The **Black Box Warning** element identifies extremely adverse drug reactions associated with the use of a particular drug.

Prototype Drug: Pr *Norepinephrine (Levophed)*
Therapeutic Class: Drug for shock **Pharmacologic Class: Sympathomimetic, vasoconstrictor**

Actions and Uses: Norepinephrine is indicated for acute hypotension, septic shock, and cardiac arrest. It acts directly on alpha-adrenergic receptors in the smooth muscle of blood vessels to immediately raise blood pressure. Its stimulation of $beta_1$-receptors in the heart increases the force of contraction and increases cardiac output. It is given by the IV route and has a duration of only 1 to 2 minutes after the infusion is terminated.

Adverse Effects and Interactions: Norepinephrine is a powerful vasoconstrictor; thus, continuous monitoring of blood pressure is required to prevent the development of hypertension. When first administered, reflex bradycardia is sometimes experienced. It also has the ability to produce various types of dysrhythmias.

Because of its potent effects on the ca
should be used with great caution in pati
Norepinephrine interacts with many
and beta blockers, which may decrea
pressure. Conversely, ergot alkaloids a
sants may increase vasopressor effects.

BLACK BOX WARNING:
Following extravasation, the affected a
trated immediately with 5–10 mg of ph
adrenergic blocker.

Table 22.3 Vasoconstrictors and Inotropic Drugs for Shock

Drug	Rate and Adult Dose	Remarks
digoxin (Lanoxin, Lanoxicaps) (see the Prototype Drug box in Core Concept 20.7)	IV: digitalizing dose 2.5–5 mcg every 6 hours for 24 hours; maintenance dose 0.125–0.5 mg/day	Doses are highly individualized for each patient; also for dysrhythmias and heart failure
dobutamine (Dobutrex)	IV: infused at a rate of 0.5–15 mcg/kg/min (max: 40 mcg/kg/min)	Selective to $beta_1$-adrenergic receptors; for cardiac decompensation
Pr dopamine (Intropin)	IV: 2–5 mcg/kg/min initial dose; may be increased to 20–50 mcg/kg/min	May activate dopaminergic, $beta_1$- or $alpha_1$-adrenergic receptors, depending on dose
Pr epinephrine (Adrenalin)	Subcutaneous: 0.1–0.5 mL of 1;100 every 10–15 min; IV: 0.1–0.25 mL of 1:1000 every 10–15 min	Nonselective adrenergic drug; available by other routes for cardiac arrest and asthma and as an adjunct to local anesthesia
isoproterenol (Isuprel)	IV: 0.02-0.06 mg bolus followed by 5mcg/min infusion	Nonselective beta-adrenergic drug; also to reverse acute bronchospasm caused by anesthesia

Drug tables provide the most important information for each drug in a user-friendly format. Drugs profiled within that chapter are also identified with a **Prototype icon** Pr.

Highlights Key Information for Safe, Effective Nursing Care

Nursing Process Focus charts provide a succinct, easy-to-read view of the most important nursing actions for the commonly prescribed drug classes. Need-to-know nursing actions are presented in the charts; they also include patient education and discharge planning.

Nursing Process Focus Patients Receiving Thrombolytic Therapy

ASSESSMENT	POTENTIAL NURSING DIAGNOSES
Prior to administration: • Obtain complete health history including cardiovascular, renal, and liver conditions; recent surgeries or trauma; allergies; drug history (especially cardiovascular and OTC); and possible drug interactions. • Acquire the results of a complete physical examination, including vital signs, height, and weight. • Evaluate laboratory blood findings: CBC, electrolytes, clotting factors (activated partial thromboplastin time, thromboplastin time, platelet count), and renal and liver function studies.	• *Deficient Knowledge* related to lack of information about drug therapy • *Risk for Injury* (bleeding) related to adverse effects of thrombolytic therapy • *Risk for Decreased Cardiac Tissue Perfusion* related to increase in size of thrombus and altered blood flow

PLANNING: PATIENT GOALS AND EXPECTED OUTCOMES

The patient will:
- Experience therapeutic effects (dissolving of preexisting blood clot(s)).
- Be free from or experience minimal adverse effects from drug therapy.
- Verbalize an understanding of the drug's use, adverse effects, and required precautions.

IMPLEMENTATION

Interventions and Rationales	Patient Education/Discharge Planning
• Administer medication correctly; have IV lines initiated or Foley catheter inserted *prior* to beginning therapy. (The	• Instruct the patient about procedures and why they are necessary prior to beginning thrombolytic therapy.

Patients Need to Know

Patients treated for dysrhythmias need to know the following recommendations:

In General

1. Monitor blood pressure regularly during treatment.
2. Monitor for a decreased heart rate and changes in rhythm while taking antidysrhythmic drugs. Report changes to a healthcare provider.
3. Do not discontinue the medication suddenly. It should be stopped gradually under the supervision of a healthcare provider

The nursing student needs to learn how to teach drug administration to patients and families. Each drug chapter contains concise **Patients Need to Know** boxes that help students teach patients and families about drug information and administration.

Safety Alerts highlight potential medication errors and The Joint Commission National Patient Safety Goals.

Safety Alert Drug-Food Interactions

Certain drug-food interactions can be very dangerous. For example, the combination of grapefruit juice and certain blood pressure-lowering drugs or some cholesterol-lowering drugs can cause toxic levels of the drug in the blood. It is advisable for patients to keep medications in their original, labeled containers so that instructions are readily available. The nurse should ensure that patients are fully informed about how to take their drugs by providing both oral and written instructions.

tolerated by most patients. As with other antidysrhythmics, patients monitored for bradycardia and hypotension. Because their cardiac entical to those of beta-adrenergic blockers, patients concurrently taking asses are especially at risk for bradycardia and possible heart failure. nts often have multiple cardiovascular disorders, such as HTN, heart thmias, it is not unusual for them to be taking drugs from multiple

Lifespan and Diversity

The healthcare provider should carefully monitor older adults with preexisting heart failure because these patients are particularly at risk from the cardiac effects of potassium channel blockers.

Lifespan and Diversity features provide important **pediatric, older adult, and specific disorder considerations** for drug therapy, so students understand variations in nursing care and drug actions.

CAM (Complementary and Alternative Medicine) Therapy boxes present popular herbal or dietary supplements that may be considered along with conventional drugs.

CAM Therapy | Grape Seed Extract for Hypertension

Grapes and grape seeds have been used to enhance wellness for thousands of years. Their primary use has been for cardiovascular conditions such as HTN, high blood cholesterol, and atherosclerosis, and to improve circulation. Some claim that grape seed extract improves wound healing, prevents cancer, and lowers the risk for the long-term consequences of diabetes.

Fast Facts Myocardial Infarction

- About 1.5 million Americans experience a new or recurrent MI each year.
- About one third of patients experiencing an MI will die; half the deaths occur prior to arrival at the hospital.
- About 60% of patients who died suddenly of MI had no previous symptoms of the disease.
- Mortality from MI is three times higher in men than in women.
- More than 20% of men and 40% of women will die from an MI within 1 year of being diagnosed.

The **Fast Facts** feature puts the disease in a social and economic perspective.

New Drug Focus boxes cover how new emerging drugs work, how they may be used, and how they may be better than what was used in the past.

New Drug Focus

NEW APPROACH FOR TREATING HEART FAILURE

A new class of drugs, the neprilysin inhibitors, is able to slow the progression of HF with minimal side effects. Neprilysin is an enzyme normally present in the body that breaks down natriuretic peptides (see Section 20.9) and other substances that affect fluid balance. By blocking neprilysin, the concentration of natriuretic peptides in the blood increases and cardiac efficiency improves. The new drug is Entresto, a

End-of-Chapter Review Resources

Student practical and vocational nurses from around the country told us that they start their chapter reading from the end of the chapter. So, to ensure students' success in the classroom, on the NCLEX-PN® exam, and in the workplace, we put dynamite review resources at the end of each chapter.

Core Concepts Summaries repeat the important points at the end of the chapter and provide a brief summary.

Chapter Review

Core Concepts Summary

27.1 Pathogens are organisms that cause disease by invading tissues or secreting toxins.

Pathogens can overwhelm natural immune defenses by growing extremely rapidly and invading normal tissues or by producing potent toxins. Bacteria are classified on the basis of their staining ability and structural and functional characteristics.

27.2 Anti-infective drugs are classified by their chemical structures or by their mechanisms of action.

Because of the large number of anti-infectives available, it is advantageous for the student to understand how to classify these drugs because medications in the same class exhibit similar pharmacologic activity. Anti-infective drugs are classified based on similarities in their chemical structures or by their mechanisms of action.

27.3 Anti-infective drugs act by selectively targeting a pathogen's metabolism or life cycle.

Bacteria multiply rapidly, and drugs have been designed to take advantage of this characteristic. Anti-infectives may be bactericidal or bacteriostatic, or both, depending on the organism and dose.

27.4 Acquired resistance is a major clinical problem that is worsened by improper use of anti-infectives.

Errors during replication result in random mutations of the bacterial DNA. Although rare, an occasional mutation may confer antibiotic resistance to a bacterium. Therapy with antibiotics kills the affected bacteria, leaving the resistant ones to multiply and spread within the patient. To limit this problem, antibiotics should be prescribed only when

27.7 The cephalosporins are similar in structure and function to the penicillins and are one of the most widely prescribed anti-infective classes.

The cephalosporins consist of a large class of antibiotics, classified by generation, that are considered alternatives to penicillin. In general, they are used for serious gram-negative infections and for patients who are resistant to or cannot tolerate the penicillins.

27.8 The tetracyclines have broad spectrums but are preferred drugs for few diseases.

The tetracyclines have a broader spectrum of action and produce more adverse effects than the penicillins. Their use is limited to a small number of diseases, such as Rocky Mountain spotted fever, typhus, cholera, Lyme disease, and chlamydial infections.

27.9 The macrolides are safe alternatives to penicillin for many infections.

The macrolides are generally prescribed when a patient is allergic to penicillin or has a penicillin-resistant infection. They produce few adverse effects.

27.10 The aminoglycosides are narrow-spectrum drugs that have the potential to cause serious toxicity.

The aminoglycosides are usually reserved for severe gram-negative infections of the urinary tract because they have the potential to cause serious adverse effects. Most of them are poorly absorbed from the GI tract and must be given parenterally.

27.11 Fluoroquinolones have wide clinical applications

REVIEW Questions

Answer the following questions to assess your knowledge of the chapter material, and go back and review any material that is not clear to you.

1. The patient is taking amoxicillin (Amoxil). Which of the following statements by the patient demonstrates that additional instruction is needed?
   1. "I will take this medication until it is gone."
   2. "I will call my doctor if I develop a fever or a rash."
   3. "Before I take my medication, I will avoid orange juice."
   4. "I will take the medication until I feel better."
2. Before administering cefazolin (Ancef), the nurse checks for a previous allergic reaction to:
   1. Yeasts.
   2. Penicillins.
   3. Sulfonamides.
   4. Macrolides.
6. A patient has been diagnosed with MRSA and is prescribed vancomycin. What information should be provided to the patient about possible adverse effects?
   1. Vancomycin may cause flushing.
   2. Adverse effects are infrequent.
   3. Vacomycin does not cause rashes.
   4. During therapy, hypertension may occur.
7. The patient with tuberculosis is taking isoniazid (INH). Which laboratory test should the nurse monitor?
   1. PT and PTT
   2. CBC
   3. BUN
   4. Liver enzymes
8. The most common adverse effects of penicillin G include(s): (Select all that apply.)
   1. Diarrhea.

Review Questions serve as a post-test for the chapter and prepare students for the NCLEX-PN®. Tests include additional practice in calculating the correct dosage.

Case Study Questions help the student apply pharmacology and nursing care to a specific client scenario.

CASE STUDY Questions

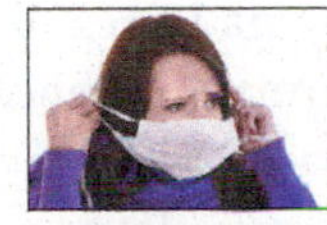

Remember Ms. Jackson, the patient introduced at the beginning of the chapter? Now read the remainder of the case study. Based on the information you have learned in this chapter, answer the questions that follow.

Ms. Shelly Jackson is a new patient at your clinic. Six months ago, she had a kidney transplant and is taking immunosuppressant drugs. Recently, she has been experiencing repeated bacterial infections due to resistant strains and has been switched to different antibiotics throughout the past 6 months. The healthcare provider suspects a kidney infection.

1. Ms. Jackson is admitted to the hospital and is administered gentamicin 300 mg daily by IV infusion. The nurse monitors which of the following tests?
   3. Nausea and vomiting.
   4. Liver failure.
3. Ms. Jackson is showing signs of hearing loss due to gentamicin therapy and the healthcare provider is going to switch her antibiotic. The nurse anticipates which of the following medications being ordered?
   1. Sulfacetamide (Klaron)
   2. Silver sulfadiazine
   3. Trimethoprim–sulfamethoxazole (Septra)
   4. Vancomycin (Vancocin)
4. The adverse effects of sulfonamides include: (Select all that apply.)
   1. Increased sensitivity of skin to sunlight.

REFERENCES

Centers for Disease Control and Prevention. (2012). *Self-study modules on tuberculosis: Module 9: Patient adherence to tuberculosis treatment.* Retrieved from http://www.cdc.gov/tb/education/ssmodules/module9/ss9reading2.htm

Herdman, T. H., & Kamitsuru, S. (Eds.). (2014). *NANDA International nursing diagnoses: Definitions and classification, 2015–2017.* Oxford, United Kingdom: Wiley-Blackwell.

SELECTED BIBLIOGRAPHY

Centers for Disease Control and Prevention. (2013). *CDC fact sheet: Incidence, prevalence and cost of sexually transmitted infections in the*

Custodio, H. T. (2014). *Hospital-acquired infections.* Retrieved from http://emedicine.medscape.com/article/967022-overview

References and Selected Bibliography

Acknowledgments

We are grateful to all the educators who reviewed the manuscript of this text. Their insights and suggestions helped us prepare a more relevant and useful book, one that focuses on the essential components of learning in the field of pharmacology. In particular, we would like to thank Teri Zak, our Development Editor, for guiding the authors through the many detailed steps necessary in producing a quality revision of this text.

Textbook Reviewers

Harriet Adedoyin-Tuyo, MSN, ANP, WHNP-BC
Faculty
Houston Community College
Vocational Nursing Program
Houston, Texas

Carla G. Birt, BSN, MSN, RN
Associate Professor of Nursing
Southern Maine Community College
South Portland, Maine

Jenna Boothe, DNP, RN
Associate Professor
Hazard Community & Technical College
Hazard, Kentucky

Kendreia Durant, CphT, BS
Pharmacy Technology Program Director
Ogeechee Technical College
Statesboro, Georgia

Judi Dzuba, RDH, MS Ed
Clinical/Adjunct Instructor for Dental Hygiene Department
Adjunct Instructor/Academic Advisor for Health Science Department
SUNY Broome Community College
Binghamton, New York

Stephanie Garthrite
Pharmacy Technology Program Director
Polaris Career Center
Middleburg Heights, Ohio

Margaret M. Gingrich, MSN, CRNP
Professor of Nursing
Harrisburg Area Community College
Harrisburg, Pennsylvania

Brittany W. Hendrix, RN
Nurse Aide Insrtuctor
Ogeechee Technical College
Statesboro, Georgia

Jennifer Houghtalen, RN, MS, FNP-BC, CNE
Nursing Department, Interim Chair
SUNY Broome Community College
Binghamton, New York

Richard Keegan, DNP, FNP-BC, RN
Assistant Professor/Clinical Faculty
Undergraduate Coordinator
California State University
Sacramento, California

Sharyn Ketcham, MBA, MHSA
Medical Assisting
Phoenix College
Phoenix, Arizona

Ellen Ketcherside, RN, CCRN, MA
Nursing Professor
Mineral Area College
Park Hills, Missouri

Holly Lofland, CPht, RPT, MS
Pharmacy Technician Program Coordinator
Tallahassee Community College
Tallahassee, Florida

Shawna Lopez, BAAS, MS, CPhT
Pharmacy Technology Program Director
Amarillo College
Amarillo, Texas

Gloria Madison, MS, RHIA, CHDA, CHTS-IM
Health Information Technology Program Director
Moraine Park Technical College
West Bend, Wisconsin

Nikki A. Marhefka, EdM, MT(ASCP), CMA(AAMA)
Medical Assisting Program Director
Central Penn College
Summerdale, Pennsylvania

Michelle C. McCranie, A.A.S., CPhT, CMA (AAMA)
Medical Assisting Instructor
Ogeechee Technical College
Statesboro, Georgia

Kimberly B. Mclain, Ph.D., RN, LMHC, NCC
Assistant Professor, Medical Assisting & Health Studies Department
SUNY Broome Community College
Binghamton, New York

Nancy Miles
Associate Professor
Southeast Kentucky Community and Technical College
Pineville, Kentucky

Toby Ann Nishikawa, MSN, RN
Assistant Professor
Weber State University
Odgen, Utah

Gwen Rogers, DBA, RN, CIC
Adjunct Instructor
Southern Maine Community College
South Portland, Maine

Cynthia Sebastiani, RN, MSN
Nursing Instructor
Mid-State Technical College
Wisconsin Rapids, Wisconsin

Audrey Smith, MS, PA-C, DFAAPA
Pharmacology Coordinator/Clinical Assistant Professor
D'Youville College, Physician Assistant Department
Buffalo, New York

Kim Smith, MSN, BSN, RN
Level 1 Coordinator for Vocational Nursing Program
Amarillo College
Amarillo, Texas

Latasha Smith, PhD
Research Fellow
Endocrinology, Metabolism, & Nutrition
Mayo Clinic—St. Mary's Campus
Rochester, Michigan

Rox Ann Sparks, RN, MSN, MICN, LNC
Retired Assistant Director of the Vocational Nursing Program and Adjunct Faculty for Fresno Pacific University RN to BSN Program
Merced College and Fresno Pacific University
Merced, California

Christine Tannious, MHA, ADS, R.PhT
Pharmacy Technician Coordinator
West Los Angeles College
Culver City, California

Judith M. Thompson, RN, MN
Practical Nursing Instructor
Richmond Community College
Hamlet, North Carolina

About the Authors

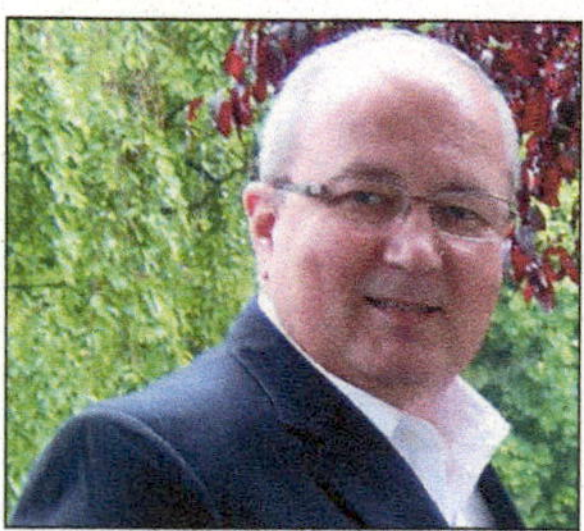

LELAND NORMAN HOLLAND, JR., PHD (NORM), over 20 years ago, started out like many scientists, planning for a career in basic science research. Quickly he was drawn to the field of teaching in higher medical education, where he has spent most of his career since that time. Among the areas where he has been particularly effective are preparatory programs in nursing, medicine, dentistry, pharmacy, and allied health. Dr. Holland is both an affiliate and a supporter of nursing and allied health education nationwide. He brings to the profession a depth of knowledge in biology, chemistry, and medically related subjects such as microbiology, biological chemistry, and pharmacology. Dr. Holland's doctoral degree is in Medical Pharmacology. He is very much dedicated to the success of students and their preparation for work–life readiness. He continues to motivate students in the lifelong pursuit of learning.

I would like to acknowledge the willful encouragement of Farrell and Norma Jean Stalcup. I dedicate this book to my beloved wife, Karen, and my three wonderful children, Alexandria Noelle, my double-deuce daughter; Caleb Jaymes, my number one son; and Joshua Nathaniel, my number three "O"!

—LNH

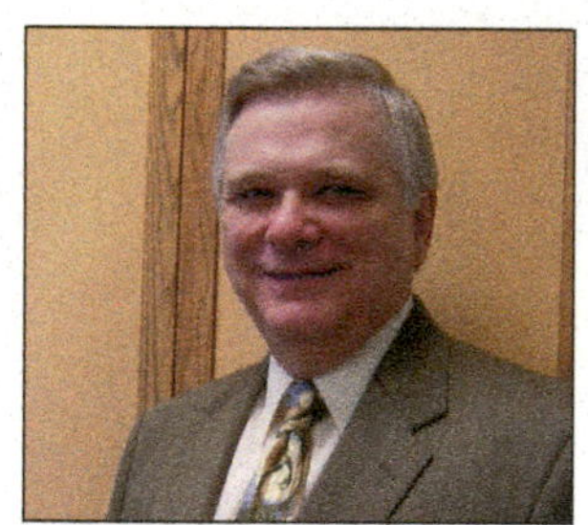

MICHAEL PATRICK ADAMS, PHD, RT(R), is an accomplished educator, author, and national speaker. The National Institute for Staff and Organizational Development in Austin, Texas, named Dr. Adams a Master Teacher. He has published two other textbooks with Pearson Publishing: *Pharmacology for Nurses: A Pathophysiologic Approach* and *Pharmacology: Connections to Nursing Practice.*

Dr. Adams obtained his master's degree in Pharmacology from Michigan State University and his Doctorate in Education at the University of South Florida. Dr. Adams was on the faculty of Lansing Community College and was Dean of Health Professions at Pasco-Hernando State College for over 15 years. He is currently Adjunct Professor of biological sciences at Pasco State College and Hillsborough Community College.

I dedicate this book to nursing educators, who contribute every day to making the world a better and more caring place.

—MPA

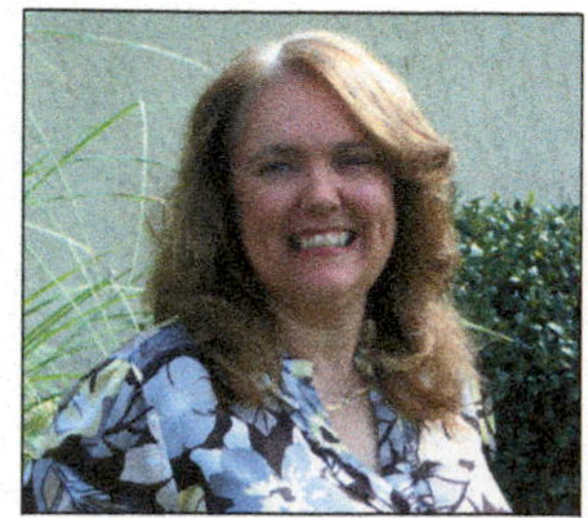

JEANINE L. BRICE, RN, MSN, has been a nurse for over 30 years, initially graduating from the registered nursing program at Charles County Community College and continuing her nursing education, receiving a BS from the University of Maryland and an MSN from Bowie State University, specializing in nursing education and community health practice. Her clinical experience includes acute medical-surgical care, obstetrics, neonatology, and pediatric public health.

Ms. Brice has been involved in nursing/technical health education for over 26 years, formerly holding the positions of Professor of Nursing, Assistant Dean of Nursing Programs, and Coordinator of Technical Health Programs at Pasco-Hernando Community College. She currently is employed at St. Petersburg College and Hillsborough Community College as an adjunct professor of biological/health sciences.

I dedicate this book to my parents, William and Helen Davis, whom I had the privilege to care for during their final days … and to all those who will need the care of a nurse. May the information contained in this book help them receive competent and compassionate nursing care.

—JLB

Contents

Unit 1

Basic Concepts in Pharmacology

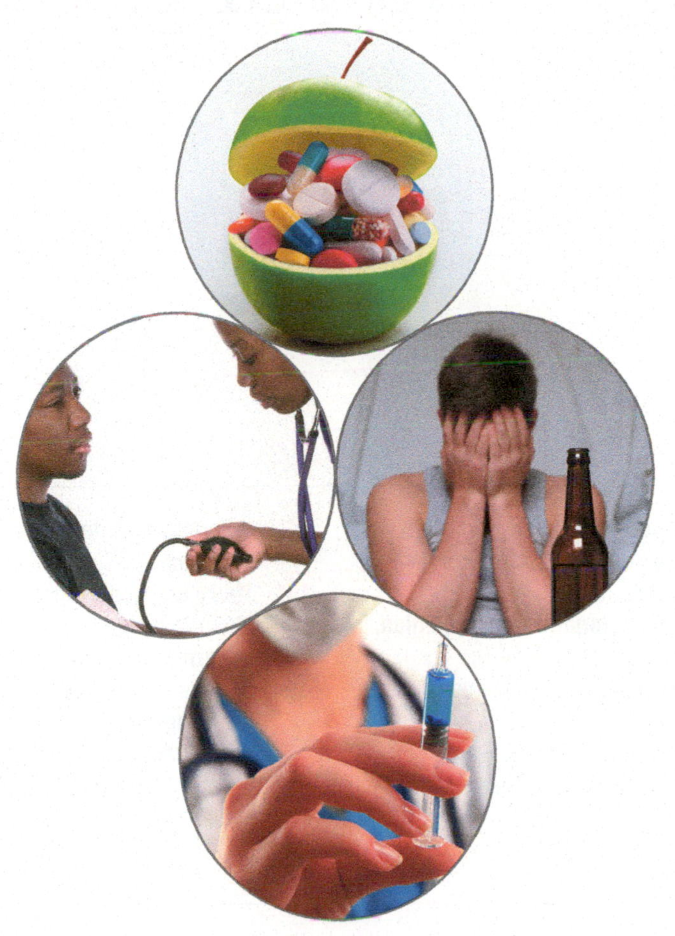

Unit Contents

Chapter 1

Introduction to Pharmacology: Drug Regulation and Approval

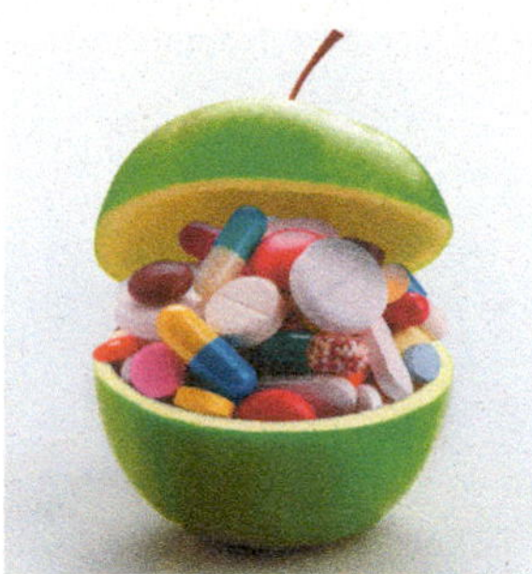

Core Concepts

1.1 Pharmacology is an expansive and challenging topic.
1.2 For healthcare providers, the fields of pharmacology and therapeutics are connected.
1.3 Medicines are classified as traditional drugs, biologics, and natural alternatives.
1.4 Medications are available by prescription or over the counter.
1.5 Pharmaceutics is the science of pharmacy.
1.6 Drug regulations were created to protect the public from drug misuse.
1.7 U.S. drug standards have become increasingly complex.
1.8 There are four stages of approval for therapeutic and biologic drugs.
1.9 Governmental agencies face the dual challenge of increasing the speed of drug approval while still ensuring the safety of new drugs.
1.10 Healthcare providers must be prepared to deal with the threat of biological and chemical attack.

Learning Outcomes

After reading this chapter, the student should be able to:

1. Explain the expansive nature of pharmacology, and give examples of interrelated subject areas needed to master the discipline.
2. Identify professions in which knowledge of pharmacology is important, and explain how the disciplines of therapeutics and pharmacology are interconnected.
3. Compare and contrast traditional drugs, biologics, and natural alternative therapies.
4. Identify the advantages and disadvantages of prescription and over-the-counter drugs.
5. Distinguish between pharmaceutics and pharmacology.
6. Discuss the history of U.S. standards, acts, and organizations leading to the requirement that drug safety must be proven before marketing.
7. Discuss the emerging roles and responsibilities of the U.S. Department of Health and Human Services and the U.S. Food and Drug Administration (FDA) with its branches in determining the safety of drugs and whether they may be used for therapy.

8. Identify four stages of approval for therapeutic and biologic drugs.
9. Discuss current challenges facing the FDA in approving new drugs for market.
10. Discuss the challenges facing healthcare providers in view of modern-day pandemic and bioterrorist threats.

Key Terms

biologics (beye-oh-LOJ-iks)
bioterrorism (beye-oh-TEH-or-izm)
black box warnings
clinical pharmacology
complementary and alternative medicine (CAM) therapies
formularies (FOR-mew-LEH-reez)
medications
natural alternative therapies
off-label use
pandemic
pathophysiology (PATH-oh-fiz-ee-OL-oh-jee)
pharmaceutics (far-mah-SOO-tiks)
pharmacology (far-mah-KOL-oh-jee)
pharmacopoeia (far-mah-KOH-pee-ah)
pharmacotherapeutics (far-mah-koh-THER-ah-PEW-tiks)
pharmacy (FAR-mah-see)
therapeutics (ther-ah-PEW-tiks)

More drugs are being administered to consumers than ever before. Because of the number of new drugs available for therapy, experts are concerned that patients might be harmed if drugs are not thoroughly tested. The purpose of this chapter is to introduce the subject of pharmacology and to emphasize the role of the government in ensuring that drugs and natural alternatives are safe and effective for public use. It addresses the role that drug therapy has in fighting disease as governmental regulators, consumers, and healthcare professionals face new challenges in the years ahead. Drugs are the most powerful weapons we have against diseases and worldwide epidemics.

In addition, bioterrorist threats have led to widespread governmental changes in emergency preparedness planning. This chapter briefly introduces the role of pharmacology in the prevention and treatment of diseases or conditions that might develop due to global biological, chemical, or nuclear threats.

Pharmacology is an expansive and challenging topic.

◀ **Core Concept 1.1**

The word **pharmacology** is derived from two Greek words: *pharmakon*, which means "medicine," and *logos*, which means "study." Thus, *pharmacology* is defined as "the study of medicine."

pharmaco = *medicine*
ology = *the study of*

Healthcare providers practice the discipline of pharmacology to study how drugs improve the health of the human body. If applied properly, drugs can dramatically improve patients' quality of life. If applied improperly, the consequences of drug action can be devastating.

The subject of pharmacology is an expansive topic ranging from a study of how drugs enter and travel throughout the body to the actual responses they produce. To learn the discipline well, students must master concepts from several interrelated areas, including anatomy, physiology, microbiology, chemistry, and **pathophysiology** (study of disease and functional changes that occur as a result of disease). The useful application of drugs depends on knowledge from at least these areas.

patho = *disease*
physio = *the nature of*
ology = *the study of*

Currently there are more than 10,000 brand and generic varieties of drugs available with many different names, interactions, adverse effects, and complicated mechanisms of action. Keeping up with the numbers of drugs is a huge challenge. Many drugs may be prescribed for more than one disease, and most produce multiple effects in the body. Further complicating the study of pharmacology is the fact that drugs may cause different responses depending on factors such as gender, age, health status, body mass, and genetics.

For healthcare providers, the fields of pharmacology and therapeutics are connected.

◀ **Core Concept 1.2**

It is obvious that a thorough knowledge of pharmacology is important to those health professionals who prescribe drugs on a daily basis. This group includes physicians, physician assistants, dentists, and advanced registered nurse practitioners (ARNPs). A second group of professions includes nurses and allied health workers who do not prescribe medications but are directly involved with drug administration as well as with issues related to drug education and management, and enforcement of drug laws. All of these occupations have in common direct contact with patients and other healthcare providers. In this text, we refer to these professionals as *healthcare providers*.

Some healthcare providers, such as nurses, may administer drugs on a daily basis, whereas others may administer drugs occasionally. An extensive knowledge of pharmacology is necessary to properly educate and advise patients regarding their healthcare needs. This knowledge is also essential to communicate effectively with other healthcare providers, who rely heavily on nurses and allied health professionals to gather medical data from their patients and to follow up on results of therapy.

For healthcare providers studying pharmacology, it becomes apparent early in training that the fields of pharmacology and therapeutics are connected. **Therapeutics** is the branch of medicine concerned with the treatment of disease and suffering. **Pharmacotherapeutics** is the use of medicine to treat disease.

Core Concept 1.3 ▶

Medicines are classified as traditional drugs, biologics, and natural alternatives.

Drugs are chemicals that produce biologic responses within the body. From this perspective, drugs may be considered part of the body's normal activities, from the essential gases that people breathe to the foods they eat. Yet it is necessary to separate drugs from agents such as foods, household products, and cosmetics. Many products, including antiperspirants, sunscreens, toothpastes, and shampoos, might alter the body's normal activities, but they are not considered to be medically therapeutic, as drugs taken for a medical disorder would be. Indeed substances designed to prevent or treat diseases are referred to as **medications**.

Therapeutic drugs are sometimes classified on the basis of how they are produced, either chemically or naturally. Most traditional drugs are chemically produced or synthesized in a laboratory. **Biologics** are agents naturally produced in animal cells, in microorganisms, or by the body itself. **Natural alternative therapies** are herbs, natural extracts, vitamins, minerals, or dietary supplements. Table 1.1 shows a summary of characteristics associated with traditional drug therapies, biologics, and natural alternative therapies. Although drugs may be described in many ways, this text limits its focus to agents used for therapy in a clinical or home setting. Traditional drugs and drug classes are discussed more thoroughly in Chapter 2. Natural alternatives are discussed more thoroughly in Chapter 7.

When studying the various approaches for therapy, the healthcare provider may encounter the category of treatment called **complementary and alternative medicine (CAM) therapies**. In addition to the herbs, vitamins, or supplements just described, CAM therapies include manipulative and body-based practices such as physical therapy, occupational therapy, massage, biofeedback, hypnosis, and acupuncture. Although some CAM therapies are effective for certain conditions, traditional therapeutic drugs and biologics remain the primary focus of this text. Many chapters include a feature called *CAM Therapy* that highlights a specific herbal product or dietary supplement.

Table 1.1 Characteristics of Traditional Therapeutic Drugs, Biologics, and Natural Alternative Therapies

Traditional Drug Therapies	• Synthetically produced in a laboratory • Routinely prescribed or administered by healthcare providers
Biologics	• Naturally produced by the body itself, in animal cells, or in microorganisms • Include hormones, monoclonal antibodies, and vaccines • Routinely prescribed or administered by healthcare providers
Natural Alternative Therapies	• Naturally produced • Include herbs, extracts, vitamins, minerals, or dietary supplements • Recommended, depending on the healthcare provider

Medications are available by prescription or over the counter.

◀ Core Concept 1.4

Legal medications are obtained either with a prescription or by purchasing them over the counter (OTC). There are differences between the two methods of dispensing. To obtain prescription drugs, patients must get a healthcare provider's order authorizing them to receive the drugs. The advantages to this are numerous. Healthcare providers have an opportunity to examine their patients and determine a specific diagnosis. They can maximize therapy by ordering the proper drug for their patients' conditions and controlling the specific amount and frequency of the drug to be dispensed. In addition, healthcare providers may give instructions on how to use the drug properly and what adverse effects to expect.

A drug's safety is related to its effectiveness. The difference between its usual effective dose and a dose that produces severe adverse effects is called its *margin of safety*. When drugs have been used over long periods without unfavorable reactions—that is, they are considered very safe and effective—regulators sometimes change them from being prescription drugs to being OTC drugs. Many drugs appear to demonstrate a wide margin of safety, but with their prolonged use, consumers and regulators may observe safety concerns. Unlike prescription drugs, OTC drugs do not require an order from a healthcare practitioner.

Patients may treat themselves safely if they carefully follow instructions included with OTC drugs. Patients must have an understanding of their own health to follow the guidelines accurately. If patients do not follow the guidelines, OTC drugs can have serious adverse effects.

Patients prefer to take OTC medications for many reasons. OTC drugs can be obtained more easily than prescription drugs. Patients do not have to make an appointment with a healthcare provider, which saves time and money. Without training, however, choosing the proper medication for a specific problem may be difficult. OTC drugs may react with foods, herbal products, and prescription or other OTC drugs. Patients may not be aware that some medications can impair their ability to function safely. Self-treatment is sometimes ineffective, and the potential for injury is much greater if the disease is allowed to progress without proper treatment.

Pharmaceutics is the science of pharmacy.

◀ Core Concept 1.5

Pharmaceutics is the science of **pharmacy** (the preparation and dispensing of drugs) and is a very important part of pharmacotherapy. The general public often confuses pharmaceutics with pharmacology, or they recognize the root *pharm* and assume that *pharmacology* is the same as *pharmacy*. Correctly put, *pharmaceutics* is the science of pharmacy, and it involves dispensing a drug to a patient after he or she has been examined by a licensed healthcare provider. *Pharmacists* are the experts who catalogue signs, symptoms, adverse effects, and drug interactions. They often act as drug advisors to patients, making sure that they receive the proper medication and educating them about undesirable symptoms or interactions.

CONCEPT REVIEW 1.1

- Explain the meaning of this statement: "Pharmacotherapy involves the science of therapeutics and pharmaceutics."

Drug regulations were created to protect the public from drug misuse.

◀ Core Concept 1.6

For many years, there were no standards or guidelines to protect the public from drug misuse. Patients could not be assured that available medicines were not a form of quackery. The archives of drug regulatory agencies are filled with examples of early medicines, such as rattlesnake oil for rheumatism. It became quite clear that drug regulations were needed to protect the public.

The first standards commonly used by pharmacists were early **formularies**, or lists of drugs and drug recipes. In 1820, the first comprehensive publication of drug standards, called the *U.S. Pharmacopoeia (USP)*, was established. (See the timeline in Figure 1.1.) A **pharmacopoeia** is a medical reference summary indicating standards of drug purity and strength, and directions for synthesis. In 1852, a national professional society of pharmacists—the American Pharmaceutical Association (APhA)—was founded. From 1852 until 1975, two major sources maintained drug standards in the United States: the USP and the APhA's *National Formulary (NF)*. All drug substances and products were covered in the USP; the *NF* focused on pharmaceutical ingredients. In 1975, the two organizations merged and created a single publication named the *U.S. Pharmacopoeia-National Formulary (USP-NF)*. Official updates for the *USP-NF* are published regularly. Today, the USP label can be found on some medication containers verifying the exact ingredients found within the container,

TIMELINE	REGULATORY ACTS, STANDARDS, AND ORGANIZATIONS
1820	A group of healthcare providers established the first comprehensive publication of drug standards called the **U.S. Pharmacopoeia (USP).**
1852	A group of pharmacists founded a national professional society called the **American Pharmaceutical Association (APhA).** The APhA then established the **National Formulary (NF),** a standardized publication focusing on pharmaceutical ingredients. The *USP* continued to catalogue all drug-related substances and products.
1862	This was the beginning of the **Federal Bureau of Chemistry,** established under the administration of President Lincoln. Over the years and with added duties, it gradually became the Food and Drug Administration (FDA).
1902	Congress passed the **Biologics Control Act** to control the quality of serums and other blood-related products.
1906	**The Pure Food and Drug Act** gave the government power to control the labeling of medicines.
1912	**The Sherley Amendment** made medicines safer by prohibiting the sale of drugs labeled with false therapeutic claims.
1938	Congress passed the **Food, Drug, and Cosmetic Act.** It was the first law preventing the marketing of drugs not thoroughly tested. This law now provides for the requirement that drug companies must submit a New Drug Application (NDA) to the FDA prior to marketing a new drug.
1944	Congress passed the **Public Health Service Act,** covering many health issues, including biologtic products and the control of communicable diseases.
1975	The *U.S. Pharmacopoeia* and *National Formulary* announced their union. The **USP-NF** became a single standardized publication.
1986	Congress passed the **Childhood Vaccine Act.** It authorized the FDA to acquire information about patients taking vaccines, to recall biologics, and to recommend civil penalties if guidelines regarding biologic use were not followed.
1988	The **FDA** was officially established as an agency of the **U.S. Department of Health and Human Services.**
1992	Congress passed the **Prescription Drug User Fee Act.** It required that nongeneric drug and biologic manufacturers pay fees to be used for improvements in the drug review process.
1994	Congress passed the **Dietary Supplement Health and Education Act** that requires clear labeling of dietary supplements. This act gives the FDA the power to remove supplements that cause a significant risk to the public.
1997	The **FDA Drug Modernization Act** reauthorized the Prescription Drug User Fee Act. This act represented the largest reform effort of the drug review process since 1938.
2002	The **Bioterrorism Act** implemented guidelines for registration of selected toxins that could pose a threat to human, animal, or plant safety and health.
2007	Dietary Supplement and Nonprescription Drug Consumer Protection Act
2007	The **FDA Amendments Act** reviewed, expanded, and reaffirmed legislation to allow for additional comprehensive reviews of new drugs and medical products. This extended the reforms imposed from 1997. The **FDA's Critical Path Initiative** was a part of this reform.
2011	Provisions of the **Health Care Reform** law allowed the FDA to approve generic versions of biologic drugs. Additional drug rebates and benefits were provided to the American public. The **FDA Food Safety Modernization Act** represents the largest reform effort of food safety review since 1938.
2012	Renewal of the **Prescription Drug User Fee Act.**

FIGURE 1.1 Historical timeline of regulatory acts, standards, and organizations.

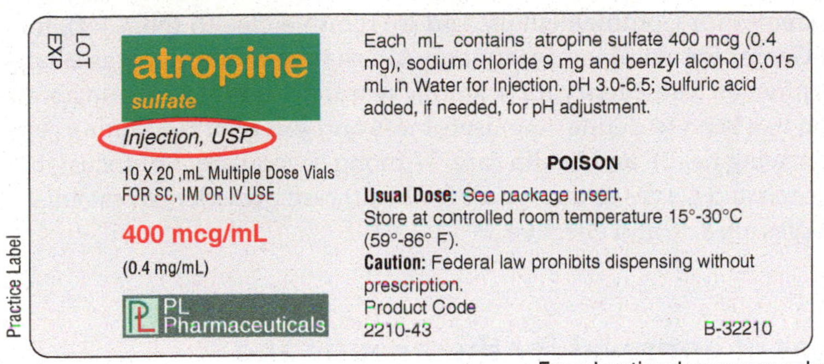

For educational purposes only

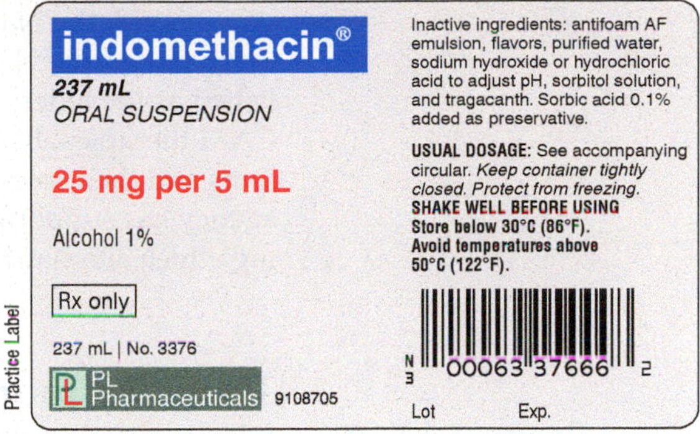

FIGURE 1.2 Some drug labels show the USP symbol; others do not.

as shown in Figure 1.2. Although there is a lot of good information on the label of a drug container, newer labeling guidelines are being proposed in an effort to promote patient safety and to reduce drug misuse.

In the early 1900s, to protect the public, the government began to develop and enforce tougher drug legislation. In 1902, the Biologics Control Act was passed to standardize the quality of serums and other blood-related products. The Pure Food and Drug Act of 1906 gave the government power to control the labeling of medicines. In 1912, the Sherley Amendment prohibited the sale of drugs labeled with false therapeutic claims intended to cheat the consumer. In 1938, Congress passed the Food, Drug, and Cosmetic Act. This was the first law preventing the marketing of drugs that had not been thoroughly tested prior to marketing. According to the provisions of this law, drug companies were required to prove the safety and *efficacy* (i.e., effectiveness) of any drug before it could be sold within the United States.

U.S. drug standards have become increasingly complex.

◀ **Core Concept 1.7**

Much has changed in the regulation of drugs since 1938. In 1988, the U.S. Food and Drug Administration (FDA) was officially established as an agency of the U.S. Department of Health and Human Services. Today, the Center for Drug Evaluation and Research (CDER), a branch of the FDA, has powerful control over whether prescription and OTC drugs may be used for therapy. The CDER states its mission as "facilitating the availability of safe effective drugs, keeping unsafe or ineffective drugs off the market, improving the health of Americans, and providing clear, easily understandable drug information for safe and effective use." Any pharmaceutical laboratory, whether private, public, or academic, must obtain FDA approval before marketing any drug. Another branch of the FDA, the Center for Biologics Evaluation and Research (CBER), regulates the use of biologics, including serums, vaccines, and products found in the bloodstream. In 1997, the FDA created *boxed warnings* to regulate drugs with "special problems." At the time no precedent had been established to monitor drugs with a potential for causing death or serious injury. **Black box warnings**, named after the black label appearing around drug safety information on package inserts, eventually became one of the primary alerts for identifying extreme adverse drug reactions discovered during and after review. The healthcare provider must be increasingly mindful about the level of precaution necessary to promote safety, including medication verification and special alerts. Because of their importance, black box warnings are included for all prototype drugs in this text.

The FDA also oversees administration of herbal products and dietary supplements, but the Center for Food Safety and Applied Nutrition (CFSAN) regulates use of these substances. Herbal products and dietary supplements are regulated by the Dietary Supplement Health and Education Act of 1994. This act does not provide the same degree of protection as the Food, Drug, and Cosmetic Act of 1938. For example, herbal and dietary supplements can be marketed without prior approval from the FDA; however, all package inserts and information are monitored once products have gone to market. The regulation of herbal products and dietary supplements is discussed in more detail in Chapter 7.

▶ Lifespan and Diversity

One historical achievement involving biologics is the 1986 Childhood Vaccine Act. This act authorized the FDA to acquire information about patients taking vaccines, to recall biologics, and to recommend civil penalties if guidelines regarding biologics were not followed.

In 1998, the National Center for Complementary and Integrative Health (NCCIH), formerly called the National Center for Complementary and Alternative Medicine, was established as the federal government's lead agency for scientific research and information about CAM therapies. Its mission has been to define "the usefulness and safety of CAM interventions and their roles in improving health and health care." Among several areas of focus, this agency has supported research and serves as a resource for healthcare providers in establishing which alternative therapies are safe and effective.

Core Concept 1.8 ▶

There are four stages of approval for therapeutic and biologic drugs.

The amount of time spent in the review and approval process for both prescription and OTC drugs depends on several checkpoints in a well-developed and organized plan. Most therapeutic drugs and biologics are reviewed in four stages, which are summarized in Figure 1.3. These stages are (1) preclinical investigation, (2) clinical investigation, (3) submission of a new drug application (NDA) with review, and (4) postmarketing studies.

Preclinical Investigation

Preclinical investigation involves basic science research. Scientists perform many tests on cells grown in the laboratory (a process called *culture*) or on animals to examine the effectiveness of a range of drug doses and to look for any adverse effects. Laboratory tests on cells and animals are important, because they assist in predicting whether drugs will cause harm in humans. Because laboratory tests do not always reflect the way a human responds, preclinical investigation results are always inconclusive.

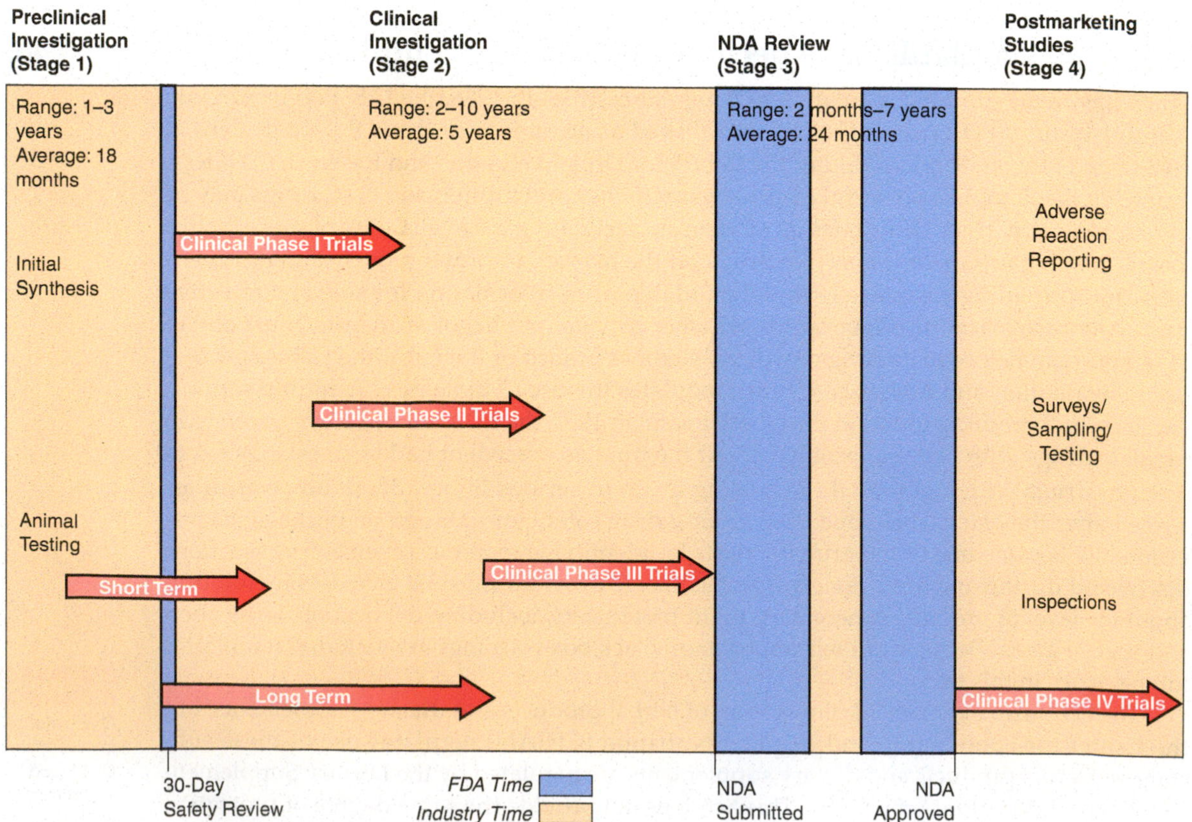

FIGURE 1.3 The approval of a new drug is a four-stage process: (1) preclinical investigation, (2) clinical investigation, (3) NDA submission and review, and (4) postmarketing studies. Within the second stage (clinical investigation), three phases of trials are conducted over two to ten years. Postmarketing studies, also called *clinical phase IV trials* or *postmarketing surveillance*, continue in large patient groups during the fourth stage of drug approval.

Clinical Investigation

Clinical investigation, the second stage of drug approval, takes place in three different phases, termed *clinical phase trials*. This is the longest part of the drug approval process and involves **clinical pharmacology**, an area of medicine devoted to the evaluation of drugs used for human benefit. During the three phases, clinical pharmacologists, researchers, and healthcare providers examine data from volunteers and large groups of selected patients with certain diseases. Together, scientists and healthcare providers establish drug doses, evaluate drug efficacy, and try to identify adverse effects. Clinical investigators address concerns such as whether the drug worsens other medical conditions, interacts unsafely with existing medications patients are taking, or affects one type of patient more than others.

CLINICAL PHASE TRIALS

Clinical phase trials are essential because responses among patients vary. If a drug appears to be effective without causing serious adverse effects, approval for marketing may be accelerated, or the drug may be used for treatment immediately in special cases with careful monitoring. If the drug shows promise but some minor problems are noted, the approval process is delayed until concerns are addressed. In any case, an NDA must be submitted before a drug is allowed to proceed to the next stage of the approval process. The three phases of clinical trials are:

- Phase I: Researchers test a new drug or treatment in a small group of people to evaluate its safety, determine a safe dosage range, and identify side effects.
- Phase II: The drug or treatment is given to a larger group of people to see if it is effective and to further evaluate its safety.
- Phase III: The drug or treatment is given to large groups of people to confirm its effectiveness, monitor side effects, compare it to commonly used treatments, and collect information that will allow the drug or treatment to be used safely.

Submission of a New Drug Application With Review

A review of the NDA is the third stage of drug approval. During this stage, clinical phase III trials and animal testing may continue, depending on the results obtained from preclinical testing. If the NDA is approved, the process continues to the final stage. If the NDA is rejected, the process stops until concerns are addressed.

Postmarketing Studies

Postmarketing surveillance is the fourth stage of the drug approval process. It is considered the last phase (phase IV) of clinical trials. It takes place after the NDA review process has been completed. Testing in humans is continued to check for any new harmful effects in larger and more diverse populations. Some adverse effects take longer to appear and are not identified until a drug is used by large numbers of patients. This phase is described as:

- Phase IV: Studies are done after the drug or treatment has been marketed to gather information on the drug's effect in various populations and any side effects associated with long-term use.

Examples of this process include approval of COX-2 selective nonsteroidal anti-inflammatory drugs (NSAIDs), which were evaluated by the FDA during 2004 and 2005. Manufacturers of valdecoxib (Bextra), celecoxib (Celebrex), and rofecoxib (Vioxx) were originally asked to revise their labeling owing to emerging concerns that some NSAIDs exhibited extreme cardiovascular and gastrointestinal risks. In September 2004, manufacturers of rofecoxib voluntarily withdrew their product from the market due to safety concerns of heart attack and stroke. In April 2005, the FDA asked the manufacturers of valdecoxib to remove their product from the market due to similar concerns. Celecoxib has remained on the market, but the FDA announced that it would continue to analyze reports of COX-2 inhibitors to determine safety profiles and patient impact. In addition, it added a black box warning for celecoxib and later to every NSAID drug insert alerting consumers to be aware of cardiovascular and gastrointestinal risks associated with use of drugs in this class.

The FDA holds annual public meetings to hear comments from patients and professional and pharmaceutical organizations about the effectiveness and safety of new drug therapies. If the FDA discovers a serious problem, it will require that a drug be withdrawn from the market and its use discontinued.

Core Concept 1.9 ▶ Governmental agencies face the dual challenge of increasing the speed of drug approval while still ensuring the safety of new drugs.

The public once criticized the FDA and other regulatory agencies for being too slow in bringing new, potentially lifesaving drugs to the consumer. In the early 1990s, organized consumer groups and drug manufacturers pressured governmental officials to speed up the drug review process. Reasons for delays in the FDA drug approval process were outdated guidelines, poor communication, and agency understaffing.

In 1992, FDA officials, members of Congress, and representatives from pharmaceutical companies negotiated the Prescription Drug User Fee Act on a five-year trial basis. This act required drug and biologic manufacturers to pay substantial application fees at the time of an NDA to fund the approval process. This act requires that the FDA meet certain benchmarks, mostly related to speeding up the NDA process. With this extra income, the FDA hired more employees and restructured its organization to handle the greater number of drug applications more efficiently. Restructuring was a resounding success. From 1992 to 1996, the FDA approved double the number of drugs while cutting some review times by as much as half. In 1997, the FDA Modernization Act was passed, reauthorizing the Prescription Drug User Fee Act. It allowed drug companies to give healthcare providers information about *FDA-unapproved* uses of certain drugs. For example, sometimes drugs are approved to treat one condition, but not others; however, healthcare providers may discover that the drug is useful in treating a different problem. When such a benefit is found frequently, a drug company is allowed to share accurate information with other providers about the drug's "unapproved" but effective use in treating another condition. When a drug is being prescribed for a condition for which it is not FDA-approved, it said to be an **off-label use**.

In recent years, the FDA has made more drugs available to the U.S. public and with a faster process of review using four general approaches. *Priority Review* has focused on specific drugs that can be developed successfully within 6 months. *Breakthrough Therapy* designates that additional drugs may be explored that show substantial improvement over existing treatments. *Accelerated Approval* allows for faster authorization of therapeutic drugs that fill a challenging or unmet medical need. *Fast Track* approval means that important criteria such as accelerated and more frequent meetings can facilitate faster development and review of drugs to treat more serious medical conditions.

One current concern is that drugs are being developed at a faster rate than risks can be assessed. This is especially true for those drugs targeted to treat certain cancers. Officials have continued to call for patients, pharmacists, allied health workers, nurses, physicians, hospitals, and pharmaceutical companies to work together to minimize risks. Because of the faster rate at which drugs are being approved for therapy, the potential for adverse drug–drug and drug–herbal interactions is greater than ever before.

CONCEPT REVIEW 1.2

- Can you recall the major U.S. acts, standards, and organizations leading up to the present time? When was the FDA established? What current U.S. laws regulate how drugs are approved for marketing?

Core Concept 1.10 ▶ Healthcare providers must be prepared to deal with the threat of biological and chemical attacks.

Throughout most of the history of the United States, concern about epidemic diseases mainly focused on the possible spread of traditional infectious diseases such as influenza, tuberculosis, cholera, and human immunodeficiency virus (HIV). Healthcare providers were also concerned about widespread food poisoning and sexually transmitted infections other than HIV. Uncommon diseases such as anthrax produced fewer fatalities, so less attention was given to them.

However, after the September 11, 2001, terrorist attacks, the healthcare community became more aware of the possibility of **bioterrorism**—the intentional use of infectious biological agents, chemical substances, or radiation to cause widespread harm or illness. Such federal agencies as the Centers for Disease Control and Prevention (CDC) and the U.S. Department of Defense increased efforts to inform, educate, and prepare the public for disease outbreaks caused by bioterrorism. In 2002, the U.S. Department of Homeland Security was organized to provide additional security and defense for the United States in a terrorist attack. The department also prioritized the important issue of citizen preparedness, educating families how best to prepare for natural emergencies and disasters.

bio = *living organisms*
terrorism = *to induce fear*

In 2014, an Ebola outbreak in West Africa rapidly became an area of concern for citizens in the United States. Three important cases were initially discovered: one involving the death of a man who had traveled to West Africa, and two locally acquired cases where healthcare workers had cared for an Ebola patient in Dallas, Texas. After treatment, the healthcare workers recovered and were discharged from the hospital. Later, a medical aid worker who had volunteered in Guinea was diagnosed with Ebola and hospitalized in New York City. After a monitoring period, the patient recovered and was released from the hospital. Following these incidents, the CDC issued updated advice to state and local officials. When treating patients with infectious diseases, healthcare providers were reminded to practice meticulous infection control procedures. The CDC also recommended that hospital workers implement a 21-day monitoring period.

▶ Lifespan and Diversity

The Ebola virus causes death by hemorrhagic fever in up to 90% of the patients who show clinical symptoms of infection.

Pandemic events or diseases of epidemic proportion that spread across human populations are considered a significant threat. These along with terrorist attacks have prompted the healthcare community to expand its awareness to outbreaks and interventions.

pan = *all*
demic = *people or population*

Among the goals of a bioterrorist are to create widespread public panic and cause as many casualties as possible. The list of agents that can be used for this purpose is long. Some of these agents are easily obtainable and require little or no specialized knowledge to spread. The most worrisome threats are:

- Acutely infectious diseases such as anthrax, smallpox, plague, and hemorrhagic viruses
- Incapacitating chemicals such as nerve gas, cyanide, and chlorinated agents
- Nuclear and radiation emergencies.

One can easily imagine what devastation would be caused if laboratories and healthcare providers were not able to identify, isolate, and treat widespread diseases caused by pandemic events or bioterrorism. The following chapters contain important information related to these areas: Chapter 27 reviews the topic of antibiotics for infectious diseases. The treatment of chemical nerve warfare agents is discussed in Chapter 9. Chapter 33 includes a discussion of the treatment of radiation exposure.

Chapter Review

Core Concepts Summary

1.1 Pharmacology is an expansive and challenging topic.

Pharmacology, the study of medicine, is a subject devoted to proper drug treatment and health of the human body. It is an expansive topic utilizing concepts from human biology, pathophysiology, and chemistry.

1.2 For healthcare providers, the fields of pharmacology and therapeutics are connected.

Therapeutics is the science associated with the treatment of suffering and the prevention of disease. *Pharmacotherapeutics* is the useful application of drugs for the purpose of fighting disease. The study of pharmacology is important to health professionals from many different fields.

1.3 Medicines may be classified as traditional drugs, biologics, and natural alternatives.

Drugs are chemical agents used to treat disease by producing biologic responses within the body. Therapeutic drugs are classified as substances produced chemically or naturally. Biologics are natural agents produced by animal cells or microorganisms. Alternative therapies include natural herbs, plant extracts, or dietary supplements.

1.4 Medications are available by prescription or over the counter.

There are two major methods of dispensing drugs. Prescription drugs require a healthcare provider's order; OTC drugs do not. There are advantages and disadvantages to both dispensing methods.

1.5 Pharmaceutics is the science of pharmacy.

Pharmaceutics involves the successful dispensation of drugs for therapeutic purposes. Dispensing medication safely is a major challenge for healthcare providers and patients.

1.6 Drug regulations were created to protect the public from drug misuse.

The first drug laws were acts created by Congress to protect patients from wrongful therapeutic claims. These and other standards form the basis of modern drug regulation agencies and organizations, such as the U.S. Department of Health and Human Services, the FDA, and publications such as the *U.S. Pharmacopoeia-National Formulary*.

1.7 U.S. drug standards have become increasingly complex.

The FDA is the primary agency regulating drug safety. Three branches of the FDA control policies regarding drug therapies: the Center for Drug Evaluation and Research (CDER), the Center for Biologics Evaluation and Research (CBER), and the Center for Food Safety and Applied Nutrition (CFSAN). Black box warnings were enacted by the FDA. The National Center for Complementary and Integrative Health (NCCIH) was established for scientific research and information about alternative therapies.

1.8 There are four stages of approval for therapeutic and biologic drugs.

Drug approval occurs in four stages: preclinical investigation, clinical investigation, submission of a new drug application (NDA) with review, and postmarketing studies. Clinical phase trials must be completed before drugs are approved for public use.

1.9 Governmental agencies face the dual challenge of increasing the speed of drug approval while still ensuring the safety of new drugs.

FDA officials, members of Congress, and pharmaceutical company representatives negotiated the Prescription Drug User Fee Act and FDA Modernization Act. These acts have sped up the approval process and require drug and biologic manufacturers to provide yearly product user fees. The concern now is that drugs are being approved at a rate faster than risks can be assessed.

1.10 Healthcare providers must be prepared to deal with the threat of biological and chemical attack.

Drugs are among the most powerful weapons to combat pandemic events and bioterrorism. Federal agencies have taken an active role in educating and preparing the public and the healthcare community about unexpected disease outbreaks.

REVIEW Questions

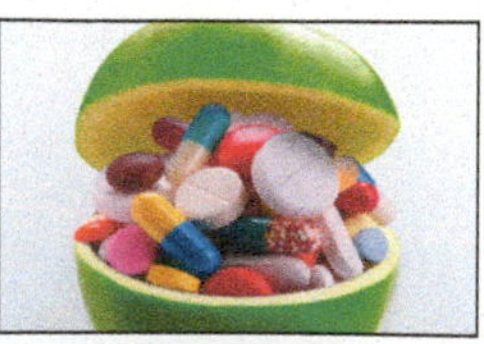

Answer the following questions to assess your knowledge of the chapter material, and go back and review any material that is not clear to you.

1. Pathophysiology is defined as the study of:
   1. How drugs enter and travel throughout the body and the responses they produce
   2. How drugs improve the health of the human body
   3. Drugs and how they elicit different responses
   4. Diseases and functional changes occurring as a result of disease
2. Biologics are:
   1. Produced in nature and include herbs, natural extracts, vitamins, and minerals
   2. Chemically produced in a laboratory
   3. Naturally produced in animal cells, microorganisms, or by the body itself
   4. Not used routinely by healthcare providers
3. Healthcare providers, such as Licensed Practical Nurses (LPNs) and Licensed Vocational Nurses (LVNs), are directly involved with drug administration and all of the following activities except:
   1. Prescribing medications
   2. Educating patients about their medications
   3. Enforcing drug laws
   4. Helping patients with medication management
4. What precautions should patients be aware of when taking over-the-counter (OTC) drugs? (Select all that apply.)
   1. Self-treatment is sometimes ineffective.
   2. OTC drugs may react with foods, herbal products, and prescription or other OTC drugs.

3. All OTC drugs are safe or they would not be available without a prescription.
4. Instructions included with the medications should be read and followed as directed.
5. Drugs recommended by friends are the best for the patient's situation.

5. Dispensing of drugs to patients after they have been examined by a licensed healthcare provider is:
   1. Pharmacology
   2. Pharmaceutics
   3. Therapeutics
   4. Healthcare

6. The act that prevents the marketing of drugs that have not been thoroughly tested is the:
   1. Pure Food and Drug Act (1906).
   2. Food, Drug, and Cosmetic Act (1938).
   3. Prescription Drug User Fee Act (1992).
   4. FDA Modernization Act (1997).

7. The longest part of the drug approval process is typically the:
   1. Preclinical investigation.
   2. Clinical investigation.
   3. New drug application submission and review.
   4. Postmarketing studies.

8. The legislation responsible for cutting new drug application review times as much as 50% is the:
   1. Pure Food and Drug Act.
   2. Sherley Amendment.
   3. Public Health Services Act.
   4. Prescription Drug User Fee Act.

9. Black box warnings are:
   1. Used to inform the consumer about general medication information.
   2. A list of ingredients within the medication.
   3. Located on the drug container label.
   4. The primary alert for notifying consumers of potential extreme adverse drug effects.

10. Which of the following is considered a bioterrorist threat? (Select all that apply.)
    1. Anthrax contamination
    2. Incapacitating chemicals
    3. Radiation exposure
    4. Viruses that cause the common cold
    5. Sexually transmitted infections

Answers and complete rationales for the Review Questions appear in Appendix A.

SELECTED BIBIOGRAPHY

Banks, L. (2013). Caring for elderly adults during disasters: Improving health outcomes and recovery. *Southern Medical Journal, 106*, 94–98. doi:10.1097/SMJ.0b013e31827c5157

Centers for Disease Control and Prevention. (n.d.) *Emergency preparedness & response: Bioterrorism agent/diseases*. Retrieved from http://emergency.cdc.gov/agent/agentlist.asp

Centers for Disease Control and Prevention. (2015) *Infection prevention and control recommendations for hospitalized patients under investigation (PUIs) for Ebola virus disease (EVD) in U.S. hospitals*. Retrieved from http://www.cdc.gov/vhf/ebola/hcp/infection-prevention-and-control-recommendations.html

Dörr, H., Baier, T., Hoebbel, M., & Meineke, V. (2013). Database SEARCH: Radiation induced skin reactions and gastrointestinal signs and symptoms as prognostic factors of the acute radiation syndrome. In *Challenge CBRN Medical Defense International, April 2013*, p. 22. Retrieved from http://media.bsbb.de/Conrad/CHALLENGE-Abstracts-ConRad.pdf

National Institutes of Health, U.S. National Library of Medicine. (n.d.). *Clinical trial phases*. Retrieved from https://www.nlm.nih.gov/services/ctphases.html

Pegg, D. (2013). *25 deadliest diseases in human history . . . not surprising, Ebola is one of them*. Retrieved from http://list25.com/25-deadliest-diseases-in-human-history

Peterson, K., McDonagh, M., Thakurta, S., Dana, T., Roberts, C., Chou, R., & Helfand, M. (2010). *Drug class review: Nonsteroidal anti-inflammatory drugs (NSAIDs): Final update 4 report*. Retrieved at http://www.ncbi.nlm.nih.gov/pubmedhealth/PMH0009765

World Health Organization. (2015). *Ebola situation report, 20 January 2016*. Retrieved from http://www.who.int/csr/disease/ebola/situation-reports/en

Chapter 2

Drug Classes, Schedules, and Categories

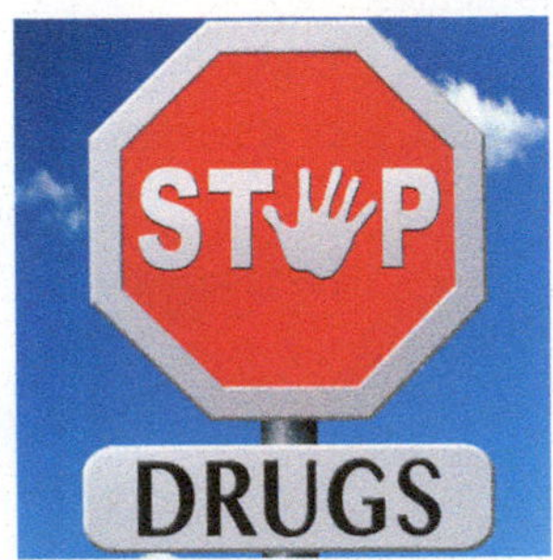

Core Concepts

2.1 **Drugs may be organized by their therapeutic and pharmacologic classifications.**

2.2 **Drugs have more than one name.**

2.3 **The differences between trade name drugs and their generic equivalents include price, formulations, and, most importantly, bioavailability.**

2.4 **Drugs with a potential for misuse and abuse are categorized into schedules.**

2.5 **In order to assess fetal risks, all prescription drugs are classified according to safety in pregnancy categories.**

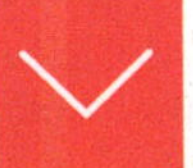

Learning Outcomes

After reading this chapter, the student should be able to:

1. Discuss the prototype approach to drug classification and the basis for which drugs are placed into therapeutic and pharmacologic classes.
2. Distinguish between a drug's chemical name, generic name, and trade name.
3. Explain how trade name drugs are different from generic equivalent drugs.
4. Discuss why drugs are sometimes placed on a restrictive list and referred to as *scheduled drugs* or *controlled substances*.
5. Identify the five pregnancy categories and explain what each category represents.

Key Terms

bioavailability (BEYE-oh-ah-VALE-ah-BILL-ih-TEE)
bioequivalence (BEYE-oh-ee-KWIV-oh-LENZ)
chemical name
combination drugs
controlled substance
generic name (je-NARE-ik)
mechanism of action
pharmacologic classification (FAR-mah-koh-LOJ-ik)
prototype drug (PRO-toh-type)
scheduled drugs
teratogen (tare-AT-oh-jen)
therapeutic classification (ther-ah-PEW-tik)
therapeutic interchange
trade name

Because of the large number of drugs available, healthcare providers and consumers must have a system for identifying drugs and determining the limitations of their use. This chapter covers the methods by which drugs may be organized—by therapeutic or pharmacologic classification. This chapter also discusses drug schedules and pregnancy categories.

Drugs may be organized by their therapeutic and pharmacologic classifications.

◀ **Core Concept 2.1**

Drugs may be classified in two major ways. They may be organized by *therapeutic usefulness*. This is referred to as a **therapeutic classification**. Drugs may also be categorized by **mechanism of action** or *how they work pharmacologically*. This is referred to as a **pharmacologic classification**. Both methods are widely used in pharmacology, even though healthcare providers often do not make the distinction when the primary purpose of drug therapy is to improve the health of their patients.

Table 2.1 shows the method of therapeutic classification, using cardiac care as the example. The cardiovascular system is concerned with the proper functioning of the heart and blood vessels. Different types of drugs affect specific cardiovascular functions. Some drugs influence blood clotting, whereas others lower blood cholesterol or prevent the onset of stroke. Drugs may be used to lower blood pressure, treat heart failure, correct abnormal heart rhythm, alleviate chest pain, and treat or prevent circulatory shock. Drugs that affect cardiac disorders may be placed in numerous therapeutic classes. Drugs that influence blood clotting are called *anticoagulants*; those that lower blood cholesterol are called *antihyperlipidemics*; and those that lower blood pressure are called *antihypertensives*.

A therapeutic classification need not be complicated. For example, it is appropriate to classify a medication simply as "a drug used for stroke" or "a drug used for shock." The key to therapeutic classification is to state clearly what a particular drug does clinically. A few additional examples of therapeutic classification are antiemetics (to prevent vomiting or emesis), antacids (to reduce gastrointestinal [GI] acid), anti-inflammatory drugs (to reduce inflammation), and antibiotics (to fight infective microorganisms).

Pharmacologic classification addresses *how* the medication produces its effects within the body. This method most directly applies to the foundational areas of science study, including principles of cellular and molecular biology.

Table 2.2 shows various types of pharmacologic classifications using high blood pressure (hypertension) as an example. A *diuretic* is a class of drug used to treat hypertension by lowering plasma volume. Thus, lowering plasma volume is the mechanism of action by which diuretics work. *Calcium channel blockers* treat hypertension by limiting the force of heart contractions. Other drugs, such as angiotensin-converting enzyme (ACE) inhibitors, block components of the hormonal network called the *renin-angiotensin pathway*, thereby reducing hypertension. Notice that each example describes *how* hypertension may be controlled. Thus, the drug's pharmacologic classification is more specific than its therapeutic classification and requires application of human biochemical and physiological principles.

Table 2.1 Organizing Drugs by Therapeutic Classification

Therapeutic Focus	
Cardiac care: Drugs affecting cardiovascular function	
Therapeutic Usefulness	**Therapeutic Classification***
influencing blood clotting	anticoagulant
lowering blood cholesterol	antihyperlipidemic
lowering blood pressure	antihypertensive
treating abnormal heartbeat	antidysrhythmic
treating chest pain (angina)	antianginal drug

*Note: Although the names of some therapeutic classifications may sound complicated, drug terminology will become more familiar as you study drugs and drug classes. When studying this topic, always refer to a medical dictionary and a drug guide.

Table 2.2 Organizing Drugs by Pharmacologic Classification

Focusing on Physiological Action	
Therapy for high blood pressure may be achieved by:	
Mechanism of Action	**Pharmacologic Classification**
lowering plasma volume	diuretic
blocking heart calcium channels	calcium channel blocker
blocking enzyme activity	ACE inhibitor
blocking stress-related activity	adrenergic blocker (drug that inhibits actions of the sympathetic nervous system)
dilating peripheral blood vessels	vasodilator

Before studying a particular drug's mechanism of action, it is recommended that students first become comfortable with the broad drug classes and then gradually move to more specific examples. Prototype drugs are an excellent place to start. A **prototype drug** is the well-understood drug model to which other medications in a pharmacologic class are compared. By learning the prototype drug, students may then predict the actions and adverse effects of other drugs in the same class. For example, by knowing the effects of penicillin V, students can apply this knowledge to the other drugs in the penicillin antibiotic class. *Students should be aware, however, that in many cases the original drug prototype is not the most widely used drug in its class.* As new drugs are developed, features such as antibiotic resistance, fewer side effects, or a more precise site of action might be factors that sway healthcare providers away from using the older drugs. Therefore, to master the subject of pharmacology, it is essential not only to be familiar with the well-established drug prototypes but also to keep up with newer and more popular drugs as they are developed and used for effective therapy. For all prototype drugs featured in this text, both therapeutic and pharmacologic classifications are provided to help students organize drug information.

CONCEPT REVIEW 2.1

- What is the difference between a therapeutic classification and a pharmacologic classification? What is a *prototype drug*, and how is the prototype drug similar to and different from other drugs within the same pharmacologic or therapeutic class?

Core Concept 2.2 ▶

Drugs have more than one name.

A major challenge when studying pharmacology is learning thousands of drug names. Adding to this difficulty is the fact that most drugs have multiple names. The three basic types of drug names are chemical, generic, and trade.

A **chemical name** is assigned using standard nomenclature established by the International Union of Pure and Applied Chemistry (IUPAC). A drug has only one chemical name, which is helpful in predicting its physical and chemical properties. Although chemical names convey a clear and concise meaning about the nature of a drug, they are often very complicated and difficult to pronounce or remember. For example, the chemical name of diazepam is 7-chloro-1,3-ciphydro-1-methyl-5-phenyl-2H-1,4-benzodiazepin-2-one. In only a few cases, usually when the name is brief and easily remembered, are chemical names commonly used. Examples of brief (and therefore useful) chemical names include lithium carbonate, calcium gluconate, and sodium chloride.

More practically, drugs are sometimes classified by *a portion* of their chemical structure, known as the chemical group name. Examples are antibiotic drugs, such as the fluoroquinolones and beta-lactam medications. Other common examples include the phenothiazines, thiazides, and benzodiazepines. Although names like these may seem complicated at first, familiarity with chemical group names will grow, and the nomenclature will become more manageable as the student becomes more proficient and communicates with fellow healthcare providers.

The **generic name** of a drug is assigned by the U.S. Adopted Name Council. With few exceptions, generic names are less complicated and easier to remember than

Table 2.3 Trade Name Products Containing Popular Generic Drugs

Generic Drugs	Trade Names
aspirin	Acuprin, Anacin, Aspergum, Bayer, Bufferin, Ecotrin, Empirin, Magnaprin, Miniprin, Ridiprin, Sloprin, Uni-Buff, Uni-Tren, Zorprin
diphenhydramine	Aler-Dryl, Allergia-C, Benadryl, Compoz Nighttime Sleep Aid, Diphedryl, Diphenadryl, Hydramine, Nytol, Pardryl, PediaCare Children's Allergy, Sominex, Unisom
ibuprofen	Advil, Dolgesic, Genpril, Haltran, IB Pro, Midol, Motrin, Nuprin, Rufen, Tab-Profen, Ultraprin

chemical names. Many organizations, including the U.S. Food and Drug Administration (FDA), the U.S. Pharmacopoeia, and the World Health Organization, routinely describe a medication by its generic name. Because there is only one generic name for each drug, healthcare providers also routinely use this name, and pharmacology students generally must memorize it.

A drug's **trade name** is assigned by the company marketing the drug. The name is usually selected for marketability, and it is usually easy to remember. The trade name is also called the *proprietary*, *product*, or *brand* name. The term *proprietary* relates to ownership. In the United States, a drug developer is given exclusive rights to name and market a drug for 17 years after a new drug application (NDA) is submitted to the FDA. Because it takes several years before a drug can be approved, the amount of time spent in approval is subtracted from the 17 years. For example, if it takes seven years for a drug to be approved, competing companies will not be allowed to market a generic equivalent drug for another 10 years. The rationale for this is that the developing company must be allowed sufficient time to recoup the millions of dollars spent in research and the time needed to develop the new drug. After 17 years, competing companies may sell a generic equivalent drug, using a different trade name, which the FDA must approve.

Trade names may be a challenge because of the dozens of product names containing similar ingredients. In other words, there is not a one-to-one match between the generic drug name and the trade name of a drug. In addition, some **combination drugs** contain more than one active generic ingredient, making it difficult to match the trade name with only one generic drug product included. As an example, refer to Table 2.3 and consider the drug diphenhydramine (generic name), also called Benadryl (one of many trade names). Many other trade names can be matched with diphenhydramine, and the sheer numbers of examples often represent a challenge for even the brightest student. One reason for different trade names has to do with the different uses of a drug. For example, Benadryl is marketed and sold as a drug for allergic reactions, whereas Unisom is marketed and sold for the treatment of insomnia. Further, generic drug doses may not be similar among the various trade name products. The rule of thumb is that a formulation's active ingredients are listed by their generic names on the product label. In publications where drugs are catalogued, the generic name is often written in lowercase, whereas the trade name is capitalized. This is the method used in this text.

CONCEPT REVIEW 2.2

- What are the differences between a chemical, a generic, and a trade name? Which name is most often used to describe the active ingredients within a drug product?

The differences between trade name drugs and their generic equivalents include price, formulations, and, most importantly, bioavailability.

◀ **Core Concept 2.3**

Usually, generic drugs are less expensive than trade name drugs. The reason is that a pharmaceutical company determines the price of a proprietary drug during its 17 years of exclusive rights to that new drug. Because there is no competition, the price can be kept quite high. The pharmaceutical company that developed a drug can sometimes obtain FDA approval to extend its exclusive rights to the drug. The exclusive rights and the high initial cost of a trade drug help the pharmaceutical company recover expenses it incurred in conducting research and developing the new medication. Once the exclusive rights end, competing companies develop and market their own version of the generic drug for less money, and consumer savings may be considerable. In some states, pharmacists may routinely substitute a generic drug when the prescription calls for a trade name. In other states, the pharmacist must dispense drugs directly as written by the healthcare practitioner or obtain approval before providing a generic substitute.

The companies that market trade name drugs often aggressively oppose laws that might restrict the routine use of their products. They claim that significant differences exist between a trade name drug and its generic equivalent, and that switching to the generic drug may be harmful to the patient. Patient advocates, on the other hand, argue that generic substitutions should always be permitted because of the cost savings.

bio = *in the living organism*
equivalence = *same impact*

Are there real differences between a trade name drug and its generic equivalent? Despite the fact that the doses may be identical, drug formulations are not always the same. The two drugs may have different *inert* ingredients or be processed differently. For example, in a tablet form, the active ingredients may be more tightly compressed in one of the preparations than in another, and this might affect how well the body can use the drug. Although reports may state that trade name drugs and generic drugs have the same **bioequivalence**, or impact on the body, and for all intents and purposes the same medication and dose, different drug products may not have the same rate and extent of absorption. For example, thyroid disorder is a delicately balanced condition for which too much medication or not enough medication will make a difference in symptoms experienced by a patient. Levothyroxine tablets (generic drug) may differ from how much Synthroid or Levoxyl (trade names) is absorbed or circulates in the bloodstream.

bio = *in the living organism*
availability = *free to activate cellular targets*

The key to comparing trade name drugs and their generic equivalents lies in measuring the *bioavailability* of the two preparations. **Bioavailability** is the physiologic ability of the drug to reach its target cells and produce its therapeutic effect (Figure 2.1). Anything that affects absorption of a drug or its distribution to the target cells will certainly affect drug action. Measuring how long a drug takes to exert its therapeutic effect gives pharmacologists a crude measure of bioavailability. Using another example, if a patient is in circulatory shock and it takes a generic drug five minutes longer than the trade name drug to produce its effect, that difference would be significant. However, if a generic medication for arthritis pain relief takes 45 minutes to act, compared with the trade name drug that takes 40 minutes, it probably does not matter which drug is prescribed.

In some cases, pharmacists must inform or notify patients of substitutions of generics for trade names. Pharmaceutical companies and some healthcare providers have supported disclosure of substitution, claiming that generic drugs—even those that have small differences in bioavailability or bioequivalence—could adversely affect outcomes in

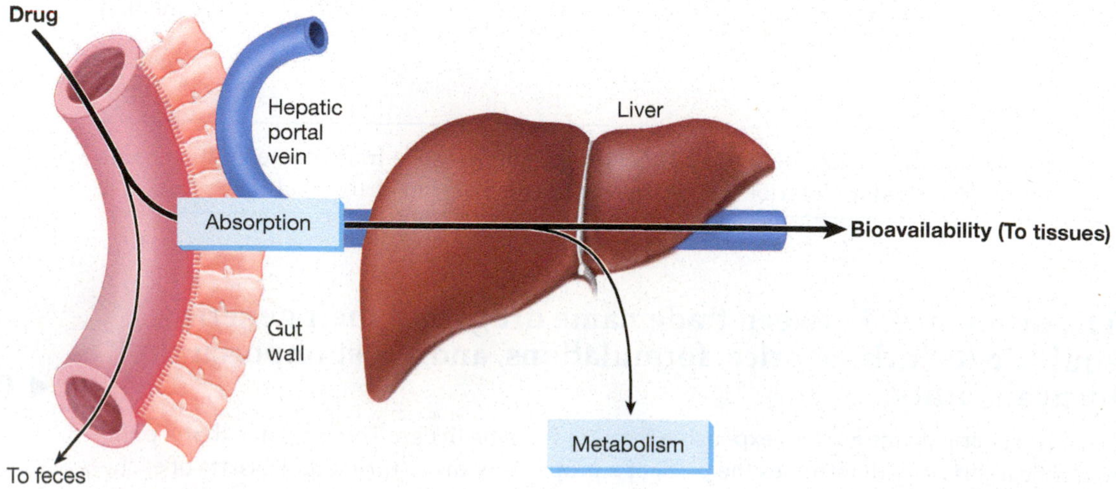

FIGURE 2.1 A drug's bioavailability will depend on the dosage form and how much will actually reach the target location.

patients with critical conditions or illnesses. Some states have compiled a *negative* formulary, a list of trade name drugs that pharmacists may *not* dispense as generic drugs. These drugs must only be dispensed exactly as written on the prescription, using the trade name drug the healthcare provider prescribed. However, laws frequently change: In many instances, the efforts of consumer advocacy groups have led to changes in or elimination of negative formulary lists.

For some long-term healthcare facilities or nursing homes, **therapeutic interchange**, or exchange of medicines within the same therapeutic or pharmacologic class, may be authorized for distribution to patients. With this approach, initiation and maintenance of treatment is interdisciplinary and involves the pharmacist, healthcare providers, clinical staff, and the patient's family. Adverse reactions and the safety of medications must be closely monitored for positive therapeutic outcomes and effectiveness.

Drugs with a potential for misuse and abuse are categorized into schedules.

◀ **Core Concept 2.4**

Some drugs are frequently abused or have a high potential for becoming addictive. Technically, *addiction* refers to the overwhelming feeling that drives someone to use a drug repeatedly. *Dependence* is a related term, often defined as a physiologic or psychological need for a substance. *Physical dependence* refers to an altered physical condition caused by the nervous system adapting to repeated drug use. In this case, when the drug is no longer available, the individual experiences physical signs of discomfort known as *withdrawal*. In contrast, when an individual is *psychologically dependent*, there are few signs of physical discomfort when the drug is withdrawn; however, the individual feels an intense compelling desire to continue drug use. These concepts are discussed in detail in Chapter 8.

Drugs that cause dependency and addiction are restricted to use in situations of medical necessity, that is, if they are allowed at all. According to law, drugs that have a significant potential for abuse are placed into five general categories called *schedules*. Additional schedules may contain drugs exempt from inclusion in the other categories. **Scheduled drugs** are classified according to their potential for abuse, dependency, and addiction: Schedule I drugs have the highest potential for abuse. They have little or no therapeutic value or are intended for research purposes only. Drugs in the remaining schedules may be dispensed only in cases when therapeutic value has been determined. Carisoprodol (Soma) may not be classified under Schedule IV in some states. Schedule V is the only category in which some drugs may be dispensed without a prescription because the quantities of the controlled drug are so low that the possibility of causing dependence is extremely remote. A few states recognize a sixth or seventh category. Schedule VI drugs are those that have no medical use and a very low risk of addiction. Marijuana may be listed as a Schedule VI drug. Butyl nitrate or "poppers" may be listed under the heading of Schedule VII. Table 2.4 shows the five major drug schedules with examples. However, not all drugs with an abuse potential are regulated or placed into schedules. Tobacco, alcohol, and caffeine are significant examples.

Table 2.4 Major Drug Schedule and Examples

Drug Schedule	Abuse Potential	Physical Dependence	Psychological Dependence	Examples
I	Very High	High	High	heroin, lysergic acid diethylamide (LSD), peyote, methaqualone, and 3,4-methylenedioxymethamphetamine ("ecstasy")
II	High	High	High	hydromorphone, methadone, meperidine, oxycodone, and fentanyl; amphetamine, methamphetamine, methylphenidate, amobarbital, glutethimide, and pentobarbital
III	Moderate	Moderate	High	products containing not more than 90 mg of codeine per dosage unit, buprenorphine products, benzphetamine, phendimetrazine, ketamine, and anabolic steroids
IV	Low	Low	Low	carisoprodol, clonazepam, clorazepate, diazepam, lorazepam, midazolam, temazepam, and triazolam
V	Very Low	Low	Low	cough preparations containing not more than 200 mg of codeine per 100 mL

Source: Data from List of controlled substances, U.S. Department of Justice, Drug Enforcement Administration, Office of Diversion Control, n.d.

In the United States, a **controlled substance** is a drug restricted by the Controlled Substances Act of 1970 and later revisions. The Controlled Substances Act is also called the Comprehensive Drug Abuse Prevention and Control Act. This act has several implications for the drugs in the controlled substances schedules. Hospitals and pharmacies must register with the U.S. Drug Enforcement Administration (DEA) and use their assigned registration numbers to purchase scheduled drugs. They must maintain complete records of all quantities purchased and sold. Drugs with higher abuse potential have more restrictions. For example, orders in a hospital must be written and signed by the healthcare provider. Most of the time, a computer system is used to obtain Schedule II drugs. Telephone orders to a pharmacy are not permitted. In an outpatient setting, refills for Schedule II drugs are not permitted, and patients must visit their healthcare providers first and then provide an originally signed prescription written or printed on paper. Even emergency departments have specific policies regarding treatment of patients with Schedule II drugs. Those convicted of unlawful manufacturing, distributing, and dispensing of controlled substances face severe penalties.

Core Concept 2.5 ▶

In order to assess fetal risks, all prescription drugs are classified according to safety in pregnancy categories.

terato = *severe deformity*
gen = *something that produces*

A major concern of expectant parents is whether a drug will harm their developing baby. Any substance that will harm a developing fetus or embryo is referred to as a **teratogen**. Pregnant patients should never take any prescribed, illegal, or OTC drug or any herbal or dietary supplement without the advice of their healthcare providers.

To protect the fetus from the teratogenic effects of prescription drugs, the FDA has implemented a category system for classifying drugs based on how safe they are for the mother and the developing baby. According to this system, drugs are placed into one of five *pregnancy categories*, labeled as A, B, C, D, and X. These labels appear within package inserts and identify levels of risk to women and the fetus. The levels are based on degrees to which a drug has been proven to cause birth defects in laboratory animals or in human beings. These categories are summarized in Table 2.5.

Consumers sometimes question whether the testing of laboratory animals is an effective way to predict harm to a developing human fetus or embryo. Results from animal testing are not always transferable to the human body. In fact, results from animal experimentation often vary from species to species. For this reason, consumers should always be cautious, even when there is reasonable assurance that a drug is safe.

The FDA is in the process of establishing new rules for assessing pregnancy risk. The proposed system will discard the current categories and instead require drug companies to

Table 2.5 Categories of Safety in Pregnancy

Safety Category	Explanation	Examples
A Lowest Risk	Studies have not shown a risk to women or to the fetus.	ferrous fumarate (Ferranol), levothyroxine (Synthroid), potassium chloride (KCl), potassium gluconate (Kaon Tablets), prenatal multivitamins, thyroglobulin (Proloid)
B	Animal studies have not shown a risk to the fetus or, if they have, studies in women have not confirmed this risk.	amoxicillin (Amoxil), fluoxetine (Prozac), insulin (Humulin R), loperamide (Imodium), penicillins, ranitidine (Zantac)
C	Animal studies have shown a risk to the fetus, but controlled studies have not been performed in women.	acyclovir (Zovirax), amitryptiline (Elavil), furosemide (Lasix), hydrochlorothiazide (HydroURIL), iron dextran (K FeRON), mineral oil (Fleet Mineral Oil), senna (Senokot)
D	Use of this drug category may cause harm to the fetus, but it may provide benefit to the mother in a life-threatening situation or when a safer therapy is not available.	ACE inhibitors, alcohol, cortisone acetate (Cortistan), nonsteroidal anti-inflammatory drugs in the third trimester, tetracyclines
X Highest Risk	Studies have shown a significant risk to women and to the fetus.	castor oil (Purge), isotretinoin, methotrexate, most oral contraceptives, norethindrone (Norlutin), oxymetholone (Anadrol), progesterone (oral forms), statins, warfarin (Coumadin)

list specific risks caused by the drug, such as structural abnormalities of the embryo or fetus, or increased infant mortality caused by taking the drug during pregnancy. The new labeling will also include possible lactation risks to the baby if a drug is taken while breastfeeding.

Chapter Review

Core Concepts Summary

2.1 Drugs may be organized by their therapeutic and pharmacologic classifications.

Two common ways to classify drugs are by therapeutic classification and pharmacologic classification. Therapeutic classes are based on a drug's clinical usefulness. Pharmacologic classes are based on a drug's mechanism of action. Prototype drugs are used to compare drugs within the same classification. Knowing about prototype drugs can help students understand other, similar drugs.

2.2 Drugs have more than one name.

Drugs may be described by a chemical, generic, or trade name. There are advantages and disadvantages to each naming method.

2.3 The differences between trade name drugs and their generic equivalents include price, formulations, and, most importantly, bioavailability.

In most states, generic drugs may be substituted for trade name products if the prescribing healthcare provider does not object. When generic drugs are substituted, differences in bioavailability may affect the safety and effectiveness of drug therapy.

2.4 Drugs with a potential for misuse and abuse are categorized into schedules.

Drugs that have the potential for abuse or dependency are placed into schedules. Schedule I is the most restrictive category. Schedule V is the least restrictive category. In some states, marijuana is classified as Schedule VI. The DEA handles drug misuse.

2.5 In order to assess fetal risks, all prescription drugs are classified according to safety in pregnancy categories.

In the United States, all drugs are placed into one of five pregnancy categories: A, B, C, D, and X. Drugs in category A are the safest; those in category X are the most harmful.

REVIEW Questions

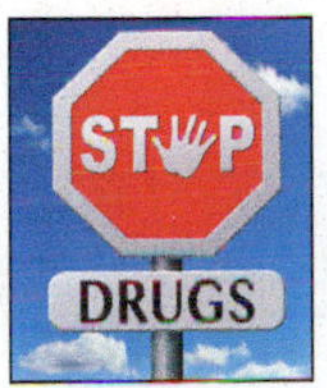

Answer the following questions to assess your knowledge of the chapter material, and go back and review any material that is not clear to you.

1. Which of the following types of drug classification focuses on what a drug does clinically?
   1. Therapeutic
   2. Pharmacologic
   3. Chemical
   4. All of the above

2. *How* a medication produces its effects in the body is referred to as a drug's:
   1. Therapeutic usefulness.
   2. Mechanism of action.
   3. Model for other drugs combating similar diseases.
   4. Clinical focus.

3. In which of the following categories does a drug have only one name?
   1. Chemical name
   2. Generic name
   3. Trade name
   4. Both 1 and 2

4. Which of the following statements is correct?
   1. Because chemical drug names are often complicated and difficult to remember or pronounce, the chemical structure of a drug is rarely considered in pharmacotherapy.
   2. Matching one active ingredient with one trade name product is not a particularly challenging job for the healthcare provider.

3. When referring to a drug, the generic name is usually capitalized, whereas the trade name is written in lowercase.
4. The drug trade name is sometimes called the proprietary name, suggesting ownership.

5. When examining the question, "Are there real differences between trade name drugs and their generic equivalents?" the answer that emerges from reading this chapter is:
1. Drug formulations for trade name drugs are the same as their generic equivalents.
2. Trade name drugs are always more tightly compressed than generic drugs.
3. Generic drugs are always best because they generally cost less.
4. Trade name drugs are sometimes preferred because of differences in bioavailability compared to generic equivalents.

6. Which of the following are true statements about a negative formulary list of trade name drugs? (Select all that apply.)
1. It is a list of trade name drugs that cannot be substituted with generic drugs.
2. It is consistent throughout the United States.
3. The drugs on the list must be dispensed by the pharmacist using the drug's trade name as written on the prescription.
4. It was formed because of concern over the bioavailability of generic drugs and possible adverse effects on patient outcomes.
5. Some consumer advocacy groups have led to changes in the lists.

7. An altered physical condition caused by the nervous system adapting to repeated drug use is:
1. Addiction.
2. Physical dependence.
3. Psychological dependence.
4. Withdrawal.

8. The Controlled Substances Act of 1970 and later revisions enable the DEA to do which of the following?
1. Introduce drugs into the marketplace.
2. Restrict the use of drugs that have a significant potential for abuse.
3. Restrict the use of all drugs that have an abuse potential.
4. Allow patients to obtain Schedule II drug refills without visiting their healthcare provider first.

9. The drug schedule that allows therapeutic use of a drug with a prescription but contains drugs with relatively lower abuse and dependency potential than other scheduled drugs is:
1. Schedule II.
2. Schedule III.
3. Schedule IV.
4. Schedule V.

10. When preparing to administer medications to pregnant patients, nurses should know that their patients:
1. Are not at risk if they take drugs placed into pregnancy safety category X.
2. Can take herbal or dietary supplements without fear of teratogenic effects to their developing baby.
3. Are relatively safe if they take medications within pregnancy safety category B.
4. Should never take drugs classified as pregnancy safety category D.

Answers and complete rationales for the Review Questions appear in Appendix A.

REFERENCE

U.S. Department of Justice, Drug Enforcement Administration, Office of Diversion Control. (n.d.) *List of controlled substances.* Retrieved from http://www.deadiversion.usdoj.gov/schedules/index.html

SELECTED BIBLIOGRAPHY

Gunatilake, R., & Patil, A. S. (2013). *Drugs in pregnancy.* Retrieved from http://www.merckmanuals.com/professional/gynecology-and-obstetrics/drugs-in-pregnancy/drugs-in-pregnancy

Keenum, A. J., Devoe, J. E., Chisolm, D. J., & Wallace, L. S. (2012). Generic medications for you, but brand-name medications for me. *Research in Social and Administrative Pharmacy, 8*, 574–578. doi:10.1016/j.sapharm.2011.12.004

McCormack, J., & Chmelicek, J. T. (2014). Generic versus brand name: The other drug war. *Canadian Family Physician, 60*(10), 911.

Medical Board of California. (2014) *Guidelines for prescribing controlled substances for pain.* Retrieved from http://www.mbc.ca.gov/licensees/prescribing/pain_guidelines.pdf

Sitler, B., & Hughes, G. (2014, February). Healthcare analytics: Patient engagement—What can we learn from other industries? *Patient Safety & Quality Healthcare.* Retrieved from http://psqh.com/january-february-2014/healthcare-analytics-patient-engagement-what-can-we-learn-from-other-industries

Chapter 3

Principles of Drug Administration

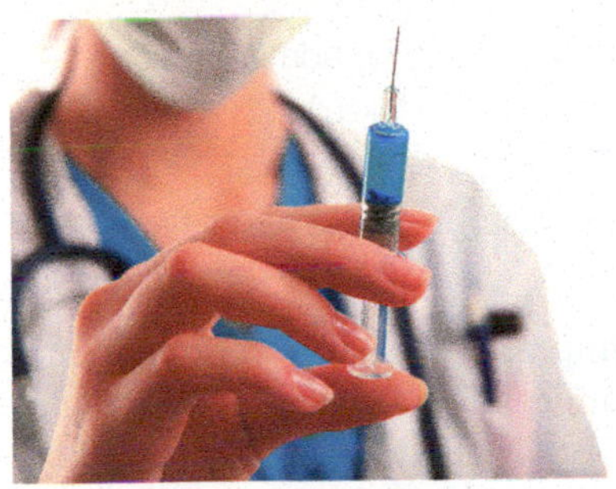

Core Concepts

3.1 A major goal in pharmacotherapy is to limit the number and severity of drug adverse events.
3.2 The rights of drug administration form the basis of proper drug delivery.
3.3 Successful pharmacotherapy depends on patient compliance.
3.4 Healthcare providers may use accepted abbreviations to communicate the directions and times for drug administration.
3.5 Three systems of measurement are used in pharmacology: metric, apothecary, and household.
3.6 Certain protocols and techniques are common to all methods of drug administration.
3.7 Enteral drugs are given orally or via nasogastric or gastrostomy tubes.
3.8 Topical drugs are applied locally to the skin and associated membranes.
3.9 Parenteral administration refers to dispensing medications by routes other than oral or topical.

Learning Outcomes

After reading this chapter, the student should be able to:

1. Discuss drug administration as a component of safe and effective healthcare, including the responsibilities of nurses, nursing assistants, therapists, and technicians.
2. Explain how the six rights of drug administration affect patient safety.
3. Give specific examples of how the healthcare provider can increase patient compliance in taking medications.
4. Interpret abbreviations used in drug administration practices.
5. Compare and contrast the three systems of measurement used in pharmacology.
6. List guidelines common to all methods of drug administration.
7. Explain the proper methods to administer enteral drugs.
8. Explain the proper methods to administer topical drugs.
9. Explain the proper methods to administer parenteral drugs.

Key Terms

adverse drug effect
adverse event
allergic reaction
anaphylaxis (ANN-ah-fah-LAX-iss)
apothecary system (ah-POTH-eh-kare-ee)
astringent effect (ah-STRIN-jent)
buccal route (BUCK-ahl)
compliance (kom-PLY-ans)
contraindications (CON-trah-EN-deh-KAY-shuns)
enteral route (EN-tur-ul)
enteric-coated (in-TARE-ik)
household systems
intradermal (ID) route (IN-trah-DERM-ul)
intramuscular (IM) route (IN-trah-musk-u-lar)
intravenous (IV) route (IN-trah-VEE-nus)
metric system
orally disintegrating tablets (ODTs)
parenteral route (pah-REN-tur-ul)
prn order
routine orders
side effect
single order
six rights of drug administration
standing order
STAT order
subcutaneous route (sub-kew-TAY-nee-us)
sublingual (SL) route (sub-LIN-gwal)
sustained-release (SR)
three checks of drug administration
topical route (TOP-ik-ul)
transdermal (trans-DER-mul)
transmucosal (trans-mew-KOH-sul)

Drug administration is an important part of providing comprehensive care to the patient. During drug administration, members of the healthcare team collaborate closely with pharmacists, physicians, their patients, and each other to ensure the safe delivery of prescribed medications. The purpose of this chapter is to introduce the roles and responsibilities of nurses and other healthcare providers, to define the practice of secure and effective distribution of medications, and to provide a basic overview of the major routes of drug administration.

Core Concept 3.1 ▶

A major goal in pharmacotherapy is to limit the number and severity of drug adverse events.

Whether administering drugs, supervising drug use, or providing assistance, the healthcare provider is expected to be familiar with the general principles of drug delivery. The large number of different drugs and the potential consequences of medication errors make this an enormous task.

The main responsibilities of the nurse include knowing and understanding the following:

- What drug is ordered
- Name (generic and trade) and drug classification
- Intended or proposed use
- Expected therapeutic effects on the body
- Situations under which drugs should not be used, or **contraindications**
- Special considerations (e.g., the effects of age, weight, body fat distribution, possible environmental assaults such as photosensitivity, individual pathophysiological states on pharmacotherapeutic response)
- Unwanted nontherapeutic effects (*side effects*)
- Why the medication has been prescribed for this particular patient
- How the medication is supplied by the pharmacy
- How the medication should be administered, including dosage ranges
- Conditions under which dosage ranges should be modified or the drug discontinued (*adverse drug reactions*)
- What nursing process considerations related to the medication apply to this patient.

contra = *opposing*
indications = *useful applications*

adverse = *negative*
drug = *medication-related*
reaction = *effect*

Nursing assistants, therapists, and technicians work closely with nurses to provide care to patients. Members of the health support staff who do not administer medications but who have an equally important role in providing care to patients have a slightly different list of tasks than nurses. These tasks provide opportunities to monitor patients and make sure no unusual reactions or undesirable effects result from the medication. Examples of tasks include:

- Monitoring blood pressure, pulse rate, and respiration rate
- Observing the skin for changes when replacing soiled or wet clothing, wraps, or bandages

- Observing for rashes or broken skin when dressing wounds, giving massages, and caring for the skin's surface
- Preparing food trays or helping to feed patients
- Observing for changes in the ability to swallow or chew when helping to feed patients
- Observing patients and reporting significant symptoms, reactions, or changes in medical condition
- Reporting strange behaviors or habits in patients
- Helping transport patients
- Monitoring special equipment.

Before any drug is administered, healthcare staff must obtain, process, and communicate important information to one another about the patient's medical history, physical assessment, disease processes, learning needs, and capabilities. They must consider growth and developmental factors and remember that many variables can influence how a patient responds to medications. Understanding these variables can increase the success of pharmacotherapy.

An **adverse event** (AE) is any undesirable experience associated with the use of a medical product in a patient. AEs are generally described in terms of intensity (e.g., mild, moderate, severe, life threatening). The term *serious adverse event (SAE)* is used to define threat of death or immediate risk of death. Some patients may experience AEs with a particular drug, whereas others may not. An AE resulting from drug administration is often termed an *adverse drug reaction* or **adverse drug effect**. Most health professionals simply refer to an unfavorable drug reaction as an *adverse effect*. Adverse effects warrant either lowering the dosage of the drug or discontinuing the drug. They are generally perceived as negative. A **side effect** is another term often confused with adverse effect. The difference is that side effect describes a *nontherapeutic reaction to a drug*. Side effects may be transient, but this is not always the case. They may require intervention, although most of the time they are perceived as tolerable. Both drug reactions have a nature and intensity that is documented and included in the published literature (e.g., drug guides, safety reports).

adverse = *negative*
event = *incident*

Allergic and anaphylactic reactions are particularly serious effects that must be carefully monitored and prevented, when possible. An **allergic reaction** is an acquired hyperresponse of body defenses to a foreign substance (allergen). Signs of allergic reactions vary in severity and include skin rash with or without itching, edema, nausea, diarrhea, runny nose, or reddened eyes with tearing. On discovering that a patient is allergic to a product, it is the nurse's responsibility to first alert the charge nurse and the patient's healthcare provider of the reaction in case it is necessary to give the patient medications to reverse the reaction. Next the nurse should document the allergy in the medical record. Many locations have electronic medical records, so there may no longer be a need to apply labels to the chart and medical administration record (MAR). All healthcare personnel, however, should follow the institution's policy for documenting the allergy so that everyone is made aware. An agency-approved allergy bracelet should be placed on the patient. The pharmacist should also be told so that the medication can be checked for cross-sensitivity with other pharmacologic products. The pharmacotherapy of allergic reactions is covered in Chapter 26.

Anaphylaxis is a severe type of allergic reaction in which massive amounts of histamine and other chemical mediators of inflammation are released throughout the body. It can lead to life-threatening shock. Symptoms of anaphylaxis are severe shortness of breath, a sudden drop in blood pressure, and tachycardia. These symptoms require immediate attention. The pharmacotherapy of anaphylaxis is covered in Chapter 22.

The rights of drug administration form the basis of proper drug delivery.

◀ **Core Concept 3.2**

The traditional **six rights of drug administration** form the operational basis for the safe delivery of medications and are recognized by such organizations as the Institute for Safe Medication Practices (ISMP). The six rights are simple and practical guidelines for nurses to use during drug preparation, delivery, and administration. The six rights are as follows:

- Right patient
- Right medication
- Right dose

- Right route of administration
- Right time of delivery
- Right documentation.

Additional rights have been added over the years, depending on particular academic curricula or agency policies. Additions to the six rights include the right to refuse medication, the right to receive drug education, right history and assessment, and the right drug–drug interaction evaluation.

The **three checks of drug administration** that nurses use with the six rights help to ensure patient safety and drug effectiveness. These checks include checking the medication label as follows:

- Checking the drug label with the MAR or medication information system when removing it from the medication drawer, refrigerator, or controlled substance locker
- Checking the drug label with the MAR when preparing it, pouring it, taking it out of the unit dose container, or connecting the IV tubing to the bag
- Checking the drug label with the MAR once more before administering it to the patient.

Despite the use of these checks and rights to provide safe drug delivery, errors still occur, and some of them are fatal. Although the nurse is accountable for preparing and administering medications, many individuals—including physicians, pharmacists, and other healthcare providers—are also responsible for safe drug practices.

Core Concept 3.3 ▶ Successful pharmacotherapy depends on patient compliance.

Patient adherence or **compliance** is another major factor affecting the success of pharmacotherapy. Compliance means taking a medication in the way it was prescribed by the practitioner or, in the case of over-the-counter (OTC) drugs, following the instructions on the label. Patient noncompliance can include not taking the medication at all, taking it at the wrong time, or taking it in the wrong way.

Even when healthcare providers conscientiously use all the principles of effective drug administration, patients may not agree that the prescribed drug regimen is worthwhile. Before administering the drug, the nurse should use the nursing process to develop a personalized care plan that will allow the patient to be an active participant in his or her care. Support staff can help ensure that the care plan works. It is important to remember that a responsible, well-informed adult always has the legal option to refuse any medication. This right allows the patient to accept or reject the pharmacotherapy based on accurate information presented in a way the patient can understand.

Fast Facts Potentially Fatal Drug Reactions

Stevens-Johnson Syndrome (SJS)

- Skin sloughing of 10% of the body
- Generalized blister-like lesions following within a few days
- Usually signaled initially by nonspecific upper respiratory infection with chills, fever, and malaise

Toxic Epidermal Necrolysis (TEN)

- Skin sloughing of 30% or more of the body (caused by skin cell breakdown)
- Severe and deadly allergic reaction caused by a drug
- Occurs when the liver fails to properly break down a drug, which then cannot be excreted normally
- Risk of death decreased if the drug is quickly withdrawn and supportive care is maintained

In the plan of care, it is important to address information that the patient must know about the prescribed medications. This includes the name of the drug; why it was ordered; its expected actions; its possible side effects; and its potential interactions with other medications, foods, herbal supplements, or alcohol. Patients need to be reminded that they have an active role in ensuring the effectiveness and safety of their medications.

Many factors influence whether patients comply with pharmacotherapy. The drug may be too expensive or may not be approved by the patient's health insurance plan. Patients may try to spread out their medication so that it lasts longer.

Patients sometimes forget doses of medications, especially when they must be taken three or four times per day. Patients often stop using drugs that have annoying side effects or that affect lifestyle. Adverse effects such as headache, dizziness, nausea, diarrhea, or impotence often cause noncompliance. Patients sometimes self-adjust their doses. Some patients believe that if one tablet is good, two must be better. Others believe that they will become dependent on the medication if it is taken as prescribed, and so they take only half the required dose. Patients usually do not want to admit or report noncompliance to the nurse because they are embarrassed or fear being reprimanded. Because there are many reasons for noncompliance, the nurse must carefully question patients about their medications. When pharmacotherapy fails to produce the expected outcomes, noncompliance should be considered as a possible reason.

Lifespan and Diversity

Many older adults take at least three different drugs each day, with some taking as many as eight or more. This leads to poor compliance among older patients. Noncompliance can be even greater for patients with dementia or Alzheimer disease.

Healthcare providers may use accepted abbreviations to communicate the directions and times for drug administration.

Core Concept 3.4

Table 3.1 lists common abbreviations that are used to give directions about drug administration. A **STAT order** refers to a medication that should be given immediately and only once. This order is often used with emergency medications that are needed for life-threatening situations. The healthcare provider normally notifies the nurse of any STAT order, so it can be obtained from the pharmacy and administered immediately.

A **single order** is for a drug that is to be given only once and at a specific time. An example is a preoperative order. A **prn order** is administered as required by the patient's condition. The nurse makes the judgment, based on patient assessment, as to when the medication should be administered. Orders not written as single, STAT, or prn are called **routine orders**. These are usually carried out within two hours of the time the order is written by the healthcare provider, but the exact timing is defined by each facility. A **standing order** is written in advance of a situation and should be carried out under specific circumstances. An example of a standing order is a set of postoperative prn

Table 3.1 Drug Administration Abbreviations*

Abbreviation	Meaning	Abbreviation	Meaning
ac	before meals	PO	by mouth
ad lib	as desired/as directed	prn	when needed/necessary
AM	morning	qid	four times per day
bid	twice per day	q2h	every 2 hours (even or when first given)
cap	capsule	q4h	every 4 hours (even)
gtt	drop	q6h	every 6 hours (even)
h or hr	hour	q8h	every 8 hours (even)
IM	intramuscular	q12h	every 12 hours
IV	intravenous	Rx	take
no	number	STAT	immediately; at once
pc	after meals; after eating	tab	tablet
PM	afternoon	tid	three times per day

**Note:* The Institute for Safe Medical Practices recommends the following abbreviations be avoided because they can lead to medication errors: q: instead use "every"; qh: instead use "hourly" or "every hour"; qd: instead use "daily" or "every day"; qhs: instead use "nightly"; qod: instead use "every other day." For these and other recommendations, see the official Joint Commission "Do Not Use List" at http://www.jointcommission.org/assets/1/18/dnu_list.pdf

prescriptions that are written for all patients who have undergone a specific surgical procedure. A common standing order for patients who have had a tonsillectomy is "Tylenol elixir 325 mg PO q6h prn sore throat." Because of the legal implications of putting all patients into a single treatment category, standing orders are no longer permitted in some facilities.

Fast Facts **Grapefruit Juice and Drug Interactions**

- Grapefruit juice may not be safe for people who take certain medications.
- Chemicals in grapefruit juice lower the activity of specific enzymes in the intestinal tract that normally break down medications. This allows a larger amount of medication to reach the bloodstream, resulting in increased drug activity.
- Drugs that may be affected by grapefruit juice include certain sedative-hypnotic drugs, antibiotics, drugs that lower blood cholesterol, some antihistamines, and antifungal agents.
- Grapefruit juice should be consumed at least two hours before or five hours after taking a medication that may interact with it.
- Some drinks that are flavored with fruit juice could contain grapefruit juice, even if grapefruit is not part of the name of the drink. Check the ingredients label.

Agency policies dictate that drug orders be reviewed by the attending healthcare provider within specific time frames, usually at least every seven days. Prescriptions for narcotics and other scheduled drugs are often automatically stopped after 72 hours, unless specifically reordered by the healthcare provider. Automatic stop orders do not generally apply when the number of doses or an exact period of time is specified.

Some medications must be taken at specific times. If a drug causes stomach upset, it is usually administered with meals to prevent epigastric pain, nausea, or vomiting. Other medications should be administered between meals because food interferes with absorption. Some central nervous system drugs and antihypertensives are best administered at bedtime because they may cause drowsiness. Others, such as sildenafil (Viagra), should be taken 30 to 60 minutes prior to sexual intercourse to achieve an erection. The nurse must pay careful attention when educating patients about when and how to take their medications to increase compliance and therapeutic success.

Once medications are administered, the nurse must correctly document that the medications have been given to the patient. Depending on the facility, documentation is done on the computer using a special program for medication administration or on a paper copy of the MAR. Either way, it is necessary that the drug name, dosage, time administered, and any assessments data be documented. For computer documentation, the identification of the nurse administering the medication is done when he or she logs on using an assigned password. On the paper copy of the MAR, the nurse must initial and sign his or her name. If a medication is refused or not given as ordered, this fact (along with the reasons) must be recorded on the appropriate form within the medical record.

Core Concept 3.5 ▶

Three systems of measurement are used in pharmacology: metric, apothecary, and household.

Dosages are labeled and dispensed according to their weight or volume. The most common system of drug measurement uses the **metric system**. The volume of a drug is expressed in terms of a liter (L) or a milliliter (mL). The abbreviation "cc" for cubic centimeter, a measurement of volume that is equivalent to 1 mL of fluid, is no longer recommended for use in medicine. The metric weight of a drug is stated in terms of kilograms (kg), grams (g), milligrams (mg), or micrograms (mcg). At one time, the abbreviation "µg" was used for micrograms, but this is no longer recommended. It is now recommended that "micrograms" and other small unusual measurements be spelled out.

Table 3.2 Metric, Apothecary, and Household Approximate Measurement Equivalents

Metric	Apothecary	Household
1 mL	15–16 minims	15–16 drops
4–5 mL (cc)	1 fluid dram	1 teaspoon or 60 drops
15 mL	4 fluid drams	1 tablespoon or 3–4 teaspoons
30 mL	8 fluid drams or 1 fluid ounce	2 tablespoons
240 mL	8 fluid ounces (1/2 pint)	1 glass or cup
500 mL	1 pint	2 glasses or 2 cups
1 L	32 fluid ounces or 1 quart	4 glasses or 4 cups or 1 quart
1 mg	1/60 grain	–
60–65 mg	1 grain	–
300–325 mg	5 grains	–
1 g	15–16 grains	–
1 kg	–	2.2 pounds

To convert grains to grams: divide grains by 15 or 16. To convert grams to grains: multiply grams by 15 or 16. To convert minims to milliliters: divide minims by 15 or 16.

The **apothecary system** and **household systems** are older systems of measurement. Although most physicians and pharmacies use the metric system, these older systems may still be seen. Until the metric system totally replaces the other systems, the healthcare provider must recognize dosages based on all three systems of measurement. Approximate equivalents among metric, apothecary, and household units of volume and weight are listed in Table 3.2.

Because Americans are familiar with the teaspoon, tablespoon, and cup, it is important for the nurse to be able to convert between the household and metric systems of measurement. In the hospital, a glass of fluid is measured in milliliters—an 8-ounce glass of water is recorded as 240 mL. If a patient being discharged is ordered to drink 2400 mL of fluid per day, the nurse may instruct the patient to drink ten 8-ounce glasses or 10 cups of fluid per day. Likewise, when a child is to be given a drug that is administered in elixir form, the nurse should explain that 5 mL of the drug is the same as one teaspoon. The nurse should encourage the use of accurate medical dosing devices at home, such as oral dosing syringes, oral droppers, cylindrical spoons, and medication cups. These are preferred over the traditional household measuring spoon because they are more accurate. Eating utensils that are commonly referred to as teaspoons or tablespoons often do not hold the volume that their names imply.

Certain protocols and techniques are common to all methods of drug administration.

◀ **Core Concept 3.6**

enteral = *ingestion*
topical = *surface*
parenteral = *equivalent to ingestion (as, for example, by intravenous route)*

The three general routes of drug administration are enteral, topical, and parenteral, with subcategories among each general route. Each route has both advantages and disadvantages. Although some drugs are formulated to be given by several routes, others are made to be given by only one route. Pharmacokinetic considerations, such as how the route of administration affects drug absorption and distribution, are discussed in Chapter 4. Certain protocols and techniques are common to all methods of drug administration. The student should refer to the drug administration guidelines in the following list before reading about specific routes of administration in Table 3.3.

- Review the medication order and check for drug allergies.
- Perform hand hygiene and apply gloves, if indicated.
- Use aseptic technique when preparing and administering medications.

- Identify the patient by asking the person to state his or her full name (or, if the patient is confused, by asking the parent or guardian), checking the patient's identification band, and comparing this information with the MAR.
- Ask the patient about known allergies, and check to see if he or she is wearing an allergy identification band.
- Ensure that the proper equipment and supplies, such as water and cups, are available at the bedside.
- Tell the patient what drug you are administering, the purpose of the drug, and how you will give it.
- Position the patient for the appropriate route of administration.
- If the drug is prepackaged as a unit dose, remove it from the packaging at the bedside.
- Unless specifically instructed to do so in the orders, do not leave drugs at the patient's bedside.
- Document the medication administration and any important patient responses on the MAR.

Table 3.3 Enteral Drug Administration

Drug Form	Administration Guidelines
A. Tablet, capsule, or liquid	**1.** Assist the patient into a sitting position. **2.** Check to be sure that the patient is alert and can swallow. **3.** Place tablets or capsules into a medication cup. **4.** If the medication is liquid, shake the bottle to mix the agent, and measure the dose into the cup at eye level. **5.** Hand the patient the medication cup. **6.** Offer a glass of water to facilitate swallowing the medication. Milk or juice may be offered (if not contraindicated). **7.** Remain with the patient until all medication is swallowed.
B. Sublingual	**1.** Check that the patient is alert and can hold the medication under the tongue. **2.** Instruct the patient not to chew or swallow the tablet, or move it around with the tongue. **3.** Instruct the patient to allow the tablet to dissolve completely before swallowing saliva. **4.** Place the sublingual tablet under the patient's tongue. **5.** Remain with the patient to make sure that all of the medication has dissolved. **6.** Offer the patient a glass of water.
C. Buccal	**1.** Check that the patient is alert and can hold the medication between the gums and the cheek. **2.** Instruct the patient to allow the tablet to dissolve completely before swallowing saliva. **3.** Instruct the patient not to chew or swallow the tablet or move it around with the tongue. **4.** Place the buccal tablet between the gum line and the cheek. **5.** Remain with the patient to be sure that all of the medication has dissolved. **6.** Offer the patient a glass of water.
D. Nasogastric and gastrostomy	**1.** Administer liquid forms of the medication when possible to avoid clogging the tube. **2.** If the medication is solid, crush it into a fine powder and mix it thoroughly with at least 30 mL of warm water until dissolved. Undissolved medications may clog the tube. **3.** Turn off the feeding tube, if applicable. **4.** Verify tube placement. The most reliable way to determine verification is by x-ray, but it can be done by aspirating stomach contents and testing pH. Verification is also done by injecting 10–30 mL of air and listening for gurgling sounds with a stethoscope over the stomach area. This method does not guarantee tube position. **5.** **Check for** *gastric residual volume.* Attach a syringe (30 or 60 mL) with plunger. Aspirate the patient's stomach contents and measure the volume. If it is greater than 100 mL (for an adult), check the facility's policy. **6.** Attach the syringe without plunger. Return the residual contents by allowing it to flow back into the tube via gravity. Flush the tube with about 10 mL (two teaspoons) of tap water. Amount of water may vary according to agency policy or healthcare provider's order. **7.** Pour the medication into the syringe barrel, also allowing it to flow into the tube by gravity. Give each medication separately, flushing between each with water. **8.** Keep the head of the bed elevated at a 45° angle for one hour to prevent aspiration. **9.** Reestablish continuous feeding, as scheduled.

Enteral drugs are given orally or via nasogastric or gastrostomy tubes.

◀ **Core Concept 3.7**

The **enteral route** includes drugs given orally and those administered through nasogastric (NG) or gastrostomy tubes. Oral drug administration (abbreviated PO, which refers to the Latin *per os*, meaning "by mouth") is the most common, most convenient, and usually the least costly of all routes. It is also considered the safest route because the skin's protective barrier is not broken. In cases of overdose, medications remaining in the stomach can be retrieved by causing vomiting. Oral preparations are available in tablet, capsule, caplet, and liquid forms. Medications administered by the enteral route take advantage of the large absorptive surfaces of the oral mucosa, stomach, or small intestine.

Tablets and Capsules

Tablets and capsules are the most common forms of drugs. Patients prefer tablets or capsules over other forms because they are easy to use. In some cases, tablets may be scored so they can easily be broken if the dose needs to be made smaller for a specific patient. **Orally disintegrating tablets (ODTs)** and oral soluble films are newer types of drug formulation that allows for quick dissolving and absorption of medications in the mouth or cheek. This approach is especially beneficial to patients who have difficulty swallowing (e.g., pediatric and geriatric patients) and for noncompliant patients (e.g., patients with psychiatric disorders).

▶ Lifespan and Diversity

For children and older patients, as well as those who may have trouble swallowing, the nurse can sometimes crush tablets or open capsules and sprinkle the drug over food or mix it with juice to make it easier to swallow and to hide its taste. It is also possible to get some medications in liquid form if swallowing is an issue for the patient.

The nurse should always check the manufacturer's instructions for administering the medication to be sure that crushing or opening is allowed. Some tablets and capsules should not be crushed or opened because their ingredients are inactivated by doing so. Other medications can severely irritate the stomach mucosa and cause nausea or vomiting. Some drugs should not be crushed because they irritate the oral mucosa, are extremely bitter, or contain dyes that stain the teeth. Most drug guides provide lists of drugs that may not be crushed. Guidelines for administering tablets or capsules are given in Table 3.3A.

The strongly acidic contents in the stomach can destroy some medications. To overcome this problem, tablets may have a hard, waxy coating that protects the medicine from acidity. These **enteric-coated** tablets are designed to dissolve in the alkaline environment of the small intestine. It is important that the nurse not crush enteric-coated tablets because the medication would then be directly exposed to the stomach environment.

Studies have clearly shown that patients are less compliant when they must take more than one dose of medicine per day, particularly if the number is three doses or more. With this in mind, pharmacologists have tried to design new drugs that need to be administered only once or twice daily. **Sustained-release (SR)** tablets or capsules are designed to dissolve very slowly. They release medication over a longer time, which increases the drug's duration of action (or length of time the medication works). Also called extended-release (XR) or long-acting (LA), medications, these forms allow convenient once or twice daily dosing. These slow and extended-release medications must not be crushed or opened because the entire dose would be absorbed too quickly, resulting in toxicity.

Giving medications by the oral route has some disadvantages. The patient must be conscious and able to swallow properly. In addition, children and some adults do not like to swallow large tablets and capsules or take oral medications that are distasteful. Certain types of drugs, including proteins, are inactivated by digestive enzymes in the stomach and small intestine. Medications absorbed from the stomach and small intestine first travel to the liver, where they may be inactivated before they ever reach their target organs. This process, called *first-pass metabolism*, is discussed in Chapter 4. The significant variation in the motility of the gastrointestinal (GI) tract among patients and in the tract's ability to absorb medications can create differences in bioavailability.

Sublingual and Buccal Drug Administration

For sublingual and buccal administration, the patient does not swallow the tablet but instead keeps it in the mouth until it dissolves. The mucosa of the oral cavity contains a rich blood supply that provides an excellent absorptive surface for certain drugs. Medications

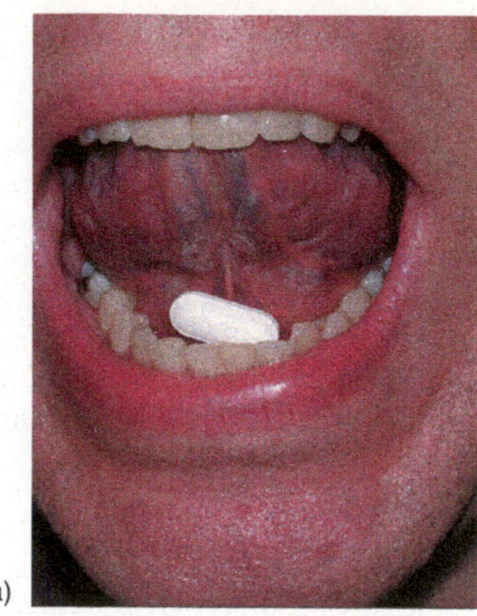

(a)

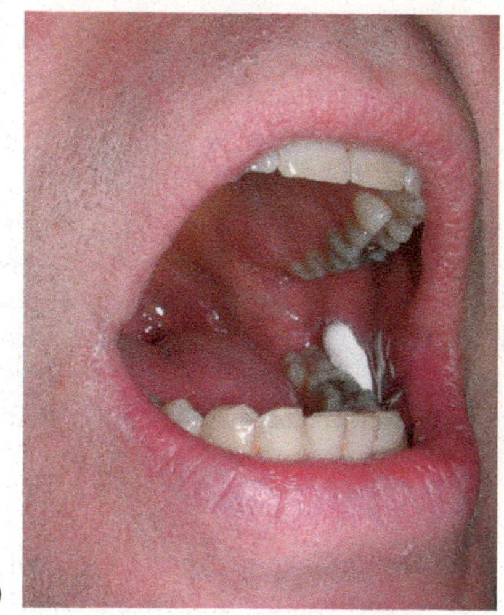

(b)

FIGURE 3.1 (a) Sublingual (under the tongue) drug administration; (b) buccal (between the gums and cheek) drug administration.

given by this route are not destroyed by digestive enzymes nor do they undergo first-pass metabolism in the liver.

For the **sublingual (SL) route**, the medication is placed under the tongue and allowed to dissolve slowly. The rich blood supply under the tongue results in a rapid onset of drug action. SL dosage forms are most often formulated as rapidly disintegrating tablets or as soft gelatin capsules filled with liquid drug.

When multiple drugs have been ordered, the SL preparations should be administered after the oral medications have been swallowed. The patient should be instructed not to move the drug with the tongue or to eat or drink anything until the medication has completely dissolved. The sublingual mucosa is not suitable for extended-release formulations because it is a relatively small area and is constantly being bathed by saliva. Table 3.3B and Figure 3.1a present important points about SL drug administration.

To administer by the **buccal route**, the tablet, capsule, lozenge, or troche is placed in the oral cavity between the gum and the cheek. The patient must be instructed not to touch the medication with the tongue, because it could get moved to the sublingual area, where it would be more rapidly absorbed, or to the back of the throat, where it could be swallowed. Medications are absorbed more slowly from the buccal mucosa than from the sublingual area. The buccal route is preferred over the sublingual route for sustained-release delivery because of its greater mucosal surface area. Drugs formulated for buccal administration generally do not cause irritation and are small enough to not cause discomfort to the patient. Table 3.3C and Figure 3.1b provide important guidelines for buccal drug administration.

Nasogastric and Gastrostomy Drug Administration

Patients with a nasogastric (NG) tube or enteral feeding system such as a gastrostomy (G) tube may have their medications administered through these devices. The soft, flexible NG tube is inserted by way of the nasopharynx or oropharynx, with the tip lying in the stomach. A G tube is surgically placed directly into the patient's stomach. Generally, the NG tube is used for short-term treatment, whereas the G tube is inserted for patients who require long-term care. Drugs administered through these tubes are usually in liquid form. Although solid drugs can be crushed or dissolved, they tend to clog the tubes. Sustained-release drugs should not be crushed and administered through NG or G tubes. Drugs administered by this route are exposed to the same physiologic processes as those given orally. If a drug is ordered to be given through either tube, and the drug should not be crushed, the nurse will need to contact the healthcare provider for an appropriate replacement medication. Table 3.3D gives important guidelines for administering drugs through NG or G tubes.

Topical drugs are applied locally to the skin and associated membranes.

◀ **Core Concept 3.8**

The **topical route** involves applying drugs locally to the skin or the membranous linings of the eye, ear, nose, respiratory tract, urinary tract, vagina, and rectum. These applications include the following:

- *Dermatologic preparations* These drugs are applied to the skin using formulations that include creams, lotions, gels, powders, and sprays. The skin is the most common topical route.
- *Instillations and irrigations* These drugs are applied into body cavities or orifices, including the eyes, ears, nose, urinary bladder, rectum, and vagina.
- *Inhalations* Inhalers, nebulizers, or positive-pressure breathing apparatuses are used to apply drugs to the respiratory tract. The most common indication for inhaled drugs is bronchoconstriction due to bronchitis or asthma. Many illegal, abused drugs are taken by this route because it provides a very rapid onset of drug action.

Drugs can be applied topically to produce a local or a systemic effect. Many drugs are applied topically to produce a local effect. For example, antibiotics may be applied to the skin to treat skin infections. Antineoplastic agents may be infused into the urinary bladder via a catheter to treat tumors of the bladder mucosa. Corticosteroids are sprayed into the nostrils to reduce inflammation of the nasal mucosa due to allergic rhinitis. Local, topical delivery of these drugs produces fewer side effects than oral or parenteral delivery of the same drugs. When these drugs are given topically, they are absorbed very slowly, and only small amounts reach the general circulation.

Other drugs are given topically to ensure slow release and absorption of the drug in the general circulation. These agents are given for their systemic (system-wide) effects. For example, a nitroglycerin patch is not applied to the skin to treat a local skin condition, but to treat chest pain caused by coronary artery disease. Likewise, prochlorperazine (Compazine) suppositories are inserted rectally not to treat a disease of the rectum but to alleviate nausea. The distinction between topical drugs given for local effects and those given for systemic effects is an important one for the nurse to know. In the case of local drugs, absorption is undesirable and may cause side effects. For systemic drugs, absorption is necessary for the therapeutic action of the drug. With either type of topical agent, drugs should not be applied to abraded or denuded skin, unless the directions so indicate.

▶ Lifespan and Diversity

Although the procedure for administering ophthalmic drugs is the same with a child as with an adult, it is advisable to enlist the help of an adult caregiver. In some cases, the infant or toddler may need to be immobilized, with the arms wrapped to prevent accidental injury to the eye during administration. For the young child, demonstrating the procedure using a doll helps gain the child's cooperation and decreases the level of anxiety.

Transdermal Delivery System

Transdermal patches are an effective means of delivering certain medications. Examples include nitroglycerin for angina pectoris and scopolamine (Transderm-Scop) for motion sickness. Although transdermal patches contain a specific amount of drug, the rate of delivery and the actual dose received may vary. Patches are changed on a regular basis, using a site rotation routine, which should be documented in the MAR. Before applying a transdermal patch, the healthcare provider should verify that the previous patch has been removed and disposed of appropriately. Drugs to be administered by this route avoid the first-pass effect in the liver and bypass digestive enzymes. Table 3.4A and Figure 3.2 illustrate the major points of transdermal drug delivery.

Ophthalmic Administration

The ophthalmic route is used to treat local conditions of the eye and surrounding structures. Common indications include excessive dryness, infections, glaucoma, and dilation of the pupil during eye examinations. Ophthalmic drugs are available in the form of eye irrigations, drops, ointments, and medicated disks. Figure 3.3 and Table 3.4B give guidelines for adult administration.

▶ Lifespan and Diversity

Administration of otic drugs to infants and young children must be performed carefully to avoid injury to sensitive structures of the ear. Otic drops should be at room temperature before adding them to the ear. When giving otic drugs to children under 3 years of age, gently pull the pinna down and back. When giving otic drugs to older children and adults, gently pull the pinna up and back.

Otic Administration

The otic route is used to treat local conditions of the ear, including infections and soft blockages of the auditory canal. Otic medications include eardrops and irrigations, which are usually ordered for cleaning. Figure 3.4 and Table 3.4C present key points in administering otic medications.

Table 3.4 Topical Drug Administration

Drug Form	Administration Guidelines
A. Transdermal	**1.** Obtain the transdermal patch, and read the manufacturer's guidelines. The application site and frequency of changing differ according to medication. **2.** Apply gloves before handling the patch to avoid absorbing any medication. **3.** Label the patch with the date, time, and your initials. **4.** Remove the previous medication or patch, and cleanse the area. **5.** If using a transdermal ointment, apply the ordered amount of medication in an even line directly on the premeasured paper that accompanies the medication tube. **6.** Press the patch or apply the medicated paper to clean, dry, and hairless skin. **7.** Rotate the sites to prevent skin irritation.
B. Ophthalmic	**1.** Instruct the patient to lie supine or sit with the head slightly tilted back. **2.** With your nondominant hand, pull the patient's lower lid down gently to expose the conjunctival sac, creating a pocket. **3.** Ask the patient to look upward. **4.** Hold the eyedropper 1/4 to 1/8 inch above the conjunctival sac. Do not hold the dropper over the patient's eye because this may stimulate the blink reflex. **5.** Instill the prescribed number of drops into the center of the pocket. Avoid touching the eye or conjunctival sac with the tip of the eyedropper. **6.** If applying ointment, follow steps 1–3, then apply a thin line of ointment evenly along the inner edge of the lower lid margin, from inner to outer canthus. **7.** Instruct the patient to gently close the eye. Apply gentle pressure with your finger to the nasolacrimal duct at the inner canthus for one to two minutes to avoid overflow drainage into the nose and throat. This minimizes the risk of absorption into the systemic circulation. **8.** With a tissue, remove the excess medication from around the patient's eye. **9.** Replace the dropper. Do not rinse the eyedropper.
C. Otic	**1.** Instruct the patient to lie on his or her side or to sit with the head tilted so that the affected ear is facing up. **2.** If necessary, use a clean washcloth to clean the pinna of the ear and the meatus to prevent any discharge from being washed into the ear canal during the instillation of the drops. **3.** Hold the dropper 1/4 inch above the ear canal, and instill the prescribed number of drops into the side of the ear canal, allowing the drops to flow downward. Avoid placing the drops directly on the tympanic membrane. **4.** Gently apply intermittent pressure to the tragus of the ear three or four times. **5.** Instruct the patient to remain on his or her side for up to 10 minutes to prevent loss of medication. **6.** If cotton ball is ordered, follow steps 1–2, then presoak with medication and insert it into the outermost part of ear canal. **7.** Wipe off any solution that may have dripped from the ear canal with a tissue.
D. Nasal drops	**1.** Ask the patient to blow his or her nose to clear the nasal passages. Have the patient lie supine. **2.** Draw up the correct volume of drug into the dropper. **3.** Instruct the patient to open and breathe through the mouth. **4.** Hold the tip of the dropper just above the patient's nostril, and without touching the nose with the dropper, direct the solution laterally toward the midline of the superior concha of the ethmoid bone—not at the base of the nasal cavity, where it will run down the throat and into the eustachian tube. **5.** Ask the patient to remain in this position for five minutes. **6.** Discard any remaining solution that is in the dropper.
E. Vaginal	**1.** Instruct the patient to assume a dorsal recumbent position with her knees bent and separated. **2.** Apply gloves; open the suppository, and lubricate the rounded end of the suppository and the gloved forefinger of your dominant hand with a water-soluble lubricant. **3.** Expose the vaginal orifice by separating the labia with your non-dominant hand. **4.** Insert the rounded end of the suppository about 8–10 cm along the posterior wall of the vagina, or as far as it will pass. **5.** If using a cream, jelly, or foam, gently insert the applicator 5 cm along the posterior vaginal wall and slowly push the plunger until empty. Remove the applicator and place on a paper towel. **6.** Ask the patient to lower her legs and remain lying in the dorsal recumbent position for five to ten minutes following insertion. Offer the patient a perineal pad.
F. Rectal suppositories	**1.** Instruct the patient to lie on the left side (Sims' position). **2.** Apply gloves; open the suppository and lubricate the rounded end. **3.** Lubricate the gloved forefinger of your dominant hand with water-soluble lubricant. **4.** Inform the patient when the suppository is to be inserted; instruct the patient to take slow, deep breaths and deeply exhale during insertion to relax the anal sphincter. **5.** Gently insert the lubricated end of the suppository into the rectum, beyond the anal-rectal ridge to ensure retention. **6.** Instruct the patient to remain in the Sims' position or lie supine to prevent expulsion of the suppository. **7.** Instruct the patient to retain the suppository for at least 30 minutes to allow absorption, unless the suppository is administered to stimulate defecation.

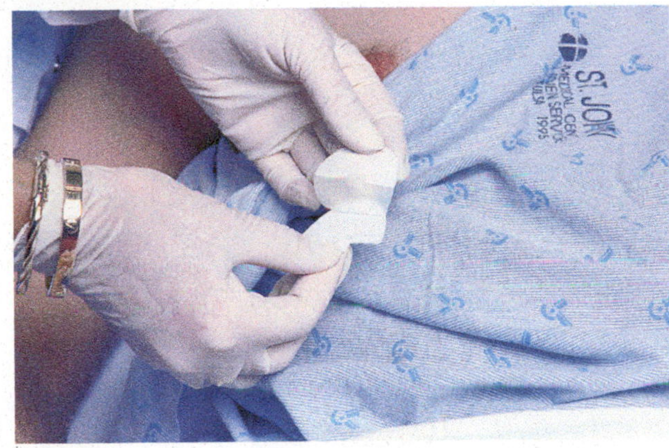

(a)

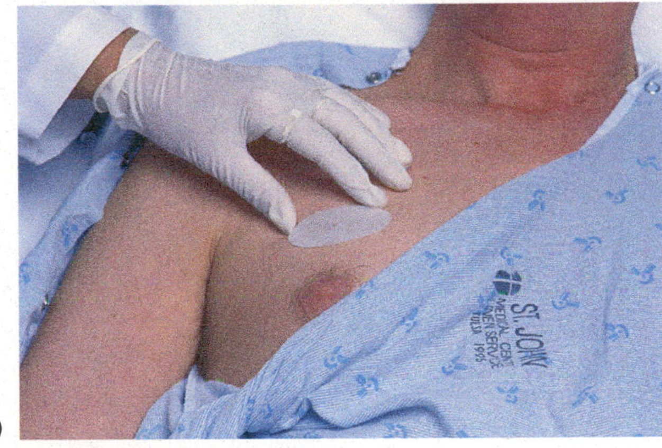

(b)

FIGURE 3.2 Transdermal patch administration: Apply gloves before handling the patch, and read the manufacturer's directions. Label the patch with the date, time, and your initials. Remove any previous medication or patch, and cleanse the area. (a) Remove the protective coating from the patch, and (b) apply the patch immediately to clean, dry, hairless skin.

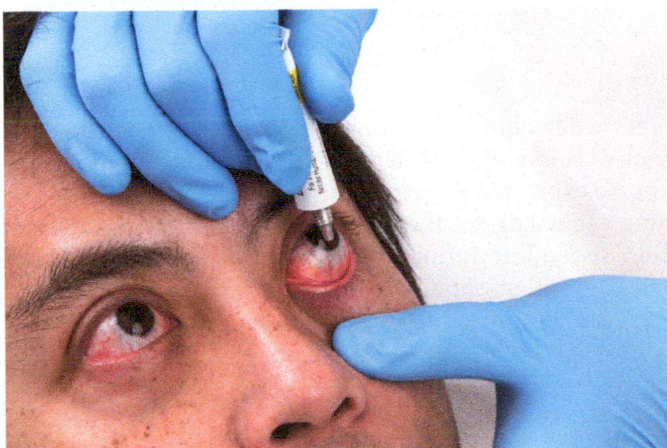

FIGURE 3.3 Ophthalmic drug administration: Instilling eye drops into the lower conjunctival sac.

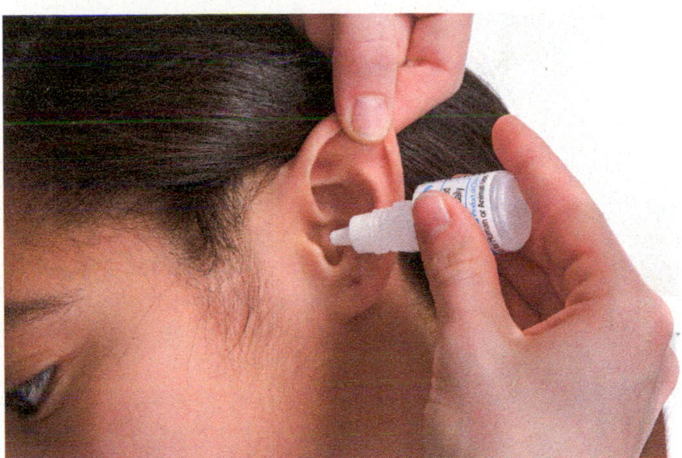

FIGURE 3.4 Otic drug administration: Instilling eardrops.
Source: Andy Crawford/DK Images

Nasal Administration

The nasal route, a **transmucosal** method of drug delivery, is used for both local and systemic drug administration. The nasal mucosa provides an excellent absorptive surface for certain medications. Advantages of this route include ease of use and avoidance of the first-pass effect in the liver and the digestive enzymes. Nasal spray formulations of corticosteroids have revolutionized the treatment of allergic rhinitis because the medication is very safe when administered by this route.

Although the nasal mucosa provides an excellent surface for drug delivery, there is the potential for damage to the cilia within the nasal cavity, and mucosal irritation is common. In addition, unpredictable mucous secretion in some individuals may affect drug absorption from this site.

Drops or sprays are often used for their local **astringent effect**, which is to shrink swollen mucous membranes or to loosen secretions and facilitate drainage. This brings immediate relief from the nasal congestion caused by the common cold. The nose also provides the route to reach the nasal sinuses and the eustachian tube. Proper positioning of the patient prior to giving nose drops for sinus disorders depends on which sinuses are being treated. The same holds true for treatment of the eustachian tube. Table 3.4D and Figure 3.5 illustrate important facts related to nasal drug administration.

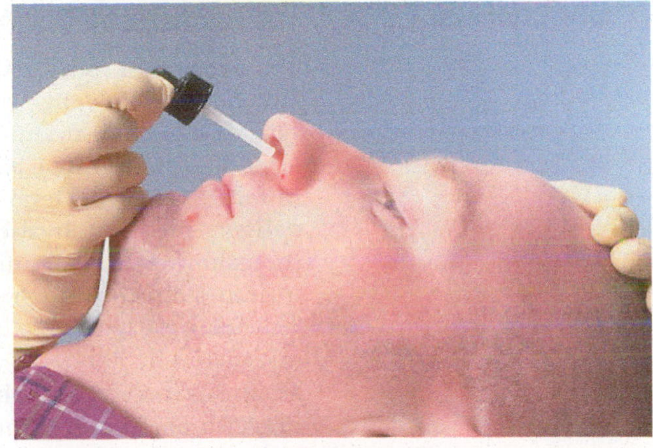

FIGURE 3.5 Nasal drug administration.

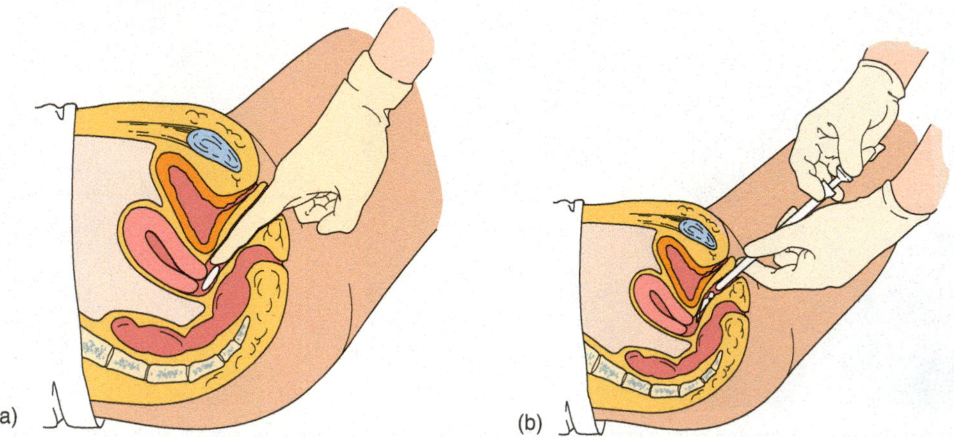

FIGURE 3.6 Vaginal drug administration: (a) instilling a vaginal suppository; (b) using an applicator to instill a vaginal cream.

Vaginal Administration

The vaginal route is used to deliver medications for treating local infections and to relieve vaginal pain and itching. Vaginal medications are inserted as suppositories, creams, jellies, or foams. It is important that the nurse explains the purpose of treatment and provides privacy for the patient. Before inserting vaginal drugs, the nurse should instruct the patient to empty her bladder. This lessens both discomfort during treatment and the possibility of irritating or injuring the vaginal lining. The patient should be offered a perineal pad following administration. Table 3.4E and Figure 3.6 provide guidelines regarding vaginal drug administration.

Rectal Administration

The rectal route may be used for either local or systemic drug administration. It is a safe and effective means of delivering drugs to patients who are comatose or who are experiencing nausea and vomiting. Rectal drugs are normally in suppository form, although a few laxatives and diagnostic agents are given via enema. Although absorption is slower than by other routes, it is steady and reliable as long as the medication can be retained by the patient. Venous blood from the lower rectum is not transported by way of the liver. Therefore, the first-pass effect is avoided, as are the digestive enzymes of the upper GI tract. Table 3.4F gives details about rectal drug administration.

Core Concept 3.9 ▶

Parenteral administration refers to dispensing medications by routes other than oral or topical.

The **parenteral route** delivers drugs via a needle into the skin layers, subcutaneous tissue, muscles, or veins, with the needle inserted at different degrees, depending on the type of injection, as shown in Figure 3.7. More advanced parenteral delivery includes administration into arteries, body cavities (such as intrathecal), and organs (such as intracardiac). Parenteral drug administration is much more invasive (meaning that the delivery method "invades" the barrier that the skin provides to protect the body) than topical or enteral administration. Because of the possibility of introducing pathogenic microbes directly into the blood or body tissues, aseptic techniques must be strictly used. The nurse is expected to identify and use appropriate materials for parenteral drug delivery, including specialized equipment and techniques involved in the preparation and administration of injectable products. The nurse must know the correct anatomical locations for parenteral administration and safety procedures regarding hazardous equipment disposal.

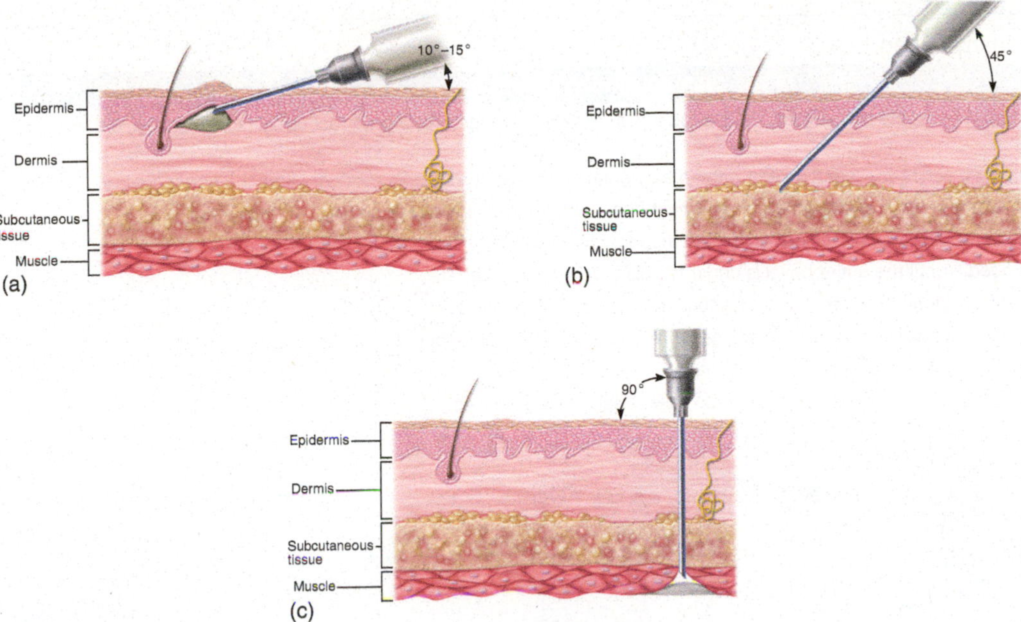

FIGURE 3.7 Parenteral drug administration: Wear gloves at all times. (a) Intradermal administration is into the dermis at a 10–15° angle. See Figure 3.8. (b) Subcutaneous administration is into the subcutaneous tissue at a 45° angle. See Figure 3.9. (c) During intramuscular administration, a drug is injected into the muscle at a 90° angle. See Figure 3.10. Intravenous drug administration (not shown here) is given directly into the bloodstream.

Intradermal and Subcutaneous Administration

Injection into the skin delivers drugs to the blood vessels that supply the layers of the skin. Drugs may be injected either intradermally or subcutaneously. The major difference between these methods is the depth of injection, which is controlled by the angle of needle placement (see Figure 3.7). An advantage of both methods is that they offer a means of administering drugs to patients who are unable to take them orally. Drugs administered by these routes also avoid the first-pass effect in the liver and the digestive enzymes. Disadvantages are that only small volumes can be administered, and injections can cause pain and swelling at the injection site.

An **intradermal (ID) route** injection is administered into the dermis layer of the skin. Because the dermis contains more blood vessels than the deeper subcutaneous layer, drugs are more easily absorbed. This route is usually used for allergy and disease screening or for local anesthetic delivery prior to venous cannulation. Only very small volumes of drug, usually 0.1 mL, can be given by ID injections. The usual sites for ID injections are the nonhairy skin surfaces of the upper back, superficial areas overlying the scapulae, the superior upper chest, and the anterior forearm. Guidelines for intradermal injections are given in Table 3.5A and Figure 3.8.

A **subcutaneous route** injection is delivered to the deeper tissue layer under the skin. Insulin, heparin, vitamins, some vaccines, and other medications are given in this area because the sites are easy to reach and provide rapid absorption. Body sites that are ideal for subcutaneous injections include the following:

- Posterior upper arm (above the triceps muscle)
- Middle two thirds of the anterior thigh area
- Subscapular areas of the upper back
- Upper dorsogluteal and ventrogluteal areas
- Abdominal areas, above the iliac crest and below the diaphragm, 2 inches out from the umbilicus and 1 inch away from moles or scars.

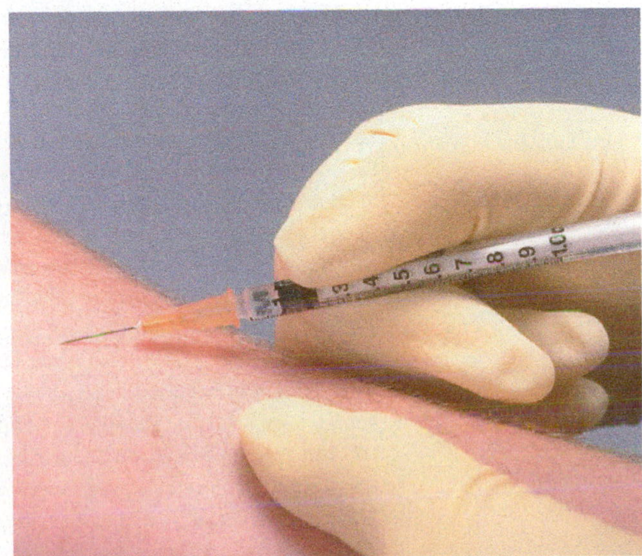

FIGURE 3.8 Intradermal drug administration: The needle is inserted, bevel up, at a 10–15° angle.

Table 3.5 Parenteral Drug Administration

Drug Form	Administration Guidelines
A. Intradermal route	**1.** Verify the order and prepare the medication in a tuberculin or 1- mL syringe with a preattached 26- to 27-gauge, 3/8–5/8 inch needle. **2.** Apply gloves and cleanse the injection site with an antiseptic swab, using a circular motion. Allow the site to air dry. **3.** With the thumb and index finger of your nondominant hand, spread the patient's skin taut. **4.** Insert the needle, with the bevel facing upward, at an angle of 10°–15°. **5.** Advance the needle until the entire bevel is under the skin; do not aspirate. **6.** Slowly inject the medication to form a small wheal or bleb (small raised area). **7.** Withdraw the needle quickly, and pat the site gently with a sterile 2×2 gauze pad. Do not massage the area. **8.** Instruct the patient not to rub or scratch the area. **9.** Draw a circle around the perimeter of the injection site. Read in 48–72 hours.
B. Subcutaneous route	**1.** Verify the order and prepare the medication in a 1- to 3-mL syringe using a 23- to 25-gauge, 1/2–5/8 inch needle. For heparin, the recommended needle is 3/8 inch and 25–26 gauge. **2.** Choose the site, avoiding bony areas, major nerves, and blood vessels. For heparin, check your facility's policy for the preferred injection sites. **3.** Check the previous rotation sites, and select a new area for injection. **4.** Apply gloves, and cleanse the injection site with an antiseptic swab using a circular motion. **5.** Allow the site to air dry. **6.** Bunch the skin between the thumb and index finger of the nondominant hand. **7.** Insert the needle at a 45° or 90° angle, depending on the patient's body size and the length of the needle you are using: 90° angle for patients with obesity; 45° angle for patients of normal weight. **8.** Inject the medication slowly. **9.** Remove the needle quickly. Gently depress the skin with an antiseptic swab. *Do not massage the site after injecting heparin or low molecular weight heparin because tissue damage may occur.*
C. Intramuscular route: ventrogluteal site	**1.** Verify the orider and prepare the medication using a 20- to 23- gauge, 1- to 1.5 inch needle. (Needle size may vary depending on the site and patient size.) **2.** Apply gloves, and cleanse the injection site with an antiseptic swab using a circular motion. Allow the site to air dry. **3.** Locate the site by placing your hand with the heel on the greater trochanter and your thumb pointing toward the umbilicus. Point to the anterior iliac spine with your index finger, spreading your middle finger to point toward the iliac crest (forming a V). Inject the medication within the V-shaped area of the index and third finger. **4.** Insert the needle with a smooth, dartlike movement at a 90° angle within the V-shaped area. **5.** Depending on agency policy and type of drug, aspirate, and observe for blood. If blood appears, withdraw the needle, discard the syringe, and prepare a new injection. **6.** Inject the medication slowly and with smooth, even pressure on the plunger. **7.** Remove the needle quickly. **8.** Apply pressure to the site with a dry, sterile 2×2 gauze and gently massage to promote absorption of the medication into the muscle.
D. Intravenous route	**1.** To add a drug to an IV fluid container: **a.** Verify the order and compatibility of the drug with the IV fluid. **b.** Prepare the medication in a 5- to 20- mL syringe using a 1- to 1.5-inch, 19- to 21-gauge needle from the original medication vial or ampule. If a needleless system is used, use the appropriate syringe or tip required per the system use. **c.** Apply gloves and assess the injection site for signs of inflammation or extravasation (oozing of tissue). **d.** Locate the medication port on the IV fluid container and cleanse it with an antiseptic swab. **e.** Carefully insert the needle or needleless access device into the port and inject the medication. **f.** Withdraw the needle, and mix the solution by rotating the container end to end. **g.** Hang the container, and check the infusion rate. **2.** To administer an IV bolus (IV push) using an existing IV line or IV lock (reseal): **a.** Verify the order and compatibility of the drug with the IV fluid. **b.** Determine the correct rate of infusion. **c.** Determine whether IV fluids are infusing at the proper rate (IV line) and that the IV site is adequate. **d.** Prepare the drug in a syringe with a 19- to 21-gauge needle. **e.** Apply gloves, and assess the IV insertion site for signs of inflammation or extravasation (oozing of fluid within the tissue). **f.** Select an injection port on the tubing that is closest to the insertion site (IV line). **g.** Cleanse the tubing or lock port with an antiseptic swab and insert the needle into the port. **h.** If administering medication through an existing IV line, occlude the tubing by pinching it just above the injection port. **i.** Slowly inject the medication over the designated time (which is not usually faster than 1 mL/min, unless otherwise specified). **j.** Withdraw the syringe. Release the tubing and ensure the proper IV infusion if using an existing IV line. **k.** If using an IV lock, check your facility's policy for use of saline flush before and after injecting medications.

Subcutaneous doses are small in volume, usually ranging from 0.5 to 1 mL, and are given at a 45° (patient of normal weight) to 90° angle (patient with obesity). The needle size varies with the patient's quantity of body fat but is usually 1/2 to 5/8 inch. The needle length is usually one-half the size of a pinched skinfold that can be grasped between the thumb and forefinger. Insulin is administered using a special syringe that has "unit" markings made specifically for insulin. Tuberculin syringes are 1 mL syringes and are typically used when administering other medications less than 1 mL. Note that tuberculin syringes and insulin syringes are not interchangeable and should not be substituted for each other. It is important to rotate injection sites in an orderly and documented manner, to promote absorption, minimize tissue damage, and alleviate discomfort. For insulin, rotation should be within an anatomical area that promotes reliable absorption and maintains consistent blood glucose levels.

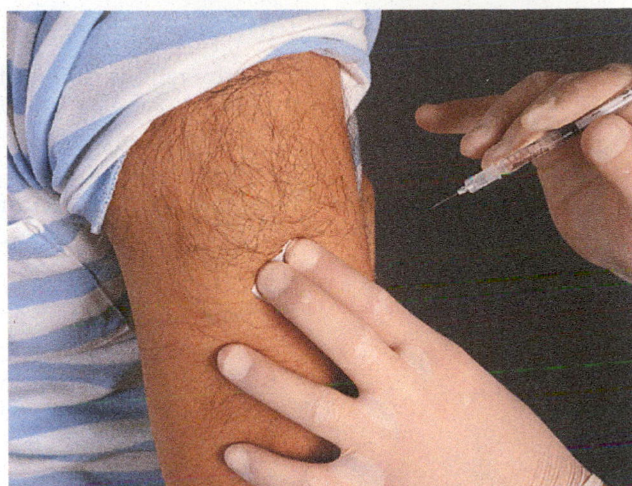

FIGURE 3.9 Subcutaneous drug administration: Skin is pinched, and depending on the amount of subcutaneous tissue, the needle is inserted at a 45° or 90° angle.

When performing subcutaneous injections, it is usually not necessary to aspirate prior to the injection. It depends on what is being injected and the patient's anatomy. Aspiration might prevent inadvertent administration into a vein or artery in a thin person. Heparin and low molecular weight heparin, such as enoxaparin (Lovenox), should never be aspirated because of the drug's anticoagulant properties. Aspiration can cause bleeding, bruising, and possible damage to the surrounding tissue. Massage after injection is also not recommended for the same reasons. Table 3.5B and Figure 3.9 include important information regarding subcutaneous drug administration.

Intramuscular Administration

An **intramuscular (IM) route** injection delivers medication into specific muscles. Because muscle tissue has a rich blood supply, medication moves quickly into blood vessels to produce a more rapid onset of action than with oral, ID, or subcutaneous administration. The anatomical structure of muscle permits this tissue to receive a larger volume of medication than the subcutaneous region. An adult with well-developed muscles can safely tolerate up to 5 mL of medication in a large muscle, although only 2 to 3 mL is recommended. The deltoid and triceps muscles should receive a maximum of 1 mL.

A major consideration for the nurse regarding IM drug administration is the selection of an appropriate injection site. Injection sites must be located away from bones, large blood vessels, and nerves. Both the size and length of the needle are determined by body size and muscle mass, the type of drug to be administered, the amount of adipose (fat) tissue overlying the muscle, and the age of the patient. Information regarding IM injections is given in Table 3.5C and Figure 3.10. The four common sites for IM injections are as follows:

▶ Lifespan and Diversity

The vastus lateralis is the preferred site for IM injections in pediatric patients.

- *Ventrogluteal site.* This area provides the greatest thickness of gluteal muscles, contains no large blood vessels or nerves, is sealed off by bone, and contains less fat than the buttock area, thus eliminating the need to determine the depth of subcutaneous fat.
- *Deltoid site.* This area is used in well-developed teens and adults for volumes of medication not to exceed 2 mL.
- *Dorsogluteal site.* This area is used for adults and for children who have been walking for at least six months. The site is rarely used due to the potential for damage to the sciatic nerve.
- *Vastus lateralis site.* Usually thick and well developed in both adults and children, the middle third of the muscle is the site for IM injections.

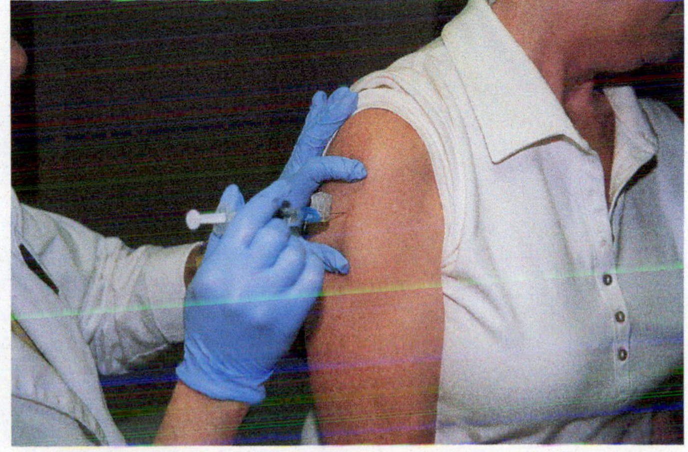

FIGURE 3.10 Intramuscular drug administration: Skin is spread taut between the thumb and forefinger, and the needle is inserted at a 90° angle.

Intravenous Administration

The **intravenous (IV) route** enables administration of medications and fluids directly into the bloodstream and allows their immediate availability for use by the body. The IV route is used when a very rapid onset of action is desired. Like other parenteral routes, IV medications bypass the enzymes of the digestive system and the first-pass effect of the liver. The three basic types of IV administration are as follows:

- *Large-volume infusion.* This type of infusion is used for fluid maintenance, replacement, or supplementation. Compatible drugs may be mixed into a large-volume IV container with fluids such as normal saline or Ringer's lactate. Table 3.5D and Figure 3.11 illustrate this technique.
- *Intermittent infusion* A small amount of IV solution is "piggy-backed" (added) to the primary large-volume infusion. This type of infusion, also illustrated in Figure 3.11, is used to give additional medications, such as antibiotics or analgesics, over a short time.
- *IV bolus (push) administration* A concentrated single dose of medication is delivered directly to the circulation via syringe. Bolus injections may be given through an intermittent injection port or by direct IV push. Details on the bolus administration technique are given in Table 3.5D and Figure 3.12.

Although the IV route provides the fastest onset of drug action, it is also the most dangerous. Once injected, the medication cannot be retrieved. If the drug solution or the needle

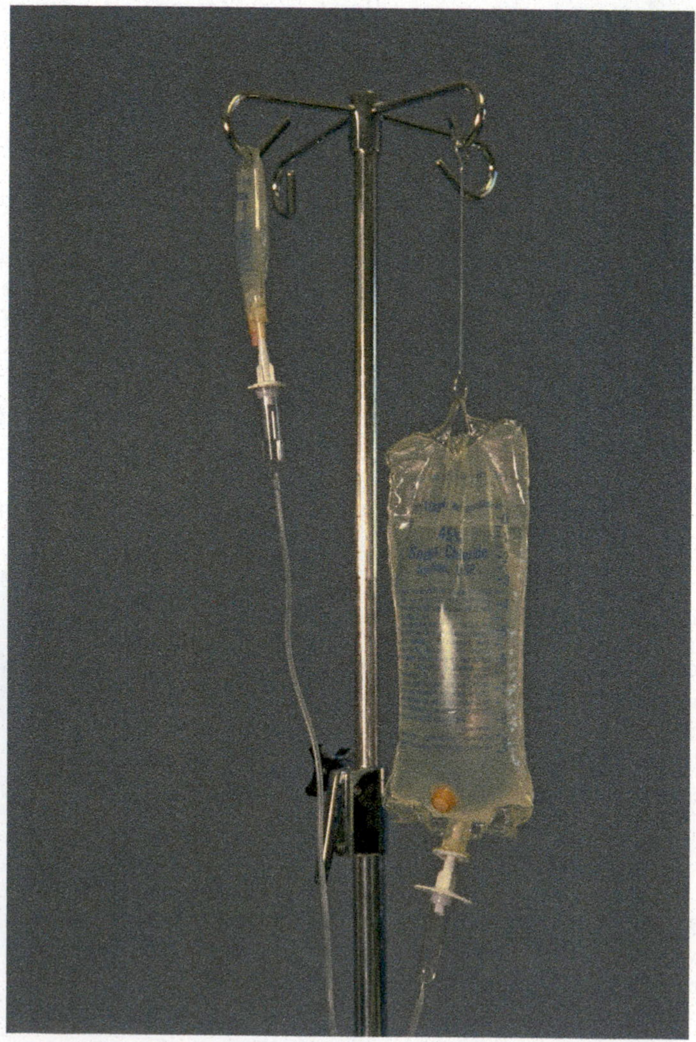

FIGURE 3.11 Administration of intravenous fluids: A large volume IV infusion bag with intermittent infusion bag "piggy-backed" into primary tubing.

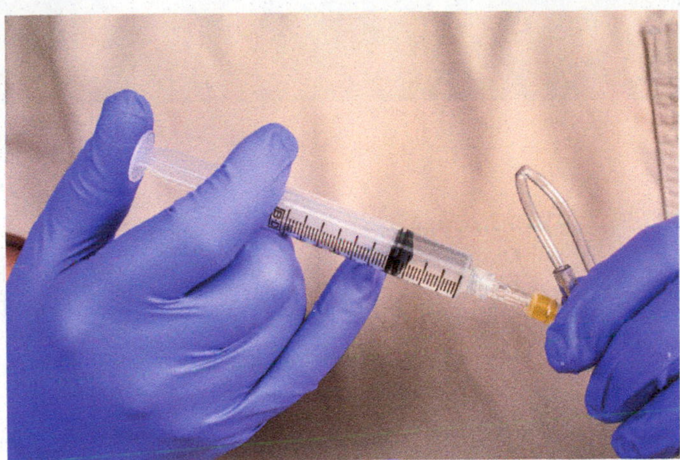

FIGURE 3.12 Injecting a medication by IV push to an existing IV tube using a needleless system.
Source: Carol Q. Urban

is contaminated, pathogens have a direct route to the bloodstream and body tissues. Patients who are receiving IV injections must be closely monitored for adverse reactions. Some adverse reactions occur immediately after injection; others may take hours or days to appear. Antidotes for drugs that can cause potentially dangerous or fatal reactions must always be readily available. Several types of needleless IV systems are also available and have been shown to greatly reduce the chance of needlestick injuries among healthcare professionals.

Safety Alert: Medication Administration Error–Mistaken Patient Identity

It is the responsibility of the nurse to check the patient's identification band, ask the patient to state name and date of birth, and verify that these pieces of information match those listed on the patient's MAR. Consider the evening nurse who entered Ms. Brown's room to administer medications. Ms. Brown was already in bed and asleep. The nurse gently shook her and said, "I have your 10 p.m. medication, Ms. Brown." Although the patient responded, she was not fully awake. She took the medication and quickly returned to sleep. Upon leaving, however, the nurse noticed the room number and realized that medication had just been given to Ms. Crown in the room next to Ms. Brown. This situation could have been avoided if the nurse had checked the identification band, asked the patient for identification information, and cross-checked the data against the MAR.

Patients Need to Know

Patients need to know the following:

1. Always ask the healthcare provider or pharmacist which medications may be taken with food and water to reduce nausea and stomach irritation.
2. Do not crush or cut into pieces enteric coated, extended-release, or sustained-release tablets or capsules. In addition, do not take enteric-coated tablets with alkaline substances, such as antacids.
3. Establish a routine for taking medications by selecting a familiar time of the day, usually on the hour. Special organizers can be obtained to properly store medicines according to times, days, and dosages.
4. Follow the dosing times exactly. If a medication is missed, do not try to "catch up" on the next scheduled dose. If remembered soon after the scheduled time, it is appropriate to take the medicine. Otherwise, wait until the next scheduled dose. An exception would be if the next dose is not scheduled until the next day. For answers to specific questions, consult a healthcare provider.
5. Store medications in a safe, dry place. Discard them if they become old or outdated.
6. Use the measuring device provided by the drug manufacturer to take medications. Do not rely on kitchen utensils to judge the exact recommended dose.

Chapter Review

Core Concepts Summary

3.1 A major goal in pharmacotherapy is to limit the number and severity of drug adverse events.

Healthcare staff must be familiar with the general principles of drug delivery. The nurse must have a comprehensive knowledge of the actions and side effects of drugs before they are administered to limit the number and severity of drug adverse events. Allergic and anaphylactic reactions are serious effects that must be carefully monitored and prevented, when possible.

3.2 The rights of drug administration form the basis of proper drug delivery.

The six rights and three checks are guidelines to safe drug administration, which involves a collaborative effort among nurses, physicians, and other healthcare professionals. The six rights are right patient, right medication, right dose, right route of administration, right time of delivery, and right documentation. The three checks are checking the MAR, checking the drug during preparation, and checking the drug before administering it to the patient.

3.3 Successful pharmacotherapy depends on patient compliance.

Pharmacologic compliance requires patients to understand and personally accept the value of the prescribed drug regimen. Understanding the reasons for noncompliance can help the healthcare team increase pharmacotherapeutic success.

3.4 Healthcare providers may use accepted abbreviations to communicate the directions and times for drug administration.

There are established orders and time schedules by which medications are routinely administered. The single order (such as a preoperative order) is for a drug that is to be given only once and at a specific time. A prn order is administered as required by the patient's condition. Orders not written as single, STAT, or prn are called routine orders. A standing order is written in advance of a situation and is to be carried out under specific circumstances. Documenting drug administration and reporting side effects are important responsibilities of the nurse.

3.5 Three systems of measurement are used in pharmacology: metric, apothecary, and household.

Healthcare professionals must recognize dosages based on all three systems of measurement: metric, apothecary, and household. The nurse must be able to convert between household and metric systems of measurement.

3.6 Certain protocols and techniques are common to all methods of drug administration.

The student should understand drug administration guidelines before proceeding to study specific drug administration routes. The three general routes of drug administration are enteral, topical, and parenteral.

3.7 Enteral drugs are given orally or via nasogastric or gastrostomy tubes.

Drugs administered via the enteral route are given orally or through nasogastric (NG) or gastrostomy (G) tubes. The enteral route is the most effective way to administer drugs.

3.8 Topical drugs are applied locally to the skin and associated membranes.

Topical drugs are applied locally to the skin or membranous linings of the eye, ear, nose, respiratory tract, urinary tract, vagina, and rectum.

3.9 Parenteral administration refers to dispensing medications by routes other than oral or topical.

Parenteral administration is the dispensing of medications via a needle, usually into the skin layers (ID), subcutaneous tissue, muscles (IM), or veins (IV).

REVIEW Questions

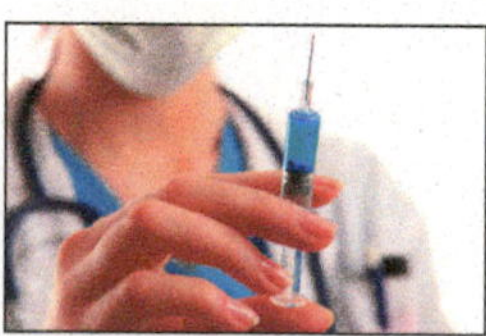

Answer the following questions to assess your knowledge of the chapter material, and go back and review any material that is not clear to you.

1. A nurse enters the patient's room with medication along with a stethoscope, a fairly large-looking syringe, and a container of water. In the course of administering the medication, the nurse will use all of these items. Which of the following routes will the nurse likely use?
   1. Transdermal
   2. Intravenous (parenteral)
   3. Nasogastric (enteral)
   4. Rectal

2. The nurse will not crush the extended-release medications ordered for the patient because:
   1. They are very distasteful, and this reduces patient compliance.
   2. Crushing alters the rate of absorption and medication delivery.
   3. Multiple drug pieces cause obstructive symptoms.
   4. Crushed oral medications have reduced bioavailability.

3. The reason why it is necessary to aspirate during an IM injection is to:
   1. Avoid placement of the needle into a blood vessel.
   2. Produce an air pocket for better drug distribution.
   3. Avoid nerve puncture.
   4. Remove air from the syringe.
4. Which of the following routes of drug administration has the fastest onset of action?
   1. Transdermal
   2. Intramuscular
   3. Intravenous
   4. Ophthalmic
5. The healthcare provider's order indicates that the medication is to be given immediately. This type of order is a:
   1. STAT order.
   2. Single order.
   3. prn order.
   4. Standing order.
6. The nurse checks the medication label three times during the course of administering a medication: while getting the medication out of the container or drawer, before placing it into the medication cup, and before administering the medication. Of the six rights of drug administration, this nurse is checking for the right:
   1. Medication.
   2. Documentation.
   3. Patient.
   4. Time of delivery.
7. When administering medications, the nurse's main responsibilities are to know and understand:
   1. The medication being ordered.
   2. The intended use of the medication.
   3. Any special considerations, such as the patient's age or pathophysiologic state.
   4. Any possible side effects or adverse drug effects the medication may cause.
   5. All of the above are important to know and understand when administering medications.
8. Which information is not listed in the medication administration record (MAR)?
   1. Date of medication administration
   2. Route of drug administration
   4. Dose of medication
   5. Drug classification
9. The healthcare provider ordered 5 mL of an oral decongestant twice a day for a pediatric patient. When teaching the mother of the patient about how much medication to give, the nurse tells her that 5 mL is equal to:
   1. Two (2) teaspoons.
   2. One (1) tablespoon.
   3. 1/4 of a cup.
   4. One (1) teaspoon.
10. The following statements are true regarding topical medication applications *except:*
    1. For a local effect, it is important that the medication stay within the area of application.
    2. The medication can be absorbed into the nurse's skin if gloves are not worn.
    3. It is never desirable for topical drugs to be absorbed into the systemic system.
    4. Topical medication applied to the skin comes in the form of creams, lotions, gels, powders, and sprays.

Answers and complete rationales to the Review Questions appear in Appendix A.

REFERENCE

Institute for Safe Medical Practices. (2015). *List of error-prone abbreviations, symbols, and dose designations.* Retrieved from http://www.ismp.org/Tools/errorproneabbreviations.pdf

SELECTED BIBLIOGRAPHY

Berman, A. J., Snyder, S., & Frandsen, G. (2016). *Kozier & Erb's fundamentals of nursing: Concepts, process, and practice* (10th ed.). Hoboken, NJ: Pearson.

Buck, M. L. (2013). *Alternative forms of oral drug delivery for pediatric patients.* Retrieved from http://www.medscape.com/viewarticle/807030_1

Olsen, J. L., Giangrasso, A. P., & Shrimpton, D. M. (2016). *Medical dosage calculations: A dimensional analysis approach* (11th ed.). Hoboken, NJ: Pearson.

The Joint Commission. (2015). *Facts about the official "do not use" list of abbreviations.* Retrieved from http://www.jointcommission.org/facts_about_do_not_use_list

U.S. Food and Drug Administration. (2014). *Medication errors related to drugs.* Retrieved from http://www.fda.gov./drugs/DrugSafety/MedicationErrors/default.htm

U.S. Food and Drug Administration. (2015). *MedWatch: The FDA safety information and adverse event reporting program.* Retrieved from http://www.fda.gov/Safety/MedWatch

Chapter 4

What Happens After a Drug Has Been Administered

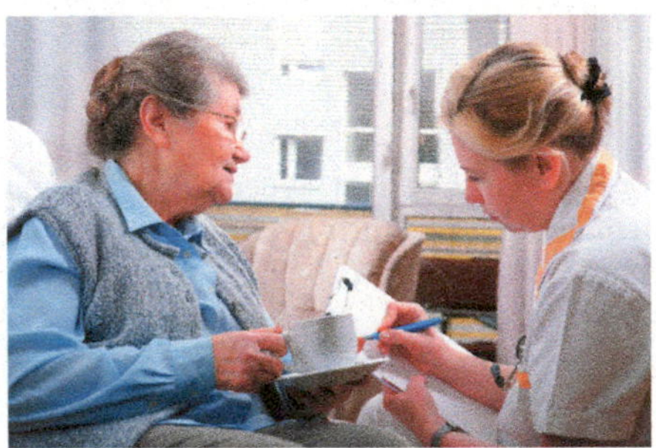

Core Concepts

4.1 Pharmacokinetics focuses on what the body does to the drugs.
4.2 Absorption is the first step in drug transport.
4.3 Distribution refers to how drugs are transported throughout the body.
4.4 Metabolism is a process whereby drugs are made less or more active.
4.5 Excretion processes remove drugs from the body.
4.6 The rate of elimination and half-life characteristics influence drug responsiveness.
4.7 Pharmacodynamics focuses on what the drugs do to the body.
4.8 Drugs activate specific receptors to produce a response.
4.9 *Potency* and *efficacy* are terms often used to describe the ability of drug therapy to reduce or resolve symptoms.

Learning Outcomes

After reading this chapter, the student should be able to:

1. Identify the four major processes of pharmacokinetics.
2. Discuss the factors affecting drug absorption.
3. Explain the significance of the blood-brain barrier, blood-placental barrier, and blood-testicular barrier, and describe how plasma proteins affect drug distribution.
4. Explain the importance of the first-pass effect, metabolic enzymes, and intermediate products of drug metabolism to the success of drug therapy.
5. Identify the major processes by which drugs are eliminated from the body, including the importance of enterohepatic recirculation.
6. Explain how rate of elimination and plasma half-life ($t_{1/2}$) are related to the duration of drug action.
7. Discuss how successful pharmacotherapy depends on principles of pharmacodynamics.
8. Explain the significance of the receptor theory and how "blockers" of drug action work.
9. Compare and contrast the therapeutic terms *potency* and *efficacy*.

Key Terms

absorption (ab-SORP-shun)
agonists (AG-on-ists)
antagonists (an-TAG-oh-nists)
biotransformation (BEYE-oh-trans-for-MAY-shun)
distribution (dis-tree-BU-shun)
duration of drug action
efficacy (EFF-ik-ah-see)
enterohepatic recirculation (EN-ter-oh-HEE-pah-tik)
excretion (eks-KREE-shun)
first-pass effect
half-life ($t_{1/2}$)
metabolism (meh-TAHB-oh-liz-ehm)
minimum effective concentration
onset of drug action
peak plasma level
pharmacodynamics (FAR-mah-koh-deye-NAM-iks)
pharmacokinetics (FAR-mah-koh-kee-NET-iks)
potency (POH-ten-see)
prodrugs
receptor (ree-SEP-tor)
receptor theory
termination of drug action
therapeutic (THARE-ah-PEW-tick) range
toxic concentration

Drugs do not affect all patients the same way. Whether a drug achieves or falls short of achieving a therapeutic response is an important concern to patients and healthcare providers. Within a population, a dose of medication may produce a dramatic response in one patient while having no effect in another.

Many factors determine a drug's response. Patients sometimes take medications under conditions that interfere with drug activity. This interference is called a *drug interaction.* Food–drug interactions may occur when patients take their medication with certain foods or beverages. Patients often take more than one medication at the same time. After drugs have been absorbed, the effectiveness of drug therapy may be altered by drug–drug interactions in the bloodstream. To understand the impact that drug interactions have on drug safety and effectiveness, one must understand concepts from two important areas: pharmacokinetics and pharmacodynamics.

Pharmacokinetics focuses on what the body does to the drugs.

◀ Core Concept 4.1

As the root words indicate, **pharmacokinetics** focuses on four processes: absorption, distribution, metabolism, and excretion, as shown in Figure 4.1. A thorough knowledge of pharmacokinetics enables the healthcare provider to understand the therapeutic effects of a drug, as well as to predict potential adverse effects of drug therapy.

pharmaco = *drug related*
kinetics = *movement*

Absorption is the first step in drug transport.

◀ Core Concept 4.2

Absorption is the first step in how the body handles a drug. Absorption is a process involving the movement of a substance from its site of administration across one or more body membranes. A drug may be absorbed locally and produce a biologic effect at a remote site. Absorption may occur across the skin and associated mucous membranes, or drugs may move across membranes that line blood vessels. Ultimately, most drugs move across many membranes to reach their target cells. Many basic science textbooks cover the ways that foods and drugs are absorbed, including passive transport and energy-requiring transport processes. The presence of food in the digestive tract slows the absorption of drugs administered orally.

Distribution refers to how drugs are transported throughout the body.

◀ Core Concept 4.3

Distribution is the process by which drugs are transported after they have been absorbed or administered directly into the bloodstream. Between the site of drug administration and the target tissue, many factors affect drug movement. One important example is the *binding* that occurs between drugs and other substances, such as plasma proteins, already present in the bloodstream. When a drug binds with a plasma protein such as albumin, the drug is held by the plasma protein in the bloodstream, where it is unable to reach its target cells. Often, a second drug will interfere with this binding by displacing the first drug from the plasma protein. In this case, the first drug's activity is intensified. The term *bioavailability* is often used to describe how much of a drug will be available after administration to produce a biological effect.

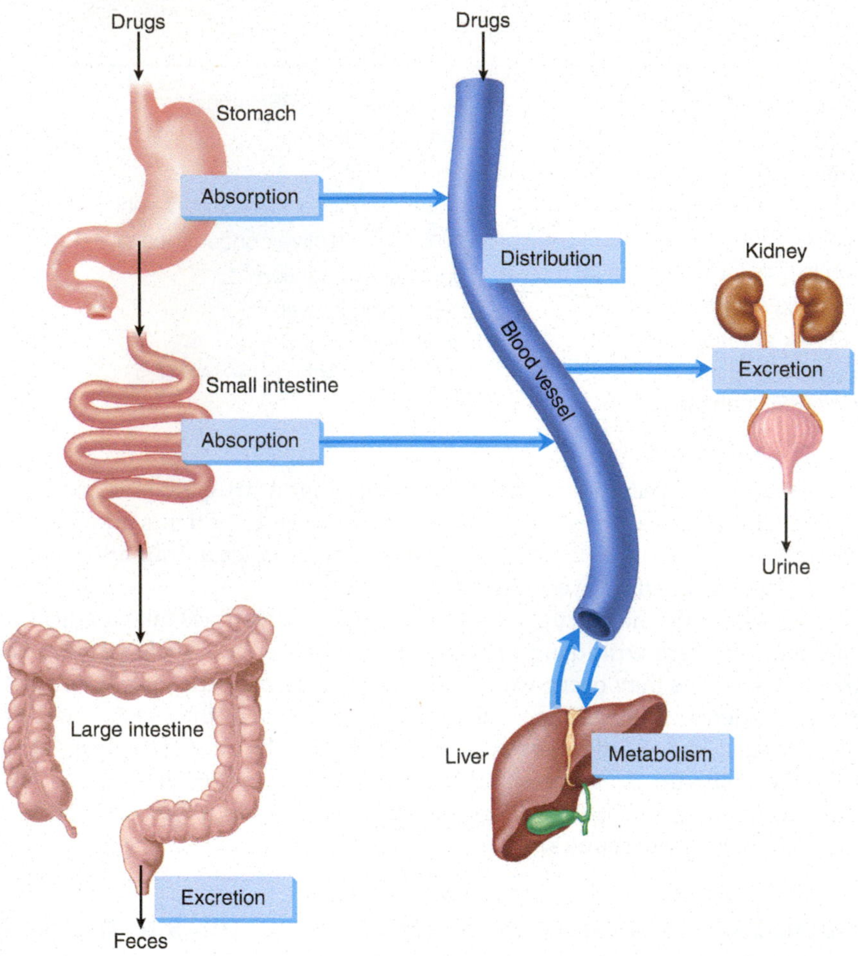

FIGURE 4.1 The four processes of pharmacokinetics (drug movement) are absorption, metabolism, distribution, and excretion.

Even if a drug is not bound by plasma proteins, it still may not be able to reach all body tissues. Three important organs contain anatomic barriers that prevent some drugs from gaining access. These are the brain, the placenta, and the testes. Even though these organs have a larger blood supply compared to most other organs in the body, their cellular barriers only allow fat-soluble substances to cross. These special barriers are called the *blood-brain barrier*, *blood-placental barrier*, and *blood-testicular barrier*.

Some drugs are able to cross the blood-brain barrier without difficulty. These include antianxiety drugs, sedatives (sleep-inducing), and psychoactive (mind-altering) drugs. Other medications, such as many antibiotics and anticancer medications, are absorbed easily in the gastrointestinal (GI)) tract but do not easily cross into the brain.

The blood-placental barrier serves an important protective function because it regulates which substances pass from the mother's bloodstream to the fetus. However, many potentially damaging agents, such as cocaine and alcohol, and even some prescription and over-the-counter (OTC) medications, easily cross this barrier. This is an extremely important issue. All food items and therapeutic drugs should be evaluated to assess their adverse effects on pregnant women and their unborn children, as discussed in Chapter 2. In males, the blood-testicular barrier prevents many drugs from reaching the testes, making it difficult to treat testicular disorders.

Core Concept 4.4 ▶

Metabolism is a process whereby drugs are made less or more active.

bio = *biologic*
transformation = *changing process*

Metabolism is the next step in pharmacokinetics. It is often described as the total of all chemical reactions in the body. Metabolism occurs in almost every cell and organ—including the GI tract and kidneys—but the liver is the primary site. The individual chemical reactions of metabolism are called **biotransformation** reactions: They are the chemical conversion of

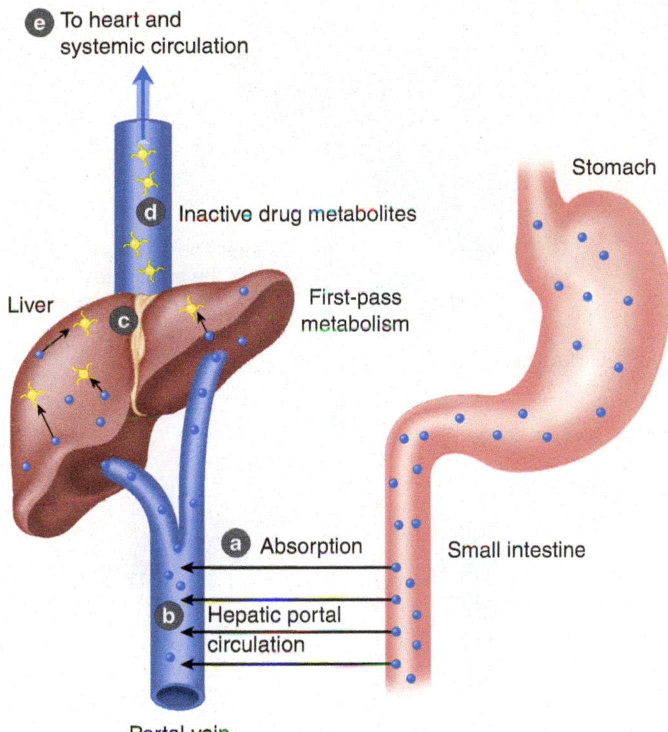

FIGURE 4.2 First-pass effect: Drugs given orally are absorbed (a) through the intestinal wall and enter the hepatic portal circulation (b). Absorbed drugs are taken directly to the liver (c) for metabolism (d) before reaching the heart and circulating throughout the rest of the body (e).

drugs from one form to another that may result in increased or decreased activity. Metabolism is important to drug therapy because these chemical reactions deactivate most drugs. For this reason, patients with liver disease usually receive much lower doses than normal because their liver is unable to metabolize the drug to a safe, active form.

Certain drugs called **prodrugs** require metabolism to make them active. In these cases, as the drug is broken down by chemical reactions of metabolism, the products formed by the breakdown produce a more intense response than does the original drug. An example of such a prodrug is sulfasalazine (Azulfidine), which is not active in its original form taken orally. Azulfidine is taken for the condition of ulcerative colitis. It is broken down by bacteria in the colon into two products that become active. Such cases of prodrugs are infrequent. Usually, metabolism is affected by the use of other drugs or the presence of other diseases.

pro = *before*
drug = *medication form*

An important mechanism that affects metabolism and drug action is the **first-pass effect.** Substances absorbed across the intestinal wall enter blood vessels known as the *hepatic portal circulation*, which carries blood directly to the liver (Figure 4.2). Drugs administered orally are absorbed into the hepatic portal circulation and are taken directly to the liver for metabolism. The liver may then metabolize the drug to a less active form before it is distributed to the rest of the body and target organs. In some cases, this first-pass effect can inactivate more than 90% of an orally administered drug before it can reach the general circulation.

Many patients differ in how efficiently their metabolic enzymes work to metabolize drugs. Age, kidney and liver disease, genetics, gender, body mass index, and other factors can dramatically affect metabolism. Some patients metabolize drugs very slowly, others very quickly.

▶ Lifespan and Diversity

In general, metabolic enzyme activity is reduced in very young and older patients. Therefore, pediatric and geriatric patients are usually more sensitive to medications than are other patients. Drug doses to the youngest and oldest age groups are often reduced to compensate for these differences.

Excretion processes remove drugs from the body.

◀ Core Concept 4.5

The last step of pharmacokinetics is **excretion**. Most substances that enter the body are removed by urination, exhalation, defecation, or sweating. Drugs are normally removed from the body by the kidneys, the respiratory tract, the GI tract, bile, or glandular activity.

The main organ of excretion is the kidney. The major role of the kidneys is to remove all nonnatural and harmful agents in the bloodstream while maintaining a balance of other natural substances. Most drugs are excreted by the kidneys. Therefore, kidney damage can

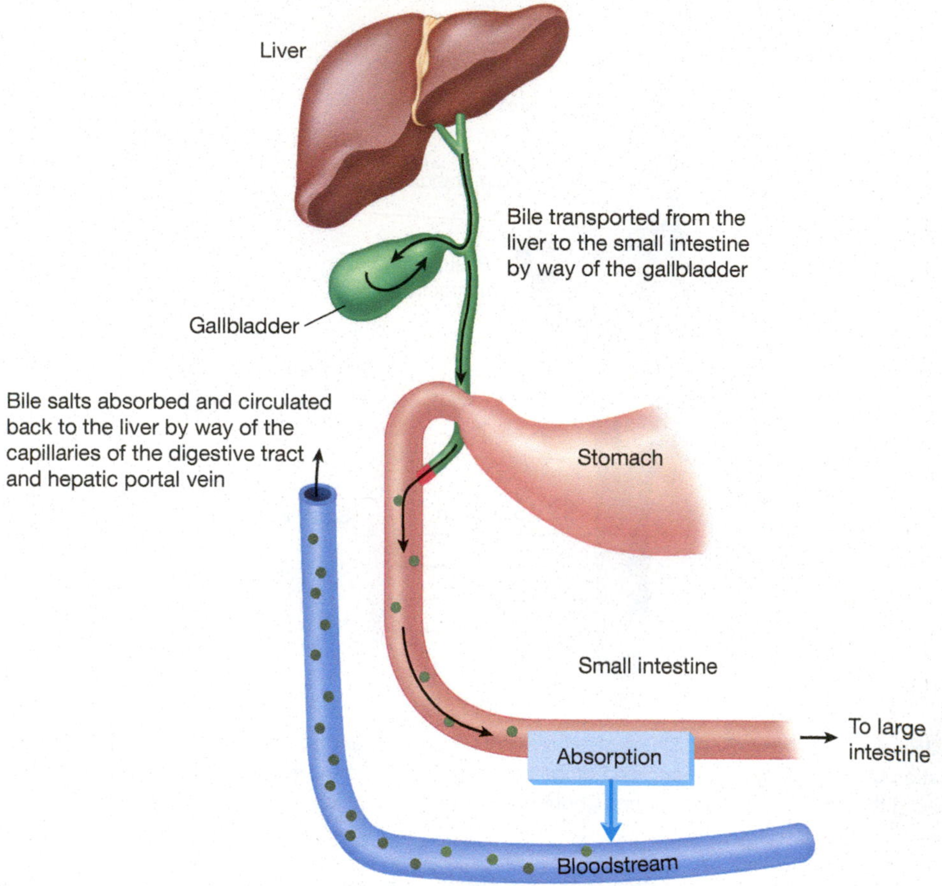

FIGURE 4.3 In the process of enterohepatic recirculation, bile is circulated back to the liver, where contained drugs are metabolized and then excreted by the kidneys. Elimination of drugs through the bile may result in prolonged drug action.

significantly prolong drug action and is a common cause of adverse reactions. Therapeutic drugs that affect kidney function are presented in Chapter 18.

Drugs that are easily changed into gaseous form are especially suited for excretion by the respiratory system. The rate of respiratory excretion is dependent on the many factors that affect gas exchange, including diffusion, gas solubility, and blood flow. The greater the blood flow into lung capillaries, the greater the excretion. In contrast to other methods of excretion, the lungs excrete most drugs in their original unmetabolized form.

Some drugs are excreted through bile. However, most components of bile are circulated back to the liver by a process known as **enterohepatic recirculation**, as shown in Figure 4.3. Recirculating drugs are then metabolized by the liver and excreted by the kidneys. The fraction of drug that is not recirculated continues on its way to the feces. Because of recirculation, elimination of drugs through bile may continue for several weeks after therapy has stopped, resulting in prolonged drug action.

Glands that produce body fluids, such as saliva and sweat, are less effective at excreting drugs. Most of the substances that are secreted in saliva and perspiration, such as urea or other waste products, are natural products. However, the mammary (breast) glands can secrete any drug capable of crossing these membranes. Therefore, a breastfeeding mother should always check with her healthcare provider before taking any prescription medication, OTC drug, herbal product, or dietary supplement.

CONCEPT REVIEW 4.1

- What does the term *pharmacokinetics* mean? Describe the four major parts of pharmacokinetics.

The rate of elimination and half-life characteristics influence drug responsiveness.

◀ **Core Concept 4.6**

Elimination, which is another term for *excretion,* is often measured so that dosages of drugs can be determined more accurately. The term *rate of elimination* refers to the amount of drug removed per unit of time from the body by normal physiologic processes. The rate of elimination is helpful in determining how long a particular drug will remain in the bloodstream, and is thus an indicator of how long a drug will produce its effect.

The **half-life ($t_{1/2}$)** of a drug is a related measurement used to ensure that maximum therapeutic dosages are administered. Half-life is the length of time required for a drug's concentration in the plasma (i.e., in circulation) to decrease by one half. It is an indicator of how long a drug will produce its effect in the body. The larger the half-life value, the longer it takes for a drug to be eliminated. Some drugs have a half-life of just a few minutes, whereas others have a half-life of several hours or days. A drug with a half-life of 10 hours will take longer to be eliminated from the body than a drug with a half-life of five hours. Drugs with longer half-lives may be given less frequently—for example, once per day.

When a patient has a renal or hepatic disease, the plasma half-life of a drug increases. This reflects the important relationship of half-life to metabolism and excretion.

Several important pharmacokinetic principles can be illustrated by measuring the serum level of a drug following a single-dose administration. These pharmacokinetic values are shown graphically in Figure 4.4. This figure demonstrates two plasma drug levels. First is the **minimum effective concentration**, the amount of drug required to produce a therapeutic effect. Second is the **toxic concentration**, the level of drug that will result in serious adverse effects. The plasma drug concentration *between* the minimum effective concentration and the toxic concentration is called the **therapeutic range** of the drug. The **onset of drug action** represents the amount of time it takes to produce a therapeutic effect after drug administration. Factors that affect drug onset may be many, depending on numerous pharmacokinetic variables. As the drug is absorbed and then begins to circulate throughout the body, the level of medication reaches its peak. The **peak plasma level** occurs when the medication has reached its highest concentration in the bloodstream. Depending on accessibility of medications to their targets, peak drug levels are not necessarily associated with optimal therapeutic effects. Multiple doses of medication may be necessary to reach therapeutic drug levels. **Duration of drug action** is the amount of time it takes for a drug to maintain its desired effect. **Termination of drug action** is when the drug effect stops.

CONCEPT REVIEW 4.2

- Why are rate of elimination and half-life ($t_{1/2}$) important to the healthcare provider?

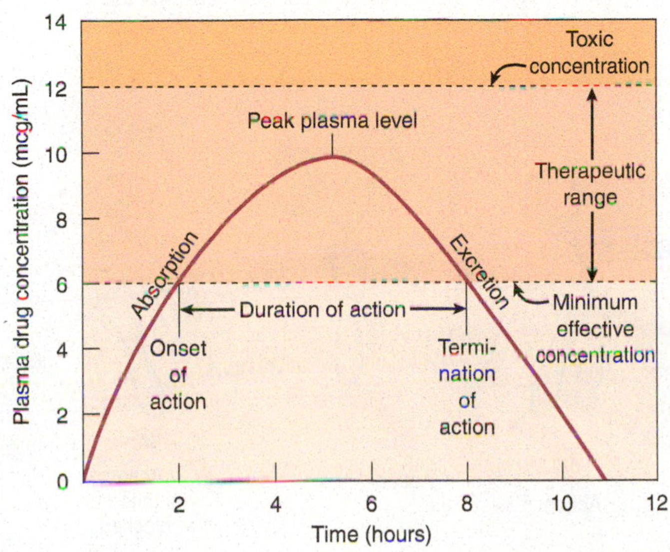

FIGURE 4.4 Single-dose drug administration: Pharmacokinetic values for this drug are as follows: onset of action = two hours; duration of action = six hours; termination of action = eight hours after administration; peak plasma concentration = 10 mcg/mL; time to peak drug effect = five hours; $t_{1/2}$ = four hours.

Table 4.1 Factors That Influence the Effectiveness of Drug Therapy

Absorption rate	Frequency of drug dosing
Changing medical condition (liver or kidney disease)	Food–drug interactions
Concentration (dose) of administered drug	Genetics
Drug–drug interactions	Half-life ($t_{1/2}$) of administered drug
Excretion rate (rate of elimination)	Metabolic rate (lower in children and older adults)

Core Concept 4.7 ▶

Pharmacodynamics focuses on what the drugs do to the body.

As discussed already, many variables influence the effectiveness of drug therapy, such as rate of administration, frequency of drug dosing, and changing medical condition. Some of these factors are listed in Table 4.1.

Successful pharmacotherapy depends on these variables as well as how effectively the body responds to drugs at specific target locations. This leads to another important core area of pharmacology: the field of pharmacodynamics. The field of pharmacodynamics is complex and requires extensive knowledge of human physiology and biochemistry. **Pharmacodynamics** deals with the mechanisms of drug action, or how the drug exerts its effects. As the root words suggest, drugs have a powerful influence on body processes. The remaining part of this chapter is devoted to a few basic pharmacodynamic principles.

pharmaco = *drug related*
dynamics = *powerful change*

Core Concept 4.8 ▶

Drugs activate specific receptors to produce a response.

Successful pharmacotherapy is based on the principle that in order to treat a disorder, a drug must interact with specific receptors in its target tissue. The **receptor theory** is a classic theory referring to the cellular mechanism by which most drugs can change body processes. A **receptor** is any structural component of a cell to which a drug binds in a dose-related manner. Receptors can be located on the plasma membrane or in the cytoplasm or nucleus of the cell. The drug or natural body substance attaches to its receptor much like a thumb drive to a computer docking port (Figure 4.5). Some drug actions are not linked to a receptor, but are connected directly with cell function, such as changing the membrane excitability of a nerve or muscle cell.

recept = *receiving*
or = *entity*

The terms *agonist* and *antagonist* are often used to describe drug action at the receptor level. **Agonists** are drugs capable of binding with receptors and causing a cellular response; these are *facilitators* of cellular action. When they are present in the bloodstream, agonists cause the tissue to respond, resulting in a therapeutic action. **Antagonists** are drugs that inhibit or block the responses of natural substances. Antagonists are called *blockers*.

ant = *against*
agonist = *activator*

therapeu = *healing treatment*
tic = *pertaining to*

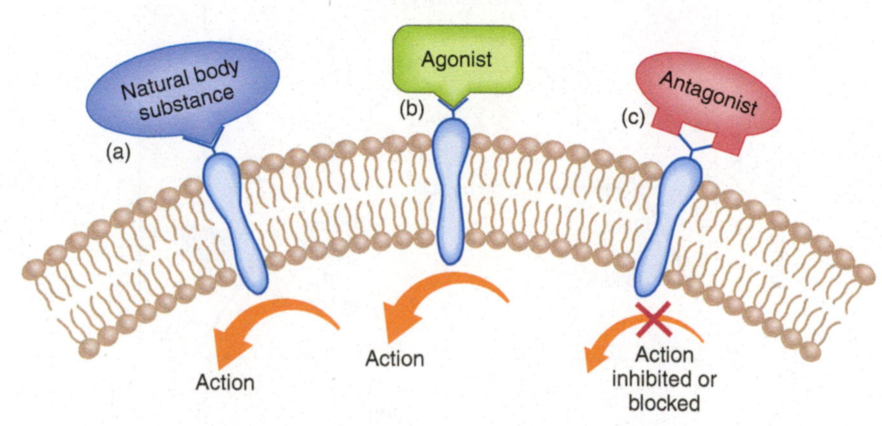

FIGURE 4.5 Cellular receptors: (a) A *neurotransmitter* or *hormone* binds to the receptor. A drug is a close "mimic" of the neurotransmitter or hormone and initiates a response by binding to the same receptor site. (b) An *agonist* is a drug that facilitates the pharmacologic response. (c) An *antagonist* is a drug that temporarily blocks or depresses the pharmacologic response.

Potency and *efficacy* are terms often used to describe the ability of drug therapy to reduce or resolve symptoms.

◀ **Core Concept 4.9**

potency = *power quality*

Potency refers to a drug's strength at a certain concentration or dose. As shown in Figure 4.6, *dose-response curves* are used to compare potencies of different drugs. If drug A has a higher potency than drug B, it means that drug A will produce a more intense effect than drug B if both drugs are given at the same dose (Figure 4.6a). A higher potency also means that a much smaller dose of the medication will be needed to produce the same effect as another drug, as shown by the shift to the left of the dose-response curve for drug A in Figure 4.6a.

efficacy = *effectiveness*

Another core concept is **efficacy**. Efficacy refers to the ability of a drug to produce a more intense response as its concentration is increased. As an example, consider Figure 4.6b. If the doses of two similarly acting drugs (A and B) are increased, they will both produce a more intense effect, but drug B will have a maximum intensity that is lower than drug A. The drug reaching a lower maximum intensity compared to another drug is said to have a lower efficacy.

In pharmacotherapeutics, it is generally more important to have a drug with higher efficacy than one with higher potency. For example, at recommended doses ibuprofen (200 mg) and aspirin (650 mg) are equally effective at relieving a headache; thus, they have the *same efficacy*. The fact that ibuprofen relieves pain at a lower dose indicates that this agent is *more potent* than aspirin. If the patient is experiencing severe pain, however, neither aspirin nor ibuprofen has sufficient efficacy to bring relief. In this instance,

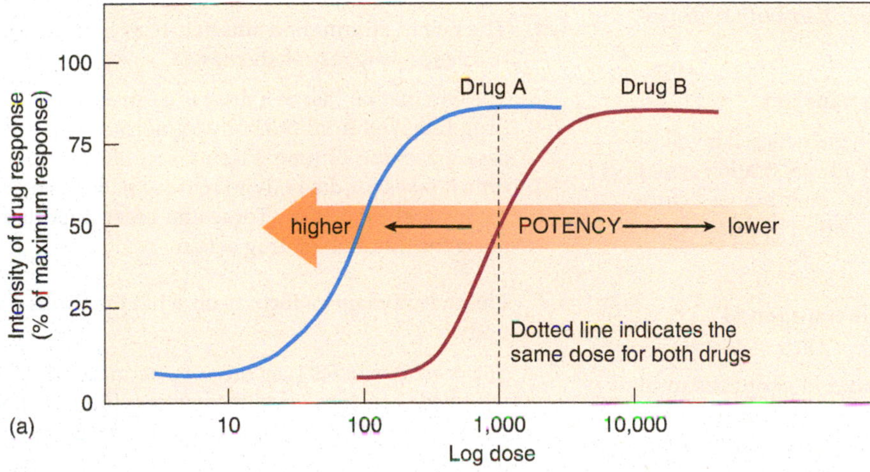

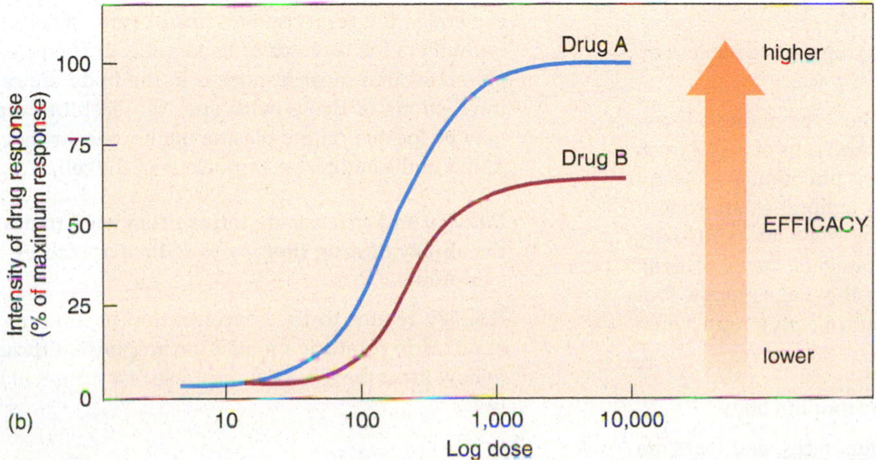

FIGURE 4.6 Potency and efficacy: (a) Drug A has a higher potency than drug B; (b) drug A has a higher efficacy than drug B.

morphine has a greater efficacy than aspirin or ibuprofen and can effectively treat this type of pain. In this example, the average dose is unimportant to the patient, but efficacy—the ability of the pain medication to bring essential relief—is crucial.

CONCEPT REVIEW 4.3

- What does the term *pharmacodynamics* mean? Identify the importance of receptors, agonists, and antagonists in influencing drug action. What is the difference between a drug's potency and its efficacy?

Chapter Review

Core Concepts Summary

4.1 Pharmacokinetics focuses on what the body does to the drugs.

Pharmacokinetics is an area of pharmacology dealing with how drugs move throughout the body. There are four components of drug transport: absorption, distribution, metabolism, and excretion.

4.2 Absorption is the first step in drug transport.

Absorption is the first step in pharmacokinetics. It involves movement of a drug from its site of administration across body membranes. Drugs cross many membranes before reaching target organs. Drug absorption is affected by many factors.

4.3 Distribution refers to how drugs are transported throughout the body.

Distribution begins after absorption and continues until drug action. Drugs bound to plasma proteins may be isolated in the plasma and prevented from reaching their target cells. The blood-brain barrier, blood-placental barrier, and blood-testicular barrier all represent areas in the body where drug distribution may be limited.

4.4 Metabolism is a process whereby drugs are made less or more active.

Metabolic processes take place in the liver, and to a lesser extent, in organs such as the kidney and cells of the GI tract. The first-pass effect is an important phenomenon. Many drugs absorbed across intestinal membranes are routed directly to the liver. Metabolic liver enzymes are usually less active in younger and in older patients; therefore, drug effects will most likely be greater in these age groups. Prodrugs are agents converted to a more active form when they are metabolically changed.

4.5 Excretion processes remove drugs from the body.

Urine, sweat, saliva, exhalation, bile, feces, and tears are the pathways the body uses to eliminate drugs and their metabolites The main organ involved with excretion is the kidney. Enterohepatic recirculation is a unique type of mechanism responsible for recirculating bile back into the bloodstream from the GI tract.

4.6 The rate of elimination and half-life characteristics influence drug responsiveness.

The elimination rate of a drug is defined as the amount of drug removed from the body by normal physiologic processes per unit of time. Plasma half-life is the amount of time it takes for the body to remove half of the drug from the general circulation. These and other important factors affect the duration of drug action.

4.7 Pharmacodynamics focuses on what the drugs do to the body.

Pharmacodynamics is an area of pharmacology concerned with how drugs produce responses within the body. Successful drug therapy depends on the effectiveness of these responses.

4.8 Drugs activate specific receptors to produce a response.

Generally, the response of a drug begins when the agent encounters the receptor of its target cell. The receptor theory states that most responses in the body are caused by interactions of drugs with specific receptors. Receptors may be located on the plasma membrane, or they may be found in the cytoplasm or nucleus of the cell.

4.9 *Potency* and *efficacy* are terms often used to describe the ability of drug therapy to reduce or resolve symptoms.

Potency relates to the concentration or amount of drug required to produce a maximum response. Efficacy refers to how great the maximal response of a drug will be.

REVIEW Questions

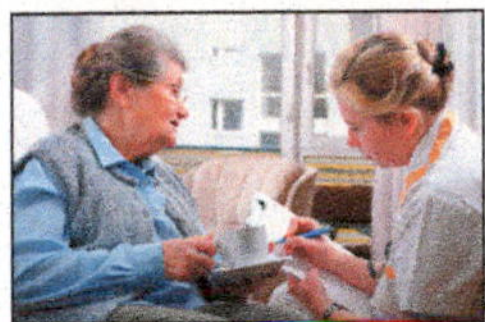

Answer the following questions to assess your knowledge of the chapter material, and go back and review any material that is not clear to you.

1. Patients with liver disorders would most likely have problems with which pharmacokinetic phase?
   1. Absorption
   2. Distribution
   3. Metabolism
   4. Excretion
2. The patient asks why the medication must be taken twice a day instead of just once. The best response would be:
   1. "Taking it once a day is fine as long as it is taken at the same time every day."
   2. "Taking it twice a day ensures that maximum concentrations are maintained within the body."
   3. "You will need to speak to your healthcare provider about this."
   4. "The first dose of the medication is blocked by deactivation, and the second dose is metabolized by the body."
3. Which of the following principles are true about how medications work? (Select all that apply.)
   1. For a drug to be effective, it must be potent.
   2. For drug efficacy to occur, a lower dose must be administered.
   3. Antagonists bind to receptors and produce responses to block agonists.
   4. The agonist-receptor interaction causes a cellular response, resulting in a therapeutic action.
   5. All drugs that have the same dose have the same efficacy.
4. A drug that binds with a receptor to produce a therapeutic response is called a(n):
   1. Antagonist.
   2. Facilitator.
   3. Agonist.
   4. Blocker.
5. If a patient takes an oral medication on a full stomach, the nurse is aware that the medication will be:
   1. Absorbed more rapidly.
   2. Absorbed more slowly.
   3. Neutralized by gastric enzymes.
   4. Activated by gastric enzymes.
6. When planning care for a patient, the nurse takes into consideration which of the following factors that could directly influence the effectiveness of drugs that will be given? (Select all that apply.)
   1. Drug–drug interactions
   2. Food–drug interactions
   3. Route of administration
   4. Time of administration within the day
   5. Diseases of the liver or kidney
7. An antibiotic has been ordered for the patient with a brain abscess. The nurse understands that:
   1. There are no antibiotics effective to treat brain abscesses because they cannot cross the blood-brain barrier.
   2. Only fat-soluble substances will pass the blood-brain barrier so the antibiotic will need to be fat-soluble.
   3. The half-life of the antibiotic will be decreased when crossing the blood-brain barrier.
   4. The gastrointestinal tract will prevent absorption from occurring.
8. When orally administered drugs are extensively metabolized by the liver, with only part of the drug dose reaching target organs, this is known as:
   1. Half-life.
   2. Potency.
   3. First-pass effect.
   4. Rate of elimination.
9. A patient asks how the body will "get rid of all the drugs" she is taking. You would respond by saying: (Select all that apply.)
   1. "Drugs are normally removed from the body by the kidneys."
   2. "Some drugs are removed from the body through some glands."
   3. "Some drugs can be more effectively excreted through the sweat glands."
   4. "Some drugs are changed into a gaseous form and are excreted by the lungs."
   5. "Drugs are excreted through the skin."
10. An older patient has reduced metabolic activity. The nurse may expect to see what change in the dosage of a drug given to this patient?
    1. Increase the medication dosage.
    2. Increase the number of times the patient has to take the medication.
    3. Decrease the medication dosage.
    4. Reduce the number of times the patient has to take the medication.

Answers and complete rationales for the Review Questions appear in Appendix A.

SELECTED BIBLIOGRAPHY

Blumenthal, D. K., & Garrison, J. C. (2011). Pharmacodynamics: Molecular mechanisms of drug action. In B. A. Chabner, L. L. Brunton, & B. C. Knollman (Eds.), *Goodman and Gilman's the pharmacological basis of therapeutics* (12th ed.). New York, NY: McGraw-Hill.

Buxton, I. L., & Benet, L. Z. (2011). Pharmacokinetics: The dynamics of drug absorption, distribution, metabolism, and elimination. In B. A. Chabner, L. L. Brunton, & B. C. Knollman (Eds.), *Goodman and Gilman's the pharmacological basis of therapeutics* (12th ed.). New York, NY: McGraw-Hill.

Chan, L. N., & Anderson, G. D. (2014). Pharmacokinetic and pharmacodynamics drug interactions with ethanol (alcohol). *Clinical Pharmacokinetics, 53*, 1115–1136. doi:10.1007/s40262-014-0190-x

Linares, O. A., Fudin, J., Daly-Linares, A., Boston, R. C. (2015). Individualized hydrocodone therapy based on phenotype, pharmacokinetics, and pharmacokinetic dosing. *Clinical Journal of Pain, 31*, 1026-1035. doi:10.1097/AJP.0000000000000214

Merck Manual Professional Edition. (2013). *Clinical pharmacology*. Retrieved at http://www.merckmanuals.com/professional/clinical-pharmacology

Chapter 5

The Nursing Process in Pharmacology

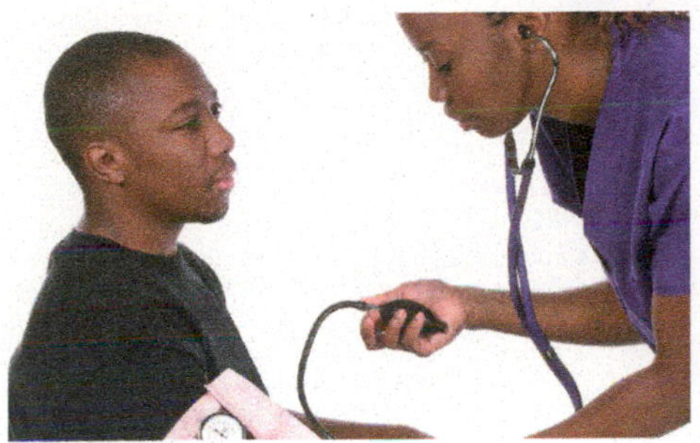

Core Concepts

5.1 The first step of the nursing process is the assessment phase.

5.2 Nursing diagnoses are based on the data gathered in the assessment phase.

5.3 In the planning phase, the nurse creates an individualized plan of care for a patient based on the identified nursing diagnoses and etiologies.

5.4 The implementation phase puts the plan of care into action.

5.5 In the evaluation phase, the nurse obtains data to determine if the goal or outcome has been achieved.

Learning Outcomes

After reading this chapter, the student should be able to:

1. Identify how the assessment phase of the nursing process can be used to gather data pertinent to medication administration.
2. Explain how nursing diagnoses can be used to improve medication administration.
3. Describe the steps in the planning phase of the nursing process.
4. Identify pharmacology applications included in the implementation phase of the nursing process.
5. Explain the importance of the evaluation phase in the nursing process as applied to pharmacotherapy.

Key Terms

assessment phase
data collection
etiologies (e-tee-OL-o-gees)
evaluation criteria
evaluation phase
goal
implementation phase
interventions
nursing diagnosis
nursing process
outcome
planning phase

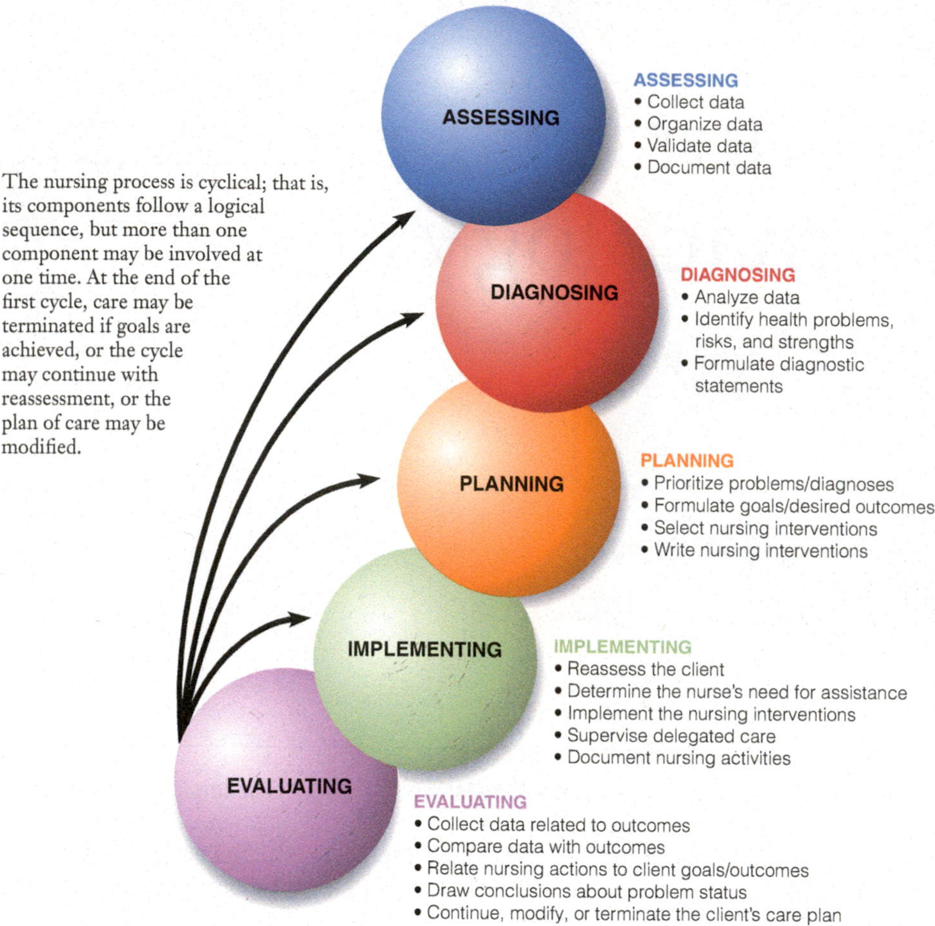

FIGURE 5.1 The five overlapping phases of the nursing process. Each phase depends on the accuracy of the other phases. Each phase involves critical thinking.
Source: From Kozier & Erb's *Fundamentals of Nursing: Concepts, Process, and Practice,* 10e by Audrey T Berman; Geralyn Frandsen. Copyright © 2016 by Pearson Education, Inc.

The **nursing process**, a systematic method of problem solving, forms the foundation of all nursing practice. The use of the nursing process is particularly essential during medication administration. By using the steps of the nursing process, nurses can ensure that the interdisciplinary practice of pharmacology results in safe, effective, and individualized medication administration and outcomes for all patients under their care.

The nursing process is an ongoing activity involving five distinct phases: assessment, diagnosis, planning, implementation, and evaluation. The nursing process is cyclical and each phase is related to all the others; they are not separate entities but overlap. The licensed practical nurse (LPN) or licensed vocational nurse (LVN) contributes to each phase of the process under the direction of the registered nurse (RN). In this chapter, each phase is briefly reviewed, and each phase's use in pharmacology is emphasized. A summary of the phases is shown in Figure 5.1.

Core Concept 5.1 ▶ The first step of the nursing process is the assessment phase.

The **assessment phase** of the nursing process, referred to as **data collection** within the scope of practice of the LPN/LVN, is the systematic collection, organization, validation, and documentation of patient data. The assessment phase serves two purposes. The first is to gather data that will enable the nurse to identify health challenges and problems that the patient is at particular risk for developing. This data will eventually be used to identify appropriate nursing diagnoses and to develop a plan of care.

The second purpose of the assessment phase is to gather initial *baseline data* on the patient that will be compared to subsequent data during the evaluation phase of the nursing process. These comparisons will indicate to what extent the treatment goals have been achieved. When applying the nursing process to pharmacology, baseline data are necessary for the nurse to be able to evaluate therapeutic drug effects and adverse drug effects. For example, a common adverse effect of many antibiotics is the risk for allergic reaction, often identified by a skin rash. To determine whether the rash is due to a medication, the nurse must first assess that a rash was not present prior to initiating drug therapy. As another example, if a patient is exhibiting elevated liver enzymes during hospitalization, the nurse will use baseline assessment data to determine whether the patient had this condition on admission, or whether it is a sign of a recent adverse drug reaction.

Data collected in the assessment phase come from many sources. These include the patient, caregivers, medical records, and other healthcare professionals. *Subjective* data include what the patient says or perceives, such as pain, anxiety, or nausea. Whenever possible, the subjective data are verified by *objective* data that are gathered through physical examination, medical history, laboratory tests, and other diagnostic sources.

Assessment must always include a comprehensive health history that includes the patient's use of prescription drugs, over-the-counter (OTC) agents, dietary supplements, and herbal products. The nurse should inquire about past and current tobacco, alcohol, and recreational drug use because these may influence treatment outcomes. Any allergic or unusual reactions to drugs should be documented, including serious adverse drug reactions that may have occurred to close family members.

The initial health history gathered during the assessment phase is used to determine whether the patient has a contraindication that would present a risk for drug therapy. For example, the nurse may discover during assessment that the patient is pregnant and should not receive isotretinoin (Accutane) for her acne because it is a pregnancy category X drug. The nurse may discover that the patient has a history of allergy to penicillin, and therefore should not be prescribed ampicillin due to the potential for cross-allergy. A thorough assessment is the best way to prevent adverse drug effects.

CONCEPT REVIEW 5.1

- What types of assessments would be important for the nurse to perform on patients who will be required to self-administer their medications at home?

Nursing diagnoses are based on the data gathered in the assessment phase.

◀ **Core Concept 5.2**

During the diagnosis phase of the nursing process, the nurse analyzes assessment data, identifies health problems, and formulates diagnostic statements. A **nursing diagnosis** is a clinical judgment of a patient's response to an actual or potential health problem, a problem that is within the nurse's scope of practice to address. It is the responsibility of the RN to identify the appropriate diagnosis and develop a plan of care. The LPN/LVN contributes to this phase by collecting data and collaborating with the RN.

dia = *through or complete*
gnosis = *knowledge*

Nursing diagnoses differ from medical diagnoses, which are determined by healthcare providers. Whereas the medical diagnosis remains constant during a patient's hospital stay, nursing diagnoses are in constant flux as the patient responds to treatments. Nursing diagnoses address changes in the patient's condition—for example, alterations in mobility, nutritional intake, urinary elimination, knowledge, ability for self-care, and risk for injury. These nursing diagnoses are used to set goals and plan care.

Nursing diagnoses are often stated as a problem, or the risk for a problem, followed by a "related to" clause that identifies the **etiologies**, or those conditions that have caused or contributed to the problem. By altering one or more of these etiologies, nurses are able to effect improvements in the diagnosed problem. This is accomplished by planning and implementing **interventions**, which are actions that the nurse takes to achieve patient goals. The nurse chooses interventions that are patient focused and target the etiologies of the problem. NANDA International has developed standard wording, known as the nursing diagnosis, for identifying actual and potential patient health problems. For example, a nursing diagnosis may be, "*Activity Intolerance* related to acute knee pain." The nurse designs interventions to address the etiology (acute knee pain) that may include the administration of pain medications, heat, or ice packs.

etio = *cause*
ology = *study of*

Table 5.1 Common Nursing Diagnoses in Pharmacotherapy

Acute Confusion related to substance abuse
Risk for Acute Confusion related to drug effects
Impaired Comfort related to drug effects
Deficient Fluid Volume related to drug effects
Excess Fluid Volume related to drug effects
Noncompliance related to lack of knowledge of drug therapy
Risk for Infection related to adverse drug effects
Risk for Injury related to adverse drug effects
Insomnia related to drug effects
Imbalanced Nutrition: Less Than Body Requirements related to drug-induced nausea
Ineffective Health Maintenance related to drug therapy regimen
Activity Intolerance related to drug effects
Deficient Knowledge related to a lack of information about new drug therapy

*Other nursing diagnoses may be applicable depending on patient assessment and type of medication being used.

Source: Herdman, T.H. & Kamitsuru, S. (Eds.), *Nursing Diagnoses: Definitions & Classification 2015–2017*. Copyright © 2014, 1994–2014 *NANDA International*. Used by arrangement by John Wiley & Sons, Inc. Companion website: www.wiley.com/go/nursingdiagnoses.

Nursing diagnoses are prioritized by their level of importance and immediacy to the patient's clinical condition. For example, alterations in breathing would likely take precedence over the potential for skin breakdown. A primary nursing role is to enable patients to become active participants in their own care. Patients need to vocalize, to the extent possible, their priorities for care, which should be considered by the nurse when diagnoses are prioritized. By including patients when identifying needs, the nurse encourages them to take a more active role in working toward meeting the identified goals.

When applied to pharmacotherapy, the diagnosis phase of the nursing process addresses three main areas of concern:

- Promoting therapeutic drug effects
- Minimizing adverse drug effects and toxicity
- Maximizing the ability of the patient for self-care, including the knowledge, skills, and resources necessary for safe and effective drug administration.

The teaching of patients is one of the basic roles of nursing, and careful attention to drug teaching can promote therapeutic outcomes as well as minimize adverse effects. Examples of nursing diagnoses that involve drug teaching include *Deficient Knowledge*, related to a lack of information about new drug therapy, and *Noncompliance*, related to not taking the prescribed medication. The teaching of patients is discussed further in the planning phase. See Table 5.1 for selected nursing diagnoses for pharmacotherapy. For a complete list, the student should refer to a nursing fundamentals textbook.

Core Concept 5.3 ▶

In the planning phase, the nurse creates an individualized plan of care for a patient based on the identified nursing diagnoses and etiologies.

After a nursing diagnosis has been established, the nurse begins to plan ways to assist the patient to establish an optimal level of wellness. In the **planning phase** of the nursing process, the nurse prioritizes diagnoses, formulates desired goals, and selects nursing interventions.

There are two main steps of the planning phase. The first step is to identify the desired **goal**, or **outcome** to be achieved, and the specific **evaluation criteria** that will be used to determine if that goal has been met. The outcome may be a short-term or long-term goal, should include the time frame whenever possible, and must be realistic for the patient to achieve. The evaluation criteria should be specific and measurable. These criteria are often indicated by the abbreviation AEB (as evidenced by). The outcome should directly address the problem identified in the nursing diagnosis. For example, if the nursing diagnosis is *Risk for Dysfunctional Gastrointestinal Motility* related to opioid analgesic use, a goal might be: the absence of altered bowel elimination, AEB regular bowel evacuation, absence of difficulty passing stool, and absence of abdominal bloating or discomfort. Notice how this plan includes a clear goal as well as specific evaluation criteria.

The second step of the planning phase is to develop a list of interventions. The interventions are specific nursing actions designed to help move the patient toward the established goal.

When planning interventions the nurse should consider the specific health problem and etiologies, current practice guidelines, acceptability to the patient, and the nurse's own capabilities. In addition, the chosen nursing interventions should be safe and appropriate for the patient's age, health, and condition; congruent with the patient's values, beliefs, and culture; and appropriate to the other ordered therapies. The choice of nursing interventions will also depend on what is realistic and practical to the situation in terms of equipment availability, financial status of the patient, and available resources, including staff, agency, family, or community resources.

With respect to pharmacotherapy, the planning phase involves two main issues: drug administration and patient teaching. For the first issue, the nurse must plan how and when to administer the drug. For oral medications, does it need to be given with food or on an empty stomach? Is it more effective if administered at a certain time of day? Can it be crushed or split? For all medications, the nurse will plan interventions to enhance therapeutic outcomes and minimize or prevent adverse drug effects.

When planning patient drug teaching, the projected length of pharmacotherapy influences the amount and type of teaching provided by the nurse. Is the drug to be given for a short time during an acute care hospitalization, or is pharmacotherapy going to be long term and self-administered following discharge? If a drug is to be given short term, the patient should be told the name of the drug and its basic actions, why the patient is receiving it, and some of the drug's most common and major adverse effects, including any that should be promptly reported to the nurse or healthcare provider.

For drugs that will be taken after discharge, patient teaching should be comprehensive and be provided both orally and in writing. This teaching should include the drug name (both generic and trade), the drug class and its major effects, why the drug is being prescribed, the therapeutic effects and when they should occur, how and when to take the drug, the common and major adverse effects and which ones should be reported to the prescriber, the types of follow-up monitoring needed, potential drug interactions, the duration of drug therapy, the activities to avoid while taking the drug, and what to do if a dose is missed or forgotten. Table 5.2 gives tips for effective patient teaching that can be used for patients of all ages.

Table 5.2 Teaching Throughout the Lifespan

Patient teaching is an essential component of the nursing process. To be effective, oral and written teaching must be age appropriate. The following are some tips for effective teaching.

Children

- Use family-centered approaches when providing drug teaching for children and adolescents.
- Engage young children and toddlers by using interactive strategies.
- Use simple, nonthreatening language.
- Provide a developmentally appropriate environment when teaching adolescents.
- Encourage problem solving to help adolescents make effective choices.

Adults

- Adult learners are independent; the nurse should facilitate learning.
- Adults learn best when the topic is of immediate value, and when new material is connected to previous experiences.
- Adults vary widely in their learning styles and preferences; teaching and learning is enhanced when patient learning styles are considered.
- Consider the literacy level of learners. It is recommended that written materials be on a fifth-grade reading level.
- Employ multiple methods of delivering information; a combination of verbal and written material is best.

Older Adults

- Plan several short learning sessions; repeat and review material covered; time needed for learning often increases with age.
- Relate new learning to the patient's real-life experiences.
- Provide printed material, videos, pictures, and diagrams that the patient can refer to at a later time.
- Modify teaching methods to sensory-perceptual deficits or cognitive decline. Ensure that the patient has the necessary aids (glasses, magnifying glass, hearing aid) to maximize the learning experience.
- Offer opportunities for practice of psychomotor skills related to administering medications.

Core Concept 5.4 ▶ The implementation phase puts the plan of care into action.

The **implementation phase** is when the nurse applies the knowledge, skills, and principles of nursing care to help move the patient toward the desired goal and optimal wellness. Implementation involves action on the part of the nurse or patient: administering a drug, providing patient teaching, and initiating actions identified by the nursing diagnoses and plan of care. The implementation phase should be designed to maximize therapeutic drug responses and prevent adverse reactions.

It must be remembered that implementation of the plan of care is subject to modification based on the patient's evolving condition. In implementing pharmacotherapy, an important decision that the nurse must make is whether it is appropriate to administer the drug at the planned time. To make this decision, the nurse needs to understand the drug's therapeutic and adverse effects well enough to know the circumstances under which it is appropriate, or not appropriate, to give the drug. After assessing a current vital sign, a laboratory result, a new health problem, or a physical assessment finding, it may be appropriate for the nurse to delay administration of an ordered drug until the prescriber can be contacted. For example, if the patient's current serum potassium level is below the normal range, and the nurse has an order to administer furosemide (Lasix), it would be an error for the nurse to administer the drug. Carrying out the order would cause serum potassium to fall, which could trigger cardiac dysrhythmias. Likewise, a patient who has a scheduled dose of morphine for pain relief but currently has a respiratory rate of less than eight should not receive the drug because it may cause respiratory failure.

As pharmacotherapy progresses, the nurse must be aware of circumstances that might require modification of the implementation phase. The patient may develop new symptoms that contraindicate the use of the drug being administered. For example, the patient may begin to show signs of a developing rash, changes in blood pressure, or alterations in mental status that call for discontinuation of the drug until the prescriber can be contacted. These examples help illustrate the cyclic nature of the nursing process: the importance of continuous assessment and the revision of the planning and implementation phases.

Implementation also includes patient teaching (Figure 5.2). Table 5.2 gives tips for effective patient teaching that can be used for patients of all ages. Patient drug teaching should start with what the patient already knows about a drug and build from there. The specific topics to include in this teaching are developed in the planning phase. When preparing to carry out the teaching, other factors that the nurse should consider are the patient's readiness to learn and whether it is an appropriate time for teaching. Patients who are in pain, sleepy, anxious, or distracted are less likely to understand instructions. Drug teaching should be tailored to the patient's developmental level, learning capacity, and preferred learning style. Patients may prefer that a family member or caregiver be present during the teaching. This is especially important for patients with limited English proficiency, pediatric patients, older adults with cognitive deficits, and patients with mental illnesses who may be incapable of safe self-administration. Patient teaching is sometimes a collaborative effort, requiring coordination with other medical disciplines as part of the sessions. Often a registered dietitian, physical therapist, pharmacist, occupational therapist, or diabetes educator collaborates in the patient teaching. When teaching, always allow sufficient time to address any areas of concern for the patient.

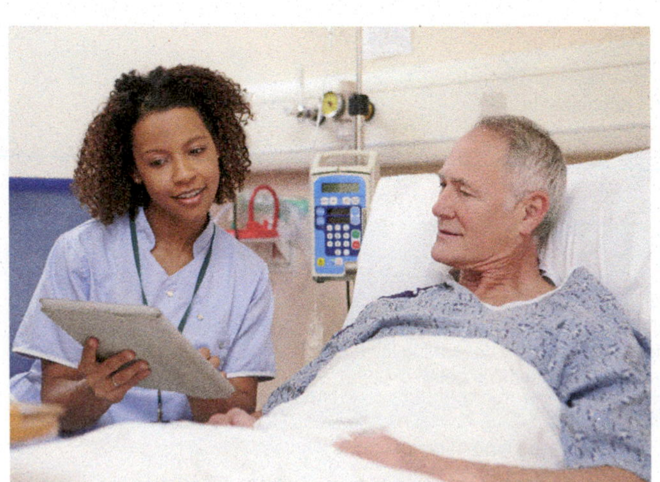

FIGURE 5.2 Teaching patients about drugs and their effects is an important step in the nursing process.
Source: Monkey Business/Fotolia

Finally, documentation is an essential part of the implementation phase. This includes a thorough reporting of the interventions carried out, the drugs that were given (or withheld), the teaching that took place, and the patient's responses to the interventions.

In the evaluation phase, the nurse obtains data to determine if the goal or outcome has been achieved.

◀ Core Concept 5.5

The **evaluation phase** compares the patient's current health status with the established outcome to determine if the plan of care is appropriate or if it needs revision. Essentially, the evaluation phase is used to determine if the goal or outcome has been met. If it has been met, the plan of care was appropriate. If the goal was partially met, the nurse may determine that the interventions may need to be continued for a longer time or otherwise modified to better resolve the health problem.

As it relates to pharmacotherapy, evaluation is used to determine whether the therapeutic effects of the drug have been achieved as well as whether adverse effects have been prevented or kept to acceptable levels. For example, if a drug is given for symptoms of pain, has the pain subsided? If an antibiotic is given for an infection, have the signs of that infection improved? If the evaluation data show no improvement in health status over the baseline data, the interventions will likely need to be revised, drug doses may need to be adjusted, more time may be needed to achieve a therapeutic drug response, or a different or additional drug may be needed. The data gathered during the evaluation phase becomes part of the assessment data and continues the cycle of nursing process as outcomes and interventions are revised. The evaluation data needs to be documented in the patient's record to ensure proper communication of the patient's response to the nursing interventions.

In an outpatient setting, lack of drug response determined during the evaluation phase may be caused by patient noncompliance with the drug regimen. During the assessment phase, the nurse must determine if the patient is taking the drug as prescribed. If noncompliance is discovered, the nurse must plan and implement strategies for increasing compliance, which includes identifying reasons for the noncompliance. Additional patient teaching is critical to obtain maximum patient compliance with the drug regimen: The nurse must help the patient to value pharmacotherapy as important to the improvement of the patient's health.

▶ Lifespan and Diversity

When evaluating the success of drug therapy in older adults, the healthcare provider should understand that noncompliance may be due to physical or other limitations. The inability to open childproof containers or to read the instructions on the label are possible causes of noncompliance. Older adults may depend on caregivers to obtain or administer their medications on a regular basis. In many cases, simply forgetting to take a medication is a cause of lack of drug effect. The healthcare provider should assist older patients in overcoming these limitations so that pharmacotherapy can be optimized.

CONCEPT REVIEW 5.2

- What strategies might the nurse implement to improve compliance with drug therapy for a geriatric patient?

CAM Therapy | Medication Errors and Dietary Supplements

Some herbal and dietary supplements have powerful effects on the body that can influence the outcomes of prescription drug therapy. In some cases, OTC supplements can enhance the effects of prescription drugs, whereas in other instances supplements may cancel the therapeutic effects of medications. For example, many patients with heart disease take garlic supplements in addition to warfarin (Coumadin) to prevent clots from forming. Because garlic and warfarin are both anticoagulants, taking them together could cause excessive bleeding. As another example, high doses of calcium supplements can cancel the beneficial antihypertensive effects of drugs, such as nifedipine (Procardia), a calcium channel blocker.

Chapter Review

Core Concepts Summary

5.1 The first step of the nursing process is the assessment phase.

Assessment is the careful, systematic collection of patient data. During this phase, the nurse gathers data that identify patient health challenges.

5.2 Nursing diagnoses are based on the data gathered in the assessment phase.

Nursing diagnoses are clinical judgments based on a patient's response to actual or potential patient problems; they include the etiologies of the health problem. These etiologies are factors that can be addressed by nursing interventions to address the health challenges of the patient.

5.3 In the planning phase, the nurse creates an individualized plan of care for a patient based on the identified nursing diagnoses and etiologies.

The first step of the planning phase is identification of a goal or outcome for the patient, including the evaluation criteria that will be used to determine whether the goal has been achieved. The second step is the formulation of nursing interventions to be used to help move the patient toward the established goal.

5.4 The implementation phase puts the plan of care into action.

When applied to pharmacology, the implementation phase involves administering the drug and providing patient drug teaching that maximizes therapeutic effects and minimizes side effects.

5.5 In the evaluation phase, the nurse obtains data to determine if the goal or outcome has been achieved.

By comparing the evaluation data to baseline data, the nurse is able to determine whether the established goal was met. Evaluation data are used to develop revised goals, plans, or interventions that will better resolve the health challenges of the patient.

REVIEW Questions

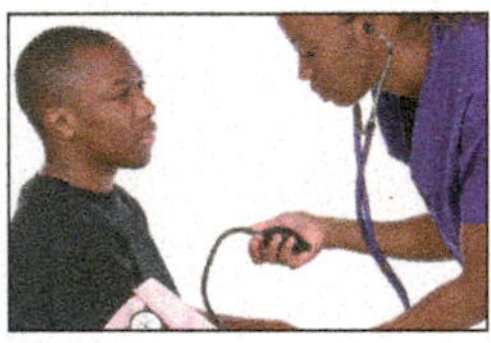

Answer the following questions to assess your knowledge of the chapter material, and go back and review any material that is not clear to you.

1. The nurse reviews a patient record for drug allergies, current medications, and disease states that could affect drug responses. These actions are part of which phase of the nursing process?
   1. Assessment/Data collection
   2. Planning
   3. Implementation
   4. Evaluation

2. The implementation phase of the nursing process involves which two main activities related to pharmacology?
   1. Developing and performing nursing interventions
   2. Providing and evaluating patient teaching
   3. Administering drugs and providing patient education
   4. Assessing and evaluating adverse drug effects

3. Which of the following would be most important for the nurse in the evaluation phase of the nursing process?
   1. Patient satisfaction with drug therapy
   2. Evidence of therapeutic drug effects
   3. Development of minor adverse drug effects
   4. The possibility of noncompliance with drug therapy

4. Which of the following is appropriate information to gather in the assessment/data collection phase of the nursing process? (Select all that apply.)
   1. Drug allergies
   2. Therapeutic response to the drug
   3. History of renal or hepatic disease
   4. The patient's physical examination information
   5. The ability to swallow if an oral medication is to be given

5. Ms. Smith is complaining of pain in her lower back. After asking Ms. Smith about her pain level, the nurse prepared the pain medication as ordered and is about to administer it to her. What phase of the nursing process is the nurse using?
   1. Assessment/Data collection
   2. Planning
   3. Implementation
   4. Evaluation

6. The second phase of the nursing process involves analyzing data and identifying health problems, such as *Activity Intolerance* related to pain. This phase is known as:
   1. Assessment/Data Collection.
   2. Implementation.
   3. Nursing diagnosis.
   4. Planning.

7. The nursing process, as it relates to pharmacology, can best be described as a:
   1. Way of determining whether a patient should use a cane or crutches when walking.
   2. Method of documentation that nurses use in their daily practice.
   3. Problem-solving method that encourages nurses to rely solely on their textbook knowledge of a patient's condition before determining a course of action.
   4. Systematic approach to problem solving that ensures the safe and effective administration of medication.

8. The role of the LPN/LVN is to:
   1. Work independently of the RN and other healthcare providers when establishing a plan of care for a patient.
   2. Assist the healthcare provider in establishing a patient's plan of care.
   3. Contribute to each phase of the process under the direction of the RN.
   4. Rely completely on the RN to utilize the nursing process when caring for patients.

9. A male patient has just been diagnosed with diabetes mellitus. The interdisciplinary team, including the LPN/LVN, is in the process of developing a schedule of teaching sessions with him on subjects such as glucose monitoring, insulin injections, and signs of hypoglycemia. What phase of the nursing process does this represent?
   1. Assessment/Data Collection
   2. Planning
   3. Implementation
   4. Evaluation

10. The nursing diagnosis statement is *Insomnia* related to anxiety as manifested by difficulty falling and staying asleep. The etiology of the problem is:
    1. Insomnia.
    2. Anxiety.
    3. Difficulty falling asleep.
    4. Difficulty staying asleep.

Answers and complete rationales for the Review Questions appear in Appendix A.

REFERENCES

Berman, A., Snyder, S., & Frandsen, G. (2016). *Kozier & Erb's fundamentals of nursing: Concepts, process, and practice* (10th ed.). Upper Saddle River, NJ: Pearson Education.

Herdman, T. H., & Kamitsuru, S. (2014). *NANDA International nursing diagnoses: Definitions and classification, 2015–2017*. Oxford, United Kingdom: Wiley-Blackwell.

BIBLIOGRAPHY

Burke, K., Mohn-Brown, E. L., & Eby, L. (2016). *Medical-surgical nursing care:* (4th ed.). Upper Saddle River, NJ: Pearson Education.

Byrne, M., Callahan, B., Carlson, K., Daley, L., Magorian, K., Phillips, P., Wilhelm, S. (2015). *Nursing: A concept-based approach to learning* (2nd ed.). Upper Saddle River, NJ: Pearson Education

NANDA International. (n.d.). *Glossary of terms: Nursing diagnosis*. Retrieved from http://www.nanda.org/nanda-international-glossary-of-terms.html

Wilkinson, J. M. (2014). *Pearson Nursing diagnosis handbook* (10th ed.). Upper Saddle River, NJ: Pearson Education.

Chapter 6

Preventing Medication Errors

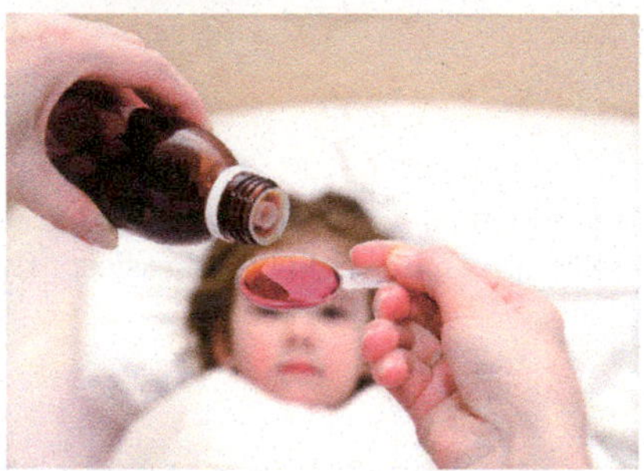

Core Concepts

6.1 **Medication errors are preventable events that may significantly impact treatment outcomes.**

6.2 **Both healthcare providers and patients can contribute to medication errors.**

6.3 **Medication errors may affect patient health and should be documented.**

6.4 **Healthcare providers use multiple strategies for reducing medication errors.**

Learning Outcomes

After reading this chapter, the student should be able to:

1. Define medication error.
2. Identify factors that contribute to medication errors.
3. Explain the impact of medication errors on patients and why errors should be documented.
4. Describe strategies that healthcare providers can implement to reduce medication errors.

Key Terms

medication error

medication error index

sentinel event

Whether they are prescribing, administering, or monitoring medication use, healthcare providers have ethical and legal responsibilities to ensure that pharmacotherapy is delivered in a safe and effective manner. Because pharmacotherapy requires multiple complex steps by pharmacists, nurses, other healthcare providers, and patients, medication administration may never be 100% error-free. The purpose of this chapter is to examine the reasons for medication errors and explore strategies used to prevent them.

Core Concept 6.1 ▶

Medication errors are preventable events that may significantly impact treatment outcomes.

According to the National Coordinating Council for Medication Error Reporting and Prevention (NCC MERP), a **medication error** is defined as the following:

> any preventable event that may cause or lead to inappropriate medication use or patient harm while the medication is in the control of the health care professional, patient, or

consumer. Such events may be related to professional practice, healthcare products, procedures, and systems, including prescribing; order communication; product labeling, packaging, and nomenclature; compounding; dispensing; distribution; administration; education; monitoring; and use. (NCC MERP, 2016)

NCC MERP also classifies medication errors by using a **medication error index** (Figure 6.1). This index places medication errors into nine categories based on the extent of the harm an

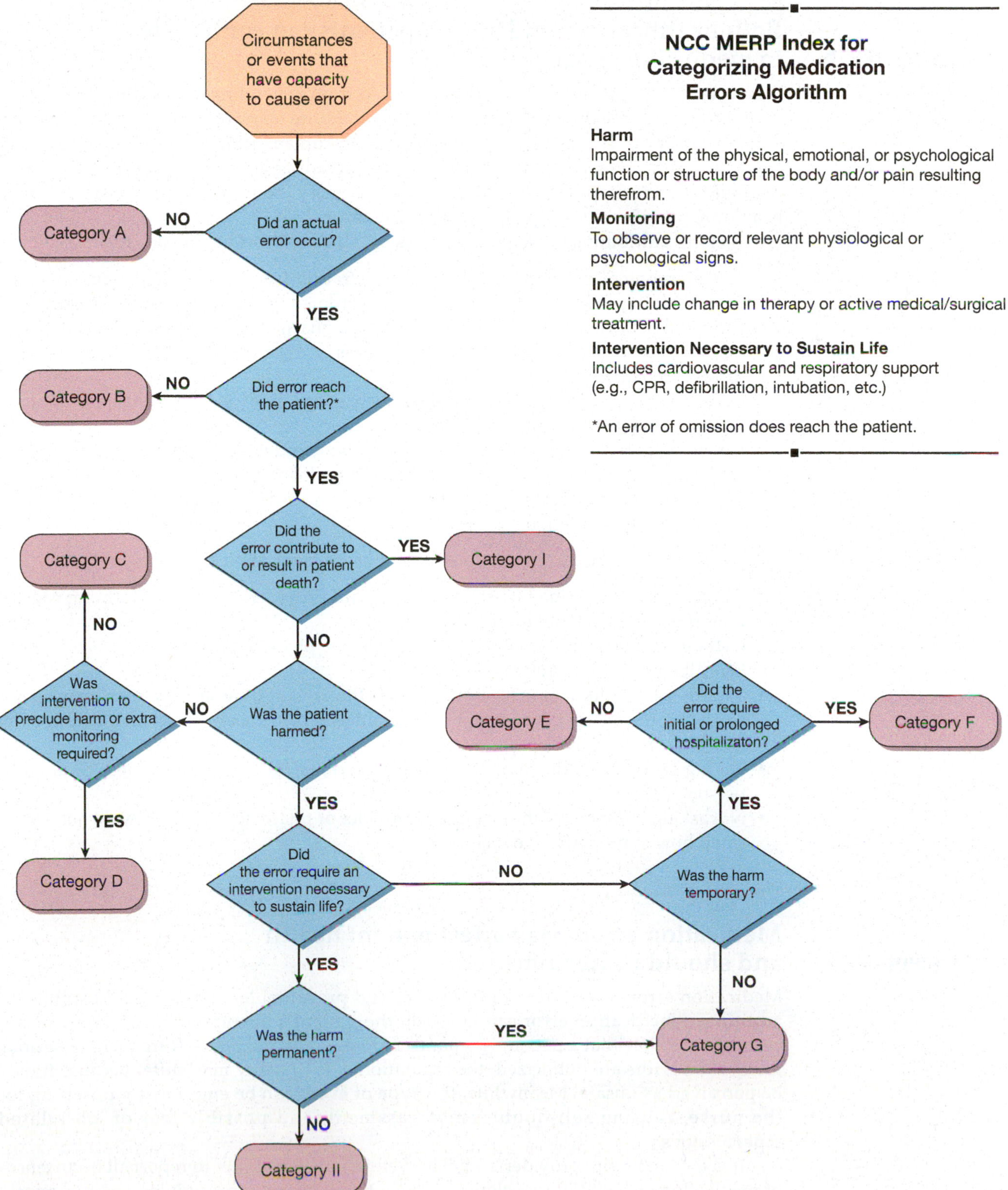

FIGURE 6.1 Index for categorizing medication errors algorithm.

Source: NCC MERP Index for Categorizing Medication Errors Algorithm from *National Coordinating Council for Medication Error Reporting and Prevention.*

error can cause. For example, Category A is a medication error in which no harm occurred to the patient, whereas category H is a medication error that resulted in permanent harm.

It is important to note that the NCC MERP definition of a medication error encompasses a large number of potential errors, some of which are not controlled by healthcare providers or patients. For example, medication errors also include mistakes in product labeling, manufacturing, and distribution.

Core Concept 6.2 ▶

Both healthcare providers and patients can contribute to medication errors.

When considering the number of steps involved from generating the medication order to administration of the drug to (or by) the patient, there are many opportunities for a medication error to occur. The majority of errors stem from human factors such as deficient knowledge and prescribing or administration errors, including errors of omission. One useful method for understanding medical errors is to classify them as being the result of either healthcare provider error or patient or caregiver error.

Factors contributing to medication errors by *healthcare providers* include the following:

- Omitting one of the rights of drug administration (see Chapter 3). Common errors include giving an incorrect dose, omitting an ordered dose, and giving the wrong drug.
- Failing to perform an agency system check. The pharmacist and nurse must collaborate on checking the accuracy and appropriateness of drug orders prior to administering drugs to a patient.
- Failing to account for patient variables such as age, body size, diminished cognitive function, and impairment in renal or hepatic function.
- Giving medications based on verbal orders, phone orders, incomplete orders, or illegible orders, which may be misinterpreted or go undocumented.
- Administering medications when the healthcare provider is unsure of the correct drug, dosage, or administration method.

Patients or their caregivers may also contribute to medication errors by:

- Taking drugs prescribed by several healthcare providers without informing each of their providers about all prescribed medications.
- Getting their prescriptions filled at more than one pharmacy.
- Not filling their prescriptions.
- Taking medications in incorrect doses, at the wrong time of day, or otherwise not following the instructions given by the healthcare provider, or those on the label of an over-the-counter (OTC) drug.
- Taking leftover medications that were prescribed for a previous illness or another person.
- Not asking questions of the healthcare provider or pharmacist when they do not understand how to properly take their medication.

Core Concept 6.3 ▶

Medication errors may affect patient health and should be documented.

Medication errors are a cause of morbidity and preventable death within hospitals. In addition, a medication error can lengthen the patient's hospital stay, which increases costs and the time that a patient is separated from family members. If frequent or serious medication errors are publicized, the reputation of the facility may suffer because it may be perceived as unsafe. Meanwhile, this type of event can be emotionally upsetting for the nurse, causing self-doubt, embarrassment, and possible fear of job-related repercussions.

It is the healthcare provider's legal and ethical responsibility to report all occurrences of medication errors. Within a clinical setting, the primary or prescribing healthcare provider should be notified first. The nurse manager or charge nurse should also be notified. After these notifications and any new patient orders have been fulfilled, a critical incident or occurrence report should be completed. In addition, when a medication error has occurred, the patient should be monitored for any adverse effects, some of which may require the initiation of lifesaving interventions for the patient, follow-up supervision, and medical treatments. All errors, whether or not they harm the patient, should be reported and investigated with the goal of identifying ways to improve the medication administration process to prevent future errors (Figure 6.2).

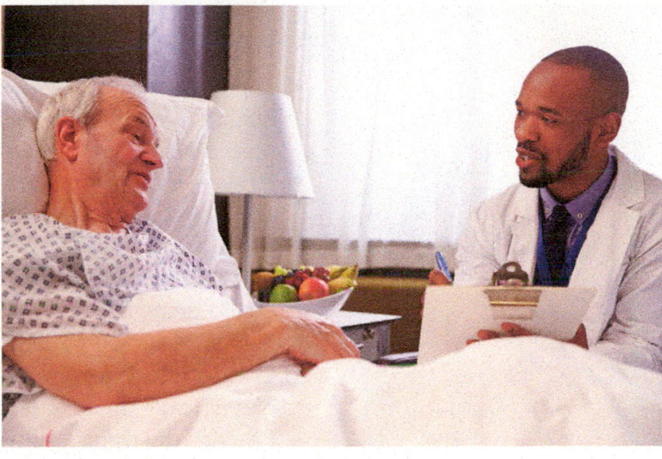

FIGURE 6.2 Obtaining a thorough history of drug allergies and current medications taken by the patient is a means of preventing some types of medication errors.
Source: Monkey Business/Fotolia

It is necessary for healthcare facilities to have risk-management departments that evaluate risks and make recommendations to reduce medication errors. Risk-management plans are specific to the type of healthcare agency, such as an acute care hospital, long-term care facility, or outpatient walk-in clinic. Using a process known as root-cause analysis (RCA), risk-management committees, which include nursing personnel, investigate incidents, track data, and identify problems by asking three questions: What happened? Why did it happen? What can be done to prevent it from happening again? Using this process, healthcare agencies can help ensure safe and effective patient care.

The Joint Commission, which accredits healthcare agencies, recognizes a specific type of event known as a **sentinel event**. A sentinel event is one that results in an unexpected, serious, or fatal injury following the administration (or lack of administration) of a medication. The serious injury may be physical or psychological, and it may occur at the time of the drug administration or place the patient at risk to a future injury. Because of the grave nature of a sentinel event, it is *always* investigated and interventions put in place to ensure that it does not recur.

At the federal level, two agencies have coordinated medication error reporting systems. The U.S. Food and Drug Administration (FDA) Safety Information and Adverse Event Reporting Program, known as *MedWatch*, allows healthcare providers and members of the public to report medication errors. The service provides a voluntary reporting form, which can be used by anyone observing or experiencing an adverse drug event. The service also provides a mandatory reporting form for healthcare agencies and pharmaceutical manufacturers, who are required by law to report certain adverse drug events caused by medication errors. MedWatch also provides up-to-date clinical information about safety issues involving prescription and OTC drugs, biologics, and special nutritional products. This includes public access to patient medication guides and access to current drug prescribing information.

The other reporting system is the Vaccine Adverse Event Reporting System (VAERS). The VAERS is a postmarketing surveillance program conducted by the Centers for Disease Control and Prevention (CDC) and the FDA. Voluntary reports may be submitted to the VAERS by patients and parents as well as healthcare providers. Vaccine manufacturers are required to report any adverse effects of which they are aware. This system serves as an important, central repository of information for identifying potential adverse effects to vaccines.

Healthcare providers use multiple strategies for reducing medication errors.

◀ **Core Concept 6.4**

The most common medication errors are administering an improper dose, giving the wrong drug, and using the wrong route of administration. There is an increased risk for errors in older adults because they often take numerous medications, have multiple healthcare providers, and are experiencing normal age-related changes in physiology. Children are another vulnerable population because they receive medication dosages based on weight (which increases the possibility of dosage miscalculations), and the nurse must accommodate for the reduced dosages.

What can the healthcare provider do in the clinical setting to avoid medication errors and promote safe drug administration? Here are some strategies for prevention:

- Positively verify the identity of each patient, such as by asking for the name and date of birth and confirming with the information on the ID wristband, before administering a medication.
- Always ask the patient about allergies to food or medications, current health concerns, and use of OTC medications and herbal supplements.
- Be aware of impairments in cognitive function and in kidney, liver, and other body systems that could affect pharmacotherapy.
- Avoid using abbreviations that can be misunderstood.
- Never administer a medication without being familiar with its uses and side effects.
- Contact the prescribing healthcare provider to clarify illegible medication orders.
- Never leave medication at the patient's bedside or give to anyone other than the patient.
- Practice the rights of medication administration: right patient, right time and frequency of administration, right dose, right route of administration, and right drug.
- Properly document the medication administration process according to institutional policy.
- Check drug calculations and measure medication doses carefully.
- Be alert for long-acting dosage forms with indicators such as *LA*, *XL*, and *XR*. These types of medications should not be crushed, chewed, or broken in half, because they would be absorbed too quickly, resulting in toxicity .
- Be alert for drugs whose names look or sound alike.

In addition, to minimize the potential for medication errors, the nurse should teach the patients or caregivers the following:

- The names of all medications they are taking, the uses, the doses, and when and how they should be taken
- The medications' adverse effects, especially those that need to be reported immediately
- To read the label prior to taking a medication and to use the medication device that comes with liquid medications rather than household measuring spoons
- To carry a list of all medications, including OTC drugs, as well as herbal and dietary supplements that are being taken. If possible, use one pharmacy for all prescriptions.
- To ask questions. Healthcare providers want to be partners in maintaining safe medication usage.

Chapter Review

Core Concepts Summary

6.1 Medication errors are preventable events that may significantly impact treatment outcomes

A medication error is any preventable event that may cause or lead to inappropriate medication use or patient harm while the medication is in the control of the healthcare provider or patient.

6.2 Both healthcare providers and patients can contribute to medication errors.

Numerous factors contribute to medication errors, including mistakes in the five rights of drug administration, failing to consider patient variables, and giving medications based on verbal, incomplete, or illegible orders. Patients also contribute to errors by using more than one pharmacy, not informing healthcare providers of all medications they are taking, or not following instructions.

6.3 Medication errors may affect patient health and should be documented.

The nurse is legally and ethically responsible for reporting medication errors—whether or not they cause harm to a patient—in the patient's medical record and on an incident report. The FDA provides a means for reporting medication errors.

6.4 Healthcare providers use multiple strategies for reducing medication errors.

Healthcare providers use many means to reduce or prevent medication errors, including verifying patient names, assessing for drug allergies and patient conditions that could affect drug action, and calculating doses accurately.

REVIEW Questions

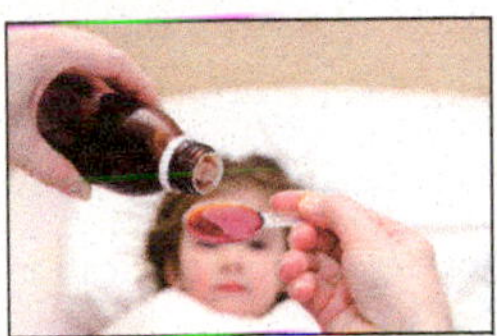

Answer the following questions to assess your knowledge of the chapter material, and go back and review any material that is not clear to you.

1. A healthcare provider has written an order for digoxin, but the nurse cannot read whether the order is for 0.25 mg, 0.125 mg, or 125 mg because there is no "zero" and the decimal point may be a "one." What action would be the best to prevent a medication error?
   1. Check the dosage with another nurse.
   2. Consult a drug handbook, and administer the normal dose.
   3. Contact the hospital pharmacist about the order.
   4. Contact the healthcare provider to clarify the illegible order.
2. The nurse administers a medication to the wrong patient. What are the appropriate nursing actions required? (Select all that apply.)
   1. Monitor the patient for adverse reactions.
   2. Document the error if the patient has an adverse reaction.
   3. Report the error to the healthcare provider.
   4. Notify the hospital legal department of the error.
   5. Document the error in a critical incident or occurrence report.
3. The nurse is teaching a postoperative patient about the medications ordered for use at home. Because this patient also has a primary care provider in addition to the surgeon, what strategy should the nurse include in this teaching session that might prevent a medication error in the home setting?
   1. Encourage the patient to consult the internet about possible side effects.
   2. Delay taking any new medications prescribed by the surgeon until the next visit with the primary provider.
   3. Have all prescriptions filled at one pharmacy.
   4. Insist on using only trade-name drugs because they are easier to remember than generic names.
4. As the nurse enters a room to administer medications, the patient states, "I'm in the bathroom. Just leave my pills on the table and I'll take them when I come out." What is the nurse's best response?
   1. Leave them on the table as requested, and check back with the patient later to verify they were taken.
   2. Leave the medications with the patient's visitors so they can verify that they were taken.
   3. Inform the patient that the medications must be taken now; otherwise they must be documented as "refused."
   4. Inform the patient that the nurse will return in a few minutes when the patient is available to take the medications.
5. The nurse is administering medications and the patient states, "I've never seen that blue pill before." What would be the nurse's most appropriate action?
   1. Verify the order and double-check the drug label.
   2. Administer the medication in the existing form.
   3. Instruct the patient that different brands are frequently used and may account for the change of color.
   4. Recommend that the patient discuss the medication with the provider, and give the medication.
6. The healthcare agency is implementing the use of root-cause analysis (RCA) to reduce the occurrence of medication errors. What areas does RCA analyze in order to prevent errors from recurring?
   1. Why the medication was ordered, whether it was the correct medication, and whether the patient experienced therapeutic results
   2. What happened, why it happened, and what can be done to prevent it from happening again
   3. What the cost of the medication was, whether it was the most appropriate medication to order, or whether there is a better alternative
   4. Whether the medication was documented in the provider's orders, the patient's medication administration record, and the pharmacy
7. Assessment or data collection is an important step of the nursing process in preventing medication errors. During this phase, the nurse would:
   1. Advise the patient to question the nurse about medications.
   2. Have the patient state the outcome of the medication.
   3. Obtain allergy and medication history information.
   4. Plan the correct times for the patient to take medications.
8. When administering medications, the nurse makes sure that: (Select all that apply.)
   1. The correct drug is given.
   2. The correct dose was calculated.
   3. The drug is given using the correct route of administration.
   4. The patient's name is verified prior to drug administration.
   5. The patient's home address is correct in the facility records.

9. A nurse has given the wrong dose of a medication. She follows agency policy by completing an incident report. The primary purpose of following this procedure for reporting errors is to:
   1. Determine who is to blame.
   2. Gather information for risk management procedures.
   3. Prevent future medication errors.
   4. Determine the competence of the nurse.

10. While administering the 12 p.m. (noon) medications, the nurse discovers that the 6 a.m. dose was not given. What should be the nurse's first action?
    1. Document this finding on the patient's chart.
    2. Complete an incident report
    3. Give both the 6 a.m. and the 12 p.m. doses.
    4. Notify the healthcare provider.

Answers and complete rationales for the Review Questions appear in Appendix A.

REFERENCE

National Coordinating Council for Medication Error Reporting and Prevention. (2016). *About medication errors: What is a medication error?* Retrieved from http://www.nccmerp.org/about-medication-errors

BIBLIOGRAPHY

Fanus, K., Huddleston, R., Wisotzkey, S., & Hempling, R. (2014). Embracing a culture of safety by decreasing medication errors. *Nursing Management, 45*(3), 16–19. doi:10.1097/01.NUMA.0000443940.60879.fa

Garrouste-Orgeas, M., Philippart, F., Bruel, C., Max, A., Lau, N., & Misset, B. (2012). Overview of medical errors and adverse events. *Annals of Intensive Care, 2*(1), 2. doi:10.1186/2110-5820-2

The Joint Commission. (2016). Sentinel events (SE). *Comprehensive Accreditation Manual for Hospitals.* Retrieved from http://www.jointcommission.org/assets/1/6/CAMH_24_SE_all_CURRENT.pdf

Keers, R. N., Williams, S. D., Cooke, J., Walsh, T., & Ashcroft, D. M. (2014). Impact of interventions designed to reduce medication administration errors in hospitals: A systematic review. *Drug Safety, 37*, 317–332. doi:10.1007/s40264-014-0152-0

Kong, M., & Mondul, A. (2014). Medication error. In Abha Agrawal (Ed.), *Patient safety* (pp. 103–114). New York, NY: Springer. doi:10.1007/978-1-4614-7419-7_7

National Coordinating Council for Medication Error Reporting and Prevention. (2016). *About NCC MERP.* Retrieved from http://www.nccmerp.org/vision-and-mission

Raban, M. Z., & Westbrook, J. I. (2014). Are interventions to reduce interruptions and errors during medication administration effective? A systematic review. *BMJ Quality & Safety, 23*, 414–421. doi:10.1136/bmjqs-2013-002118

U.S. Food and Drug Administration. (2016). *Medwatch: The FDA safety information and adverse event reporting program.* Retrieved from http://www.fda.gov/Safety/MedWatch/default.htm

Westbrook, J. I., Woods, A., Rob, M. I., Dunsmuir, W. T. M., & Day, R. O. (2010). Association of interruptions with an increased risk and severity of medication administration errors. *Archives of Internal Medicine, 170*, 683–690. doi:10.1001/archinternmed.2010.65

Chapter 7

The Role of Complementary and Alternative Therapies in Pharmacology

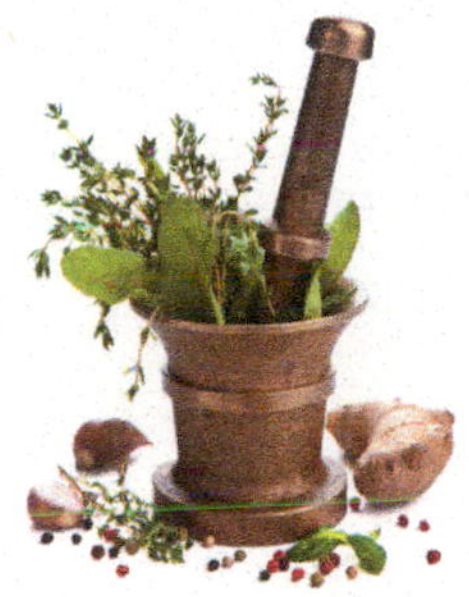

Core Concepts

7.1 Complementary and alternative medicine focuses on treating the whole person using natural products and mind–body therapies.

7.2 Herbal products have been used as medicines for thousands of years.

7.3 Many herbal products are standardized with respect to a specific active ingredient.

7.4 Herbs can have significant pharmacologic actions and may interact with conventional drugs.

7.5 Specialty supplements are nonherbal products that are widely used to promote wellness.

7.6 Dietary supplements are not regulated in the same manner as prescription medications.

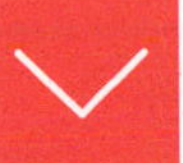

Learning Outcomes

After reading this chapter, the student should be able to:

1. Compare and contrast complementary and alternative medicine therapies to conventional medical therapies.
2. Discuss the reasons why herbal products and dietary supplements have steadily increased in popularity.
3. Explain why it is important to standardize herbal products based on specific active ingredients.
4. Describe drug interactions and adverse effects that may be caused by herbal and dietary supplements.
5. Explain how a specialty supplement differs from an herbal product.
6. Describe strengths and weakness of legislation governing the use of dietary supplements.

Key Terms

complementary and alternative medicine (CAM)
dietary supplements
Dietary Supplement and Nonprescription Drug Consumer Protection Act
Dietary Supplement Health and Education Act (DSHEA)
herb
integrative healthcare
specialty supplements

Complementary and alternative therapies represent a multibillion-dollar industry: Sales of dietary supplements exceed $32 billion annually (Garcia-Cazarin, Wambogo, Regan, & Davis, 2014). Consumers have turned to these treatments for a wide variety of reasons. Some people have the impression that natural substances have more healing power than synthetic medications. The ready availability of over-the-counter (OTC) herbal and specialty supplements at a reasonable cost, combined with effective marketing strategies, has convinced many people to try them. This chapter examines the role of herbal and specialty supplements in the prevention and treatment of disease.

Core Concept 7.1 ▶

Complementary and alternative medicine focuses on treating the whole person using natural products and mind–body therapies.

Complementary and alternative medicine (CAM) comprises a diverse set of therapies and healing systems that are considered to be outside of mainstream healthcare. Most CAM systems share the following characteristics:

- Focus on treating each person as an individual
- Consider the health of the whole person
- Emphasize the integration of mind and body
- Promote disease prevention, self-care, and self-healing
- Recognize the role of spirituality in health and healing.

Because of the widespread use of CAM, scientific attention has focused on determining the effectiveness, or lack of effectiveness, of these therapies. Although some research into these alternative systems has been conducted, few CAM therapies have been subjected to rigorous clinical and scientific study. It is likely that some of these therapies will become mainstream treatments, whereas others will be found ineffective. The line between what is defined as an alternative therapy and what is considered mainstream is constantly changing. Increasing numbers of healthcare providers now recommend CAM therapies to their patients. Table 7.1 describes some of these therapies.

Fast Facts CAM Therapies in America

One of the largest studies of Americans' use of complementary therapies conducted by the National Center for Complementary and Integrative Health (NCCIH, 2012) surveyed over 45,000 people. Findings of this study included the following:

- Thirty-three percent of adults and about 12% of children are currently using CAM.
- The most frequent condition treated with CAM was pain.
- The most commonly used supplement reported by both adults and children was fish oil.
- The percentage of adults practicing yoga has increased from 5% in 2002 to almost 10% in 2012.

Healthcare providers have long known the value of CAM therapies in preventing and treating disease. For example, prayer, meditation, massage, and yoga have been used for centuries to treat body, mind, and spirit. From a pharmacology perspective, the value of CAM therapies is their ability to reduce the need for medications. If a patient can find anxiety relief through massage or biofeedback therapy, for example, the use of antianxiety drugs may be reduced or eliminated. Reduction of drug dose leads to fewer adverse effects and better compliance with drug therapy. Applying both conventional and complementary approaches to healing the patient is called **integrative healthcare**.

This chapter focuses on products used as dietary supplements, **Dietary supplements** are products available OTC that are intended to add to or supplement the nutritional value

Table 7.1 Complementary and Alternative Therapies

Healing Method	Examples
Alternate healthcare systems	Naturopathy, homeopathy, chiropractic, Native American medicine (e.g., sweat lodges, medicine wheel), Chinese traditional medicine (e.g., acupuncture, Chinese herbs)
Biologic therapies	Herbal therapies, nutritional supplements, special diets
Energy therapies	Therapeutic touch, Reiki, craniosacral, qigong, biofield energy healing
Manual healing	Massage therapy, physical therapy, pressure-point therapies
Mind–body interventions	Yoga, meditation, hypnotherapy, guided imagery, biofeedback, movement-oriented therapies (e.g., music, dance)
Spiritual	Faith and prayer, shamanism

of the diet. The two subcategories of dietary supplements presented in this chapter include herbal products and specialty supplements. Vitamins and minerals, also considered dietary supplements, are presented in Chapter 32.

CONCEPT REVIEW 7.1

- How does the healing philosophy of complementary and alternative medicine differ from that of conventional mainstream medicine?

HERBAL PRODUCTS

The number of people seeking herbal alternatives to conventional medical therapies has steadily increased over the past three decades. Many herbs are used by patients to supplement traditional pharmacotherapy.

Herbal products have been used as medicines for thousands of years.

◀ **Core Concept 7.2**

Technically, an herb is a plant that lacks woody stems or bark. Over time, the term **herb** has come to refer to any plant product with a useful application, either as a food enhancer (such as a flavoring) or as a medicine. Herbs are sometimes called botanicals.

The use of herbs in the treatment of disease has been recorded for thousands of years. One of the earliest recorded uses was a prescription for garlic in 3000 B.C. Eastern and Western medicine have recorded thousands of herbs and herb combinations claimed to have therapeutic value. Some of the more popular herbs and their primary uses are shown in Table 7.2.

The public's interest in herbal medicine began to decline when the pharmaceutical industry was born in the late 1800s. Drugs could be standardized and produced more cheaply than natural herbal products. In the early 1900s, regulatory agencies required that medicines be safe and effective. The focus of healthcare shifted to treating specific diseases, rather than promoting wellness and holistic care. Information about most herbal and alternative therapies was no longer taught in medical schools; these healing techniques were criticized as being unscientific relics of the past.

Beginning in the 1970s and continuing to the present, herbal therapies have experienced a remarkable comeback. The majority of adult Americans are either currently taking herbal products on a regular basis or have taken them in the past. This increase in popularity is due to a number of factors, including increased availability of herbal products, aggressive marketing by the herbal industry, increased attention to natural alternatives, and renewed interest in preventive medicine. The gradual aging of the population has led to more patients seeking therapeutic alternatives for chronic conditions such as pain, arthritis, prostate

▶ Lifespan and Diversity

A wide range of dietary supplements, such as herbs and other specialty products, are being used to treat children. Unfortunately, the use of these therapies in children has not been well studied. Just as with conventional medicine, children may react differently than adults to herbal and other CAM therapies. The healthcare provider should assess for the use of supplements in all pediatric patients. It is important to ensure that caregivers know the importance of an accurate diagnosis from a licensed healthcare provider and that supplements or other CAM products should not replace or delay conventional medical care. In addition, caregivers should be taught to store all herbs and dietary supplements away from children, use only as directed, and report any side effects to the child's healthcare provider.

Table 7.2 Popular Herbal Products

Common Name	Medicinal Part	Primary Use(s)
Aloe	Leaves	Treat skin ailments (topical) and constipation (oral)
Bilberry	Berries, leaf	Terminate diarrhea, improve and protect vision
Black cohosh	Roots	Relieve symptoms of premenstrual syndrome and menopause
Cranberry	Berries, juice	Prevent urinary tract infection
Echinacea	Entire plant	Enhance immune system, reduce inflammation
Evening primrose	Oil extracted from seeds	Relieve pain and inflammation
Flaxseed	Ground seeds and oil	Reduce blood cholesterol, laxative
Garlic	Bulbs	Reduce blood cholesterol and blood pressure, as an anticoagulant
Ginger	Root	Relieve gastrointestinal (GI) upset and nausea associated with pregnancy or motion sickness, as an anti-inflammatory
Ginkgo biloba	Leaves and seeds	Improve memory, reduce dizziness
Ginseng	Root	Relieve stress, enhance immune system, decrease fatigue
Green Tea	Leaves	As an antioxidant to lower LDL cholesterol; to prevent cancer, relieve GI upset, nausea, vomiting
Milk thistle	Seeds	As an antitoxin to protect against liver disease
Saw palmetto	Ripe fruit/berries	Relieve urinary symptoms related to benign prostatic hyperplasia
Soy	Beans	Source of protein, vitamins, and minerals; relieve menopausal symptoms; prevent cardiovascular disease
St. John's wort	Flowers, leaves, stems	Reduce depression and anxiety, as an anti-inflammatory
Valerian	Roots	Relieve stress, promote sleep

difficulties, and the need for hormone replacement. In addition, the high cost of prescription medicines has driven many people to seek less expensive alternatives.

Core Concept 7.3 ▶

Many herbal products are standardized with respect to a specific active ingredient.

The active substances in an herb may be present in only one specific part of the plant or in all parts. For example, the active chemicals in saw palmetto are in the berries. For ginger and black cohosh, the roots are used for their healing properties.

Most modern drugs contain only one active ingredient. This chemical is standardized and accurately measured so that the amount of drug received by the patient is precisely known. It is a common misconception that herbal products also contain one active ingredient, which can be extracted and delivered to patients in exact amounts, like drugs. Herbs, however, may contain dozens of active chemicals, many of which have not yet been isolated, studied, or even identified. It is possible that some of these substances work together synergistically and may not have the same activity if isolated. Furthermore, the strength of an herbal preparation often varies from batch to batch depending on where the herb was grown and how it was collected, prepared, and stored.

To achieve consistency, scientists have attempted to standardize the strength or dose of herbal products. Some of these standardizations are shown in Table 7.3. Until science can better characterize these substances, however, it is best to view the active ingredient of an herb as being the entire herb. An example of standardization—the ingredients of ginkgo biloba—is shown in Figure 7.1.

The two basic formulations of herbal products are solid and liquid. Solid products include pills, tablets, and capsules made from dried herbs. Other solid products are salves and ointments that are administered topically. Liquid formulations are made by extracting the active chemicals from the plant and include teas, infusions, tinctures, and extracts. Some formulations of ginkgo biloba, one of the most popular herbals, are illustrated in Figure 7.2.

Table 7.3 Standardization of Selected Herb Extracts

Herb	Standardization	Percent
Black cohosh	Triterpene glycosides	2.5
Echinacea	Echinacosides	4
Ginger	Pungent compounds (gingerols)	Greater than 10
Ginkgo leaf	Flavone glycosides	24–25
	Terpene lactones	6
Ginseng root	Ginseosides	5–15
Milk thistle root	Silymarin	80
St. John's wort	Hypericins	0.3–0.5
	Hyperforin	3–5
Saw palmetto	Fatty acids and sterols	80–90

GINKGO BILOBA
Dietary Supplement
Natures
Herbal
Harvest
200 Capsules
175 mg
† May support memory and concentration
† May help to maintain circulation
Supplement Facts
Serving Size: 1 capsule
Amount Per Serving
Ginkgo biloba leaf 175 mg*
Standardized to:
24% Flavonglycosides
6% Terpene lactones
*Daily value not established.
Recommended Dose: 1 capsule per day with a meal as a food supplement.
†This statement has not been evaluated by the Food and Drug Administration. This product is not intended to diagnose, treat, cure or prevent any disease.

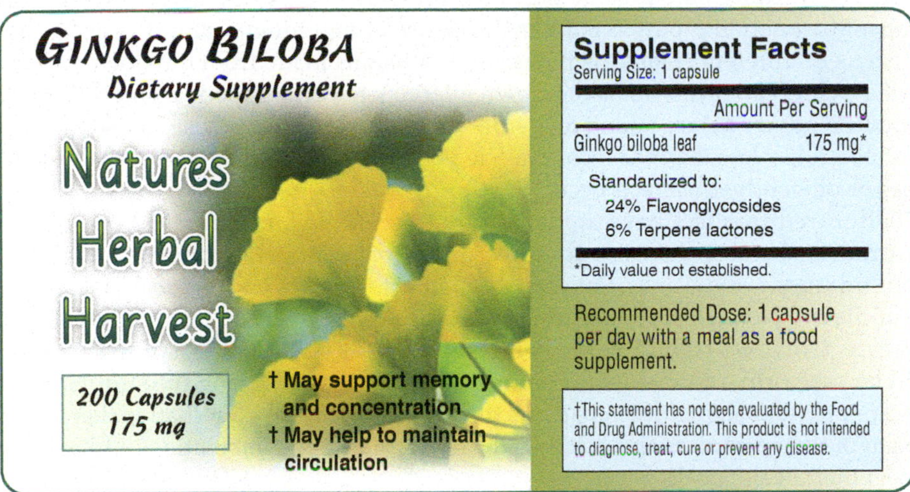

FIGURE 7.1 This ginkgo biloba label indicates the product is standardized to percent flavonglycosides and percent terpenes, active substances that are found in the ginkgo leaf. Also note the health claims on the label, which have not been evaluated by the FDA.

HERB TEA
Ginkgo Blend
GINKGO
BILOBA

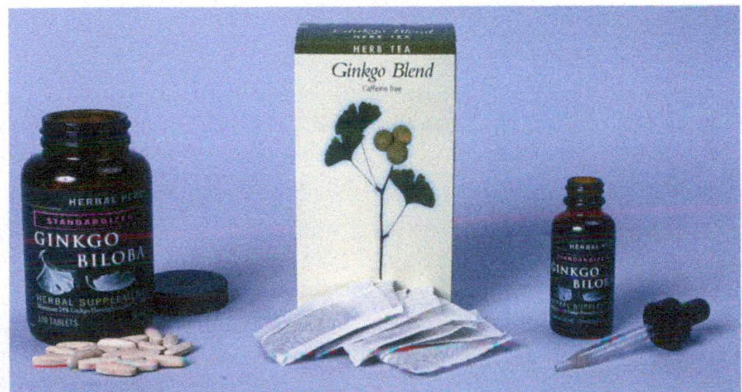

FIGURE 7.2 Three different ginkgo formulations: tablets, tea bags, and liquid extract.

Herbs can have significant pharmacologic actions and may interact with conventional drugs.

◀ **Core Concept 7.4**

A key concept to remember when dealing with natural therapies is that "natural" does not always mean better or safe. There is no question that some herbs contain active chemicals as powerful as, and perhaps more effective than, currently approved medications. Thousands of years of experience, combined with current scientific research, have shown that some herbal remedies have therapeutic actions. Because a substance comes from a natural product, however, does not make it either safe or effective. For example, poison ivy is natural, but it certainly is not safe or therapeutic. Herbal products may not offer an improvement over conventional therapy in treating certain disorders and, indeed, may be of no value whatsoever. Most importantly, a patient who substitutes an unproven alternative therapy for an established, effective medical treatment may delay healing, suffer harmful effects, and endanger his or her health.

Most herbal products are safe when taken in low to moderate doses as directed on the label. Some herbal products, however, contain ingredients that may interact with prescription drugs. For example, patients taking medications with potentially serious adverse effects, such as insulin, warfarin (Coumadin), or digoxin (Lanoxin), should be warned never to take any dietary supplement without first discussing their needs with their healthcare provider. Pregnant or lactating women should consult with their healthcare provider before taking herbal products. The healthcare professional should also remember that the potential for any drug interaction increases in older adults, especially those with hepatic or renal impairment. Although the true extent of herb–drug interactions is largely unknown, some of the documented interactions are shown in Table 7.4.

Another warning that must be heeded with natural products is to beware of allergic reactions. Most herbal products contain a mixture of ingredients, and it is not unusual to find dozens of different chemicals in teas and infusions made from the flowers, leaves, or roots of a plant. Patients who have known allergies to certain foods or medicines should seek medical advice before taking an herbal product. It is always wise to take the smallest amount possible—less than the recommended dose—when starting herbal therapy to see if allergies or other adverse effects occur.

Healthcare providers have an obligation to seek the latest medical information on herbal products because there is a good possibility that their patients are using them to supplement traditional medicines. Patients should be advised to be skeptical of claims on the labels of dietary supplements and to seek their health information from reputable sources. Healthcare providers should never condemn patients' use of alternative therapies, but instead be supportive and seek to understand their goals for taking the supplements. The healthcare provider should teach patients the appropriate role of alternative therapies in the treatment of their disorders and discuss which treatments or combination of treatments will best meet their health goals.

Table 7.4 Selected Herb–Drug Interactions

Common Name	Interacts With	Comments
Echinacea	Amiodarone, anabolic steroids, ketoconazole, methotrexate	Possible increased hepatotoxicity
Garlic	Aspirin and other nonsteroidal anti-inflammatory drugs (NSAIDs), warfarin (Coumadin)	Increased bleeding risk
	Insulin, oral hypoglycemic agents	Additive hypoglycemic effects
Ginger	Aspirin and other NSAIDs, heparin, warfarin	Increased bleeding risk
Ginkgo biloba	Anticonvulsants	Possible decreased anticonvulsant effectiveness
	Aspirin and NSAIDs	Increased bleeding potential
	Heparin and warfarin (Coumadin)	Increased bleeding potential
	Tricyclic antidepressants	Possible decreased seizure threshold
Ginseng	Central nervous system (CNS) depressants	Increased sedation
	Digoxin (Lanoxin)	Increased toxicity
	Diuretics	Possible weakened diuretic effects
	Insulin and oral hypoglycemic agents	Increased hypoglycemic effects
	Warfarin	Decreased anticoagulant effects
St. John's wort	CNS depressants and opiates	Increased sedation
	Cyclosporine (Sandimmune)	Possible decreased cyclosporine levels
	Oral contraceptives	Decreased drug effectiveness
	Selective serotonin reuptake inhibitors , tricyclic antidepressants	Possible serotonin syndrome (headache, dizziness, sweating, agitation)
	Warfarin (Coumadin)	Decreased anticoagulant effects
Valerian	Barbiturates, benzodiazepines, and other CNS depressants	Increased sedation

SPECIALTY SUPPLEMENTS

Specialty supplements are a type of dietary supplement that includes products such as *probiotics, fish oils, amino acids, and enzymes*. Like herbal therapies, they are available OTC and are widely used by patients to enhance wellness.

Specialty supplements are nonherbal products that are widely used to promote wellness.

◀ Core Concept 7.5

Specialty supplements are dietary products *intended to enhance (or complement) a specific function in the body, such as supporting joint health or immune function.* The actions of specialty supplements are often more specific than those of herbs, and they are generally targeted for one or a small number of specific conditions. Popular specialty supplements are listed in Table 7.5.

In general, specialty supplements have a legitimate rationale for their use. For example, chondroitin and glucosamine are natural substances in the body necessary for cartilage growth and maintenance. Amino acids are natural building blocks of muscle protein. Fish oils contain omega fatty acids that have been shown to reduce the risk of heart disease in certain patients.

Unfortunately, the link between most specialty supplements and their intended benefits is unclear. In some cases, the body already has sufficient quantities of the substance; therefore, taking additional amounts may be of no benefit. In other cases, the supplement is marketed for conditions for which it has no proven effect (Figure 7.3). The good news is that these substances, when taken in amounts stated on the label, are generally not harmful. The bad news, however, is that they can give patients false hopes of an easy cure for a chronic condition such as heart disease or the pain of arthritis. As with herbal products, the healthcare provider should advise patients to be cautious about the health claims regarding the use of specialty supplements.

CONCEPT REVIEW 7.2

- Explain the differences between an herbal product and a specialty supplement.

Dietary supplements are not regulated in the same manner as prescription medications.

◀ Core Concept 7.6

Since the passage of the Food, Drug, and Cosmetic Act of 1935, Americans have come to expect that all prescription and OTC drugs have passed rigid standards of safety prior to being marketed. Furthermore, it is assumed that the effectiveness of these drugs has been

Table 7.5 Popular Specialty Supplements

Name	Common Uses
Amino acids	Build protein, muscle strength, and endurance
Carnitine	Enhance energy and sports performance, heart health, memory, immune function, and male fertility
Coenzyme Q10	Prevent heart disease, as an antioxidant
Dehydroepiandrosterone (DHEA)	Boost immune functions and memory
Fish oil	Reduce blood cholesterol, enhance brain function, increase visual acuity (due to presence of omega-3 fatty acids)
Glucosamine and chondroitin	Reduce symptoms of arthritis and other joint problems
Lactobacillus acidophilus	Maintain intestinal health
Melatonin	Restore normal sleep patterns
Methyl sulfonyl methane (MSM)	Reduce allergic reactions to pollen and foods, relieve pain and inflammation of arthritis and similar conditions
Red yeast rice extract	Reduce blood cholesterol
S-adenosylmethione (SAM-e)	Reduce pain of osteoarthritis and fibromyalgia; also as an antidepressant

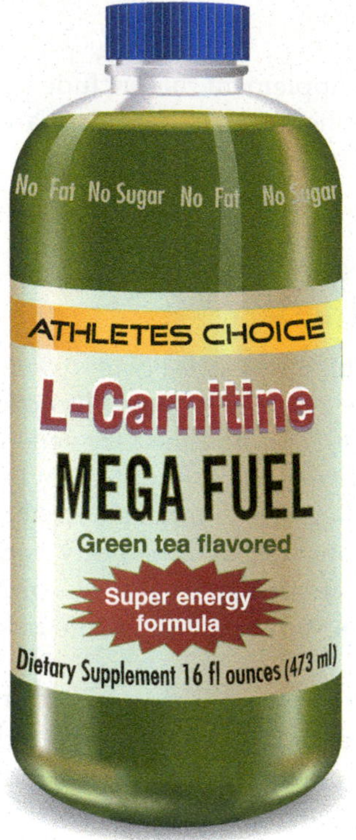

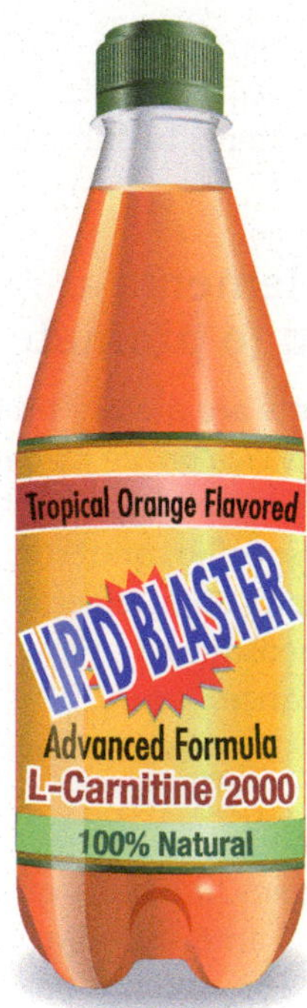

FIGURE 7.3 L-carnitine is a popular dietary supplement. Notice the claims of improving athletic performance and weight loss, neither of which has been supported by the scientific literature.

tested, and that they truly provide the therapeutic benefits claimed by the manufacturer. Indeed, most people would be outraged if they found out that the drug they purchased for pain relief or to cure an infectious disease was totally ineffective. Unfortunately, herbal products and specialty supplements are regulated by a far less rigorous law, the **Dietary Supplement Health and Education Act (DSHEA)** of 1994.

The DSHEA exempts dietary supplements from the Food, Drug, and Cosmetic Act, the legislation that regulates prescription drugs. They are not classified as drugs or approved by the U.S. Food and Drug Administration (FDA).

One strength of the legislation is that it gives the FDA the power to remove from the market any dietary supplement that poses a "significant or unreasonable" risk to the public. The DSHEA also requires such products to be clearly labeled as dietary supplements. Figure 7.1 shows the label for ginkgo biloba clearly stating that the herbal product is not approved by the FDA to treat any medical condition.

Unfortunately, the DSHEA has significant weaknesses that have led to a lack of standardization in the dietary supplement industry and to less protection of the consumer. These flaws include:

- Effectiveness does not have to be demonstrated by the manufacturer prior to marketing.
- Safety does not have to be proven by the manufacturer. It is the government's job to prove that the dietary supplement is *unsafe* and to take the necessary steps to remove it from the market.
- Labels must clearly state that the dietary supplement is not intended to diagnose, treat, cure, or prevent any disease. However, claims about a product's effect on body structure and function are allowed, including the following:
  - Helps promote healthy immune systems
  - Reduces anxiety and stress
  - Helps to maintain cardiovascular function
  - May reduce pain and inflammation.
- The DSHEA does not regulate the *accuracy* of the label; the product may or may not contain the product listed in the amounts claimed.

Several steps have been taken to address the lack of purity and mislabeling of dietary supplements. In an attempt to protect consumers, Congress passed the **Dietary Supplement and Nonprescription Drug Consumer Protection Act** of 2007. Companies marketing herbal and specialty supplements are now required to include contact information (address and phone number) on the product labels for consumers to use in reporting adverse events. Companies must notify the FDA of a serious adverse event, which is defined as any adverse reaction resulting in death, a life-threatening experience, inpatient hospitalization, a persistent or significant disability, or a birth defect. Companies must notify the FDA of any serious adverse event reports within 15 days of receiving such reports.

The FDA now requires that manufacturers of dietary supplements evaluate the identity, purity, potency, and composition of their products. The labels must accurately reflect what is in the product, which must be free of contaminants such as pesticides, toxins, glass, or heavy metals. The FDA may take action on any misbranded or adulterated product after it reaches the market.

CONCEPT REVIEW 7.3

- How does the federal regulation of an herb by the DSHEA differ from the federal regulation of a prescription drug?

Chapter Review

Core Concepts Summary

7.1 Complementary and alternative medicine focuses on treating the whole person using natural products and mind–body therapies.

Complementary and alternative medicine (CAM) is a set of therapies and healing systems used by many patients for disease prevention and self-healing. Complementary therapies offer nonpharmacologic alternatives to promote health and healing. They focus on the holistic treatment of the individual patient, integrating natural products and mind–body therapies, often in conjunction with conventional therapies.

7.2 Herbal products have been used as medicines for thousands of years.

Thousands of herbal therapies are recorded in Eastern and Western history. The popularity of alternative herbal remedies has steadily increased in recent years.

7.3 Many herbal products are standardized with respect to a specific active ingredient.

Many herbal products are standardized extracts of specific chemicals, while others contain whole herbs. Unlike drugs, herbs contain numerous chemicals that may act in a coordinated manner to produce a therapeutic effect. The active ingredients may be in the flowers, leaves, stems, or roots of an herb.

7.4 Herbs can have significant pharmacologic actions and may interact with conventional drugs.

Just because a substance comes from a natural product does not make it safe or effective. Although herbal supplements may have therapeutic applications, they may not be the best product for treating the disease and may interact with prescription medicines.

7.5 Specialty supplements are nonherbal products that are widely used to promote wellness.

Specialty supplements include nonherbal therapies that are used to enhance a specific aspect of wellness. These products usually have a rational basis for therapy, although their benefits have not been conclusively proven.

7.6 Dietary supplements are not regulated in the same manner as prescription medications.

The DSHEA loosely regulates dietary supplements. Specialty supplements and herbal products can be marketed without any proof that they are safe or effective. The labels of dietary supplements must be accurate, and the manufacturers must document the purity, potency, and composition of their products.

REVIEW Questions

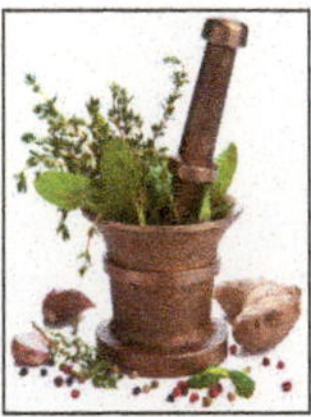

Answer the following questions to assess your knowledge of the chapter material, and go back and review any material that is not clear to you.

1. The patient is to be started on warfarin (Coumadin) therapy. It is important for the nurse to check for the use of which herbs? (Select all that apply.)
   1. Ginseng
   2. Ginger
   3. St. John's wort
   4. Valerian
   5. Echinacea
2. Patients often use herbal therapies for which of the following reasons?
   1. To prevent overuse of prescription medications
   2. To increase feelings of wellness and promote holistic treatment
   3. Because herbal therapies are much more regulated than prescription drugs
   4. Because herbal therapies are so much safer than man-made drugs
3. It is important that nurses ensure that their patients receive education regarding herbal products because:
   1. Herbal products are approved under strict FDA regulations.
   2. Labeling is not always reliable, and herbal products should be used with caution.
   3. There are so few side effects, and they can be purchased without a prescription.
   4. The manufacturer has repeatedly demonstrated effectiveness.
4. An example of a specialty supplement is:
   1. *Lactobacillus acidophilus.*
   2. Ginseng.
   3. Garlic.
   4. Ginkgo biloba.
5. Why is it important for the nurse to collect information from the patient about the use of complementary and alternative medicine (CAM)?
   1. Patients must be warned that most CAM therapies are dangerous.
   2. Additional treatment may not be needed.
   3. CAM therapies could interact with prescription and OTC medications.
   4. Most CAM therapies are totally ineffective.
6. The nurse understands that specialty supplements are used:
   1. For a diverse range of disease conditions.
   2. For treatment of a specific condition.
   3. When prescriptive medications are no longer effective.
   4. When the body no longer makes sufficient quantities of the substance.
7. The Dietary Supplement Health and Education Act (DHSEA) is responsible for:
   1. Strict herbal product testing.
   2. Ensuring that herbal products are labeled as "dietary supplements."
   3. Sending the herbal product to the FDA for evaluation.
   4. Ensuring safety of the product.
8. The patient is admitted with digoxin (Lanoxin) toxicity. The nurse checks for the use of which of the following herbal products?
   1. St. John's wort
   2. Valerian
   3. Fish oil
   4. Ginseng
9. The patient requests information on alternative treatments for arthritis. The nurse provides information on which of the following supplements?
   1. Garlic and soy
   2. Fish oil
   3. Chondroitin and glucosamine
   4. DHEA
10. Which of the following herbal products is commonly used to enhance the immune system?
    1. Soy
    2. Saw palmetto
    3. Cranberry
    4. Echinacea

Answers and complete rationales for the Review Questions appear in Appendix A.

REFERENCES

Garcia-Cazarin, M. L., Wambogo, E. A., Regan, K. S., & Davis, C. D. (2014). Dietary supplement research portfolio at the NIH, 2009–2011. *The Journal of Nutrition, 144*, 414–418. doi:10.3945/jn.113.189803

National Center for Complementary and Integrative Health. (2012). *Use of complementary health approaches in the U.S.* Retrieved from https://nccih.nih.gov/research/statistics/NHIS/2012/key-findings

SELECTED BIBLIOGRAPHY

Alissa, E. M. (2014). Medicinal herbs and therapeutic drugs interactions. *Therapeutic drug monitoring, 36,* 413–422. doi:10.1097/FTD.0000000000000035

American Botanical Council. (2014). *Herbal dietary supplement retail sales up 7.9% in 2013.* Retrieved from http://cms.herbalgram.org/press/2014/2013_Herb_Market_Report.html

Arkowitz, H., & Lilienfeld, S. O. (2013). Can herbs ease anxiety and depression? *Scientific American Mind, 24*(3), 72–73. doi:10.1038/scientificamericanmind0713-72

Chawla, R., Thakur, P., Chowdhry, A., Jaiswal, S., Sharma, A., Goel, R., . . . Arora, R. (2013). Evidence based herbal drug standardization approach in coping with challenges of holistic management of diabetes: A dreadful lifestyle disorder of 21st century. *Journal of Diabetes and Metabolic Disorders, 12,* 35. doi:10.1186/2251-6581-12-35

Dante, G., Bellei, G., Neri, I., & Facchinetti, F. (2014). Herbal therapies in pregnancy: What works? *Current Opinion in Obstetrics and Gynecology, 26,* 83–91. doi:10.1097/GCO.0000000000000052

Lindquist, R., Snyder, M., & Tracy, M. F. (Eds.). (2013). *Complementary & alternative therapies in nursing.* New York, NY: Springer.

Posadzki, P., Watson, L. K., & Ernst, E. (2013). Adverse effects of herbal medicines: An overview of systematic reviews. *Clinical Medicine, 13,* 7–12. doi:10.7861/clinmedicine.13-1-7

Prasad, K., Sharma, V., Lackore, K., Jenkins, S. M., Prasad, A., & Sood, A. (2013). Use of complementary therapies in cardiovascular disease. *The American Journal of Cardiology, 111,* 339–345. doi:10.1016/j.amjcard.2012.10.010

Ravindran, A. V., & da Silva, T. L. (2013). Complementary and alternative therapies as add-on to pharmacotherapy for mood and anxiety disorders: A systematic review. *Journal of Affective Disorders, 150,* 707–719. doi:10.1016/j.jad.2013.05.042

Smeriglio, A., Tomaino, A., & Trombetta, D. (2014). Herbal products in pregnancy: Experimental studies and clinical reports. *Phytotherapy Research, 28,* 1107–1116. doi:10.1002/ptr.5106

Chapter 8

Substance Abuse

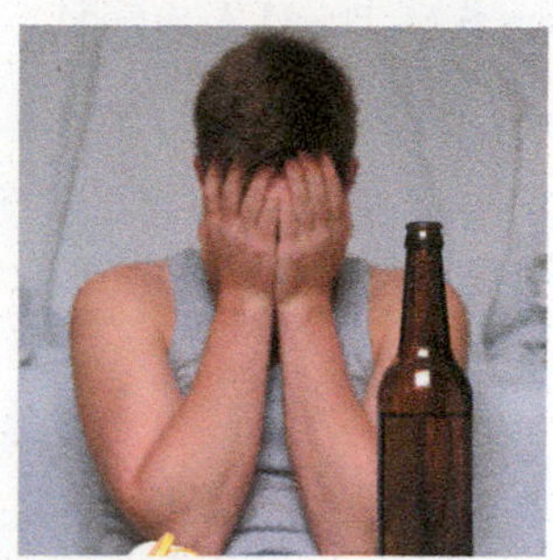

Core Concepts

8.1 **Abused and misused substances belong to many different chemical classes.**
8.2 **Addiction depends on multiple, complex, and interacting variables.**
8.3 **Substance dependence is classified as physical dependence or psychological dependence.**
8.4 **Withdrawal results when an abused substance is no longer available.**
8.5 **Tolerance occurs when higher and higher doses of a drug are needed to achieve the initial response.**
8.6 **Central nervous system (CNS) depressants decrease the activity of the central nervous system.**
8.7 **Marijuana produces little physical dependence or tolerance.**
8.8 **Hallucinogens cause an altered state of thought and perception similar to that found in dreams.**
8.9 **CNS stimulants increase the activity of the central nervous system.**
8.10 **Nicotine is powerful and highly addictive.**
8.11 **Healthcare providers strive to remain free from impairment due to alcohol and drug addiction.**

Learning Outcomes

After reading this chapter, the student should be able to:

1. Discuss the various classes in which abused substances are found.
2. Explain underlying causes of addiction.
3. Compare and contrast psychological and physical dependence.
4. Compare and contrast classic and conditioned withdrawal.
5. Explain the significance of drug tolerance to pharmacotherapy.
6. Explain the major characteristics of abuse, dependence, and tolerance resulting from central nervous system depressants, including sedatives, sedative-hypnotics, benzodiazepines, opioids, and ethyl alcohol.
7. Explain characteristics of physical dependence and tolerance with the use of marijuana.
8. Explain examples and characteristics of hallucinogenic drug misuse.
9. Explain the major characteristics of abuse, dependence, and tolerance resulting from CNS stimulants, including amphetamine, methylphenidate, and methamphetamine-related drugs; and cocaine and caffeine.
10. Explain the powerfully addictive properties of nicotine.
11. List the reasons why healthcare providers may have problems with alcohol and substance or drug use.

Key Terms

addiction (ah-DIK-shun)
alcohol intoxication (AL-ku-hol in-tak-su-KA-shun)
analgesics (AN-ahl-GEE-siks)
attention-deficit/hyperactivity disorder (ADHD)
club drugs
cross-tolerance (krause TOL-er-ans)
delta 9-tetrahydrocannabinol (THC) (TEH-trah-HEYE-droh-cah-NAB-in-ol)
designer drugs (de-ZEYE-ner drugs)
drug abuse
drug misuse
narcolepsy (NAR-koh-lep-see)
opioids (OH-pee-oyds)
physical dependence (FI-zi-kul dee-PEN-dens)
psychedelics (seye-keh-DEL-iks)
psychological dependence (seye-koh-LOJ-i-kul dee-PEN-dens)
substance abuse
substance dependence
tolerance (TOL-er-ans)
withdrawal syndrome (with-DRAW-ul SIN-drom)

Substance abuse is the self-administration of a drug in a way that culture or society views as abnormal and not acceptable. Throughout history, individuals have consumed both natural and prescription drugs to increase physical or mental performance, cause a relaxed feeling, change a psychological state, or simply fit in with the crowd. Substance abuse has a tremendous economic, social, and public health impact on society. **Drug abuse** is the recurrent use of legal or illegal drugs, or the improper use of prescription or over-the-counter drugs with negative consequences. **Drug misuse** refers to the use of a drug for purposes for which it was not intended or using a drug in excessive quantities.

Abused and misused substances belong to many different chemical classes.

◀ **Core Concept 8.1**

Substances from a wide variety of chemical classes are abused and can be taken by many different routes. Abused and misused substances have in common an ability to affect the nervous system, particularly the brain. Some agents, such as opium, marijuana, cocaine, nicotine, caffeine, and alcohol, are obtained from natural sources. Others agents are synthetic or **designer drugs** that are created in illegal laboratories solely for making money in illegal drug trafficking. **Club drugs** are substances taken at dance clubs, all-night parties, and raves.

Although the public often connects substance use with illegal drugs, this is not necessarily the case: Alcohol and nicotine are the two most commonly used drugs. Marijuana use for medicinal and recreational purposes is becoming fairly commonplace nationwide. Legal prescription medications such as oxycodone (OxyContin), methamphetamine, and alprazolam (Xanax) have become frequent drugs of misuse. Volatile inhalants, found in common household products such as aerosols and paint thinners, are also often misused. Aerosols will make a user high with the practice of "huffing." Other frequently used substances include **analgesics** or *pain-reducing* drugs, sedatives, hallucinogens like lysergic acid diethylamide (LSD), and club drugs such as Ecstasy and flunitrazepam (Rohypnol), a powerful benzodiazepine depressant.

an = *without*
algesics = *causing pain*

Several drugs once used therapeutically are now illegal because of their high potential for abuse. Cocaine was once widely used as a local anesthetic, but today all cocaine purchased and used in the private sector is illegal. LSD is now illegal, although in the 1940s and 1950s it was used in psychotherapy. Phencyclidine (PCP) was popular in the early 1960s as an anesthetic but was taken off the market in 1965 because patients reported hallucinations, delusions, and anxiety after recovering from anesthesia. Many of the amphetamines, once prescribed for bronchodilation, were stopped in the 1980s after psychotic episodes were reported. Some commonly abused and misused substances are summarized in Table 8.1.

sedatives = *causing sedation*
hallucinogens = *causing hallucinations*

Table 8.1 Commonly Abused and Misused Substances

	Natural Substances	Therapeutic Applications
LEGAL SUBSTANCES WITHOUT PRESCRIPTION		
Aerosol inhalants	Solvents, varnishes	
Caffeine	Coffee	Over-the-counter (OTC) drugs
Ethyl alcohol	Drinking alcohol	OTC drugs
Nicotine	Tobacco	Smoking cessation drugs
LEGAL SUBSTANCES WITH PRESCRIPTION		
Amphetamines, methamphetamines, and methylphenidate (Ritalin)	Not applicable	CNS stimulants
Anabolic steroids		Weight or muscle gain products
Barbiturates		Sedatives; CNS depressants
Benzodiazepines		Sedatives; CNS depressants
Dextromethorphan (DMX)		OTC cough suppressants
Gamma hydroxybutyrate (GHB)		Anesthetic
Ketamine		Anesthetic
Opioid Analgesics		Pain therapy
ILLEGAL SUBSTANCES OR HAVING THERAPEUTIC APPLICATIONS		
Cannabinoids (THC)*	Marijuana	Glaucoma and other conditions
LSD	Rye/grain fungus	Psychiatric therapy
Mescaline	Peyote	
Opioids	Opium	Heroin
Phencyclidine (PCP)*		Anesthetic
Cocaine	Coca plant	Local anesthetic
Psilocybin	Mushrooms	
CLUB DRUGS WITH NO MEDICINAL USE—DESIGNER DRUGS		
MDA*	Not applicable	Not applicable
MMDA* (Ecstasy)		
DOM* (STP)		

*Chemical names are complicated and extensive; see Core Concepts 8.7 and 8.8 for more information.

Fast Facts **Substance Abuse in the United States**

- Over 94 million Americans have admitted using illicit drugs at least once.
- For grades 8 through 12, use of illicit drugs was 27.2% in 2014, down from its peak at 34.1% in 1997.
- About one in five Americans has lived with an alcoholic relative while growing up. Children of alcoholic parents are four times more likely to become alcoholics than children of nonalcoholic parents.
- Alcohol is an important factor in 68% of manslaughters, 54% of murders, 48% of robberies, and 44% of burglaries.
- Among youth between the ages of 12 and 17, approximately 7.2 million have drunk alcohol at least once. Girls are as likely as boys to drink alcohol.
- Thirty-three percent of 10th graders and 44% of 12th graders have reported using marijuana and hashish.
- Eleven percent of age 18- to 25-year-olds have abused cocaine; 17% of 26-year-olds and above have abused cocaine.
- Over 2 million Americans have used cocaine on a monthly basis; over one-half a million have used crack cocaine.
- Approximately 70% of the cocaine entering the United States comes from Colombia and passes through south Florida.
- Thirty percent of all Americans are cigarette smokers, including over 25% who are between the ages of 12 and 25.
- Nine out of ten adult smokers start by the age of 18 years. Use of e-cigarettes in 2014 was reported by 8% of 8th graders, 16% of 10th graders, and 17% of 12th graders.
- Three percent of 12th graders have reported using Ecstasy (MDMA).
- LSD is one of the most potent drugs known, with only 25–150 mcg constituting a dose. Use of hallucinogens among high school students has been declining (1.8% in 2014 down from 3.4% in 2013).

Core Concept 8.2 ▶

Addiction depends on multiple, complex, and interacting variables.

addict = *given over*

Addiction, the progressive and chronic abuse of a substance, is an overwhelming desire that drives someone to use a drug repeatedly despite serious health and social consequences. It is impossible to predict accurately whether a person will become an addict.

Scientists have used psychological profiles and investigated genetic links in an attempt to predict a person's addictive tendency, but no firm connections have been found. Addiction depends on multiple, complex, and interacting variables. These variables fall into the following categories:

- *Agent or drug factors* Cost, availability, dose, method of administration (e.g., oral, IV, inhalation), speed of onset or duration of effect, and length of drug use
- *User factors* Genetic factors (e.g., metabolic enzymes, natural tolerance), tendency toward risk-taking behavior, prior experiences with drugs, disease that may require a scheduled drug
- *History of trauma, or physical or sexual abuse* Correlated to later substance abuse in represented groups (e.g. children, women, men)
- *Environmental factors* Social and community *norms* (behavior accepted within a community), role models, peer influences, educational opportunities, underprivileged population groups

Addiction may begin with a real need for pharmacotherapy. For example, narcotic analgesics may be prescribed for pain, or sedatives for a sleep disorder. A favorable experience of pain relief or being able to fall asleep may cause a patient to want to repeat these positive experiences.

It is a common misunderstanding, even among some health professionals, that the therapeutic use of scheduled drugs creates large numbers of patients with addiction. In fact, prescription drugs rarely cause addiction when used as prescribed. The risk of addiction for prescription medications is mostly a function of the dose and the length of therapy. For this reason, medications having a potential for abuse are usually prescribed at the lowest effective dose for the shortest time necessary to treat the medical problems (see Chapter 15 for more information on pain management). As mentioned in Chapters 1 and 2, numerous laws have been passed in an attempt to limit drug abuse and addiction.

Substance dependence is classified as physical dependence or psychological dependence.

◀ **Core Concept 8.3**

Whether a substance is addictive relates to how easily an individual can stop taking it repeatedly. When a person has an overwhelming desire to take a drug and cannot stop, it is referred to as **substance dependence**. Substance dependence is classified into two categories: physical dependence and psychological dependence.

Physical dependence is an altered physical condition caused by the nervous system adapting to repeated substance use. Over time, the body's cells are tricked into believing that it is normal for the substance to continually be present. With physical dependence, uncomfortable symptoms, known as **withdrawal syndrome**, occur when the agent is stopped. Often, the fear of withdrawal is sufficient to thwart continued addictive behavior. **Opioids**, such as morphine and heroin, may produce physical dependence rather quickly with repeated doses, particularly when taken intravenously. Alcohol, sedatives, some stimulants, and nicotine are other examples of substances that may easily produce physical dependence with repeated use.

In contrast to physical dependence, **psychological dependence** causes no apparent signs of physical discomfort after the agent is stopped. The person, however, will have an intense craving and will display an overwhelming desire to continue using the substance even if there are obvious negative economic, physical, or social consequences. The intense craving may be associated with the individual's home environment or social contacts. Strong psychological cravings for a substance may continue for months or even years and is often responsible for *relapse* (return to the original drug-seeking behavior) during substance abuse therapy. In some cases, psychological dependence may develop very quickly, after only one use, such as with crack cocaine—a potent, inexpensive form of cocaine.

re = *again*
lapse = *fall back*

Core Concept 8.4 ▶ Withdrawal results when an abused substance is no longer available.

Once an individual becomes physically dependent and the substance is stopped, withdrawal syndrome will occur. Symptoms of withdrawal syndrome may be severe for patients who are physically dependent on alcohol and sedatives. Helping a patient withdraw from these agents is best done in a substance abuse treatment facility. Examples of withdrawal syndromes related to different abused and misused substances are listed in Table 8.2.

Prescription drugs may be used to reduce the severity of withdrawal symptoms. For example, alcohol withdrawal can be treated with a benzodiazepine such as diazepam (Valium), and opioid withdrawal might be treated with methadone. Another drug used in the treatment of opioid dependence is buprenorphine. Buprenorphine may be dispensed alone or in combination with opioid-blocking drugs. Opioid-blocking drugs block the euphoric and pain-relieving effects of heroin and other opioids. Thus, naltrexone may be administered, or buprenorphine may be administered in combination with naloxone. Examples include buccal film (Bunavail), sublingual film (Suboxone), or sublingual tablets (Subutex, Zubslov). Opioids and opioid-blocking drugs are discussed in Chapter 15. Symptoms of nicotine withdrawal may be relieved by nicotine replacement therapy (NRT) in the form of patches or chewing gum and the use of bupropion (Wellbutrin). No specific pharmacologic treatments are indicated for withdrawal from CNS stimulants, hallucinogens, marijuana, or inhalants.

With chronic substance abuse, patients will often associate their conditions and surroundings—including social contacts with other users—with use of the drug. Users tend to return to drug-seeking behavior when they interact with other substance abusers. Counselors often encourage patients to stop associating with past social contacts or having relationships with other substance abusers to lessen the possibility of relapse. With the assistance of 12-step self-help groups such as Alcoholics Anonymous and Narcotics Anonymous, some patients are able to move to a drug-free lifestyle by making friends with new people who are drug- and alcohol-free.

Core Concept 8.5 ▶ Tolerance occurs when higher and higher doses of a drug are needed to achieve the initial response.

Tolerance is a biological condition that occurs when the body adapts to a substance after it is repeatedly administered. Over time, higher doses of the agent are needed to produce the

Table 8.2 Selected Drugs of Abuse and Misuse: Withdrawal Symptoms and Signs of Toxicity

Drug	Withdrawal Symptoms	Signs of Toxicity
Alcohol	Tremors, fatigue, anxiety, abdominal cramping, hallucinations, confusion, seizures, delirium tremens	Extreme somnolence, severe CNS depression, diminished reflexes, respiratory depression
Barbiturates	Insomnia, anxiety, weakness, abdominal cramps, tremor, anorexia, seizures, skin hypersensitivity reactions, hallucinations, delirium	Severe CNS depression, tremor, diaphoresis, vomiting, cyanosis, tachycardia, Cheyne–Stokes respirations
Benzodiazepines	Insomnia, restlessness, abdominal pain, nausea, sensitivity to light and sound, headache, fatigue, muscle twitches	Somnolence, confusion, diminished reflexes, coma
Cocaine and amphetamines	Mental depression, anxiety, extreme fatigue, hunger	Dysrhythmias, lethargy, skin pallor, psychosis
Hallucinogens	Rarely observed; dependent on specific drug	Panic reactions, confusion, blurred vision, increase in blood pressure, psychotic-like state
Marijuana	Irritability, restlessness, insomnia, tremor, chills, weight loss	Euphoria, paranoia, panic reactions, hallucinations, psychotic-like state
Nicotine	Irritability, anxiety, restlessness, headaches, increased appetite, insomnia, inability to concentrate, decrease in heart rate and blood pressure	Heart palpitations, tachyarrhythmias, confusion, depression, seizures
Opioids	Excessive sweating, restlessness, pinpoint pupils, teary eyes, agitation, goose bumps, tremor, violent yawning, nausea, vomiting, constipation, abdominal cramps and pain, muscle spasms with kicking movements, weight loss	Respiratory depression, cyanosis, extreme somnolence, coma

initial effect. For example, at the start of pharmacotherapy, a patient may find that 2 mg of a sedative is effective for causing sleep. After taking the medication for several months, the patient notices that it takes 4 mg or perhaps 6 mg to fall asleep. Development of drug tolerance is common for substances that affect the nervous system. Tolerance should be thought of as a natural consequence of continued drug use and not be considered evidence of addiction or substance abuse.

Tolerance does not develop at the same rate for all actions of a drug. For example, patients usually develop tolerance to the nausea and vomiting produced by narcotic analgesics after only a few doses. Tolerance to the mood-altering effects of these drugs and to their ability to reduce pain develops more slowly but eventually may be complete. Tolerance never develops to the ability of these drugs to constrict the pupils. Patients will often put up with annoying side effects of drugs, such as the sleepiness caused by antihistamines, if they know that tolerance to these effects will develop quickly.

Once tolerance develops to one substance, it often also occurs with use of closely related drugs. This reaction is known as **cross-tolerance**. For example, a heroin addict will be tolerant to the analgesic effects of other opioids such as morphine or meperidine. Patients who have developed tolerance to alcohol will show tolerance to other CNS depressants such as barbiturates, benzodiazepines, and some general anesthetics. This is important to know because doses of related medications may need to be adjusted so that the patient receives maximum therapeutic benefit.

The terms *immunity* and *resistance* are often confused with *tolerance*. These terms more correctly refer to the immune system and infections, and they should not be used to mean tolerance. For example, microorganisms become *resistant* to the effects of an antibiotic; they do not become *tolerant*. Patients become *tolerant* to the effects of pain relievers; they do not become *resistant*. Therefore, it is incorrect to say that patients are *immune* to drug therapy.

CAM Therapy | Milk Thistle for Liver Damage

Milk thistle is a plant found growing in the Mediterranean region that has been used as an herbal medicine for centuries. The active ingredient in the milk thistle plant (*Silybum marianum*), silymarin, has been thought to protect the liver against injury. Some studies have indeed shown that silymarin is able to neutralize the effects of alcohol and actually stimulate liver regrowth. It acts as an antioxidant and free-radical scavenger. It is typically taken for liver cirrhosis, chronic hepatitis, and gallbladder disorders. The herb has few side effects other than mild diarrhea, bloating, and upset stomach.

Anti-inflammatory and anticarcinogenic properties of milk thistle have also been documented. Milk thistle has been claimed to reduce the growth of cancer cells, but this has not been confirmed by controlled research studies. Patients should be urged to report the use of this herb to their healthcare provider.

CONCEPT REVIEW 8.1

- What is the difference between physical dependence and psychological dependence? How do patients know when they are physically dependent on a substance?

Central nervous system (CNS) depressants decrease the activity of the central nervous system.

◀ **Core Concept 8.6**

depressant = *dispirited or lowered feeling*

CNS depressants form a group of drugs that cause patients to feel sedated or relaxed. Drugs in this group include barbiturates, nonbarbiturate sedative-hypnotics, benzodiazepines, alcohol, and opioids. Although the majority of these substances are legal, they are controlled because of their abuse potential.

Sedatives and Sedative-Hypnotics

tranquilizer = *causing a tranquil state*

Sedatives, sometimes referred to as *tranquilizers*, are prescribed mostly for sleep disorders and some forms of epilepsy. The two primary classes of sedatives are the barbiturates and the nonbarbiturate sedative-hypnotics. See Chapter 10 for discussion of their historic use in treating sleep disorders and Chapter 14 for their use in treating epilepsy. Their actions, indications, safety profiles, and addictive potential are generally the same. Physical dependence, psychological dependence, and tolerance develop when these agents are taken for long periods at high doses. Patients sometimes abuse these drugs by taking more doses than prescribed, sharing their medication with friends, or selling their medication. These drugs are frequently combined with other drugs of abuse such as CNS stimulants or alcohol. People with addiction often alternate between amphetamines, which keep them awake for several days, and barbiturates, which help them to relax and fall asleep. Methamphetamine, for example, is an amphetamine-like stimulant drug (Core Concept 8.9). It has the ability to keep someone awake and produce many of the signs that counter sleep such as an elevated breathing rate and heart rate, and increased blood pressure.

Many sedatives have a long duration of action. Effects may last an entire day, depending on the specific drug. Patients may appear dull or apathetic, with slurred speech and lack of motor coordination. High doses of these drugs suppress the respiratory centers in the brain, and the user may stop breathing or enter a coma. Death may result from overdose. Withdrawal symptoms from these drugs may also be life threatening.

eu = *healthy or well*
phoric = *bearing*

One drug of interest is gamma hydroxybutyric acid (GHB). GHB is approved by the U.S. Food and Drug Administration (FDA) as sodium oxybate (Xyrem) to treat patients with narcolepsy. Recreational users often abuse GHB by consuming it in high doses. Although used to produce a euphoric (pleasure) state, overdose of this drug can cause severe respiratory depression, seizures, and coma. Thus, its depressant effects warrant close attention in the nonbarbiturate sedative-hypnotic category.

Benzodiazepines

anxio = *anxiety/restlessness*
lytic = *destruction*

amnestic = *loss of memory*

Benzodiazepines are another group of CNS depressants that have a potential for abuse. They are one of the most widely prescribed classes of drugs and have largely replaced the barbiturates for certain disorders. Their primary indication is anxiety; thus, they are called *anxiolytic* drugs (see Chapter 10). They are also used for short-term treatment of seizures (see Chapter 14) and as muscle relaxants (see Chapter 13). Common benzodiazepines include alprazolam (Xanax), clonazepam (Klonopin), diazepam (Valium), temazepam (Restoril), triazolam (Halcion), and midazolam (Versed). Flunitrazepam (Rohypnol) is not approved by the FDA for any medical condition, but it is a club drug noted for its amnestic properties. Users will often feel carefree, without worry, and can even be subject to assault.

Benzodiazepines are one of the most frequently prescribed drug classes, and benzodiazepine abuse has various presentations. Individuals who abuse benzodiazepines may appear detached, sleepy, or disoriented. Death due to overdose is rare, even with high doses, unless benzodiazepines are used in combination with other CNS depressants. Abusers may combine these agents with alcohol, cocaine, or heroin to increase their drug experience. If combined with other agents, death due to overdose is very likely. Death due to seizures is a common occurrence with benzodiazepine withdrawal and with alcohol withdrawal.

Opioids

Opioids are prescribed for severe pain, persistent cough, and diarrhea. The opioid class includes opium, morphine, and codeine, which are processed from natural substances found in the unripe seeds of the poppy plant, and synthetic drugs, such as hydromorphone (Dilaudid), oxycodone (OxyContin), fentanyl (Duragesic, Sublimaze), methadone (Dolophine), and heroin. The therapeutic effects of the opioids are discussed in more detail in Chapter 15.

The effects of *oral* opioids begin within 30 minutes and may last more than a day. *Parenteral* forms produce immediate effects, including the brief, intense rush of euphoria sought by heroin addicts. Individuals experience a range of CNS effects, from extreme pleasure to slowed body activities and extreme sedation. Signs include constricted pupils, an increase in the ability to withstand pain, and respiratory depression.

Addiction to opioids can occur rapidly, and withdrawal can produce intense symptoms. Although extremely unpleasant, withdrawal from opioids is not necessarily life threatening. Methadone is a narcotic sometimes used to treat opioid addiction. Although methadone has addictive properties of its own, it does not produce the same degree of euphoria as other opioids, and its effects are longer lasting. Heroin addicts may be switched to methadone to prevent unpleasant withdrawal symptoms. Because methadone is taken orally, the serious risks associated with intravenous drug use, such as hepatitis and AIDS, are eliminated. Patients sometimes remain on methadone maintenance for their lifetimes. Withdrawal from methadone is more prolonged than from heroin or morphine, but the symptoms are less intense.

Ethyl Alcohol

Ethyl alcohol, commonly known as alcohol, is one of the most widely abused drugs. Alcohol is a legal substance for adults and is available as beer, wine, and liquor. The economic, social, and health consequences of alcohol abuse are staggering. In contrast to the many negative consequences associated with long-term abuse of alcohol, drinking small quantities of alcohol on a daily basis has been found to reduce the risk of stroke and heart attack.

Alcohol is classified as a CNS depressant, because it slows the actions of the region of the brain responsible for alertness and wakefulness. Alcohol easily crosses the blood–brain barrier, and its effects can be noticed within 5 to 30 minutes. Effects of alcohol are directly related to the amount consumed within a certain time frame and include relaxation, sedation, memory impairment, loss of motor coordination, reduced judgment, and decreased inhibition. **Alcohol intoxication** occurs when muscle coordination is lost and mental function is affected. It results in a characteristic odor to the breath and increased blood flow in certain areas of the skin, causing a flushed face, pink cheeks, or red nose. Although these symptoms are easily recognized, the nurse must be aware that other substances and disorders may cause similar effects. For example, many antianxiety agents, sedatives, and antidepressants can cause drowsiness, memory difficulties, and loss of motor coordination. Certain mouthwashes, medicines, and other substances containing alcohol can give the breath an "alcoholic" smell.

The presence of food in the stomach will slow the absorption of alcohol, thus delaying the onset of drug action. *Metabolism*, or detoxification of alcohol by the liver, occurs at a slow, constant rate, which is not affected by the presence of food. The average rate is about 15 mL per hour—equal to one alcoholic beverage per hour. If consumed at a higher rate, alcohol will accumulate in the blood and produce greater effects on the brain. Overdose of alcohol may produce vomiting, severe hypotension, respiratory failure, and coma.

Chronic alcohol consumption produces both psychological and physiologic dependence and results in a large number of adverse health effects. The organ most affected by chronic alcohol abuse is the liver. Alcoholism is a common cause of *cirrhosis*, a harmful and often fatal failure of the liver to perform its vital functions. Liver failure causes abnormalities in blood clotting and nutritional deficiencies and sensitizes the patient to the effects of all medications metabolized by the liver.

cirrh = *orange/yellow*
osis = *condition*

Alcohol withdrawal syndrome is severe and may be life threatening. The use of antiseizure medications for treating severe alcohol withdrawal symptoms is discussed in Chapter 14. Long-term treatment for alcohol abuse includes behavioral counseling and participation in self-help groups such as Alcoholics Anonymous. Disulfiram (Antabuse) may be given to discourage relapses. Disulfiram inhibits acetaldehyde dehydrogenase, the enzyme that metabolizes alcohol. If alcohol is consumed while taking disulfiram, the patient becomes violently ill within 5 to 10 minutes, with headache, shortness of breath, nausea, vomiting, and other unpleasant symptoms. Disulfiram is only effective in highly motivated patients, because the success of pharmacotherapy is entirely dependent on patient compliance. Alcohol sensitivity can continue for up to two weeks after disulfiram has been discontinued. As a pregnancy category X drug, disulfiram should never be taken during pregnancy.

In addition to disulfiram, acamprosate calcium (Campral, Forest) is an FDA-approved drug for maintaining alcohol abstinence in patients with alcohol dependence. Additional studies comparing the therapeutic benefit of disulfiram with acamprosate are ongoing. Adverse reactions to acamprosate include diarrhea, flatulence, and nausea. This drug is not recommended for patients who have impaired kidney functioning. Other anticraving drugs include opioid antagonists such as naltrexone (ReVia, Vivitrol), which reduce the intoxicating effects of alcohol and the urge to drink. Additional drugs that may help in maintaining abstinence and controlling impulsivity are the antiseizure drug, topiramate (Topamax) and the muscle relaxant, baclofen (Lioresal). The therapeutic effects of the antiseizure drugs are discussed in Chapter 14; muscle relaxants are discussed in Chapter 13.

CONCEPT REVIEW 8.2

- Compare the potential to cause coma or death of barbiturates and benzodiazepines.

Core Concept 8.7 ▶ Marijuana produces little physical dependence or tolerance.

Cannabinoids are substances obtained from the hemp plant *Cannabis sativa*, which grows in tropical climates. Cannabinoid agents are usually smoked and include marijuana, hashish, and hash oil. Although more than 61 cannabinoid chemicals have been identified, the ingredient responsible for most of the psychoactive properties is **delta-9-tetrahydrocannabinol (THC)**.

Marijuana (street names "grass," "pot," "weed," "reefer," or "dope") is a natural product obtained from *C. sativa*. As with ethyl alcohol, it is among the more commonly used drugs in the United States. Use of marijuana slows motor activity, decreases coordination, and causes disconnected thoughts, paranoia, and euphoria. It increases thirst and craving for food, particularly chocolate and other sweets. One hallmark symptom of marijuana use is red or bloodshot eyes, caused by dilation of blood vessels. THC also accumulates in the reproductive organs and may cause infertility and birth defects.

para = *beside*
noia = *mind*

When inhaled, marijuana produces effects that occur within minutes and last up to 24 hours. Because marijuana smoke is inhaled more deeply and held within the lungs for a longer time than cigarette smoke, it introduces four times more tar into the lungs than tobacco smoke. Smoking marijuana on a daily basis may increase the risk of lung cancer and other respiratory disorders. Chronic use is associated with lack of motivation and loss of productivity.

Unlike many abused substances, marijuana produces little physical dependence or tolerance. Withdrawal symptoms are mild, if they are experienced at all. Metabolites of THC, however, remain in the body for months to years, allowing laboratory specialists to determine easily whether someone has used marijuana. For several days after use, THC can also be detected in the urine.

Marijuana legalization has been a passionate topic due to strong convictions among certain members of the U.S. population. In many instances patients have been given limited approval for marijuana therapy provided they have a doctor's recommendation. Various diseases and conditions have been cited as being improved by marijuana: glaucoma, epilepsy, improved lung capacity in smokers of tobacco, benefit in cancer patients, anxiety, Alzheimer disease, multiple sclerosis, muscle spasms, lessened side-effects of hepatitis C treatment, inflammatory bowel disease, arthritis, metabolic benefits in emaciated patients, lupus, Crohn disease, Parkinson disease, posttraumatic stress disorder (PTSD), benefit to stroke victims, alcohol cessation treatment, to stimulate the appetite in chemotherapy patients, and to prevent nightmares. Although research has not demonstrated that marijuana is an effective therapy for all these conditions, over 23 states have legalized marijuana. A few states have also legalized the recreational use of this drug.

CONCEPT REVIEW 8.3

- Name three legal substances that are both used in traditional therapies and frequently abused. Are these substances natural or synthetic? Compare ethyl alcohol and marijuana in terms of common use.

Hallucinogens cause an altered state of thought and perception similar to that found in dreams.

◀ **Core Concept 8.8**

Hallucinogens consist of an assorted class of chemicals that have in common the ability to produce an altered, dreamlike state of consciousness. Sometimes called **psychedelics**, the prototype substance for this class is LSD. All hallucinogens are Schedule I drugs and have no medical use.

For nearly all drugs of abuse, predictable symptoms occur in every user. Effects from hallucinogens, however, are highly variable and depend on the mood and expectations of the user and the surrounding environment in which the substance is used. Two patients taking the same agent will report completely different symptoms, and the same patient may report different symptoms with each use. Users who take LSD or *psilocybin* (Figure 8.1) may experience symptoms such as laughter, visions, religious revelations, or deep personal insights. Common occurrences are hallucinations and afterimages (images that are projected onto people as they move). Users also report unusually bright lights and vivid colors. Some users hear voices; others report smells. Many experience a profound sense of truth and deep thoughts. Unpleasant experiences can be terrifying and may include anxiety, panic attacks, confusion, severe depression, or paranoia.

LSD (street names "acid," "the beast," "blotter acid," "California sunshine") is made from a fungus that grows on rye and other grains. LSD is almost always used in an oral form. It can be manufactured in capsules, tablets, or liquids. A common and inexpensive method for distributing LSD is to place drops of the drug on small pieces of paper that often contain images of cartoon characters or graphics related to the drug culture. After drying, the paper containing the LSD is swallowed to produce the drug's effects.

LSD is distributed throughout the body immediately after use. Effects are experienced within an hour and may last 6 to 12 hours. It affects the central and autonomic nervous systems, increasing blood pressure, elevating body temperature, dilating pupils, and increasing heart rate. Repeated use may cause memory loss and inability to reason. In extreme cases,

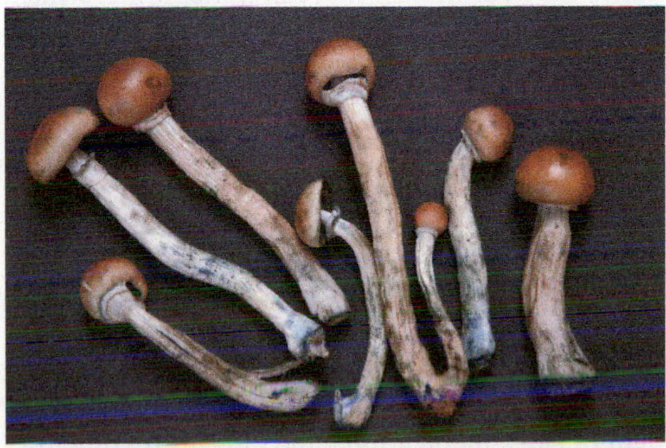

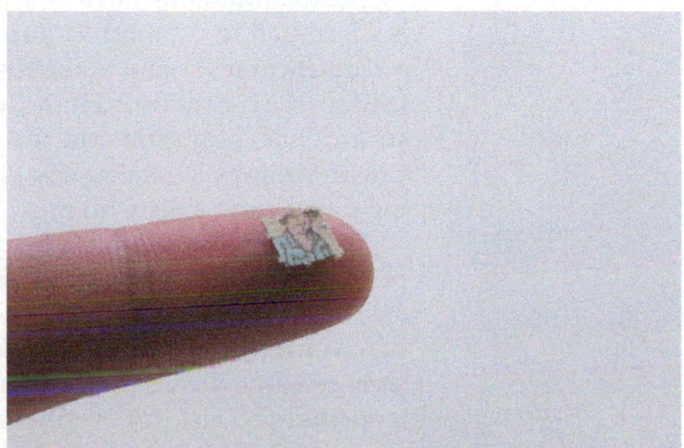

FIGURE 8.1 Comparison of psilocybin and LSD. Psilocybin is derived from a mushroom (left); an LSD blot is shown (right).
Source: (left) Janine Wiedel Photolibrary/Alamy Stock Photo, (right) Joe Bird/Alamy Stock Photo

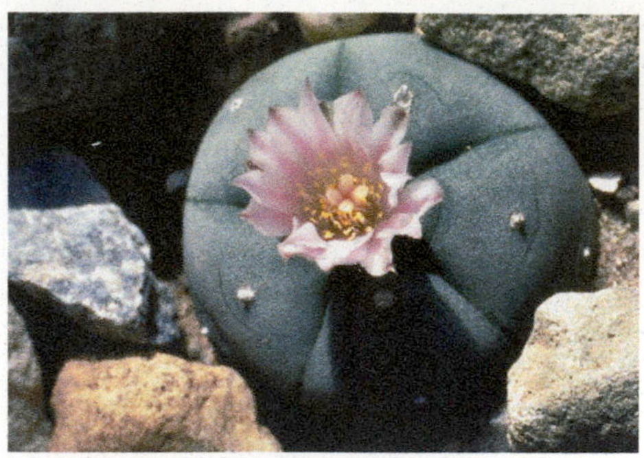

FIGURE 8.2 Mescaline is derived from the peyote plant (shown in photo).
Source: R. Konig/Jacana/Science Source

patients may develop psychoses. One unusual adverse effect is flashbacks, in which the user experiences the effects of the drug again—sometimes weeks, months, or years after the drug was initially taken. Although users may experience tolerance, they have little or no dependence with hallucinogens.

Other hallucinogenic drugs that are abused include the following:

- *Mescaline* found in the peyote cactus of Mexico and Central America (Figure 8.2)
- *MDMA (3,4-methylenedioxymethamphetamine, XTC, Ecstasy, or Molly)* an amphetamine originally created for research purposes but now extremely popular among teens and young adults
- *DOM (2,5 dimethoxy-4-methylamphetamine, STP)* a recreational drug often linked with rave parties
- *MDA (3,4-methylenedioxyamphetamine)* called the love drug because it is believed to enhance sexual desire
- *PCP (phenylcyclohexylpiperadine; also called phencyclidine; street name "angel dust")* produces a trancelike state that may last for days and results in severe brain damage; used as an animal tranquilizer
- *Ketamine (date rape drug or special coke)* produces unconsciousness and amnesia; primary legal use is as an anesthetic
- *MDPV (3,4-methylenedioxypyrovaleron; bath salts; cathinone)* a synthetic stimulant drug made from the Khat plant found in East Africa and southern Arabia; swallowed, snorted, smoked, or injected, it causes paranoia, increased sociability, increased sex drive, hallucinations and panic attacks.

CONCEPT REVIEW 8.4

- In examining and interviewing a patient, how could you determine whether he or she is under the influence of marijuana or hallucinogens?

Core Concept 8.9 ▶

CNS stimulants increase the activity of the central nervous system.

stimulant = *arousing feelings*
narco = *numbness or stupor*
lepsy = *seizure*

Stimulants include a varied family of drugs with the ability to increase the activity of the CNS. Some are available by prescription for use in the treatment of **narcolepsy** (a sleep disorder in which people fall asleep unexpectedly), obesity, and **attention-deficit/hyperactivity disorder (ADHD)**. As drugs of abuse and misuse, CNS stimulants are taken to produce a sense of exhilaration, improve mental and physical performance, reduce appetite, prolong wakefulness, or simply "get high." Stimulants include amphetamines, cocaine, methylphenidate, and caffeine.

CNS stimulants have effects similar to the neurotransmitter norepinephrine, which is discussed in Chapter 9. Norepinephrine activates neurons in a part of the brain that affects awareness and wakefulness, called the *reticular formation* (see Chapter 10 for an in-depth discussion). High doses of amphetamines give the user a feeling of self-confidence, euphoria, alertness, and empowerment. Long-term use, however, often causes feelings of restlessness, anxiety, and fits of rage, especially when the user is coming down from a drug high.

Most CNS stimulants affect cardiovascular and respiratory activities, raising blood pressure and increasing respiration rate. Other symptoms include dilated pupils, sweating, and tremors. Overdoses of some stimulants lead to seizures and cardiac arrest.

Amphetamines and dextroamphetamines were once widely prescribed for depression, obesity, drowsiness, and congestion. In the 1960s, the healthcare profession realized that the risk for amphetamine dependence outweighed the drug's therapeutic usefulness. Because of the development of safer medications, the current therapeutic uses of these drugs are extremely limited. Most substance abusers get these agents from illegal laboratories, which can easily produce amphetamines and make tremendous profits.

Dextroamphetamine (Dexedrine) may be used to treat narcolepsy and for short-term weight loss when all other attempts to lose weight have been exhausted. Adderall (formulation of dextroamphetamine and amphetamine) is used to treat narcolepsy and ADHD.

Methamphetamine (street name "ice" or "crank") is often used as a recreational drug for those who like the "rush" that it provides. It is usually administered in powder or crystal form, but it also may be smoked. Methamphetamine is a Schedule II drug marketed under the trade name Desoxyn, although most abusers obtain it from illegal methamphetamine laboratories. A drug related to methamphetamine, called methcathinone (street name "cat"), is made illegally and snorted, taken orally, or injected intravenously. Methcathinone is a Schedule I agent.

Methylphenidate (Ritalin) is a CNS stimulant (Schedule II drug) that is widely prescribed for children diagnosed with ADHD (see Chapter 11). Ritalin has a calming effect on children who are inattentive or hyperactive. It stimulates the alertness center in the brain and allows the child to focus on tasks for longer periods. Lisdexamfetamine (Vyvanse) is another amphetamine-like substance used to treat ADHD. In adults and teens, Ritalin and Vyvanse usually produce the same effects as cocaine and amphetamines and are sometimes abused by adolescents and adults seeking euphoria. The tablets are crushed and used intranasally or dissolved in liquid and injected intravenously. Ritalin is also sometimes mixed with heroin (street name "speedball").

Cocaine is a natural substance obtained from the leaves of the coca plant, which grows in the Andes Mountain region of South America. The plant has been used by Andean cultures since 2500 B.C. Natives of this region chew the coca leaves or make teas of the dried leaves. Because it is taken orally, its absorption is slow, and the leaves contain only 1% cocaine, so users do not have the ill effects caused by chemically pure extracts from the plant. In the Andean culture, the use of coca leaves is not considered substance abuse because it is part of that society's culture.

Cocaine is a Schedule II drug that produces actions similar to those of the amphetamines, although its effects are usually more rapid and intense. Similar to local anesthetic drugs, it blocks sodium channels and produces mild numbness to body surface membranes. It is the second most commonly abused illegal drug in the United States. Routes of administration include snorting, smoking, and injecting. In smaller doses, cocaine produces CNS effects of intense euphoria, a decrease in hunger, analgesia, delusions of physical strength, and increased sensory perception. Larger doses will magnify these effects and also cause rapid heartbeat, sweating, dilation of the pupils, and elevated body temperature. After euphoria diminishes, the user often feels irritable, depressed, and distrustful and usually has insomnia. Some users report the sensation that insects are crawling under their skin. Users who snort cocaine develop a chronic runny nose, a crusty redness around the nostrils, and deterioration of the nasal cartilage. Overdose can cause dysrhythmias, convulsions, stroke, or death due to respiratory arrest. The withdrawal syndrome for amphetamines and cocaine is much less intense than that from alcohol or barbiturates.

Caffeine is a natural substance found in the seeds, leaves, or fruits of more than 63 plant species throughout the world. Significant amounts of caffeine are consumed in chocolate, coffee, tea, and soft drinks (Table 8.3). Sometimes caffeine is added to over-the-counter (OTC) pain relievers to help relieve migraines and other conditions. Caffeine travels to almost all parts of the body after ingestion, and several hours are needed for the body to metabolize and eliminate the drug. Caffeine has a pronounced diuretic effect.

Caffeine is considered a CNS stimulant because it produces increased mental alertness, restlessness, nervousness, irritability, and insomnia. The physical effects of caffeine include bronchodilation, increased blood pressure, increased production of stomach acid, and changes in blood glucose levels. Repeated use of caffeine may result in physical dependence and tolerance.

CONCEPT REVIEW 8.5

- Identify three groups of stimulants discussed in this section, and give examples for each group. Identify the major systems in the body affected by these stimulants.

Table 8.3 Caffeine Content of Common Drugs, Foods, and Beverages

	Serving Size	Caffeine (mg)
OTC DRUGS		
NoDoz, maximum strength; Vivarin	1 tablet	200
Excedrin	2 tablets	130
NoDoz, regular strength	1 tablet	100
Anacin (also available in caffeine-free formulation)	2 tablets	64
COFFEES		
Coffee, brewed and instant	8 ounces	95–135
Coffee, decaffeinated	8 ounces	5
TEAS		
Tea, leaf or bag	8 ounces	50
Tea, green	8 ounces	30
Tea, instant	8 ounces	15
SOFT DRINKS		
Mountain Dew	12 ounces	55.5
Diet Coke	12 ounces	46.5
Coca-Cola Classic	12 ounces	34.5
Pepsi-Cola	12 ounces	37.5
CHOCOLATES AND CANDIES		
Hershey's Special Dark chocolate bar	1 bar (1.5 ounces)	31
Hershey Bar (milk chocolate)	1 bar (1.5 ounces)	10
Cocoa or hot chocolate	8 ounces	85

Core Concept 8.10 ▶

Nicotine is powerful and highly addictive.

Nicotine is sometimes considered a CNS stimulant because of its ability to increase alertness. However, its actions and long-term consequences place it into a class by itself. Nicotine is unique among abused substances in that it is legal, strongly addictive, and highly carcinogenic. Furthermore, use of tobacco can cause harmful effects from secondhand smoke to those in the immediate area of the smoker. Patients often do not consider tobacco use to be substance abuse. The most common method by which nicotine enters the body is through the inhalation of cigarette, pipe, or cigar smoke. Electronic smoking devices are often referred to as e-cigarettes. They heat and vaporize a solution that may contain nicotine instead of burning tobacco. Metal or plastic tubes contain a cartridge filled with a liquid that is vaporized by a battery-powered heating element. The user inhales the aerosol as they would inhale regular tobacco smoke. Regular tobacco smoke contains more than 1000 chemicals, many of which are carcinogens. The primary addictive substance in cigarette smoke and many e-cigarettes is nicotine. Effects of inhaled nicotine may last from 30 minutes to several hours.

Nicotine affects many body systems, including the nervous, cardiovascular, and endocrine systems. Nicotine stimulates the CNS directly, causing increased alertness and ability to focus, feelings of relaxation, and lightheadedness. The cardiovascular effects of nicotine include accelerated heart rate and increased blood pressure, caused by activation of nicotinic receptors located within the autonomic nervous system (see Chapter 9). These cardiovascular effects can be serious in patients taking oral contraceptives. The risk of a fatal heart attack is five times greater in smokers than in nonsmokers. Muscular tremors may occur with moderate doses of nicotine, and convulsions may result from very high doses. Nicotine affects the endocrine system by increasing the basal metabolic rate, leading to weight loss. Nicotine also reduces appetite. Chronic use may lead to bronchitis, emphysema, and lung cancer.

Both psychological and physical dependence occur relatively quickly with nicotine. Once started on tobacco, patients tend to continue their drug use for many years, despite overwhelming medical evidence that their quality of life may be adversely affected and their life span shortened. Discontinuation results in agitation, weight gain, anxiety, headache, and an extreme craving for the drug. Although NRT (such as patches or gum), bupro-prion (Zyban, Wellbutrin), and varenicline (Chantix) assist patients in dealing with the unpleasant withdrawal symptoms, users often relapse because of stress, weight gain, and unpleasant symptoms.

Healthcare providers strive to remain free from impairment due to alcohol and drug addiction.

◀ **Core Concept 8.11**

Healthcare providers play a key role in the identification, prevention, and treatment of substance abuse. Abusers are often reluctant to report their drug use for fear of embarrassment or being arrested. Healthcare staff must be knowledgeable about the signs of substance abuse and withdrawal symptoms, and develop a keen sense of perception during interaction with their patients. A trusting healthcare provider–patient relationship is essential in helping patients deal with their dependence. By using therapeutic communication skills and by demonstrating a nonjudgmental, empathetic attitude, the healthcare team can build a trusting relationship with people who need medical assistance.

Impairment due to substance abuse is not only a patient behavioral or societal problem; it is also a concern for the healthcare provider. Nurses, physicians, anesthesiologists, and pharmacists have the highest risk for drug abuse. Critical care providers are especially likely to abuse stimulants and substances like marijuana or anxiolytic medications. Overall, it is estimated that up to 15% of medical professionals will misuse drugs at some point in their career (Merlo, Singhakant, Cummings, & Cottler, 2013). Alcohol is the most commonly abused legal substance; prescription drugs are abused secondly.

Reasons for these problems seem to be increasing stress due to the demands of the healthcare profession in general; social environments among medical professionals that promote self-reliance and independence; difficulty sleeping, in particular among workers with rotating shifts; and overall fatigue. Warning signs of substance abuse are overworking habits (e.g., arriving early and staying late for many days on end), high performance followed by deteriorating performance, isolation from other working staff, and frequent excuses (unexplained or complicated variables related to the worker's professional or social life).

Obvious signs may be frequent mood swings, irritability, or tearful outbursts followed by depression. Signs of substance abuse may be the smell of alcohol on the breath covered up by mints or mouthwash, frequent absence from the unit to visit the restroom, or patients complaining of not receiving medications. For, example, patients may complain about feeling pain despite having received seemingly adequate or repeated dosing of medication.

There are organizations that focus chiefly on addiction in the nursing profession as well as psychiatric disorders among nurses and other healthcare workers. The focus need not be just on disciplinary action but also on monitoring and support services. Agencies have adopted alternative disciplinary and peer assistance programs to make sure that both patients and healthcare providers receive proper assistance.

Patients Need to Know

Patients taking medications with abuse potential need to know the following regarding:

Alcohol

1. Limit alcoholic beverage intake to two drinks per day for men or one drink per day for women.
2. Avoid alcohol use entirely if liver disease, gastric reflux, peptic ulcers, or pregnancy exists.
3. Check with your healthcare provider when combining alcohol and medications (prescription or OTC). Alcohol is considered a CNS depressant, so never combine it with other CNS depressants.
4. Consuming more than one alcoholic drink per hour will usually result in blood alcohol levels above the legal limit for operating a vehicle.

CNS Stimulants

5. Avoid sources of caffeine such as chocolate, coffee, tea, and OTC drugs with caffeine if taking CNS stimulants.
6. Always take methylphenidate (Concerta, Metadate, Ritalin) at least six hours prior to sleep to avoid insomnia.

CNS Depressants

7. Never take more CNS depressant medication than prescribed. If the prescribed dose is not providing sufficient relief, notify a healthcare provider due to the possibility of acquired tolerance.
8. Never combine CNS depressants (including alcohol) unless advised to do so by a healthcare provider.

Tobacco

9. Nicotine is a major contributor to cancer, heart disease, and stroke.
10. Secondhand smoke is dangerous, particularly to children and pregnant women.
11. If using NRT, discontinue smoking immediately and follow the instruction sheet provided with the NRT of choice.

Chapter Review

Core Concepts Summary

8.1 Abused and misused substances belong to many different chemical classes.

Some abused substances, such as alcohol and nicotine, are available without a prescription. Others, such as barbiturates, benzodiazepines, and most opioids, have legitimate medical uses. Still others, such as LSD and heroin, are illegal, having no current medical applications.

8.2 Addiction depends on multiple, complex, and interacting variables.

Addiction is an overwhelming feeling that causes someone to continue taking drugs. Although ideas about addiction have changed over the years, healthcare providers now recognize addiction as being related to drug, genetic, and environmental factors.

8.3 Substance dependence is classified as physical dependence or psychological dependence.

Dependence is an overwhelming need to take a drug on a continual basis. When physical dependence exists, the patient exhibits signs of withdrawal after the drug is discontinued. Psychological dependence is an intense craving for the drug.

8.4 Withdrawal results when an abused substance is no longer available.

When an abused drug is discontinued, patients may experience uncomfortable physical symptoms known as withdrawal syndrome. Symptoms vary depending on the specific drug of abuse and range from mild to life threatening.

8.5 Tolerance occurs when higher and higher doses of a drug are needed to achieve the initial response.

Tolerance occurs over time when patients adapt to continued drug use and require higher doses to produce the same effect. Cross-tolerance or tolerance resulting from prior exposure to a related drug also results in higher doses needed to produce the same effect.

8.6 Central nervous system (CNS) depressants decrease the activity of the central nervous system.

Substances that make patients feel relaxed and sleepy, and work by generally slowing neuronal activity in the brain, include sedatives, opioids, and ethyl alcohol. Examples of sedatives are barbiturates and benzodiazepines. Because of their abuse potential, many of these substances are controlled. Ethyl alcohol is a legal substance.

8.7 Marijuana produces little physical dependence or tolerance.

Marijuana produces less physical dependence than most other drugs and produces less tolerance. The medical value of this drug remains controversial and unproven. The risks of using this substance are lung cancer, respiratory problems, and lack of motivation.

8.8 Hallucinogens cause an altered state of thought and perception similar to that found in dreams.

Hallucinogens, also called psychedelics, have the ability to produce altered states of consciousness and dreams. They include LSD, mescaline, MDMA (Ecstasy), DOM (STP), MDA (love drug), and ketamine (an anesthetic).

8.9 CNS stimulants increase the activity of the central nervous system.

Amphetamines, methylphenidate, cocaine, and caffeine increase alertness by stimulating the central nervous system. Some substances are available by prescription and are used for narcolepsy, obesity, and attention deficit disorder. Caffeine is available in many consumer products, including chocolate, coffee, tea, soft drinks, and coffee ice cream. Cocaine is among the most commonly abused substances in America.

8.10 Nicotine is powerful and highly addictive.

Nicotine is a unique, legal, carcinogenic, and highly addictive substance. The most common method of entry into the body is by inhalation of cigarette, pipe, or cigar smoke. Important effects of inhaled nicotine include stimulation of the CNS and increased cardiovascular effects.

8.11 Healthcare providers strive to remain free from impairment due to alcohol and drug addiction.

Reasons why healthcare providers have problems with alcohol or drug abuse seem to be related to demands in the health profession, including self-reliant social and professional environments, rotating working shifts, and fatigue. Signs of impairment are frequent mood swings, irritability or depressive symptoms, smell of alcohol on the breath, frequent absences from the unit, and patients not receiving proper medications. Support groups and organizations assist with these related issues.

REVIEW Questions

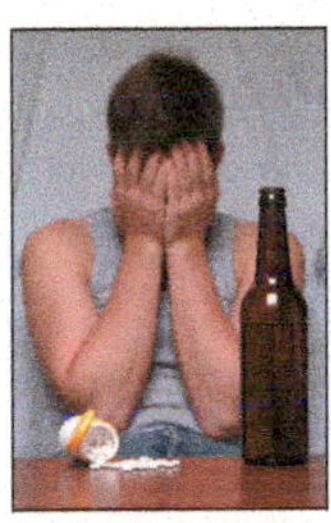

Answer the following questions to assess your knowledge of the chapter material, and go back and review any material that is not clear to you.

1. The two most commonly abused drugs are:
1. Methylphenidate (Ritalin) and meperidine (Demerol).
2. Lysergic acid diethylamide (LSD) and phencyclidine (PCP).
3. Alcohol and nicotine.
4. Opioids and inhalants.

2. A patient has been admitted to the emergency department with a diagnosis of cocaine overdose. The nurse monitors the patient for:
1. Irritability, restlessness, and abdominal cramping.
2. Dysrhythmias, convulsions, and stroke.
3. Insomnia, hallucinations, and tremors.
4. Delirium, extreme fatigue, hunger, and headaches.

3. The patient requires a higher dose of the substance to produce the initial effect. The nurse recognizes this as:
1. Toxicity.
2. Resistance.
3. Immunity.
4. Tolerance.

4. The patient has developed an opioid addiction. Which of the following medications will be used for opioid withdrawal?
1. Methadone
2. Heroin
3. Diazepam (Valium)
4. Alprazolam (Xanax)

5. Which of the following substances produces little physical dependence or tolerance?
1. Heroin
2. Marijuana
3. Alcohol
4. Cocaine

6. The nurse recognizes that methylphenidate (Ritalin) is classified as a:
1. Schedule I drug.
2. Schedule II drug.
3. Schedule III drug.
4. Schedule IV drug.

7. The nurse checks the patient and finds the following: increased heart rate, dilated pupils, elevated body temperature, and sweating. The nurse suspects:
1. Marijuana use.
2. Heroin use.
3. Cocaine use.
4. Amphetamine use.

8. Which of the following would the nurse find when monitoring the patient for use of barbiturates?
1. Drowsiness, lack of muscle coordination, decreased respirations
2. Euphoria and irritability
3. Increased pain threshold and hallucinations
4. Increased blood pressure and respirations

9. Physical dependence differs from psychological dependence in that with physical dependence:
1. There is an intense craving for the drug.
2. There is an overwhelming need to take the drug.
3. The patient exhibits signs of withdrawal after the drug is discontinued.
4. Higher doses are required to produce the initial effect of the drug.

10. The nurse educates the patient on disulfiram (Antabuse), explaining that:
   1. Only small amounts of alcohol may be ingested while on this drug.
   2. If alcohol is ingested, the patient may experience shortness of breath, nausea, vomiting, and headache.
   3. It is safe for use in pregnancy.
   4. It enhances alcohol metabolism within the body.

Answers and complete rationales for the Review Questions appear in Appendix A.

REFERENCE

Merlo, L., Singhakant, S., Cummings, S., & Cottler, L. (2013). Reasons for misuse of prescription medication among physicians undergoing monitoring by a physician health program. *Journal of Addiction Medicine, 7*, 349–353. doi: 10.1097/ADM.0b013e31829da074

SELECTED BIBLIOGRAPHY

American Academy of Child & Adolescent Psychiatry. (2011). *Facts for families guide: Alcohol use in families, No. 17, updated 2011*. Retrieved from https://www.aacap.org/AACAP/Families_and_Youth/Facts_for_Families/FFF-Guide/Children-Of-Alcoholics-017.aspx

Baumann, M. H. (2014). Awash in a sea of 'bath salts': Implications for biomedical research and public health. *Addiction, 109*, 1577–1579. doi:10.1111/add.12601

Centers for Disease Control and Prevention. (2014). *Best practices for comprehensive tobacco control programs*. Retrieved from http://www.cdc.gov/tobacco/stateandcommunity/best_practices/pdfs/2014/comprehensive.pdf

D'Apolito, K. (2013). Breastfeeding and substance abuse. *Clinical Obstetric Gynecology, 56*, 202–211. doi:10.1097/GRF.0b013e31827e6b71

Dick, D. M., & Agrawal, A. (2008). The genetics of alcohol and other drug dependence. Retrieved from http://pubs.niaaa.nih.gov/publications/arh312/111-118.pdf

Fiellin, L. E., Tetrault, J. M., Becker, W. C., Fiellin, D. A., & Hoff, R. A. (2012). Previous use of alcohol, cigarettes, and marijuana and subsequent abuse of prescription opioids in young adults. *Journal of Adolescent Health, 52*, 158–163. doi:10.1016/j.jadohealth.2012.06.010

Foundation for a Drug-Free World. (n.d.). *The truth about marijuana: International statistics*. Retrieved from http://www.drugfreeworld.org/drugfacts/marijuana/international-statistics.html

Giaconia, R. M., Reinherz, H. Z., Paradis, A. D., & Stashwick, C. K. (2003). Comorbidity of substance use disorders and posttraumatic stress disorder in adolescents. In P. Oimette, & P. J. Brown (Eds.), *Trauma and substance abuse: Causes, consequences, and treatment of comorbid disorders* (pp. 227–242). Washington, DC: American Psychological Association.

Heinzerling, K. G., Gadzhyan, J., van Oudheusden, H., Rodriguez, F., McCracken, J., & Shoptaw, S. (2013). Pilot randomized trial of bupropion for adolescent methamphetamine abuse/dependence. *Journal of Adolescent Health, 52*, 502–505. doi:10.1016/j.jadohealth.2012.10.275

Murray, R. P., Barnes, G. E., & Ekuma, O. (2005). Does personality mediate the relation between alcohol consumption and cardiovascular disease morbidity and mortality? *Addictive Behaviors, 30*, 475–488. doi:10.1016/j.addbeh.2004.06.017

National Institute on Drug Abuse. (2014). *Drugfacts: High school and youth trends*. Retrieved from http://www.drugabuse.gov/publications/drugfacts/high-school-youth-trends

National Institute on Drug Abuse. (2016). *Marijuana*. Retrieved from http://www.drugabuse.gov/drugs-abuse/marijuana

O'Brien, C. P. (2012). Drug addiction and drug abuse. In L. L. Brunton, B. Chabner, and B. Knollman (Eds.), *Goodman & Gilman's the pharmacological basis of therapeutics* (12th ed., pp. 649–668). New York, NY: McGraw-Hill.

Sabella, D. (2016). Mental health matters: Revisiting child sexual abuse and survivor issues. *American Journal of Nursing, 116*(3) 48–54. doi:10.1097/01.NAJ.0000481280.22557.45

Substance Abuse and Mental Health Services Administration. (2015). *Behavioral health barometer United States, 2014* (HHS Publication No. SMA–15–4895). Retrieved from http://www.samhsa.gov/data/sites/default/files/National_BHBarometer_2014.pdf

Substance Abuse and Mental Health Services Administration. (2015). *Population data / The national survey on drug use and health (NSDUH)*. Retrieved from http://www.samhsa.gov/data/population-data-nsduh

Substance Abuse and Mental Health Services Administration. (2015). *Risk and protective factors and initiation of substance use: Results from the 2014 national survey on drug use and health*. Retrieved from http://www.samhsa.gov/data/sites/default/files/NSDUH-DR-FRR4-2014rev/NSDUH-DR-FRR4-2014.pdf

Sznitman, S. R., & Zolotov, Y. (2015). Cannabis for therapeutic purposes and public health and safety: A systematic and critical review. *International Journal of Drug Policy, 26*, 20–29. doi:10.1016/j.drugpo.2014.09.005

Thornburg, J., Malloy, Q., Cho, S., Studabaker, W., & Lee, Y. O. (2015). *Exhaled electronic cigarette emissions: What's your secondhand exposure?* Research Triangle Park, NC: RTI Press. doi:10.3768/rtipress.2015.rb.0008.1503

USA Today. (2014). Doctors, medical staff on drugs put patients at risk. Retrieved at http://www.usatoday.com/story/news/nation/2014/04/15/doctors-addicted-drugs-health-care-diversion/7588401

Unit 2

The Nervous System

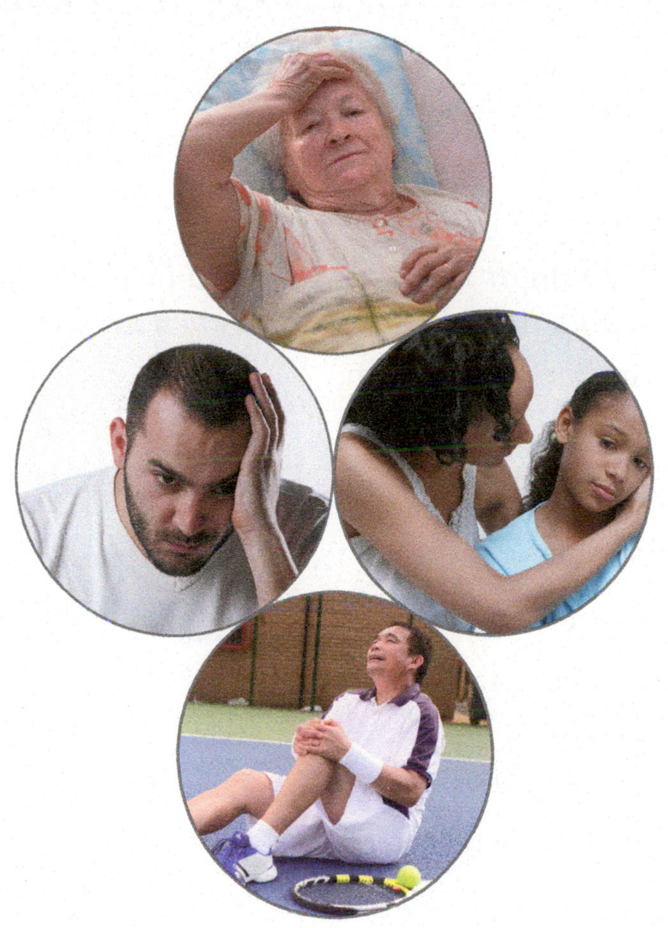

Unit Contents

Chapter 9

Drugs Affecting Functions of the Autonomic Nervous System

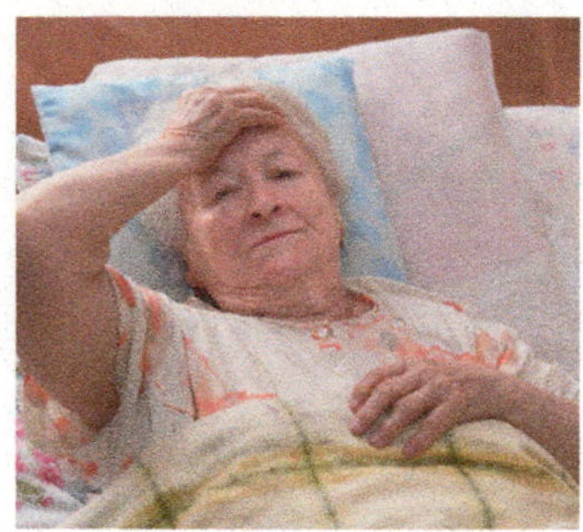

"I thought this was going to be a simple procedure. But after 4 days in bed, now I can't even urinate."

Mrs. Martha Wheaton

Core Concepts

9.1 The nervous system has two major divisions: central and peripheral.

9.2 The autonomic nervous system has sympathetic and parasympathetic branches.

9.3 Synapses are common junction sites of drug action.

9.4 Norepinephrine and acetylcholine are the two primary neurotransmitters in the autonomic nervous system.

9.5 Autonomic drugs are classified according to the receptors they stimulate or block.

9.6 Cholinergic drugs have few therapeutic uses because of their numerous adverse effects.

9.7 Cholinergic blockers are most commonly used to dry secretions and to treat asthma.

9.8 Adrenergic drugs are primarily used for their effects on the heart, bronchial tree, and nasal passages.

9.9 Adrenergic blockers are primarily used to treat hypertension, bronchial constriction, and nasal congestion.

Drug Snapshot

The following drugs are discussed in this chapter:

Drug Classes	Prototype Drugs
Cholinergic drugs	Pr bethanechol (Urecholine)
Cholinergic blockers	Pr atropine (AtroPen)
Adrenergic drugs	Pr phenylephrine (Neo-Synephrine)
Adrenergic blockers	Pr prazosin (Minipress)

Learning Outcomes

After reading this chapter, the student should be able to:

1. Identify the two primary divisions and three primary functions of the nervous system.
2. Compare and contrast actions of the sympathetic and parasympathetic branches of the autonomic nervous system.
3. Describe the basic functional unit of the nervous system, and explain how neural impulses are conducted.
4. Identify the primary neurotransmitters and types of receptors important to the functioning of the autonomic nervous system.

5. Explain autonomic drugs and the basis of how they are classified.
6. Describe the mechanisms of action, important adverse effects, and primary uses of cholinergic drugs, cholinergic-blocking drugs, adrenergic drugs, and adrenergic-drugs with representative examples.

Key Terms

acetylcholine (ACh) (ah-SEET-ul-KOH leen)
adrenergic (add-rah-NUR-jik)
adrenergic blockers
adrenergic drugs
alpha (α)-receptor
anticholinergics
beta (β)-receptor
cholinergic (kol-in-UR-jik)
cholinergic blockers
cholinergic drugs
epinephrine (EH-pin-NEF-rin)
ganglia (GANG-lee-ah)
muscarinic (MUS-kah-RIN-ik)
nicotinic (NIK-oh-TIN-ik)
norepinephrine (NE) (nor-EH-pin-NEF rin)
parasympathetic nervous system (PAIR-ah-SIM-pah-THET-ik)
parasympathomimetics (PAIR-ah-SIM-path-oh-mah-MET-iks)
sympathetic nervous system (SIM-pah-THET-ik)
sympatholytics (SIM-path-oh-LIT-iks)
sympathomimetics (SIM-path-oh-mih-MET-iks)

Neuropharmacology represents one of the largest and most complicated branches of pharmacology. Nervous system medications are used to treat a variety of neural disorders, including anxiety, depression, schizophrenia, insomnia, and seizures. They also exert a vast array of general side effects. Examples include abnormalities in heart rate and rhythm, high blood pressure, pressure within the eyeball, urination and digestion symptoms, altered breathing activity, and congestion.

Traditionally, the study of neuropharmacology begins with the autonomic nervous system. A firm grasp of autonomic pharmacology is necessary to understand and treat disorders of affected organ systems. The remaining chapters in this unit are devoted to the specific treatment of nervous system conditions.

The nervous system has two major divisions: central and peripheral.

◀ **Core Concept 9.1**

The nervous system is divided into the *central nervous system (CNS)* and the *peripheral nervous system (PNS)*. The CNS is made up of the brain and spinal cord. The PNS consists of all nervous tissue outside the CNS. The basic functions of the nervous system are to:

- Recognize stimuli in the internal and external environments
- Process and integrate these environmental stimuli
- React to the environmental stimuli with a series of actions or responses.

Figure 9.1 shows the basic divisions of the PNS. Nerves in the PNS either recognize stimuli to the environment (*sensory* subdivision) or respond to these stimuli by moving muscles or secreting chemicals (*motor* subdivision). The *somatic nervous system* consists of nerves that provide voluntary control over skeletal muscle. Nerves of the *autonomic nervous system* exert involuntary control over smooth muscle, cardiac muscle, and glands. Organs and tissues regulated by outgoing impulses of the autonomic nervous system include the heart, digestive tract, respiratory tract, reproductive tracts, arteries, salivary glands, and portions of the eye.

soma = *body*

auto = *self*
nom = *regulation*
ic = *relating to*

The autonomic nervous system has sympathetic and parasympathetic branches.

◀ **Core Concept 9.2**

The autonomic nervous system has two branches called the **sympathetic nervous system** and the **parasympathetic nervous system**. Almost all organs and glands receive nerve impulses from both branches of the autonomic nervous system.

The sympathetic nervous system is activated under conditions of stress and results in a set of reactions characterized as the *fight-or-flight response*. The parasympathetic nervous system is activated under nonstressful conditions and results in reactions characterized as

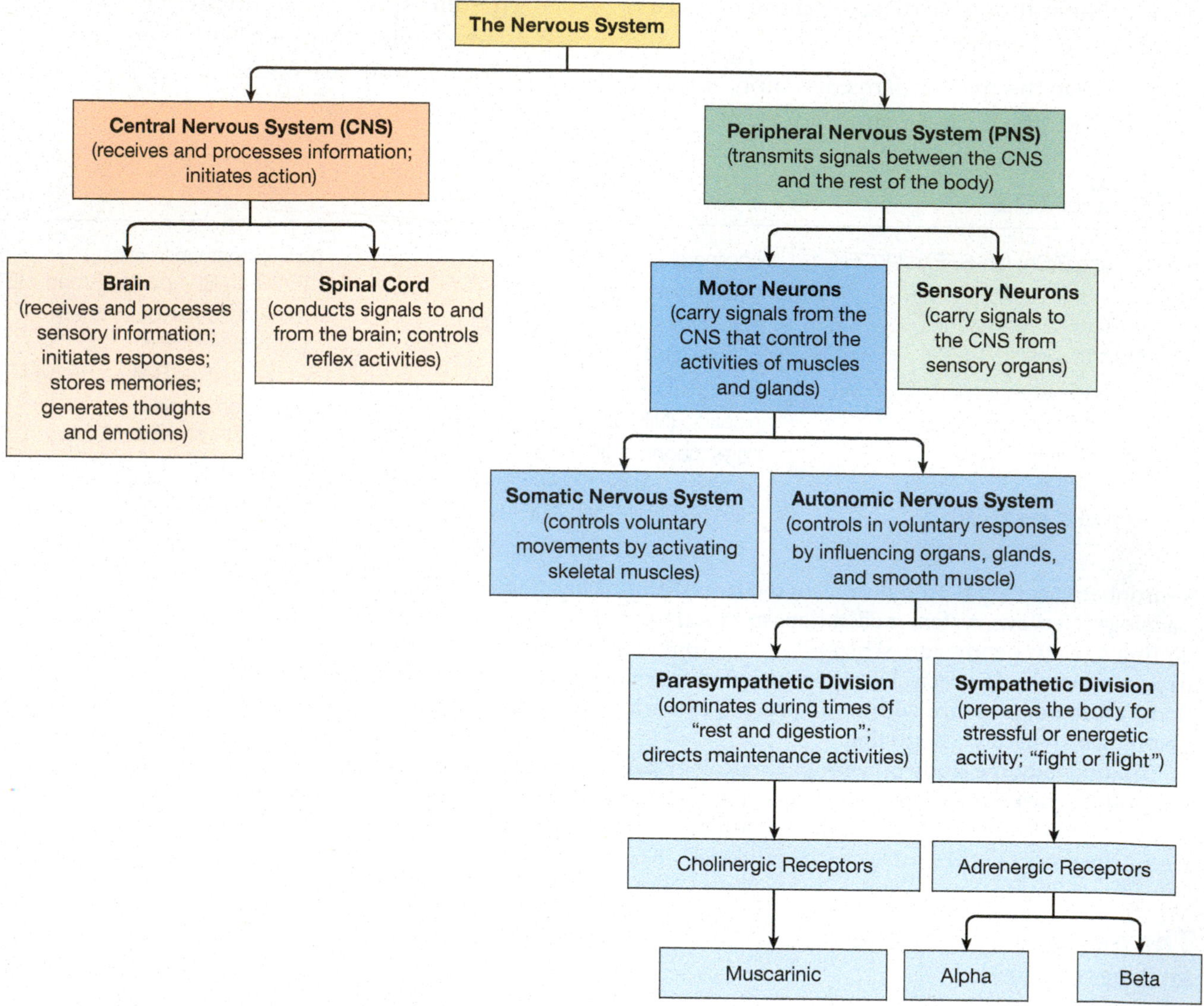

FIGURE 9.1 Functional divisions of the nervous system.

the *rest-and-digest response.* Most of the reactions of the sympathetic branch are opposite to those of the parasympathetic branch. For example, activation of sympathetic nerves increases heart rate, whereas activation of parasympathetic nerves decreases heart rate. The major actions of the two branches are shown in Figure 9.2. It is essential to learn these actions early in the study of pharmacology because knowledge of autonomic effects is used to predict the actions and adverse effects of many drugs.

CONCEPT REVIEW 9.1

- How would a person who is engaging in stressful or energetic activity benefit from the sympathetic effects of bronchodilation, slowed GI motility, and pupil dilation?

Core Concept 9.3 ▶ Synapses are common junction sites of drug action.

The basic functional unit of the nervous system is the nerve cell or *neuron.* For information to be transmitted throughout the nervous system, neurons must communicate with each other and with muscles and glands. A nerve impulse travels along a neuron to an area at the end of the neuron called the *synapse.* The synapse contains a space called the *synaptic cleft*, which must be crossed in order for impulses to reach the next neuron. The neuron generating the original impulse is called the *presynaptic neuron.* The nerve on the other side of the synapse, waiting to receive the impulse, is called the *postsynaptic neuron.* This basic structure is shown in Figure 9.3.

pre = *before*
post = *after*
synaptic = *relating to the synapse*

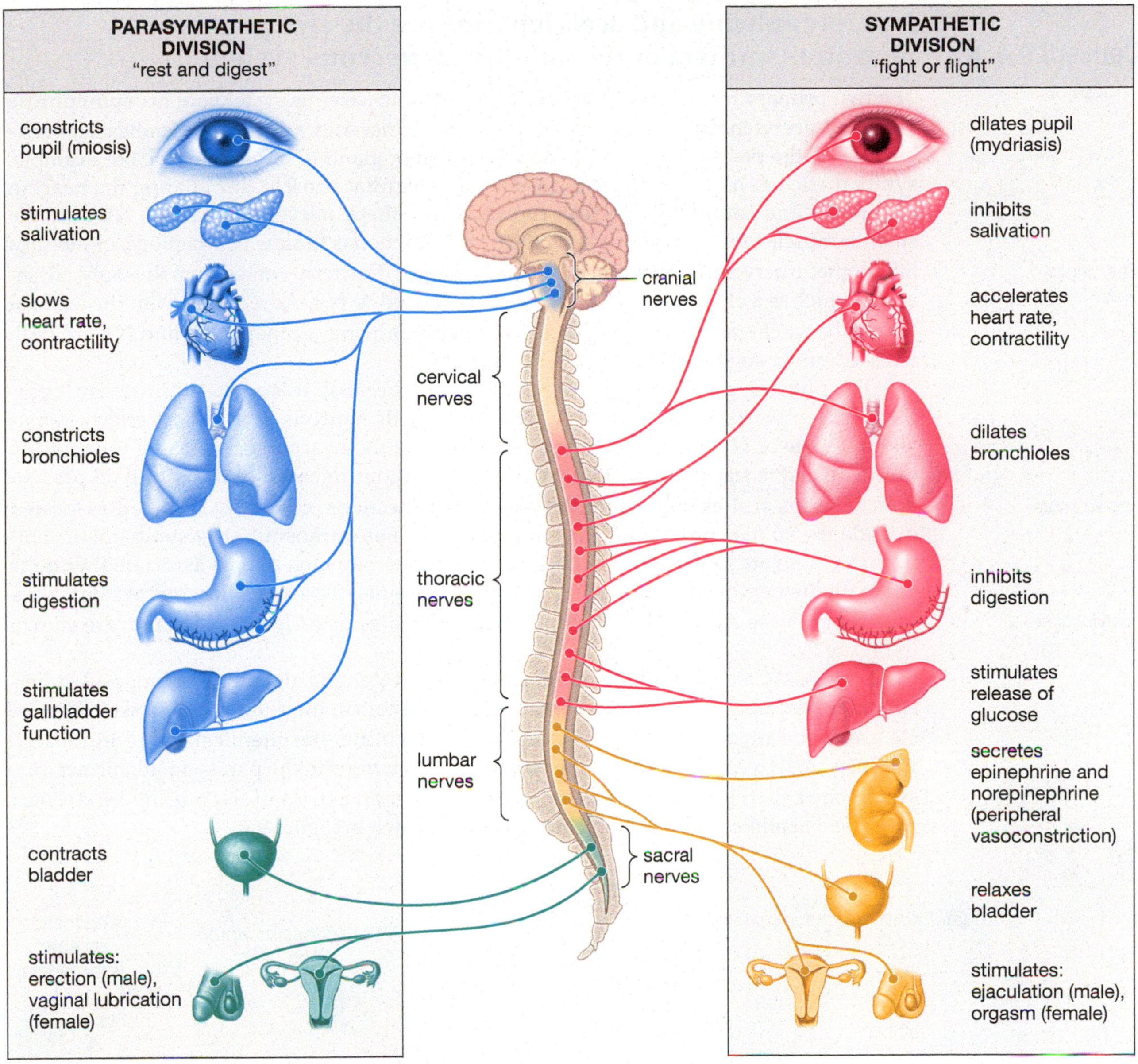

PARASYMPATHETIC DIVISION
"rest and digest"
constricts pupil (miosis)
stimulates salivation
slows heart rate, contractility
constricts bronchioles
stimulates digestion
stimulates gallbladder function
contracts bladder
stimulates: erection (male), vaginal lubrication (female)
cranial nerves
cervical nerves
thoracic nerves
lumbar nerves
sacral nerves
SYMPATHETIC DIVISION
"fight or flight"
dilates pupil (mydriasis)
inhibits salivation
accelerates heart rate, contractility
dilates bronchioles
inhibits digestion
stimulates release of glucose
secretes epinephrine and norepinephrine (peripheral vasoconstriction)
relaxes bladder
stimulates: ejaculation (male), orgasm (female)

FIGURE 9.2 Effects of the parasympathetic and sympathetic nervous systems.

Preganglionic neuron
Postganglionic neuron
Ganglionic synapse
Target tissue
Ventral spinal cord

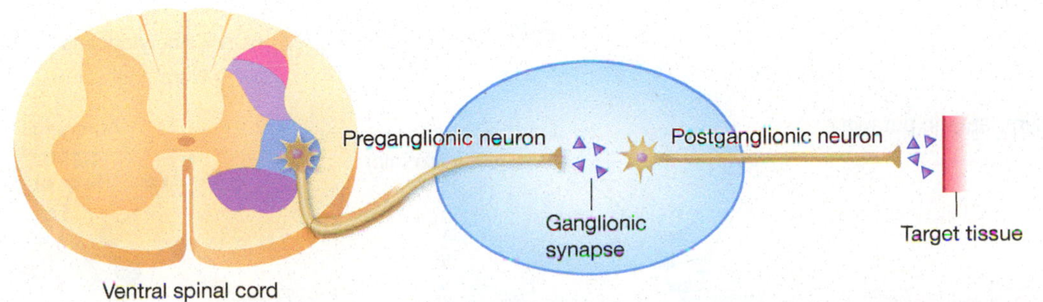

FIGURE 9.3 Basic structure of the autonomic pathway.

Chemicals called *neurotransmitters* allow nerve impulses to cross the synaptic cleft. Neurotransmitters are released into the synaptic cleft when the nerve impulse reaches the end of a presynaptic neuron. The neurotransmitter travels across the synaptic cleft to reach receptors on the postsynaptic neuron, which then regenerates the impulse. Many different types of neurotransmitters are located throughout the nervous system, each related to distinct functions. *Many drugs are identical to or have the same general structure as neurotransmitters.* Drugs alter autonomic function by either blocking or enhancing the activity of autonomic neurotransmitters.

Core Concept 9.4 ▶

Norepinephrine and acetylcholine are the two primary neurotransmitters in the autonomic nervous system.

The two primary neurotransmitters of the autonomic nervous system are **norepinephrine (NE)** and **acetylcholine (ACh)**. In the sympathetic nervous system, NE is released at the junction of the postsynaptic neuron and the organ or gland to be acted upon. For example, sympathetic nerves in the heart release NE onto cardiac muscle, stimulating the heart to beat faster and contract with greater force. Sympathetic nerves also release NE onto the smooth muscle lining of the digestive tract, and its action is to slow contractions, or motility. Sympathetic nerves are sometimes called **adrenergic**. This term comes from the word adrenaline, which is a chemical in the body closely related to NE. Adrenaline from the adrenal glands has a chemical structure identical to **epinephrine**. Epinephrine and NE are both released under conditions of extreme stress.

adren = *adrenal gland (adrenaline)*

The physiology of ACh is more complicated because it is released in several locations. When released at the ends of parasympathetic neurons, it produces effects generally opposite of NE, such as slowing the activity of the heart and increasing the motility of the digestive tract. ACh is also the neurotransmitter released at the end of all presynaptic neurons at sites called **ganglia**, which are collections of neuronal cell bodies located outside the spinal cord. In addition, ACh is also a neurotransmitter of sympathetic neurons that activate sweat glands; this is a unique case in which ACh is associated with the sympathetic nervous system rather than just the parasympathetic nervous system. Neurons that release ACh are called **cholinergic**. The sites of ACh and NE action are shown in Figure 9.4.

ganglia = *nerve knots*

cholin = *acetylcholine*
erg = *work*
ic = *relating to*

Because ACh can stimulate receptors both at the ganglia and at the organ level, different names are assigned to these receptors. ACh receptors in the ganglia and in skeletal muscle are called **nicotinic** receptors, named after nicotine, the chemical found in tobacco products. ACh receptors at the end of postsynaptic neurons in the parasympathetic nervous system are called **muscarinic** receptors, named after an extract of the mushroom *Amanita muscaria*. Nicotinic and muscarinic receptors are shown in Figure 9.4.

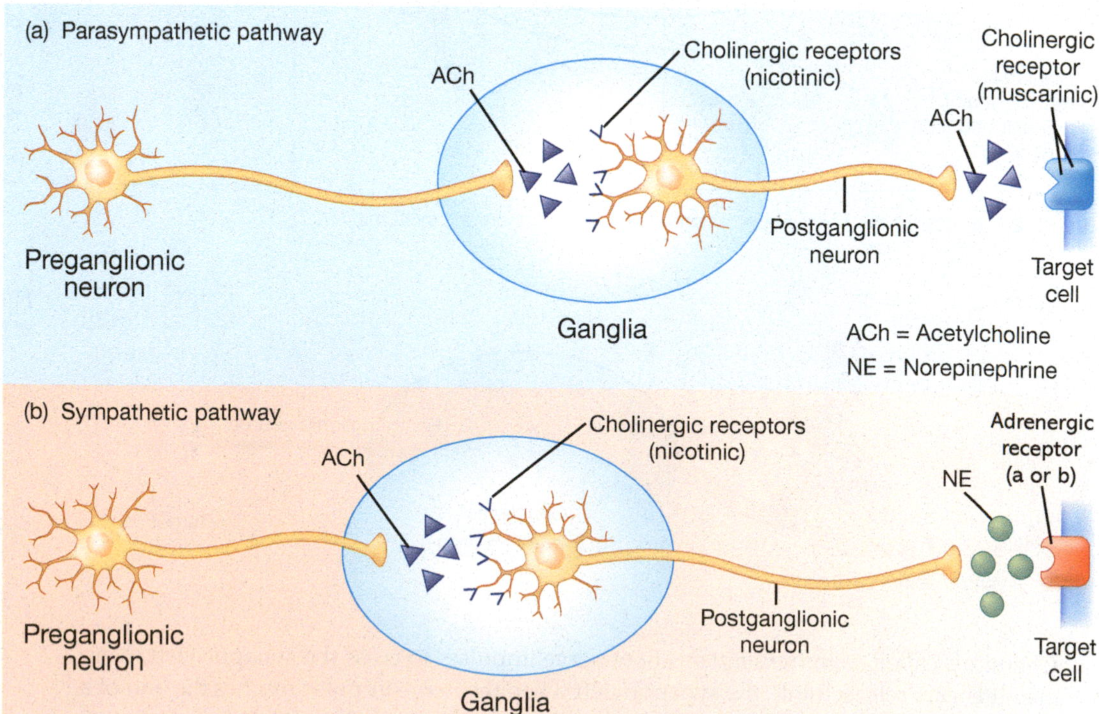

FIGURE 9.4 Acetylcholine (ACh) receptors in the ganglia and skeletal muscles (not shown here) are called *nicotinic*. ACh receptors at the ends of postganglionic neurons in the parasympathetic pathway are called *muscarinic*. Norepinephrine (NE) receptors are adrenergic receptors (α and β) in the sympathetic pathway.

Source: From *Pharmacology: Connections to Nursing Practice*, 3e by Michael Patrick Adams; Carol Urban. Copyright © 2015 by Pearson Education, Inc.

Table 9.1 Types of Autonomic Receptors

Neurotransmitter	Receptor	Primary Locations	Responses
Acetylcholine (cholinergic)	Muscarinic	Parasympathetic target: organs other than the heart	Stimulation of smooth muscle contractions and gland secretions
		Heart	Decrease in heart rate and force of contraction
	Nicotinic	Cell bodies of postganglionic neurons (sympathetic and parasympathetic pathways)	Stimulation of smooth muscle contractions and gland secretions
Norepinephrine (adrenergic)	Alpha_1	All sympathetic target organs except the heart	Constriction of blood vessels, dilation of pupils
	Alpha_2	Presynaptic adrenergic neuron terminals	Inhibition of norepinephrine release
	Beta_1	Heart and kidneys	Increase in heart rate and force of contraction; release of renin
	Beta_2	All sympathetic target organs except the heart	Inhibition of smooth muscle contractions
	Beta_3	Adipose tissue	Breakdown of fat
		Bladder	Suppress emptying of bladder

adipose = *fat*

NE receptors are of two basic subtypes: **alpha (α)-receptors** and **beta (β)-receptors.** *Alpha* and *beta* are Greek letters commonly used in naming chemical and scientific compounds. These receptors are further subdivided into beta_1, beta_2, beta_3, alpha_1, and alpha_2. Drugs may be selective and affect only one type of NE receptor, or they may affect all receptors. The type of response depends on the specific type of receptor that is activated. Drugs may also affect one type of receptor at low doses and begin to affect other receptors when the dose is increased. Table 9.1 shows a list of receptors and expected autonomic responses when receptors are activated.

Autonomic drugs are classified according to the receptors that they stimulate or block.

◀ **Core Concept 9.5**

Because they can block or activate either the sympathetic or parasympathetic nervous system, autonomic drugs are classified based on one of four possible actions:

sympatho = *sympathetic*
parasympatho = *parasympathetic*
mimetic = *to mimic*
lytic = *to undo*

1. *Activation of the sympathetic nervous system.* These drugs are called **adrenergic drugs** or **sympathomimetics**. They produce the classic symptoms of the fight-or-flight response.
2. *Activation of the parasympathetic nervous system.* These drugs are called **cholinergic drugs** or **parasympathomimetics** and produce the classic symptoms of the rest-and-digest response.
3. *Inhibition of the sympathetic nervous system.* These drugs are called **adrenergic blockers** or **sympatholytics** and produce actions opposite to those of the sympathomimetics.
4. *Inhibition of the parasympathetic nervous system.* These drugs are called **cholinergic blockers** or **anticholinergics** and produce actions opposite to those of the parasympathomimetics.

Students beginning their study of pharmacology will quickly learn that the actions and terminologies of autonomic drugs are very important. It is necessary to learn each drug class very well because the actions of other drug classes are logical extensions of the first. For example, both the adrenergic drugs and the cholinergic blockers increase heart rate and dilate the pupils. The other two drug classes, the cholinergic drugs and the adrenergic blockers, have the opposite effects of slowing heart rate and constricting the pupils. Mastering actions and terminologies of autonomic drugs will reap rewards later when the drugs are applied to various systems. See Table 9.2 for a quick review of the autonomic drug classes.

Table 9.2 Review of Autonomic Drug Classes

	Stimulation	Inhibition
Parasympathetic Nervous System	Cholinergic drugs (parasympathomimetics)	Cholinergic blockers (anticholinergics)
Sympathetic Nervous System	Adrenergic drugs (sympathomimetics)	Adrenergic blockers (sympatholytics)

Core Concept 9.6 ▶

Cholinergic drugs have few therapeutic uses because of their numerous adverse effects.

Remember the term *cholinergic* refers to neurons having ACh as the neurotransmitter. Cholinergic drugs or parasympathomimetics mimic actions of the parasympathetic nervous system. These drugs are associated with rest-and-digest responses. Because of their high potential for serious adverse effects, direct-acting cholinergic drugs are used only in a clinical setting. For instance, in ophthalmology, they are used to reduce intraocular pressure in patients with glaucoma (see Chapter 38). Others are used after anesthesia to stimulate the smooth muscles of the bowel or urinary tract. Potential adverse effects are increased salivation, sweating, abdominal cramps, and hypotension.

Indirect-acting cholinergic drugs, or drugs that inhibit the important enzyme acetylcholinesterase, have the same physiologic actions and adverse effects as direct-acting drugs including increased gland activity, sweating, increased muscle activity, and lowered heart rate. Acetylcholinesterase inhibitors facilitate the effects of the natural neurotransmitter ACh. Therefore, neostigmine (Prostigmin) and physostigmine (Antilirium) can induce actions in the body associated with the rest-and-digest response (see Figure 9.2).

Several drugs in this class are used for their effects on ACh receptors *in skeletal muscle* rather than for their parasympathetic action. For example, myasthenia gravis is an autoimmune disorder marked by destruction of cholinergic receptors found on the membranes of skeletal muscle tissue. Administration of pyridostigmine (Mestinon), neostigmine (Prostigmin), and other drugs (Table 9.3) will stimulate skeletal muscle contraction or temporarily help to restore the severe muscle weakness found in this disease. Because several drugs useful in treating Alzheimer disease are structurally similar to myasthenia drugs, the table includes drugs such as donepezil (Aricept), galantamine (Razadyne), and rivastigmine (Exelon). These drugs increase the amount of ACh binding to receptors located *within the brain* (see Chapter 13). Thus, cholinergic drugs may have effects in both the PNS *and* CNS.

Nerve agents (see Chapter 1) such as sarin and organophosphate insecticides are chemicals that inhibit acetylcholinesterase enzyme in the synaptic cleft throughout the entire

Table 9.3 Cholinergic Drugs (Parasympathomimetics)

Type	Drug	Primary Uses
Direct acting	Pr bethanechol (Urecholine)	Stimulation of urination
	cevimeline (Evoxac)	Treatment of dry mouth
	pilocarpine (Isopto Carpine, Ocusert, Salagen)	Glaucoma, treatment of dry mouth
Indirect acting (inhibitors of cholinesterase enzyme)	ambenonium (Mytelase)	Myasthenia gravis
	donepezil (Aricept) (see the Prototype Drug box in CC 13.5)	Alzheimer disease
	edrophonium (Tensilon)	Diagnosis of myasthenia gravis
	galantamine (Razadyne)	Alzheimer disease
	neostigmine (Prostigmin)	Myasthenia gravis
	physostigmine (Antilirium)	Cholinergic-blocking toxicity
	pyridostigmine (Mestinon, Regonol)	Myasthenia gravis
	rivastigmine (Exelon)	Alzheimer disease

nervous system. These agents can cause widespread and toxic parasympathomimetic effects. Symptoms are severe salivation, reduced heart rate, muscle twitching, uncontrolled urination and defecation, confusion, convulsions, hypotension, and even death. In an emergency, if nerve agents are released, Mark I injector kits containing the anticholinergic drug atropine or related medications are used to counteract toxic effects. Atropine blocks the attachment of ACh to receptor sites and prevents overstimulation caused by harmful nerve agents. In instances where too much anticholinergic activity occurs, as with atropine overdose or ingestion of poisonous substances, physostigmine (Antilirium) can be used as an antidote to counter adverse effects resulting from intense cholinergic blockade.

Prototype Drug: Pr *Bethanechol (Urecholine)*

Therapeutic Class: Urinary retention (incomplete bladder emptying) treatment **Pharmacologic Class:** Cholinergic receptor drug, parasympathomimetic

Actions and Uses: Bethanechol is a direct-acting parasympathomimetic that interacts with ACh receptors to cause actions typical of parasympathetic stimulation. It affects mostly the digestive and urinary tracts, where it stimulates smooth muscle contraction. These actions are particularly useful in stimulating the return of normal gastrointestinal (GI) and urinary tract function following general anesthesia.

Adverse Effects and Interactions: The adverse effects of bethanechol are parasympathetic actions: increased salivation, sweating, abdominal cramping, and hypotension that can lead to fainting. It should not be given to patients with suspected urinary or intestinal obstruction or those with active asthma.

Do not use with ambenonium, neostigmine, and other cholinergic drugs; mecamylamine (blocker of ACh at the ganglia) may cause abdominal symptoms and hypotension. Procainamide, quinidine, atropine, and epinephrine reduce the effects of bethanechol.

Nursing Process Focus Patients Receiving Direct- and Indirect-Acting Cholinergic Drug Therapy

ASSESSMENT	POTENTIAL NURSING DIAGNOSES*
Prior to administration: • Obtain a complete health history including cardiovascular, respiratory, GI, urinary, vision and neuromuscular conditions, allergies, and drug history for possible drug interactions. • Acquire the results of a complete physical examination including vital signs, height, weight, bowel sounds, ability to urinate, mental status, muscle strength, chewing ability, and signs such as ptosis and diplopia. • Evaluate laboratory blood findings: complete blood count (CBC), chemistry, renal and liver function studies.	• *Urinary Incontinence* related to adverse effects of direct-acting drugs • *Impaired Urinary Elimination* related to adverse effects of direct-acting drugs • *Impaired Physical Mobility* related to adverse effects of indirect-acting drugs • *Deficient Knowledge* related to a lack of information about drug therapy • *Noncompliance* related to adverse effects of drug therapy • *Risk for Injury* related to adverse effects of drug therapy

PLANNING: PATIENT GOALS AND EXPECTED OUTCOMES

The patient will:

- Experience therapeutic effects: direct acting (an increase in bowel and bladder function and tone; regain normal pattern of elimination).
- Experience therapeutic effects: indirect acting (a decrease in myasthenia gravis symptoms such as muscle weakness, ptosis, and diplopia).
- Be free from or experience minimal adverse effects from drug therapy.
- Verbalize an understanding of the drug's use, adverse effects, and required precautions.

IMPLEMENTATION

Interventions and (Rationales)	Patient Education/Discharge Planning
All Cholinergic drugs	
• Monitor for therapeutic effects dependent on the reason drug is being given. (Improvement in mental status, urinary output, and muscle strength indicates effectiveness of drug therapy.)	• Encourage patient and caregivers to practice support measures to maximize therapeutic effects, e.g., adequate rest periods and assistance with activities of daily living (ADLs).

(*Continued*)

Nursing Process Focus (*continued*)

Interventions and (Rationales)	Patient Education/Discharge Planning
• Monitor for adverse effects and notify healthcare provider if pulse drops below 60 beats per minute or blood pressure is below approved parameters. (These drugs may decrease heart rate and blood pressure, which may indicate cholinergic crisis that requires atropine.)	• Instruct the patient to immediately report any of the following symptoms to the healthcare provider: nausea, vomiting, diarrhea, rash, jaundice, change in color of stool, feeling faint, tremors, or changes in behavior.
• Monitor liver enzymes at the start of therapy and weekly for six weeks. (Drugs may cause liver toxicity.)	• Instruct the patient to adhere to laboratory testing regimen for serum blood level tests of liver enzymes as directed.
• Administer medication correctly and evaluate the patient's knowledge of proper administration. (Proper administration helps to prevent complications.)	Instruct the patient to: • Take the drug as directed on regular schedule to maintain serum levels and control symptoms. • Not chew or crush sustained-release tablets. • Take oral cholinergic drugs on an empty stomach to lessen incidence of nausea and vomiting and to increase absorption.
DIRECT ACTING	
• Monitor intake and output ratio. Palpate the abdomen for bladder distention. (Frequent monitoring will detect early signs of therapeutic or adverse effects. Drug onset of action is within 60 minutes, stimulating the smooth muscle of the bladder to contract and causing urination.)	• Advise the patient to be near bathroom facilities after taking these drugs.
• Provide for eye comfort such as adequately lighted areas and continue to monitor vision. (A cholinergic effect may cause blurred vision and difficulty seeing in low light.)	Advise the patient: • That blurred vision is a possible adverse effect and to take appropriate safety precautions. • Not to drive or engage in potentially hazardous activities until the drug's effects are known.
• Help patients to rise from a lying to sitting or standing position until drug effects are determined. (Cholinergic drugs may cause orthostatic hypotension.)	• Instruct the patient to avoid abrupt position changes and to avoid prolonged standing in one place.
INDIRECT ACTING	
• Monitor neuromuscular status including muscle strength, ptosis, diplopia, and chewing. (Improvement demonstrates therapeutic effects.)	• Instruct patients to report to their healthcare provider any difficulty with vision or swallowing.
• Schedule the medication around mealtimes. Check drug reference material on administration with or without food. (Some drugs should be taken with food and others on an empty stomach.)	• Instruct the patient about the appropriate time to take medications.
• Schedule activities to avoid fatigue. (Excess fatigue can lead to cholinergic crisis.)	Instruct the patient to: • Plan activities according to muscle strength and fatigue. • Take frequent rest periods to avoid fatigue.
• Monitor for muscle weakness after dose is given. (Depending on time of onset, it may indicate cholinergic crisis—overdose or myasthenic crisis—underdose.)	Instruct the patient to: • Report any severe muscle weakness that occurs 1 hour after administration of medication. • Report any muscle weakness that occurs three or more hours after medication administration because this is a major symptom of myasthenic crisis.

EVALUATION OF OUTCOME CRITERIA

Evaluate the effectiveness of drug therapy by confirming that patient goals and expected outcomes have been met (see "Planning"). *See Table 9.3 for a list of drugs to which these nursing actions apply.*

*Herdman, T.H. & Kamitsuru, S. (Eds.), *Nursing Diagnoses: Definitions & Classification* 2015–2017. Copyright © 2014, 1994–2014 NANDA International. Used by arrangement by John Wiley & Sons, Inc. Companion website: www.wiley.com/go/nursingdiagnoses.

Cholinergic blockers are most commonly used to dry secretions and to treat asthma.

◀ **Core Concept 9.7**

Cholinergic blockers are drugs that have actions opposite those of the parasympathetic nervous system. They mimic the fight-or-flight response. Although the term *anticholinergic* is commonly used, a better term for this class of drugs would be *muscarinic blockers*, which more accurately describes blockade of the muscarinic receptor. Most therapeutic uses of the cholinergic blockers relate to their autonomic actions: dilation of pupils, increase in heart rate, drying of secretions, treating an overactive bladder (incontinence), and dilation of the bronchi. Cholinergic blockers have been widely used in medicine for many disorders. A relatively high incidence of adverse effects and the development of safer, and sometimes more effective, medications has limited the current use of cholinergic blockers. For example, cholinergic blockers were once drugs of choice in treating peptic ulcers, but they have been replaced by proton-pump inhibitors and H_2-receptor blockers (see Chapter 31). Two important adverse effects that limit their usefulness include tachycardia (fast heart rate) and the tendency to cause urinary retention in men with prostate disorders.

incontinence = *not controlled (usually digestive or urinary)*

tachy = *rapid*
cardia = *heart beat*

Some cholinergic blockers are used for their effects *in the CNS*, rather than their autonomic actions. Scopolamine (Hyoscine, Transderm-Scop) is used to produce sedation and prevent motion sickness (see Chapter 7); benztropine (Cogentin) and trihexyphenidyl (Artane) are prescribed to reduce the muscular tremor and rigidity associated with Parkinson disease (see Chapter 13). Some of the more common cholinergic blockers and their primary uses are listed in Table 9.4.

Table 9.4 Cholinergic-Blocking Drugs (Anticholinergics)

Drug	Primary Uses
aclidinium (Tudorza Pressair)	Chronic obstructive pulmonary disease (COPD)
Pr atropine (AtroPen)	Poisoning with anticholinesterase agents; to increase heart rate, dilate pupils
benztropine (Cogentin) (see the Prototype Drug box in Core Concept 13.3)	Parkinson disease, neuroleptic side effects
cyclopentolate (Cyclogyl)	Dilation of pupils
darifenacin (Enablex)	Overactive bladder
dicyclomine (Bentyl, others)	Irritable bowel syndrome
donepezil (Aricept)	Alzheimer disease
fesoterodine (Toviaz)	Prevention of urgent, frequent, or uncontrolled urination
glycopyrrolate (Cuvposa, Robinul)	Production of a dry field prior to anesthesia, reduced salivation, peptic ulcers
ipratropium (Atrovent)	Asthma
methscopolamine (Pamine)	Motion sickness, ulcers
oxybutynin (Ditropan, Oxytrol)	Incontinence
propantheline (Pro-Banthine)	Irritable bowel syndrome, peptic ulcer
scopolamine (Hyoscine, Transderm-Scop)	Motion sickness, irritable bowel syndrome, adjunct to anesthesia
solifenacin (Vesicare)	Overactive bladder
tiotropium (Spiriva)	Asthma
tolterodine (Detrol)	Overactive bladder with symptoms of urge urinary incontinence, urgency, and frequency
trihexyphenidyl	Parkinson disease
tropicamide (Mydriacyl, Tropicacyl)	Mydriasis and cycloplegia for diagnostic procedures
trospium (Sanctura)	Overactive bladder

mydriasis = *prolonged pupil dilation*
cycloplegia = *ciliary eye muscle paralysis*

Prototype Drug: Atropine (Atropen)

Therapeutic Class: Antidote for anticholinesterase poisoning, antidysrhythmic, mydriatic (pupil dilating drug)

Pharmacologic Class: Anticholinergic, cholinergic receptor blocker

Actions and Uses: Atropine is a natural product found in the deadly nightshade plant, or *Atropa belladonna*. By blocking ACh (muscarinic) receptors, atropine causes symptoms of the fight-or-flight response, such as increased heart rate, bronchodilation, decreased motility in the GI tract, mydriasis (pupil dilation), and decreased secretions from glands. Throughout history, atropine has been used for a variety of purposes, although its use has declined because of the development of safer, more effective medications. Atropine is used to treat hypermotility diseases of the GI tract such as irritable bowel syndrome, to suppress secretions during surgical procedures, to increase the heart rate in patients with a slow heartbeat bradycardia), to dilate the pupil during eye examinations, and to cause bronchodilation in patients with asthma. Atropine is an antidote for poisoning with nerve gas agents and organophosphate insecticides.

Adverse Effects and Interactions: The adverse effects of atropine limit its therapeutic usefulness. Adverse effects include dry mouth, constipation, urinary retention, and an increased heart rate. Atropine is usually contraindicated in patients with glaucoma because the drug may increase pressure within the eyeball.

Use of amantadine, antihistamines, tricyclic antidepressants, quinidine, disopyramide, and procainamide can increase the anticholinergic effects of atropine. Use with levodopa may decrease the effects of the latter. The antipsychotic effects of phenothiazines are generally decreased.

Nursing Process Focus Patients Receiving Cholinergic Blocker (Anticholinergic) Therapy

ASSESSMENT

Prior to administration:

- Obtain a complete health history including cardiovascular, respiratory, vision and neurological conditions, allergies, and drug history for possible drug interactions.
- Evaluate laboratory blood findings: CBC, chemistry, renal and liver function studies.
- Acquire the results of a complete physical examination including heart rate and rhythm, blood pressure, temperature, weight, bowel sounds, and elimination patterns.

POTENTIAL NURSING DIAGNOSES*

- *Deficient Knowledge* related to a lack of information about drug therapy
- *Decreased Cardiac Output* related to adverse effects of drug therapy
- *Impaired Oral Mucous Membranes* related to decrease in exocrine secretions
- *Constipation* related to adverse effect of drug therapy
- *Urinary Retention* related to adverse effects of drug therapy
- *Risk for Imbalanced Body Temperature* related to inhibited sweat gland secretions
- *Risk for Injury* related to neurological effects of medication

PLANNING: PATIENT GOALS AND EXPECTED OUTCOMES

The patient will:

- Experience therapeutic effects (a decrease in symptoms for which the medication is prescribed).
- Be free from or experience minimal adverse effects from drug therapy.
- Verbalize an understanding of the drug's use, adverse effects, and required precautions.

IMPLEMENTATION

Interventions and (Rationales)	Patient Education/Discharge Planning
• Closely monitor heart function and notify the healthcare provider if blood pressure or pulse exceeds established parameters or dysrhythmias develop. (Anticholinergic drugs stimulate heart rate, increasing the chance for dysrhythmias.)	• Instruct the patient to monitor vital signs, ensuring proper use of home equipment.
• Observe for adverse effects such as drowsiness, blurred vision, tachycardia, dry mouth, constipation, urinary hesitancy or retention, and decreased sweating. (Adverse effects are the result of the blockage of muscarinic receptors; can also be caused by an overdose of medication.)	Instruct the patient to: • Immediately report adverse effects such as palpitations, shortness of breath, or drowsiness to the healthcare provider. • Avoid driving and hazardous activities until effects of drugs are known.

Interventions and (Rationales)	**Patient Education/Discharge Planning**
• Provide comfort measures. For dry mucous membranes, apply lubricant to moisten lips and oral mucosa, and assist in rinsing mouth. Use artificial tears for dry eyes, as needed. (Adverse effects of drug therapy can include dry mucous membranes and photosensitivity.)	Instruct the patient to: • Use oral rinses, sugarless gum or candy, and frequent oral hygiene to help relieve dry mouth. • Avoid alcohol-containing mouthwashes that can further dry oral tissue. • Wear sunglasses to decrease sensitivity to bright light.
• Minimize exposure to heat or cold and strenuous exercise. (Cholinergic blockers can inhibit sweat gland secretions due to direct blockade of the muscarinic receptors on the sweat glands. Sweating is necessary for patients to cool down, so this inhibition of sweating can increase their risk for hyperthermia.)	• Advise the patient to limit activity outside when the temperature is hot. Strenuous activity in a hot environment may cause heat stroke.
• Monitor intake and output ratio. Palpate the abdomen for bladder distention. (Cholinergic blockers can cause urinary retention.)	• Instruct the patient to notify the healthcare provider if difficulty in voiding occurs.
• Monitor patients routinely for abdominal distention and auscultate for bowel sounds. (Cholinergic blockers may decrease tone and motility of the intestinal tract.)	• Advise the patient to increase fluid intake and add bulk to the diet, if constipation becomes a problem.
EVALUATION OF OUTCOME CRITERIA	
Evaluate the effectiveness of drug therapy by confirming that patient goals and expected outcomes have been met (see "Planning"). *See Table 9.4 for a list of drugs to which these nursing actions apply.*	

*Herdman, T.H. & Kamitsuru, S. (Eds.), *Nursing Diagnoses: Definitions & Classification* 2015–2017. Copyright © 2014, 1994–2014 NANDA International. Used by arrangement by John Wiley & Sons, Inc. Companion website: www.wiley.com/go/nursingdiagnoses.

Adrenergic drugs are primarily used for their effects on the heart, bronchial tree, and nasal passages.

◀ **Core Concept 9.8**

Adrenergic drugs, or sympathomimetics, have actions similar to those produced by activation of the sympathetic nervous system (the fight-or-flight response). Again, remember that the term *adrenergic* refers to neurons (nerve terminals) or body tissues (adrenal glands) containing adrenaline-like substances. The adrenergic drugs produce many of the same effects as the cholinergic blockers. However, because the sympathetic neurotransmitters activate two types of receptors, alpha- and beta-, the actions of the adrenergics have wider therapeutic applications.

Although most effects of adrenergics are predictable based on their autonomic actions, their primary effects depend on which adrenergic receptors are stimulated. Drugs such as phenylephrine (Neo-Synephrine) stimulate $alpha_1$-receptors and are often used to dry nasal secretions. Because $beta_1$-receptors are predominant in the heart, $beta_1$-drugs such as dobutamine (Dobutrex) are used to stimulate the heart rate and increase its strength of contraction. $Beta_2$-drugs such as albuterol (Proventil) cause bronchodilation and are useful in the treatment of asthma.

Some adrenergic drugs are nonselective, stimulating more than one type of adrenergic receptor. For example, epinephrine stimulates all types of adrenergic receptors and is used for cardiac arrest and asthma. Pseudoephedrine (Sudafed, others) stimulates both $alpha_1$- and $beta_2$-receptors and is used orally as a nasal decongestant. Isoproterenol (Isuprel) stimulates both $beta_1$- and $beta_2$-receptors and is used to increase the rate, force, and conduction speed of the heart and, occasionally, to treat asthma. The nonselective drugs generally also cause a wider variety of adverse effects all over the body.

Some of the more commonly used adrenergic drugs are shown in Table 9.5. Most drugs in this class are presented in other chapters of this book. For prototypes of drugs in this class, see epinephrine (Adrenalin) and norepinephrine (Levophed) in Chapter 23, and oxymetazoline (Afrin, others) and salmeterol (Serevent) in Chapter 30.

nonselective = *not specifically directed*

hyper = *elevated*
tension = *blood pressure*

anaphylactic = *itchy rash, low blood pressure, swollen throat*

obstructive = *narrowed*
pulmonary = *lung passage*

dys = *abnormal*
rhythmias = *heart rhythms*

Table 9.5 Adrenergic Drugs (Sympathomimetics)

Drug	Primary Receptor Subtype	Primary Uses
albuterol (Proventil, Ventolin, VoSpire)	$Beta_2$	Asthma
clonidine (Catapres)	$Alpha_2$ in CNS	Hypertension
dobutamine (Dobutrex)	$Beta_1$	Cardiac stimulant
dopamine (Intropin) (see the Prototype Drug box in Core Concept 22.5)	$Alpha_1$ and $beta_1$	Shock
droxidopa (Northera)	$Beta_3$	Orthostatic hypotension
epinephrine (Adrenalin, others) (see the Prototype Drug box in Core Concept 22.6)	Alpha and beta	Cardiac arrest, asthma; anaphylactic and allergic reactions
formoterol (Foradil, Performist)	$Beta_2$	Asthma, COPD
isoproterenol (Isuprel)	$Beta_1$ and $beta_2$	Asthma, dysrhythmias, heart failure
metaproterenol	$Beta_2$	Asthma
methyldopa (Aldomet)	$Alpha_2$ in CNS	Hypertension
midodrine (ProAmatine)	Alpha	Hypertension
mirabegron (Myrbetriq)	$Beta_3$	Urinary incontinence
norepinephrine (Levophed) (see the Prototype Drug box in Core Concept 22.4)	Alpha and $beta_1$	Shock
olodaterol (Striverdi, Respimat)	$Beta_2$	COPD
oxymetazoline (Afrin and others) (see the Prototype Drug box in Core Concept 30.6)	Alpha	Nasal congestion
Pr phenylephrine (Neo-Synephrine)	Alpha	Maintain blood pressure, nasal congestion
pseudoephedrine (Sudafed and others)	Alpha and beta	Nasal congestion
salmeterol (Serevent)	$Beta_2$	Asthma
terbutaline	$Beta_2$	Asthma

CONCEPT REVIEW 9.2

- Why do the adrenergic drugs produce many of the same symptoms as the cholinergic blockers?

Prototype Drug: Pr *Phenylephrine (Neo-Synephrine)*

Therapeutic Class: Nasal decongestant, mydriatic agent, antihypotensive **Pharmacologic Class:** Adrenergic drug, $alpha_1$-adrenergic drug

Actions and Uses: Phenylephrine is a selective alpha-adrenergic drug that is available in several formulations, including intranasal, ophthalmic, IM, subcutaneous, and IV. All of its actions and indications result from sympathetic stimulation. When applied intranasally by spray or drops, it reduces nasal congestion by constricting small blood vessels in the nasal mucosa. Applied topically to the eye during ophthalmic examinations, phenylephrine can dilate the pupil without causing significant paralysis of the eye muscles (cycloplegia). The parenteral administration of phenylephrine can reverse acute hypotension caused by spinal anesthesia or vascular shock. Because it lacks beta-adrenergic activity, it produces relatively few cardiac adverse effects at therapeutic doses. Its longer duration of activity and lack of significant cardiac effects gives phenylephrine some advantages over epinephrine or norepinephrine in treating acute hypotension.

Adverse Effects and Interactions: When used topically or intranasally, adverse effects are uncommon. Prolonged intranasal use can cause burning of the mucosa and rebound congestion. Ophthalmic preparations can cause narrow-angle glaucoma because of their mydriatic effect. High doses can cause reflex bradycardia due to the elevation of blood pressure caused by stimulation of $alpha_1$-receptors. When given parenterally, the drug should be used with caution in patients with advanced coronary artery disease or hypertension. Anxiety, restlessness, and tremor may occur due to the drug's stimulatory effect on the CNS. Patients with hyperthyroidism may experience a severe increase in basal metabolic rate, resulting in increased blood pressure and tachycardia. Drug interactions may occur with monoamine oxidase inhibitors (MAOIs), causing a hypertensive crisis. Increased effects may also occur with tricyclic antidepressants. This drug is incompatible with iron preparations (ferric salts).

BLACK BOX WARNING:
Severe reactions, including death, may occur with IV infusion even when appropriate dilution is used to avoid rapid diffusion. Therefore, restrict IV use for situations in which other routes are not feasible.

Nursing Process Focus Patients Receiving Adrenergic Drug Therapy

ASSESSMENT	POTENTIAL NURSING DIAGNOSES*
Prior to administration: • Obtain a complete health history including cardiovascular, respiratory, vision and liver conditions, allergies, and drug history for possible drug interactions. • Obtain data regarding treatment of nasal congestion and current status of nasal mucosa for changes such as excoriation or bleeding. • Acquire the results of a complete physical examination including vital signs, height, weight, cardiac and urinary output. • Evaluate laboratory blood findings: CBC, chemistry, renal and liver function studies.	• *Deficient Knowledge* related to a lack of information about drug therapy • *Decreased Cardiac Output* related to bradycardia (disorder) • *Ineffective Breathing Pattern* related to nasal congestion • *Disturbed Sleep Pattern* related to adrenergic stimulation and drug-induced excitation • *Risk for Decreased Cardiac Tissue Perfusion* related to bronchoconstriction (disorder) • *Risk for Injury* related to adverse effects of drug therapy

PLANNING: PATIENT GOALS AND EXPECTED OUTCOMES

The patient will:
- Experience therapeutic effects (a decrease in symptoms for which the drug is being given).
- Be free from or experience minimal adverse effects from drug therapy.
- Verbalize an understanding of the drug's use, adverse effects, and required precautions.
- Demonstrate proper nasal or ophthalmic medication instillation technique.

IMPLEMENTATION

Interventions and (Rationales)	Patient Education/Discharge Planning
• Administer medication correctly and evaluate the patient's knowledge of proper administration. If drug is being administered IV, closely monitor IV insertion sites for extravasation and use an infusion pump to deliver medication. Use a tuberculin syringe when administering subcutaneous doses that are extremely small. For metered-dose inhalation, shake the container well, and wait at least two minutes between medications. Instill only the prescribed number of drops when using ophthalmic solutions.	Instruct the patient to: • Use the drug as prescribed and not "double up" on doses. • Take the medication early in the day to avoid insomnia. • Keep drug on hand for emergencies if using rescue inhalers or epinephrine kits; notify healthcare provider immediately after use.
• Monitor the patient for adverse effects. (Adverse effects of adrenergic drugs may be serious and limit therapy.)	Instruct the patient to: • Immediately report shortness of breath, palpitations, dizziness, chest or arm pain or pressure, or other angina-like symptoms to the healthcare provider. • Consult the healthcare provider before attempting to use adrenergic drugs to treat nasal congestion or eye irritation. • Monitor blood pressure, pulse, and temperature to ensure proper use of home equipment.
• Monitor breathing patterns and observe for shortness of breath or audible wheezing. Provide supportive nursing measures such as proper positioning for patients with dyspnea. (Monitoring provides information about effects of medication. Patients with respiratory problems should consult their healthcare provider to ensure the correct medication is being used for their condition.)	Instruct the patient: • To immediately report any difficulty breathing. • With a history of asthma to consult a healthcare provider before using over-the-counter (OTC) drugs to treat nasal stuffiness.
• Observe the patient's responsiveness to light. (Some adrenergic drugs cause photosensitivity.)	• Instruct patients using ophthalmic adrenergic drugs that transient stinging and blurred vision on instillation is normal. Headache and/or brow pain may also occur.
• Provide eye comfort by reducing exposure to direct bright light in the environment; shield the eyes with a rolled washcloth or eye bandages for severe photosensitivity. (Adrenergic drugs can cause mydriasis and sensitivity to light.)	• Instruct the patient to avoid driving and other activities requiring visual acuity until blurring subsides.

(*Continued*)

Nursing Process Focus (*continued*)

Interventions and (Rationales)	Patient Education/Discharge Planning
• For patients receiving nasal adrenergic drugs, observe the nasal cavity. Monitor for rhinorrhea and epistaxis. (Vasoconstriction may cause transient stinging, excessive dryness, or bleeding.)	Instruct the patient to: • Observe the nasal cavity for signs of excoriation or bleeding before instilling nasal spray or drops; review procedure for safe instillation of nasal sprays or eyedrops. • Limit usage of OTC adrenergic drugs; inform the patient about rebound nasal congestion.

EVALUATION OF OUTCOME CRITERIA

Evaluate the effectiveness of drug therapy by confirming that patient goals and expected outcomes have been met (see "Planning"). *See Table 9.5 for a list of drugs to which these nursing actions apply.*

Core Concept 9.9 ▶ Adrenergic blockers are primarily used to treat hypertension, bronchial constriction, and nasal congestion.

Adrenergic blockers inhibit the actions of the sympathetic nervous system. These drugs produce many of the same responses as the cholinergic drugs, but they are more widely used. Because the sympathetic nervous system has alpha- and beta-receptors, the actions of adrenergic blockers are selective and have wide therapeutic applications. In fact, they are the most widely prescribed class of autonomic drugs. Many of the adrenergic blockers are shown in Table 9.6.

vaso = *smooth muscle (blood vessel)*
dilation = *enlargement of diameter*

hypo = *lowered*
tensive = *blood pressure*

Alpha-adrenergic blockers, or simply *alpha blockers*, are primarily used for their effects on vascular smooth muscle. By relaxing vascular smooth muscle in small arteries, $alpha_1$ blockers such as doxazosin (Cardura) cause vasodilation, which results in decreased blood pressure (hypotensive effect). Their primary use is in the treatment of hypertension, either alone or in combination with other drugs.

Table 9.6 Adrenergic-Blocking Drugs (Sympatholytics)

Drug	Primary Receptor Subtype	Primary Uses
acebutolol (Sectral)	$Beta_1$	Hypertension, dysrhythmias, angina
alfuzosin (UroXatral)	$Alpha_1$	Benign prostatic hyperplasia (BPH)
atenolol (Tenormin) (see the Drug Prototype box in Core Concept 21.6)	$Beta_1$	Hypertension, angina
betaxolol (Betaoptic, Kerlone)	$Beta_1$	Hypertension, glaucoma
carteolol (Cartrol)	$Beta_1$ and $beta_2$	Hypertension, glaucoma
carvedilol (Coreg) (see the Prototype Drug box in Core Concept 20.8)	$Alpha_1$, $beta_1$, and $beta_2$	Hypertension, heart failure
doxazosin (Cardura) (see the Prototype Drug box in Core Concept 19.10)	$Alpha_1$	Hypertension
esmolol (Brevibloc)	$Beta_1$	Hypertension, dysrhythmias
metoprolol (Lopressor, Toprol)	$Beta_1$	Hypertension, migraine prevention
nadolol (Corgard)	$Beta_1$ and $beta_2$	Hypertension
phentolamine (Regitine)	Alpha	Severe hypertension
Pr prazosin (Minipress)	$Alpha_1$	Hypertension
propranolol (Inderal, Innopran XL) (see the Prototype Drug box in Core Concept 23.7)	$Beta_1$ and $beta_2$	Hypertension, dysrhythmias, heart failure
silodosin (Rapaflo)	$Alpha_1$	BPH
sotalol (Betapace)	$Beta_1$ and $beta_2$	Dysrhythmias
tamsulosin (Flomax)	$Alpha_1$	BPH
terazosin (Hytrin)	$Alpha_1$	Hypertension
timolol (Blocadren, Timoptic) (see the Prototype Drug box in Core Concept 38.5)	$Beta_1$ and $beta_2$	Hypertension, angina, glaucoma

Some drugs in this class selectively block $beta_1$-receptors. Because $beta_1$-receptors are only present in the heart, the effects of drugs such as atenolol (Tenormin) are often called *cardioselective.* By slowing the heart rate, they lower blood pressure, which is their primary use.

Some beta blockers, such as propranolol (Inderal, InnoPran XL), are nonselective, blocking both $beta_1$- and $beta_2$-receptors. The nonselective beta blockers are used to treat hypertension, angina, and cardiac rhythm abnormalities. Their nonselective actions generally result in more adverse effects than the selective beta blockers. Prototypes of adrenergic blockers can be found for doxazosin (Cardura) in Chapter 19, carvedilol (Coreg) in Chapter 20, propranolol (Inderal, InnoPran XL) in Chapter 23, and atenolol (Tenormin) in Chapter 21.

cardio = *the heart*
selective = *directed (toward)*
benign = *gentle*
prostatic = *prostate-related*
hyperplasia = *enlargement*

angina = *chest pain*

CONCEPT REVIEW 9.3

- Both cholinergic drugs and adrenergic blockers produce similar actions. Why are adrenergic blockers used to treat hypertension, but cholinergic drugs are not used for this purpose?

Prototype Drug: *Prazosin (Minipress)*

Therapeutic Class: Antihypertensive **Pharmacologic Class:** Sympatholytic, $alpha_1$-adrenergic blocker

Actions and Uses: Prazosin is a selective $alpha_1$-adrenergic blocker that competes with NE at its receptors on vascular smooth muscle in arterioles and veins. Its major action is a rapid decrease in peripheral resistance that reduces blood pressure. It has little effect on cardiac output or heart rate, and it causes less reflex tachycardia than some other drugs in this class. Tolerance to its antihypertensive effect may occur. Its most common use is in combination with other drugs, such as beta blockers or diuretics, in the pharmacotherapy of hypertension. Prazosin has a short half-life and is often taken two or three times per day.

Adverse Effects and Interactions: Like other alpha blockers, prazosin has a tendency to cause orthostatic hypotension due to $alpha_1$-inhibition in vascular smooth muscle. In rare cases, this hypotension can be so severe as to cause unconsciousness about 30 minutes after the first dose. This is called the *first-dose phenomenon*. To avoid this situation, the first dose should be very low and given at bedtime. Dizziness, drowsiness, or lightheadedness may occur as a result of decreased blood flow to the brain due to the drug's hypotensive action. Reflex tachycardia may occur due to the rapid falls in blood pressure. The alpha blockade may also result in nasal congestion or inhibition of ejaculation.

Drug interactions include increased hypotensive effects with concurrent use of antihypertensives and diuretics.

Nursing Process Focus Patients Receiving Adrenergic Blocker Therapy

ASSESSMENT	POTENTIAL NURSING DIAGNOSES*
Prior to administration: • Obtain a complete health history including neurological, liver, GI and genitourinary conditions; allergies; and drug history for possible drug interactions. • Acquire the results of a complete physical examination including vital signs, height, weight. For BPH (obtain urinary pattern and output). • Evaluate laboratory blood findings: CBC, chemistry, renal and liver function studies.	• *Deficient Knowledge* related to a lack of information about drug therapy • *Impaired Urinary Elimination (frequency)* related to adverse effects of drug therapy • *Sexual Dysfunction* related to adverse effects of drug therapy • *Risk for Injury* related to dizziness, syncope

PLANNING: PATIENT GOALS AND EXPECTED OUTCOMES

The patient will:
- Experience therapeutic effects (a decrease in blood pressure or ease of urination).
- Be free from or experience minimal adverse effects from drug therapy.
- Verbalize an understanding of the drug's use, adverse effects and required precautions.

IMPLEMENTATION

Interventions and (Rationales)	Patient Education/Discharge Planning
• In patients with BPH, monitor for urinary hesitancy/feeling of incomplete bladder emptying, and interrupted urinary stream.	• Instruct the patient to report increased difficulty with urination to a healthcare provider.

(Continued)

Nursing Process Focus (*continued*)

Interventions and (Rationales)	Patient Education/Discharge Planning
• Monitor for syncope. (Alpha-adrenergic blockers produce first-dose syncope phenomenon and may cause loss of consciousness.)	Instruct the patient to: • Take this medication at bedtime, and to take the first dose *immediately* before getting into bed. • Avoid abrupt changes in position; warn the patient about first-dose phenomenon and reassure that this effect diminishes with continued therapy.
• Take vital signs and notify healthcare provider if pulse or blood pressure drops below approved parameters. Monitor for dizziness, drowsiness, or lightheadedness. (These drugs can cause severe hypotension. Dizziness is a sign of decreased blood flow to the brain due to the drug's hypotensive action.)	Instruct the patient to: • Monitor vital signs, especially blood pressure, ensuring proper use of home equipment and when to consult the nurse regarding "reportable" blood pressure readings. • Rise from lying to sitting or standing slowly to avoid dizziness. • Report dizziness or syncope that persists beyond the first dose, as well as paresthesias and other neurologic changes.
• Monitor level of consciousness and mood. (Adrenergic blockers can exacerbate existing mental depression.)	• Instruct the patient to immediately report any feelings of depression. • Interview the patient regarding suicide potential; obtain a "no-self harm" verbal contract from the patient.
• Observe for adverse effects that may include blurred vision, tinnitus, epistaxis, and edema.	Inform the patient: • That nasal congestion may be an adverse effect. • To report any adverse reactions to the healthcare provider. • About the potential danger of concomitant use of OTC nasal decongestants.
• Monitor liver function. (These drugs increase the risk for liver toxicity.)	Instruct the patient: • To adhere to a regular schedule of laboratory testing for liver function as ordered by the healthcare provider. • To report signs and symptoms of liver toxicity: nausea, vomiting, diarrhea, rash, jaundice, abdominal pain, tenderness or distention, or change in color of stool. • About the importance of ongoing medication regimen compliance and follow-up.

EVALUATION OF OUTCOME CRITERIA

Evaluate the effectiveness of drug therapy by confirming that patient goals and expected outcomes have been met (see "Planning"). *See Table 9.6 for a list of drugs to which these nursing actions apply.*

*Herdman, T.H. & Kamitsuru, S. (Eds.), *Nursing Diagnoses: Definitions & Classification* 2015–2017. Copyright © 2014, 1994–2014 NANDA International. Used by arrangement by John Wiley & Sons, Inc. Companion website: www.wiley.com/go/nursingdiagnoses.

Patients Need to Know

Patients treated with autonomic medications need to know the following:

In General

1. Do not take any OTC cold, cough, or sinus drugs without seeking medical advice because these likely contain autonomic drugs, which could increase your risk for adverse effects.
2. Report any palpitations, shortness of breath, chest pain, or large changes in blood pressure immediately to a healthcare provider. Some of the most serious adverse effects of autonomic drugs relate to the cardiovascular system.
3. Notify a healthcare provider before taking autonomic drugs if the following conditions are present: thyroid disease, diabetes mellitus, dysrhythmias, or hypertension. Such medications have the potential to cause serious adverse effects in individuals with these conditions.
4. Move slowly when changing from a supine or sitting to an upright position to avoid dizziness and perhaps fainting. Many of the autonomic medications affect blood pressure.
5. Notify a healthcare provider if any significant change in bowel habits or abdominal cramping or constipation occurs after taking autonomic drugs.
6. Inform a healthcare provider before taking cholinergic blockers (anticholinergics) if urinating difficulty is present or if the diagnosis of BPH has been made.

7. Chew gum or suck on hard candies if dry mouth is experienced when taking autonomic drugs. Proper oral hygiene is important to avoid dental caries.

Regarding Adrenergic Blockers

8. Do not discontinue the use of beta blockers abruptly because doing so can result in chest pain or rebound hypertension.
9. Alpha blockers can sometimes cause impotence as an adverse effect. If there are difficulties with ejaculation, notify a healthcare provider so that other drug options can be explored.

Chapter Review

Core Concepts Summary

9.1 The nervous system has two major divisions: central and peripheral.

The central nervous system consists of the brain and spinal cord. The peripheral nervous system consists of a sensory portion and a motor portion. Outgoing motor signals are characterized as voluntary (somatic) or involuntary (autonomic).

9.2 The autonomic nervous system has sympathetic and parasympathetic branches.

Stimulation of sympathetic nerves causes symptoms of the fight-or-flight response. Stimulation of parasympathetic nerves induces the rest-and-digest response. With few exceptions, the actions of the two divisions oppose each other.

9.3 Synapses are common junction sites of drug action.

Synapses consist of a presynaptic nerve and a postsynaptic nerve with a space between them called the synaptic cleft. Neurotransmitters cross this synaptic cleft to regenerate the nerve impulse.

9.4 Norepinephrine and acetylcholine are the two primary neurotransmitters in the autonomic nervous system.

Norepinephrine is the neurotransmitter at the organ level in the sympathetic nervous system. Norepinephrine receptors may be alpha or beta subtypes. Acetylcholine is the neurotransmitter at the end of all presynaptic nerves (ganglia), at sweat glands, and in skeletal muscle. Acetylcholine receptors may be nicotinic or muscarinic.

9.5 Autonomic drugs are classified according to the receptors that they stimulate or block.

Adrenergic drugs stimulate sympathetic target organs, and cholinergic drugs primarily stimulate parasympathetic target organs. Adrenergic blockers inhibit actions of the sympathetic nervous system, whereas cholinergic blockers inhibit actions of the parasympathetic nervous system.

9.6 Cholinergic drugs have few therapeutic uses because of their numerous adverse effects.

Cholinergic drugs are used to treat glaucoma and to stimulate the urinary or digestive tracts following general anesthesia. Toxic nerve agents are cholinergic drugs, producing harmful effects in the body.

9.7 Cholinergic blockers are most commonly used to dry secretions and to treat asthma.

The use of cholinergic blockers has declined due to their numerous adverse effects. They are used to dry secretions, dilate the bronchi, and dilate the pupils.

9.8 Adrenergic drugs are primarily used for their effects on the heart, bronchial tree, and nasal passages.

Adrenergic drugs may stimulate one or several subtypes of adrenergic receptors. Uses include increasing the heart rate, dilating the bronchi, and drying excess secretions caused by colds.

9.9 Adrenergic blockers are primarily used to treat hypertension, bronchial constriction, and nasal congestion.

Adrenergic blockers are the most commonly prescribed autonomic drugs. They may be selective for only one receptor subtype, such as the $beta_1$-blockers, or nonselective, inhibiting several subtypes. Hypertension is their primary indication.

REVIEW Questions

Answer the following questions to assess your knowledge of the chapter material, and go back and review any material that is not clear to you.

1. While assisting the RN with the development of a plan of care for a patient with glaucoma, the LPN recognizes that which of the following drugs would be contraindicated for the patient?
   1. Pilocarpine (Carpine)
   2. Betaxolol (Betoptic)
   3. Timolol (Timoptic)
   4. Atropine

2. The patient diagnosed with glaucoma would most likely be prescribed which of the following drugs?
   1. Adrenergic drugs
   2. Cholinergic drugs
   3. Adrenergic blockers
   4. Cholinergic blockers

3. The nurse informs the patient that rebound congestion can occur with long-term use of this adrenergic drug:
   1. Albuterol (Proventil)
   2. Neostigmine (Prostigmin)
   3. Salmeterol (Serevent)
   4. Phenylephrine (Neo-Synephrine)

4. The patient is diagnosed with urinary bladder urgency and incontinence. Which of the following cholinergic blockers does the healthcare provider order for these conditions?
   1. Dicyclomine (Bentyl)
   2. Ipratropium (Atrovent)
   3. Oxybutynin (Ditropan)
   4. Scopolamine (Transderm-Scop)

5. A patient being given an alpha$_1$-adrenergic blocker asks what this drug does. The nurse tells him that alpha-adrenergic blockers cause: (Select all that apply.)
   1. Vasodilation.
   2. Decreased blood pressure.
   3. Increased blood pressure.
   4. Vasoconstriction.
   5. Dizziness

6. While obtaining a patient's medication history, the patient tells the nurse, "I'm on metoprolol (Lopressor)." The nurse knows that this drug is a(n):
   1. Alpha blocker.
   2. Beta blocker.
   3. Cholinergic.
   4. Cholinergic blocker.

7. Prior to administering atenolol (Tenormin), the nurse assesses:
   1. Respirations and blood pressure.
   2. Respirations and heart rate.
   3. Heart rate and blood pressure.
   4. Temperature and blood pressure.

8. The healthcare provider orders metaproterenol 20 mg by mouth three times a day. The pharmacy sends metaproterenol sulfate syrup, 10 mg/5 mL. The nurse will administer ________ per day.
   1. 20 mL
   2. 60 mL
   3. 30 mL
   4. 40 mL

9. A patient has been prescribed phenylephrine to help relieve nasal congestion. The nurse informs the patient that prolonged use of this drug can cause:
   1. Decreased heart rate.
   2. Decreased blood pressure.
   3. Drowsiness.
   4. Rebound congestion.

10. The nurse suspects that the cholinergic blocker the patient is taking is causing which one of the following adverse effects?
    1. Diaphoresis
    2. Confusion
    3. Dry mouth
    4. Increased urination

CASE STUDY Questions

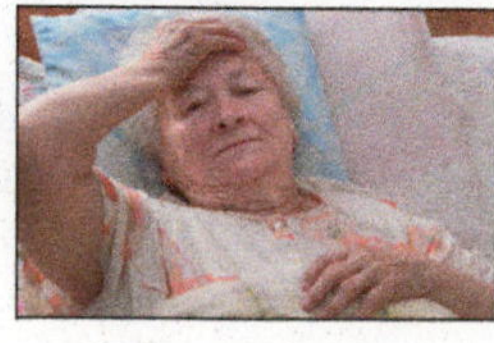

Remember Mrs. Wheaton, the patient introduced at the beginning of the chapter? Now read the remainder of the case study. Based on the information you have learned in this chapter, answer the questions that follow.

Mrs. Martha Wheaton, an 80-year-old woman, has been having problems with nonobstructive urinary retention following surgery, a retropubic urethral suspension. She required a Foley catheter for four days but was unable to void after removal of the catheter. The healthcare provider ordered bethanechol (Urecholine) for Mrs. Wheaton.

1. Mrs. Wheaton asks why the healthcare provider ordered bethanechol. The nurse explains that:
   1. It causes the kidneys to produce more urine, which increases the pressure within the bladder, forcing her to urinate.
   2. It inhibits smooth muscle contractions, causing the bladder to relax.
   3. It stimulates smooth muscle contractions, causing the bladder to function normally.
   4. It decreases the amount of urine produced in the kidneys so as not to put as much pressure on the bladder.

2. What information about bethanechol does the nurse provide for Mrs. Wheaton? (Select all that apply.)
   1. No adverse effects are significant to report when taking this medication.
   2. The patient should avoid abrupt position changes.
   3. Salivation and sweating may increase.
   4. The patient should be near a bathroom after taking this medication.

A couple of months later, Mrs. Wheaton has been diagnosed with severe hypertension and is prescribed prazosin (Minipress).

3. The nurse informs Mrs. Wheaton that prazosin is a type of:
   1. Cholinergic drug.
   2. Cholinergic blocker.
   3. Adrenergic drug.
   4. Adrenergic blocker.
4. Mrs. Wheaton asks the nurse if there are any precautions she should know about. The nurse informs her that alpha adrenergic blockers may cause: (Select all that apply.)
   1. Dizziness when changing positions.
   2. Possible increased heart rate.
   3. Nasal congestion.
   4. Nausea.

Answers and complete rationales for the Review and Case Study Questions appear in Appendix A.

REFERENCE

Herdman, T. H., & Kamitsuru, S. (Eds.). (2014). *NANDA International nursing diagnoses: Definitions and classification, 2015–2017*. Oxford, United Kingdom: Wiley-Blackwell.

SELECTED BIBLIOGRAPHY

Becker, D. E. (2012) Basic and Clinical Pharmacology of Autonomic Drugs. *Anesthesia Progress, 59*(4), 159–169. doi:10.2344/0003-3006-59.4.159

Biaggioni, I., & Robertson, D. (2015). Adrenoceptor agonists & sympathomimetic drugs. In B. G. Katzung, S. B. Masters, & A. J. Trevor (Eds.), *Basic and Clinical Pharmacology* (13th ed., pp. 133–151). New York, NY: McGraw-Hill.

Cazzola, M., & Matera, M. G. (2012). Tremor and β(2)-adrenergic agents: Is it a real clinical problem? *Pulmonary Pharmacology and Therapeutics, 25*, 4–10. doi:10.1016/j.pupt.2011.12.004

De Lima, L. G., Saconato, H., Atallah, A. N., & da Silva, E. M. (2014). Beta-blockers for preventing stroke recurrence. *Cochrane Database of Systematic Reviews, 10*, Article No.: CD007890. doi:10.1002/14651858.CD007890.pub3

Katzung, B. G. (2015). Introduction to autonomic pharmacology. In B. G. Katzung & A. J. Trevor (Eds.), *Basic and Clinical Pharmacology* (13th ed., pp. 87–104). New York, NY: McGraw-Hill.

Larochelle, P., Tobe, S. W., & Lacourcière, Y. (2014). β-Blockers in hypertension: Studies and meta-analyses over the years. *Canadian Journal of Cardiology, 30*(5 Suppl), S16–S22. doi:10.1016/j.cjca.2014.02.012

Madhuvrata, P., Cody, J. D., Ellis, G., Herbison, G. P., & Hay-Smith, E. J. (2012). Which anticholinergic drug for overactive bladder symptoms in adults. *Cochrane Database of Systematic Reviews, 1*, Art. No.: CD005429. doi:10.1002/14651858.CD005429.pub2

Pappano, A. J. (2015). Cholinoceptor-blocking drugs. In B. G. Katzung & A. J. Trevor (Eds.), *Basic and clinical pharmacology* (13th ed., pp. 121–132). New York, NY: McGraw-Hill.

Sellers, D. J., & Chess-Williams, R. (2012). Muscarinic agonists and antagonists: Effects on the urinary bladder. *Handbook of Experimental Pharmacology, 208*, 375–400.

Westfall, T. C., & Westfall, D. P. (2011). Neurotransmission: The autonomic and somatic motor nervous systems. In L. L. Brunton, B. A. Chabner, & B. C. Knollmann (Eds.), *Goodman and Gilman's the pharmacological basis of therapeutics* (12th ed.). New York, NY: McGraw-Hill.

Chapter 10

Drugs for Anxiety and Insomnia

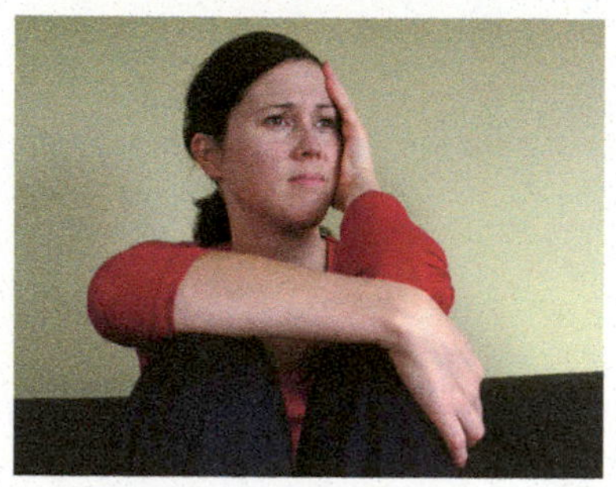

"I'm so nervous all the time; I can't even care for my children. All I can think of is that terrible accident."
Ms. Cynthia Reynolds

Core Concepts

10.1 **Anxiety disorders fall into many categories, including generalized anxiety, panic disorder, and anxiety due to fearful, recurrent, and traumatic life events.**

10.2 **Regions of the cerebral cortex, diencephalon, and brain stem are responsible for anxiety and wakefulness.**

10.3 **Anxiety is managed with both pharmacologic and nonpharmacologic strategies.**

10.4 **An inability to sleep is linked with anxiety.**

10.5 **Anxiety and insomnia are treated with many types of central nervous system (CNS) drugs.**

10.6 **When taken properly, antidepressants reduce symptoms of panic and anxiety.**

10.7 **Benzodiazepines are useful for the short-term treatment of anxiety and insomnia.**

10.8 **Barbiturates depress CNS function and cause drowsiness.**

10.9 **Additional drugs provide therapy for anxiety-related symptoms and sleep disorders.**

Drug Snapshot

The following drugs are discussed in this chapter:

Drug Classes	Prototype Drugs
Antidepressants	Pr escitalopram (Lexapro)
Benzodiazepines	Pr lorazepam (Ativan)
Barbiturates	
Nonbenzodiazepine, Nonbarbiturate CNS Drugs	Pr zolpidem (Ambien)

Learning Outcomes

After reading this chapter, the student should be able to:

1. Identify the major categories of anxiety disorders.
2. Identify areas of the brain responsible for feelings of emotion and restlessness.
3. Explain the pharmacologic and nonpharmacologic strategies used to manage anxiety and anxiety-related symptoms.
4. Discuss why we sleep and how normal sleep patterns can be interrupted.
5. Identify the four categories of central nervous system drugs used to treat anxiety and sleep disorders.
6. Introduce the major classes of antidepressants and describe how they control anxiety.

7. Identify the role benzodiazepines play in treating anxiety disorders and insomnia, their mechanisms of action, primary actions, and important adverse effects.
8. Explain the sedative-hypnotic properties of barbiturates and their historic role in treating anxiety and restlessness.
9. Identify anti-anxiety drugs chemically unrelated to benzodiazepines or barbiturates.

Key Terms

antidepressants (AN-tee-dee-PRESS-ahnts)
anxiety
anxiolytics (ANG-zee-oh-LIT-iks)
barbiturates (bar-bi-CHUR-ates)
benzodiazepines (ben-zo-di-AZ-eh-peenz)
black box warning
CNS depressants (dee-PRESS-ahnts)
generalized anxiety disorder (GAD)
hypothalamus (HEYE-po-THAL-ah-mus)
insomnia (in-SOM-nee-uh)
limbic system (LIM-bik)
obsessive–compulsive disorder (OCD)
panic disorder
phobias (FO-bee-ahs)
post-traumatic stress disorder (PTSD)
rebound insomnia
reticular activating system (RAS)
reticular formation (re-TIK-u-lurr)
sedative-hypnotic (SED-ah-tiv hip-NOT-ik)
sedatives (SED-ah-tivs)
social anxiety disorder

Patients experience nervousness and tension more often than any other symptoms. Seeking relief from these symptoms, patients often turn to a variety of pharmacologic and alternative therapies. Most healthcare providers agree that even though drugs do not cure the underlying problem, they can provide short-term help to calm patients who are experiencing acute anxiety or who have simple sleep disorders. This chapter discusses drugs that treat anxiety, cause sedation, or help patients sleep.

ANXIETY

According to the *International Classification of Diseases*, 10th edition (ICD-10), **anxiety** is a state of apprehension, tension, or uneasiness that stems from the anticipation of danger, the source of which is largely unknown or unrecognized. The "dominant symptoms are highly variable, but complaints of continuous feelings of nervousness, trembling, muscular tension, sweating, lightheadedness, palpitations, dizziness, and epigastric discomfort are common." Anxious individuals can often identify at least some factors that bring on their symptoms. Most people state that their feelings of anxiety are disproportionate to any factual dangers.

Anxiety disorders fall into many categories, including generalized anxiety, panic disorder, and anxiety due to fearful, recurrent, and traumatic life events.

◀ **Core Concept 10.1**

The anxiety experienced by people faced with a stressful environment or situations is called *situational anxiety*. To a certain degree, situational anxiety is beneficial because it motivates people to accomplish tasks in a prompt manner—if for no other reason than to end the source of nervousness. Situational stress may be intense, but many people often learn to cope with this kind of stress without seeking conventional medical intervention.

According to the *Diagnostic and Statistical Manual of Mental Disorders*, 5th edition (DSM-5) (American Psychiatry Association, 2013), anxiety disorders are classified into the following general areas:

- Separation Anxiety Disorder
- Selective Mutism
- Specific Phobia
- Social Anxiety Disorder (Social Phobia)

- Panic Disorder
- Panic Attack (Specifier)
- Agoraphobia
- Generalized Anxiety Disorder
- Substance/Medication-Induced Anxiety Disorder
- Anxiety Disorder Due to Another Medical Condition
- Other Specified Anxiety Disorder
- Unspecified Anxiety Disorder.

Generalized anxiety disorder (GAD) is difficult-to-control, excessive anxiety that lasts six months or more. It occurs in response to a variety of life events or activities, and it interferes with normal, day-to-day functions. It is by far the most common type of stress disorder routinely observed by healthcare providers. Symptoms include restlessness, fatigue, muscle tension, nervousness, inability to focus or concentrate, an overwhelming sense of dread, and sleep disturbances. Autonomic signs of sympathetic nervous system activation involve sweating, blood pressure elevation, heart palpitations, varying degrees of respiratory change, and dry mouth. Parasympathetic responses may involve abdominal cramping, diarrhea, and urinary urgency. Additional motor symptoms experienced by the patient may include increased reflexes and numbness and tingling of the extremities. Women are slightly more likely to experience GAD, and its prevalence is highest in those ages 20 to 35.

A second category of anxiety, called **panic disorder**, is characterized by intense feelings of immediate apprehension, fearfulness, terror, or impending doom, accompanied by increased autonomic nervous system activity. Although panic attacks usually last less than 10 minutes, patients may describe them as seemingly endless. As many as 5% of the population will experience one or more panic attacks during their lifetimes, and women are affected about twice as often as men.

phobia = *fear*

Among the other categories of anxiety are phobias, obsessive-compulsive disorder, and post-traumatic stress disorder. **Phobias** are fearful feelings attached to specific objects or situations. Attacks may occur when a person feels trapped, embarrassed, or unable to escape. Fear of crowds is termed **social anxiety disorder**, or *social phobia*. Performers may experience feelings of dread, nervousness, or apprehension termed *performance anxiety*. Some anxiety is normal when a person faces a crowd or performs for a crowd, but extreme fear is not normal. Phobias compel a patient to avoid the fearful stimulus entirely, to the point that his or her behavior is unnatural. **Obsessive–compulsive disorder (OCD)** involves recurrent, intrusive

Fast Facts Anxiety Disorders

- Millions of Americans experience anxiety every year.
- Other illnesses commonly coexist with anxiety, including depression, eating disorders, and substance abuse.
- Major categories of anxiety are:
  - Phobias
    - About 15% of the U.S. population has a specific phobia.
    - Specific phobias usually begin in childhood and last for many years.
    - Over 2% of adult Americans have severe *social phobia*.
    - About 0.8% of adult Americans have *agoraphobia*, an intense fear of situations or places that might cause them to panic, or feel trapped, helpless, or embarrassed.
  - Generalized anxiety disorder (GAD)
    - More than 3% of the U.S. population is diagnosed with GAD in a given year.
    - Generalized anxiety symptoms are most prevalent between childhood and middle age.
  - Post-traumatic stress disorder (PTSD)
    - About 3% of the U.S. population has PTSD.
    - PTSD can develop at any age, although the average time of onset is early adulthood.
  - Panic Disorder
    - About 3% of the U.S. population have panic disorder.
    - Panic attacks often begin in late adolescence or early adulthood.
    - Not everyone who experiences panic attacks will develop panic disorder.
  - Obsessive–compulsive disorder (OCD)
    - One percent of the U.S. population has OCD.
    - Almost 51% of OCD cases are classified as severe.
    - The first symptoms of OCD usually begin in the late teenage years.
- For details, see the National Institute of Mental Health website.

thoughts or repetitive behaviors that interfere with normal activities or relationships. Common examples include fear of exposure to germs and repetitive hand washing. **Post-traumatic stress disorder (PTSD)** is a type of extreme situational anxiety that develops in response to reexperiencing a previous life event. Traumatic life events such as war, physical or sexual abuse, natural disasters, or homicidal situations may lead to a sense of helplessness and reexperiencing of the traumatic event. War, terrorist attacks, and weather events such as major hurricanes are examples of situations that trigger PTSD. Economic changes, global recession, and unemployment have been responsible for much persistent anxiety. People who experience lingering effects from traumatic life events are at risk for developing signs and symptoms of PTSD.

Regions of the cerebral cortex, diencephalon, and brain stem are responsible for anxiety and wakefulness.

◀ **Core Concept 10.2**

The emotional areas of the brain responsible for anxiety and restlessness are mostly the limbic system, the hypothalamus, and the reticular activating system (Table 10.1). The **limbic system** is an area of the *cerebral cortex* responsible for emotional expression, learning, and memory. Signals routed through the limbic system connect with the hypothalamus, an area of the brain referred to as the *diencephalon*. Emotional states associated with this connection include anxiety, fear, anger, aggression, remorse, depression, euphoria, and changes in appetite and sexual drive.

Table 10.1 Areas of the Brain Responsible for Anxiety and Restlessness

Major Brain Regions	Specific Brain Regions	Role in Anxiety Symptoms
Cerebral cortex	Parahippocampal gyrus and cingulate gyrus (limbic areas), reticular activating system	Responsible for emotional expression, learning, memory, anxious feelings, fear, dread, restlessness, and alertness
Diencephalon	Hypothalamus	Triggers unconscious responses to extreme stress (fight-or-flight response)
Brainstem	Reticular formation	Responsible for overall level of heightened alertness

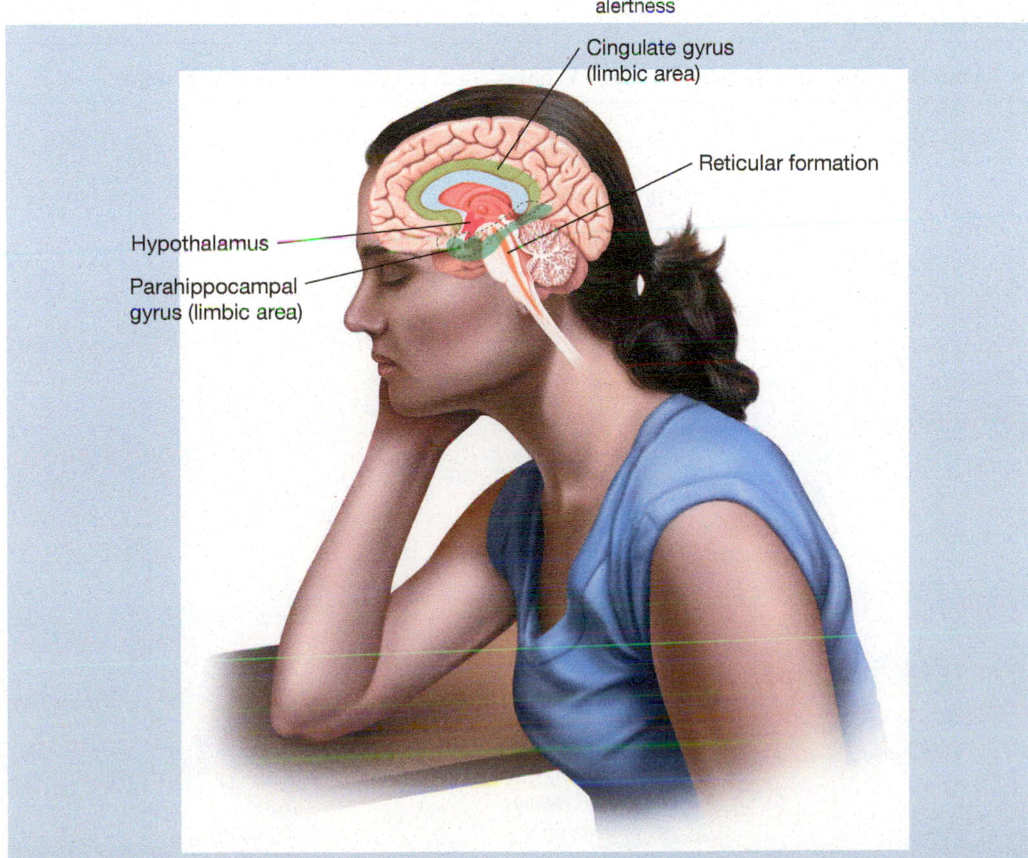

The **hypothalamus** is an important center that triggers unconscious responses to extreme stress, such as increased blood pressure, elevated breathing rate, and dilated pupils. These are responses connected with the fight-or-flight response of the autonomic nervous system (see Chapter 9). The endocrine functions of the hypothalamus are discussed in Chapter 33.

The hypothalamus also connects with the **reticular formation**, a network of neurons found along the entire length of the *brainstem*. Stimulation of the reticular formation causes increased alertness and arousal; inhibition causes drowsiness and sleep.

The larger area to which the reticular formation is connected is called the **reticular activating system (RAS)**. The RAS controls sleeping and wakefulness and performs an alerting function for the cerebral cortex. It also helps a person focus attention on individual tasks by transmitting information to higher brain centers. The RAS is the neural mechanism thought to be responsible for emotions such as anxiety and fear. It is also the mechanism associated with restlessness and an interrupted sleeping pattern.

Core Concept 10.3 ▶ Anxiety is managed with both pharmacologic and nonpharmacologic strategies.

Although stress itself may be incapacitating, it is often only a symptom of an underlying disorder. Uncovering and addressing the cause of the anxiety is more productive than merely treating the symptoms with medications. Patients should be encouraged to explore and develop nonpharmacologic coping strategies to deal with the underlying causes. Such strategies may include personal counseling, behavioral therapy, biofeedback techniques, meditation, and other complementary and alternative therapies. One model for anxiety management is shown in Figure 10.1.

anxio = *anxiety*
lytic = *to dissolve away; break*

When anxiety becomes severe enough to significantly interfere with activities of daily living (ADLs), pharmacotherapy is indicated. In most types of stress, **anxiolytics**, or drugs having the ability to relieve anxiety, are quite effective. These include medications in a number of therapeutic categories, involving drugs for depression (see Chapter 11) and seizures (see Chapter 14). Anxiolytics provide treatment for GAD, panic disorder, phobias, PTSD, and OCD.

CONCEPT REVIEW 10.1

- What does the term *anxiolytic* mean? What disorders do anxiolytic drugs treat?

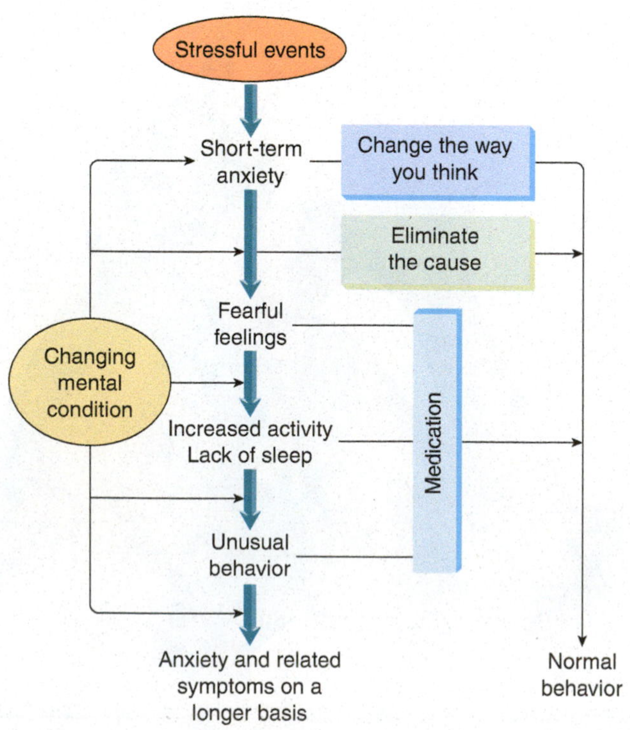

FIGURE 10.1 This model shows how stressful events can lead to anxiety. Nonpharmacologic coping strategies often help to eliminate short-term anxiety, whereas medication may be needed if anxiety and related symptoms begin to occur on a longer basis.

INSOMNIA

Insomnia is a condition characterized by a patient's inability to fall asleep or remain asleep. Pharmacotherapy may be needed if the sleeplessness interferes with ADLs.

in = *not (without)*
somnia = *sleep*

An inability to sleep is linked with anxiety.

◀ **Core Concept 10.4**

Why is it that we need sleep? During an average lifetime, about 33% of our time is spent sleeping or trying to sleep. Insufficient sleep is associated with increased workplace and driving accidents. Although it is well established that sleep is essential for wellness, scientists are unsure of its function or how much is needed. Following are some theories:

- Inactivity during sleep gives the body time to grow and repair.
- Sleep is a function that evolved as a protective mechanism. Throughout history, nighttime was the safest time of day, so deep rest (sleep) occurred during those hours.
- Sleep deals with "electrical" charging and discharging of the brain. The brain needs time for processing and filing new information collected throughout the day. When this is done without interference from the environment, these vast amounts of data can later be retrieved through memory.

Fast Facts **Insomnia**

- One-third of the world's population has trouble sleeping during part of the year.
- Insomnia is a common problem with night-shift workers and alternating shift workers.
- Insomnia is more common in women than in men.
- Patients older than 65 years old sleep less than patients in any other age group.
- Only about 70% of people with insomnia ever report this problem to their healthcare provider.
- People buy over-the-counter (OTC) sleep medications and combination drugs with sleep additives (e.g., the antihistamine diphenhydramine) more than any other drug category. Trade name products include Advil PM, Excedrin PM, Nytol, Equate Nighttime Sleep-Aid, Sominex, Compoz, Tylenol PM, and Unisom.
- As a natural alternative for sleep, some people take melatonin, kava kava, or valerian.

The acts of sleeping and waking are synchronized with many different bodily functions. Body temperature, blood pressure, hormone levels, and respiration fluctuate cyclically throughout the 24-hour day. When this cycle is impaired, pharmacologic or other interventions may be needed to readjust it. Increased levels of the neurotransmitter serotonin help initiate the various processes of sleep.

Insomnia, or sleeplessness, is a disorder associated with anxiety. There are several major types of insomnia. *Short-term* or *behavioral insomnia* may be attributed to stress caused by a hectic lifestyle or the inability to resolve day-to-day conflicts within the home or workplace. Worries about work, marriage, children, and health are common reasons for short-term sleep loss. When stress interrupts normal sleeping patterns, patients cannot sleep because their minds are too active. *Long-term insomnia* may be caused by more intense emotional and mood-related illnesses such as depression, manic disorders, or chronic pain.

Foods or beverages containing stimulants such as caffeine may interrupt sleep. Patients may also find that using tobacco products makes them restless and edgy. Alcohol, although often enabling a person to fall asleep, may produce vivid dreams and frequent awakening that prevent restful sleep. Eating a large meal—especially one high in protein and fat—close to bedtime may interfere with sleep because metabolism increases to digest the food. Certain medications cause central nervous system (CNS) stimulation, and these should not be taken immediately before bedtime. Stressful conditions—for example, too much light, an uncomfortable room temperature (especially one that is too warm), snoring, sleep apnea, and recurring nightmares—also interfere with sleep.

▶ **Lifespan and Diversity**

Older adults are more likely to experience problems with sedatives and medications designed to help them sleep. For the first night or two, drugs may seem to help the insomnia of an older patient, but as the medication accumulates in the system, it produces generalized brain dysfunction. The agitated patient may then be mistakenly overdosed with higher doses of medication.

Nonpharmacologic means of relieving insomnia are usually tried before drug therapy, because long-term use of sleep medications will likely worsen insomnia and may cause physical or psychological dependence. Some patients experience a phenomenon called **rebound insomnia**. This effect occurs when a sedative drug is stopped abruptly or when it has been taken for a long time and drug dependence occurs. Alcohol abuse can also cause rebound insomnia.

CONCEPT REVIEW 10.2

- Why might a patient not be able to enjoy normal sleep? Why is long-term drug therapy for lack of sleep not a good idea?

Core Concept 10.5 ▶

Anxiety and insomnia are treated with many types of central nervous system (CNS) drugs.

CNS drugs are used to alter brain activity in patients with anxiety or sleep disorders. These medications are grouped into four major classes: (1) antidepressants, (2) benzodiazepines, (3) barbiturates, and (4) nonbarbiturate and nonbenzodiazepine CNS drugs.

anti = *against*
depressant = *depressed neuronal function*

Antidepressants have an ability to enhance mood by altering the levels of two important neurotransmitters in the brain—norepinephrine and serotonin. By restoring the balance of these neurotransmitters, antidepressants can reduce the symptoms associated with depression, panic, OCD, and phobia. Antidepressants used to treat anxiety and insomnia include selective serotonin reuptake inhibitors (SSRIs), atypical antidepressants (such as serotonin–norepinephrine reuptake inhibitors [SNRIs]), tricyclic antidepressants (TCAs), and monoamine oxidase inhibitors (MAOIs). Use of the latter two types of drugs has declined in recent years. The mechanisms of action and important considerations of these drugs are covered in Chapter 11.

Another approach to relieving anxiety is the use of **CNS depressants** that slow neuronal activity in the brain. These drugs range from those that relax, to those that sedate, to those that cause sleep and anesthesia. Coma and death are the end stages of CNS depression. Some drug classes can produce the full range of CNS depression from relaxation to full anesthesia, whereas others are less effective across this range. Medications that depress the CNS are sometimes called **sedatives** because of their ability to sedate or relax a patient. At higher doses, many of the same drugs can cause sleep and therefore are called *hypnotics*. The term **sedative-hypnotic** is often used to describe a drug with the ability to produce a calming effect at lower doses and sleep at higher doses. *Tranquilizer* is an older term used to describe a drug that produces a soothing or tranquil feeling.

sedative = *calming*
hypnotic = *sleep-inducing*

tranquilizer = *drug that soothes or makes you tranquil*

CNS depressants used for anxiety and sleep disorders are categorized into three major classes: antidepressants, benzodiazepines, and barbiturates. An additional category consists of miscellaneous drugs chemically unrelated to the other drug groups. These miscellaneous antianxiety drugs are presented in Section 10.9.

As discussed in Chapter 8, long-term use of many CNS depressants can lead to physical or psychological dependence. The withdrawal syndrome for some CNS depressants can cause life-threatening neurologic reactions, including fever, psychosis, and seizures. Other withdrawal symptoms include increased heart rate and lowered blood pressure; loss of appetite; muscle cramps; impaired memory, concentration, and orientation; abnormal sounds in the ears and blurred vision; and insomnia, agitation, anxiety, and panic. Noticeable withdrawal symptoms typically last 2 to 4 weeks. Subtle ones can last months.

CONCEPT REVIEW 10.3

- Describe what each of the following terms means in relation to anxiety and alertness: CNS depressants, sedatives, hypnotics, sedative-hypnotics, and tranquilizers.

Core Concept 10.6 ▶

When taken properly, antidepressants reduce symptoms of panic and anxiety.

Antidepressants not only treat symptoms of major depressive disorder termed *clinical depression* (see Chapter 11); they also to treat symptoms of anxiety associated with panic disorders, OCD, social phobia, and PTSD. Because many of the features observed in patients with depressive disorder overlap with anxiety disorders, methods of intervention are often the same.

For most patients, panic symptoms come in two stages. The first stage is called *anticipatory anxiety*, when the patient begins to think about an upcoming challenge and starts to feel dread. The second stage is when physical symptoms such as shortness of breath, rapid heart rate, and muscle tension begin. Many of the stressful symptoms are associated with activation of the autonomic nervous system. The strategy in treating panic attacks is to help the patient face the fear and suppress symptoms during one or both of these stages. Drugs can lessen the negative thoughts associated with anticipating the panic, thereby reducing the stress. Drugs also decrease neuronal activity and suppress functions of the autonomic nervous system, helping the patient to remain calm. The patient can then use self-help skills to control behavior.

Antidepressants, which reduce persistent symptoms of panic and anxiety, are summarized in Table 10.2. SSRIs and atypical antidepressants effectively treat symptoms of panic disorder, PTSD, OCD, and phobias. SSRIs and SNRIs produce fewer major adverse effects than the TCAs or MAOIs.

Table 10.2 Antidepressants for Anxiety Disorders

Drug	Route and Adult Dose	Remarks
SELECTIVE SEROTONIN REUPTAKE INHIBITORS (SSRIs)		
citalopram (Celexa)	PO: start at 20 mg/day, may increase to 40 mg/day if needed	For depression, anxiety disorders (off-label)
Pr escitalopram (Lexapro)	PO: 10 mg/day, may increase to 20 mg/day if needed after 1 week	For depression, GAD
fluoxetine (Prozac)	PO: 20 mg/day, may increase by 20 mg/day (max: 80 mg/day); 20 mg/day; when stable may switch to 90 mg sustained-release capsule every week (max: 90 mg/week)	For depression, OCD, panic disorder, premenstrual dysphoric disorder
fluvoxamine (Luvox)	PO: Start with 50 mg/day, may increase slowly up to 300 mg/day or divided two times/day	For depression, social anxiety, OCD, panic disorder, GAD, PTSD
paroxetine (Paxil)	PO: 20–60 mg/day	For depression, GAD, social anxiety, panic disorder, OCD, PTSD, and premenstrual dysphoric disorder
sertraline (Zoloft) (see the Prototype Drug box in Core Concept 11.3)	PO: Begin with 50 mg/day, gradually increase every few weeks according to response (max: 200 mg)	For depression, social anxiety, panic disorder, OCD, PTSD, premenstrual dysphoric disorder
ATYPICAL ANTIDEPRESSANTS		
duloxetine (Cymbalta)	PO: 40–60 mg/day in one or two divided doses	For depression, GAD, neuropathic pain, fibromyalgia
mirtazapine (Remeron)	PO: 15 mg/day in a single dose; may increase every 1–2 weeks (max: 45 mg/day)	For depression, PTSD (off-label)
trazodone (Oleptro)	PO: 150 mg/day in divided doses, may increase by 50 mg/day every 3–4 days (max: 400–600 mg/day)	For depression, insomnia (off-label), GAD (off-label)
venlafaxine (Effexor)	PO: Start with 37.5 mg immediate release every day and increase to 75–225 mg/day extended release	For depression, social anxiety, GAD, neuropathic pain (off-label)
TRICYCLIC ANTIDEPRESSANTS (TCAs)		
amitriptyline (Elavil)	PO: 75–100 mg/day, may gradually increase to 150–300 mg/day	For depression
clomipramine (Anafranil)	PO: 75–100 mg/day in divided doses	For OCD, depression
desipramine (Norpramin)	PO: 75–100 mg/day in divided doses, may gradually increase to 150–300 mg/day	For depression
doxepin (Silenor)	PO: 30–150 mg/day in divided doses, may gradually increase to 300 mg/day	For depression
imipramine (Tofranil) (see the Prototype Drug box in Core Concept 11.3)	PO: 75–100 mg/day in divided doses (max: 300 mg/day)	For depression, GAD
nortriptyline (Aventyl, Pamelor)	PO: 25 mg three times/day or four times/day, gradually increased to 100–150 mg/day	For depression
trimipramine (Surmontil)	PO: 75–100 mg/day (max: 300 mg/day) in divided doses	For depression
MONOAMINE OXIDASE INHIBITORS (MAOIs)		
phenelzine (Nardil) (see the Prototype Drug box in Core Concept 11.3)	PO: 15 mg three times/day, increase to at least 60 mg/day, may need up to 90 mg/day	For depression
tranylcypromine (Parnate)	PO: 30 mg/day in divided doses, may increase by 10 mg/day at 3-week intervals (max: 60 mg/day)	For depression

As with all CNS drugs, precautions must be taken to make sure that medications are effective. Because of adverse reactions, some patients might find antidepressant treatment unacceptable. In 2004, the U.S. Food and Drug Administration (FDA) issued an advisory warning (**black box warning**) pointing out the potential warning signs of suicide in adults and children at the beginning of antidepressant therapy and when doses are changed. In the course of treatment, it is possible that several signs that are the focus of anxiety therapy—for example, irritability, panic attacks, agitation, insomnia, and hostility—may emerge. See Chapter 11 for more detailed primary actions and adverse effects of these drugs. Following is a brief introduction to important considerations for each type of antidepressant:

- *SSRIs* These drugs are safer than the other classes of antidepressants and result in fewer occurrences of unfavorable sympathomimetic and anticholinergic effects (see Chapter 9). Because serotonin is thought to play a role in mood, these medications have received more attention in recent years. SSRIs can cause weight gain and sexual dysfunction. Excessive doses of these medications can cause confusion, anxiety, restlessness, hypertension, tremors, sweating, fever, blurred vision, constipation, and muscle incoordination. Serotonin syndrome is a potentially life-threatening reaction when taking too-high doses of SSRIs or taking SSRIs with other antianxiety or antidepressive drugs that increase serotonin levels. Patients taking these drugs should avoid alcohol. SSRIs are often the preferred drugs for anxiety.
- *Atypical antidepressants* These are chemically unrelated to the other antidepressants. Their adverse effects are generally similar to those of SSRIs. SNRIs inhibit the reuptake of both serotonin and norepinephrine; therefore, these drugs are included here. Common adverse effects are headache, insomnia, nervousness, dry mouth, dizziness, weight loss, sexual dysfunction, and chills.
- *TCAs* These are not recommended in patients with a history of heart attack, heart block, or abnormal heart rhythm. Patients often have annoying anticholinergic effects (see Chapter 9). Most TCAs are pregnancy category C or D. These drugs should not be used with alcohol or other CNS depressants. Patients with asthma, gastrointestinal disorders, alcoholism, schizophrenia, or bipolar disorder should use TCAs with extreme caution.
- *MAOIs* Patients should strictly avoid foods containing tyramine (a form of the amino acid tyrosine) and caffeine. MAOIs intensify the effects of insulin and other diabetes drugs. Common adverse effects include orthostatic hypotension, hypertensive crisis, headache, and diarrhea. MAOIs are rarely prescribed due to food-drug interactions and serious adverse effects. Serotonin syndrome is a potentially life-threatening drug reaction when taking too-high doses of MAOIs.

hyper = *elevated*
thermia = *temperature*

dia = *across (through pores)*
phoresis = *to carry (implying sweat)*

neuro = *nerve*
leptic = *locked (seized up)*

malignant = *aggressive harm*
syndrome = *abnormal characteristic*

Prototype Drug: Pr *Escitalopram (Lexapro)*

Therapeutic Class: Antidepressant; anxiolytic **Pharmacologic Class:** Selective serotonin reuptake inhibitor (SSRI)

Actions and Uses: Escitalopram is an SSRI. Selective inhibition of serotonin reuptake results in antidepressant activity without adverse autonomic effects such as increased heart rate or hypertension. This medication is indicated for generalized anxiety and depression. Off-label uses include the treatment of panic disorders.

Adverse Effects and Interactions: Serious reactions include dizziness, nausea, insomnia, somnolence, confusion, and seizures if taken in overdose. MAOIs should be avoided due to serotonin syndrome, marked by autonomic hyperactivity, hyperthermia, rigidity, diaphoresis, and neuroleptic malignant syndrome. Combination with MAOIs could result in hypertensive crisis, hyperthermia, and autonomic instability. Escitalopram will increase plasma levels of metoprolol and cimetidine. Concurrent use of alcohol and other CNS depressants may enhance CNS depressant effects; patients should avoid alcohol when taking this drug. Use caution with herbal supplements such as St. John's wort, which may cause serotonin syndrome and increase the effects of escitalopram.

BLACK BOX WARNING:
Antidepressants increase the risk of suicidal thinking and behavior in children, adolescents, and young adults with major depressive disorder and other psychiatric disorders.

Benzodiazepines are useful for the short-term treatment of anxiety and insomnia.

◀ **Core Concept 10.7**

The **benzodiazepines** are one of the most widely prescribed drug classes. The root word *benzo* refers to an aromatic compound, one having a carbon ring structure attached to different atoms or to another carbon ring. Two nitrogen atoms incorporated into the ring structure are the reason for the *diazepine* portion of the name.

benzo = *aromatic or ring structure*
di = *two*
azepine = *nitrogen containing*

The benzodiazepines are used for panic disorder, generalized anxiety, phobias, and insomnia (Table 10.3). Since the introduction of the first benzodiazepines—chlordiazepoxide (Librium) and diazepam (Valium)—in the 1960s, the class has become one of the most widely prescribed in medicine. Although newer benzodiazepines are available, all have the same actions and adverse effects. They differ primarily in their onset and duration of action. Some, such as the induction drug midazolam (Versed), have a rapid onset time of 15 to 30 minutes; others, such as oxazepam (Serax), take 2 to 3 hours to reach peak blood levels. In cases in which the benzodiazepines are used for insomnia therapy, this is important because *time of onset* translates to *time until sleep* for the patient. Duration of action translates to *time of anticipated sleep* or *drowsiness*. The benzodiazepines are categorized as Schedule IV drugs, although they produce considerably less physical dependence and result in less tolerance than the barbiturates.

These drugs intensify the effect of gamma-aminobutyric acid (GABA), which is a natural inhibitory neurotransmitter found throughout the brain. Most are metabolized in the liver to active metabolites and excreted primarily in urine. Death with routine use of benzodiazepines is unlikely, unless the benzodiazepines are taken in combination with other CNS depressants, or the patient suffers from sleep apnea.

Most benzodiazepines are given orally. Those that can be given parenterally, such as diazepam (Valium) and lorazepam (Ativan), should be monitored carefully because of their rapid onset of CNS effects and possible respiratory depression. Due to the possibility of dependence, benzodiazepines may be inappropriate for patients who have a diagnosis of substance abuse.

Because of their greater safety, the benzodiazepines are primarily used for the short-term treatment of insomnia caused by anxiety. Benzodiazepines shorten the length of time it takes to fall asleep and reduce the frequency of interrupted sleep. Although most

Table 10.3 Benzodiazepines for Anxiety and Insomnia

Drug	Route and Adult Dose	Remarks
ANXIETY		
alprazolam (Xanax)	Panic disorder (extended release): PO: 0.5-1 mg/day Anxiety (immediate release): PO: 0.25–0.5 mg three times/day	For GAD, phobias, social anxiety, panic disorder
chlordiazepoxide (Librium)	Mild anxiety: PO: 5–25 mg three or four times/day	For phobias, alcohol withdrawal
clonazepam (Klonopin)	PO: 1–2 mg/day in divided doses (max: 4 mg/day)	For phobias, social anxiety, seizures, panic disorder
clorazepate (Tranxene)	PO: 15 mg/day (max: 4 mg/day)	For alcohol withdrawal, seizures
diazepam (Valium) (see the Prototype Drug box in Core Concept 14.6)	PO: 2–10 mg two times/day	For alcohol withdrawal, seizures, muscle spasms, induction of anesthesia
Pr lorazepam (Ativan)	Anxiety: PO: 2–6 mg/day in divided doses (max: 10 mg/day)	For panic disorder, phobias, alcohol withdrawal, seizures, induction of anesthesia
oxazepam (Serax)	PO: 10–30 mg three or four times/day	For phobias, alcohol withdrawal
INSOMNIA		
estazolam	PO: 1 mg at bedtime (max: 2 mg/day)	For insomnia: 15–60 min onset and medium duration
flurazepam (Dalmane)	PO: 15–30 mg at bedtime	For insomnia: 30–60 min onset and long duration
quazepam (Doral)	PO: 7.5–15 mg at bedtime	For insomnia: 20–45 min onset and long duration
temazepam (Restoril)	PO: 7.5–30 mg at bedtime	For insomnia: 45–60 min onset and medium duration
triazolam (Halcion)	PO: 0.125–0.25 mg at bedtime (max: 0.5 mg/day)	For insomnia: 15–30 min onset and short duration

benzodiazepines increase total sleep time, some reduce Stage IV sleep, and some affect REM sleep. In general, the benzodiazepines used to treat short-term insomnia are different from those used to treat GAD (see Table 10.3).

Benzodiazepines have a number of other important indications. Diazepam (Valium) is featured as a prototype drug in Chapter 14 for its use in treating seizure disorders. Other uses include treatment of alcohol withdrawal symptoms (see Chapter 8), central muscle relaxation (see Chapter 13), and as induction drugs in general anesthesia (see Chapter 16).

Nursing Process Focus Patients Receiving Antianxiety Therapy

ASSESSMENT	POTENTIAL NURSING DIAGNOSES*
Prior to administration: • Obtain a complete health history including cardiovascular, neurologic, and renal and liver conditions; allergies, drug history, likelihood of drug dependency, and possible drug interactions. • Identify factors that precipitate anxiety or insomnia and actions that have been previously tried to decrease symptoms. • Acquire baseline vital signs and neurologic status including level of consciousness (LOC) and stress and coping patterns. • Evaluate laboratory blood findings: renal and liver function studies.	• *Acute Confusion* related to adverse effects of drug therapy • *Deficient Knowledge* related to a lack of information about administration and adverse effects of drug therapy • *Ineffective Coping* related to anxiety or drug dependence • *Insomnia* related to anxiety or adverse effects of drug therapy • *Risk for Injury* related to sedative effect of drug

PLANNING: PATIENT GOALS AND EXPECTED OUTCOMES

The patient will:
- Experience therapeutic effects (an increase in psychological comfort, normal sleep patterns).
- Be free from or experience minimal adverse effects from drug therapy (absence of physical and behavioral manifestations of anxiety).
- Verbalize an understanding of the drug's use, adverse effects, and required precautions.

IMPLEMENTATION

Interventions and (Rationales)	Patient Education/Discharge Planning
• Monitor vital signs. Observe respiratory patterns, especially during sleep, for evidence of apnea or shallow breathing. (Benzodiazepines can reduce the need to breathe in susceptible patients.)	Instruct the patient: • To consult a healthcare provider before taking this drug if snoring is a problem (snoring may indicate an obstruction in the upper respiratory tract, resulting in hypoxia). • Regarding methods to monitor vital signs at home, especially respirations.
• Monitor neurologic status, especially LOC. (Confusion or lack of response may indicate overmedication.)	• Instruct the patient to report extreme lethargy, slurred speech, disorientation, or ataxia to the healthcare provider.
• Ensure patient safety (i.e., nurses call light within reach). (Drug may cause excessive drowsiness.)	Instruct the patient to: • Not drive or perform hazardous activities until the effects of the drug are known. • Request assistance when getting out of bed and walking until the effect of the medication is known.
• Monitor the patient's intake of stimulants, including caffeine (in beverages such as coffee, tea, cola, and other soft drinks and in OTC analgesics such as Excedrin), nicotine from tobacco products, and any drugs such as alcohol that produce drowsiness. (These products can enhance or reduce the drug's effectiveness.)	Instruct the patient to: • Avoid drinking or eating drinks or food with caffeine, especially before bedtime. • Avoid taking alcohol or OTC sleep-inducing antihistamines such as diphenhydramine. • Consult a healthcare provider before self-medicating with any OTC preparation.

Interventions and (Rationales)	Patient Education/Discharge Planning
• Monitor effect and emotional status. (Drug may increase risk of mental depression, especially in patients with suicidal tendencies.)	Instruct the patient to: • Report significant mood changes, especially depression. • Avoid consuming alcohol or taking other CNS depressants while on benzodiazepines because these increase the depressant effect.
• Administer medication correctly, and evaluate the patient's knowledge of proper administration. Avoid abrupt discontinuation of therapy. (Withdrawal symptoms, including rebound anxiety and sleeplessness, are possible with abrupt discontinuation after long-term use.)	Instruct the patient: • To take the drug exactly as prescribed. Discontinuation of medication must be done gradually. • To keep all follow-up appointments as directed by the healthcare provider to monitor response to the medication. • About nonpharmacologic methods for reestablishing sleep regimen.

EVALUATION OF OUTCOME CRITERIA

Evaluate effectiveness of drug therapy by confirming that patient goals and expected outcomes have been met (see "Planning"). *See Table 10.1 and 10.2 for a list of drugs to which these nursing actions apply.*

*Herdman, T.H. & Kamitsuru, S. (Eds.), *Nursing Diagnoses: Definitions & Classification* 2015–2017. Copyright © 2014, 1994–2014 NANDA International. Used by arrangement by John Wiley & Sons, Inc. Companion website: www.wiley.com/go/nursingdiagnoses.

Prototype Drug: Pr *Lorazepam (Ativan)*

Therapeutic Class: Sedative-hypnotic, anxiolytic, anesthetic adjunct **Pharmacologic Class: Benzodiazepine, GABA receptor drug**

Actions and Uses: Lorazepam is a benzodiazepine that acts by increasing the effects of GABA, an inhibitory neurotransmitter in the CNS. It is one of the most potent benzodiazepines. It has an extended half-life of 10 to 20 hours that allows for once or twice a day oral dosing. In addition to its use as an anxiolytic, lorazepam is used as a preanesthetic medication to provide sedation and for the management of status epilepticus.

Adverse Effects and Interactions: The most common adverse effects of lorazepam are drowsiness and sedation, which may decrease with time. When given in higher doses or by the intravenous (IV) route, more severe effects may be observed, such as amnesia, weakness, disorientation, ataxia, sleep disturbance, blood pressure changes, blurred vision, double vision, nausea, and vomiting.

Lorazepam interacts with multiple drugs; for example, concurrent use of CNS depressants, including alcohol, increases sedation effects and the risk of respiratory depression and death. Lorazepam may contribute to digoxin toxicity by increasing the serum digoxin level. Symptoms include visual changes, nausea, vomiting, dizziness, and confusion.

Lorazepam should be used with caution with herbal supplements. For example, sedation-producing herbs such as kava, valerian, chamomile, or hops may have an additive effect with medication. Stimulant herbs such as gotu-kola and ma huang may reduce the drug's effectiveness.

Barbiturates depress CNS function and cause drowsiness.

◀ **Core Concept 10.8**

barbiturate = *barbituric acid compound*

Barbiturates are drugs derived from barbituric acid. Until the discovery of the benzodiazepines, barbiturates were used extensively for anxiety and insomnia treatment (Table 10.4). Although barbiturates are still indicated for several conditions, they are rarely prescribed for treating anxiety or insomnia because of their significant adverse effects and the availability of more effective medications. Most barbiturates are used for procedural sedation, pre-anesthesia, or uncontrolled convulsions. The risk of psychological and physical dependence is high—barbiturates are Schedule II, III, and IV drugs. The withdrawal syndrome from barbiturates is extremely severe and can be fatal. Overdose results in profound respiratory depression, hypotension, and shock. Signs of overdose are difficulty breathing, heart palpitations, sweating, nausea and vomiting, and loss of consciousness. People have used barbiturates to commit suicide. Addiction and death due to overdose is not uncommon.

Barbiturates are capable of depressing CNS function at all levels. Like benzodiazepines, barbiturates act by binding to GABA receptor–chloride channel molecules, intensifying the effect of GABA throughout the brain. At low doses, they reduce anxiety and cause drowsiness. At moderate doses, they inhibit seizure activity (see Chapter 14) and promote sleep, probably by inhibiting brain impulses traveling through the limbic system and the RAS. At higher doses, some barbiturates can produce anesthesia (see Chapter 16).

Table 10.4 Sedative–Hypnotic Barbiturates

Drug	Route and Adult Dose	Remarks
SHORT ACTING		
pentobarbital (Nembutal)	Sedative: PO: 20–30 mg two or three times/day Hypnotic: PO: 120–200 mg	For acute convulsive episodes, limited usefulness as a hypnotic, Schedule III
secobarbital (Seconal)	Sedative: PO: 100–300 mg/day in three divided doses Hypnotic: PO: 100–200 mg	For surgery, prior to anesthesia, limited usefulness as a hypnotic, Schedule II
INTERMEDIATE ACTING		
butabarbital (Butisol)	Sedative: PO: 15–30 mg three or four times/day Hypnotic: PO: 50–100 mg at bedtime	Pre-surgical anesthetic to induce drowsiness, limited usefulness as a hypnotic, Schedule III
LONG ACTING		
phenobarbital (Luminal) (see the Prototype Drug box in Core Concept 14.6)	Sedative: PO: 30–120 mg/day	Anticonvulsant with hypnotic properties, Schedule IV

When taken for prolonged periods, barbiturates stimulate the microsomal enzymes in the liver that metabolize medications. Thus, barbiturates can stimulate their own metabolism as well as that of hundreds of other drugs that use these enzymes for their breakdown. With repeated use, tolerance develops to the sedative effects of these drugs, and cross-tolerance to other CNS depressants such as the opioids. Tolerance does not develop, however, to the respiratory depressant effects.

CONCEPT REVIEW 10.4

- Identify the major drug classes used for sedation and insomnia. Why are CNS depressants especially dangerous if administered in high doses?

Core Concept 10.9 ▶

Additional drugs provide therapy for anxiety-related symptoms and sleep disorders.

The final group of CNS drugs used for anxiety and sleep disorders consists of miscellaneous drugs that are chemically unrelated to the antidepressants, benzodiazepines, or barbiturates. These include the antiseizure medication valproate (Depakote) and the beta blockers atenolol (Tenormin) and propranolol (Inderal). Drugs used mainly for insomnia therapy include eszopiclone (Lunesta), zaleplon (Sonata), and zolpidem (Ambien). Buspirone (BuSpar) and zolpidem (Ambien) are commonly prescribed for their anxiolytic effects. Zolpidem (Ambien), ramelteon (Rozerem), and eszopiclone (Lunesta) are used primarily for their hypnotic effects. Dexmedetomidine (Precedex) is primarily used as an adjunctive medication during short surgical procedures (Table 10.5).

cognitive = *thinking, remembering, and reasoning*

motor = *producing motion or action*

The mechanism of action for buspirone (BuSpar) is unclear but appears to be related to D_2 dopamine receptors in the brain. The drug has profound effects on presynaptic dopamine receptors and a high attraction for serotonin receptors. Buspirone is less likely than benzodiazepines to affect cognitive and motor performance and rarely interacts with other CNS depressants. Common adverse effects include dizziness, headache, and drowsiness. Dependence and withdrawal problems are less of a concern with buspirone. Therapy may take several weeks to achieve optimal results.

The antiseizure medication valproate/valproic acid (Depakene, Depakote) is an important drug used to treat a variety of seizure types. Common uses include treatment for all partial and generalized seizures (see Chapter 14), the control of symptoms in patients with bipolar disorder (see Chapter 11), and to prevent migraine headaches (see Chapter 15). For these reasons, valproic acid is listed as one medication that might be helpful in reducing

Table 10.5 Nonbenzodiazepine, Nonbarbiturate CNS Drugs for Anxiety and Insomnia

Drug	Route and Adult Dose	Remarks
ANXIETY THERAPY		
Sedatives		
buspirone (BuSpar)	PO: 7.5–15 mg in divided doses, may increase by 5 mg/day every 2–3 days (max: 60 mg/day)	For GAD, OCD
dexmedetomidine (Precedex)	IV: Loading dose 1 mcg/kg over 10 min; maintenance dose 0.2–0.7 mcg/kg/hr	Adjunctive medication during surgery, induction in anesthesia
Antiseizure Medication		
valproate/valproic acid (Depakene, Depakote)	Mania: PO: 250 mg three times/day (max: 60 mg/kg/day)	For panic disorder, seizures, smoking, bipolar disorder, prevention of migraines
Beta Blockers		
atenolol (Tenormin) (see the Prototype Drug box in Core Concept 21.7)	PO: 25–100 mg once/day	For performance anxiety, social anxiety
propranolol (Inderal, InnoPran XL) (see the Prototype Drug box in Core Concept 23.7)	Trembling: PO: 40 mg two times/day (max: 320 mg/day)	For performance anxiety, social anxiety
INSOMNIA THERAPY		
Nonbenzodiazepines		
eszopiclone (Lunesta)	PO: 1–2 mg at bedtime (max: 3 mg/day)	60 min onset and medium duration
zaleplon (Sonata)	PO: 10 mg at bedtime (max: 20 mg)	15–30 min onset and short duration
Pr zolpidem (Ambien, Edular, others)	PO: 5–10 mg at bedtime	30 min onset and short (medium CR) duration
Melatonin Receptor Drug		
ramelteon (Rozerem)	PO: 8 mg at bedtime	30 min onset and short duration
tasimelteon (Hetlioz)	PO: 20 mg/day at bedtime, at the same time every night	30 min onset and short duration
Orexin Receptor Blocker		
suvorexant (Belsomra)	PO: 10 mg at bedtime (max: 20 mg/day)	30–120 min onset and long duration.
Antihistamines		
diphenhydramine (Nytol and Sominex)	OTC medication	60–180 min onset and long duration
doxylamine (Unisom)	OTC medication	60–120 min onset and long duration

anxiety symptoms among patients predisposed to panic disorders, mood swings, or intense headaches. Adverse gastrointestinal effects such as nausea and vomiting are common. Rare life-threatening hepatotoxicity and pancreatitis are a concern.

Beta blockers were covered in Chapter 9 and are covered more thoroughly as they pertain to management of hypertension (see Chapter 19), angina (see Chapter 21), and cardiac dysrhythmias (see Chapter 23). Sweating, heart palpitations, and shaking are expected signs of situational, social, and performance anxiety. Low doses of beta blockers reduce symptoms connected with panic, tension, and excitement.

Zolpidem (Ambien) is a Schedule IV controlled substance limited to the short-term treatment of insomnia. It is highly specific to the GABA receptor and produces muscle relaxation (see Chapter 13) and antiseizure effects (see Chapter 14) only at doses much higher than hypnotic doses. As with other CNS depressants, zolpidem should be used cautiously in patients with respiratory impairment, in older persons, and in conjunction with other CNS depressants. Lower dosages may be necessary. In 2011, the FDA issued a statement saying that sleeping pills containing the drug zolpiden were dosed too high, especially for women, and related to incidences of car crashes and other injuries. Ambien taken in recommended doses (5-10 mg) has been shown to decrease sleep latency for up to 35 days in controlled clinical studies. Also, because of the rapid onset of this drug (within 30 minutes), zolpidem should be taken just prior to expected sleep. Adverse reactions are usually minimal (mild nausea, dizziness, diarrhea, daytime drowsiness). Rebound insomnia may occur when the drug is discontinued.

Prototype Drug: Pr Zolpidem (Ambien, Edluar, Others)

Therapeutic Class: Sedative-hypnotic **Pharmacologic Class:** Nonbenzodiazepine, nonbarbiturate CNS depressant, GABA receptor drug

Actions and Uses: Although it is a nonbenzodiazepine, zolpidem acts in a similar fashion to facilitate GABA-mediated CNS depression in the brain. The only indication for zolpidem is short-term insomnia management (2 to 6 weeks). It is available in immediate-release, extended-release, orally disintegrating tablet, and spray forms. Zolpidem is pregnancy category B (immediate release) or C (extended release).

Adverse Effects and Interactions: Adverse effects include daytime sedation, confusion, amnesia, dizziness, depression, nausea, and vomiting. The drug should be used with caution in depressed patients or those with a potential for suicide ideation. The most common long-term risks of zolpidem use are dependence and addiction. Ambien should not be taken longer than 4 weeks. With continued use patients may experience withdrawal symptoms including sleeplessness, anxiety, headaches, muscle pain, tremors, and seizures.

Drug interactions with zolpidem include an increase in sedation when used concurrently with other CNS depressants, including alcohol. When taken with food, absorption is slowed significantly and the onset of action may be delayed.

CAM Therapy | Valerian for Anxiety and Insomnia

Valerian (*Valeriana officinalis*) is a perennial plant that grows in Europe, Asia, and North America. Valerian has several substances in its roots that affect the CNS; the exact active chemical has yet to be identified. This herb has been used to treat nervousness, anxiety, and insomnia for thousands of years and is one of the most widely used herbal CNS depressants. The herb appears to have effects similar to benzodiazepines such as diazepam (Valium). The major side effects of valerian are extensions of its therapeutic effects: drowsiness and decreased alertness. Valerian should not be combined with alcohol or other drugs that cause sedation or drowsiness because excessive drowsiness may occur.

Although structurally unrelated to other drugs used to treat insomnia, eszopiclone (Lunesta) has properties similar to those of zolpidem (Ambien). Eszopiclone's longer elimination half-life, about twice as long as that of zolpidem, may give it an advantage in maintaining sleep and decreasing early-morning awakening. Eeszopiclone is more likely to cause daytime sedation.

Zaleplon (Sonata) may be useful for people who desire to fall asleep but need to awake early in the morning. It is sometimes used for travel purposes and has been advertised by pharmaceutical companies for this purpose.

Ramelteon is a melatonin receptor drug, which has been shown to speed the onset of sleep. It has a relatively short onset of action (30 minutes), and its duration is comparable to the noncontrolled release form of zolpidem. The FDA indications for remelteon or zolpidem are not limited to short-term use because they do not appear to produce dependence or tolerance to dose.

In 2014, tasimelteon (Hetlioz) was approved by the FDA as a second melatonin receptor agonist. This drug is indicated for the treatment of non-24-hour sleep-wake disorder. The most common adverse effects of tasimelteon, although minor in occurrence, have been headaches and abnormal dreams. Mild toxicity or reduced effectiveness could occur if tasimelteon is taken in combination with fluvoxamine (Luvox) or rifampin (Rifadin).

Also in 2014, the FDA approved a new drug in its own class. Suvorexant (Belsomra) tablets are approved for difficulty in falling and staying asleep. Suvorexant is a receptor antagonist that blocks the action of orexin, a chemical involved in the sleep-wake cycle in the brain. The expected action of orexin is uninterrupted sleep lasting for about 7 hours. Suvorexant is taken within 30 minutes of bedtime.

Drugs included in Table 10.5 without dosing information are diphenhydramine (Nytol and Sominex) and doxylamine (Unisom). These are OTC sleep aids. Antihistamines also produce drowsiness and are beneficial in calming patients. They offer the advantage of not causing dependence, although their use is often limited by anticholinergic adverse effects. Diphenhydramine is a common component of antihistamine combinations available OTC for allergic rhinitis and cough and for allergic reactions in general (see Chapter 26).

CONCEPT REVIEW 10.5

- What are the major drug classes used to treat GAD, panic disorder, and anxiety symptoms caused by fearful, recurrent, and traumatic life events?
- Name popular drugs used to treat symptoms of anxiety and insomnia.

Patients Need to Know

Patients taking anxiolytics and CNS depressants need to know the following:

1. Stimulants such as coffee, tea, and chocolate should be avoided because they counteract anxiolytics and sedatives and may worsen anxiety symptoms.
2. Exercise, progressive muscle relaxation, and slow, deep breathing can assist with anxiety relief.
3. Alcohol, antihistamines, and other CNS depressants can increase the effects of anxiolytics. They should be avoided to decrease the risk of accidental depressant overdose and death.
4. Anxiolytics can cause drowsiness. Until effects of these drugs have been established, assistance with getting out of bed and driving may be needed and operation of machinery should be avoided.
5. Anxiolytics and sedatives should be stored in a secure place to avoid accidental ingestion by children and animals.
6. Avoid abrupt discontinuation of medication because withdrawal symptoms may occur after long-term use.
7. Immediately report any significant changes in mood, especially thoughts of suicide, to the healthcare provider.
8. Do not take any OTC medications without first consulting the healthcare provider.
9. Smoking and nicotine dependence are increased in patients with anxiety disorders. Thus, it is believed that smoking and pharmacotherapy for anxiety-related disorders are counter effective. Quitting smoking can reduce anxiety.

Safety Alert: Interpreting Medication Orders

It is extremely important for nurses to know their patients' needs and to clarify with the healthcare provider any medication order that is difficult to interpret or is questionable. For example, an error could be made if an order to discontinue "SSRI," intended to mean "sliding scale regular insulin," is misinterpreted as an order to discontinue the "selective serotonin reuptake inhibitor."

Chapter Review

Core Concepts Summary

10.1 Anxiety disorders fall into many categories, including generalized anxiety, panic disorder, and anxiety due to fearful, recurrent, and traumatic life events.

Major types of anxiety disorders are generalized anxiety, panic disorder, phobias, obsessive–compulsive disorder, and post-traumatic stress disorder.

10.2 Regions of the cerebral cortex, diencephalon, and brain stem are responsible for anxiety and wakefulness.

The limbic system, hypothalamus, and reticular activating system control anxiety and wakefulness. Neural signals passing between these brain regions and involving the brainstem, diencephalon, and cerebral cortex are responsible for anxiety, fear, restlessness, and an interrupted sleep pattern.

10.3 Anxiety is managed with both pharmacologic and nonpharmacologic strategies.

Patients should be encouraged to explore and develop coping strategies for dealing with stress. In cases when anxiety becomes too severe, anxiolytics are an effective treatment.

10.4 An inability to sleep is linked with anxiety.

There are many reasons why a patient might experience sleeplessness. Stress is one factor in short-term insomnia.

Others include caffeine, nicotine, room temperature, light, snoring, and sleep apnea. In long-term insomnia, psychological and physiological factors may be involved.

10.5 Anxiety and insomnia are treated with many types of central nervous system (CNS) drugs.

Antidepressants treat symptoms of stress by altering levels of norepinephrine and serotonin in the brain. *Sedatives, sedative-hypnotics, and CNS depressants* are terms used to describe benzodiazepines, barbiturates, and other drugs. These drugs suppress impulses traveling through the limbic and reticular activating systems, thereby reducing symptoms of stress, producing drowsiness, and promoting sleep.

10.6 When taken properly, antidepressants reduce symptoms of panic and anxiety.

Several classes of antidepressants treat panic and anxiety symptoms: tricyclic antidepressants (TCAs), monoamine oxidase inhibitors (MAOIs), selective serotonin reuptake inhibitors (SSRIs), and atypical antidepressants. The new SSRIs are preferred because they produce fewer sympathomimetic and anticholinergic effects.

10.7 Benzodiazepines are useful for the short-term treatment of anxiety and insomnia.

Benzodiazepines are commonly prescribed for insomnia. Several drugs are used; in general, they differ from the ones used to treat anxiety. Onset and duration of action help determine therapeutic application.

10.8 Barbiturates depress CNS function and cause drowsiness.

Barbiturates are rarely, if ever, prescribed for insomnia. The primary role of this class of drugs is pre-anesthetic sedation and for treatment of convulsions. They depress CNS function by binding to GABA receptors and causing drowsiness. Higher doses of barbiturates cause hypnosis.

10.9 Additional Drugs Provide Therapy for Anxiety-Related Symptoms and Sleep Disorders.

Miscellaneous drugs provide relief from anxiety and anxiety-related symptoms. These include CNS depressants, antiseizure medications, and beta blockers. Additional drugs employed for insomnia therapy involve nonbenzodiazepines, melatonin receptor drugs, a new class of drugs called orexin receptor blockers, and antihistamines (usually diphenhydramine found in many OTC products).

REVIEW Questions

Answer the following questions to assess your knowledge of the chapter material, and go back and review any material that is not clear to you.

1. After eight months of use, the patient abruptly discontinues his zaleplon (Sonata). The patient is now complaining of anxiety and inability to sleep. The nurse suspects:
   1. A panic disorder.
   2. Long-term insomnia.
   3. Behavioral insomnia.
   4. Rebound insomnia.

2. Your patient was started on buspirone (BuSpar) for anxiety disorder 3 days ago. The patient now calls the healthcare provider's office stating that it "just isn't working." Your best response would be:
   1. "BuSpar should give you immediate relief. I will notify the healthcare provider that this medication is not effective."
   2. "It may take several weeks for BuSpar to be fully effective."
   3. "You may need an increased dose of BuSpar for it to work."
   4. "You will need additional medications to ease your anxiety."

3. The hospitalized patient is sleeping at the time the next sedative is ordered. The nurse should:
   1. Wake the patient and administer the next dose of sedative.
   2. Notify the healthcare provider.
   3. Hold the dose and document the reason.
   4. Hold this dose and administer it with the next dose.

4. The nurse informs the patient on zolpidem (Ambien) that it:
   1. Will take a week for the medication to be effective.
   2. May be taken two to three hours before bedtime.
   3. Should be taken just prior to going to bed.
   4. Must be used long term to be effective.

5. The patient has been taking barbiturates for the last few months for difficulty sleeping. The nurse's main concern for the patient who suddenly stops taking the barbiturate would be:
   1. Respiratory depression.
   2. Severe withdrawal.
   3. Hypotension.
   4. Shock.

6. Which of the following nursing interventions would be most appropriate for a patient who has just been administered a sedative?
   1. Orient to surroundings.
   2. Assess for respiratory dysfunction.
   3. Shut off the lights and close the door.
   4. Make sure the call light is within the patient's reach.

7. Anxiety and insomnia are treated with which of the following? (Select all that apply.)
   1. Benzodiazepines
   2. Antidepressants

3. Antipsychotics
4. Barbiturates
5. OTC antihistamine sleep aids

8. It is important to ensure the patient knows to avoid ______, which can increase the effects of central nervous system depressants.
   1. Nicotine
   2. Alcohol
   3. Chocolate
   4. Tea

9. Which of the following is indicated for the treatment of generalized anxiety disorder?
   1. Alprazolam (Xanax)
   2. Estazolam
   3. Clonazepam (Klonopin)
   4. Lorazepam (Ativan)

10. The patient taking lorazepam (Ativan) is monitored for which of the following adverse effects?
    1. Ataxia
    2. Euphoria
    3. Astigmatism
    4. Tachypnea

CASE STUDY Questions

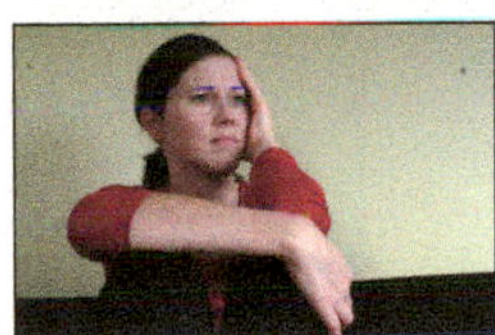

Remember Ms. Reynolds, the patient introduced at the beginning of the chapter? Now read the remainder of the case study. Based on the information you have learned in this chapter, answer the questions that follow.

Ms. Cynthia Reynolds is a 34-year-old interior designer who witnessed and was nearly involved in a fatal car crash on her way to a patient's house about 6 months ago. Since that time she has been having dreams about the accident, and during the day she often thinks about the events and the injured people she saw. She is fearful of driving and does all she can to avoid leaving her home-based office. When she hears a siren, she feels immediate anxiety and terror. After seeing a healthcare provider, Ms. Reynolds is diagnosed with PTSD and is given an SSRI to help relieve her anxiety.

1. There are a couple of SSRIs indicated for the signs and symptoms of PTSD. The nurse would expect Ms. Reynolds to take:
   1. Celexa.
   2. Lexapro.
   3. Prozac.
   4. Paxil.

2. While taking the SSRI, Ms. Reynolds is monitored for:
   1. Diarrhea.
   2. Hypotension.
   3. Hallucinations.
   4. Weight gain.

Answers and complete rationales for the Review and Case Study Questions appear in Appendix A.

REFERENCES

American Psychiatry Association. (2013). *DSM-5 development*. Retrieved at http://www.dsm5.org/Pages/Default.aspx

Herdman, T. H., & Kamitsuru, S. (Eds.). (2014). *NANDA International nursing diagnoses: Definitions and classification, 2015–2017*. Oxford, United Kingdom: Wiley-Blackwell.

National Institute of Mental Health. (n.d.). *Any anxiety disorder among adults*. Retrieved from http://www.nimh.nih.gov/health/statistics/prevalence/any-anxiety-disorder-among-adults.shtml

World Health Organization. (2016). *The ICD-10 classification of mental and behavioural disorders: Clinical descriptions and diagnostic guidelines*. Geneva, Switzerland: Author.

SELECTED BIBLIOGRAPHY

American Sleep Association. (n.d.). *About insomnia*. Retrieved from https://www.sleepassociation.org/patients-general-public/insomnia/insomnia

Boelen, P. A., & Carleton, R. N. (2012). Intolerance of uncertainty, hypochondriacal concerns, obsessive-compulsive symptoms, and worry. *The Journal of Nervous and Mental Disease, 200*, 208–213. doi:10.1097/NMD.0b013e318247cb17

Centers for Disease Control and Prevention. (2016) *Getting enough sleep?* Retrieved from http://www.cdc.gov/features/getting-enough-sleep/index.html

Ghafoori, B., Barragan, B., Tohidian, N., & Palinkas, L. (2012). Racial and ethnic differences in symptom severity of PTSD, GAD, and depression in trauma-exposed, urban, treatment-seeking adults. *Journal of Traumatic Stress, 25*, 106–110. doi:10.1002/jts.21663

Gonçalves, D. C., & Byrne, G. J. (2013). Who worries most? Worry prevalence and patterns across the lifespan. *International Journal of Geriatric Psychiatry, 28*, 41–49. doi:10.1002/gps.3788

Grandner, M. A., Martin, J. L., Patel, N. P., Jackson, N. J., Gehrman, P. R., Pien, G., . . . Gooneratne, N. S. (2012). Age and sleep disturbances among American men and women: Data from the U.S. Behavioral Risk Factor Surveillance System. *Sleep, 35*(3), 395–406. doi:10.5665/sleep.1704

Maercker, A., Brewin, C. R., Bryant, R. A., Cloitre, M., Reed, G. M., van Ommeren, M., . . . Saxena, S. (2013). Proposals for mental disorders specifically associated with stress in the International Classification of Diseases-11. *Lancet, 381*, 1683–1685. doi:10.1016/S0140-6736(12)62191-6

National Institute of Mental Health. (2016). *Anxiety disorders*. Retrieved from http://www.nimh.nih.gov/health/topics/anxiety-disorders/index.shtml

Roh, J. H., Jiang, H., Finn, M. B., Stewart, F. R., Mahan, T. E., Cirrito, J. R., . . . Holtzman, D. M. (2014). Potential role of orexin and sleep modulation in the pathogenesis of Alzheimer's disease. *The Journal of Experimental Medicine, 211*, 2487–2496. doi:10.1084/jem.20141788

Takayanagi, Y., Spira, A. P., Bienvenu, O. J., Hock, R. S., Carras, M. C., Eaton, W. W., & Mojtabai, R. (2015). Antidepressant use and lifetime history of mental disorders in a community sample: Results from the Baltimore Epidemiologic Catchment Area Study. *Journal of Clinical Psychiatry, 76*, 40–44. doi:10.4088/JCP.13m08824

Torres, R., Kramer, W. G., Baroldi, P. (2015). Pharmacokinetics of the dual melatonin receptor agonist tasimelteon in subjects with hepatic or renal impairment. *Journal of Clinical Pharmacology, 55*, 525–533. doi:10.1002/jcph.440

Vázquez, G. H., Baldessarini, R. J., Tondo, L. (2014). Co-occurrence of anxiety and bipolar disorders: Clinical and therapeutic overview. *Depression and Anxiety, 31*, 196–206. doi:10.1002/da.22248

Chapter 11

Drugs for Emotional, Mood, and Behavioral Disorders

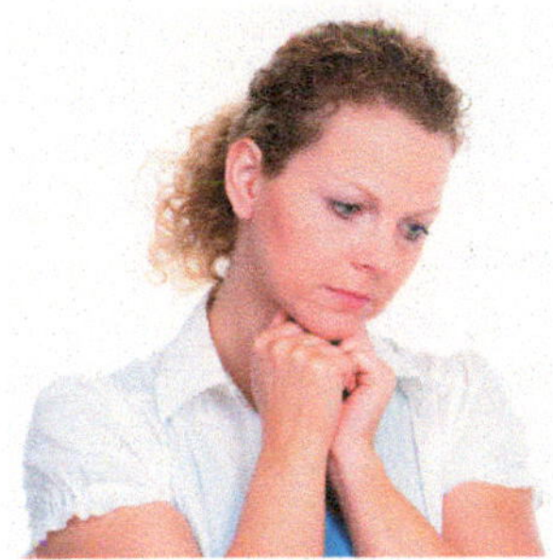

"I hate my job. And my family is constantly nagging me about sleeping too much and eating too little. I don't know what's wrong with me."

Mrs. Rachel Coxilean

Core Concepts

11.1 People suffer from depression for many reasons.

11.2 For best results, treatment of severe depression requires both medication and psychotherapy.

11.3 Antidepressants enhance mood by boosting the actions of neurotransmitters, including norepinephrine, dopamine, and serotonin.

11.4 Patients with bipolar disorder may experience emotions ranging from depression to extreme agitation.

11.5 Mood stabilization in patients with bipolar disorder is accomplished with lithium and other drugs.

11.6 Attention-deficit/hyperactivity disorder presents challenges for children and adults.

11.7 Central nervous system stimulants have been the main course of treatment for ADHD.

Drug Snapshot

The following drugs are discussed in this chapter:

Drug Classes	Prototype Drugs
Antidepressants	
Selective serotonin reuptake inhibitors (SSRIs)	Pr sertraline (Zoloft)
Atypical antidepressants	
Tricyclic antidepressants (TCAs)	Pr imipramine (Tofranil)
Monoamine oxidase inhibitors (MAOIs)	Pr phenelzine (Nardil)
Drugs for Bipolar Disorder	
Mood stabilizers	
Antiseizure drugs	
Atypical antipsychotic drugs	
Drugs for Attention-Deficit/Hyperactivity Disorder (ADHD)	
CNS stimulants	Pr methylphenidate (Ritalin)
Nonstimulant drugs for ADHD	

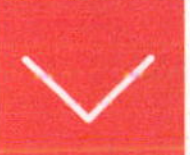

Learning Outcomes

After reading this chapter, the student should be able to:

1. Explain the situational and biological causes of major depressive disorder.
2. Discuss the pharmacologic management and psychotherapeutic approaches to treatment of severe depression.
3. Explain the antidepressant drug classes and how they restore chemical imbalances of neurotransmitters in the brain.
4. Identify symptoms of bipolar disorder and extreme mania.

5. Discuss the pharmacologic management of severe depression and when patients display extreme shifts to mania.
6. Identify symptoms of ADHD.
7. Discuss CNS stimulants and nonstimulant drugs for ADHD.

Key Terms

antidepressants (AN-tee-dee-PRESS-ahnts)
antipsychotic drugs
attention-deficit/hyperactivity disorder (ADHD)
bipolar disorder (bi-PO-ler)
clinical depression
depression (dee-PRESS-shun)
disruptive mood dysregulation disorder (dis-REG-you-lay-shun)
dysthymic disorder (dis-THIGH-mick)
major depressive disorder
monoamine oxidase inhibitors (MAOIs) (mon-oh-AHM-een OK-se-daze)
mood stabilizers
postpartum depression
premenstrual dysphoric disorder (dis-FOR-ick)
psychotic depression
seasonal affective disorder (SAD)
selective serotonin reuptake inhibitors (SSRIs) (sir-eh-TO-nin)
serotonin–norepinephrine reuptake inhibitors (SNRIs)
serotonin syndrome (SES)
situational depression
tricyclic antidepressants (TCAs) (treye-SICK-lick)

Inappropriate or intense emotions over a prolonged period of time are associated with mental health disorders. Although mood changes are a normal part of life, when those changes become severe and impair functioning within the family, work environment, or interpersonal relationships, an individual may be diagnosed as having a mood disorder. The two major categories of mood disorders are depression and bipolar disorder. A third behavioral disorder, attention-deficit/hyperactivity disorder (ADHD), is also included in this chapter.

DEPRESSION

Depression is an emotional disorder characterized by many symptoms, which include changes in sleeping, eating, and daily activities, and persistent mood changes such as feeling constant sadness, shame, and guilt (Table 11.1).

Core Concept 11.1 ▶ People suffer from depression for many reasons.

In some cases, depression may be situational or reactive, meaning that it results from challenging circumstances such as severe physical illness, loss of a job, death of a loved one, divorce, or financial difficulties coupled with inadequate psychosocial support. In other

Table 11.1 Situational and Biological Causes of Depression

Situational Causes of Depression
• Unpleasant life circumstances—grief, divorce, loss of or dissatisfaction with a job, financial difficulty, excessive stress or responsibilities, childhood history of emotional or sexual abuse • Negative thinking patterns—an environment that is likely to cause an individual to feel as if any attempts to escape or correct a situation are hopeless; poor self-image or lack of support from family or friends • Substance abuse—substances that produce unpleasant adverse effects or withdrawal symptoms, such as opiates, alcohol, or other CNS depressants • Medications—unfavorable adverse effects from medication intended to treat a medical disorder (e.g., some antihypertensive drugs and oral contraceptives)
Biological Causes of Depression
• Genetic—history of depression in one's family • Hormonal changes in the body—fluctuations of reproductive or metabolic hormones • Neurobiological dysfunction—chemical disturbances in the brain; usually related to abnormal functioning or release of neurotransmitters (e.g., dopamine, norepinephrine, serotonin, or melatonin) • Symptoms from a second disorder—almost any debilitating disorder, including head trauma, dementia, brain stroke or tumors, chronic pain, or thyroid dysfunction

cases, the depression may be biological or physiological in origin, associated with dysfunction of neurologic processes associated with an imbalance of neurotransmitters. Family history of depression increases the risk of biological depression. In many cases genetics seems to play a role in expression of this disorder. This has been surmised based on the variation of treatment responses among members of the population.

Among the most common forms of mental illness, **major depressive disorder** or **clinical depression** is estimated to affect 5% to 10% of adults in the United States. The American Psychiatric Association's *Diagnostic and Statistical Manual of Mental Disorders*, 5th edition (DSM-5, 2013), describes the following criteria for diagnosis of a major depressive disorder: a depressed affect plus at least five of the following symptoms lasting for a minimum of two weeks:

- Difficulty sleeping or sleeping too much
- Extreme fatigue; without energy
- Abnormal eating patterns (eating too much or not enough)
- Vague physical symptoms (gastrointestinal [GI] pain, joint or muscle pain, or headaches)
- Inability to concentrate or make decisions
- Feelings of despair, guilt, and misery; lack of self-worth
- Obsessed with death (expressing a wish to die or to commit suicide)
- Avoiding psychosocial and interpersonal interactions
- Lack of interest in personal appearance or sex
- Delusions or hallucinations.

The majority of depressed patients are not found in psychiatric hospitals but in mainstream society. For proper diagnosis and treatment to occur, recognition of depression is often a collaborative effort among healthcare providers. For example, it might be the pharmacist who recognizes that a customer is depressed when the customer buys natural or over-the-counter (OTC) remedies to control anxiety symptoms or to induce sleep. **Situational depression** may be the result of circumstances in a person's life. **Dysthymic disorder** is a chronic condition persisting for at least 2 years that is characterized by moderate depressive symptoms of an unknown origin that prevents a person from feeling happiness or functioning normally. **Disruptive mood dysregulation** is characterized in children by severe and recurrent temper tantrums that exceed conditions warranted by the situation. **Premenstrual dysphoric disorder** is a condition in which women express signs of irritability and tension before menstruation. Disruptive mood dysregulation and premenstrual dysphoric disorder are relatively new diagnoses in the mental health field. The process from recognizing depression to properly diagnosing and treating patients should be a collective attempt among healthcare providers. All staff members should be alert for signs and symptoms of depression in patients they treat.

dys = *ill*
thymic = *mind*

meno = *monthly*
pause = *stop*

pre = *before*
menstrual = *menstruation*

Some women experience intense mood shifts associated with pregnancy, childbirth, and menopause. For example, up to 80% of women experience **postpartum depression** during the first several weeks after their baby is born. Many women face additional stresses such as responsibilities both at work and home, single parenthood, and caring for children and aging parents. If mood is severely depressed and persists long enough, many women will likely benefit from medical treatment.

post = *after*
partum = *delivery*

Because of the possible consequences of perinatal mood disorders, some state agencies mandate that all new mothers receive information about mood shifts prior to their discharge after giving birth. Healthcare providers in obstetricians' offices, pediatric outpatient settings, and family medicine centers are encouraged to conduct routine screening for symptoms of perinatal mood disorders.

peri = *around*
natal = *birth*

During the dark winter months, some patients experience **seasonal affective disorder (SAD)**. This type of depression is associated with a reduced release of the brain neurohormone melatonin. Exposing patients on a regular basis to specific wavelengths of light may relieve SAD depression and prevent future episodes.

Psychotic depression is another condition characterized by the expression of mood shifts and unusual behaviors. Intense behaviors include hallucinations, combativeness, and disorganized speech patterns. For patients with psychosis and for patients with extreme mood swings, unusual behaviors are often treatable with antipsychotic drugs (see Chapter 12).

▶ Lifespan and Diversity

Depression is the most common mental health disorder of older patients, encompassing a variety of physical, emotional, cognitive, and social considerations.

Core Concept 11.2 ▶

For best results, treatment of severe depression requires both medication and psychotherapy.

The first step in treating depression is a complete health assessment. Drugs such as corticosteroids, levodopa, and oral contraceptives can cause symptoms of depression, and the healthcare provider should rule out this possibility. Medical and neurologic disorders, ranging from vitamin B deficiencies to thyroid gland disorders to early Alzheimer disease, can mimic depression. Once physical causes for depression are ruled out, a psychological evaluation may be performed by a psychiatrist or psychologist to confirm the diagnosis.

During the health assessment, inquiries should be made about alcohol and drug use, and whether the patient has had thoughts about death or suicide. In addition, because depression is sometimes associated with heredity, the health history should include questions about whether other family members have had a depressive illness and, if treated, what therapies they received and which of them were effective.

After healthcare providers assess for symptoms of depression, it is necessary to determine the course of treatment. In general, severe depressive illness, particularly that which recurs, requires treatment with both medication and psychotherapy to achieve the best response. Counseling therapies help patients gain insight into and resolve their problems through verbal interaction with the therapist. Behavioral therapies help patients learn how to obtain more satisfaction and rewards through their own actions and how to unlearn the behavioral patterns that contribute to or result from their depression.

Two short-term psychotherapies that are helpful for some forms of depression are interpersonal and cognitive-behavioral therapies. *Interpersonal therapy* focuses on the patient's disturbed personal relationships that both cause and worsen the depression. *Cognitive-behavioral therapy* helps the patient change the negative styles of thought and behavior that are often associated with depression. *Psychodynamic therapies*, often postponed until the depressive symptoms are significantly improved, focus on resolving the patient's internal conflicts.

In patients with serious and life-threatening mood disorders that are unresponsive to pharmacotherapy, electroconvulsive therapy (ECT) has been the traditional treatment. Although ECT has been found to be safe, there may be serious complications related to the anesthesia that is used and to the potential seizure activity caused by ECT. Studies suggest that repetitive transcranial magnetic stimulation (rTMS) may improve mood in major depressive disorder. In contrast to ECT, it has minimal effects on memory, does not require general anesthesia, and produces its effects without a generalized seizure.

trans = *across*
cranial = *head*

Even with the best professional care, the patient with depression may take a long time to recover. Individuals with major depression may have multiple bouts of the illness over the course of their lifetime. This can take its toll on the patient's family, friends, and other caregivers who may sometimes feel exhausted, frustrated, and even depressed themselves. They may experience episodes of anger toward the depressed loved one, only to subsequently suffer reactions of guilt about being angry. Such feelings can be distressing, and the caregiver may not know where to turn for help. It is often the healthcare provider who is best able to assist the family members of a person suffering from depression.

Core Concept 11.3 ▶

Antidepressants enhance mood by boosting the actions of neurotransmitters, including norepinephrine, dopamine, and serotonin.

Antidepressants are medications that combat depression by enhancing mood. Depression is thought to be associated with an imbalance of neurotransmitters in certain regions of the brain. Although medication does not completely restore these chemical imbalances, it does help to reduce depressive symptoms while the patient develops effective means of coping. Remember that antidepressants are often used off-label to treat a greater variety of symptoms, including anxiety and restlessness (see Chapter 10); so, many areas of the CNS are potentially targeted by this drug class. Antidepressants may also be used in pain management.

There is one important warning about antidepressants: The U.S. Food and Drug Administration (FDA) has issued a black box warning to be included in drug package inserts and drug information sheets. The advisory is issued to patients, families, and healthcare providers to closely monitor adults and children who are taking antidepressants for warning signs of suicide, especially at the beginning of treatment. In these cases, doses may be changed. The FDA further advises that signs of anxiety, panic attacks, agitation, irritability, insomnia, impulsivity, hostility, and mania may be expected with some patients. Children, adolescents, and young adults are at a greater risk for suicidal ideation than older adults.

There are two major ways in which most antidepressants work: (1) by blocking the enzymatic breakdown of norepinephrine and dopamine, and (2) by slowing the reuptake of serotonin (chemical name, 5-hydroxytryptamine [5-HT]) and norepinephrine. The primary classes of antidepressant drugs, also shown in Table 11.2, are as follows:

- Selective serotonin reuptake inhibitors (SSRIs)
- Atypical antidepressants
- Tricyclic antidepressants (TCAs)
- Monoamine oxidase inhibitors (MAOIs).

Table 11.2 Antidepressants

Drug	Route and Adult Dose	Remarks
SELECTIVE SEROTONIN REUPTAKE INHIBITORS (SSRIs)		
citalopram (Celexa)	PO: Start at 20 mg/day (max: 40 mg/day)	Does not mimic the sympathetic response; has no acetylcholine blocking properties
escitalopram (Lexapro) (see the Prototype Drug box in Core Concept 10.6)	PO: 10 mg daily, may increase to 20 mg after 1 week	For generalized anxiety disorder (GAD)
fluoxetine (Prozac)	PO: 20 mg/day in the a.m. (max: 80 mg/day)	For obsessive–compulsive disorder (OCD), panic disorder, and eating disorders
fluvoxamine (Luvox)	PO: Start with 50 mg/day (max: 300 mg/day)	For OCD; no severe adverse cardiovascular effects; fewer acetylcholine blocking effects
paroxetine (Paxil, Pexeva)	Depression: PO: 10–50 mg/day (max: 80 mg/day); OCD: PO: 20–60 mg/day; panic attacks: PO: 40 mg/day	For OCD, GAD, post-traumatic stress disorder (PTSD), and panic attacks
Pr sertraline (Zoloft)	Adult: PO: Start with 50 mg/day, gradually increase every few weeks to a range of 50–200 mg; Geriatric: Start with 25 mg/day	Does not mimic sympathetic response; has no acetylcholine blocking properties
vilazodone (Viibryd)	Adult: PO: Start with 10 mg/day for 7 days; follow with 20 mg once daily for an additional 7 days; increase to 40 mg once daily	For major depression; thought not to cause significant weight gain or decreased sexual desire
ATYPICAL ANTIDEPRESSANTS		
bupropion (Wellbutrin, Zyban)	PO: 75–100 mg tid (greater than 450 mg/day increases risk for adverse reactions)	For changing moods, schizoaffective disorders, and as an aid to quit smoking; increased risk for seizures; weaker blocker of serotonin and norepinephrine uptake
duloxetine (Cymbalta)	PO: 40–60 mg/day in one or two divided doses	For major depression, GAD, neuropathic pain, chronic fatigue syndrome, stress urinary incontinence, and fibromyalgia
mirtazapine (Remeron)	PO: 15 mg/day in a single dose at bedtime, may increase every 1–2 weeks (max: 45 mg/day)	Potent blocker of 5-HT_2 and 5-HT_3 receptor subtypes; blocks presynaptic $alpha_2$-receptors, enhancing norepinephrine release
nefazodone	PO: 50–100 mg bid, may increase up to 300–600 mg/day	Minimal cardiovascular effects; fewer effects in blocking acetylcholine; less sedation; less sexual dysfunction compared to other antidepressants
trazodone	PO: 150 mg/day, may increase by 50 mg/day every 3–4 days. (max: 400–600 mg/day for regular release)	Increases total sleep time; reduces night awakenings; has anxiolytic effects
venlafaxine (Effexor)	PO: Start with 37.5 mg immediate release every day and increase to 75–225 mg sustained release per day	For major depression, situational depression, GAD, social anxiety, and neuropathic pain
vortioxetine (Trintellix)	PO: 5–20 mg/day once daily	For major depression

(Continued)

Table 11.2 Antidepressants (*continued*)

Drug	Route and Adult Dose	Remarks
TRICYCLIC ANTIDEPRESSANTS (TCAs)		
amitriptyline (Elavil)	Adult: PO: 75–100 mg/day (may gradually increase to 150–300 mg/day)	For biological depression; inhibits gastric acid secretion by blocking histamine-2 receptors in the body
amoxapine (Asendin)	Adult: PO: Start with 100 mg/day, may increase to 300 mg/day	For situational and biological depression; not associated with cardiotoxicity
clomipramine (Anafranil)	PO: 75–300 mg/day in divided doses	For depression accompanying OCD
desipramine (Norpramin)	PO: 75–100 mg/day, may increase to 150–300 mg/day	Active metabolite of imipramine
doxepin (Sinequan)	PO: 30–150 mg/day, may gradually increase to 300 mg/day	For depression accompanying anxiety or alcohol dependence
Pr imipramine (Tofranil)	PO: 75–100 mg/day (max: 300 mg/day)	For biological depression or alcohol or cocaine dependence; may cause cardiac dysfunction and abnormal blood cell count; may control bed-wetting in children
maprotiline	PO: Start at 75 mg/day and gradually increase every 2 weeks to 150 mg/day (max: 300 mg/day)	For a broad range of depression from mild to severe
nortriptyline (Pamelor)	PO: 25 mg tid or qid; may increase to 100–150 mg/day	For biological depression; interactions similar to imipramine
protriptyline (Vivactil)	PO: 15–40 mg/day in three to four divided doses (max: 60 mg/day)	For symptoms of depression; few sedative qualities; causes increased heart rate
trimipramine (Surmontil)	PO: 75–100 mg/day (max: 300 mg/day)	For depression accompanied by a sleep disorder (has strong sedative effects)
MONOAMINE OXIDASE INHIBITORS (MAOIs)		
isocarboxazid (Marplan)	PO: 10–30 mg/day (max: 30 mg/day)	For patients who have not responded to other medications; may cause peripheral edema and high blood pressure
Pr phenelzine (Nardil)	PO: 15 mg tid (max: 90 mg/day)	May cause a hypertensive crisis or respiratory depression; use cautiously in patients with epilepsy or diabetes, or who are likely to abuse drugs and alcohol
selegiline (Emsam)	Transdermal patch: Applied to dry, intact skin once every 24 hours; recommended starting dose and target dose is 6 mg/24 hours	Skin patch used to treat major depressive disorder, designed to deliver medication over a 24-hour period
tranylcypromine (Parnate)	PO: 30 mg/day may increase by 10 mg/day at 3-week intervals up to 60 mg/day	For severe depression in patients who have not responded to other medications

CONCEPT REVIEW 11.1

- What are the major causes of depression? Identify symptoms of major depressive disorder. What name is used to describe drugs that treat depression?

Selective Serotonin Reuptake Inhibitors

Selective serotonin reuptake inhibitors (SSRIs) are drugs that slow the reuptake of serotonin into presynaptic nerve terminals. They have become preferred drugs for the treatment of depression.

In the 1970s, it became increasingly clear that serotonin had a more substantial role in depression than once thought. Researchers knew that some drugs altered the sensitivity of serotonin to receptors in the brain, but they did not know how this was connected to depression. Ongoing efforts to find antidepressants with fewer adverse effects led to the development of the SSRIs.

Serotonin (also called 5-HT) is a natural neurotransmitter in the CNS and is found in high concentrations in neurons of the hypothalamus, limbic system, medulla oblongata, and spinal cord. Serotonin is important to several body activities, including the cycling between nonrapid eye movement (NREM) and rapid eye movement (REM) sleep, pain perception, and emotional states (see Chapter 10). Lack of adequate serotonin in the CNS can lead to depression. Serotonin is metabolized to a less active substance by an enzyme located in presynaptic terminals called *monoamine oxidase (MAO)*. A second enzyme, *catecholamine O-methyl transferase (COMT)*, metabolizes serotonin in the synaptic cleft.

Increased levels of serotonin in the synaptic cleft cause complex neurotransmitter changes in presynaptic and postsynaptic neurons in the brain. Presynaptic receptors become less sensitive, whereas postsynaptic receptors become more sensitive. This concept is illustrated in Figure 11.1.

SSRIs have approximately the same efficacy at relieving depression as the TCAs and the MAOIs. The major advantage of the SSRIs, and the one that makes them first-line drugs, is their greater safety profile. Sympathomimetic effects (increased heart rate and hypertension) and anticholinergic effects (dry mouth, blurred vision, urinary retention, and constipation) are less common with this drug class. Sedation is also experienced less frequently and cardiotoxicity is not observed. All drugs in the SSRI class have equal efficacy and similar side effects. In general, SSRIs elicit a therapeutic response more quickly than TCAs.

One of the most common adverse effects of SSRIs relates to sexual dysfunction. Up to 70% of both men and women may experience decreased libido and lack of ability to reach orgasm. In men, delayed ejaculation and impotence may occur. For patients who are sexually active, these adverse effects may result in noncompliance with pharmacotherapy. Other common adverse effects of SSRIs include weight gain, nausea, headache, anxiety, and insomnia.

Serotonin syndrome (SES) is an adverse event that may occur when a patient is taking an SSRI and an additional medication that affects the metabolism, synthesis, or reuptake of serotonin. The result is that serotonin accumulates in the body. Symptoms can begin as early as two hours or as late as several weeks after taking the first dose. SES can be produced by the administration of an SSRI with an MAOI, a TCA, lithium, or a number of other medications. Symptoms of SES include mental status changes (confusion, anxiety, and restlessness), hypertension, tremors, sweating, fever, and lack of muscular coordination. Conservative treatment is to discontinue the SSRI and provide supportive care. In severe cases, mechanical ventilation and muscle relaxants may be necessary. If left untreated, death may occur.

mono = *one*
amine = *NH2 chemical formula*
oxidase = *water-forming enzyme (hydrogen reacts with oxygen)*

catecholamine = *sympathomimetic amine (dopamine, epinephrine, or norepinephrine)*
O-methyl transferase = *special CH_3 transferring enzyme (O = ortho position [chemical term])*

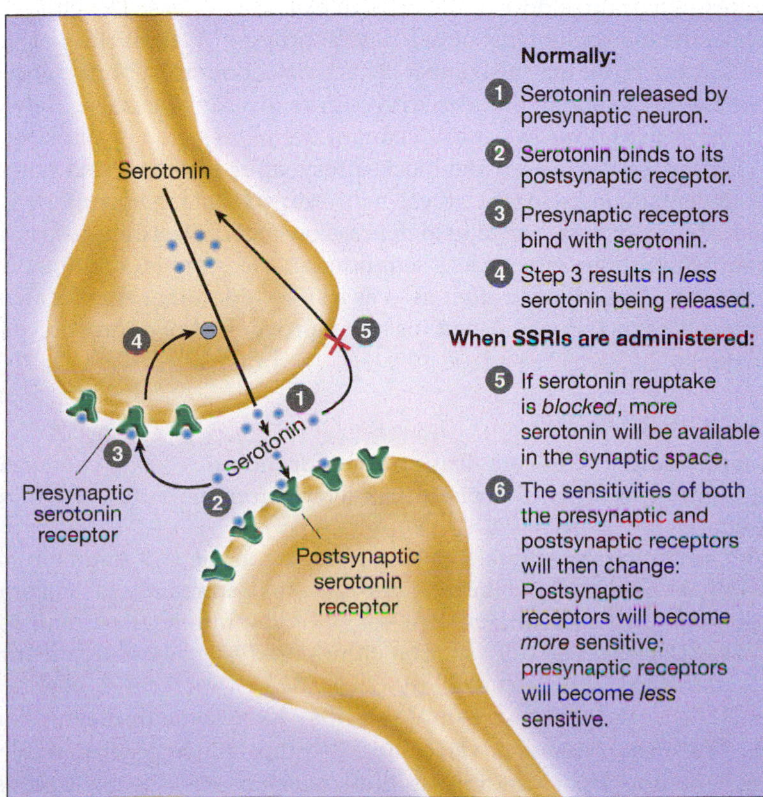

FIGURE 11.1 SSRIs selectively inhibit the reuptake of serotonin, causing complex changes in the presynaptic and postsynaptic neurons.

Prototype Drug: Sertraline (Zoloft)

Therapeutic Class: Antidepressant **Pharmacologic Class:** Selective serotonin reuptake inhibitor (SSRI)

Actions and Uses: Sertraline is used for the treatment of depression, anxiety, OCD, and panic disorder. The antidepressant and anxiolytic properties of this drug can be attributed to its ability to inhibit the reuptake of serotonin in the brain. Other uses include premenstrual dysphoric disorder, PTSD, and social anxiety disorder. Therapeutic actions include enhancement of mood and improvement of affect with maximum effects observed after several weeks.

Adverse Effects and Interactions: Adverse effects include agitation, insomnia, headache, dizziness, somnolence, and fatigue. Take extreme precautions in patients with cardiac disease, hepatic impairment, seizure disorders, suicidal ideation, mania, or hypomania. Antabuse should be avoided because of the alcohol content of the drug concentrate. Highly protein-bound medications such as digoxin and warfarin should be avoided due to risk of toxicity and increased blood concentrations leading to increased bleeding. MAOIs may cause neuroleptic malignant syndrome, extreme hypertension, and serotonin syndrome, characterized by headache, agitation, dizziness, fever, diarrhea, sweating, and shivering. Use cautiously with other centrally acting drugs to avoid adverse CNS effects. Patients should use caution if taking St. John's wort or L-tryptophan to avoid SES.

BLACK BOX WARNING:
Antidepressants can increase the risk of suicidal thinking and behavior, especially in children, adolescents, and young adults with major depressive disorder and other psychiatric disorders.

Atypical Antidepressants

a = *not*
typical = *characteristic*

In terms of classification, the atypical antidepressants do not fit conveniently into the other antidepressant drug classes. Thus, "atypical" in this case really refers to the unique chemical structures represented in the group.

Duloxetine (Cymbalta) and venlafaxine (Effexor), sometimes considered to be in their own subgroup, are the **serotonin–norepinephrine reuptake inhibitors (SNRIs)**. They specifically inhibit the reabsorption of serotonin and norepinephrine and elevate mood by increasing the levels of these neurotransmitters in the CNS. In many cases, levels of dopamine are also affected with the SNRIs. In addition to being approved for the treatment of major depression, duloxetine (Cymbalta) is also approved for the treatment of GAD and for neuropathic pain characteristic of fibromyalgia and diabetic neuropathy. Venlafaxine (Effexor), approved to treat depression and GAD, is available in an intermediate-release form that requires two or three doses a day and an extended-release (XR) form that allows the patient to take the medication just once a day. Bupropion (Wellbutrin) not only inhibits the reuptake of serotonin but may also affect the activity of norepinephrine and dopamine. It should be used with caution in patients with seizure disorders because it lowers the seizure threshold. Bupropion is marketed as Zyban for use in cessation of smoking. Mirtazapine (Remeron) is used for depression and blocks presynaptic serotonin and norepinephrine receptors, thereby enhancing release of these neurotransmitters. Nefazodone is similar to Remeron. It was originally designed to treat depression, and causes minimal cardiovascular effects, fewer anticholinergic effects, less sedation, and less sexual dysfunction than the other antidepressants. Trazodone is often used as a sleep aid, rather than as an antidepressant. The high levels of trazodone needed for the improvement of depression causes sedation in many patients.

Tricyclic Antidepressants

tri = *three*
cyclic = *rings*

Tricyclic antidepressants (TCAs) are drugs named for their three-ring chemical structure. They were the mainstay of depression pharmacotherapy from the early 1960s until the 1980s and are still used.

pre = *before*
post = *after*
synaptic = *the synapse*

TCAs act by inhibiting the reuptake of both norepinephrine and serotonin into presynaptic nerve terminals, as shown in Figure 11.2. TCAs are used mainly for major depressive disorder and occasionally for situational depression. Clomipramine (Anafranil) is approved for treatment of OCD, and other TCAs are sometimes used as off-label treatments for panic attacks (see Chapter 10).

ortho = *standing up*
static = *still*
hypo = *reduced*
tension = *blood pressure*

enuresis = *urination*

Although TCAs treat depressive symptoms, they have some unpleasant and serious adverse effects. The most common adverse effect is orthostatic hypotension (feeling dizzy when changing to an upright or standing position), which occurs due to vasoconstriction of

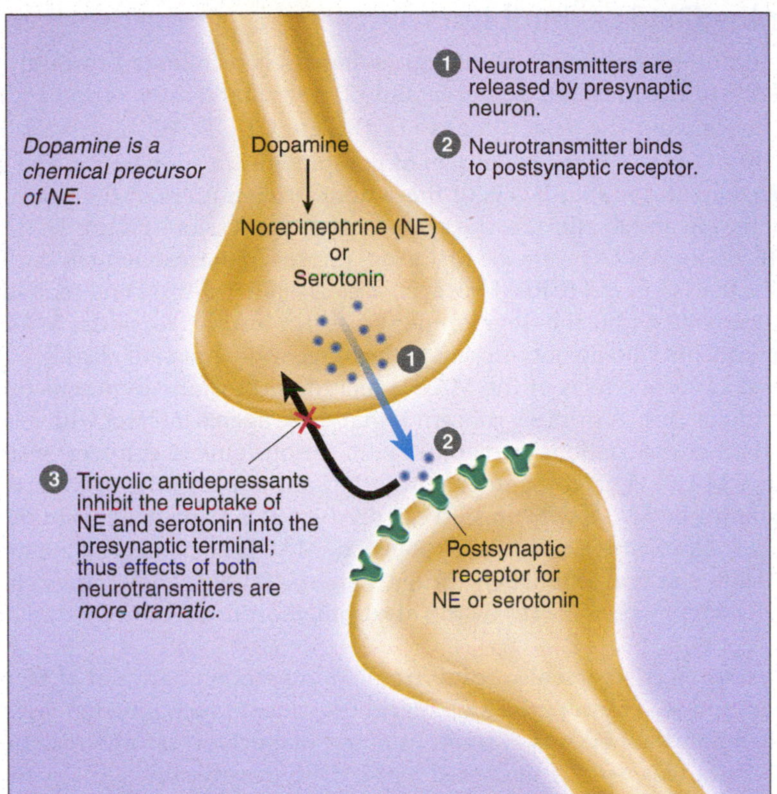

FIGURE 11.2 TCAs inhibit the reuptake of both norepinephrine and serotonin.

blood vessels. Sedation is a frequently reported complaint at the beginning of therapy, but patients usually become tolerant to this effect after several weeks of treatment. Most TCAs have a long half-life, which increases the risk of adverse effects for patients with delayed excretion. Anticholinergic effects, such as dry mouth, constipation, urinary retention, blurred vision, and tachycardia, are common (see Chapter 9). Significant drug interactions can occur with CNS depressants, sympathomimetics, anticholinergics, and MAOIs. Since the discovery of newer antidepressants, TCAs are less frequently used as first-line drugs in the treatment of anxiety mixed with depression.

Lifespan and Diversity

TCAs can cause heart block and other adverse cardiac effects. They must be used cautiously in older adults or those with cardiac disease.

Prototype Drug: *Imipramine (Tofranil)*

Therapeutic Class: Antidepressant **Pharmacologic Class:** Tricyclic antidepressant, serotonin and norepinephrine reuptake inhibitor

Actions and Uses: Imipramine blocks the reuptake of serotonin and norepinephrine into nerve terminals. It is mainly used for major depressive disorder, although it is occasionally used for the treatment of nocturnal enuresis in children. The nurse may find imipramine prescribed for a number of off-label uses, including intractable pain, anxiety disorders, and withdrawal syndromes from alcohol and cocaine.

Adverse Effects and Interactions: Adverse effects include sedation, drowsiness, blurred vision, dry mouth, and cardiovascular symptoms such as dysrhythmias, heart block, and orthostatic hypotension. Agents that mimic the action of norepinephrine or serotonin should be avoided because imipramine inhibits their metabolism and may produce toxicity. Some patients may experience photosensitivity. Concurrent use of other CNS depressants, including alcohol, may cause sedation. Cimetidine (Tagamet) may inhibit the metabolism of imipramine, leading to increased serum levels and possible toxicity. Clonidine may decrease its antihypertensive effects and increase risk for CNS depression. Use of oral contraceptives may increase or decrease imipramine levels. Disulfiram may lead to delirium and tachycardia.

Imipramine should be used with caution with herbal supplements, such as evening primrose oil or ginkgo biloba, because they may lower the seizure threshold. St. John's wort used with imipramine may cause SES.

BLACK BOX WARNING:
Antidepressants can increase the risk of suicidal thinking and behavior, especially in children, adolescents, and young adults with major depressive disorder and other psychiatric disorders. This drug is not approved for use in pediatric patients.

Monoamine Oxidase Inhibitors

The action of norepinephrine at adrenergic synapses is terminated through two means: (1) reuptake into the presynaptic nerve and (2) enzymatic destruction by the enzyme MAO. By decreasing the effectiveness of the enzyme MAO, **monoamine oxidase inhibitors (MAOIs)** limit the breakdown of norepinephrine, dopamine, and serotonin in the CNS. This creates higher levels of these neurotransmitters in the brain to facilitate neurotransmission and to alleviate the symptoms of depression (Figure 11.3).

In the 1950s, the MAOIs were the first drugs approved to treat depression. They are just as effective as the TCAs and SSRIs. However, because of drug–drug and food–drug interactions, hepatotoxicity, and the development of safer antidepressants, MAOIs are now reserved for patients who do not respond to the other antidepressant classes.

Common adverse effects of the MAOIs include orthostatic hypotension, headache, insomnia, and diarrhea. A primary concern is that these agents interact with a large number of foods and other medications, sometimes with serious effects. A hypertensive crisis can occur when a MAOI is used together with other antidepressants or sympathomimetic drugs. Combining an MAOI with an SSRI can produce SES. If given with antihypertensives, the patient can experience excessive hypotension. MAOIs also increase the hypoglycemic effects of insulin and oral antidiabetic drugs. Extreme fever is known to occur in patients taking MAOIs with meperidine (Demerol), dextromethorphan (Pedia Care and others), and TCAs.

A hypertensive crisis can also result from an interaction between MAOIs and foods containing tyramine, a form of the amino acid tyrosine. In fact, tyrosine is a precursor to norepinephrine in the nervous system. In many respects, tyramine resembles norepinephrine. Tyramine is usually degraded by MAO in the intestines. If a patient is taking MAOIs, however, tyramine enters the bloodstream in high amounts and displaces norepinephrine in presynaptic nerve terminals. The result is a sudden increase in norepinephrine, causing acute hypertension. Symptoms usually occur within minutes of ingesting the food and include occipital headache, stiff neck, flushing, palpitations, profuse sweating, and nausea. Calcium channel blockers may be given as an antidote to

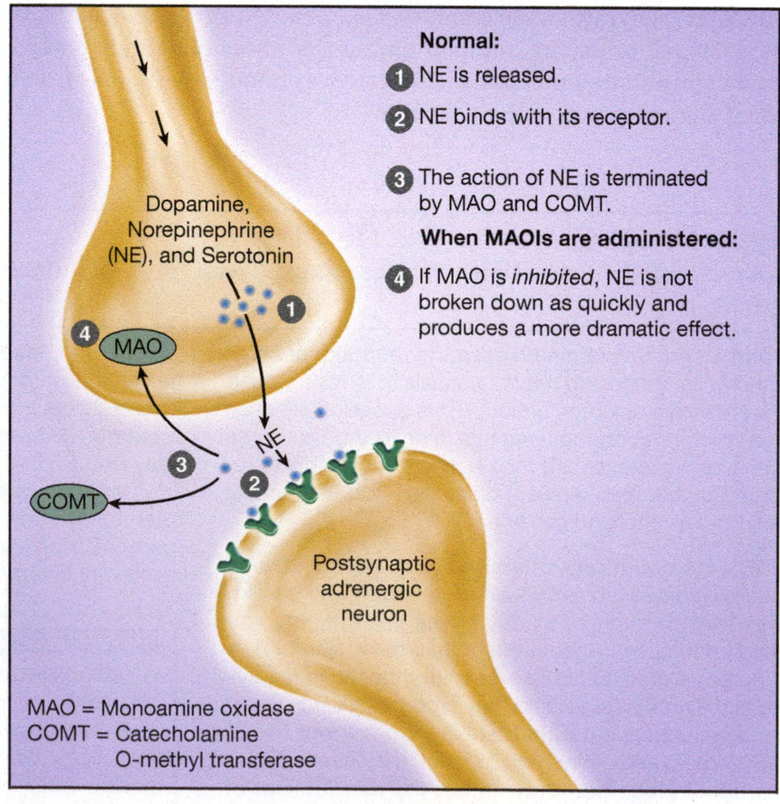

FIGURE 11.3 MAOIs inhibit monoamine oxidase, an enzyme that stops the actions of neurotransmitters such as dopamine, norepinephrine, and serotonin.

reduce blood pressure. Examples of foods containing tyramine include smoked or pickled meats, most cheeses, yogurt, soy sauce, yeast, avocados, chocolate, pineapple and alcoholic beverages.

Prototype Drug: Pr *Phenelzine (Nardil)*

Therapeutic Class: Antidepressant **Pharmacologic Class:** Monoamine oxidase inhibitor (MAOI)

Actions and Uses: Phenelzine produces its effects by irreversible inhibition of MAO; therefore, it intensifies the effects of norepinephrine in adrenergic synapses. It is used to manage symptoms of depression not responsive to other types of pharmacotherapy, and it is occasionally used for panic disorder. Drug effects may continue for two to three weeks after therapy is discontinued.

Adverse Effects and Interactions: Common adverse effects are constipation, dry mouth, orthostatic hypotension, insomnia, nausea, and loss of appetite. It may increase heart rate and neural activity, leading to delirium, mania, anxiety, and convulsions. Severe hypertension may occur when ingesting foods containing tyramine. Seizures, respiratory depression, circulatory collapse, and coma may occur in cases of severe overdose. Many other drugs affect the action of phenelzine. Use with TCAs and SSRIs should be avoided, because the combination can cause temperature elevation and seizures. Opiates, including meperidine, should be avoided due to increased risk of respiratory failure or hypertensive crisis.

Phenelzine should be used with caution with herbal supplements such as ginseng, which could cause headache, tremors, mania, insomnia, irritability, and visual hallucinations. Concurrent use of ephedra could cause hypertensive crisis.

BLACK BOX WARNING:
Antidepressants can increase the risk of suicidal thinking and behavior, especially in children, adolescents, and young adults with major depressive disorder and other psychiatric disorders.

CONCEPT REVIEW 11.2

- Name the major classes of antidepressants. Name representative drugs within each class, and describe how each drug works pharmacologically.

Nursing Process Focus Patients Receiving Antidepressant Therapy

ASSESSMENT

Prior to drug administration:

- Obtain a complete health history including cardiovascular, thyroid, renal and liver conditions, allergies, drug history, likelihood of drug dependency, and possible drug interactions.
- Evaluate laboratory blood findings: complete blood count (CBC), chemistry, clotting factors, glucose, renal and liver function studies.
- Determine neurologic status, including history of mental previous disorders, seizure activity, level of consciousness, and identification of recent mood and behavior patterns.
- Identify factors that may have precipitated the depressive episode and actions that have been previously tried to decrease symptoms.

POTENTIAL NURSING DIAGNOSES*

- *Ineffective Coping* related to inadequate level of confidence in ability to cope
- *Deficient Knowledge* related to a lack of information about drug therapy
- *Noncompliance* related to length of time before medication reaches therapeutic levels and adverse effects of drug therapy
- *Urinary Retention* related to adverse anticholinergic effects of drug
- *Risk for Injury* related to adverse effects of medications and depressive state

PLANNING: PATIENT GOALS AND EXPECTED OUTCOMES

The patient will:

- Experience therapeutic effects (mood elevation) and effectively engage in activities of daily living.
- Be free from or experience minimal adverse effects from drug therapy.
- Verbalize an understanding of the drug's use, adverse effects, and required precautions.

(Continued)

Nursing Process Focus (*continued*)

IMPLEMENTATION

Interventions and (Rationales)	Patient Teaching/Discharge Planning
• Administer the medication correctly and evaluate the patient's knowledge of proper administration. (Proper administration helps to increase the effectiveness of drugs and prevent severe adverse effects.)	Instruct the patient to: • Take exactly as prescribed, and use the prescribed drug produced by the same manufacturer, if possible, each time the prescription is refilled. • Take a missed dose as soon as it is noticed but do not take double or extra doses to catch up. • Take with food to decrease GI upset. • Not abruptly discontinue taking medication. • Practice reliable contraception and notify the healthcare provider if pregnancy is planned or suspected.
• Monitor vital signs, especially pulse and blood pressure. Notify the healthcare provider if pulse or blood pressure drop below approved parameters. (TCAs may cause orthostatic hypotension.)	Instruct the patient to: • Report any change in sensorium, particularly impending syncope. • Avoid abrupt changes in position. • Monitor vital signs (especially blood pressure), ensuring proper use of home equipment. • Consult the healthcare provider regarding "reportable" blood pressure readings (e.g., lower than 80/50 mmHg).
• Observe for SES in SSRI use: confusion, anxiety, restlessness, hypertension, tremors, diaphoresis, fever, lack of muscular coordination, and possibly death (usually occurs with concurrent use of St. John's wort or MAOIs). If suspected, discontinue the drug and initiate supportive care. Respond according to intensive care unit or emergency department protocols.	Inform the patient: • That overdosage may result in SES, which can be life threatening. • To seek immediate medical attention for dizziness, headache, tremor, nausea, vomiting, anxiety, disorientation, lack of muscle coordination, sweating, and fever. • To seek medical attention if an increase in sweating is associated with nausea, vomiting, or chest pain.
• Monitor cardiovascular status. Observe for hypertension and signs of impending stroke or myocardial infarction and heart failure. (Cardiovascular symptoms may be a result of the sympathomimetic effects of MAOIs and TCAs.)	• Instruct the patient to immediately report severe headache, dizziness, paresthesias, bradycardia, chest pain, tachycardia, nausea, vomiting, or diaphoresis.
• Monitor neurologic status. Observe for somnolence and seizures. (TCAs may cause somnolence related to CNS depression and may reduce the seizure threshold.)	Instruct the patient to: • Report any significant changes in neurologic status, such as seizures, extreme lethargy, slurred speech, disorientation, or ataxia to the healthcare provider, and to discontinue the drug. • Take the dose at bedtime to avoid daytime sedation.
• Monitor mental and emotional status. Observe for suicidal ideation. (Therapeutic benefits may be delayed. Outpatients should have no more than a 7-day medication supply.) Also monitor for underlying or concomitant psychoses such as schizophrenia or bipolar disorders (may trigger manic states).	Instruct the patient: • To immediately report dysphoria or suicidal impulses • To commit to a "no-self harm" verbal contract • That it may take a couple of weeks before improvement is noticed, and about one month to achieve full therapeutic effect
• Monitor sleep–wake cycle. Observe for insomnia or daytime somnolence. (Sleep disturbances can be an effect of disease processes or use of certain antidepressants such as MAOIs.)	Instruct the patient to: • Take the drug very early in the morning to promote normal timing of sleep onset. • Avoid driving or potentially hazardous activities until the effects of the drug are known. • Take at bedtime if daytime drowsiness persists. • Take in the morning if insomnia persists.
• Monitor renal status and urinary output. (Medications may cause urinary retention due to muscle relaxation in the urinary tract. Imipramine is excreted through the kidneys. Fluoxetine is slowly metabolized and excreted, increasing the risk of organ damage.)	Instruct the patient to: • Monitor fluid intake and output. • Notify the healthcare provider of edema, dysuria (hesitancy, pain, diminished stream), changes in urine quantity or quality (e.g., cloudy, with sediment). • Report fever or flank pain that may indicate a urinary tract infection related to urine retention.

Interventions and (Rationales)	Patient Teaching/Discharge Planning
• Use cautiously with older or young patients. (Diminished kidney and liver function related to aging can result in higher serum drug levels and may require lower doses. Children, due to an immature CNS, respond paradoxically to CNS-active drugs.)	Instruct the patient that: • Older patients may be more prone to adverse effects such as hypertension and dysrhythmias. • Children on imipramine for nocturnal enuresis may experience mood alterations.
• Monitor GI status. Observe for abdominal distention. (Muscarinic blockade reduces tone and motility of intestinal smooth muscle and may cause paralytic ileus.)	Instruct the patient to: • Exercise, drink adequate amounts of fluids, and add dietary fiber to promote stool passage. • Consult the healthcare provider regarding a bulk laxative or stool softener if constipation becomes a problem.
• Continue to monitor laboratory studies, including CBC, clotting factors, and liver enzymes. Observe for signs and symptoms of liver toxicity. (Some antidepressants may cause liver toxicity or GI bleeding. Antidepressants need to be used cautiously in patients with a history of liver disease.)	Instruct the patient to: • Report nausea, vomiting, diarrhea, rash, jaundice, epigastric or generalized abdominal pain or tenderness, and change in color of stool to the healthcare provider. • Comply with the laboratory testing regimen for blood tests and urinalysis as directed.
• Observe for signs of bleeding. (Imipramine may cause blood dyscrasias. Use with warfarin may increase bleeding time.)	Instruct the patient to: • Report excessive bruising, fatigue, pallor, shortness of breath, visible bleeding, or tarry stools to the healthcare provider. • Conduct guaiac testing on stool for occult blood.
• Monitor for signs of dehydration. (Dehydration may cause lithium toxicity.)	• Inform the patient about the importance of staying well hydrated. • Instruct the patient to report any nausea, emesis, diarrhea, weakness, lack of muscle coordination, confusion, lethargy, polyuria, or seizures (signs of lithium toxicity) to the healthcare provider.
• Monitor immune and metabolic status. Use with caution in patients with diabetes mellitus or hyperthyroidism. (If given in hyperthyroidism, this drug can cause agranulocytosis. Imipramine may either increase or decrease serum glucose. Fluoxetine may cause initial anorexia and weight loss, but prolonged therapy may result in weight gain of up to 20 pounds.)	Instruct the patient: • With diabetes to monitor glucose level daily and to consult the nurse regarding reportable serum glucose levels. • To monitor weight. Possible anorexia and weight loss will diminish with continued therapy.
• Observe for extrapyramidal symptoms and anticholinergic effects. In overdosage, 12 hours of anticholinergic activity is followed by CNS depression. Do not treat overdosage with quinidine, procainamide, atropine, or barbiturates. (Quinidine and procainamide can increase the possibility of dysrhythmia; atropine can lead to severe anticholinergic effects; and barbiturates can lead to excess sedation.)	Instruct the patient to: • Immediately report any involuntary muscle movement of the face or upper body (e.g., tongue spasms), fever, anuria, lower abdominal pain, anxiety, hallucinations, psychomotor agitation, visual changes, dry mouth, and difficulty swallowing to the healthcare provider. • Relieve dry mouth with (sugar-free) hard candies, by chewing gum, and by drinking fluids. • Avoid alcohol-containing mouthwashes, which can further dry oral mucous membranes.
• Monitor visual acuity. Use with caution in narrow-angle glaucoma. (Imipramine may cause an increase in intraocular pressure. Anticholinergic effects may produce blurred vision.)	Instruct the patient to: • Report any visual changes, headache, or eye pain to the healthcare provider. • Inform an eye care professional of imipramine therapy.
• Ensure patient safety. (Dizziness caused by orthostatic hypotension increases the risk of fall injuries.)	Instruct the patient to: • Call for assistance before getting out of bed or attempting to ambulate alone. • Avoid driving or performing hazardous activities until blood pressure is stabilized and effects of the drug are known.

EVALUATION OF OUTCOME CRITERIA

Evaluate the effectiveness of drug therapy by confirming that patient goals and expected outcomes have been met (see "Planning"). *See Table 11.2 for a list of drugs to which these nursing actions apply.*

BIPOLAR DISORDER

bi = *two*
polar = *extremes*

Bipolar disorder is characterized by extreme and opposite moods. Patients may display signs of euphoria and depression or feelings of excitement and calm.

Core Concept 11.4 ▶ Patients with bipolar disorder may experience emotions ranging from depression to extreme agitation.

Once known as *manic depression*, bipolar disorder is characterized by extreme and opposite moods, such as euphoria and depression. Although the moods of patients may shift between extremes, usually patients will remain in one mood for a while, or they may remain in a normal mood for prolonged times.

dys = *difficulty (as in illness)*
phoric = *bearing*
mania = *excessively intense or excited mood*

Depressed and slightly depressed or *dysphoric* signs and symptoms are the same as those described earlier in this chapter. Patients with bipolar disorder also display signs of *mania*, an emotional state characterized by high psychomotor activity and irritability. Symptoms of mania are shown in the following list; these are generally the opposite of depressive symptoms.

- Disordered sleep patterns
- Activity for days without rest and without appearing tired
- Easy agitation and aggression
- Feelings of exaggerated confidence
- Making choices without regard for a long-term plan or consequences of action
- Attention seeking
- Unusual interest in sex
- Drug abuse, including alcohol, cocaine, or sleeping medications
- Denial that the behavior is a problem

CONCEPT REVIEW 11.3

- Identify the symptoms of mania. How do manic symptoms generally compare with depressive symptoms?

Core Concept 11.5 ▶ Mood stabilization in patients with bipolar disorder is accomplished with lithium and other drugs.

anti = *against*
psychotic = *psychosis, mental state*
seizure = *to take hold*

Drugs for bipolar disorder are called **mood stabilizers** because they have the ability to moderate extreme shifts in emotions between mania and depression. Currently, lithium, antiseizure drugs, and atypical antipsychotic drugs are still used for mood stabilization in patients with bipolar disorder. Table 11.3 lists selected drugs used to treat bipolar disorder.

For years, the traditional treatment of bipolar disorder was lithium (Eskalith) used as monotherapy or in combination with other drugs. Lithium was approved in the United States in 1970. With lithium, serum levels must be checked every 1 to 3 days when

CAM Therapy | St. John's Wort for Depression

One of the most popular herbs in the United States, St. John's wort (*Hypericum perforatum*) grows throughout Asia, Europe, and North America. Its modern use is as an antidepressant. It gets its name from a legend that red spots once appeared on its leaves on the anniversary of the beheading of St. John the Baptist. The word *wort* is a British term for "plant."

Research suggests that substances found in St. John's wort selectively inhibit serotonin reuptake in certain brain neurons. A number of clinical studies suggest that St. John's wort is an effective treatment for mild to moderate depression, and that it may be just as effective as TCAs and SSRIs. Recent analyses also suggest that the herb may be effective for major depression and that it causes fewer adverse effects than traditional drugs. St. John's wort may interact with many medications, including oral contraceptives, warfarin, digoxin, and cyclosporine. It should not be taken concurrently with antidepressant medications.

St. John's wort is well tolerated, producing mild adverse effects such as GI distress, fatigue, and allergic skin reactions. The herb contains compounds that photosensitize the skin; thus patients should be advised to apply sunscreen or wear protective clothing when outdoors.

Table 11.3 Drugs for Bipolar Disorder: Mood Stabilizers

Drug	Route and Adult Dose	Remarks
lithium (Eskalith)	PO: Initial 600 mg tid, maintenance 300 mg tid (max: 2.4 g/day)	For mania and depressive symptoms; used cautiously for epilepsy and psychosis
ANTISEIZURE DRUGS		
carbamazepine (Tegretol)	PO: 200 mg bid, gradually increased to 800–1200 mg/day in three to four divided doses	For manic depressive and schizoaffective symptoms; also used as antiseizure medication
lamotrigine (Lamictal)	PO: 50 mg/day for 2 weeks, may increase gradually to 300–500 mg/day (max: 700 mg/day)	Antiseizure medication; fatal rash has been reported in children less than 16 years old
valproate (Depakote)/valproic acid (Depakene) (see the Prototype Drug box for valproic acid in Core Concept 14.7)	PO: 250 mg tid (max: 60 mg/kg/day) PO (Depakote ER): 10–60 mg	For mania and prevention of migraines; also used as an antiseizure medication
ATYPICAL ANTIPSYCHOTIC DRUGS		
aripiprazole (Abilify)	PO: 10–15 mg/day (max: 30 mg/day)	For add-on treatment in adults with major depression; mania or mixed episodes of bipolar disorder; schizophrenia; irritability associated with autistic disorder in pediatric patients
asenapine (Saphris)	Adult: 10 mg sublingually bid (monotherapy); 5 mg sublingually bid (adjunct to lithium or valproic acid therapy)	For acute mania or mixed episodes associated with bipolar disorder in adults; taken alone or with a mood stabilizer (lithium or valproate)
cariprazine (Vraylar)	PO: 1.5–6 mg once daily	Newer drug for bipolar disorder and schizophrenia
olanzapine (Zyprexa)	Adult: PO: Start with 5–10 mg/day (max: 20 mg/day)	For schizophrenia and manic episodes of bipolar disorder
quetiapine (Seroquel)	PO: Start with 25 mg bid; may increase to a target dose of 300–400 mg/day in divided doses	For acute depressive episodes associated with bipolar disorder
risperidone (Risperdal) (see the Prototype Drug box inCore Concept 12.5)	PO: 1–6 mg bid; increase by 2 mg daily to an initial target dose of 6 mg/day	For schizophrenia; episodes of mania or mixed episodes of bipolar disorder; behavior problems such as aggression, self-injury, and sudden mood changes in teenagers and children with autism
ziprasidone (Geodon)	PO: 20 mg bid (max: 80 mg bid)	For acute mania or mixed episodes associated with bipolar disorder; maintenance treatment of bipolar disorder when added to lithium or valproate; schizophrenia

beginning therapy, and every two to three months thereafter. To ensure therapeutic action, concentrations of lithium in the blood must remain within the range of 0.6 to 1.5 mEq/L. Close monitoring encourages compliance and helps to avoid toxicity. Lithium is taken as a salt, so it mixes in the bloodstream like sodium chloride. Therefore, conditions in which sodium is lost (e.g., excessive sweating or increased urination, which leads to dehydration) can cause the kidneys to reabsorb the lithium salts back into the blood, producing elevated serum levels of lithium known as lithium toxicity. Lithium overdose may be treated with hemodialysis and supportive care.

For the most complete control of bipolar disorder, it is not unusual for other drugs to be used in combination with lithium. During the depressed state, a TCA or an atypical antidepressant such as bupropion (Wellbutrin) may be necessary. During manic phases, a benzodiazepine will moderate manic symptoms (see Chapter 10). In cases of extreme agitation, delusions, or hallucinations, antipsychotic drugs may be indicated (see Chapter 12). Continued patient compliance is essential to achieving successful pharmacotherapy because some patients do not perceive their condition as abnormal.

Today, antiseizure drugs (see Chapter 14) and atypical **antipsychotic drugs** (see Chapter 12) have emerged as the most effective agents for mood stabilization. For example, valproic acid (Depakene, Depakote), carbamazepine (Tegretol), and lamotrigine (Lamictal) are the antiseizure drugs most often used in the treatment of rapidly cycling and mixed states of bipolar disorder. Several atypical antipsychotics are very effective for the treatment of extreme mania. Important antipsychotic drugs for bipolar disorder are aripiprazole (Abilify), asenapine (Saphris), olanzapine (Zyprexa), quetiapine (Seroquel), risperidone (Risperdal), and ziprasidone (Geodon). Longer term stabilization of extreme and unusual behaviors with atypical antipsychotics is covered in Chapter 12. Lithium has remained effective for purely manic or purely depressive states.

CONCEPT REVIEW 11.4

- Give the general name of drugs used to treat bipolar disorder. What has been the main drug used to treat bipolar disorder, and how does it work pharmacologically? What other drugs treat bipolar disorder?

ATTENTION-DEFICIT/HYPERACTIVITY DISORDER

A condition characterized by poor attention span, behavior control issues, and hyperactivity is called **attention-deficit/hyperactivity disorder (ADHD)**. Although the condition has most often been diagnosed in childhood, symptoms of ADHD may extend into adulthood, and an increasing number of adults are being evaluated for ADHD.

Core Concept 11.6 ▶

Attention-deficit/hyperactivity disorder presents challenges for children and adults.

▶ Lifespan and Diversity

ADHD affects as many as 5% of all children. Most children diagnosed with this condition are between the ages of 3 and 7 years, and boys are four to eight times more likely to be diagnosed than girls.

ADHD is characterized by developmentally inappropriate behaviors involving difficulty in paying attention or focusing on tasks. ADHD may be diagnosed when a child's hyperactive behaviors significantly interfere with normal play, sleep, or learning activities. Hyperactive children usually have increased motor activity shown by a tendency to be fidgety and impulsive and to interrupt and talk excessively during their developmental years; therefore, they may not be able to interact with others appropriately at home or school. In boys, the activity levels are usually more overt. Girls show less aggression and impulsiveness but may show more anxiety, mood swings, social withdrawal, and cognitive and language delays. Girls also tend to be older at the time of diagnosis, so problems and setbacks related to the disorder exist for a longer time before treatment interventions are undertaken. Symptoms of ADHD are shown in the following list:

- Easy distractibility
- Failure to receive or follow instructions properly
- Inability to focus on one task at a time and tendency to jump from one activity to another
- Difficulty remembering
- Frequent loss or misplacing of personal items
- Excessive talking and interrupting other children in a group
- Inability to sit still when asked repeatedly
- Impulsiveness
- Sleep disturbances.

Most children with ADHD have associated challenges. Many find it difficult to concentrate on tasks assigned in school. Even if they are gifted, their grades may suffer because they have difficulty following a conventional routine. Discipline may also be a problem. Teachers are often the first to suggest that a child should be examined for ADHD and receive medication when behaviors in the classroom escalate to the point of interfering with learning. A diagnosis is based on psychological and medical evaluations.

Fast Facts ADHD

- ADHD is the major reason why children are referred for mental health treatment.
- About 50% of children are also diagnosed with oppositional defiant or conduct disorder.
- Anxiety disorder is diagnosed in 25% of children.
- About one-third are also diagnosed with depression.
- Learning disabilities are present in about 20% of children.

The cause of ADHD is not clear. Evidence suggests that hyperactivity may be related to a deficit or dysfunction of dopamine, norepinephrine, and serotonin in the reticular activating system of the brain (see Chapter 10). ADHD was once thought to be caused by sugar, chocolate, high-carbohydrate foods and beverages, and certain food additives, but these have been disproved as causing or aggravating ADHD.

One-third to one-half of children diagnosed with ADHD also experience symptoms of attention dysfunction in their adult years. Symptoms of ADHD in adults appear similar to those of mood disorders and include anxiety, mania, restlessness, and depression, which can also cause difficulties in interpersonal relationships. Attention dysfunction in adults is often linked with poor self-esteem, diminished social success, and introverted behaviors. Patients may have mood swings similar to bipolar disorder.

Central nervous system stimulants have been the main course of treatment for ADHD.

◀ **Core Concept 11.7**

Traditional therapies for ADHD include CNS stimulants. Newer therapies have added non-CNS stimulants.

CNS Stimulants

These drugs stimulate specific areas of the CNS that heighten alertness and increase focus. In 2002, a nonstimulant was first approved to treat ADHD. Agents for treating ADHD are listed in Table 11.4.

Stimulants reverse many of the symptoms and help patients to focus on tasks. The most widely prescribed drug for ADHD is methylphenidate (Ritalin). Other less prescribed CNS stimulants include d- and 1-amphetamine racemic mixtures (Adderall), dextroamphetamine (Dexedrine), or methamphetamine (Desoxyn). More recently, extended-release forms have been made available: dextroamphetamine mixture (Adderall XR), dexmethylphenidate (Focalin XR), and slow-releasing methylphenidate (Ritalin, LA/SR). Lisdexamfetamine (Vyvanse) is a psychostimulant prodrug of phenethylamine and amphetamine. It is a once-daily prescription medication that helps increase attention and decrease impulsiveness and hyperactivity.

Table 11.4 Drugs for Attention-Deficit/Hyperactivity Disorder

Drug	Route and Adult Dose	Remarks
CNS STIMULANTS		
amphetamine (Adderall, Adderall-XR)	3–5 years old: PO: 2.5 mg one to two times/day 6 years old: PO: 5 mg daily to bid (max: 40 mg/day); Adult: 10 mg/day extended release (max: 30 mg/day)	For daytime sleep disorder (narcolepsy); high potential for abuse
dexmethylphenidate (Focalin, Focalin-XR)	6 years old to adult: PO: 2.5 mg bid (max: 20 mg/day); 5 mg/day extended release	For ADHD; mild stimulant to the CNS
dextroamphetamine (Dexedrine)	3–5 years old: PO: 2.5 mg daily to bid, 6 years old: PO: 5 mg daily to bid (max: 40 mg/day)	Potent appetite suppressant; for short-term treatment of ADHD; safety in children less than 3 years old has not been established
lisdexamfetamine (Vyvanse)	6 years old to adult: PO: 20–70 mg once daily (max: 70 mg/day)	Prodrug of dextroamphetamine
methamphetamine (Desoxyn)	6 years old: PO: 2.5–5 mg daily to bid (max: 20–25 mg/day)	Abuse potential high in adults
Pr methylphenidate (Concerta, Daytrana, Metadate, Methylin, Ritalin, Quillivant XR)	6 years old: PO: 5–10 mg bid (max: 60 mg/day) Adult: PO: 5–20 mg (prompt-release tablets) bid to tid; may switch to extended release once the maintenance dose is determined; doses vary depending on drug formulation	Most widely used drug for ADHD; more dramatic effect on attention deficit than hyperactivity; also for narcolepsy; once-daily extended release liquid form available
NONSTIMULANTS		
atomoxetine (Strattera)	Children less than 70 kg: PO: Start with 0.5 mg/kg/day; may increase to target dose of 1.2 mg/kg/day (max dose: 1.4 mg/kg/day or 100 mg) Adult: PO: Start with 40 mg, may increase to target dose of 80 mg/day (max: 100 mg/day)	Inhibits reuptake of norepinephrine; safety and efficacy in children less than 6 years old has not been established
clonidine (Kapvay)	6 years old to 17 years old: PO: Start with 0.1 mg/day (max: 0.4 mg/day)	Sometimes prescribed when patients are aggressive, active, or have difficulty sleeping; stimulates alpha$_2$-receptors in the brain
guanfacine (Intuniv)	6 years old to 17 years old: PO: Start with 1 mg/day (max: 4 mg/day)	For high blood pressure; used alone or together with other ADHD medicines

Patients taking CNS stimulants must be carefully monitored because the drugs may cause paradoxical hyperactivity. Adverse reactions include insomnia, nervousness, anorexia, and weight loss. Occasionally, a patient may suffer from dizziness, depression, irritability, nausea, or abdominal pain. These drugs are Schedule II controlled substances and pregnancy category C.

Prototype Drug: Pr *Methylphenidate (Ritalin)*

Therapeutic Class: Drug for attention-deficit/hyperactivity disorder (ADHD), narcolepsy drug

Pharmacologic Class: Central nervous system stimulant, norepinephrine and dopamine releasing agent

Actions and Uses: Methylphenidate activates the reticular activating system, causing heightened alertness in various regions of the brain, particularly those centers associated with focus and attention. Activation is partially achieved by the release of neurotransmitters such as norepinephrine, dopamine, and serotonin. Impulsiveness, hyperactivity, and disruptive behavior are usually reduced within a few weeks. These changes promote improved psychosocial interactions and academic performance.

Adverse Effects and Interactions: In a patient with no ADHD, methylphenidate causes nervousness and insomnia. All patients are at risk for irregular heartbeat, high blood pressure, and liver toxicity. Methylphenidate is a Schedule II drug, indicating its potential to cause dependence when used for extended periods. Periodic drug-free holidays are recommended to reduce drug dependence and to assess the patient's condition.

Methylphenidate interacts with many drugs. For example, it may decrease the effectiveness of anticonvulsants, anticoagulants, and guanethidine. Use with clonidine may increase adverse effects. Antihypertensives or other CNS stimulants could increase the vasoconstrictive action of methylphenidate. MAOIs may produce hypertensive crisis.

BLACK BOX WARNING:
Methylphenidate is a Schedule II drug with high abuse potential. Administration for long periods of time may lead to drug dependence. Misuse may cause sudden death or a serious cardiovascular adverse event.

Non-CNS Stimulants

Nonstimulants are now approved for treatment of ADHD. This is an advantage because they have no abuse potential. A common form of treatment for ADHD in children and adults is atomoxetine (Strattera). Although its exact mechanism is not known, it is classified as a norepinephrine reuptake inhibitor. Efficacy appears to be equivalent to methylphenidate (Ritalin). Patients taking atomoxetine have demonstrated an improved ability to focus on tasks and reduced hyperactivity. Common adverse effects include headache, insomnia, upper abdominal pain, decreased appetite, and cough. Unlike methylphenidate, it is not a scheduled drug; thus, parents who are hesitant to place their child on stimulants have a reasonable alternative.

Clonidine (Kapvay) is sometimes prescribed when patients are extremely aggressive, active, or have difficulty falling asleep. Clonidine improves clinical symptoms of ADHD and is a centrally acting alpha$_2$-adrenergic drug. The extended-release tablet offers the advantage of once-daily dosing. Blood pressure should be monitored during therapy due to hypotensive effects caused by clonidine.

Guanfacine (Intuniv) was approved in 2011, for use in combination therapy with stimulants. Because the drug is a known antihypertensive, blood pressure should always be monitored during therapy. Sedation is common especially at the initiation of drug therapy.

CONCEPT REVIEW 11.5

- What are the symptoms experienced by patients with ADHD? Which drug is most often used in the treatment of these symptoms?

Patients Need to Know

Patients taking antidepressants need to know the following:

In General

1. Avoid driving or operating machinery until response to the medication is known. Its sedating effects can increase the risk for injury.
2. Do not stop taking the medication without consulting your healthcare provider.
3. Antidepressants may take 1 to 4 weeks to become fully effective.

4. Some antidepressants can increase the risk of suicidal thinking and behavior, especially in children, adolescents, and young adults.

Regarding TCAs

5. Tricyclics may increase appetite, cause dizziness upon rapid change of position, and be sedating. Report dry mouth, constipation, urinary retention, increase in heart rate and palpitations, or blurred vision if they occur.
6. Avoid the use of alcohol; it increases sedative effects.

Regarding MAOIs

7. MAOIs may cause problems with sleep, agitation, orthostatic hypotension, and dangerous interactions with other medications. Eating foods high in tyramine can cause a hypertensive crisis. Such foods include aged cheeses, wine, luncheon meats, and sausages.
8. Report any of the following adverse effects to your healthcare provider: increased heart rate or lightheadedness when changing positions.
9. Monitor weight; an increase or a decrease may occur.
10. A decrease in sexual interest or performance may occur. Discuss a change in medication with your healthcare provider.

Regarding SSRIs

11. SSRIs may cause GI upset, dizziness, skin rash, and headache. Report these signs and symptoms to your healthcare provider.
12. Avoid foods containing large amounts of tryptophan, such as cottage cheese, poultry, peanuts, and sesame seeds.
13. Do not combine MAOIs and SSRIs. Do not take St. John's wort with any antidepressant. These combinations, such as confusion, mania, headache, respiratory problems, kidney failure, and possibly death, can cause serious adverse effects, termed SES.
14. If insomnia is a problem, take the medication in the morning.
15. If nausea is a problem, take the medication with food, unless otherwise instructed.

For ADHD

16. Many drugs used for the treatment of ADHD are controlled substances.
17. Dependence may occur due to the high abuse potential of CNS stimulants.
18. Monitor blood pressure closely. CNS stimulants often increase blood pressure; nonstimulants may reduce blood pressure.
19. Take drugs at least six hours before bedtime to avoid insomnia.
20. Avoid giving drinks containing caffeine to children who are seizure prone and those with diabetes. (CNS stimulants lower the threshold in patients with seizure disorders and alter insulin needs in patients with diabetes.)
21. Monitor height and weight in children with prolonged therapy.
22. Take drugs after meals to reduce appetite-suppressive effects.
23. Do not take these medications for the purpose of combating fatigue.
24. Even though atomoxetine (Strattera) is a nonstimulant medication, it has many of the same adverse effects as the other ADHD medications.

Chapter Review

Core Concepts Summary

11.1 People suffer from depression for many reasons.

Depression involves both situational and biological causes. The major categories of mood disorders are major depressive disorder and dysthymic disorder. Disruptive mood dysregulation disorder and premenstrual dysphoric disorder are conditions having dysthymic and depressive components. The recognition of depressive symptoms is a collaborative effort among healthcare providers.

11.2 For best results, treatment of severe depression requires both medication and psychotherapy.

After a health examination is performed to rule out physical causes of depression, a psychological evaluation may be performed. Patients diagnosed with a major depressive disorder have at least five symptoms of recognized depression. Treatment may include medication in addition to a number of other approaches, including counseling and behavioral therapy, short-term psychotherapies, interpersonal therapy, psychodynamic therapies, and in extreme cases, electroconvulsive therapy (ECT) and repetitive transcranial magnetic stimulation (rTMS). Most therapeutic approaches involve a long-term commitment from patients, healthcare providers, and family.

11.3 Antidepressants enhance mood by boosting the actions of neurotransmitters, including norepinephrine, dopamine, and serotonin.

Drugs for depression are called antidepressants. The major classes of antidepressants are selective serotonin reuptake inhibitors (SSRIs), atypical antidepressants, tricyclic antidepressants (TCAs), and monoamine oxidase inhibitors (MAOIs). All drug classes work by increasing the amount of serotonin, dopamine, and norepinephrine in the nerve synapse, thereby intensifying neurotransmitter action and enhancing mood.

11.4 Patients with bipolar disorder may experience emotions ranging from depression to extreme agitation.

Bipolar disorder is characterized by extreme and opposite moods, such as euphoria and depression. During the depressive states, patients express signs of depression. Patients may then change to signs of mania or a state of high psychomotor activity and irritability.

11.5 Mood stabilization in patients with bipolar disorder is accomplished with lithium and other drugs.

Drugs for bipolar disorder are called mood stabilizers. Lithium (Eskalith) may be used alone or in combination with other drugs, including antidepressants and antianxiety agents. Antiseizure drugs and atypical antipsychotic drugs have emerged as more effective drug treatments for bipolar disorder. Drugs are selective for extreme mania, extreme depression, or cycling of mood that occurs between extreme emotional states.

11.6 Attention-deficit/hyperactivity disorder presents challenges for children and adults.

ADHD is a condition characterized by poor attention span, behavior control issues, and hyperactivity. It is normally diagnosed in childhood, although one-third to one-half of children with symptoms experience them into adulthood. As adults, patients with ADHD have symptoms similar to mood disorders.

11.7 Central nervous system stimulants have been the main course of treatment for ADHD.

The traditional drugs used to treat ADHD in children have been the CNS stimulants. Patients taking CNS stimulants must be carefully monitored to avoid adverse reactions. Nonstimulants include atomoxetine (Strattera), which has been used as a reasonable alternative to existing Schedule II controlled substances.

REVIEW Questions

Answer the following questions to assess your knowledge of the chapter material, and go back and review any material that is not clear to you.

1. Patient education for the patient started on a selective serotonin reuptake inhibitors would include:
   1. The avoidance of tyramine-containing foods.
   2. The signs and symptoms of hypertension crisis.
   3. That tremors are a common adverse effect.
   4. That sexual dysfunction is one of the most common adverse effects.

2. A patient is taking a monoamine oxidase inhibitor for depression. In planning care for this patient, the nurse knows that a hypertensive crisis may be possible and plans on having what drug on hand as an antidote?
   1. Meperidine (Demerol)
   2. Dextromethorphan
   3. Calcium channel blockers
   4. Carbamazepine (Tegretol)

3. The nurse informs the patient to remain well hydrated while taking lithium because dehydration can lead to:
   1. Lower serum lithium levels.
   2. Increased effectiveness.
   3. The need to increase the lithium dosage.
   4. Lithium toxicity.

4. The patient on methylphenidate (Ritalin) should be monitored for:
   1. Signs of weight loss.
   2. Hypotension.
   3. Renal toxicity.
   4. Extreme euphoria.

5. Which of the following symptoms would indicate that a patient may be at risk for lithium toxicity?
   1. Increased urination and sweating
   2. Dry mouth, vomiting, hypotension
   3. Constipation, blurred vision, hypertension
   4. Increased appetite, increased energy, memory loss

6. Imipramine (Tofranil) has been ordered for a patient experiencing depression. The nurse ensures the patient knows about which of the following?
   1. The use of alcohol is permitted with this drug.
   2. Avoid standing up too quickly.
   3. Effectiveness occurs within a few hours of administration.
   4. If a dose is missed, double up on the next dose.

7. The patient is taking phenelzine (Nardil). The nurse advises the patient to avoid eating:
   1. Eggs.
   2. Aged cheeses.
   3. Onions.
   4. Apples.

8. An older patient has a prescription for sertraline (Zoloft) 25 mg/day, PO, to be taken for 1 week and then increased to 50 mg/day the second week. The pharmacy gives the patient 50-mg tablets. How many tablets will the patient take per day during the first week?
   1. One-quarter of the tablet
   2. One tablet
   3. Half tablet
   4. One and one-half tablets

9. The nurse is providing education material to a patient just prescribed duloxetine (Cymbalta) for depression. The patient states that he has heard this medication is also used for: (Select all that apply.)
   1. Phobias.
   2. Generalized anxiety.
   3. Neuropathic pain.
   4. Seizures.
   5. Schizophrenia

10. A patient asks how most antidepressants work. The nurse responds by saying that antidepressants improve mood by increasing levels of:
    1. Epinephrine and norepinephrine.
    2. Reticular formation.
    3. Norepinephrine and serotonin.
    4. GABA and serotonin.

CASE STUDY Questions

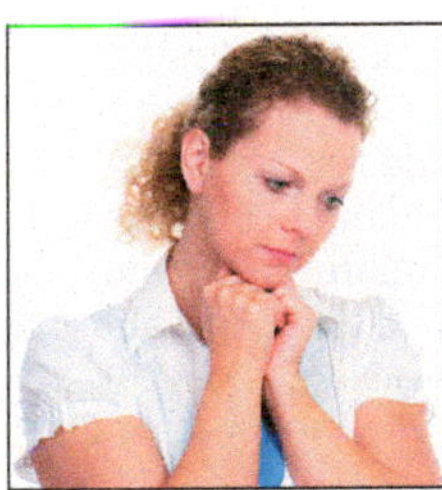

Remember Mrs. Coxilean, the patient introduced at the beginning of the chapter? Now read the remainder of the case study. Based on the information you have learned in this chapter, answer the questions that follow.

Mrs. Rachel Coxilean, a 32-year-old woman, visits her healthcare provider and explains that lately she has been experiencing frequent headaches, disinterest in eating and sex, and a hard time "keeping focused." For the past 2 years, she has been taking OTC medication to help her sleep. Two times within the past year, she missed work because of extreme fatigue. Mrs. Coxilean does not drink alcohol and admits, "The stress is almost overwhelming sometimes." Mrs. Coxilean is diagnosed with major depressive disorder.

1. During the planning process, it is determined that the main reason why Mrs. Coxilean would not be treated with mood stabilizers is the lack of:
   1. Complaints from the patient, suggesting ADHD.
   2. Toxicity concerns for this class of drug.
   3. Evidence that the patient feels her condition is normal.
   4. Extreme shifts between mania and depression.

2. The healthcare provider is thinking of prescribing henelzine (Nardil). If Mrs. Coxilean were to take this medication, the nurse would most likely tell her:
   1. "Avoid reducing your salt intake. It increases excretion of this medication."
   2. "Avoid chocolate and some other foods when taking this medication."
   3. "You can take herbal supplements without any risks."
   4. "You can continue to take OTC medication for sleep, but monitor the frequency."

3. After considering Mrs. Coxilean's symptoms and noting that her laboratory values were normal, the nurse would expect that she would be started on which medication?
   1. Doxepin (Sinequan)
   2. Tranylcypromine (Parnate)
   3. Sertraline (Zoloft)
   4. Bupropion (Wellbutrin)

4. An SSRI was prescribed for Mrs. Coxilean. Which of the following effects might still remain a problem? (Select all that apply.)
   1. Headaches
   2. Loss of appetite
   3. Poor sexual activity
   4. Ability to focus

Answers and complete rationales for the Review and Case Study Questions appear in Appendix A.

REFERENCES

American Psychiatric Association. (2013). *Diagnostic and statistical manual of mental disorders* (5th Ed.; DSM-5). Arlington, VA.: Author. doi.org/10.1176/appi.books.9780890425596

Herdman, T. H., & Kamitsuru, S. (Eds.). (2014). *NANDA International nursing diagnoses: Definitions and classification, 2015–2017.* Oxford, United Kingdom: Wiley-Blackwell.

SELECTED BIBLIOGRAPHY

Berlim, M. T., Van den Eynde, F., & Daskalakis, Z. J. (2013). High-frequency repetitive transcranial magnetic stimulation accelerates and enhances the clinical response to antidepressants in major depression: A meta- analysis of randomized, double-blind, and sham-controlled trials. *Journal of Clinical Psychiatry, 74*(2), e122–e129. doi:10.4088/JCP.12r07996

Centers for Disease Control and Prevention. (2013). *Mental health surveillance among children—United States, 2005–2011*. Retrieved from http://www.cdc.gov/mmwr/preview/mmwrhtml/su6202a1.htm

Coelho L. F., Barbosa, D. L., Rizzutti, S., Muszkat, M., Bueno, O. F., & Miranda, M. C. (2015). Use of cognitive behavioral therapy and token economy to alleviate dysfunctional behavior in children with attention-deficit hyperactivity disorder. *Frontiers in Psychiatry, 6*, 167. doi:10.3389/fpsyt.2015.00167

Del Vecchio, V. (2014). Following the development of ICD-11 through *World Psychiatry* (and other sources). *World Psychiatry, 13*, 102–104. doi:10.1002/wps.20095

Diagnostic and Statistical Manual of Mental Disorders (5th Ed.; DSM-5). (2013). *Disruptive mood dysregulation disorder.* Retrieved from http://www.dsm5.org/Documents/Disruptive%20Mood%20Dysregulation%20Disorder%20Fact%20Sheet.pdf

Huang, Y-S., & Tsai, M-H. (2011). Long-term outcomes with medications for attention-deficit hyperactivity disorder: Current status of knowledge. *CNS Drugs, 25*, 539–554. doi:10.2165/11589380-000000000-00000

Karaosmanoğlu, A. D., Butros, S. R., & Arellano, R. (2013). Imaging findings of renal toxicity in patients on chronic lithium therapy. *Diagnostic and Interventional Radiology, 19, 299-303.* doi:10.5152.dir.2013.097

Krasowski, M. D., & Blau, J. L. (2011). Drug interactions with St. John's wort. In A. Dasgupta & C. A. Hammett-Stabler (Eds.), *Herbal supplements: Efficacy, toxicity, interactions with Western drugs, and effects on clinical laboratory tests*. Hoboken, NJ: John Wiley & Sons. doi:10.1002/9780470910108.ch12

Lentz, G. M. (2012). Primary and secondary dysmenorrhea, premenstrual syndrome, and premenstrual dysphoric disorder: etiology, diagnosis, management. In V. L. Katz, , G. M. Lentz, R. A. Lobo, & D. M. Gershenson (Eds.), *Comprehensive gynecology* (6th ed.). Philadelphia, PA: Elsevier.

Lin E., & Lane H-Y. (2015). Genome-wide association studies in pharmacogenomics of antidepressants. *Pharmacogenomics, 16*(5), 555–566. doi:10.2217/pgs.15.5

Lu, D. Y., Lu, T. R., Zhu, P. P., & Che, J. Y. (2016). The efficacies and toxicities of antidepressant drugs in clinics, building the relationship between chemo-genetics and socio-environments. *Central Nervous System Agents in Medicinal Chemistry, 16*, 12–18. doi:10.2174/1871524915666150430131511

Palasik, B., Sieluk, J., dos Reis, S., & Doshi, P. (2015). Stimulant use and cardiovascular risk among children and adolescents with ADHD: What product labeling does, or does not, tell us. *Value in Health, 18*(7), A747. doi:10.1016/j.jval.2015.09.2884

Regier, D. A., Kuhl, E. A., & Kupfer, D. J. (2013). The DSM-5: Classification and criteria changes. *World Psychiatry, 12*, 92–98. doi:10.1002/wps.20050

Sanders-Bush, E., & Hazelwood, L. (2015). 5-Hydroxytryptamine (serotonin) and dopamine. In L. L. Brunton, B. A. Chabner, & B. C. Knollmann (Eds.), *Goodman & Gilman's the pharmacological basis of therapeutics* (12th ed., pp. 381–417). New York, NY: McGraw-Hill

Shapero, B. G., Black, S. K., Liu, R. T., Klugman, J., Bender, R. E., Abramson, L. Y., & Alloy, L. B. (2014). Stressful life events and depression symptoms: The effect of childhood emotional abuse on stress reactivity. *Journal of Clinical Psychology, 70*, 209–223. doi:10.1002/jclp.22011

Chapter 12

Drugs for Psychoses

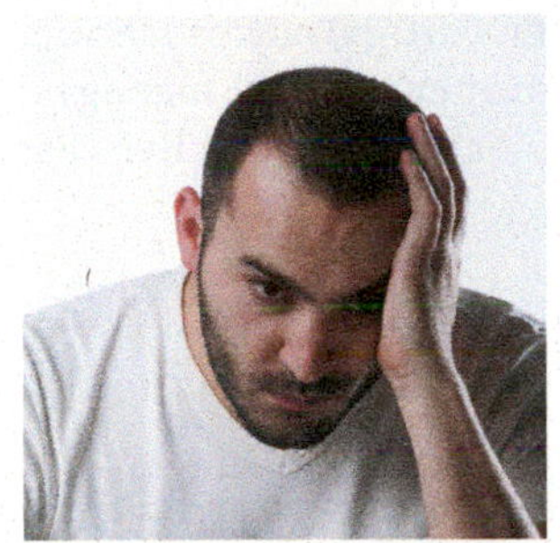

"I don't need medication. What I need is for you to tell those FBI and CIA agents to stop looking in my windows every night."

—Mr. Jeremy Wayne

Core Concepts

12.1 **Most psychoses have no identifiable cause and require long-term drug therapy.**

12.2 **Patients with schizophrenia experience many different symptoms that may change over time.**

12.3 **The experience and skills of the healthcare provider are critical to the successful pharmacologic management of psychoses.**

12.4 **Conventional antipsychotic drugs include the phenothiazines, phenothiazine-like drugs, and nonphenothiazines.**

12.5 **Atypical antipsychotic drugs address the needs of patients with psychoses.**

Drug Snapshot

The following drugs are discussed in this chapter:

Drug Classes	Prototype Drugs
Conventional (First-Generation) Antipsychotics	
Phenothiazines	Pr chlorpromazine
Nonphenothiazines	Pr haloperidol (Haldol)
Atypical (Second-Generation) Antipsychotics	Pr risperidone (Risperdal)
Dopamine System Stabilizers (Third-Generation Antipsychotics)	

Learning Outcomes

After reading this chapter, the student should be able to:

1. Identify the signs characteristic of psychosis, and describe how psychotic episodes are controlled.
2. Compare and contrast the positive and negative symptoms of schizophrenia, and explain the cause of schizophrenia and related behaviors.
3. Discuss factors important to the successful management of psychosis, including the major generations of antipsychotics.
4. Explain the goals of conventional, atypical, and third-generation antipsychotic drugs; identify representative drugs, and explain their mechanisms of drug action, primary actions, and important adverse effects including extrapyramidal symptoms.

Key Terms

akathisia (ACK-ah-THEE-shea)
cognitive symptoms
delirium (dee-LEAR-ee-um)
dementia (dee-MEN-she-ah)
extrapyramidal symptoms (EPS) (peh-RAM-ed-el)
negative symptoms
neuroleptic malignant syndrome (NMS) (noo-roh-LEP-tik)

neuroleptics (noo-roh-LEP-ticks)
secondary parkinsonism
positive symptoms
schizoaffective disorder (SKIT-soh-ah-FEK-tiv)
schizophrenia (SKIT-soh-FREN-ee-uh)
tardive dyskinesia (TAR-div dis-ki-NEE-zee-uh)

Severe mental illness can be incapacitating for the patient and intensely frustrating for family members dealing with the patient on a regular basis. Before the 1950s, patients with acute mental dysfunction were institutionalized, often for their entire lives. With the introduction of chlorpromazine in the 1950s and the development of subsequent drugs, antipsychotic drugs have revolutionized the treatment of mental illness. With proper medical management, patients with serious mental disorders can now lead normal or near-normal lives as functional members of society.

Core Concept 12.1 ▶

Most psychoses have no identifiable cause and require long-term drug therapy.

Patients with psychoses often are unable to distinguish what is real from what is illusion. Because of this, patients may be viewed as medically and legally incompetent. The following signs are characteristic of psychosis:

- *Delusions* (strong beliefs in something that is false or not based on reality); for example, the patient may believe that someone is planting thoughts in their head.
- *Hallucinations* (seeing, hearing, or feeling something that is not there); for example, the patient may hear voices or see spiders crawling on walls that others nearby do not hear or see.
- *Illusions* (distorted or misleading perceptions of something that is actually real); for example, the patient may see a shadow and believe it is really a person.
- *Disorganized behavior* For example, the patient may wear clothes in an entirely inappropriate manner and for no apparent reason, such as dressing up with layers of clothes, including a hat, sunglasses, and several pairs of socks over the hands and feet.
- *Difficulty relating to others* For example, the patient may become withdrawn from other people in the room, showing signs of distress, maybe even turning combative if confronted or questioned. Behavior may range from total inactivity to extreme agitation.
- *Paranoia* (suspicion and mistrust without justification or evidence); for example, the patient may have an extreme suspicion that he is being followed, or that someone is trying to kill him.

Psychosis may be classified as *acute* or *chronic*. Acute psychotic episodes occur over hours or days, whereas chronic psychoses develop over months or years. Sometimes a cause may be attributed to the psychosis, such as trauma, brain damage, overdoses of certain medications, extreme depression, chronic alcoholism, or drug addiction. Genetic factors are known to play a role in some psychoses. Unfortunately, the vast majority of psychoses have no identifiable cause.

People with psychosis are usually unable to function in society without long-term drug therapy. Patients must see their healthcare provider periodically, and medication must be taken for life. Family members and social support groups are important sources of help for patients who cannot function without continuous drug therapy.

SCHIZOPHRENIA

schizo = *split*
phrenia = *mind*

Schizophrenia is a type of psychosis characterized by abnormal thoughts and thought processes, disordered communication, withdrawal from other people and the outside environment, and a high risk for suicide. Several subtypes of schizophrenic disorders are based on clinical presentation.

Core Concept 12.2 ▶

Patients with schizophrenia experience many different symptoms that may change over time.

Schizophrenia is the most common psychotic disorder, affecting 1% to 2% of the population. Symptoms generally begin to appear in early adulthood, with a peak incidence in men 15 to 24 years of age and in women 25 to 34 years of age. Patients experience a variety of symptoms that may change over time.

When observing patients with schizophrenia, healthcare workers should look for both positive and negative symptoms. **Positive symptoms** are those that *add on* to normal behavior. These include hallucinations, delusions, and disorganized thoughts or speech. **Negative symptoms** are those that *subtract from* normal behavior. These include lack of interest, motivation, responsiveness, or pleasure in daily activities. Proper diagnosis of positive and negative symptoms is important for selecting the most appropriate antipsychotic drug for treatment. Similar to negative symptoms, **cognitive symptoms** may be difficult to recognize as part of schizophrenia. Often, they are detected when specific tests are performed by healthcare providers. With poor cognition, patients have trouble adjusting to real life situations, and this is a distressing part of their ability to fit into society. The following symptoms may appear quickly or take several months or years to develop:

POSITIVE SYMPTOMS

- Hallucinations, delusions, or paranoia
- Strange behavior, such as talking in rambling statements or making up words
- Strange or irrational actions
- Changes from stupor to extreme hyperactivity

NEGATIVE SYMPTOMS

- Attitude of indifference toward or detachment from life activities
- Neglect of personal hygiene, job, and school
- Noticeable withdrawal from social activities and relationships
- Changes from extreme hyperactivity to stupor

COGNITIVE SYMPTOMS

- Poor ability to make decisions and to understand information
- Problems applying information once learning has occurred
- Trouble paying attention.

CONCEPT REVIEW 12.1

- What are the characteristic signs of schizophrenia? What distinguishes a positive symptom from a negative symptom?

Fast Facts Psychosis

- Symptoms of psychosis are often associated with other mental health problems, including substance abuse, depression, and dementia.
- More than 2.4 million Americans have schizophrenia.
- Patients with psychosis often develop symptoms between the ages of 13 and the early 20s.
- As many as 46% of homeless people in America have schizophrenia, severe mental illness, or substance use disorders.
- The probability of developing schizophrenia is 1 in 100 for the general population, 1 in 10 if one parent has the disorder, and 4 in 10 if both parents are schizophrenic.

Schizoaffective disorder is a related condition in which the patient exhibits symptoms of both schizophrenia and mood disorder. For example, an acute schizoaffective reaction may include distorted perceptions, hallucinations, and delusions, followed by extreme depression. Over time, both positive and negative psychotic symptoms appear.

schizo = *schizophrenia*
affective = *mood*

Many conditions can cause bizarre behavior, and these should be distinguished from schizophrenia. Bipolar disorder, organic or drug-induced psychosis, delusional disorder, and postpartum psychosis are among the unique situations where psychotic symptoms may develop. Chronic use of amphetamines, marijuana, or cocaine can create a paranoid syndrome. Certain complex partial seizures (see Chapter 14) can cause unusual symptoms that are sometimes mistaken for psychoses. Brain neoplasms, infections, or hemorrhage can also cause bizarre, psychotic-like symptoms.

The cause of schizophrenia has not been determined, although several theories have been proposed. There appears to be a genetic component, because many schizophrenic patients have family members who have been afflicted with the same disorder. Another theory suggests that the disorder is caused by imbalances of neurotransmitters in specific brain regions. This theory suggests the possibility of overactive dopaminergic pathways in the basal nuclei, an area of the brain responsible for motor activity. Neurons in the substantia nigra project to the caudate nucleus and putamen, which are regions of the corpus striatum. The corpus striatum is responsible for synchronized motor activity, actions such as the starting and stopping of leg and arm motions during walking. Also, ventral tegmental neurons project to the hippocampus, nucleus accumbens, and areas of the frontal cortex. Tegmental neurons are thought to precipitate an interest in sights, sounds, ideas, and thoughts. Collectively, neuronal pathways seem to be associated with reinforcement learning and motivational behavior. Important dopaminergic pathways are depicted in Figure 12.1.

Symptoms of schizophrenia seem to be connected with dopamine type 2 (D_2) receptors. The basal nuclei are particularly rich in D_2 receptors, whereas areas of the frontal cortex are filled with reverberating subcortical circuits contingent on dopamine levels. Neural circuitries project back to the origin of dopamine synthesis and stimulate the release of more dopamine. All antipsychotic drugs act by entering dopaminergic synapses and compete with the binding of dopamine to receptors. By blocking a majority of the D_2 receptors, antipsychotic drugs reduce positive feedback-type impulses and lessen symptoms of schizophrenia.

CONCEPT REVIEW 12.2

- What are the major types of psychoses, and how are they differentiated? How are the symptoms of schizophrenia reduced?

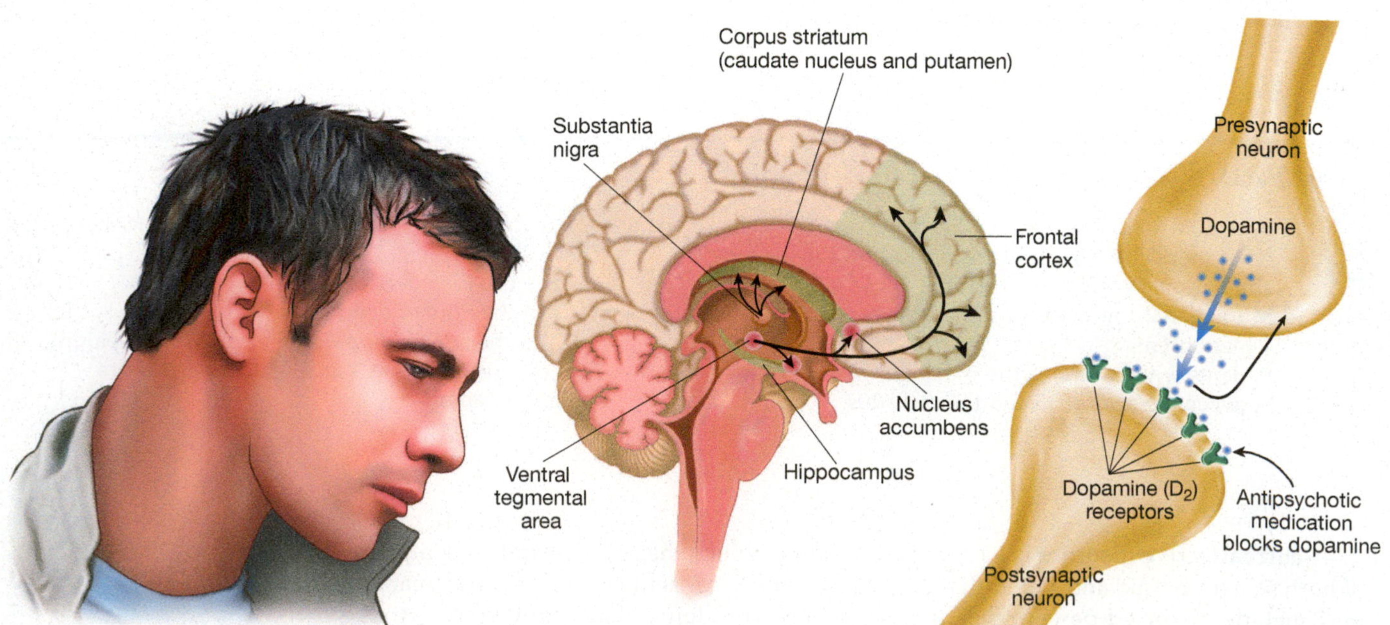

FIGURE 12.1 Overactive dopaminergic pathways in the substantia nigra and ventral tegmental area may be responsible for schizophrenia symptoms; antipsychotic drugs occupy D_2 receptors, preventing dopamine from stimulating postsynaptic neurons.

Source: Pharmacology for Nurses: A Pathophysiologic Approach (5th Ed.), by M. Adams, N. Holland, & C. Urban, 2017. Reprinted and electronically reproduced by permission of Pearson Education, Inc., Hoboken, New Jersey.

The experience and skills of the healthcare provider are critical to the successful pharmacologic management of psychoses.

◀ **Core Concept 12.3**

The patient's caregiver can be an essential partner in helping the healthcare team manage severe mental illness and the challenges accompanying antipsychotic drug therapy. Often patients will display signs of cognitive impairment (reduced ability to think and remember) accompanied by hallucinations (seeing things that are not there) or delusions (obvious false beliefs). These signs will dictate the form of therapy and whether the patient should be diagnosed with psychosis along with aspects of **dementia** (a degenerative disorder characterized by progressive memory loss, confusion, and inability to think or communicate effectively) or **delirium** (erratic behavior involving hallucinations). Agitation often accompanies these behaviors.

The medical management of severe mental illness is extremely challenging. Many patients do not see their behavior as abnormal and have difficulty understanding the need for medication. If their medication produces undesirable adverse effects, such as severe muscle twitching or loss of sexual function, patient compliance diminishes and symptoms of their pretreatment illness quickly return. Agitation, distrust, and extreme frustration are common, because patients cannot comprehend why others are unable to think and see the same as they do.

The primary goal of pharmacotherapy for patients with schizophrenia is to reduce psychotic symptoms to a level that allows the patient to maintain satisfactory social relationships, as well as self-care and keeping a job. From a pharmacologic perspective, therapy has both a positive and a negative side. Although many symptoms of psychoses can be managed with current drugs, adverse effects are common and often severe. The antipsychotic drugs do not cure mental illness, and symptoms remain in remission only as long as the patient chooses to take the drug. The relapse rate for patients who discontinue their medication is 60% to 80%.

The pharmacotherapy of psychosis has undergone three major generations. The first generation appeared in the early 1950s when the original drugs for treating severe mental illnesses were discovered. These drugs included *typical* or *conventional* antipsychotics such as chlorpromazine. The second-generation or *atypical* antipsychotic drugs were discovered in the 1970s and 1980s and are more frequently prescribed because they produce significantly fewer adverse effects. Risperidone (Risperdal) is an example of an atypical antipsychotic. Aripiprazole (Abilify) and brexpripazole (Rexulti) are two additional examples thought to reduce the risk of hyperglycemia and type 2 diabetes that may occur with longer-term use of some antipsychotics. These two drugs are grouped as *third-generation antipsychotics*. Third-generation antipsychotics began to be recognized in 2002, when the U.S. Food and Drug Administration (FDA) approved Abilify for the treatment of schizophrenia. Because antipsychotic drugs treat a nervous state of mind, they are sometimes referred to as **neuroleptics**.

neuro = *nervous*
leptic= *state of mind*

In terms of effectiveness, there is little difference among the various antipsychotic drugs. In other words, there is no single drug of choice for schizophrenia. Selection of a specific drug is based on clinician experience, the occurrence of adverse effects, and the needs of the patient. For example, patients with psychosis due to a degenerative disease may need an antipsychotic with minimal extrapyramidal symptoms (EPS). These are motor impulses or nerve signals that may cause intense skeletal muscle contractions. Those who operate machinery need a drug that does not cause sedation. Patients who are sexually active may want a drug without negative sexual effects. Specific drugs may be chosen to reduce the risk of impaired glucose tolerance and type 2 diabetes.

extra = *outside*
pyramidal = *brain stem pyramids*

CONVENTIONAL (FIRST-GENERATION) ANTIPSYCHOTICS

Conventional antipsychotic drugs include the phenothiazines, phenothiazine-like drugs, and nonphenothiazines.

◀ **Core Concept 12.4**

The conventional antipsychotics include the phenothiazines and phenothiazine-like drugs listed in Table 12.1. Within each category, drugs are named by their chemical structure. Both groups have similar actions and are considered first-generation antipsychotics.

Table 12.1 Conventional Antipsychotics: Phenothiazines

Drug	Route and Adult Dose	Remarks
Pr chlorpromazine	PO: 25–100 mg tid or qid (max: 1000 mg/day) IM/IV: 25–50 mg (max: 600 mg every 4–6 hours)	For agitated patients; strong sedative properties; controls nausea and vomiting, dementia, and hiccups not treated by any other means;
fluphenazine	PO: 0.5–10 mg/day (max: 20 mg/day)	Also for dementia; available in IM or subcutaneous forms
perphenazine	PO: 4–16 mg bid to qid (max: 64 mg/day)	Also for dementia and nausea; available in IM and IV forms
prochlorperazine (Compazine)	PO: 0.5–10 mg/day (max: 20 mg/day)	Antiemetic drug used to treat nausea and vomiting
thioridazine (Mellaril)	PO: 50–100 mg tid (max: 800 mg/day)	For moderate to severe depression and dementia; strong sedative properties
trifluoperazine	PO: 1–2 mg bid (max: 20 mg/day)	Also for dementia; use cautiously in patients with seizure disorders; available in IM form

Prototype Drug: Pr *Chlorpromazine*

Therapeutic Class: Conventional antipsychotic, schizophrenia agent **Pharmacologic Class: Phenothiazine, D_2 dopamine receptor blocker**

Actions and Uses: Chlorpromazine provides symptomatic relief of positive symptoms of schizophrenia and controls manic symptoms in patients with schizoaffective disorder. Many patients must take chlorpromazine for 7 or 8 weeks before they experience improvement. Extreme agitation may be treated with IM or IV injections, which begin to act within minutes. Chlorpromazine can also control severe nausea and vomiting.

Adverse Effects and Interactions: Strong blockade of alpha$_2$-adrenergic receptors and weak blockade of cholinergic receptors explain some of chlorpromazine's adverse effects. Common adverse effects are dry mouth, blurred vision, dizziness, drowsiness, impotence, tachycardia, and orthostatic hypotension. Disruption of body movements may include acute dystonia, akathisia, secondary parkinsonism, and tardive dyskinesia. EPS occur mostly in older adult patients, women, and pediatric patients who are dehydrated. **Neuroleptic malignant syndrome (NMS)** as described in Table 12.2 may also occur. Patients taking chlorpromazine and exposed to warmer temperatures should be monitored more closely for symptoms of NMS.

Chlorpromazine interacts with several drugs. For example, use with sedative medications such as phenobarbital should be avoided. Taking chlorpromazine with tricyclic antidepressants can elevate blood pressure. Use of chlorpromazine with antiseizure medication can lower the seizure threshold.

Use with caution with herbal supplements, such as kava and St. John's wort, which may increase the risk and severity of dystonia.

BLACK BOX WARNING:
Older adult patients with dementia-related psychosis are at increased risk for death when taking conventional antipsychotics.

Phenothiazines and Phenothiazine-Like Drugs

The phenothiazines are most effective at treating the positive symptoms of schizophrenia, such as hallucinations and delusions, and have been the treatment of choice for psychoses for 50 years.

The first effective drug used to treat schizophrenia was the low-potency phenothiazine chlorpromazine, approved by the FDA in 1954. Other phenothiazines are now available to treat mental illness. All block the excitement associated with the positive symptoms of schizophrenia, although they differ in their potency and adverse effect profiles. Hallucinations and delusions often begin to diminish within days. Other symptoms, however, may require as long as 7 to 8 weeks of pharmacotherapy to improve. Because of the high rate of recurrence of psychotic episodes, pharmacotherapy should be considered long term, usually for the life of the patient. Phenothiazines are thought to act by preventing both dopamine and serotonin from occupying critical neurologic receptor sites.

Although the phenothiazines once revolutionized treatment of severe mental illness, they exhibit numerous adverse effects that can limit pharmacotherapy. General adverse effects are listed in Table 12.2. Anticholinergic effects such as dry mouth, orthostatic hypotension, and urinary retention are common. Ejaculation disorders occur in a high percentage of patients; delay in achieving orgasm (in both men and women) is a common cause for noncompliance. Menstrual disorders are common. Each phenothiazine has a slightly different spectrum of adverse effects.

Table 12.2 Adverse Effects of the Conventional Antipsychotics

Effect	Description
Acute dystonias	Severe spasms, particularly the back, tongue, and facial muscles; twitching movements
Akathisia	Constant pacing with repetitive, compulsive movements
Secondary parkinsonism	Tremor, muscle rigidity, stooped posture, and shuffling gait
Tardive dyskinesia	Bizarre tongue and face movements such as lip smacking and wormlike motions of the tongue; puffing of cheeks, uncontrolled chewing movements
Neuroleptic malignant syndrome	Symptoms include high fever, confusion, muscle rigidity, and elevated serum creatine kinase levels; NMS can be fatal
Orthostatic hypotension	Particularly severe when moving quickly from a recumbent position to an upright position
Sedation	Usually diminishes with continued therapy
Sexual dysfunction	Impotence and diminished libido

Unlike many other drugs whose primary action is on the central nervous system (CNS) (e.g., amphetamines, barbiturates, anxiolytics, alcohol), antipsychotic drugs do not cause physical or psychological dependence. They also have a wide safety margin between a therapeutic dose and a lethal dose; deaths due to overdoses of antipsychotic drugs are uncommon.

Extrapyramidal symptoms (EPS) are a particularly serious set of adverse reactions to antipsychotic drugs. EPS include acute dystonias, akathisia, secondary parkinsonism, and tardive dyskinesia. Acute *dystonias* (see Chapter 13) occur early in the course of pharmacotherapy and involve severe muscle spasms, particularly of the back, neck, tongue, and face. **Akathisia**, the most common EPS, is an inability to rest or relax. The patient paces, has trouble sitting or remaining still, and has difficulty sleeping. Symptoms of phenothiazine-induced **secondary parkinsonism** include tremor, muscle rigidity, stooped posture, bradykinesia, and a shuffling gait. Secondary parkinsonism results from abnormal neuronal activity in areas of the corpus striatum and substantia nigra mainly due to medications, such as those used to treat psychosis, major psychiatric disorders, or nausea. Other causes of secondary parkinsonism may be repeated head trauma, neurodegenerative disorders such as palsy, brain lesions, exposure to toxins, metabolic disorders, and some forms of dementia. Long-term use of phenothiazines may lead to **tardive dyskinesia**, which is characterized by unusual tongue and face movements such as lip smacking and wormlike motions of the tongue. If EPS are reported early and the drug is withdrawn or the dosage is reduced, the adverse effects can be reversible. With higher doses given for prolonged periods, the EPS may become permanent.

dys = *abnormal*
tonia = *muscle tone*

a = *without*
kathisia = *sitting*

brady = *slow*
kinesia = *movement*

corpus = *body*
striatum = *striped*

substantia = *substance*
nigra = *black*

tardive = *late*
dys = *abnormal*
kinesia = *movement*

With the conventional antipsychotics, it is not always possible to control the disabling symptoms of schizophrenia without producing some degree of EPS. In these patients, drug therapy may be warranted to treat EPS. Concurrent pharmacotherapy with an anticholinergic drug may prevent some of the EPS (see Chapter 13). For acute dystonia, benztropine (Cogentin) may be given parenterally. Levodopa medications are usually avoided, because of their ability to increase dopamine function and thus antagonize the action of the phenothiazines. Beta-adrenergic blockers and benzodiazepines are sometimes given to reduce signs of akathisia.

Nonphenothiazine Drugs

The nonphenothiazine antipsychotic class consists of drugs whose chemical structures are dissimilar to the phenothiazines (Table 12.3). Introduced shortly after the phenothiazines, the nonphenothiazines were initially expected to produce fewer adverse effects. Unfortunately, this appears not to be the case. The spectrum of adverse effects for the nonphenothiazines is identical to that for the phenothiazines, although the degree to which a particular effect occurs depends on the specific drug. In general, the nonphenothiazine drugs cause

non = *not having*
pheno = *chemical ring structure*
thiazine = *sulfur and nitrogen around four carbon atoms*

Table 12.3 Conventional Antipsychotics: Nonphenothiazines

Drug	Route and Adult Dose	Remarks
Pr haloperidol (Haldol)	PO: 0.2–5 mg bid or tid	For severe psychosis, dementia, and Tourette syndrome; available in IM form
loxapine (Loxitane)	PO: Start with 20 mg/day and increase to 60–100 mg/day (max: 250 mg/day)	Also for dementia
pimozide (Orap)	PO: 1–2 mg/day and increase to 7–16 mg/day (max: 10 mg/day)	For Tourette syndrome; use cautiously in patients with seizure disorders
thiothixene (Navane)	PO: 2 mg tid; may increase up to 15 mg/day (max: 60 mg/day)	Also for dementia; off-label use as an antidepressant

less sedation and fewer anticholinergic adverse effects than chlorpromazine but exhibit an equal or even greater incidence of EPS. Concurrent therapy with other CNS depressants must be carefully monitored because of the potential additive effects.

Drugs in the nonphenothiazine class have the same therapeutic effects and effectiveness as the phenothiazines. They are also believed to act by the same mechanism as the phenothiazines—that is, by blocking postsynaptic D_2 dopamine receptors. As a class, they offer no significant advantages over the phenothiazines in the treatment of schizophrenia.

Prototype Drug: Pr *Haloperidol (Haldol)*

Therapeutic Class: Conventional antipsychotic, schizophrenia agent **Pharmacologic Class:** Nonphenothiazine, D_2 dopamine receptor blocker

Actions and Uses: Haloperidol is classified chemically as a butyrophenone. Its primary use is for the management of acute and chronic psychotic disorders. It may be used to treat patients with Tourette syndrome and children with severe behavior problems such as unprovoked aggressiveness and explosive hyperexcitability. It is approximately 50 times more potent than chlorpromazine but has equal efficacy in relieving symptoms of schizophrenia. Haldol LA is a long-acting preparation that lasts for approximately 3 weeks following IM or subcutaneous administration. This is particularly beneficial for patients who are uncooperative or unable to take oral medications.

Adverse Effects and Interaction: Haloperidol produces less sedation and hypotension than chlorpromazine, but the incidence of EPS is high. Older adults are more likely to experience adverse effects and often are prescribed half the adult dose until the adverse effects of therapy can be determined. Although NMS is rare, it may occur.

Haloperidol interacts with many drugs. For example, the following drugs decrease the effects and absorption of haloperidol: aluminum- and magnesium-containing antacids, levodopa (also increases chances of levodopa toxicity), lithium (increases chance of severe neurologic toxicity), phenobarbital, phenytoin (also increases chances of phenytoin toxicity), rifampin, and beta blockers (may increase blood levels of haloperidol, thus leading to possible toxicity). Haloperidol inhibits the action of centrally acting antihypertensives.

Use with caution with herbal supplements such as kava, which may increase the effect of haloperidol.

BLACK BOX WARNING:

Older patients with dementia-related psychosis are at increased risk for death when taking conventional antipsychotics.

Nursing Process Focus Patients Receiving Phenothiazines and Nonphenothiazine Therapy

ASSESSMENT

Prior to administration:

- Obtain a complete health history including cardiovascular, renal and liver conditions, allergies, drug history, and possible drug interactions.
- Acquire baseline vital signs and electrocardiogram (ECG), laboratory blood levels (complete blood count [CBC], chemistry, drug screening, renal and liver function studies), and urine specimens for laboratory analysis.
- Determine neurological status (altered thought processes, level of consciousness (LOC), mental status, and identification of recent mood and behavior patterns).
- Identify patient support system(s).

POTENTIAL NURSING DIAGNOSES*

- *Ineffective Therapeutic Regimen Management* related to noncompliance with medication regimen, presence of adverse effects, and need for long-term medication use
- *Anxiety* related to symptoms of psychosis and adverse effects of drug therapy
- *Noncompliance* related to length of time before medication reaches therapeutic levels and adverse effects of drug therapy
- *Deficient Knowledge* related to a lack of information about disease process and drug therapy
- *Risk for Injury* related to adverse effects of drug therapy and thought processes

PLANNING: PATIENT GOALS AND EXPECTED OUTCOMES

The patient will:
- Experience therapeutic effects (reduction of psychotic symptoms).
- Be free from or experience minimal adverse effects from drug therapy.
- Verbalize an understanding of the drug's use, adverse effects, and required precautions.
- Adhere to recommended treatment regimen.

IMPLEMENTATION

Interventions and (Rationales)	Patient Education/Discharge Planning
• Administer medication correctly and evaluate the patient's knowledge of proper administration. (Ensuring proper administration helps to avoid unnecessary adverse effects and interactions with other medications while determining effectiveness.)	Instruct the patient: • Not to take any other medication or herbal therapies unless approved by the healthcare provider. • That it may take up to 8 weeks for full therapeutic effects to be seen.
• Monitor for therapeutic effects, e.g., decreased psychotic symptoms. (If the patient continues to exhibit symptoms of psychosis, he or she may not be taking the drug as ordered, may be taking an inadequate dose, or may not be affected by the drug; it may need to be discontinued and another antipsychotic begun.)	Instruct the patient to: • Notice increases or decreases of symptoms of psychosis, including hallucinations, abnormal sleep patterns, social withdrawal, delusions, or paranoia. • Contact the healthcare provider if no decrease of symptoms occurs over a 6-week period.
• Monitor for adverse effects of medications such as drowsiness, dizziness, lethargy, headaches, blurred vision, skin rash, diaphoresis, nausea, vomiting, anorexia, diarrhea, anuresis, depression, hypotension, or hypertension.	Instruct the patient: • Regarding the adverse effects specific to the type of antipsychotic medication being taken. • To report adverse effects to their healthcare provider.
• Monitor for anticholinergic adverse effects such as orthostatic hypotension, constipation, anorexia, genitourinary problems, respiratory changes, and visual disturbances.	Instruct the patient to: • Avoid abrupt changes in position. • Not drive or perform hazardous activities until the effects of the drug are known. • Report vision changes. • Comply with required laboratory tests. • Increase dietary fiber, fluids, and exercise to prevent constipation. • Relieve symptoms of dry mouth with sugarless hard candy or gum and frequent drinks of water. • Notify the healthcare provider immediately if urinary retention occurs.
• Monitor for EPS such as those associated with tardive dyskinesia, dystonia, akathisia, secondary parkinsonism. (Presence of EPS may be sufficient reason for the patient to discontinue the antipsychotic. Monitor for NMS, which is life threatening and must be reported and treated immediately.)	Instruct the patient to: • Recognize that EPS such as the development of tremors, involuntary repetitive movements, decreased muscle tone, or increased restlessness may occur and not to stop taking medication until healthcare provider is seen. • Immediately seek treatment for elevated temperature, unstable blood pressure, profuse sweating, dyspnea, muscle rigidity, incontinence.
• Monitor for weight gain, menstrual irregularities, impotence, and gynecomastia. (Some antipsychotic drugs may cause weight gain and have pituitary effects.)	• Instruct the patient and caregivers to weigh the patient weekly and to report a weight gain of 2 pounds (1 kg) or more per week to the healthcare provider. • Instruct the patient to talk to healthcare provider about sexual concerns.
• Monitor for alcohol or illegal drug use. (Patient may decide to use alcohol or illegal drugs as a means of coping with symptoms of psychosis, and may stop taking the antipsychotic. Concurrent use will cause increased CNS depressant effect.)	• Instruct the patient to refrain from alcohol and illegal drug use. Refer the patient to community support groups such as Alcoholics Anonymous (AA) or Narcotics Anonymous (NA) as appropriate.
• Monitor caffeine use. (Use of caffeine-containing substances will negate effects of antipsychotics.)	Instruct the patient to: • Avoid caffeine. • Recognize common caffeine-containing products and assist in finding acceptable substitutes, such as decaffeinated coffee and tea, and caffeine-free colas.

(*Continued*)

Nursing Process Focus (*continued*)

Interventions and (Rationales)	Patient Education/Discharge Planning
• Continue to monitor vital signs, especially blood pressure and heart rate. Monitor for cardiovascular changes, including hypotension, tachycardia, and ECG changes. (Haloperidol has fewer cardiotoxic effects than other antipsychotics and may be preferred for patients with existing cardiovascular problems.)	• Instruct the patient that dizziness and falls, especially on sudden position changes, may indicate cardiovascular changes. • Provide information on safety measures such as slowly rising from a sitting position.
• Monitor for smoking. (Heavy smoking may decrease metabolism of haloperidol, leading to decreased effectiveness.)	• Instruct the patient to stop or decrease smoking. Refer to smoking cessation programs, if indicated.
• Monitor older adult patients closely. (Older patients may need lower doses and a more gradual dosage increase. Older women are at greater risk for developing tardive dyskinesia.)	Instruct the patient: • To look for unusual reactions such as confusion, depression, and hallucinations and for symptoms of tardive dyskinesia, and to report them immediately. • On ways to counteract anticholinergic effects of medication while taking into account any other existing medical problems.
• Monitor laboratory results, including CBC and drug levels.	• Advise the patient of the necessity of having regular laboratory studies done.
• Monitor for use of medication. (All antipsychotics must be taken as ordered for therapeutic results to occur.)	• Instruct the patient that medication must be continued as ordered, even if no therapeutic benefits are felt, because it may take several months for full therapeutic benefits to take effect.
• Monitor for seizures. (Drug may lower seizure threshold.)	• Instruct the patient that seizures may occur, and review appropriate safety precautions.
• Monitor the patient's environment. (Drug may cause blurred vision, change in color vision, and interfere with the ability to regulate body temperature.)	Instruct the patient to: • Report to healthcare provider as soon as possible any change in vision. • Avoid temperature extremes.

EVALUATION OF OUTCOME CRITERIA

Evaluate the effectiveness of drug therapy by confirming that patient goals and expected outcomes have been met (see "Planning"). *See Tables 12.1 and 12.3 for lists of the drugs to which these nursing actions apply.*

ATYPICAL (SECOND-GENERATION) ANTIPSYCHOTICS

Atypical antipsychotics treat both positive and negative symptoms of schizophrenia. They have become preferred drugs for treating psychoses. Researchers have continued to look for drugs in this class with equal or better effectiveness, thus introducing the dopamine system stabilizers or dopamine partial agonists.

Core Concept 12.5 ▶

Atypical antipsychotic drugs address the needs of patients with psychoses.

The approval of clozapine (Clozaril), the first atypical antipsychotic, marked the first major advance in the pharmacotherapy of psychoses since the discovery of chlorpromazine decades earlier. Clozapine and the other drugs in this class are called *second generation* or *atypical,* because they have a broader spectrum of action than the conventional antipsychotics, controlling both the positive and the negative symptoms of schizophrenia (Table 12.4). Furthermore, at therapeutic doses they exhibit their antipsychotic actions without producing the major EPS effects of the conventional drugs. Some atypical drugs, such as clozapine and risperidone, are especially useful for patients in whom other drugs have proved unsuccessful. Unfortunately, however, clozapine and other atypical antipsychotics can cause neutropenia (decreased neutrophil count) and agranulocytosis (*decreased* white blood cells [WBCs] with granules).

neutro = *neutrophil*
penia = *deficiency*

a = *without/deficiency*
granulo = *granular*
cyto = *blood cell*
sis = *condition*

Table 12.4 Atypical Antipsychotic Drugs

Drug	Route and Adult Dose	Remarks
asenapine (Saphris)	Sublingual: 5 mg bid (max: 10 mg bid)	For acute management of mania or mixed episodes associated with bipolar disorder in adults
clozapine (Clozaril)	PO: Start at 25–50 mg/day and increase to a target dose of 50–450 mg/day (max: 900 mg/day)	For schizophrenia (adults older than 16 years); causes neutropenia and agranulocytosis
iloperidone (Fanapt)	PO: 12–24 mg/day administered bid	For schizophrenia (adults older than 16 years)
lurasidone (Latuda)	PO: 40 mg once daily (max: 80 mg/day)	For schizophrenia; once-a-day oral medication
olanzapine (Zyprexa)	PO adult: Start with 5–10 mg/day, (max: 20 mg/day)	Blocks alpha receptors and acetylcholine
paliperidone (Invega)	PO: 6 mg/day (max: 12 mg/day)	For schizophrenia; schizoaffective disorder in adults and adolescents (12–17 years old)
primavanserin (Nuplazid)	PO: 17 mg bid	Newer drug for hallucinations and delusions associated with Parkinson disease
quetiapine (Seroquel)	PO (regular release): Start with 25 mg bid, may increase to a target dose of 300–400 mg/day in divided doses PO (extended release): 300 mg daily (max: 800 mg/day)	For schizophrenia; also used for depression; patients may experience orthostatic hypotension; use cautiously in older adults
Pr risperidone (Risperdal)	PO: 1–6 mg bid, increase to an initial target dose of 6 mg/day IM: 25 mg once every 2 weeks (max: 50 mg)	For schizophrenia and bipolar disorder; off-label use in behavioral disturbances (patients with intellectual and developmental disabilities)
ziprasidone (Geodon)	PO: 20 mg bid (max: 80 mg bid) IM: 10–20 mg every 2–4 hours (max: 40 mg/ day)	For schizophrenia and bipolar disorder; off-label use for Tourette syndrome; patients may experience orthostatic hypotension

Atypical antipsychotics are thought to act by blocking several receptor types in the brain. Like the phenothiazines, they block dopamine D_2 receptors. However, the atypicals also block serotonin and alpha$_2$-adrenergic receptors, which is thought to account for some of their properties. Because the atypical drugs are loosely bound to D_2 receptors, they produce fewer extrapyramidal adverse effects than the conventional antipsychotics.

Although there are fewer adverse effects with atypical antipsychotics, adverse effects are still significant, and patients must be carefully monitored. Most antipsychotics cause

Prototype Drug: Pr *Risperidone (Risperdal)*

Therapeutic Class: Atypical antipsychotic, schizophrenia agent, psychotic depression agent

Pharmacologic Class: Serotonin (5-HT) receptor antagonist, D_2 dopamine receptor antagonist (weaker affinity)

Actions and Uses: Therapeutic effects of risperidone include treatment and prevention of schizophrenia relapse and expression of bipolar mania symptoms. Risperidone also treats symptoms of irritability in children with autism. Expected results are a reduction of excitement, paranoia, or negative behaviors associated with psychosis. Effects result from blockade of dopamine type 2, serotonin type 2, and alpha$_2$-adrenergic receptors located within the CNS. For a full range of effectiveness, the drug is sometimes combined with lithium (Eskalith) or valproic acid (Depakene). Risperidone is a long-acting preparation, which, following IM administration, releases only a small amount. After a 3-week lag, the rest of the drug releases and lasts for approximately 4 to 6 weeks. PO preparations release sooner and have a 1- to 2-week onset of action.

Adverse Effects and Interactions: If older patients with dementia-related psychoses are given risperidone, they are at an increased risk for heart failure, pneumonia, or sudden death. Patients with underlying cardiovascular disease may be especially prone to dysrhythmias and hypotension. Risperidone should be avoided in patients with a history of seizures, suicidal ideations, or kidney or liver disease. This medication may cause hyperglycemia and worsen glucose control in patients with diabetes. It is not known whether risperidone passes into breast milk or if it could harm a nursing baby. Due to its category C classification, safety in pregnancy has not been established.

Common adverse effects are EPS (involuntary shaking of the head, neck, and arms), hyperactivity, fatigue, nausea, dizziness, visual disturbances, fever, and orthostatic hypotension. Risperidone may cause weight gain.

Patients taking risperidone should avoid CNS depressants such as alcohol, antihistamines, sedative-hypnotics, and opioid analgesics. These can increase some of the adverse effects of risperidone. Due to inhibition of liver enzymes, other drugs that increase the adverse effects of risperidone include the selective serotonin reuptake inhibitors (SSRIs) such as paroxetine, sertraline, and fluoxetine (Prozac), and antifungal drugs such as fluconazole, itraconazole, and ketoconazole. Risperidone may interfere with elimination by the kidneys of clozapine, also increasing the risk of adverse reactions.

Kava, valerian, or chamomile may increase risperidone's CNS depressive effects.

BLACK BOX WARNING:

Older adult patients with dementia-related psychosis are at increased risk for death when taking conventional antipsychotics.

Table 12.5 Dopamine System Stabilizers (Third-Generation Antipsychotics)

Drug	Route and Adult Dose	Remarks
aripiprazole (Abilify)	PO: 10–15 mg daily (max: 30 mg/day)	For major depressive disorder, bipolar disorder, and schizophrenia; may cause loss of glycemic control in patients with diabetes
brexpiprazole (Rexulti)	PO: 2–4 mg daily (max 4 mg/day IM: 441–882 mg every 4–6 weeks	For major depressive disorder and schizophrenia; akathisia and slight weight gain may occur

weight gain, and the atypical drugs are associated with obesity and its risk factors. Risperidone (Risperdal) and some of the other antipsychotic drugs increase prolactin levels, which can lead to menstrual disorders, decreased libido, and osteoporosis in women. In men, high prolactin levels can cause lack of libido and impotence. There is also concern that some atypical drugs alter glucose metabolism, which can lead to type 2 diabetes.

DOPAMINE SYSTEM STABILIZERS (THIRD-GENERATION ANTIPSYCHOTICS)

In 2002, due to side effects caused by conventional and atypical antipsychotic medications, a new drug class was developed to better meet the needs of patients with psychoses. This class, sometimes considered to be an atypical antipsychotic, is the dopamine-serotonin system stabilizer (DSS) or dopamine partial agonists. Aripiprazole (Abilify) was the first drug in this group. Brexpiprazole (Rexulti) was approved in 2015. These medications control both the positive and negative symptoms of schizophrenia. They are listed in Table 12.5. Dopamine partial agonists are generally well tolerated in patients with schizophrenia. In particular, their use seems to be associated with a lower incidence of EPS than haloperidol and fewer weight-gain issues than other atypical antipsychotics, for example, olanzapine.

Anticholinergic adverse effects are virtually nonexistent. In fact, the incidence of adverse effects compared to the other atypical antipsychotic drugs is very low. Aripiprazole is also used to treat bipolar disorder and mixed episodes of mania and depression, as monotherapy or adjunctive (add–on) therapy. For major depressive disorder, aripiprazole and brexpiprazole are used as adjunctive therapy. Notable side effects, however, include headache, nausea and vomiting, fever, constipation, and anxiety.

Nursing Process Focus Patients Receiving Atypical and Third-Generation Antipsychotic Therapy

ASSESSMENT

Prior to administration:
- Obtain a complete health history including cardiovascular, renal and liver conditions, allergies, drug history, and possible drug interactions.
- Acquire baseline vital signs and ECG, laboratory blood levels (CBC, chemistry, drug screening, renal and liver function studies) and urine specimens for laboratory analysis.
- Determine neurological status (altered thought processes, hallucinations, LOC, mental status, and identification of recent mood and behavior patterns).
- Identify patient support system(s).

POTENTIAL NURSING DIAGNOSES*

- *Ineffective Therapeutic Regimen Management* related to noncompliance with medication regimen, presence of adverse effects, and need for long-term medication use
- *Anxiety* related to symptoms of psychosis
- *Noncompliance* related to length of time before drug reaches therapeutic levels, desire to use alcohol or illegal drugs
- *Deficient Knowledge* related to a lack of information about disease process and drug therapy
- *Risk for Injury* related to adverse effects of drug therapy, and thought processes

PLANNING: PATIENT GOALS AND EXPECTED OUTCOMES

The patient will:
- Experience therapeutic effects (reduction of psychotic symptoms).
- Be free from or experience minimal adverse effects from drug therapy.
- Verbalize an understanding of the drug's use, adverse effects and required precautions.
- Adhere to recommended treatment regimen.

IMPLEMENTATION	
Interventions and (Rationales)	**Patient Education/Discharge Planning**
• Administer medication correctly and evaluate the patient's knowledge of proper administration. (Ensuring proper administration helps to avoid unnecessary adverse effects and interactions with other medications while determining effectiveness.)	Instruct the patient: • Not to take any other medication or herbal therapies unless approved by the healthcare provider. • That it may take up to 6 weeks for full therapeutic effects to be seen.
• Monitor red blood cell [RBC] and WBC counts. (Agranulocytosis [WBCs below 3500] can be a life-threatening adverse effect of these medications, which may also suppress bone marrow and lower infection-fighting ability.)	Instruct the patient to: • Keep appointments for laboratory testing. • Report any sore throat, signs of infection, fatigue without apparent cause, or bruising to the healthcare provider.
• Observe for adverse effects. (These drugs may affect blood pressure, heart rate, and other autonomic functions.)	• Instruct the patient to report any adverse effects such as drowsiness, dizziness, depression, anxiety, tachycardia, hypotension, nausea, vomiting, excessive salivation, changes in urinary frequency or urgency, incontinence, weight gain, muscle pain or weakness, rash, and fever to the healthcare provider.
• Monitor for anticholinergic adverse effects. (These medications may cause dry mouth, constipation, or urinary retention.)	Instruct the patient to: • Increase dietary fiber, fluids, and exercise to prevent constipation. • Relieve symptoms of dry mouth with sugar-free hard candy or chewing gum and frequent drinks of water. • Immediately notify the healthcare provider if urinary retention occurs. Possible catheter placement may be necessary.
• Monitor for therapeutic effects, e.g., decrease of psychotic symptoms. (Decreased symptoms indicate an effective dose and type of medication.)	Instruct the patient to: • Notice increases or decreases of symptoms of psychosis, including hallucinations, abnormal sleep patterns, social withdrawal, delusions, or paranoia. • Contact the healthcare provider if symptoms do not decrease over a 6-week period.
• Monitor for alcohol or illegal drug use. (Used concurrently, these will cause increased CNS depression. The patient may decide to use alcohol or illegal drugs as a means of coping with symptoms of psychosis and may stop taking the drug.)	• Instruct the patient to avoid alcohol or illegal drug use. Refer the patient to AA, NA, or other support group as appropriate.
• Monitor caffeine use. (Use of caffeine-containing substances inhibits the effects of antipsychotics.)	Instruct the patient about: • Common caffeine-containing products. • Acceptable substitutes, including decaffeinated coffee and tea, and caffeine-free soda.
• Monitor for smoking. (Heavy smoking may decrease blood levels of the drug.)	• Instruct the patient to stop or decrease smoking. Refer to smoking cessation programs if indicated.
• Monitor older adult patients closely. (Older patients may be more sensitive to anticholinergic adverse effects.)	• Instruct older patients on ways to counteract anticholinergic effects of the medication while taking into account any other existing medical problems.

EVALUATION OF OUTCOME CRITERIA

Evaluate the effectiveness of drug therapy by confirming that patient goals and expected outcomes have been met (see "Planning"). *See Tables 12.4 and 12.5 for a list of drugs to which these nursing actions apply.*

*Herdman, T.H. & Kamitsuru, S. (Eds.), *Nursing Diagnoses: Definitions & Classification* 2015–2017. Copyright © 2014, 1994–2014 NANDA International. Used by arrangement by John Wiley & Sons, Inc. Companion website: www.wiley.com/go/nursingdiagnoses.

CONCEPT REVIEW 12.3

- What is a neuroleptic drug? What are the general classes of drugs used to treat psychoses? How does each drug category generally affect positive or negative symptoms of schizophrenia?

Patients Need to Know

Patients being treated for psychoses need to know the following:

1. It is important to report the development of tremors, muscle spasms, involuntary repetitive movements, decreased muscle tone, or increased restlessness to the healthcare provider. These symptoms may indicate serious adverse effects that can be reversed if medication is changed soon after they start.
2. Consult a healthcare provider if dry mouth, rapid heart rate, constipation, or urinary retention occurs. An additional medication may be prescribed to relieve these signs and symptoms.
3. Avoid taking antacids with antipsychotics because they delay or decrease antipsychotic absorption.
4. Avoid alcohol or other sedatives while taking antipsychotics; it increases the depressant effects.
5. Extra protection from the sun is necessary; wear a hat and sunscreen.
6. Avoid driving or operating machinery until response to the medication is known. Its sedating effects can increase the risk for injury.
7. Contact a healthcare provider for guidance if symptoms get worse or are not relieved by the medication. Do not stop the medication unless directed to do so.
8. Patients may have trouble with balance and an unsteady gait. Healthcare providers and family members should monitor patients for a potential increase in falls.

Chapter Review

Core Concepts Summary

12.1 Most psychoses have no identifiable cause and require long-term drug therapy.

Psychosis is characterized by delusions, hallucinations, illusions, disorganized behavior, difficulty relating to others, and paranoia. Psychoses may be classified as acute or chronic. Sometimes a cause can be found for the psychosis, but the vast majority of cases have no identifiable cause. Most patients with psychoses are not able to function normally in society without long-term drug therapy.

12.2 Patients with schizophrenia experience many different symptoms that may change over time.

Schizophrenia is the most common psychiatric disorder; it is characterized by abnormal thoughts, disordered communication, withdrawal, and suicidal risk. Patients with schizophrenia exhibit positive (adding) or negative (subtracting) symptoms. Proper diagnosis of these symptoms is important for selecting the appropriate antipsychotic drug. The cause of schizophrenia has not been determined. Symptoms seem to be associated with neural dopamine type 2 (D2) receptors found in the basal nuclei. Schizoaffective disorders are characterized by symptoms of both schizophrenia and mood disorder.

12.3 The experience and skills of the healthcare provider are critical to the successful pharmacologic management of psychoses.

Managing severe mental illness is difficult. Many patients do not see themselves as abnormal and have difficulty understanding the need for medication. Although many symptoms of psychosis can be controlled with current drug therapy, adverse effects are common and often severe. Skills of the healthcare team are particularly valuable to achieving successful drug treatment.

12.4 Conventional antipsychotic drugs include the phenothiazines, phenothiazine-like drugs, and nonphenothiazines.

Antipsychotic drugs are sometimes called *neuroleptics*. The two basic categories of drugs for psychosis are conventional antipsychotics and atypical antipsychotics. With conventional antipsychotics, it is not always possible to control extrapyramidal symptoms (EPS), which include muscle spasms (dystonia), inability to remain seated (akathisia), and unusual tongue and facial movements (tardive dyskinesia). Phenothiazines, phenothiazine-like drugs, and nonphenothiazines treat positive signs of schizophrenia, but all have unpleasant adverse effects.

12.5 Atypical antipsychotic drugs address the needs of patients with psychoses.

Atypical antipsychotic drugs treat both positive and negative signs of schizophrenia and have become preferred drugs for treating psychoses. Like the phenothiazine drugs, atypical drugs block D_2 receptors. Although there are fewer adverse effects with atypical drugs, they are still significant, and patients must be carefully monitored. Dopamine system stabilizers (DSS) or dopamine partial agonists represent the third-generation class of antipsychotics developed to better meet the needs of patients with psychoses.

REVIEW Questions

Answer the following questions to assess your knowledge of the chapter material, and go back and review any material that is not clear to you.

1. While caring for a patient taking an antipsychotic drug, the nurse understands that:
   1. Antipsychotic medications cure mental illnesses.
   2. Some adverse effects of antipsychotic drugs can lead to noncompliance.
   3. Antipsychotic medications are only administered when the patient is symptomatic.
   4. Antipsychotic drugs improve symptoms within hours of administration.

2. Family members of a patient diagnosed with schizophrenia are being educated on the adverse effects of phenothiazines. Which of the following would the nurse include? (Select all that apply.)
   1. The patient may experience a sedative effect that usually diminishes with continued therapy.
   2. Severe muscle spasms may occur early in therapy.
   3. Tardive dyskinesia can occur with long-term therapy.
   4. Medications can be given to help prevent some adverse effects.
   5. Monitor the patient's blood pressure because phenothiazines are known to cause hypertension.

3. Which of the following symptoms is an anticholinergic effect of chlorpromazine?
   1. Hallucinations, illusions, paranoia
   2. Hypertension, polyuria, increased salivation
   3. Dry mouth, tachycardia, blurred vision
   4. High fever, confusion, muscle rigidity

4. The patient on thioridazine (Mellaril) has developed muscle spasms, difficulty sleeping, and a shuffling gait. The nurse recognizes this as:
   1. Anticholinergic effects.
   2. Cholinergic effects.
   3. Extrapyramidal symptoms.
   4. Serotonin syndrome.

5. The patient states that he has not taken his antipsychotic drug for the past 2 weeks because it was causing sexual dysfunction. The nurse explains that it is important to continue taking his medication as prescribed because:
   1. Hypertensive crisis may occur with abrupt withdrawal.
   2. Muscle twitching may occur.
   3. Noncompliance may bring on secondary parkinsonism.
   4. Symptoms of psychosis are likely to return.

6. When evaluating the effects of certain antipsychotic medications, neuroleptic malignant syndrome is most likely to occur with use of which of the following drug?
   1. Chlorpromazine
   2. Aripiprazole (Abilify)
   3. Risperidone (Risperdal)
   4. Clozapine (Clozaril)

7. The nurse understands that haloperidol (Haldol) may be ordered for which of the following reasons?
   1. Seizures
   2. Unprovoked aggressiveness
   3. Severe mental depression
   4. Alcoholism

8. The nurse monitors the patient taking which of the following drug groups because it can lead to type 2 diabetes?
   1. Phenothiazines
   2. Nonphenothiazines
   3. Atypical antipsychotics
   4. All antipsychotics

9. The nurse is speaking to a patient diagnosed with schizophrenia and his family about the use of herbal supplements. She warns them about a possible interaction with conventional antipsychotic medication and which herbal supplement?
   1. Echinacea
   2. St. John's wort
   3. Black cohosh
   4. Saw palmetto

10. A patient is taking aripiprazole (Abilify). Which patient effects should the nurse observe to determine whether the drug is having a therapeutic effect?
    1. Elevated mood and coping skills
    2. Orthostatic hypotension and sedation
    3. Decreased delusional thinking and hallucinations
    4. Improved sleep and dietary habits

CASE STUDY Questions

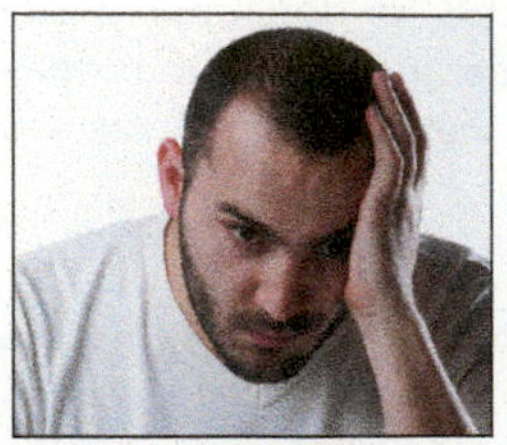

Remember Mr. Wayne, the patient introduced at the beginning of the chapter? Now read the remainder of the case study. Based on the information you have learned in this chapter, answer the questions that follow.

Mr. Jeremy Wayne, age 38, has been diagnosed with a psychosis characterized by the following symptoms: reports of seeing people who are not there, talking about government agents who are trying to kill him, and communicating with "double agents" about suspicious behavior. This patient has been in and out of the hospital for the past 4 weeks. Mr. Wayne's family reports difficulty in controlling him because he has not been taking his medication. Members in the community have seen Mr. Wayne pacing up and down the highway for several weeks. It becomes necessary to temporarily confine Mr. Wayne for medical treatment. He has had this disorder for 15 years and has a strong, supportive family (mother and father).

1. The symptoms described for Mr. Wayne are called _________ symptoms and respond best to treatment with which class of antipsychotic medication?
   1. Positive; conventional or typical antipsychotic
   2. Negative; conventional or typical antipsychotic
   3. Positive; atypical antipsychotic
   4. Negative; atypical antipsychotic
2. Mr. Wayne has been taking risperidone (Risperdal) for the past 10 years and decided to stop taking his medication about a month ago. He is placed back on his medication, so the nurse monitors him closely for which of the following adverse effects? (Select all that apply.)
   1. Hyperactivity
   2. Spasms (shaking of head/neck)
   3. Fatigue
   4. Fever
   5. Weight loss
3. According to the healthcare provider's order, the nurse gives Mr. Wayne which of the following medications to help reduce the incidence of dystonia (spasms)?
   1. Levodopa (Larodopa)
   2. Benztropine (Cogentin)
   3. Thioridazine (Mellaril)
   4. Trifluoperazine
4. The healthcare provider orders the long-acting preparation of fluphenazine 15 mg subcutaneously. The pharmacy supplies fluphenazine 25 mg/mL. The nurse administers _______.
   1. 0.4 mL.
   2. 1.4 mL.
   3. 0.6 mL.
   4. 1.6 mL.

Answers and complete rationales for the Review and Case Study Questions appear in Appendix A.

REFERENCE

Herdman, T. H., & Kamitsuru, S. (Eds.). (2014). *NANDA International nursing diagnoses: Definitions and classification, 2015–2017.* Oxford, United Kingdom: Wiley-Blackwell.

SELECTED BIBLIOGRAPHY

Correll, C. U., Skuban, A., Ouyang, J., Hobart, M., Pfister, S., McQuade, R., . . . Eriksson, H. (2015). Efficacy and safety of brexpiprazole for the treatment of acute schizophrenia: A 6-week randomized, double-blind, placebo-controlled trial. *The American Journal of Psychiatry, 172,* 870–880. doi:10.1176/appi.ajp.2015.14101275

de Araújo, A. N., de Sena, E. P., de Oliveira, I. R., & Juruena, M. F. (2012). Antipsychotic agents: Efficacy and safety in schizophrenia. *Drug Healthcare Patient Safety Journal, 4,* 173–180. doi:10.2147/DHPS.S37429

Dunlop, J., & Brandon, N. J. (2015). Schizophrenia drug discovery and development in an evolving era: Are new drug targets fulfilling expectations? *Journal of Psychopharmacology, 29,* 230–238. doi:10.1177/0269881114565806

Gareri, P., Segura-García, C., Manfredi, V. G. L., Bruni, A., Ciambrone, P., Cerminara, G., . . . De Fazio, P. (2014). Use of atypical antipsychotics in the elderly: A clinical review. *Clinical Interventions in Aging, 9,* 1363–1373. doi:10.2147/CIA.S63942

Gierisch, J. M., Nieuwsma, J. A., Bradford, D. W., Wilder, C. M., Mann-Wrobel, M. C., McBroom, A. J., . . . Williams, J. W. (2013). Interventions to improve cardiovascular risk factors in people with serious mental illness. *Comparative Effectiveness Reviews,* No. *105.* Retrieved from http://www.ncbi.nlm.nih.gov/books/NBK138237/?

Haggerty, J. (2016). *Do people inherit schizophrenia?* Retrieved from http://psychcentral.com/lib/do-people-inherit-schizophrenia

Leucht, S., Cipriani, A., Spineli, L., Mavridis, D., Orey, D., Richter, F., . . . Davis, J. M. (2013). Comparative efficacy and tolerability of 15 antipsychotic drugs in schizophrenia: A multiple-treatments metaanalysis. *Lancet, 382,* 951–962. doi:10.1016/S0140-6736(13)60733-3

Maeda, K., Lerdrup, L., Sugino, H., Akazawa, H., Amada, N., McQuade, R., . . . Kikuchi, T.. (2014). Brexpiprazole II: Antipsychotic-like and procognitive effects of a novel serotonin-dopamine activity modulator. *Journal of Pharmacology and Experimental Therapeutics, 350,* 605–614. doi:10.1124/jpet.114.213819

Murri, M. B., Guaglianone, A., Bugliani, M., Calcagno, P., Respino, M., Serafini, G., . . . Amore, M. (2015). Second-generation antipsychotics and neuroleptic malignant syndrome: Systematic review and case report analysis. *Drugs in Research and Development, 15,* 45–62. doi:10.1007/s40268-014-0078-0

National Alliance of Mental Illness. (n.d.). *Mental illness facts and numbers*. Retrieved from http://www2.nami.org/factsheets/mentalillness_factsheet.pdf

National Institute of Mental Health. (n.d.). *Any anxiety disorder among adults*. Retrieved from http://www.nimh.nih.gov/health/statistics/prevalence/any-anxiety-disorder-among-adults.shtml

Seida, J. C., Schouten, J. R., Mousavi, S. S., Hamm, M., Beaith, A., Dryden, D. M., . . . Carrey, N. (2012). First- and second-generation antipsychotics for children and young adults. *Comparative Effectiveness Reviews*, No. 39. Rockville, MD: Agency for Healthcare Research and Quality. Retrieved from http://www.effectivehealthcare.ahrq.gov/ehc/products/147/835/CER39_Antipsychotics-Children-Young-Adults_20120221.pdf

Steinberg, M., & Lyketsos, C. G. (2012). Atypical antipsychotic use in patients with dementia: Managing safety concerns. *American Journal of Psychiatry*, *169*, 900–906. doi:10.1176/appi.ajp.2012.12030342

Chapter 13

Drugs for Degenerative Diseases and Muscles

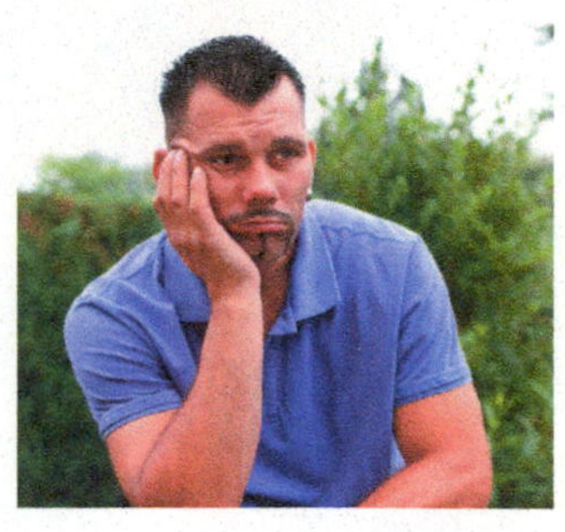

"It's hard to face the future, knowing what MS does to you."
Mr. Robert Wingate

Core Concepts

13.1 **Medications are unable to cure most degenerative diseases of the central nervous system (CNS).**

13.2 **Parkinson disease is progressive, with the occurrence of full symptoms taking many years.**

13.3 **Antiparkinson drugs act on the brain to restore the balance between dopamine and acetylcholine.**

13.4 **Patients with Alzheimer disease experience a dramatic loss of ability to perform tasks that require acetylcholine as the CNS neurotransmitter.**

13.5 **Alzheimer disease is treated with acetylcholinesterase inhibitors and other drugs.**

13.6 **Symptoms of multiple sclerosis result from demyelination of CNS nerve fibers.**

13.7 **Drugs for multiple sclerosis reduce immune attacks in the brain and treat unfavorable symptoms.**

13.8 **Muscle spasms are caused by injury, overmedication, hypocalcemia, and debilitating neurologic disorders.**

13.9 **Muscle spasms may be treated with pharmacologic and nonpharmacologic therapies.**

13.10 **Many muscle relaxants treat muscle spasms by inhibiting upper motor neuron activity, causing sedation, or altering simple reflexes.**

13.11 **Effective treatment for spasticity includes both physical therapy and medications.**

13.12 **Some drugs for spasticity provide relief by acting directly on muscle tissue, interfering with the release of calcium ions.**

13.13 **Neuromuscular blocking drugs block the effect of acetylcholine at the receptor.**

Drug Snapshot

The following drugs are discussed in this chapter:

Drug Classes	Prototype Drugs
Drugs for Parkinson Disease	
Dopaminergic drugs	Pr levodopa, carbidopa, and entacapone (Stalevo)
Cholinergic blockers (anticholinergics)	Pr benztropine (Cogentin)
Drugs for Alzheimer Disease	
Acetylcholinesterase inhibitors	Pr donepezil (Aricept)
Other drugs that slow progression of AD	
Drugs that treat behavioral symptoms of AD	
Drugs for Multiple Sclerosis	
Drugs for Muscle Spasms	
Centrally acting muscle relaxants	Pr cyclobenzaprine (Amrix, Flexeril)
Drugs for Spasticity	
Direct-acting antispasmodics	Pr dantrolene (Dantrium)
Neuromuscular blocking drugs	
Nondepolarizing blockers	
Depolarizing blockers	

Learning Outcomes

After reading this chapter, the student should be able to:

1. Identify the most common degenerative diseases of the CNS.
2. Describe progressive symptoms of Parkinson disease, and explain its neurological basis.
3. Explain the goals of pharmacotherapy for Parkinson disease, and categorize drugs used in its treatment based on drug classes, actions, and important adverse effects.
4. Describe the symptoms of Alzheimer disease and dementia.
5. Explain the goals of pharmacotherapy for Alzheimer disease and categorize drugs used in its treatment based on drug classes, actions, and important adverse effects.
6. Describe symptoms of multiple sclerosis.
7. Describe the pharmacologic management of multiple sclerosis.
8. Describe muscle spasms and how these injuries occur.
9. Discuss pharmacologic and nonpharmacologic strategies used to treat muscle spasms and spasticity.
10. Explain the roles of centrally acting skeletal muscle relaxants in treating muscle spasms.
11. Discuss the approaches for spasticity treatment, including regular and consistent physical therapy.
12. Explain the roles of direct-acting antispasmodics in treating muscle spasticity.
13. Discuss the pharmacology of neuromuscular blocking drugs.

Key Terms

acetylcholinesterase (AChE) (AS-ee-til-KOH-lin-ES-ter-ays)
Alzheimer disease (AD) (ALLZ-heye-mers)
dystonia (diss-TONE-ee-ah)
multiple sclerosis (MS) (skle-ROH-sis)
neuromuscular blocking drugs (NEWR-oh-musc-you-lahr)
parkinsonism
spasticity (spas-TISS-ih-tee)

Central degenerative diseases and muscle disorders affect a patient's ability to perform activities of daily living (ADLs) and most often lead to immobility. Appropriate body movement depends on intact neural pathways and proper muscle functioning. Without medical intervention, neurologic disorders can result in major sensory, cognitive, or motor problems. Parkinson disease (PD), Alzheimer disease (AD), and multiple sclerosis (MS) are three common debilitating and progressive neurologic disorders. Although medications are unable to stop or reverse the progressive nature of these diseases, therapy can often slow down the disorders and offer symptomatic relief. Common muscle disorders are muscle spasms and spasticity. This chapter focuses on the pharmacotherapy of neurodegenerative diseases and muscle disorders as well as treatments involving the neuromuscular junction.

Medications are unable to cure most degenerative diseases of the central nervous system (CNS).

◀ **Core Concept 13.1**

Degenerative diseases of the central nervous system (CNS) include a variety of disorders with different causes and outcomes. Amyotrophic lateral sclerosis (ALS) is a progressive muscle weakness disorder affecting approximately 6400 people in the United States every year. Some disorders, such as Huntington chorea, are quite rare, affect younger patients,

Table 13.1 Degenerative Diseases of the Central Nervous System

Disease	Description
Alzheimer disease (AD)	Progressive loss of brain function characterized by memory loss, confusion, and dementia (a degenerative disorder characterized by progressive memory loss, confusion, and inability to think or communicate effectively)
Amyotrophic lateral sclerosis (ALS)	Progressive weakness and wasting of muscles caused by destruction of motor neurons
Huntington chorea	Autosomal dominant genetic disorder resulting in progressive dementia and involuntary, spasmodic movements of limb and facial muscles
Multiple sclerosis (MS)	Demyelination of neurons in the CNS resulting in progressive weakness, visual disturbances, mood alterations, and cognitive deficits
Parkinson disease (PD)	Progressive loss of dopamine in the CNS causing tremor, muscle rigidity, and abnormal movement and posture

and are caused by chromosomal defects. Others, such as AD, affect millions of people, mostly older patients, and have a devastating economic and social impact. Nearly 1 million people have PD, and this disorder can occur at any age. More than 2.3 million people are affected by MS worldwide. Table 13.1 lists major degenerative diseases of the CNS.

Fast Facts Neurodegenerative Diseases

Parkinson Disease

- Most patients with PD are above the age of 50.
- Greater than 50% of patients with PD who have difficulty with voluntary movement are less than 60 years of age.
- More men than women develop this disorder.

Alzheimer Disease and Dementia

- Dementia is a group of symptoms that affect mental tasks like memory and reasoning.
- Of all patients with dementia, 60% to 70% have AD.
- AD mainly affects patients over the age of 65.

Multiple Sclerosis

- Onset of symptoms typically occurs between ages 15 and 40.
- Women are affected twice as often as men.
- MS occurs most often in Caucasians of northern European origin.
- MS is about five times more prevalent in temperate climates than in tropical climates.

The cause of most neurologic degenerative diseases is unknown. Most progress from hardly noticeable signs and symptoms early in the disease to serious neurologic and cognitive deficits. In their early stages, disorders may be difficult to diagnose. With the exception of PD, pharmacotherapy provides only minimal benefit. Currently, medication is unable to cure any of the major neurodegenerative diseases.

PARKINSON DISEASE

Parkinson disease is a degenerative disorder of the CNS caused by death of neurons that produce the brain neurotransmitter dopamine. It is the second most common degenerative disease of the nervous system, affecting many Americans. Pharmacotherapy is often successful in reducing some of the distressing symptoms of this disorder.

Core Concept 13.2 ▶ Parkinson disease is progressive, with the occurrence of full symptoms taking many years.

Parkinson disease primarily affects patients older than 50 years of age; however, even teenagers can develop the disorder. Men are affected slightly more often than women. The disease is progressive. The appearance of full symptoms often takes many years. The symptoms of PD, described as **parkinsonism**, are summarized as follows:

- *Tremors* The hands and head develop a palsy-like motion or shakiness when at rest; *pill-rolling* is a common behavior in progressive states, in which patients rub the thumb and forefinger together as if a pill were between them.

- *Muscle rigidity* Stiffness may resemble symptoms of arthritis. Patients often have difficulty bending over or moving limbs. These symptoms may not be noticeable at first but become more obvious as the disease progresses.
- *Bradykinesia* This is the most noticeable of all symptoms. Patients may have difficulty chewing, swallowing, or speaking. Patients with PD have difficulties initiating movement and controlling fine muscle movements. Walking often becomes difficult, and patients shuffle their feet without taking normal strides.
- *Postural instability* Patients may lean forward or backward slightly and may easily lose their balance. Stumbling results in frequent falls and injuries.
- *Affective flattening* Patients often have a "masked face" where there is little facial expression or blinking of the eyes.

brady = *slow*
kinesia = *movement*

affective = *body emotion*
flattening = *without expression*

Although PD is a progressive neurologic disorder primarily affecting muscle movement, other health problems often develop in these patients, including anxiety, depression, sleep disturbances, dementia, and disturbances of the autonomic nervous system (difficulty urinating and performing sexually). Several theories have been proposed to explain the development of parkinsonism. Because some patients with PD have a family history of this disorder, a genetic link is highly probable. Numerous environmental toxins, such as carbon monoxide, cyanide, manganese, chlorine, and pesticides, also have been suggested as causes, but results of studies have not proven the cause–effect link. Viral infections, head trauma, and stroke have also been proposed as causes.

Symptoms of parkinsonism develop due to the degeneration and destruction of dopamine-producing neurons found within an area of the brain known as the *substantia nigra*. When not enough dopamine is released, this neurotransmitter cannot make contact with other critical areas of the brain.

substantia = *substance*
nigra =*black*

The most critical area for dopamine contact is the *corpus striatum*, an area responsible for controlling unconscious muscle movement. Patients with PD have difficulty initiating and controlling movements. Balance, posture, muscle tone, and involuntary muscle movements depend on the proper balance between dopamine (inhibitory) and acetylcholine (stimulatory). Under normal conditions, the inhibitory effects of dopamine and the excitatory effects of acetycholine (ACh) balance one another to produce smooth, coordinated muscle movement. If dopamine is absent, ACh is able to overstimulate the corpus striatum. For this reason, drug therapy for parkinsonism focuses not only on restoring dopamine function but also on blocking the effect of ACh within this sensitive area of the brain.

corpus =*body*
striatum = *striped*

Extrapyramidal symptoms (EPS) develop in response to the same neurochemical actions that cause PD. Recall that antipsychotic drugs act by blocking dopamine receptors. Treatment with some antipsychotic drugs may cause parkinsonism-like symptoms (secondary parkinsonism) by interfering with the same neural pathway and functions affected by the lack of dopamine. Antiparkinson drugs are sometimes used to treat EPS caused by antipsychotic medications.

extra = *outside*
pyramidal = *medullary pyramidal tracts*
symptoms = *involuntary motor characteristics (e.g., EPS)*

EPS may occur suddenly and become a medical emergency. With acute EPS, patients' muscles may spasm or lock up. Fever and confusion are other signs or symptoms of this reaction. If acute EPS occur in a healthcare facility, short-term medical treatment may be provided by administering diphenhydramine (Benadryl), which is an antihistamine that has ACh-blocking properties. When symptoms are recognized outside a healthcare facility, the patient should be immediately taken to the emergency department. Untreated acute episodes of EPS can be fatal.

CONCEPT REVIEW 13.1

- PD primarily affects which body functions? What are the five major symptoms of this disorder?

Antiparkinson drugs act on the brain to restore the balance between dopamine and acetylcholine.

◀ **Core Concept 13.3**

The goal of pharmacotherapy for PD is to increase the ability of the patient to perform ADLs such as eating, walking, dressing, and bathing. Although pharmacotherapy does not cure this disorder, it can dramatically reduce symptoms in some patients.

anti = *against*
cholinergic = *acetylcholine action*

Antiparkinson drugs are given to restore the balance of dopamine and ACh within the corpus striatum of the brain. These drugs include dopaminergic drugs and anticholinergics (cholinergic blockers).

Dopaminergic Drugs

dopaminergic = *dopamine action*

Dopaminergic drugs, shown in Table 13.2, are used to increase dopamine action within critical areas of the corpus striatum. The basic ingredient in many of the preferred drugs for parkinsonism is levodopa, a dopaminergic substance that has been used more often than any other for this disorder. As shown in Figure 13.1, levodopa is a precursor (a more basic chemical form) of dopamine. Supplying the nerve terminals directly with levodopa leads to increased synthesis of dopamine. Levodopa can cross the blood-brain barrier but dopamine cannot. Therefore, dopamine by itself is not used for therapy. The effectiveness of levodopa can be enhanced by combining it with carbidopa. This combination, marketed as Parcopa and Sinemet, makes more levodopa available to enter the CNS. Carbidopa (Lodosyn) alone can also increase the concentration of dopamine and levodopa in the brain.

Levodopa is chemically similar to some amino acids. Foods high in protein use the same pathways for the absorption into the bloodstream or brain, and therefore compete with levodopa (with or without carbidopa) for absorption. If levodopa is taken with foods high in protein, the effectiveness of the medication will be reduced. In addition, levodopa is absorbed in the small intestine; therefore, any foods or conditions that delay gastric emptying will reduce drug availability.

catecholamine = *neurotransmitter group synthesized from dopamine*

O-methyl-transferase = *degrading enzyme transferring a methyl (CH_3) group (e.g., COMT)*

Other approaches to enhancing dopamine are used in treating parkinsonism. Tolcapone (Tasmar), entacapone (Comtan), rasagiline (Azilect), and selegiline (Eldepryl, Zelapar) inhibit enzymes that normally destroy levodopa and dopamine. Rasagiline and selegiline are monoamine oxidase inhibitors (MAOIs). Apomorphine (Apokyn), bromocriptine (Parlodel), pramipexole (Mirapex), and ropinirole (Requip) directly activate the dopamine receptor and are called *dopamine receptor drugs*. Amantadine (Symmetrel), an antiviral

Table 13.2 Dopaminergic Drugs Used for Parkinsonism

Drug	Route and Adult Dose	Remarks
amantadine (Symmetrel)	PO: 100 mg daily or bid	For relief of drug-induced EPS; may cause release of dopamine from nerve terminals; also for infection with influenza A virus
apomorphine	Subcutaneous: 2 mg for the first dose; may increase doses every few days (max: 6 mg); if more than 1 week passes between doses, dose should be restarted at 2 mg	Activates dopamine receptors; may improve ability to walk, talk, and move
bromocriptine (Parlodel)	PO: 1.25–2.5 mg/day up to 100 mg/day in divided doses	Also for suppression of lactation, female infertility, and overproduction of growth hormone; activates the dopamine receptor directly
entacapone (Comtan)	PO: 200 mg given with levodopa–carbidopa up to 8 times/day	Blocks synaptic enzyme catecholamine O-methyl transferase (COMT) responsible for metabolizing dopamine
levodopa–carbidopa (Parcopa, Sinemet)	PO: 1 tablet containing 10 mg carbidopa/100 mg levodopa or 25 mg carbidopa/100 mg levodopa tid (max: 6 tablets/day)	Prevents metabolism of levodopa, enhancing dopamine action
Pr levodopa–carbidopa-entacapone (Stalevo)	PO: 1 tablet containing 10 mg carbidopa/100 mg levodopa or 25 mg carbidopa/100 mg levodopa tid (max: 6 tablets/day)	Chemical precursor to dopamine combined with a dopamine enhancer and a COMT enzyme inhibitor
pramipexole (Mirapex)	PO: Start with 0.125 mg tid and increase to a target dose of 1.5 mg tid	Activates dopamine receptors; also approved to treat restless legs syndrome (RLS)
rasagiline (Azilect)	PO: 0.5–1 mg once daily	Blocks monoamine oxidase (MAO), the enzyme that degrades dopamine within brain nerve terminals
ropinirole (Requip)	PO: Start with 0.25 mg tid and increase to a target dose of 1 mg tid	Activates dopamine receptors; approved to treat RLS
rotigotine (Neupro)	Transdermal: 2-8 mg/day (one patch)	For early-stage and advancedstage PD, and RLS
selegiline (Eldepryl, Zelapar)	PO: 5 mg bid (max: 10 mg/day)	Blocks MAO; also for depression
tolcapone (Tasmar)	PO: 100 mg tid (max: 600 mg/day)	Blocks synaptic enzyme COMT

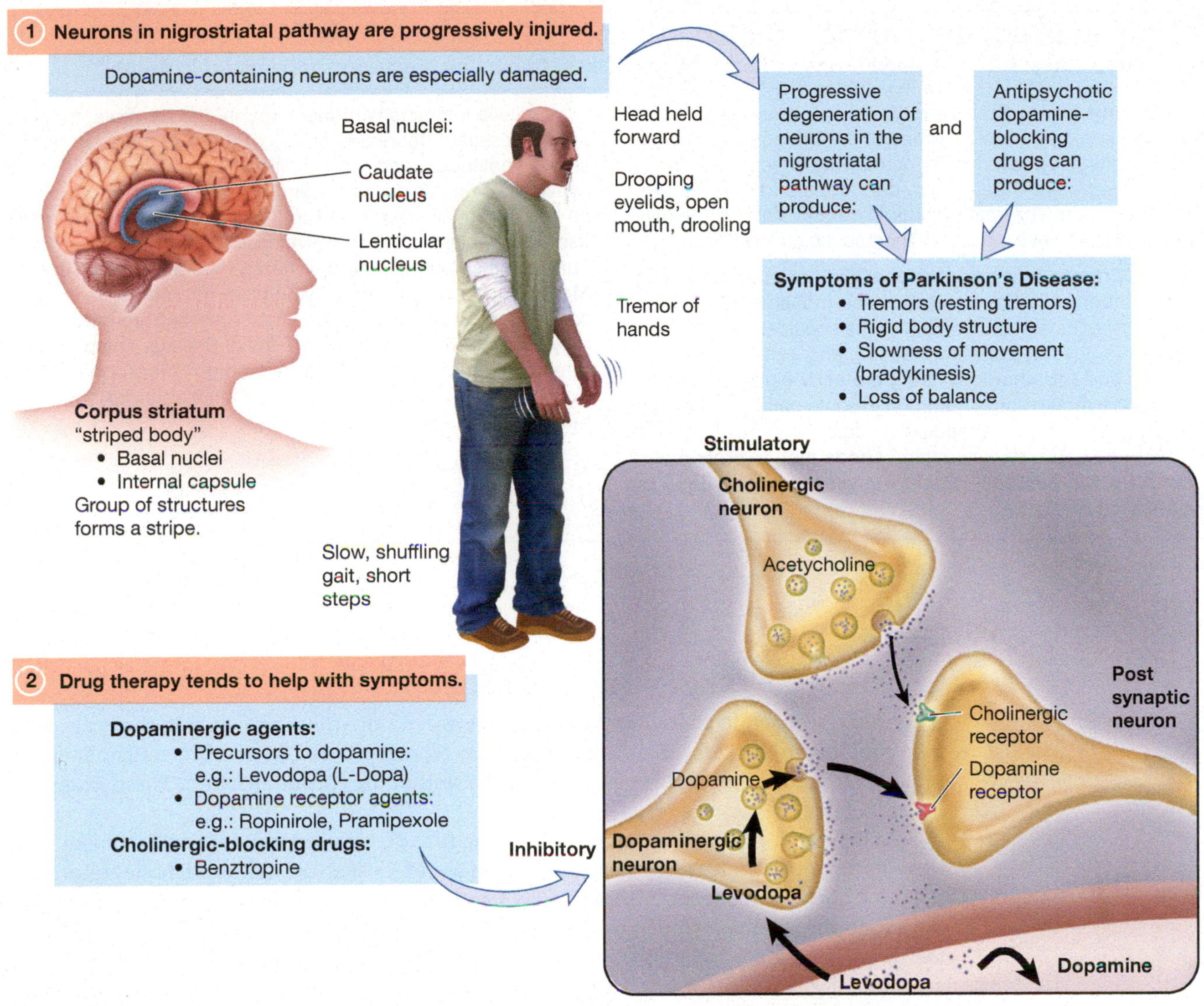

FIGURE 13.1 Dopamine cannot cross the blood–brain barrier. Levodopa, its precursor, can. Once levodopa crosses the blood–brain barrier and enters neurons, it is converted into dopamine, which normally inhibits firing of the next neuron. Natural ACh in the brain stimulates the same postsynaptic neuron. Thus, to restore normal neuronal activity, drug therapy attempts to either (a) restore dopamine inhibitory action or (b) block ACh (cholinergic) stimulatory activity.

agent, causes the release of dopamine from nerve terminals. All these drugs are considered adjuncts to the pharmacotherapy of parkinsonism because they are not as effective as levodopa. In terms of ADLs, most levodopa–carbidopa combination drugs are thought to control motor symptoms better. Pramipexole (Mirapex) and ropinirole (Requip) have proven to be safe and effective for initial sole therapy and also when combined with levodopa–carbidopa.

monoamine oxidase (MAO) = *catecholamine degrading enzyme*

Additional drugs that reduce the requirements for levodopa–carbidopa include the catechol-O-methyl transferase (COMT) inhibitors. Entacapone (Comtan) and tolcapone (Tasmar) are COMT inhibitors. Like levodopa–carbidopa, these drugs increase concentrations of existing dopamine in nerve terminals and improve motor fluctuations related to the "wearing-off" effect. Entacapone combined with carbidopa and levodopa is marketed as Stalevo. Side effects of COMT inhibitors include mental confusion, hallucinations, nausea and vomiting, cramps, headache, diarrhea, and possible liver damage.

Rotigotine (Neupro) is a dopamine receptor transdermal patch that can be applied once daily. In clinical trials, it was shown to effectively treat early PD as monotherapy and was even shown to be effective in the treatment of advanced-stage PD and RLS. The most common side effects of rotigotine for RLS are application site reactions, drowsiness, nausea, and headache.

Prototype Drug: Levodopa, Carbidopa, and Entacapone (Stalevo)

Therapeutic Class: Antiparkinson drugs **Pharmacologic Class:** Dopamine precursor, dopaminergic drugs

Actions and Uses: Stalevo restores the neurotransmitter dopamine in extrapyramidal areas of the brain, thus relieving some Parkinson symptoms. To increase its effect, levodopa is combined with two other drugs, carbidopa and entacapone, which prevent its enzymatic breakdown. Several months may be needed to achieve maximum therapeutic effects.

Adverse Effects and Interactions: Side effects of Stalevo include uncontrolled and purposeless movements such as extending the fingers and shrugging the shoulders, involuntary movements, loss of appetite, nausea, and vomiting. Muscle twitching and spasmodic winking are early signs of toxicity. Orthostatic hypotension is common in some patients. The drug should be discontinued gradually, because abrupt withdrawal can produce acute parkinsonism. Foods high in protein and vitamin B6 will decrease the effectiveness of levodopa or levodopa–carbidopa.

Stalevo interacts with many drugs. For example, tricyclic antidepressants decrease effects of Stalevo, increase orthostatic hypotension, and may increase sympathetic activity, with hypertension and sinus tachycardia. Stalevo cannot be used if an MAOI was taken within 14 to 28 days, because concurrent use may precipitate hypertensive crisis. Haloperidol taken concurrently may antagonize the therapeutic effects of Stalevo. Methyldopa may increase toxicity. Antihypertensives may cause increased hypotensive effects. Antiseizure medication may decrease the therapeutic effects of Stalevo. Antacids containing magnesium, calcium, or sodium bicarbonate may increase Stalevo absorption, which could lead to toxicity. Kava may worsen the Parkinson symptoms.

Cholinergic Blockers (Anticholinergics)

A second approach to changing the balance between dopamine and ACh in the brain is to give cholinergic blockers, or anticholinergics. By blocking the effect of ACh, anticholinergics inhibit the overactivity of this neurotransmitter within the corpus striatum. These drugs are listed in Table 13.3.

Anticholinergics such as atropine were the first drugs used to treat parkinsonism. The large number of adverse effects has limited the use of these drugs. The anticholinergics now used for parkinsonism act within the CNS and produce fewer adverse effects. However, they continue to cause unpleasant autonomic symptoms such as dry mouth, blurred vision, tachycardia, urinary retention, and constipation (very troublesome). The centrally acting anticholinergics are not as effective as levodopa in relieving severe symptoms of parkinsonism. They are used early in the course of the disease when symptoms are less severe, in patients who cannot tolerate levodopa, and in combination therapy with other antiparkinson drugs.

CONCEPT REVIEW 13.2

- Antiparkinson drugs attempt to restore the balance of which two major CNS neurotransmitters?

Table 13.3 Anticholinergic Drugs Used for Parkinsonism

Drug	Route and Adult Dose	Remarks
Pr benztropine (Cogentin)	PO: 0.5–1 mg/day (max: 6 mg/day)	Also used to relieve EPS from neuroleptic drugs; does not improve tardive dyskinesia
biperiden (Akineton)	PO: 2 mg daily to qid	Blocks ACh receptors; thus, produces actions associated with muscarinic blockade (e.g., blurred vision, dry mouth); available in IM and IV forms
diphenhydramine (Benadryl) (see the Prototype Drug box in Core Concept 30.4)	PO: 25–50 mg tid or qid (max: 300 mg/day)	Also for allergic reactions, motion sickness, sedation, and coughing; blocks cholinergic function even though it is an antihistamine; available in IM/IV forms
trihexyphenidyl (Artane)	PO: Start with 1 mg; gradually increase to 6–10 mg/day (max: 15 mg/day)	Also used to relieve EPS; off-label use for Huntington chorea and spasmodic torticollis

Prototype Drug: Pr *Benztropine (Cogentin)*

Therapeutic Class: Antiparkinson drug **Pharmacologic Class: Centrally acting cholinergic receptor blocker**

Actions and Uses: Benztropine acts by blocking excess cholinergic stimulation of neurons in the corpus striatum. It is used for relief of parkinsonism symptoms and for the treatment of EPS brought on by antipsychotic pharmacotherapy. This medication suppresses tremors but does not affect tardive dyskinesia.

Adverse Effects and Interactions: As expected from its autonomic action, benztropine can cause typical anticholinergic adverse effects such as sedation, dry mouth, constipation, and tachycardia.

Benztropine interacts with many drugs. For example, it should not be taken with alcohol, tricyclic antidepressants, MAOIs, phenothiazines, procainamide, or quinidine because of combined sedative effects. Over-the-counter (OTC) cold medicines and alcohol should be avoided. Other drugs that enhance dopamine release or activation of the dopamine receptor may produce additive effects. Haloperidol will cause decreased effectiveness.

Antihistamines, phenothiazines, tricyclics, disopyramide, and quinidine may increase anticholinergic effects, and antidiarrheals may decrease absorption.

ALZHEIMER DISEASE

Alzheimer disease (AD) affects memory, thinking, and behavior. It is one of the forms of dementia that gradually gets worse over time. As many as 50% of people are affected with AD by the age of 85. The patient generally lives 5 to 10 years following diagnosis; AD is the fourth leading cause of death. Drugs help slow down the rate at which symptoms become worse.

Dementia is a degenerative disorder characterized by progressive memory loss, confusion, and inability to think or communicate effectively. Consciousness and perception are usually unaffected. Although the cause of most dementia is unknown, it is usually associated with cerebral atrophy or other structural changes within the brain.

Structural damage within the brain of patients with AD has been well documented. *Amyloid plaques* and *neurofibrillary tangles*, found at autopsy, are present in nearly all patients with AD. It is suspected that these structural changes are caused by chronic inflammatory or oxidative cellular damage to surrounding neurons. There is a loss in both the number and function of neurons in patients with AD.

Patients with Alzheimer disease experience a dramatic loss of ability to perform tasks that require acetylcholine as the CNS neurotransmitter.

◀ Core Concept 13.4

Because ACh is a major neurotransmitter within the hippocampus (an area of the brain responsible for learning and memory) and other parts of the cerebral cortex, neuronal function within these brain areas is especially affected. Symptoms of AD include the following:

- Impaired memory and judgment
- Confusion or disorientation
- Inability to recognize family or friends
- Aggressive behavior
- Depression
- Psychoses, including paranoia and delusions
- Anxiety.

Alzheimer disease is treated with acetylcholinesterase inhibitors and other drugs.

◀ Core Concept 13.5

Drugs are used to slow memory loss and other progressive symptoms of dementia. Additional drugs may be given to treat associated symptoms such as depression, anxiety, or psychoses. The acetylcholinesterase (AChE) inhibitors are the most widely used class of drugs for treating AD. Representative drugs used for treatment of AD are listed in Table 13.4.

acetylcholinesterase (AChE) = *ACh terminating enzyme*
inhibitor = *suppressing factor*

Table 13.4 Drugs Used for Alzheimer Disease

Drug	Route and Adult Dose	Remarks
Pr donepezil (Aricept)	PO: 5–10 mg at bedtime	For mild to moderate dementia; may cause nausea, diarrhea, muscle cramps, and weight loss
galantamine (Razadyne)	PO: Start with 4 mg bid; may increase gradually to a target dose of 12 mg bid (max: 8–16 mg bid)	For mild to moderate dementia; may cause weight loss, dizziness, nausea, vomiting, and orthostatic hypotension
memantine (Namenda)	PO: Start with 5 mg once daily; may increase dose to 10 mg bid	For moderate to severe dementia; NMDA receptor blocking drug; may cause a serious skin reaction, fatigue, dizziness, headache, confusion, vomiting, coughing, constipation, pain, and difficulty in breathing
rivastigmine (Exelon)	PO: Start with 1.5 mg bid; may increase gradually to target dose 3–6 mg bid (max: 12 mg bid) Transdermal: 5 cm^2 patch (4.6mg/24 hours), 10 cm^2 patch (9.5mg/24 hours)	For mild to moderate dementia; may cause flu-like symptoms, dizziness, and weight loss

Acetylcholinesterase Inhibitors

The U.S. Food and Drug Administration (FDA) has approved only a few drugs specifically for AD. The most effective of these medications acts by intensifying the effect of ACh at the cholinergic receptor, as shown in Figure 13.2. ACh is naturally degraded in the synapse by the enzyme **acetylcholinesterase (AChE)**. When AChE is inhibited, ACh levels increase and greatly impact the receptors. As described in Chapter 9, the AChE inhibitors *indirectly* stimulate the receptors for ACh.

ADLs = *activities of daily living*

The goal of pharmacotherapy for AD is to improve function in ADLs, behavior, and cognition. Although the AChE inhibitors improve functions in all three areas, their effectiveness is limited. These drugs do not cure AD—they only slow its progression. Therapy is begun as soon as the diagnosis of AD is established. These drugs are ineffective in treating the severe stages of this disorder, probably because so many neurons have been damaged. Increasing the levels of ACh is only effective if there are functioning neurons present. Therefore, the AChE inhibitors are often discontinued as the disease progresses because their therapeutic benefit may not outweigh their expense or the risk of adverse effects. When discontinuing therapy, doses of the AChE inhibitors should be lowered gradually.

All AChE inhibitors used to treat AD are equally effective. Their adverse effects are those expected of drugs that enhance the parasympathetic nervous system (see Chapter 9). These include nausea, vomiting, and diarrhea. Rivastigmine (Exelon) is associated with weight loss, a potentially serious adverse effect in some older adults.

Prototype Drug: Pr *Donepezil (Aricept)*

Therapeutic Class: Drug for Alzheimer disease **Pharmacologic Class: Acetylcholinerase inhibitor**

Actions and Uses: Donepezil is an AChE inhibitor that improves memory in cases of mild to moderate AD dementia by enhancing the effects of ACh in neurons in the cerebral cortex that have not yet been damaged. Patients should receive pharmacotherapy for at least 6 months prior to assessing the maximum benefits of drug therapy. Improvement in memory may be observed as early as 1 to 4 weeks following medication. The therapeutic effects of donepezil are often short-lived, and the degree of improvement is modest at best. An advantage of donepezil over other drugs in its class is that its long half-life permits it to be given once daily.

Adverse Effects and Interactions: Common adverse effects of donepezil are vomiting, diarrhea, and darkened urine. CNS adverse effects include insomnia, syncope, depression, headache, and irritability. Musculoskeletal adverse effects include muscle cramps, arthritis, and bone fractures. Generalized adverse effects include headache, fatigue, chest pain, increased libido, hot flashes, urinary incontinence, dehydration, and blurred vision. Hepatotoxicity has not been observed. Patients with bradycardia, hypotension, asthma, hyperthyroidism, or active peptic ulcer disease should be monitored carefully. Anticholinergics will be less effective. Donepezil interacts with several other drugs. For example, bethanechol causes a synergistic effect. Phenobarbital, phenytoin, dexamethasone, and rifampin may speed elimination of donepezil. Quinidine or ketoconazole may inhibit metabolism of donepezil. Because donepezil acts by increasing cholinergic activity, two parasympathomimetics should not be administered at the same time.

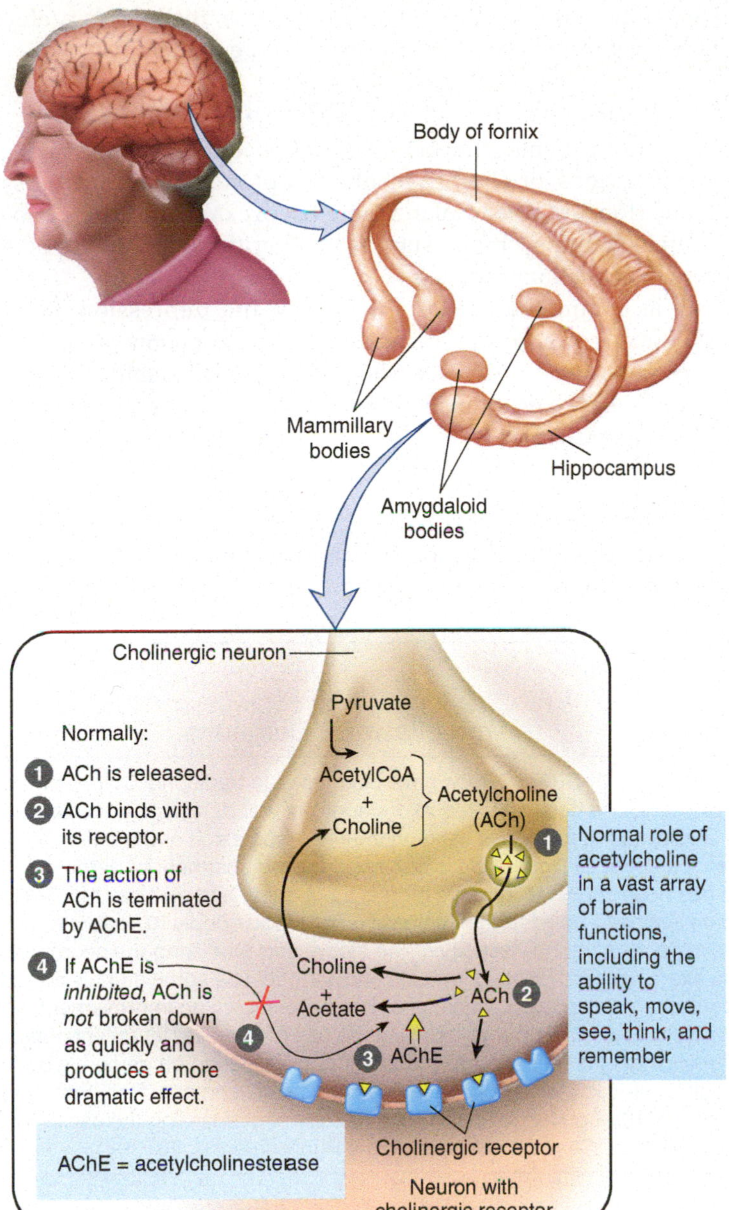

FIGURE 13.2 Alzheimer medications work by intensifying the effect of ACh at the receptor.

Other Drugs That Slow the Progression of AD

Although AChE inhibitors are the mainstay of treatment for AD dementia, several other agents have been investigated for possible benefit in delaying the progression of this disease. Because at least some of the neuronal changes in AD are caused by oxidative cellular damage, antioxidants such as vitamin E have been examined. Other drugs purported to prevent or help slow the onset of AD progression are NSAIDs and selegiline, an MAOI.

Memantine (Namenda) is approved for combination treatment of moderate to severe AD. Its mechanism of action differs from that of the AChE inhibitors. Unlike AChE inhibitors that address the cholinergic defect in the brains of patients with AD, memantine reduces the abnormally high levels of glutamate. Glutamate exerts its neural effects through interaction with the N-methyl-D-aspartate (NMDA) receptor. When bound to the receptor, glutamate causes calcium to enter neurons, producing an excitatory effect. Too much glutamate in the brain may be responsible for brain cell death. Memantine, along with AChE inhibitors such as donepezil, may have a protective function in reducing neuronal calcium overload.

Caprylidene (Axona) is a medical food approved for patients with AD. This food medication is metabolized into ketone bodies, which the brain can use for energy even when its ability to process glucose is impaired. Brain-imaging scans of older adults and those with

AD have revealed an impaired ability to take up glucose, the brain's preferred source of energy. Thus, patients with AD may benefit from this type of therapy.

Drugs That Treat Behavioral Symptoms of AD

Agitation occurs in most patients with AD. This is often accompanied by delusional behavior, paranoia, hallucinations, or other psychotic symptoms. Atypical antipsychotic drugs such as risperidone (Risperdal) and olanzapine (Zyprexa) may be used to control these episodes. Conventional antipsychotics such as haloperidol (Haldol) are occasionally prescribed, although EPS often limit their use.

Although not as common as agitation, anxiety and depression may also occur in patients with AD. Anxiolytics such as buspirone (BuSpar) or some of the benzodiazepines are used to control excessive anxiety (see Chapter 10). Mood stabilizers such as sertraline (Zoloft), citalopram (Celexa), or fluoxetine (Prozac) may be given when major depression interferes with ADLs (see Chapter 11).

CONCEPT REVIEW 13.3

- Alzheimer disease is a dysfunction of which brain neurotransmitters? How do drugs for Alzheimer disease restore neurotransmitter function and improve symptoms of dementia?

CAM Therapy | *Ginkgo biloba* for Dementia

The seeds and leaves of *Ginkgo biloba* have been used in traditional Chinese medicine for thousands of years. The tree is planted throughout the world, including the United States. In Western medicine, the focus has been on treating depression and memory loss. In Germany, an extract of *Ginkgo biloba* is approved for the treatment of dementia.

Ginkgo has been shown to improve mental functioning and stabilize AD. The mechanism of action seems to be related to increasing the blood supply to the brain by dilating blood vessels, decreasing the viscosity of the blood, and modifying the neurotransmitter system. The exact benefit of ginkgo remains unclear because some studies concluded that cognitive performance improved, whereas others have shown no improvement in the symptoms or progress of AD. Ginkgo may increase the risk of bleeding in patients taking anticoagulants. A review of nine different trials of the effects of ginkgo on dementia concluded that the supplement was more effective than a placebo (Weinmann, Roll, Schwartzbach, Vauth & Willich, 2010). Cancer concerns have been raised regarding the use of gingko as a supplement ingredient (Center for Science in the Public Interest, 2013).

MULTIPLE SCLEROSIS

oligo = *little*
dendro = *branched*
cytes = *cells*
scleroses = *thickened or hardened plaques*

Multiple sclerosis (MS) is a disorder characterized by damaged myelin located within the CNS. Antibodies produced by the patient slowly target and destroy myelin, axonal membranes, and supporting cells of the CNS, for example oligodendrocytes. As axons are destroyed, the ability of nerves to conduct electrical impulses is impaired. Inflammation accompanies damaged tissue, and multiple filamentous plaques called *scleroses* are formed.

Core Concept 13.6 ▶

Symptoms of multiple sclerosis result from demyelination of CNS nerve fibers.

neurologic = *pertaining to the nervous system*

During the early stages of MS, some damaged axons recover due to partial myelination and the development of alternative circuitry, but as antibodies continue to attack neural tissue, further damage and inflammation lead to neuronal death. Patients often have recurrent episodes of neurologic dysfunction, which progress at a fairly rapid rate.

The etiology of MS is unknown. Many clinicians and scientists suspect genetic or microbial factors due to reports that, in most cases, MS occurs in regions of colder climate. One theory proposes acquired immunological resistance against pathogenic factors in warmer climates. Microscopic pathogens such as viruses have been suggested, though there is no strong evidence for this theory.

Signs and symptoms associated with axonal injury include fatigue, heat sensitivity, neuropathic pain, spasticity, impaired cognitive ability, disruption of balance and coordination, bowel and bladder symptoms, sexual dysfunction, dizziness, vertigo, visual impairment, and slurred speech. Although the disease is progressive, the precise course of MS is unpredictable, and each patient experiences a variety of symptoms depending on the extent and localization of demyelination.

neuropathic = *nervous disease*
spasticity = *stiffness of muscle*
cognitive = *reasoning ability*
vertigo = *confusion and disorientation*

Drugs for multiple sclerosis reduce immune attacks in the brain and treat unfavorable symptoms.

◀ **Core Concept 13.7**

Like many neurodegenerative disorders, there are no drugs available that can cure MS or reverse the progressive nature of the disease. Existing drugs are only partially effective and some have serious adverse effects. Drugs are used to either modify the progression of the disease or to manage symptoms. Drugs for treating MS are shown in Table 13.5.

One approach to modify disease progression attempts to reduce inflammation and prevent attacks on the nervous system. Drugs also address impairment of movement due to demyelination of neurons. Goals are accomplished through the use of immune system modulating drugs, immunosuppressants, and drugs that block neuronal potassium channels.

The most treatable form of this disorder is *relapsing-remitting MS (RRMS)*. This condition involves unpredictable relapses (attacks) during which time new symptoms appear or existing symptoms become more severe (Figure 13.3). These symptoms can last for varying periods (days or months), followed by partial or total remission (recovery). The disease may be inactive for months or years. On average, people with RRMS have one or two attacks a year.

Immune system modulating drugs (also called *immunostimulants* [see Chapter 26]) are used to treat the underlying causes of MS and to decrease the overall relapse rate. Interferon beta-1a (Avonex, Rebif) and interferon beta-1b (Betaseron, Extavia) are first-line therapies for slowing the neuronal damage caused by MS. Peginterferon beta-1a (Plegridy) is a "pegylated" form of interferon, meaning that polyethylene glycol is attached to the interferon molecules to allow them to maintain their biologic effects for a longer time. Because the biologic effects last longer, dosing can occur at less frequent intervals. Although generally well tolerated, the interferons have unfavorable adverse effects, including flu-like symptoms (e.g., headaches, fever, chills, muscle aches), anxiety, discomfort experienced at

Table 13.5 Drugs Used for Multiple Sclerosis

Drug	Comments	Route Administered
FOR IMMUNE ATTACKS AGAINST THE CNS		
alemtuzumab (Lemtrada)	Immunosuppressant drug	IV
dalfampridine (Ampyra)	Potassium channel blocker to treat walking impairment	PO
dimethyl fumarate (Tecfidera)	Myelin oxidative stress reducer	PO
fingolimod (Gilenya)	Immune system modulator	PO
glatiramer (Copaxone)	Immune system modulator; myelin protein protectant	Subcutaneous
interferon beta-1a (Avonex, Rebif)	Immune system modulator	IM and subcutaneous
interferon beta-1b (Betaseron, Extavia)	Immune system modulator	Subcutaneous
mitoxantrone (Novantrone)	Immunosuppressant drug	IV
natalizumab (Tysabri)	Immune system modulator	IV
peginterferon beta-1a (Plegridy)	Immune system modulator	Subcutaneous
teriflunomide (Aubagio)	Immune system modulator	PO
Drug	**Comments**	**Symptoms Relieved**
FOR THE RELIEF OF MS SYMPTOMS		
amantadine (Symmetrel)	Dopaminergic drug	Fatigue, memory loss, weakness
gabapentin (Neurontin)	Antiseizure drug	Anxiety, insomnia, neuropathic pain
modafinil (Provigil)	Central adrenergic drug	Fatigue, memory loss, weakness
methylprednisolone (Solu-Medrol)	Corticosteroid medication	Myelin swelling and inflammation

Relapsing–Remitting MS (RRMS) – RRMS is the most common form of the disease. It is characterized by clearly defined acute attacks with full recovery.

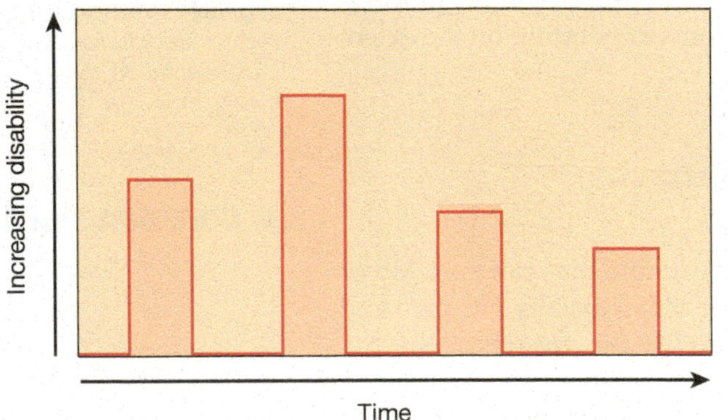

Secondary–Progressive MS (SPMS) – SPMS begins with an initial relapsing-remitting disease course, followed by progression of disability with occasional relapses and minor remissions and plateaus.

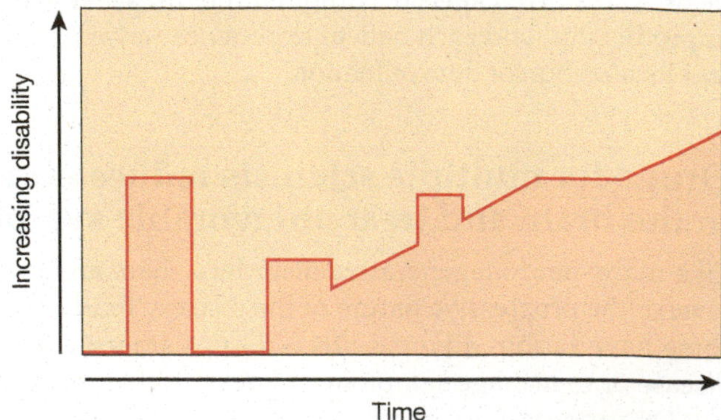

Progressive–Relapsing MS (PRMS) – PRMS, which is the least common disease course, shows progression of disability from onset but with clear acute relapses, with or without full recovery.

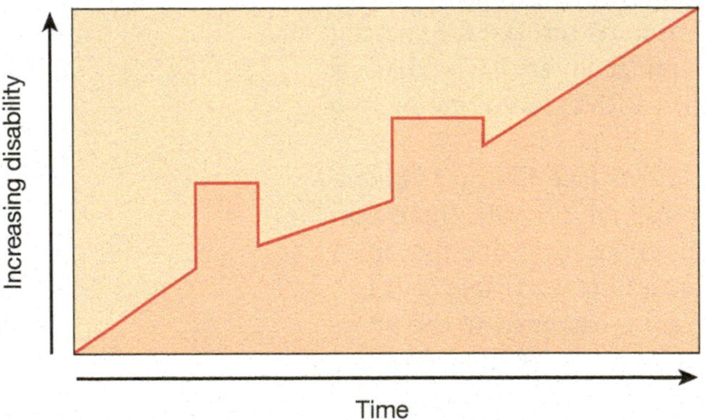

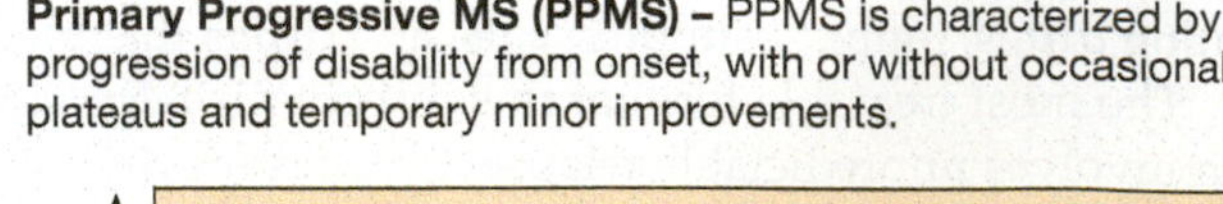
Primary Progressive MS (PPMS) – PPMS is characterized by progression of disability from onset, with or without occasional plateaus and temporary minor improvements.

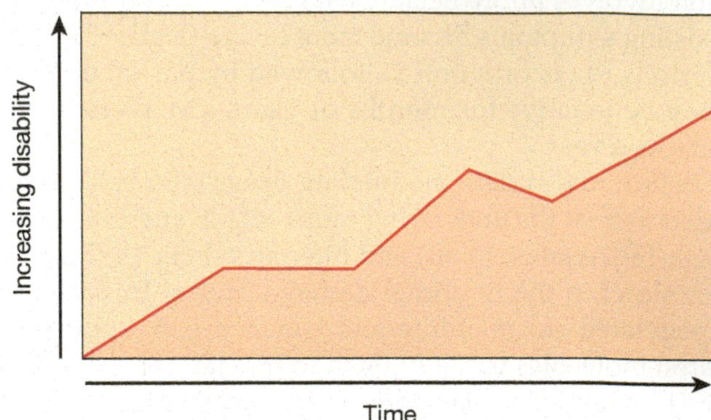

FIGURE 13.3 Four disease courses of MS.
Source: Compliments of the National Multiple Sclerosis Society.

the injection site, and liver toxicity. Due to toxicity concerns and additive effects, caution should be exercised when taking these drugs in combination with chemotherapeutic agents or bone marrow-suppressing drugs.

Another first-line drug treatment, glatiramer (Copaxone) is an immunomodulating synthetic protein that resembles myelin basic protein, an essential part of the nerve's myelin coating. Because glatiramer resembles myelin, it is thought to curb the body's attack on the myelin covering and reduce the creation of new brain lesions. Glatiramer is available in prefilled syringes that can be kept at room temperature for several days. However, patients often complain of adverse effects and having to inject themselves. Adverse effects include redness, pain, swelling, itching, or a lump at the site of injection. Flushing, chest pain, weakness, infection, pain, nausea, joint pain, anxiety, and muscle stiffness are other common adverse effects.

Mitoxantrone (Novantrone) is approved for patients with MS who have not responded to interferon or glatiramer therapy. Primarily a chemotherapeutic drug, mitoxantrone is substantially more toxic than the immune system modulating drugs. Toxicity is a concern due to irreversible cardiac injury and potential harm to a fetus. Notable adverse effects are reversible hair loss, gastrointestinal (GI) discomfort (nausea and vomiting), and allergic symptoms (itching, rash, hypotension). Some patients experience a blue-green tint to their urine, which is harmless.

Approved in 2010, fingolimod (Gilenya) is an oral medication used for treating relapsing forms of MS. Its mechanism of action is unknown, although it may work by reducing the number of circulating lymphocytes, leading to reduced migration of leukocytes into the

CNS. White blood cells cause inflammation and destruction of nerves in patients with MS. Fingolimod decreases the number of MS flare-ups and slows down the development of physical impairment caused by MS.

In 2010, dalfampridine (Ampyra) tablets were approved as the first treatment to address walking impairment in patients with MS. It exerts an effect through its broad-spectrum potassium channel blockade and has been shown to increase nerve conduction and improve walking speed. The most bothersome adverse effect of dalfampridine is increased seizure activity. Because of this concern, this drug is contraindicated in patients with a prior history of seizures.

contraindicated = *not advisable*

Teriflunomide (Aubagio) is one of the newer immunomodulator therapies for relapsing MS. Teriflunomide is the active metabolite of leflunomide (Arava), a drug previously approved to treat rheumatoid arthritis. Therapy with teriflunomide must be carefully monitored because the drug can cause severe liver damage, renal failure, and bone marrow suppression. It is contraindicated in pregnant patients due to possible teratogenic effects on the fetus.

teratogenic = *causing birth defects*

Approved for progressive forms of MS in 2014, alemtuzumab (Lemtrada) is generally reserved for people who have had inadequate responses to two or more MS therapies. The FDA originally had concerns about this medication due to risks of low platelet counts in the bloodstream, and potentially dangerous bleeding. When considering Lemtrada, women should talk to their healthcare providers if they are pregnant or planning to become pregnant. Alemtuzumab carries black box warnings regarding potentially serious adverse effects such as cytopenias, infusion reactions, infections, and malignancies.

Miscellaneous drugs used for MS include modafinil (Provigil) and amantadine (Symmetrel) for treating fatigue, memory loss, and progressive weakness symptoms. Modafinil is an alpha$_1$-adrenergic drug thought to activate receptors that respond to the brain neurotransmitter norepinephrine. This agent increases alertness and energy and improves memory. Gabapentin (Neurontin) is an antiseizure drug used for treating mood disturbances, including depression and sensitivity to pain (see Chapter 14). Methylprednisolone (Solu-Medrol) and prednisone are steroidal anti-inflammatory agents that are administered for brief periods when the patient is experiencing acute MS symptoms caused by swelling and inflammation in the brain. Other medications not found in Table 13.5 may be used routinely to help treat fatigue and neurologic symptoms due to MS (i.e., pain and discomfort).

MUSCLE SPASMS

Muscle spasms are involuntary contractions of a muscle or groups of muscles. The muscles tighten, develop a fixed pattern of resistance, and lose functioning ability.

Muscle spasms are caused by injury, overmedication, hypocalcemia, and debilitating neurologic disorders.

◀ **Core Concept 13.8**

hypo =*lowered*
calc =*calcium*
emia =*blood levels*

Muscle spasms are a common condition usually associated with overuse of and local injury to the skeletal muscle. Other causes of muscle spasms include overmedication with antipsychotic drugs (see Chapter 12), epilepsy, hypocalcemia, pain, and debilitating neurologic disorders. Patients with muscle spasms may experience inflammation, edema, and pain at the affected muscle; loss of coordination; and reduced mobility. When a muscle goes into spasm, it freezes in a contracted state. A single, prolonged contraction is called a *tonic spasm*, whereas multiple, rapidly repeated contractions are called *clonic spasms*. Treatment of muscle spasms includes use of both nonpharmacologic and pharmacologic therapies.

tonic = *single prolonged transient*
clonic = *multiple repetitive transient*
spasms = *involuntary contractions*

Muscle spasms may be treated with pharmacologic and nonpharmacologic therapies.

◀ **Core Concept 13.9**

etiology = *cause or origin*

Identifying the etiology of muscle spasms requires a careful history and a physical examination. After a determination has been made, nonpharmacologic therapies are normally used in conjunction with medications. Nonpharmacologic measures may include immobilization of the affected muscle, application of heat or cold, hydrotherapy, ultrasound, supervised exercises, massage, or manipulation.

Fast Facts Muscle Spasms

- More than 12 million people worldwide have muscle spasms.
- Muscle spasms severe enough to warrant drug therapy are often found in patients who have had other debilitating disorders, such as neurodegenerative diseases, stroke, injury, or cerebral palsy; women are more susceptible to neck muscle spasms due to architecture of the neck area.
- Cerebral palsy is usually associated with events that occur before or during birth, but it may be caused by head trauma or infection during the first few months or years of life.
- Dystonia affects about 250,000 people in the United States; it is the third most common movement disorder after PD and essential tremor.
- Researchers have recognized multiple forms of inheritable dystonia and identified at least 10 genes or chromosomal locations responsible for the various manifestations.
- Muscle spasms can be caused by a variety of factors, including pharmacologic therapy, traumatic neck injury, degenerative disc conditions, stress, inflammatory or neurologic conditions, muscle weakness, and overexertion.

Pharmacotherapy for muscle spasms may include combinations of analgesics, anti-inflammatory drugs, and centrally acting skeletal muscle relaxants. Most skeletal muscle relaxants relieve symptoms of muscular stiffness and rigidity that result from muscular injury. Drugs also help improve mobility. Therapeutic goals are to minimize pain and discomfort, increase range of motion, and improve the patient's ability to function independently.

CONCEPT REVIEW 13.4

- Give several reasons why muscle spasms develop. What is the main goal of therapy for muscle spasms?

Core Concept 13.10 ▶

Many muscle relaxants treat muscle spasms by inhibiting upper motor neuron activity, causing sedation, or altering simple reflexes.

Antispasmodic drugs relieve symptoms of muscular stiffness and rigidity. They improve mobility in patients who have restricted movements.

Many antispasmodic drugs treat muscle spasms at the level of the CNS. The exact mechanisms of action are not fully known, but it is believed that these drugs affect the brain or spinal cord by inhibiting upper motor neuron activity, causing sedation, or altering simple reflexes.

Skeletal muscle relaxants are used to treat local spasms resulting from muscular injury and may be prescribed alone or in combination with other medications to reduce pain and increase range of motion. Commonly used centrally acting medications are baclofen (Lioresal), cyclobenzaprine (Amrix, Flexeril), tizanidine (Zanaflex), and benzodiazepines such as diazepam (Valium), clonazepam (Klonopin), and lorazepam (Ativan). These drugs are listed in Table 13.6. All of the centrally acting drugs can cause sedation.

Baclofen (Lioresal) is structurally similar to the inhibitory neurotransmitter gamma amino butyric acid (GABA) and produces its effect by a mechanism that is not fully known. It inhibits neuronal activity within the brain and possibly the spinal cord. There is some uncertainty about whether the spinal effects of baclofen are associated with GABA. Baclofen may be used to reduce muscle spasms in patients with MS, cerebral palsy, or spinal cord injury. Common adverse effects of baclofen are drowsiness, dizziness, weakness, and fatigue. Baclofen is often the preferred drug because of its wide safety margin.

Tizanidine (Zanaflex) is a centrally acting alpha$_2$-adrenergic agonist that inhibits motor neurons, mainly at the spinal cord level. It also affects some neural activity in the brain, with patients receiving high doses report drowsiness. Though uncommon, one adverse effect of tizanidine is hallucinations. The drug's most frequent adverse effects are dry mouth, fatigue, dizziness, and sleepiness. Tizanidine is as effective as baclofen and is considered by some to be the preferred drug.

Table 13.6 Centrally Acting Antispasmodic Drugs

Drug	Route and Adult Dose	Remarks
SKELETAL MUSCLE RELAXANTS		
baclofen (Lioresal)	PO: 5 mg tid (max: 80 mg/day)	May be administered PO or by an implantable pump that infuses medication directly into the subarachnoid space
carisoprodol (Soma)	PO: 350 mg tid	CNS depressant; does not inhibit motor activity like other conventional muscle relaxants; muscle relaxation seems to be related to sedation
chlorzoxazone (Paraflex, Parafon Forte)	PO: 250–500 mg tid–qid (max: 3 g/day)	Depresses nerve transmission in the brain and spinal cord, possibly by sedation; not effective for cerebral palsy
Pr cyclobenzaprine (Amrix, Flexeril)	PO: 10–20 mg bid–qid (max: 60 mg/day)	Short-term relief of muscle spasms associated with acute musculoskeletal conditions; not for cerebral palsy or CNS diseases
metaxalone (Skelaxin)	PO: 800 mg tid–qid for maximum of 10 days	For acute musculoskeletal conditions; causes its effect through sedation
methocarbamol (Robaxin)	PO: 1.5 g qid for 2–3 days, then reduce to 1 g qid	Adjunct to physical therapy for acute musculoskeletal disorders and tetany
orphenadrine (Banflex, Myolin, Norflex)	PO: 100 mg bid	IM and IV forms available
tizanidine (Zanaflex)	PO: 4–8 mg tid–qid (max: 36 mg/day)	To relax muscle tone associated with spasticity; effective at the spinal cord level
BENZODIAZEPINES		
clonazepam (Klonopin)	PO: 0.5 mg tid (max: 20 mg/day)	Usually taken in combination with other drugs; for relief of skeletal muscle spasms; primarily for seizure disorders
diazepam (Valium) (see the Prototype Drug box in Core Concept 14.6)	PO: 4–10 mg bid–qid; IM/IV 2–10 mg, repeat if needed in 3–4 hours; IV pump: Administer emulsion at 5 mg/min	For relief of skeletal muscle spasms associated with cerebral palsy, partial paralysis
lorazepam (Ativan) (see the Prototype Drug box in Core Concept 10.7)	PO: 1–2 mg bid–tid (max: 10 mg/day)	For extreme muscle tension

As discussed in Chapter 14, benzodiazepines inhibit both sensory and motor neuron activities by enhancing the effects of GABA. Common adverse effects include drowsiness and ataxia (loss of coordination). Benzodiazepines are usually prescribed for muscle relaxation when baclofen and tizanidine fail to produce adequate relief.

tetany = *prolonged tightened muscles*

Prototype Drug: Pr *Cyclobenzaprine (Amrix, Flexeril)*

Therapeutic Class: Skeletal muscle relaxant, centrally acting **Pharmacologic Class: Catecholamine reuptake inhibitor**

Actions and Uses: Cyclobenzaprine relieves muscle spasms of local origin without interfering with general muscle function. This drug acts by depressing motor activity, primarily in the brainstem, with limited effects also occurring in the spinal cord. It increases circulating levels of norepinephrine, blocking presynaptic uptake. Its mechanism of action is similar to that of tricyclic antidepressants (see Chapter 11). It causes muscle relaxation in acute muscle spasticity, but it is not effective in cases of cerebral palsy or diseases of the brain and spinal cord. This medication is meant to provide therapy for only 2 to 3 weeks.

Adverse Effects and Interactions: Adverse reactions to cyclobenzaprine include drowsiness, blurred vision, dizziness, dry mouth, rash, and tachycardia. It should be used with caution in patients with myocardial infarction (MI), dysrhythmias, or severe cardiovascular disease. One reaction, although rare, is swelling of the tongue.

Alcohol, phenothiazines, and other CNS depressants may cause additive sedation. Cyclobenzaprine should not be used within 2 weeks of an MAOI because hyperpyretic crisis and convulsions may occur.

SPASTICITY

Spasticity is a condition in which muscle groups remain in a continuous state of contraction, usually as a result of damage to the CNS. The contracting muscles become stiff with increased muscle tone. Signs and symptoms may include mild to severe pain, exaggerated deep tendon reflexes, muscle spasms, scissoring (involuntary crossing of the legs), and fixed joints.

Core Concept 13.11 ▶ Effective treatment for spasticity includes both physical therapy and medications.

Spasticity usually results from damage to the motor area of the cerebral cortex, which controls muscle movement. Etiologies most commonly associated with this condition include neurologic disorders such as cerebral palsy, severe head injury, spinal cord injury or lesions, and stroke. **Dystonia**, a chronic neurologic disorder, is characterized by involuntary muscle contractions that force body parts into abnormal, occasionally painful movements or postures. It affects the muscle tone of the arms, legs, trunk, neck, eyelids, face, or vocal cords. Spasticity, whether short term or long term, can be distressing and greatly impacts an individual's quality of life. In addition to causing pain, it also impairs physical mobility, thereby influencing the person's ability to perform ADLs and diminishing their sense of independence.

Effective treatment for spasticity includes both physical therapy and medications. Medications alone are not adequate to reduce the complications of spasticity, and regular and consistent physical therapy exercises have been shown to be effective in decreasing the severity of symptoms. Types of treatment include muscle stretching to help prevent contractures, muscle group strengthening exercises, and repetitive motion exercises for improvement of accuracy. In extreme cases, surgery has been used for tendon release or to sever the nerve-muscle pathway.

CAM Therapy | Cayenne for Muscular Tension

Cayenne (*Capsicum annum*), also known as chili pepper, paprika, or red pepper, has been used as a remedy for muscle tension and associated pain. Applied in a cream base, it is commonly used to relieve muscle spasms in the shoulder and areas of the arm. Capsaicin, the active ingredient in cayenne, diminishes the chemical messengers that travel through the sensory nerves, thereby decreasing the sensation of pain. Its effect accumulates over time, so creams containing capsaicin need to be applied regularly to be effective. Although no known medical condition exists that would prevent the use of cayenne, it should never be applied over broken skin. External use of full-strength cayenne should be limited to no more than 2 days, because it may cause skin inflammation, blisters, and ulcers. It also needs to be kept away from eyes and mucous membranes to avoid burns. Hands must be washed thoroughly after usage. Commercial OTC creams containing capsaicin are available.

Core Concept 13.12 ▶ Some drugs for spasticity provide relief by acting directly on muscle tissue, interfering with the release of calcium ions.

Drugs that are effective in the treatment of spasticity include two centrally acting drugs, baclofen (Lioresal) and diazepam (Valium), and a direct-acting drug, dantrolene (Dantrium). The direct-acting drugs produce an antispasmodic effect at the level of the neuromuscular junction, as shown in Figure 13.4.

Dantrolene relieves spasticity by interfering with the release of calcium ions in skeletal muscle. Other direct-acting drugs include incobotulinumtoxin A (Xeomin), onabotulinumtoxin A (Botox), and rimabotulinumtoxin B (Myobloc). Although these botulinum toxins are generally known for their use in cosmetic procedures, in some instances they may offer temporary relief of dystonia symptoms.

Botulinum toxin is an unusual drug because in high doses it acts as a poison. *Clostridium botulinum* is the bacterium responsible for food poisoning or botulism. At lower doses, however, this drug is safe and effective as a muscle relaxant. It produces its effect by blocking the release of ACh from cholinergic nerve terminals (see Chapter 9). Botulinum can cause extreme weakness, so its use may require the addition of other therapies to improve muscle strength. To prevent major problems with mobility or posture, botulinum toxin is often applied to small muscle groups. Sometimes this drug is administered together with centrally acting oral medications to further increase the functional use of a range of muscle groups.

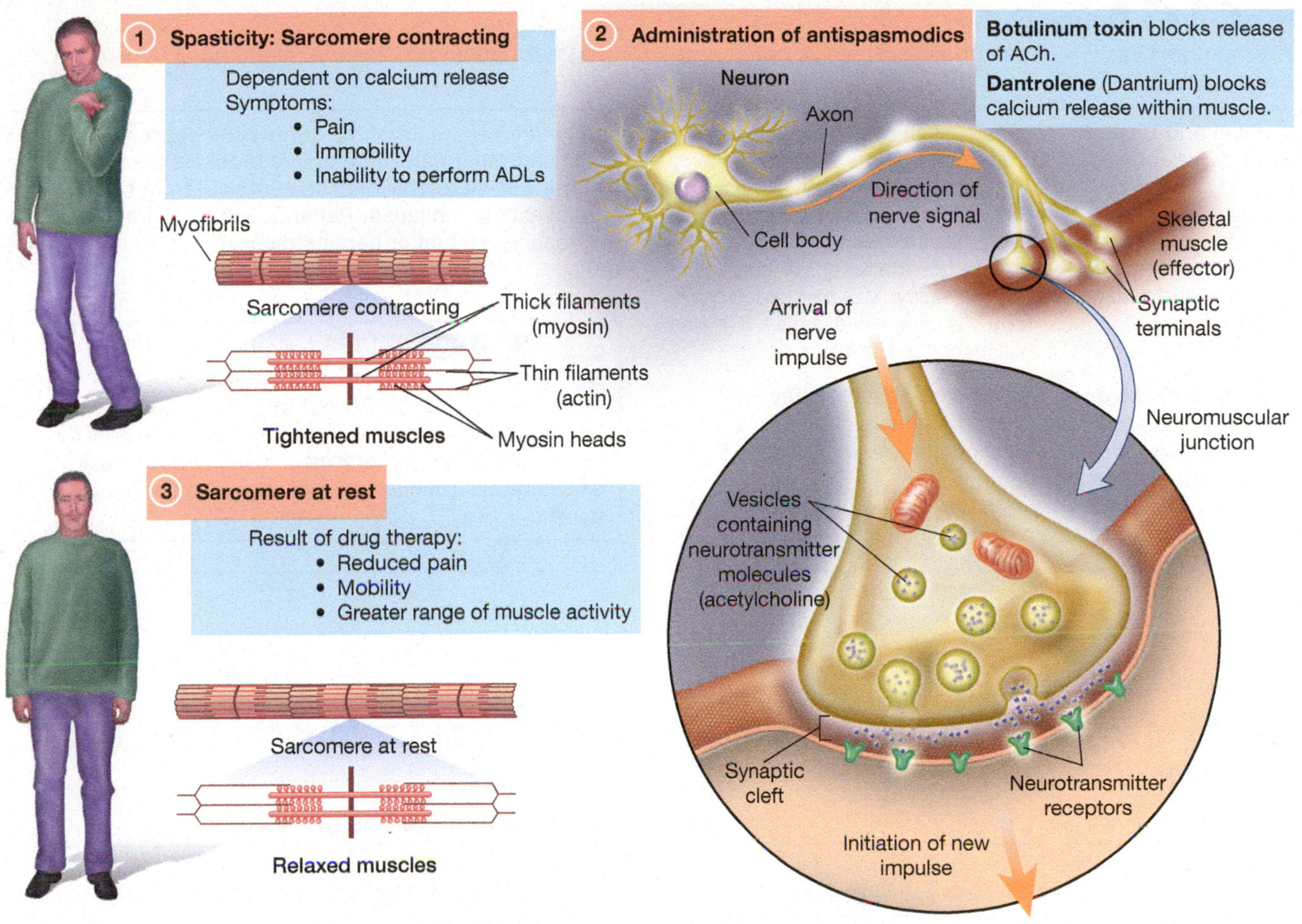

FIGURE 13.4 The use of antispasmodics, which block release of ACh or calcium, can result in less muscle tension to reduce pain as well as provide greater mobility and range of motion.

Drawbacks to botulinum therapy are its delayed and limited effects. The treatment is mostly effective within 6 weeks of administration, and its effects last for only 3 to 6 months. Another drawback is the pain of injecting botulinum directly into the muscle. Local anesthetics are usually given to block this pain. Direct-acting antispasmodic drugs are summarized in Table 13.7.

blepharospasm = *involuntary blinking of the eyelids*

Table 13.7 Direct-Acting Antispasmodic Drugs

Drug	Route and Adult Dose	Remarks
DRUGS BLOCKING THE RELEASE OF ACH		
abobotulinumtoxinA (Dysport)	50 units in five equal aliquots injected directly into target muscle	For cervical dystonia; relaxes facial muscles around the eye and forehead
incobotulinumtoxin A (Xeomin)	120 units injected per treatment session directly into target muscle	For cervical dystonia and involuntary blinking of the eyelids (blepharospasm)
onabotulinumtoxin A (Botox)	25 units injected directly into target muscle (max: 30-day dose should not exceed 200 units)	Mainly for cosmetic procedures; relaxes facial muscles around the eye and forehead; also for excessive sweating, chronic migraine, overactive bladder, and cervical dystonia
rimabotulinumtoxin B (Myobloc)	2500–5000 units/dose injected directly into target muscle; doses should be divided among muscle groups	For cervical dystonia
DRUG REDUCING SKELETAL MUSCLE TENSION		
Pr dantrolene (Dantrium)	PO: 25 mg daily, increase to 25 mg bid–qid; may increase every 4–7 days up to 100 mg bid–tid	Hydantoin-like medication; also for the treatment of malignant hyperthermia; IV form available

Prototype Drug: Dantrolene (Dantrium)

Therapeutic Class: Skeletal muscle relaxant, peripheral-acting **Pharmacologic Class:** Skeletal muscle calcium release blocker

Actions and Uses: Dantrolene is often used for spasticity, especially for spasms of the head and neck. It directly relaxes muscle spasms by interfering with the release of calcium ions from storage areas inside skeletal muscle cells. It does not affect cardiac or smooth muscle. Dantrolene is especially useful for muscle spasms when they occur after spinal cord injury or stroke and in cases of cerebral palsy, MS, and occasionally for the treatment of muscle pain after heavy exercise. It is also used for the treatment of malignant hyperthermia.

Adverse Effects and Interactions: Adverse effects include muscle weakness, drowsiness, dry mouth, dizziness, nausea, diarrhea, tachycardia, erratic blood pressure, photosensitivity, and urinary retention.

Dantrolene interacts with many other drugs. For example, it should not be taken with OTC cough preparations and antihistamines, alcohol, or other CNS depressants. Verapamil and other calcium channel blockers taken with dantrolene increase the risk of ventricular fibrillation and cardiovascular collapse. Patients with impaired cardiac or pulmonary function or hepatic disease should not take this drug.

BLACK BOX WARNING:
Dantrolene has a potential for hepatotoxicity. Liver dysfunction may be evidenced by blood chemical enzyme levels. The risk of hepatic injury is greater in females over 35 years of age and after 3 months of therapy. Therapy should be discontinued after 45 days if no observable benefit.

Nursing Process Focus Patients Receiving Drugs for Muscle Spasms or Spasticity

ASSESSMENT	POTENTIAL NURSING DIAGNOSES*
Prior to administration: • Obtain a complete health history including cardiovascular, respiratory, and neuromuscular conditions, allergies, drug history and possible drug interactions. • Acquire baseline vital signs and electrocardiogram. • Evaluate laboratory blood levels: Complete blood count, chemistry, drug screening, renal and liver function studies. • Determine neurologic status; especially level of consciousness (LOC) and neurologic effects on motor and respiratory function.	• *Pain (Acute/Chronic)* related to muscle spasms • *Impaired Physical Mobility* related to acute or chronic pain • *Deficient Knowledge* related to a lack of information about drug therapy or disease process • *Risk for Injury* related to adverse effects of drug therapy

PLANNING: PATIENT GOALS AND EXPECTED OUTCOMES

The patient will:
- Experience therapeutic effects (a decrease in pain, increase in range of motion and reduction of muscle spasms).
- Be free from or experience minimal adverse effects from drug therapy.
- Verbalize an understanding of the drug's use, adverse effects, and required precautions.

IMPLEMENTATION

Interventions and (Rationales)	Patient Education/Discharge Planning
• Monitor LOC and vital signs. (Some skeletal muscle relaxants alter the patient's LOC. Others within this class may alter blood pressure and heart rate.)	Instruct the patient to: • Avoid driving and other activities requiring mental alertness until the effects of the medication are known. • Report any significant change in sensorium, such as slurred speech, confusion, hallucinations, or extreme lethargy. • Report palpitations, chest pain, dyspnea, unusual fatigue, weakness, and visual disturbances. • Avoid using other CNS depressants such as alcohol that will intensify sedation.
• Monitor pain and provide proper medication. Determine the location, duration, and precipitating factors of the patient's pain. (Drugs should diminish the patient's pain.)	Instruct the patient to: • Report the development of new sites of muscle pain. • Take medications as ordered.

Interventions and (Rationales)	Patient Education/Discharge Planning
• Provide additional pain relief measures such as positional support, gentle massage, and moist heat or ice packs. (Drugs alone may not be sufficient in providing pain relief.)	Instruct the patient: • That complementary pain interventions such as positioning, gentle massage, and the application of heat or cold to the painful area may be helpful. • In relaxation techniques, deep breathing, and meditation methods to facilitate relaxation and reduce pain.
• Monitor muscle tone, range of motion, and degree of muscle spasm. (This helps to determine the effectiveness of drug therapy and possible need for changes in drug therapy).	Instruct the patient: • To perform gentle range of motion, only to the point of mild physical discomfort, throughout the day. • That medication may cause a decrease in muscle strength and dosage may need to be reduced.
• Monitor for adverse effects such as drowsiness, weakness, fatigue, dry mouth, dizziness, faintness, rash, blurred vision, photosensitivity, rash, tachycardia, erratic blood pressure, photosensitivity, and urinary retention. (These adverse effects may occur with common antispasmodic drugs).	Instruct the patient: • To report any adverse effects to the healthcare provider. • To take medication with food to decrease GI upset. • That frequent mouth rinses, sips of water, and sugarless candy or gum may help with dry mouth. • To report signs of urinary retention such as a feeling of urinary bladder fullness, distended abdomen, and discomfort. • To use sunscreen and protective clothing when outdoors.
• Administer medication correctly and evaluate the patient's knowledge of proper administration. Do not abruptly stop providing medication, and monitor for withdrawal symptoms. (Abrupt withdrawal of drugs such as baclofen may cause serious symptoms.)	• Advise the patient not to abruptly discontinue medication. This action may result in withdrawal reactions such as visual hallucinations, paranoid ideation, and seizures.
• Obtain liver enzyme studies as recommended for patients taking peripheral-acting skeletal muscle relaxants. (These drugs have the potential to cause hepatotoxicity.)	Instruct the patient to: • Have laboratory blood tests done as prescribed by the healthcare provider.

EVALUATION OF OUTCOME CRITERIA

Evaluate the effectiveness of drug therapy by confirming that patient goals and expected outcomes have been met (see "Planning"). *See Tables 13.6 and 13.7 for lists of drugs to which these nursing actions apply.*

NEUROMUSCULAR BLOCKING DRUGS

Neuromuscular blocking drugs bind to nicotinic receptors located on the surface of skeletal muscle fibers. Drugs called *nicotinic blocking drugs* interfere with the binding of ACh, thereby preventing voluntary muscle contraction. Nicotinic blocking drugs are *anticholinergic* (see Chapter 9).

nicotin = *nicotine*
ic = *related to*

cholin = *acetycholine*
erg = *work (action)*
ic = *related to*

Neuromuscular blocking drugs block the effect of acetylcholine at the receptor.

◀ **Core Concept 13.13**

Neuromuscular blocking drugs are classified into two major categories: nondepolarizing blockers and depolarizing blockers. *Nondepolarizing blockers* compete with ACh for the receptor. As long as drugs interfere with the binding of ACh, muscles remain relaxed. By a related mechanism, *depolarizing blockers* bind to the ACh receptor and produce a state of continuous depolarization. Remember that *depolarization* is the rapid cycling influx of sodium into neurons, propagating the electrical signal. This action first results in small fasciculations or a time of brief repeated muscle movements, followed by relaxation of muscle fibers. Relaxation is short-lived until charges across the muscle membrane are restored (repolarization). Importantly, patients treated with neuromuscular blockers are able to feel pain even though they cannot react to it. Thus, for surgical procedures, concomitant use of anesthetic agents is essential (see Chapter 16).

fascicu = *muscle fascicle (bundle)*
lation = *movement*

It is important to note that neuromuscular blocking drugs are different from *ganglionic blocking drugs* that target the autonomic nervous system. With ganglionic blocking drugs, ACh does indeed bind to nicotinic receptors, but the resulting actions of these drugs are involuntary and do not involve skeletal muscle (see Chapter 9). Ganglionic blockers dampen

ganglion = *cell bodies grouped outside CNS*

Table 13.8 Neuromuscular Blocking Drugs

Drug	Duration	Administration Route
NONDEPOLARIZING BLOCKERS		
atracurium (Tracrium)	Long duration	IV
cisatracurium (Nimbex)	Long duration	IV
mivacurium (Mivacron)	Shorter duration	IV
rocuronium (Zemuron)	Long duration	IV
tubocurarine	Longest duration; oldest of the nondepolarizing drugs	IV and IM
vecuronium (Norcuron)	Long duration	IV
DEPOLARIZING BLOCKERS		
succinylcholine (Anectine) (see the Prototype Drug box in Core Concept 16.6)	Shortest duration	IV and IM

parasympathetic tone and produce effects such as increased heart rate, dry mouth, urinary retention, and reduced GI activity. They also dampen sympathetic tone, resulting in reduced sweating and less norepinephrine being released from postsynaptic nerve terminals. As an example, mecamylamine (Inversine) is a ganglionic blocker primarily used to treat patients with essential hypertension (see Chapter 19).

The classic example of a nondepolarizing blocker is tubocurarine. Tubocurarine and related blocking drugs are used to relax the muscles of patients being prepared for lengthy surgical procedures (Table 13.8). Although not preferred for mechanical ventilation or endotracheal intubation, small doses of these drugs may be used for intermediate surgical procedures. Concerns of tubocurarine-like treatment include over-relaxation of muscles. For example, normal breathing activity (involving the diaphragm, glottic, and intercostal muscles) and swallowing activity (involving the neck and certain esophageal muscles) require skeletal muscle contraction.

malignant = *harmful*
hyper = *elevated*
thermia = *fever*

post = *after*
operative = *surgery*

Depolarizing agents are used primarily to relax the muscles of patients receiving electroconvulsive therapy (ECT) (see Chapter 14) and for brief surgical procedures (see Chapter 16). Short surgical procedures involve mechanical ventilation and endotracheal intubation. Succinylcholine (Anectine) is the prototype example of a depolarizing blocker. Adverse effects include elevated blood levels of potassium, malignant hyperthermia, and postoperative muscle pain and persistent paralysis in some patients. As a specific antidote for persistent paralysis, patients are often given AChE inhibitors.

Patients Need to Know

Patients being treated for degenerative diseases and disorders of the neuromuscular system need to know the following:

Regarding Drugs for Parkinson Disease or Dementia

1. Take levodopa–carbidopa at least 30–60 minutes before eating in order to allow the medication to be absorbed before food can interfere. Do not take with foods that contain protein, as these foods can decrease drug effectiveness.
2. Be extremely careful about getting up quickly from a seated position. Many dementia drugs cause dizziness, lightheadedness, blurred vision, and difficulty in concentrating.
3. Do not skip taking the medications, and do not take OTC preparations (especially medications for colds or pain) without checking with a healthcare provider.
4. Be aware that urine may become a little dark. This is a normal side effect of dopamine-like drugs.
5. Do not drink alcoholic beverages or take sedatives. Combined effects may be harmful.
6. Be familiar with adverse effects specific to the drugs being taken. Drugs used for PD may produce nausea, dry mouth, and diminished sweating in some cases. Drugs used for dementia may cause nausea, diarrhea, muscle cramps, weight loss, and darker urine color.

Regarding Drugs for Muscle Spasms and Spasticity

7. When receiving treatment for problems with mobility, it often takes several weeks for effectiveness to begin. Follow the advice of a healthcare provider in order to achieve full therapeutic effect.
8. Most antispasmodic drugs produce adverse effects such as drowsiness and dizziness. Therefore, avoid CNS depressants and alcohol.

Regarding Neuromuscular Blockers

9. Some patients react adversely to neuromuscular blockers. Inform the healthcare provider about any important family history, such as malignant hyperthermia, myasthenia gravis, cardiovascular disease, and any other unusual problems.
10. Be aware that unpleasant muscle pain may be associated with surgical procedures.

Chapter Review

Core Concepts Summary

13.1 Medications are unable to cure most degenerative diseases of the central nervous system (CNS).

Degenerative diseases of the CNS include Alzheimer disease (AD), multiple sclerosis (MS), and Parkinson disease (PD). The cause of most neurologic degenerative disorders is unknown. With the exception of PD, drug therapy provides only minimal benefit.

13.2 Parkinson disease is progressive, with the occurrence of full symptoms taking many years.

PD, or parkinsonism, is a degenerative disorder caused by death of neurons that produce the brain neurotransmitter dopamine. Dopamine producing neurons in the substantia nigra supply nerve signals to the corpus striatum. When dopamine is depleted, symptoms of parkinsonism, including tremors, muscle rigidity, bradykinesia (slow movement), and postural instability, occur. These symptoms are the same EPS effects caused by prolonged antipsychotic drug treatment.

13.3 Antiparkinson drugs act on the brain to restore the balance between dopamine and acetylcholine.

Balance, posture, muscle tone, and involuntary muscle movement depend on the proper balance between the neurotransmitter dopamine (inhibitory) and ACh (stimulatory) in the corpus striatum. Drug therapy for parkinsonism focuses on restoring dopamine function (dopaminergic drugs) and blocking the effect of ACh overactivity (cholinergic blockers).

13.4 Patients with Alzheimer disease experience a dramatic loss of ability to perform tasks that require acetylcholine as the CNS neurotransmitter.

AD is a devastating, progressive, degenerative disease characterized by impaired memory, confusion or disorientation, inability to recognize family or friends, aggressive behavior, depression, psychoses, and anxiety. AD is responsible for 70% of all dementia. Although the cause of AD is unknown, structural brain damage and a dramatic loss of ability to perform tasks that require ACh as the neurotransmitter have been documented.

13.5 Alzheimer disease is treated with acetylcholinesterase inhibitors and other drugs.

Only a few drugs for AD have been approved. Most drugs act by intensifying the effect of acetylcholine (ACh) at the cholinergic receptor. ACh is naturally degraded in the synapse by the enzyme acetylcholinesterase (AChE). When AChE is inhibited, ACh levels increase and produce a greater effect on the receptor. This treatment improves function in ADLs, behavior, and cognition.

13.6 Symptoms of multiple sclerosis result from demyelination of CNS nerve fibers.

MS is an autoimmune disorder of the CNS. Antibodies slowly destroy myelin in the brain and spinal cord, disrupting the ability of nerves to conduct electrical impulses. Over time, debilitating symptoms appear, including fatigue, heat sensitivity, pain, muscle cramps and spasms, impaired ability to think and reason, balance and coordination problems, and bowel and bladder symptoms.

13.7 Drugs for multiple sclerosis reduce immune attacks in the brain and treat unfavorable symptoms.

Two strategies for treating MS are reducing the immune response and relieving the symptoms. The most treatable form of MS is relapsing-remitting MS (RRMS), in which unpredictable relapses occur. Drug treatments include immune system modulating drugs, immunosuppressants, and miscellaneous drugs used for treatment of MS symptoms such as inflammation, pain, fatigue, memory loss, and progressive weakness.

13.8 Muscle spasms are caused by injury, overmedication, hypocalcemia, and debilitating neurologic disorders.

Muscle spasms, or involuntary contractions of a muscle or group of muscles, occur for many reasons, including overmedication with antipsychotic drugs, epilepsy, hypocalcemia, pain, and incapacitating neurologic disorders. Two types of muscle spasms are tonic spasms and clonic spasms.

13.9 Muscle spasms may be treated with pharmacologic and nonpharmacologic therapies.

After a thorough medical exam, nonpharmacologic therapies such as immobilization, heat or cold, hydrotherapy, ultrasound, supervised exercises, massage, and manipulation may be used along with medications. Medications include analgesics, anti-inflammatory drugs, and centrally acting skeletal muscle relaxants.

13.10 Many muscle relaxants treat muscle spasms by inhibiting upper motor neuron activity, causing sedation, or altering simple reflexes.

Skeletal muscle relaxants treat local spasms resulting from muscular injury and may be prescribed alone or in combination with medications that reduce pain and increase range of motion. These include centrally acting drugs (affecting the brain or spinal cord) that have the potential to cause sedation and alter reflex activity.

13.11 Effective treatment for spasticity includes both physical therapy and medications.

Spasticity is a condition in which certain muscle groups remain in a state of contraction. Symptoms associated with spasticity include pain, exaggerated deep tendon reflexes, muscle spasms, scissoring, and fixed joints. Medications alone are not adequate in reducing the complications of spasticity.

13.12 Some drugs for spasticity provide relief by acting directly on muscle tissue, interfering with the release of calcium ions.

Direct-acting drugs produce an antispasmodic effect at the level of the neuromuscular junction. Drugs affect either calcium release from the muscle, or they interfere with the release of ACh.

13.13 Neuromuscular blocking drugs block the effect of acetylcholine at the receptor.

Neuromuscular blocking drugs are classified as nondepolarizing blockers and depolarizing blockers. Both drugs bind to ACh receptors, relaxing muscles by slightly different mechanisms and durations of action.

REVIEW Questions

Answer the following questions to assess your knowledge of the chapter material, and go back and review any material that is not clear to you.

1. The patient taking levodopa is taught that he must wait at least 1 hour before or after eating foods high in:
   1. Vitamin C.
   2. Carbohydrates.
   3. Folic acid.
   4. Protein.

2. A patient in the early stages of Alzheimer disease was started on donepezil (Aricept) a few weeks ago. She calls the nurse at the healthcare provider's office and states that she has been experiencing what she believes to be adverse effects of the drug. Which of the following effects could the patient be experiencing? (Select all that apply.)
   1. Sleepiness
   2. Nausea
   3. Diarrhea
   4. Tinnitus
   5. Darkened urine

3. When administering levodopa to a patient with Parkinson disease, the nurse understands that this drug:
   1. Increases cholinergic stimulation within the brain.
   2. Restores acetylcholine and blocks dopamine within the brain.
   3. Restores dopamine function and blocks acetylcholine within the brain.
   4. Destroys dopamine receptors within the brain.

4. The patient with Parkinson disease is placed on haloperidol (Haldol) because of agitation and has started experiencing extrapyramidal symptoms. Which of the following drugs would be ordered?
   1. Levodopa–carbidopa drugs
   2. Risperidone (Risperdal)
   3. Benztropine (Cogentin)
   4. Cyclobenzaprine (Flexeril)

5. The patient with Alzheimer disease has been started on rivastigmine (Exelon). The patient will be evaluated for:
   1. Liver toxicity.
   2. Weight loss.
   3. Renal failure.
   4. Extrapyramidal symptoms.

6. A patient had a surgical procedure in which succinylcholine (Anectine) was used to relax the muscles. This patient would be monitored for:
   1. Hypothermia.
   2. Complaints of muscle pain.
   3. High sodium levels (hypernatremia).
   4. Low levels of potassium (hypokalemia).

7. A patient is given a prescription for carisoprodol (Soma), 350 mg, PO, three times a day. The pharmacy provides a bottle of 350 mg tablets. How many milligrams will the patient take in one day?
   1. 900 mg
   2. 1115 mg
   3. 1050 mg
   4. 1015 mg

8. An interferon is prescribed for a patient with MS. The nurse includes which of the following points when educating the patient about drug therapy?
   1. Report flu-like symptoms to the healthcare provider.
   2. Expect urine to be orange.
   3. Report the development of diarrhea.
   4. The symptoms will get better over a period of a year.

9. A patient is being seen in the emergency department after an automobile crash. She complains that her lower back hurts. After an examination and x-ray, the patient is given a diagnosis of muscle strain with associated spasms, and is placed on cyclobenzaprine (Flexeril) to help relax the muscles. In educating the patient about the drug, the nurse informs her that: (Select all that apply.)
   1. It can cause drowsiness.
   2. If taken with alcohol, additional drowsiness may occur.
   3. It is only intended for short-term use (2–3 weeks).
   4. It can cause headaches.
   5. It can cause blurred vision.

10. A patient with a spinal cord injury is experiencing muscle spasms. The healthcare provider has prescribed dantrolene to help control the spasms. The nurse informs the patient to report which of the following possible adverse effect(s) if they should occur?
   1. Excessive salivation
   2. Excessive urination
   3. Muscle weakness
   4. Insomnia

CASE STUDY Questions

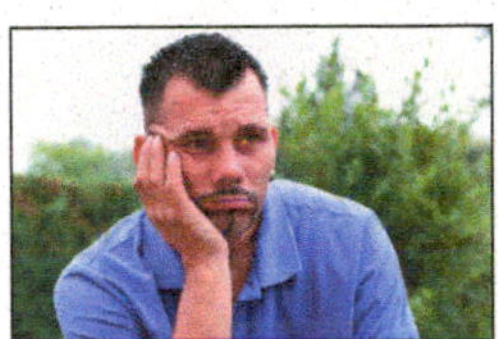

Remember Mr. Wingate, the patient introduced at the beginning of the chapter? Now read the remainder of the case study. Based on the information you have learned in this chapter, answer the questions that follow.

Mr. Robert Wingate, a 35-year-old man with MS, has persistent pain in his right hip and comes in for treatment. He explains that he has been taking enteric-coated aspirin for several weeks. He has been experiencing severe headaches and muscle twitches (multiple, rapidly repeating contractions) in his right hamstring. The muscle twitches have not been severe, but he is concerned that they may be related to his condition. Lately, he has been experiencing fatigue, and his vision is sometimes "blurry." Laboratory values show slight hypocalcemia. The patient says that he hasn't had any trouble with his diet. No abnormalities in bone structure or peripheral inflammatory symptoms are observed on examination.

1. The nurse caring for Mr. Wingate just received a medication order to administer an immune system modulator. Which of the following medications might the nurse administer?
   1. Amantadine (Symmetrel)
   2. Interferon beta-1b (Betaseron)
   3. Memantine (Namenda)
   4. Gabapentin (Neurontin)

2. After being started on the immune system modulator, Mr. Wingate asks the nurse about this class of medications. The nurse responds by saying: (Select all that apply.)
   1. "These drugs slow down the destruction of the neurons caused by multiple sclerosis."
   2. "These drugs have very few adverse effects."
   3. "There are no precautions when taking this type of drug with other drugs."
   4. "Adverse effects can include fever, chills, and muscle aches."

3. In evaluating the effectiveness of Mr. Wingate's antispasmodic therapy, the nurse would expect that the medication would:
   1. Improve Mr. Wingate's symptoms for the long term.
   2. Improve Mr. Wingate's symptoms for the short term.
   3. Make Mr. Wingate's symptoms worse.
   4. Cause Mr. Wingate to be sedated.

4. If Mr. Wingate's condition and symptoms were to progress significantly, which of the following drugs would be ordered?
   1. Selegiline (Eldepryl, Zelapar)
   2. Gabapentin (Neurontin)
   3. Mitoxantrone (Novantrone)
   4. Donepezil (Aricept)

Answers and complete rationales for the Review and Case Study Questions appear in Appendix A.

REFERENCES

Center for Science in the Public Interest. (2013). *Consumers urged to avoid ginkgo in wake of new cancer concerns*. Retrieved from http://www.cspinet.org/new/201304181.html

Herdman, T. H., & Kamitsuru, S. (Eds.). (2014). *NANDA International nursing diagnoses: Definitions and classification, 2015–2017*. Oxford, United Kingdom: Wiley-Blackwell.

National Multiple Sclerosis Society. (n.d.). *Multiple sclerosis FAQs*. Retrieved from http://www.nationalmssociety.org/What-is-MS/MS-FAQ-s

Weinmann, S., Roll, S., Schwarzbach, C., Vauth, C., & Willich, S. (2010). Effects of Ginkgo biloba in dementia: A systematic review and meta-analysis. *Biomed Central Geriatrics, 10*, 14. doi:10.1186/1471-2318-10-14

SELECTED BIBLIOGRAPHY

Alzheimer's Association. (2014). 2014 Alzheimer's disease: Facts and figures. *Alzheimer's & Dementia, 10*(2). Retrieved from http://www.alz.org/downloads/Facts_Figures_2014.pdf

Arnold, D. L., Calabresi, P. A., Kieseier, B. C., Sheikh, S. I., Deykin, A., Zhu, Y., . . . Hung, S. (2014). Effect of peginterferon beta-1a on MRI measures and achieving no evidence of disease activity: Results from a randomized controlled trial in relapsing-remitting multiple sclerosis. *BMC Neurology, 14,* 240. doi:10.1186/s12883-014-0240-x

Bruno, D., Grothe, M. J., Nierenberg, J., Zetterberg, H., Blennow, K., Teipel, S., & Pomara, N. (2015). A study on the specificity of the association between hippocampal volume and delayed primacy performance in cognitively intact elderly individuals. *Neuropsychologia, 69,* 1–8. doi:10.1016/j.neuropsychologia.2015.01.025

Drugs.com. (2015). *Carbidopa and levodopa.* Retrieved from http://www.drugs.com/pro/carbidopa-and-levodopa.html

Féger, J., & Hirsch, E. C. (2015). In search of innovative therapeutics for neuropsychiatric disorders: The case of neurodegenerative diseases. *Annales Pharmaceutiques Francaises, 73,* 3–12. doi:10.1016/j.pharma.2014.10.001

Genetics Home Reference. (2016). *Multiple sclerosis.* Retrieved from http://ghr.nlm.nih.gov/condition/multiple-sclerosis

Hagmeyer, S., Haderspeck, J. C., & Grabrucker, A. M. (2015). Behavioral impairments in animal models for zinc deficiency. *Frontiers in Behavioral Neuroscience, 8,* 443. doi:10.3389/fnbeh.2014.00443

Havrdova, E., Horakova, D., & Kovarova, I. (2015). Alemtuzumab in the treatment of multiple sclerosis: Key clinical trial results and considerations for use. *Therapeutic Advances in Neurological Disorders, 8,* 31–45. doi:10.1177/1756285614563522

Jaturapatpom, D., Isaac, M. G., McCleery, J., & Tabet, N. (2012). Aspirin, steroidal and non-steroidal anti-inflammatory drugs for the treatment of Alzheimer's disease. *Cochrane Database of Systematic Reviews, 2,* 1–115. doi:10.1002/14651858.CD006378.pub2

Milo, R. (2015). Effectiveness of multiple sclerosis treatment with current immunomodulatory drugs. *Expert Opinion on Pharmacotherapy, 16,* 659–673. doi:10.1517/14656566.2015.1002769

Parkinson's Disease Foundation. (n.d.). *Statistics on Parkinson's.* Retrieved from http://www.pdf.org/en/parkinson_statistics

Pietrangelo, A., & Higuera, V. (2015). *Multiple sclerosis by the numbers: Facts, statistics, and you.* Retrieved from http://www.healthline.com/health/multiple-sclerosis/facts-statistics-infographic

Samuel, M., Rodriguez-Oroz, M., Antonini, A., Brotchie, J. M., Chaudhuri, K. R., Brown, R. G., . . . Lang, A. E. (2015). Management of impulse control disorders in Parkinson's disease: Controversies and future approaches. *Movement Disorders, 30,* 150–159. doi:10.1002/mds.26099

Chapter 14

Drugs for Seizures

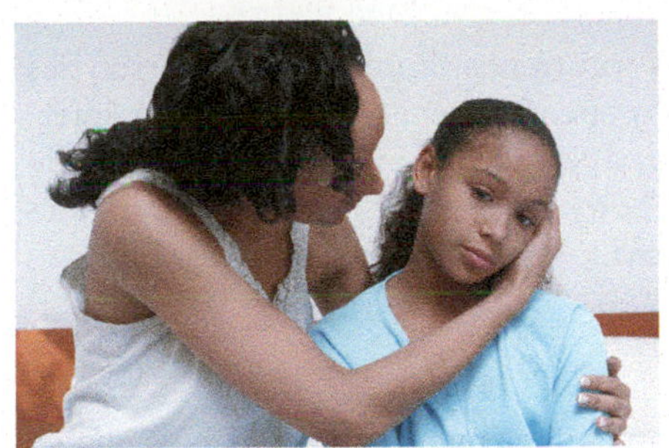

"I felt so helpless when I found out Destiny's problem was seizures. I'm glad there's a medication that will help her live a normal life."
Mrs. Kemi Anthonia

Core Concepts

14.1 Although some types of seizures involve convulsions, others do not.
14.2 Many causes of seizure activity are known; a few are not.
14.3 Epileptic seizures are typically identified as partial, generalized, or special epileptic syndromes.
14.4 Effective seizure management involves strict compliance with safe drug therapy practices.
14.5 Antiseizure pharmacotherapy is directed at controlling the movement of electrolytes across neuronal membranes or affecting neurotransmitter balance.
14.6 By increasing the effects of gamma-aminobutyric acid (GABA) in the brain, some drugs reduce a wide range of seizure types.
14.7 Hydantoin and related drugs are generally effective in treating partial seizures and tonic-clonic seizures.
14.8 Succinimides generally treat absence seizures.

Drug Snapshot

The following drugs are discussed in this chapter:

Drug Classes	Prototype Drugs
Drugs That Potentiate GABA Action	
Barbiturates	Pr phenobarbital (Luminal)
Benzodiazepines	Pr diazepam (Valium)
Other GABA-Related Drugs	
Hydantoin and Related Drugs	
Hydantoins	Pr phenytoin (Dilantin)
Phenytoin-related drugs	Pr valproic acid (Depakene)
Succinimides	Pr ethosuximide (Zarontin)

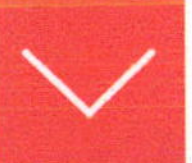

Learning Outcomes

After reading this chapter, the student should be able to:

1. Compare and contrast the terms epilepsy, seizures, and convulsions.
2. Recognize possible causes of seizures.
3. Relate signs and symptoms to specific types of seizures.
4. Explain the importance of safety and patient drug compliance in the pharmacotherapy of epilepsy and seizures.
5. Describe the pharmacologic management of epilepsy and acute seizures.
6. Explain the mechanisms of action by which barbiturates, benzodiazepines, and other GABA-related drugs control seizure activity.
7. For hydantoin-related drugs and succinimides, identify representative drugs and explain their mechanisms of drug action, primary actions, and important adverse effects.

Key Terms

action potential (poh-TEN-shial)
convulsions (kon-VULL-shuns)
eclampsia (ee-KLAMP-see-uh)
epilepsy (EPP-ih-lepp-see)
febrile seizures
generalized seizures
partial (focal) seizures
preeclampsia (pree-ee-KLAMP-see-uh)
pseudoseizures (SU-do-SEE-zhurrs)
seizure (SEE-zhurr)
status epilepticus (ep-ih-LEP-tih-kus)

epilepsy = *taking hold or to seize*

By definition, **epilepsy** is any condition characterized by recurrent seizures. When a person has had two or more seizures that have not been provoked by specific events such as trauma, infection, fever, or chemical change, he or she is considered to have epilepsy. Symptoms may include blackout, fainting spells, sensory disturbances, jerking body movements, and temporary loss of memory. This chapter examines the drug therapies used to treat different kinds of seizures.

SEIZURES

A **seizure** is a disturbance of electrical activity in the brain that may affect consciousness, motor activity, and sensation. Seizures are caused by abnormal or uncontrolled neuronal discharges. Uncontrolled charges start in one area of the brain and often move to other areas. A valuable tool in measuring uncontrolled neuronal activity, the electroencephalogram (EEG) is useful in diagnosing seizure disorders. Figure 14.1 compares normal and abnormal neuronal tracings.

Core Concept 14.1 ▶

Although some types of seizures involve convulsions, others do not.

Seizures and *convulsions* are not interchangeable terms. **Convulsions** specifically refer to involuntary, violent spasms of large skeletal muscles of the face, neck, arms, and legs. Some types of seizures involve muscle spasms; others do not.

Fast Facts Epilepsy

- Over 3 million Americans have epilepsy.
- One of every 100 teenagers has epilepsy.
- Of the U.S. population, 10% will have seizures within their lifetime.
- Most people with seizures are younger than 45 years of age.
- Epilepsy is not a mental illness, and children with epilepsy have IQ scores equivalent to those of children without the disorder.
- Famous people who had epilepsy include Julius Caesar, Alexander the Great, Napoleon, Vincent van Gogh, Charles Dickens, Joan of Arc, and Socrates.
- Among adult alcoholics receiving treatment for withdrawal, over half will experience seizures within 6 hours upon arriving for treatment.

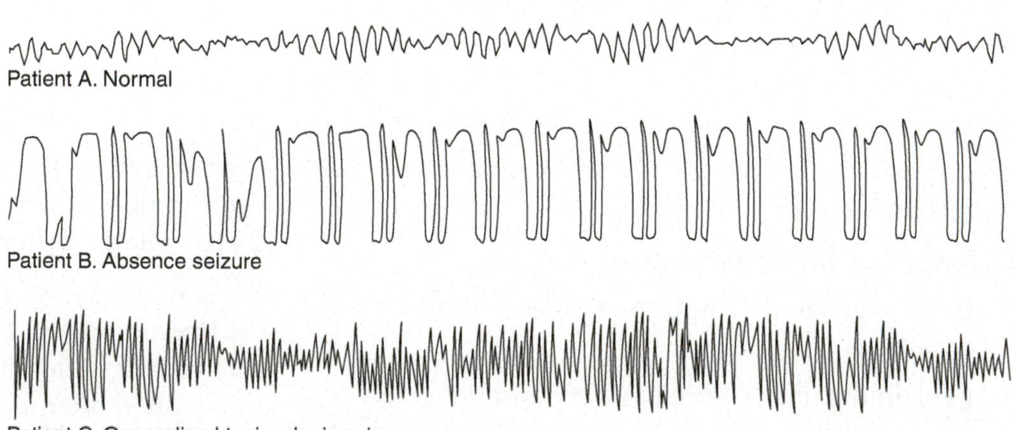

FIGURE 14.1 Tiny neural impulses are detected by an electroencephalogram (EEG), a device that captures brain-wave activity. Brain waves have characteristic patterns termed *alpha*, *beta*, *delta*, and *theta*. Alpha waves are the predominant waveform observed in patients with normal brain activity. Although interpretation of brain waves is a complex art, you can see from these examples that the EEG tracings of patients B and C are dramatically different from those of patient A, who has no seizures.

Drugs described in this chapter are generally referred to as *antiseizure drugs* rather than *anticonvulsants*. Recognizing also that antiseizure drugs are commonly called *antiepileptic drugs* (AEDs), the term *antiseizure* in this chapter applies to the treatment of all seizure-related symptoms, including signs of epilepsy.

Many causes of seizure activity are known; a few are not.

◀ **Core Concept 14.2**

A seizure is considered symptomatic of an underlying disorder, rather than the disease itself. Triggers include exposure to strobe or flickering lights or the occurrence of small fluid and electrolyte imbalances. Patients appear to have a lower tolerance to environmental triggers, and seizures often occur when patients are sleep deprived.

There are many different causes of seizure activity. In some but not all cases, the cause of seizure activity may be apparent. Seizures represent the most common serious neurologic problem affecting children prior to the age of 5, with an overall incidence from 2% to 5% for **febrile seizures** and 1% for idiopathic epilepsy. Febrile seizures are often caused by a high body temperature but not necessarily associated with an underlying health issue. Acute infection may be associated with a spike in body temperature. Medications for mood disorders, psychoses, and local anesthesia may cause seizures when given in high doses, possibly because of increased levels of stimulatory neurotransmitters or toxicity. Seizures may also occur from drug abuse, as with cocaine, or during withdrawal from alcohol or sedative–hypnotic drugs. Some seizures can occur due to extreme stress or an emotional state of mind. **Pseudoseizures** or psychogenic nonepileptic seizures (PNES) are paroxysmal (sharp recurrent) episodes that resemble and are often misdiagnosed as epileptic seizures. Family history of epilepsy is a risk factor for seizures; however, many people with epilepsy have children who never develop the disorder. Examples of childhood epilepsy that may be inherited include benign focal childhood epilepsy, childhood absence epilepsy, and juvenile myoclonic epilepsy; these types have no other known cause. Idiopathic seizures are seizures with no identifiable underlying cause.

psycho = *mind*
genic = *causing*
par = *during*
oxysmal = *suddenly sharp*

idio = *one's own arising*
pathic = *disease-related*

Seizures may present as an acute situation, or they may occur on a chronic basis. Seizures resulting from an acute complication are generally not recurrent after the situation has been resolved. On the other hand, if a brain abnormality exists such as with an acute complication, recurrent seizures are likely. The following are known causes of seizures:

- *Infectious diseases* Acute infections such as meningitis and encephalitis can cause inflammation in the brain.
- *Trauma* Physical trauma such as direct blows to the skull may increase intracranial pressure; chemical trauma such as the presence of toxic substances or the ingestion of poisons may cause brain injury.
- *Metabolic disorders* Changes in fluid and electrolytes such as hypoglycemia, hyponatremia, and water intoxication may cause seizures by altering electrical impulse transmission at the cellular level.
- *Vascular diseases* Changes in oxygenation such as those caused by respiratory hypoxia and carbon monoxide poisoning, and changes in perfusion such as those caused by hypotension, cerebral vascular accidents, shock, and cardiac dysrhythmias, may be causes.
- *Pediatric disorders* Rapid increase in body temperature may result in a febrile seizure.
- *Neoplastic disease* Tumors, especially rapidly growing ones, may occupy space, increase intracranial pressure, and damage brain tissue by disrupting blood flow.
- *Emotional, stress-related conditions* Pseudoseizures are psychological in nature; they can be psychogenic or organic (natural cause) in origin.
- *Genetics* Children of a parent with epilepsy may or may not develop seizures. Whether a family history of epilepsy increases a person's risk for seizures partly depends on the type of epilepsy.

Seizures can have a significant impact on quality of life. They may cause serious injury if they occur when a person is driving a vehicle or performing a dangerous activity. Without successful pharmacotherapy, epilepsy can severely limit participation in school, employment, or social activities and can affect self-esteem. Chronic depression may accompany poorly controlled seizures. Important considerations in healthcare include identifying patients at risk for seizures, documenting the pattern and type of seizure activity, and implementing safety precautions. In collaboration with the patient, healthcare provider, pharmacist, and all healthcare staff are instrumental in achieving positive therapeutic outcomes. Through a combination of pharmacotherapy, patient–family support, and education, effective seizure control can be achieved in the majority of patients.

Core Concept 14.3 ▶

Epileptic seizures are typically identified as partial, generalized, or special epileptic syndromes.

▶ Lifespan and Diversity

Onset of epilepsy is most common among the youngest and oldest age groups. About 50% of children have a generalized epilepsy syndrome compared with about 20% of adults. The incidence of epilepsy in older adults is greater than among the general population, perhaps because of the greater prevalence of mild strokes and cardiac arrest in this age group.

Seizure symptoms vary depending on the areas of the brain affected by the abnormal electrical activity. These symptoms range from muscle twitching or slight tremor (shaking) of a limb to sudden, violent shaking and total loss of consciousness. Staring into space, altered vision, and difficult speech are other behaviors a person may exhibit during a seizure. It is important to determine the cause of recurrent seizures in order to plan for appropriate treatment options.

Methods of classifying epilepsy have changed over time. For example, the terms *grand mal* and *petit mal* epilepsy have been replaced by more descriptive and detailed categorization. Epilepsies are typically identified using the International Classification of Epileptic Seizures. Example nomenclatures are *partial* (less used term *focal*), *generalized*, and *special epileptic syndromes*. Types of partial or generalized seizures may be recognized based on symptoms observed during a seizure episode. Some symptoms are hard to notice and reflect the simple nature of neuronal misfiring in specific areas of the brain; others are more complex.

Partial Seizures

Partial (focal) seizures involve a limited portion of the brain. Abnormal electrical activity starts on one side and travels only a short distance before it stops. The area where the abnormal electrical activity starts is known as the abnormal *focus* (plural, *foci*).

Simple partial seizures have an onset from a small, limited focus. They are usually subdivided into sensory, motor, autonomic, or psychic categories, depending on the types of symptoms. Patients may feel disoriented for a while, and they may hear and see things that are not there. Some patients smell and taste things that are not present, or have an upset stomach. Others may become emotional and experience a sense of joy, sorrow, or grief. Breathing rate and heart rate may change abruptly. The arms, legs, or face may twitch.

psycho = *mind*
motor = *motion or movement*

somno = *sleepiness*
lence = *filled with*

Complex partial seizures (formerly known as *psychomotor* or *temporal lobe seizures*) have sensory, motor, or autonomic symptoms with some degree of altered or impaired consciousness. Total loss of consciousness may not occur during a complex partial seizure, but a period of brief confusion and somnolence may follow the seizure. Such seizures are often preceded by an *aura*, sometimes described as an unpleasant odor or taste. Seizures may start with a blank stare, and patients may begin to chew or swallow repetitively. Some patients fumble with clothing; others try to take off their clothes. Most patients will not pay attention to verbal commands and will act as if they are having a psychotic episode. After a seizure, patients do not remember the seizure incident.

Generalized Seizures

bi = *two*
lateral = *sides*
sym = *same*
metrically = *measurement*

As the name suggests, **generalized seizures** are not localized to one area but travel throughout the entire brain on both sides. The seizure is thought to originate bilaterally and symmetrically within the brain.

Absence seizures (formerly known as *petit mal seizures*) most often occur in children and last only for a few seconds. Because episodes are short-lived, they are difficult to detect. Absence epilepsy often goes unrecognized, or this disorder may be mistaken for daydreaming or signs of attention deficit hyperactivity disorder (ADHD). Staring and temporary loss of responsiveness are the most common signs. There may be slight motor activity with eyelid fluttering or repetitive jerking motions. If patients stare into space for a brief time, less than about 10 seconds, they may be diagnosed with simple absence seizures. If they stare into space for less than about 20 seconds while making minor body movements, patients may be diagnosed with complex absence seizures.

Atonic seizures are sometimes called *drop attacks*. Patients retain consciousness, but they often stumble and fall for no apparent reason. Lasting for only a matter of seconds, episodes are very short.

a = *without*
tonic = *tension*

Tonic-clonic seizures (formerly known as *grand mal seizures*) are the most common type. This applies to all age groups. Seizures may be preceded by an aura (e.g., spiritual feeling, flash of light, special noise). Intense muscle contractions indicate the *tonic phase*. Due to air being forced out of the lungs, a hoarse cry may occur at the onset of the seizure. Patients may temporarily lose bladder or bowel control. Breathing may become shallow and even stop momentarily. The *clonic phase* is characterized by alternating contraction and relaxation of muscles. The seizure usually lasts 1 to 3 minutes, after which the patient becomes drowsy, disoriented, and sleeps deeply.

▶ Lifespan and Diversity

Preventing the onset of high fever is the best way to control febrile seizures in children.

Special Epileptic Syndromes

Special epileptic seizures include the febrile seizures of infancy, reflex epilepsies, and other forms of myoclonic epilepsies. Myoclonic epilepsies often go along with other neurologic abnormalities or progressively debilitating symptoms.

Febrile seizures typically cause tonic-clonic motor activity lasting for 1 to 2 minutes, with rapid return of consciousness. These occur together with a rapid rise in body temperature and usually occur only once during any given illness. Febrile seizures are most likely to occur within the 6-month to 5-year-old age group. The greatest risk is around the second year of life.

febrile = *fever*

Myoclonic seizures are characterized by large, jerking body movements. Major muscle groups contract quickly, and patients appear unsteady and clumsy. They may fall from a sitting position or drop whatever they are holding. *Infantile spasms* are an example of a type of *generalized, myoclonic seizure* and are distinguished by short-lasting muscle spasms in the trunk and extremities. Such spasms are often not identified as seizures by parents or healthcare providers because the movements are much like the normal infantile startle reflex.

myo = *muscle*
clonic = *repetitive jerking motions*

Status epilepticus is a medical emergency caused by the repeated occurrence of seizures. This state could result with any type of seizure, but usually generalized tonic-clonic seizures are observed. When generalized tonic-clonic seizures are long and continuous, hypoxia may develop. Continuous muscle contractions also lead to hypoglycemia, acidosis, and hypothermia (due to increased metabolic needs, lactic acid production, and heat loss during muscle movement). Carbon dioxide retention also leads to acidosis. If not treated, status epilepticus can cause brain damage, and ultimately, death. Medical treatment involves the IV administration of antiseizure medications. During seizure activity, steps must be taken to make sure that the airway remains open.

status = *state of*
epilepticus = *seizure activity*

hypo = *lowered*
glycemia = *blood sugar level*
thermia = *body temperature*

acid = *hydrogen ion accumulation (reduced pH; e.g., lactic acid)*
osis = *condition of*

For some people living with epilepsy, the risk of Sudden Unexpected Death in Epilepsy (SUDEP) is an important concern. SUDEP refers to deaths in people with epilepsy that are not caused by drowning, injury, or other known causes. Each year about one out of 1000 people with epilepsy succumb to SUDEP. Patients with uncontrolled or frequent seizures, generalized tonic-clonic or grand mal seizures, and children who have had recurrent seizures beginning from an early age are at highest risk for this disorder.

CONCEPT REVIEW 14.1

- What is epilepsy? What is the difference between a seizure and a convulsion? Name and identify signs of the more common types of seizures.

Core Concept 14.4 ▶ Effective seizure management involves strict compliance with safe drug therapy practices.

The choice of drug for antiseizure pharmacotherapy depends on the patient's signs, previous medical history, and associated pathologies. Once a medication is selected, the patient is placed on a low initial dose. The amount is gradually increased until seizure control is achieved or until drug adverse effects prevent additional increases in dose. Serum drug levels may be obtained to assist the healthcare provider in determining the most effective drug concentration. If seizure activity continues, a different medication is added in small-dose increments while the dose of the first drug is slowly reduced. Because seizures are likely to occur if antiseizure drugs are abruptly withdrawn, the medication is usually discontinued over a period of 6 to 12 weeks.

Antiseizure drugs with indications are shown in Table 14.1. Some of the antiseizure drugs offer advantages over others. Owing to the limited induction of drug-metabolizing enzymes, the pharmacokinetic profiles of the more recently approved antiseizure drugs seem to be less complicated. In addition, the more recently approved antiseizure drugs are generally better tolerated.

mono = *only*
therapy = *treatment*

adjunctive = *joined or added*

In most cases, effective seizure management can be obtained using only a single drug, or *monotherapy*. For some patients, two antiseizure medications may be needed, although unwanted adverse effects may appear. Some antiseizure drug combinations may actually increase the incidence of seizures. Many of the antiseizure medications are used as additional or *adjunctive* therapy.

After several years of being seizure free, patients may question the need for their medications. In general, withdrawal of antiseizure drugs should be attempted only after at least 3 years of seizure-free activity and only under close direction from the healthcare provider. Doses of medications are reduced slowly, one at a time, over a period of several months. If seizures recur during the withdrawal process, pharmacotherapy is resumed, usually with the original stabilizing drug. A good fact to remember about all antiseizure drugs is that they can have serious clinical drawbacks if not taken properly.

An important topic when discussing epilepsy and seizure treatment is birth control. Because several antiseizure drugs decrease the effectiveness of oral contraceptives,

Table 14.1 Selected Antiseizure Drugs with Indications

		Generalized Seizures		Special
Drug	Partial Seizures	Absence	Tonic–Clonic	Myoclonic
DRUGS THAT POTENTIATE GABA				
diazepam (Valium)	✓	✓	✓	✓
gabapentin (Neurontin)	✓			
lorazepam (Ativan)	✓	✓	✓	✓
phenobarbital (Luminal)	✓		✓	
pregabalin (Lyrica)	✓			
primidone (Mysoline)	✓		✓	
tiagabine (Gabitril)	✓			
topiramate (Topamax, Trokendi XR)	✓		✓	✓
HYDANTOIN AND RELATED DRUGS				
carbamazepine (Tegretol)	✓		✓	
lamotrigine (Lamictal)	✓	✓	✓	✓
levetiracetam (Keppra)	✓		✓	✓
oxcarbazepine (Trileptal, Oxtellar XR)	✓			
phenytoin (Dilantin)	✓		✓	
valproic acid (Depakene)	✓	✓	✓	✓
zonisamide (Zonegran)	✓	✓	✓	✓
SUCCINIMIDES				
ethosuximide (Zarontin)		✓		

additional barrier methods of birth control should be practiced to avoid unintended pregnancy. Prior to pregnancy and considering the serious nature of epilepsy, patients should consult with their healthcare provider to determine the most appropriate plan of action for seizure control. If patients become pregnant, extreme caution is necessary. Most antiseizure drugs are pregnancy category D. Some antiseizure drugs may cause folate deficiency, a condition correlated with fetal neural tube defects. Vitamin supplements may be necessary. **Preeclampsia** and **eclampsia** are severe hypertensive disorders of pregnancy, characterized by seizures, coma, and perinatal mortality. Eclampsia is likely to occur from around the 20th week of gestation to at least 1 week following delivery of the baby. Roughly one-fourth of patients with eclampsia experience seizures within 72 hours postpartum.

peri = *surrounding (before and after)*
natal = *birth*

post = *after*
partum = *delivery*

Additional drawbacks include the fact that some AEDs may impact early child development. In 2013, a study of children whose mothers took AEDs while pregnant indicated an increased risk of early development issues. These children were not able to interact socially compared to children whose mothers did not take AEDs. Language and motor skills of the children were also impacted. Some children developed autistic traits.

Another issue of antiseizure drug therapy relates to warnings issued by the U.S. Food and Drug Administration (FDA). Healthcare providers have been encourged to balance carefully the clinical need for antiseizure drugs against the risk for suicidality among patients taking these drugs. Patients and caregivers are encouraged to pay close attention to changes in mood and not to make changes in the antiseizure regimen without consulting with their healthcare provider.

Although antiseizure medications were originally designed for epilepsy, the nerve-calming qualities of these drugs have helped patients with migraines and neuralgia. Indeed, the usefulness of antiseizure drugs has extended beyond pain management. They actually help calm patients with behavioral and mood disturbances such as ADHD, borderline personality disorder, and post-traumatic stress disorder (PTSD). Antiseizure drugs have even helped patients with schizophrenia. Epilepsy, bipolar disorder, psychoses, and neuropathic pain (i.e., peripheral neuropathy, diabetic neuropathy) are among the disorders successfully treated with antiseizure medications.

neuro = *nerve*
algia = *pain*

neuro = *nerve*
pathic = *disease-related*

CONCEPT REVIEW 14.2

- Give the names of antiseizure drugs used for the management of specific seizure types. Match the drugs with the types of seizures they best control. Which drugs are generally used for a broader range of seizures? Which medications treat neuropathies?

Antiseizure pharmacotherapy is directed at controlling the movement of electrolytes across neuronal membranes or affecting neurotransmitter balance.

◄ **Core Concept 14.5**

In a resting state, neurons are normally surrounded by a higher concentration of sodium ions, calcium ions, and chloride ions. Potassium ion levels are higher inside the cell. An influx of sodium or calcium ions into the neuron *enhances* neuronal activity, whereas an influx of chloride ions *suppresses* neuronal activity.

The goal of antiseizure pharmacotherapy is to suppress neuronal activity just enough to prevent abnormal or repetitive firing. To this end, there are three general mechanisms by which antiseizure drugs work:

- Stimulating an influx of chloride ions, an effect associated with the neurotransmitter gamma-aminobutyric acid (GABA)
- Delaying an influx of sodium ions
- Delaying an influx of calcium ions.

Some drugs act by more than one mechanism. This has prompted drug researchers to try to understand more clearly various drug mechanisms and to develop safer and more effective AEDs. Recently a fourth mechanism has been studied: blocking of the primary excitatory neurotransmitter glutamate. Glutamate works in concert with the cell's Na^+-K^+ ATPase pump, which helps to restore ion balances across neuronal membranes after firing. Any drug that blocks glutamate activity prevents an influx of positive ions into the cell, so this is consistent with the last two mechanisms.

A related observation has been low levels of the inhibitory amino acid taurine in damaged neuronal tissue. Thus, it has been proposed that taurine stabilizes neuronal cell membranes primarily by reducing glutamate-induced positive ion (sodium and calcium) influxes. Therefore, higher levels of glutamate seem to be associated with neuronal damage. Restoring amino acid–related ion balances (e.g., dietary consideration) has been among the approaches for the general treatment of recurrent and sudden seizure attacks.

Core Concept 14.6 ▶

By increasing the effects of gamma-aminobutyric acid (GABA) in the brain, some drugs reduce a wide range of seizure types.

Several important antiseizure drugs act by increasing the action of GABA, the primary inhibitory neurotransmitter in the brain. These drugs mimic the effects of GABA by stimulating an influx of chloride ions that interact with the GABA receptor–chloride channel molecule. A model of this receptor is shown in Figure 14.2. When the receptor is stimulated, chloride ions move into the cell and suppress the firing of neurons. The predominant effect of GABA activation is central nervous system (CNS) depression.

A group of drugs, called GABA agonists, have been found to activate the GABA receptor. Drugs may bind directly to the GABA receptor through specific binding sites designated as $GABA_A$ or $GABA_B$. Most antiseizure drugs bind to the $GABA_A$ site. Drugs may also enhance GABA release, or drugs may block the reuptake of GABA into nerve cells and other supporting cells in the CNS. A few drugs have been developed that inhibit GABA degrading enzymes.

Barbiturates, benzodiazepines, and several more recently developed drugs reduce seizure activity by intensifying GABA action. These drugs are listed in Table 14.2.

The antiseizure properties of phenobarbital were discovered in 1912, and this drug is still prescribed for seizures. As a class, barbiturates generally have a low margin for safety, a high potential for dependence, and may cause significant CNS depression. Phenobarbital, however, is able to suppress abnormal neuronal discharges without causing profound sedation. It is inexpensive, long acting, and produces a low incidence of adverse effects. When the drug is given orally, it may take several weeks to achieve optimal effects. Phenobarbital is a preferred drug used in the pharmacotherapy of neonatal seizures. Primidone (Mysoline) has a pharmacologic profile similar to phenobarbital and is among the drugs used to potentiate GABA action.

neo = *new*
natal = *birth*

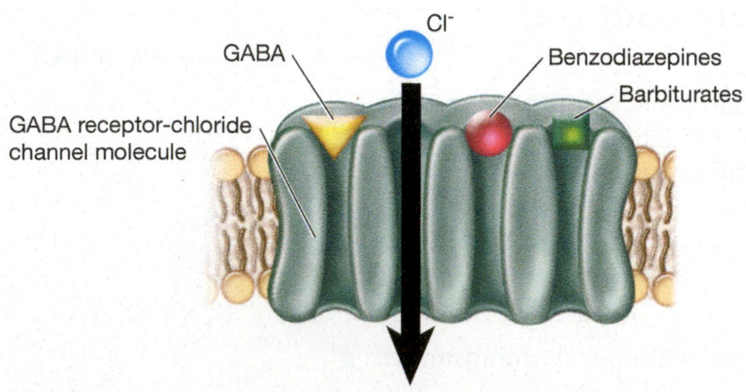

FIGURE 14.2 Model of the GABA receptor–chloride channel. The chloride selectivity filter allows the channel to open exclusively to chloride ions when GABA, benzodiazepines, or barbiturates bind to the cellular receptor (shown in green). Some antiseizure drugs are similar to the structure of GABA, or they may potentiate GABA indirectly. After the influx of chloride ions, the net result is inhibition of the neuron's action potential and suppression of the neuron's firing rate.

Like barbiturates, benzodiazepines and several other drugs intensify the effect of GABA in the brain. The benzodiazepines bind directly to the GABA receptor, suppressing abnormal neuronal firing. Benzodiazepines used in treating epilepsy include clobazam (Onfi), clonazepam (Klonopin), clorazepate (Tranxene), diazepam (Valium), and lorazepam (Ativan). Parenteral diazepam is used to terminate status epilepticus. Short-term indications of benzodiazepines include treatment of absence seizures and myoclonic seizures. Because tolerance may begin to develop after only a few months of therapy, seizures may recur unless doses are periodically adjusted. Benzodiazepines and other GABA-related drugs are generally not used alone in seizure pharmacotherapy, but instead are used in combination with other antiseizure medications.

Some of the GABA-related antiseizure drugs have been used for a variety of other conditions, including depression, migraines, and neuropathic pain

Table 14.2 Antiseizure Drugs That Potentiate GABA Action

Drug	Route and Adult Dose	Remarks
BARBITURATES		
Pr phenobarbital (Luminal)	PO: 60–200 mg/day IV/IM: 200–600 mg up to 20 mg/kg For status epilepticus: IV: 15–18 mg/kg (max: 20 mg/kg)	For tonic-clonic seizures, partial seizures, status epilepticus, and eclampsia; Schedule IV drug; see Prototype Drug box for adverse effects
primidone (Mysoline)	PO: 250 mg/day (max: 2 g/day)	Similar treatment profile to phenobarbital
BENZODIAZEPINES		
clobazam (Onfi)	PO: 5–20 mg/day (max: 20-40 mg daily	For the adjunctive treatment of seizures associated with Lennox-Gastaut syndrome (LGS) in patients aged 2 years or older
clonazepam (Klonopin)	PO: 1.5 mg/day gradually increased until seizures are controlled (max: 20 mg/day)	For absence seizures and motor seizures; also for panic disorder; Schedule IV drug; may cause drowsiness and impaired cognitive and motor performance
clorazepate (Tranxene)	PO: 7.5 mg tid (max: 90 mg/day)	For partial seizures; also for anxiety; Schedule IV drug
Pr diazepam (Valium)	IV push: administer at 5 mg/min IM/IV 5–10 mg (repeat as needed at 10–15 min intervals up to 30 mg)	For status epilepticus; also for anxiety and muscle spasms; see the Prototype Drug box for adverse effects
lorazepam (Ativan) (see the Prototype Drug box in Core Concept 10.7)	IV: 4 mg injected slowly at 2 mg/min; if inadequate response after 10 min, may repeat once	For status epilepticus; also for nausea and vomiting, preoperative sedation, anxiety, and insomnia; most potent of the available benzodiazepines Schedule IV drug
OTHER DRUGS THAT POTENTIATE GABA		
ezogabine (Potiga)	PO: Start with 100 mg tid; may gradually increase dose. Optimize effective dosage between 200 mg tid to 400 mg tid (max: 400 mg tid)	For partial onset seizures; often referred to as potassium channel openers due to their ability to suppress recurrent neuronal activity; may cause psychiatric and nervous system symptoms: confusion, memory impairment, blurred vision, balance disorder
gabapentin (Gralise, Horizant, Neurontin)	PO: Start with 300 mg and gradually increase to 1200 mg/day (400 mg tid); may increase to 1800–2400 mg/day (max: 2400 mg/day)	For partial seizures or seizures that could become generalized; also for nerve pain caused by herpesvirus or shingles (herpes zoster) and restless legs syndrome; structure similar to GABA; speeds up the release of GABA from brain neurons; may cause unsteadiness, weight gain, fatigue, dizziness
pregabalin (Lyrica)	PO: Start with 150 mg/day in divided doses, bid–tid and gradually increase (max: 600 mg/day)	For partial seizures; also for nerve pain associated with diabetes, herpesvirus or shingles (herpes zoster), and fibromyalgia; structure similar to GABA; similar adverse effects to gabapentin
tiagabine (Gabitril)	PO: Start with 4 mg/day in divided doses and gradually increase (max: 56 mg/day)	For partial seizures; inhibits uptake of GABA, prolonging GABA action; may cause confusion, stuttering, loss of sensation in the fingertips
topiramate (Topamax, Qudexy XR)	PO (regular release): Start with 50 mg/day and gradually increase (max: 1600 mg/day) PO (extended release): 200–400 mg once daily	For partial seizures; useful in trigeminal neuralgia; enhances the action of GABA; may cause weight loss, numbness and tingling of the fingers and toes, depression, agitation, hostility
vigabatrin (Sabril)	PO: For infantile spasms, begin therapy at 50 mg/kg/day bid and gradually increase (max: 150 mg/kg/day); for adults with refractory complex partial seizures, initiate therapy at 500 mg bid and gradually increase (max: (1.5 grams bid)	For infantile spasms in babies and refractory (hard to manage) complex partial seizures in adults; increases GABA in the CNS; may cause fatigue, headache, irritability, gastrointestinal (GI) disturbances, and irritated respiratory passages

associated with diabetic peripheral neuropathy, postherpetic neuralgia, fibromyalgia, and spinal cord injury. In addition, some antiseizure drugs have been used for the management of anxiety and bipolar disorder symptoms. Two antiseizure drugs, gabapentin (Neurontin) and pregabalin (Lyrica), stand out as off-label approaches for the successful management of neuropathic pain and postherpetic neuralgia. Topiramate (Topamax, Trokendi XR) may be used in the treatment of trigeminal neuralgia.

fibro = *fiber-related*
my = *muscle*
algia = *pain*

post = *after*
herpet = *herpes*
ic = *related*

Prototype Drug: Phenobarbital (Luminal)

Therapeutic Class: Antiseizure drug, sedative-hypnotic **Pharmacologic Class:** Barbiturate, $GABA_A$ receptor drug

Actions and Uses: Phenobarbital is a long-acting barbiturate used for the management of a variety of seizures. It is also used for insomnia. Phenobarbital should not be used for pain relief, because it may increase a patient's sensitivity to pain.

Phenobarbital acts biochemically in the brain by enhancing the action of the neurotransmitter GABA, which is responsible for suppressing abnormal neuronal discharges that can cause epilepsy.

Adverse Effects and Interactions: Phenobarbital is a Schedule IV drug that may cause dependence. Common adverse effects include drowsiness, vitamin deficiencies (vitamin D, folate, B_9, and B_{12}), and laryngospasms. With overdose, phenobarbital may cause severe respiratory depression, CNS depression, coma, and death. Phenobarbital is a pregnancy category D drug.

Phenobarbital interacts with many other drugs. For example, it should not be taken with alcohol or other CNS depressants. These substances potentiate the action of barbiturates, increasing the risk of life-threatening respiratory depression or cardiac arrest. Phenobarbital increases the metabolism of many other drugs, reducing their effectiveness.

Prototype Drug: Diazepam (Valium)

Therapeutic Class: Antiseizure drug, sedative-hypnotic, anxiolytic, anesthetic adjunct, skeletal muscle relaxant (centrally acting) **Pharmacologic Class:** Benzodiazepine, GABA receptor drug

Actions and Uses: Diazepam binds to GABA receptors located throughout the CNS. It produces its effects by suppressing neuronal activity in the limbic system and subsequent impulses that might be transmitted to the reticular activating system. Effects of this drug are suppression of abnormal neuronal foci that may cause seizures, calming without strong sedation, and skeletal muscle relaxation. When used orally, maximum therapeutic effects may take from 1 to 2 weeks. Tolerance may develop after about 4 weeks. When given IV, effects occur within minutes, and its anticonvulsant effects last for about 20 minutes.

Adverse Effects and Interactions: Diazepam should not be taken with alcohol or other CNS depressants because of combined sedation effects. Other drug interactions include cimetidine, oral contraceptives, valproic acid, and metoprolol, which potentiate diazepam's action, and levodopa and barbiturates, which decrease diazepam's action. Diazepam increases the levels of phenytoin in the bloodstream and may cause phenytoin toxicity. When given IV, hypotension, muscular weakness, tachycardia, and respiratory depression are common. Because of tolerance and dependency, use of diazepam is reserved for short-term seizure control or for status epilepticus.

Diazepam should be used with caution with herbal supplements, such as kava and chamomile, which may cause an increased effect.

CAM Therapy | The Ketogenic Diet for Epilepsy

The ketogenic diet may be used when seizures cannot be controlled through pharmacotherapy or when there are unacceptable adverse effects to medications. Before AEDs were developed, this diet was a primary treatment for epilepsy.

The ketogenic diet is a strict diet that is high in fat and low in carbohydrates and protein. It limits water intake and carefully controls caloric intake. Each meal has the same ketogenic ratio of 4 g of fat to 1 g of protein and carbohydrate. Extra fat is usually given in the form of cream.

Research suggests that the diet produces a high success rate for certain patients. The diet appears to be equally effective for every seizure type. The most frequently reported adverse effects include vomiting, fatigue, constipation, diarrhea, and hunger. Kidney stones, acidosis, and slower growth rates are possible risks. Those interested in trying the diet must consult with their healthcare provider; this is not a do-it-yourself diet and may be harmful if not monitored carefully by skilled professionals.

Core Concept 14.7 ▶

Hydantoin and related drugs are generally effective in treating partial seizures and tonic-clonic seizures.

Hydantoins and related drugs dampen CNS activity by delaying an influx of sodium ions across neuronal membranes. Sodium movement is the major factor that determines whether a neuron will undergo an **action potential**. Sodium channels guide the movement of sodium ions into the cell. If sodium channels are temporarily inactivated, neuronal activity will be suppressed. With hydantoin and related drugs, sodium channels are not blocked completely; they are just made to be less sensitive. If sodium channels are blocked, neuronal activity completely stops, as occurs with local anesthetic drugs (see Chapter 16).

Several drugs in this group may also affect the threshold of neuronal firing, or they may interfere with activation of the excitatory neurotransmitter glutamate. These approaches, although not directly connected with desensitization of sodium channels, result in the same effect (delayed depolarization of the neuron). Hydantoin and related drugs are listed in Table 14.3.

The antiseizure medication that has been in circulation the longest and is still commonly used is phenytoin (Dilantin). Approved in the 1930s, phenytoin is a broad-spectrum hydantoin drug, useful in treatment of all kinds of epilepsy except absence seizures. It

Table 14.3 Hydantoins and Related Drugs

Drug	Route and Adult Dose	Remarks
HYDANTOINS		
ethotoin (Peganone)	PO: Initial dose 1 g/day or less in divided doses and gradually increase. Usual maintenance dosage is 2–3 g/day	For tonic-clonic and complex partial seizures; prevents the spread of seizure activity rather than abolish the primary focus; may cause swelling of the lips, tongue, and throat; mood changes, chest pain, vision problems, fever.
fosphenytoin (Cerebyx)	For status epilepticus: Initial dose 15–20 mg PE/kg administered IV at 100–150 mg PE/min (max: 150 mg PE/min) For nonemergent loading and maintenance dosing: Initial dose 10–20 mg PE/kg administered IV no greater than 150 mg PE/min or IM; daily maintenance 4–6 mg PE/kg/day in divided doses (PE = phenytoin equivalents)	For status epilepticus; converted to phenytoin in the body; short-term substitute for oral phenytoin
Pr phenytoin (Dilantin)	PO (extended release): Start with 100 mg/week and increase gradually for seizure control up to 200 mg tid if needed	For tonic-clonic seizures, complex partial seizures, and seizures after head trauma; may cause unsteadiness and cognitive problems, cosmetic issues (abnormal growth of body and face hair, and skin blemishes), blood disorders, bone marrow suppression, gingival hyperplasia
PHENYTOIN-RELATED DRUGS		
carbamazepine (Tegretol)	PO: 200 mg bid, gradually increased to 800–1,200 mg/day	For tonic-clonic and complex partial seizures; also for trigeminal neuralgia; bipolar disorder, ADHD, schizophrenia, borderline personality disorder, and PTSD; may cause Stevens–Johnson syndrome, blood disorders, liver disease, reduced bone health
eslicarbazepine (Aptiom)	PO: Start with 400 mg/day and gradually increase to 800 mg/day; 800–1600 mg/day maintenance (max: 1200 mg/day)	Approved as an adjunctive medication to treat seizures associated with epilepsy
felbamate (Felbatol)	Partial seizures: PO: Start with 1200 mg/day in divided doses; and gradually increase (max: 3600 mg/day) Lennox-Gastaut syndrome: PO: start at 15 mg/kg/day in divided doses and gradually increase (max: 45 mg/kg/day)	For Lennox-Gastaut syndrome and partial seizures; may cause anemia and liver toxicity in some patients
lamotrigine (Lamictal)	PO: Start with 50 mg/day and gradually increase (max: 700 mg/day)	For partial seizures, generalized tonic-clonic seizures, myoclonic seizures; also for bipolar disorder; may cause dizziness, fatigue, insomnia
levetiracetam (Keppra)	PO: 500 mg twice daily (max: 3000 mg total per day)	For partial seizures; may cause drowsiness, weakness, susceptibility to infections, nasal problems, nervousness
oxcarbazepine (Oxtellar XR, Trileptal)	PO: Start with 300 mg bid and gradually increase (max: 1200 mg/day)	Similar treatment profile to carbamazepine; may cause serious skin and organ hypersensitivity reactions in some patients
rufinamide (Banzel)	PO: 400 to 800 mg/day (max: 3200 mg/day)	For the adjunctive treatment of Lennox-Gastaut syndrome in children 4 years and older and adults
Pr valproic acid (Depakene, Stavzor)**	PO or IV: 15 mg/kg/day in divided doses and gradually increase until seizures are controlled (max: 60 mg/kg/day)	Broad-spectrum AED; for absence seizures, mixed generalized types of seizures; also for bipolar disorder; see Prototype Drug box for adverse effects
zonisamide (Zonegran)	PO: 100–400 mg/day	Broad-spectrum AED; for partial seizures; it is a sulfonamide, which may cause an allergic reactions

**Other formulations of valproic acid include derivatives valproate sodium and divalproex sodium.

hematologic = *blood-related*

thrombocytopenia = *reduced platelets*

neutropenia = *reduced neutrophils*

agranulocytosis = *state of deficient granulocytes*

anemias = *red blood cell deficiencies*

provides effective seizure suppression without the potential for abuse or extreme sedative effects. Patients vary significantly in their ability to metabolize phenytoin; therefore, dosages are highly individualized. Because of the very narrow range between therapeutic dose and toxic dose, patients must be carefully monitored. Hematologic toxicities have been associated with phenytoin drug use: thrombocytopenia, leukopenia, neutropenia, agranulocytosis, anemias, and other blood disorders have been reported. In addition, liver disease, renal dysfunction, and cardiac toxicity are severe potential hazards. Phenytoin and fosphenytoin (drug converted to phenytoin) are first-line drugs in the treatment of status epilepticus.

Most drugs share a mechanism similar to the hydantoins, including carbamazepine (Tegretol), oxcarbazepine (Oxtellar, Trileptal), and valproic acid (Depakene, Stavzor), which is also available as valproate sodium (Depacon), and divalproex sodium (Depakote, Depakote ER). Because carbamazepine produces fewer adverse effects than phenytoin or phenobarbital, it is a preferred drug for treating tonic-clonic and partial seizures. Carbamazepine has been approved for the treatment of trigeminal neuralgia, a painful condition associated with nerves in the facial area. Carbamazepine may be prescribed off-label for a variety of indications, including ADHD, schizophrenia, borderline personality disorder, and PTSD. Patients should not take grapefruit juice when prescribed and should report any visual disturbances. Oxcarbazepine is a derivative of carbamazepine, so its treatment profile is similar. Oxcarbazepine is slightly better tolerated, although serious skin and organ hypersensitivity reactions have been noted. Valproic acid is a preferred drug for absence seizures and is taken in combination with other drugs for partial seizures. Valproic acid, carbamazepine, and lamotrigine are taken for bipolar disorder (see Chapter 11).

More recently approved antiseizure drugs show promise in treatment for a range of disorders, including absence seizures, partial seizures, myoclonic seizures, generalized tonic-clonic seizures, and mood disorders. The most common adverse effects of these drugs are drowsiness, dizziness, and blurred vision. Lamotrigine (Lamictal) has a broad spectrum of antiseizure activity and is FDA approved for long-term maintenance of bipolar disorder. Its duration of action is greatly affected by other drugs that inhibit or enhance hepatic metabolizing enzymes. Levetiracetam (Keppra) and zonisamide (Zonegram) are approved for adjunctive therapy of partial seizures in adults. Zonisamide (a sulfonamide) has triggered hypersensitivity reactions in some patients. Felbamate (Felbatol) has induced potentially harmful reactions, including liver toxicity and aplastic anemia.

In a severe form of epilepsy called *Lennox-Gastaut syndrome (LGS)*, valproic acid (Depakene, Depakote), lamotrigine (Lamictal), felbamate (Felbatol), topiramate (Topamax, Trokendi XR), and rufinamide (Banzel) are often used for treatment. LGS is characterized by tonic, atonic, atypical absence, and myoclonic symptoms. There is usually no single antiseizure medication that will control symptoms of this particular syndrome.

Prototype Drug: Pr *Phenytoin (Dilantin)*

Therapeutic Class: Antiseizure drug, antidysrhythmic **Pharmacologic Class: Hydantoin, sodium influx suppressing drug**

Actions and Uses: Phenytoin acts by desensitizing sodium channels in the CNS responsible for neuronal responsivity. Desensitization prevents the spread of disruptive electrical charges in the brain that produce seizures. It is effective against most types of seizures except absence seizures. Phenytoin has antidysrhythmic activity similar to lidocaine (Class IB). An off-label use is for digoxin-induced dysrhythmias.

Adverse Effects and Interactions: Phenytoin may cause dysrhythmias such as bradycardia or ventricular fibrillation, severe hypotension, and hyperglycemia. Severe CNS reactions include headache, nystagmus, ataxia, confusion, slurred speech, paradoxical nervousness, twitching, and insomnia. Peripheral neuropathy may occur with long-term use. Phenytoin can cause multiple blood dyscrasias, including agranulocytosis and aplastic anemia. It may cause severe skin reactions, such as rashes, including exfoliative dermatitis, and Stevens–Johnson syndrome. Connective tissue reactions include systemic lupus erythematosa, hypertrichosis, hirsutism, and gingival hyperplasia.

Phenytoin interacts with many other drugs, including oral anticoagulants, glucocorticoids, H_2 antagonists, antituberculin drugs, and food supplements such as folic acid, calcium, and vitamin D. It impairs the effectiveness of drugs such as digoxin, doxycycline, furosemide, estrogens and oral contraceptives, and theophylline. Phenytoin, when combined with tricyclic antidepressants, can trigger seizures.

Phenytoin should be used with caution with herbal supplements such as herbal laxatives (buckthorn, cascara sagrada, and senna), which may increase potassium loss.

Prototype Drug: Pr *Valproic Acid (Depakene)*

Therapeutic Class: Antiseizure drug, bipolar disorder drug, migraine prophylaxis **Pharmacologic Class:** Valproate, sodium influx suppressing drug, calcium influx suppressing drug, GABA potentiating drug

Actions and Uses: The mechanism of action of valproic acid is the same as phenytoin, although effects on GABA and calcium channels may cause some additional actions. It is useful for a wide range of seizure types, including absence seizures and mixed types of seizures. Other uses include treatment of bipolar disorder and prevention of migraine headaches.

Valproic acid has several trade names and formulations, which sometimes causes confusion when studying this drug. These include the following.

- Valproic acid (Depakene) is the standard form of the drug given by the oral route.
- Valproate sodium is the sodium salt of valproic acid given orally or IV (Depacon).
- Divalproex sodium (Depakote ER) is a sustained release combination of valproic acid and its sodium salt. It is given orally and is available in an enteric-coated form.

Adverse Effects and Interactions: Adverse effects include sedation, drowsiness, GI upset, and prolonged bleeding time. Other effects include visual disturbances, muscle weakness, tremor, psychomotor agitation, bone marrow suppression, weight gain, abdominal cramps, rash, alopecia, pruritus, photosensitivity, erythema multiforme, and fatal hepatotoxicity.

Valproic acid interacts with many drugs. For example, aspirin, cimetidine, chlorpromazine, erythromycin, and felbamate may increase valproic acid toxicity. Concomitant warfarin, aspirin, or alcohol use can cause severe bleeding. Alcohol, benzodiazepines, and other CNS depressants potentiate CNS depressant action. Lamotrigine, phenytoin, and rifampin lower valproic acid levels. Valproic acid increases serum phenobarbital and phenytoin levels. Use of clonazepam concurrently with valproic acid may induce absence seizures.

BLACK BOX WARNING:

May result in fatal hepatic failure, especially in children under the age of 2 years. Nonspecific symptoms often precede hepatic toxicity: weakness, facial edema, anorexia, and vomiting. Liver function tests should be performed prior to treatment and at specific intervals during the first 6 months of treatment. Valproic acid can produce life-threatening pancreatitis and teratogenic effects, including spina bifida.

Succinimides generally treat absence seizures.

◀ **Core Concept 14.8**

Neurotransmitters, hormones, and some medications bind to neuronal membranes, stimulating the entry of calcium. Without calcium influx, neuronal transmission would not be possible. Succinimides delay entry of calcium into neurons by blocking calcium channels, increasing the electrical threshold of the neuron, and reducing the likelihood of an action potential. By raising the seizure threshold, succinimides keep neurons from firing too quickly, thus suppressing abnormal foci. The succinimides are generally effective only against absence seizures. These drugs are listed in Table 14.4.

succin = *chemical related to succinic acid*
imide = *having an NH functional group*

Ethosuximide (Zarontin) is the most commonly prescribed drug in this class. It remains the preferred drug for absence seizures. It joins the other positive ion suppressing drugs that successfully treat absence seizures: valproic acid (Depakene, Depakote), lamotrigine (Lamictal), and zonisamide (Zonegran).

CONCEPT REVIEW 14.3

- Name three general drug classes introduced by the Drug Snapshot feature at the beginning of this chapter. Identify the various stated chemical categories of antiseizure medications. Based on pharmacologic mechanisms, which of the drug examples do not conveniently fit into only one drug class? Which of the drugs control a wide range of seizure types? Which of the drugs have therapeutic applications other than seizure management?

Table 14.4 Succinimides

Drug	Route and Adult Dose	Remarks
Pr ethosuximide (Zarontin)	PO: 250 mg bid, increased every 4–7 days (max: 1.5 g/day)	For absence seizures, myoclonic seizures, and akinetic epilepsy; may cause nausea, anorexia, abdominal pain, vomiting, gum overgrowth, blood disorders, behavioral changes, Stevens-Johnson syndrome
methsuximide (Celontin)	PO: 300 mg/day, may increase every 4–7 days (max: 1.2 g/day in divided doses)	For absence seizures; may be used in combination with other anticonvulsants in mixed types of seizure activity; may cause dizziness, drowsiness, blurred vision, increased risk for suicidal thoughts, fetal toxicity

Prototype Drug: Ethosuximide (Zarontin)

Therapeutic Class: Antiseizure drug **Pharmacologic Class:** Succinimide, low-threshold calcium channel blocking drug

Actions and Uses: Ethosuximide is a preferred drug for absence (petit mal) seizures. It depresses the activity of neurons in the motor cortex by elevating the neuronal threshold. It is usually ineffective against psychomotor or tonic-clonic seizures; however, it may be given in combination with other medications that better treat these conditions. It is available in tablet and flavored syrup formulations.

Adverse Effects and Interactions: Ethosuximide may impair mental and physical abilities. Psychosis or extreme mood swings, including depression with suicidal intent, can occur. Behavioral changes are more prominent in patients with a history of psychiatric illness. CNS effects include dizziness, headache, lethargy, fatigue, ataxia, sleep pattern disturbances, attention difficulty, and hiccups. Bone marrow suppression and blood dyscrasias are possible, as is systemic lupus erythematosus.

Other reactions include gingival hyperplasia and tongue swelling. Common adverse effects are abdominal distress and weight loss.

Drug interactions include carbamazepine or oxycarbamazepine, which decrease ethosuximide serum levels. Using phenytoin together with ethosuximide may increase the effects of phenytoin. Valproic acid causes ethosuximide serum levels to fluctuate (increase or decrease). Serum drug levels should be done periodically to determine drug concentration.

Nursing Process Focus Patients Receiving Antiseizure Drug Therapy

ASSESSMENT	POTENTIAL NURSING DIAGNOSES*
Prior to administration: • Obtain a complete health history including cardiovascular, renal and liver conditions, growth and developmental patterns, allergies, drug history, and possible drug interactions. • Evaluate laboratory blood findings: complete blood count (CBC), chemistry, renal and liver function studies, and drug screening. • Acquire the results of a complete physical examination including vital signs, electrocardiogram (ECG) and neurological status (level of consciousness [LOC], mental status and identification of recent seizure activity, EEG results).	• *Noncompliance* related to length of time before medication reaches therapeutic levels and adverse effects of drug therapy • *Deficient Knowledge* related to a lack of information about disease process and drug therapy • *Ineffective Therapeutic Regimen Management* related to noncompliance with medication regimen, presence of adverse effects, and need for long-term medication use • *Risk for Injury* related to effects of seizure and adverse effects of drug therapy

PLANNING: PATIENT GOALS AND OUTCOMES

The patient will:

- Experience therapeutic effects (absence of or a reduction in the number or severity of seizures).
- Be free from or experience minimal adverse effects from drug therapy.
- Verbalize an understanding of the drug's use, adverse effects, and required precautions.

IMPLEMENTATION

Interventions and (Rationales)	Patient Education/Discharge Planning
• Monitor neurologic status, especially changes in LOC or mental status, including signs or expressions of suicide. (Sedation may indicate overmedication or an adverse effect. These medications may also cause suicidality.)	Instruct the patient to report to the healthcare provider: • Any significant change in sensorium, such as slurred speech, confusion, hallucinations, or lethargy. • Any changes in seizure quality or unexpected involuntary muscle movement such as twitching, tremor, or unusual eye movement. • Any thoughts or expressions of suicide.
• Protect the patient from injury during seizure events until the therapeutic effects of the drugs are achieved.	• Instruct the patient to avoid driving and other hazardous activities until the effects of the drug are known.
• Monitor the effectiveness of drug therapy. (Observe for developmental and neurologic changes; may indicate a need for dose adjustment.)	Instruct the patient to: • Keep a seizure diary to chronicle events during symptoms phase or during dose adjustment. • Take the medication exactly as prescribed, and use the prescribed drug produced by the same manufacturer each time the prescription is refilled. (Switching brands may result in alterations in seizure control.) • Take a missed dose as soon as remembered, but do not take double doses. (Doubling doses could result in toxic serum level.)

Interventions and (Rationales)	Patient Education/Discharge Planning
• Monitor laboratory tests for drug levels: CBC, renal, and liver function studies. (Many antiseizure medications require blood testing to ensure therapeutic levels are achieved and maintained. The tests are used to determine medication dosages. Some drugs can cause liver toxicity.)	• Instruct the patient about the importance of keeping all laboratory appointments.
• Monitor for adverse effects. Observe for hypersensitivity, nephrotoxicity, and hepatotoxicity.	• Instruct the patient to report adverse effects (specific to the drug regimen) immediately to the healthcare provider.
• Monitor oral health. Observe for signs of gingival hyperplasia, bleeding, or inflammation (phenytoin specific).	Instruct the patient to: • Use a soft toothbrush and oral rinses as prescribed by a dentist. • Avoid mouthwashes containing alcohol. • Report changes in oral health, such as excessive bleeding or inflammation of the gums. • Maintain a regular schedule of dental visits.
• Monitor GI status. (Valproic acid is a GI irritant and anticoagulant.) Conduct guaiac stool testing for occult blood. (Phenytoin's CNS depressant effects decrease GI motility, producing constipation.)	Instruct the patient to: • Take the drug with food to reduce GI upset. • Immediately report any severe or persistent heartburn, upper GI pain, nausea, or vomiting to the healthcare provider. • Increase exercise, fluid intake, and fiber intake to facilitate stool passage.
• Monitor nutritional status. (Phenytoin's action on electrolytes may cause decreased absorption of folic acid, vitamin D, magnesium, and calcium. Deficiencies in these vitamins and minerals lead to anemia and osteoporosis. Valproic acid may cause an increase in appetite and weight.)	Instruct the patient: • In dietary or drug administration techniques specific to prescribed medications. • To report significant changes in appetite or weight gain.
• Obtain information and monitor use of other medications. Antiseizure medications should not be used with CNS depressants or alcohol.	• Instruct the patient to report use of any medication to the healthcare provider. • Inform the patient not to drink alcohol while taking these medications.
• Administer medication correctly, and evaluate the patient's knowledge of proper administration. Do not abruptly stop providing medication and monitor for presence of seizures. (Abrupt withdrawal of drugs can cause seizures to occur.)	• Advise the patient not to discontinue medication abruptly. This action may result in status epilepticus.

EVALUATION OF OUTCOME CRITERIA

Evaluate effectiveness of drug therapy by confirming that patient goals and expected outcomes have been met (see "Planning"). *See Tables 14.2, 14.3, and 14.4 for a list of drugs to which these nursing actions apply.*

*Herdman, T.H. & Kamitsuru, S. (Eds.), *Nursing Diagnoses: Definitions & Classification* 2015–2017. Copyright © 2014, 1994–2014 NANDA International. Used by arrangement by John Wiley & Sons, Inc. Companion website: www.wiley.com/go/nursingdiagnoses.

Patients Need to Know

Patients taking antiseizure medications need to know the following:

In General

1. Never abruptly stop taking antiseizure medication; doing so can cause seizures to return.
2. Avoid alcohol and other CNS depressants because they can increase sedation.
3. Antiseizure medications may cause drowsiness; avoid driving and the use of machinery that could lead to injury.
4. It may require several dosage adjustments over many months to find the dosage that allows performance of normal daily activities while controlling seizures.
5. It is important to keep laboratory appointments because many antiseizure medications require blood testing to ensure that the drug is at a safe and effective level in the blood.
6. Antiseizure medication may reduce effectiveness of birth control.
7. Consult a healthcare provider before trying to become pregnant; some antiseizure medications are not safe to use during pregnancy.
8. Report excess fatigue, drowsiness, agitation, confusion, or suicidal thoughts to a healthcare provider.

Regarding Hydantoins and Related Medications

9. Report the following adverse effects to a healthcare provider: gum overgrowth (gingival hyperplasia), skin rash, tremors, weight gain, diarrhea, irregular menses, dizziness, nausea, or oversedation.

10. Hydantoins and related medications interact with many other drugs; do not add any other prescription, over-the-counter (OTC) drugs, or herbal supplements until a healthcare provider is consulted. Do not consume alcohol while taking these medications.

Regarding Succinimides

11. Report the following adverse effects to a healthcare provider: hiccups or epigastric pain with ethosuximide (Zarontin), drowsiness, or increased bleeding time.

Chapter Review

Core Concepts Summary

14.1 Although some types of seizures involve convulsions, others do not.

Epilepsy is any disorder characterized by more than two recurrent seizures. *Seizures* are abnormal and uncontrolled neuronal brain discharges. *Convulsions* are uncontrolled muscle contractions that accompany some major seizures. Drugs used to treat epilepsy are often referred to as *antiseizure drugs* or *antiepileptic drugs* (AEDs), rather than anticonvulsants.

14.2 Many causes of seizure activity are known; a few are not.

A seizure is considered a symptom of epilepsy rather than a disorder itself. In some cases, the exact cause of seizures is not known; however, there are many known causes. Seizures are the most common neurologic problem. Through a combination of pharmacotherapy, patient–family support, and education, effective seizure control can be achieved by most patients.

14.3 Epileptic seizures are typically identified as partial, generalized, or special epileptic syndromes.

Epilepsies are identified using the International Classification of Epileptic Seizures nomenclature, as partial (focal), generalized, or special epileptic syndromes. Partial seizures are further described as simple or complex seizures. Generalized seizures are described as absence seizures, atonic seizures, or tonic-clonic seizures. Special epileptic syndromes include febrile seizures, myoclonic seizures, and status epilepticus.

14.4 Effective seizure management involves strict compliance with safe drug therapy practices.

The choice of drug for epilepsy pharmacotherapy depends on the type of seizures the patient is experiencing, the patient's previous medical history, diagnostic studies, and the pathologic processes causing the seizures. In most cases, a single drug can effectively control seizures. In some patients, two antiseizure medications may be necessary. When discussing antiseizure medications, suicidality, developmental issues of children, birth control, and pregnancy are important topics for consideration.

14.5 Antiseizure pharmacotherapy is directed at controlling the movement of electrolytes across neuronal membranes or affecting neurotransmitter balance.

There are three general mechanisms by which antiseizure drugs work: stimulating an influx of chloride ions (an effect associated with the neurotransmitter GABA), delaying an influx of sodium, and delaying an influx of calcium. Antiseizure drugs are represented by these and possibly additional overlapping mechanisms: blocking of the excitatory neurotransmitter, glutamate, and delaying an efflux of potassium ions across neuronal membranes.

14.6 By increasing the effects of gamma-aminobutyric acid (GABA) in the brain, some drugs reduce a wide range of seizure types.

Some antiseizure drugs mimic the effects of GABA by stimulating an influx of chloride ions. Drugs may bind directly to the GABA receptor, enhance GABA release, block the reuptake of GABA into nerve cells and glia, or inhibit GABA degrading enzymes. Barbiturates, benzodiazepines, and recently-approved GABA-related drugs reduce seizure activity by potentiating GABA action.

14.7 Hydantoin and related drugs are generally effective in treating partial seizures and tonic-clonic seizures.

This class of drugs depresses CNS activity by desensitizing sodium channels and also by affecting the threshold of neuronal firing. Several widely used drugs, including phenytoin (Dilantin), carbamazepine (Tegretol), and valproic acid (Depakene), work by this mechanism. Some drugs act by more than one mechanism. Additional antiseizure drugs may be used alone in therapy or as adjunctive drugs.

14.8 Succinimides generally treat absence seizures.

Succinimides delay entry of calcium into neurons by blocking calcium channels, increasing the electrical threshold, and reducing the likelihood that an action potential will be generated. Ethosuximide (Zarontin) is the most commonly prescribed drug in this class.

REVIEW Questions

Answer the following questions to assess your knowledge of the chapter material, and go back and review any material that is not clear to you.

1. A young woman with a diagnosed seizure disorder asks the nurse about getting pregnant. In planning her response, the nurse knows that most antiseizure medications fall under which pregnancy category?
   1. A
   2. B
   3. C
   4. D

2. The patient on phenytoin (Dilantin) asks why she must have her laboratory tests checked. Your best response would be:
   1. "Dilantin can cause problems with the blood's plasma."
   2. "You will need to ask your doctor."
   3. "We are checking to make sure you are getting enough but not too much medication."
   4. "We must see if you are developing any adverse effects of the medication."

3. The patient on antiseizure medication wants to know how long he or she must take the medication before being cured. Your best response would be:
   1. "You should be totally seizure free in 1 to 2 weeks."
   2. "We may need to add additional medications before you are cured."
   3. "It may take up to 3 years before you are cured."
   4. "The goal of therapy is to control seizure activity."

4. A patient who has had repeated tonic-clonic seizures is admitted to the hospital. He has had a history of status epilepticus. In preparation for the possibility that status epilepticus may happen again, the nurse will have which drug available to terminate this serious type of seizure?
   1. Diazepam (Valium)
   2. Gabapentin (Neurontin)
   3. Clorazepate (Tranxene)
   4. Clonazepam (Klonopin)

5. The nurse is reviewing a patient's chart and reads that the patient experienced a generalized seizure involving alternating contractions and relaxation of the muscles. The nurse knows that this phase of the seizure is called the ______ phase.
   1. Absence
   2. Clonic
   3. Febrile
   4. Myoclonic

6. One of the most common adverse effects of the recently developed antiseizure drugs is:
   1. Gastrointestinal upset.
   2. Spasms.
   3. Drowsiness.
   4. Dry mouth.

7. A nurse is teaching a patient the importance of taking the antiseizure medication, phenobarbital (Luminal), every day at the same time. She informs the patient not to take more of this medication than prescribed because it may cause: (Select all that apply.)
   1. Severe respiratory depression.
   2. Coma.
   3. Confusion.
   4. Death.
   5. Tachycardia.

8. The nurse collects data on a patient taking ethosuximide (Zarontin) for which of the following possible adverse effects?
   1. Urinary dysfunction
   2. Gingival hyperplasia
   3. Tremors
   4. Depression

9. The nurse monitors for the occurrence of gingival hyperplasia for the patient who is taking which antiseizure medication?
   1. Valproic acid (Depakene)
   2. Carbamazepine (Tegretol)
   3. Phenytoin (Dilantin)
   4. Primidone (Mysoline)

10. The nurse checks a patient's phenytoin serum levels because, in addition to taking phenytoin, the patient is also taking:
    1. Ethosuximide (Zarontin).
    2. Phenobarbital (Luminal).
    3. Carbamazepine (Tegretol).
    4. Valproic acid (Depakene).

CASE STUDY Questions

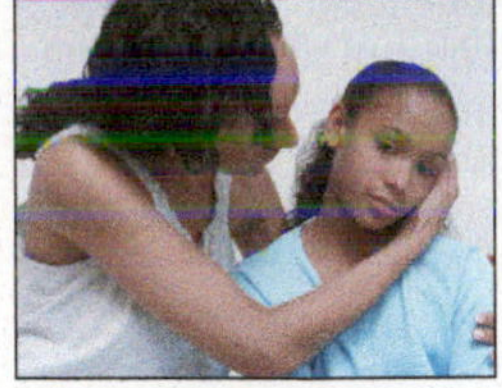

Remember Mrs. Anthonia and her daughter, Destiny, who were introduced at the beginning of the chapter? Now read the remainder of the case study. Based on the information you have learned in this chapter, answer the questions that follow.

Mrs. Kemi Anthonia and her 9-year-old daughter, Destiny, recently visited the family healthcare provider. Mrs. Anthonia was concerned that Destiny's development might be stunted. Several complaints were noted: "Destiny sometimes acts very unusually, like she is not paying attention . . . on occasion she is unresponsive and bats her eyes . . . this sometimes lasts for a few seconds and everything appears normal again . . . lately she has been waking up a lot during the night." After a complete neurologic exam and set of laboratory tests, the provider prescribed ethosuximide (Zarontin) for Destiny to be taken in gradually increased doses over 7 days and then for a sustained period at the same dose. The provider then scheduled a return visit to the clinic in 7 days.

1. The maintenance dose of ethosuximide is usually based on 20 mg/kg/day in divided doses. Destiny weighs 66 pounds. How many kg does she weigh? How many milligrams will she receive in a day? The nurse calculates the medication dosage and determines that Destiny weighs:
   1. 33 kg and will receive 600 mg/day.
   2. 30 kg and will receive 660 mg/day.
   3. 30 kg and will receive 600 mg/day.
   4. 30 kg and will receive 630 mg/day.
2. Mrs. Anthonia asks the nurse how ethosuximide (Zarontin) works to help her daughter's condition. The nurse replies that ethosuximide will:
   1. Enhance the release of a neurotransmitter called GABA, which suppresses the firing of neurons.
   2. Delay the amount of sodium going into the nerves, decreasing the ability of nerve impulses to travel.
   3. Delay the entry of calcium into nerves keeping them from firing too quickly.
   4. Activate the receptors that receive the neurotransmitter GABA.
3. The nurse lets Mrs. Anthonia know that Destiny will need to return to the clinic to:
   1. Be reexamined because Destiny's medication has a high potential for dependence.
   2. Be reexamined because Destiny's medication can cause anemia.
   3. Check serum drug levels to determine the most effective drug concentration.
   4. Check the welfare of Destiny because her medication has a low margin of safety.
4. Which of the following medications, if prescribed for Destiny as a second medication, would cause ethosuximide (Zarontin) serum levels to fluctuate?
   1. Phenobarbital (Luminal)
   2. Diazepam (Valium)
   3. Pregabalin (Lyrica)
   4. Valproic acid (Depakene)

Answers and complete rationales for the Review and Case Study Questions appear in Appendix A.

REFERENCE

Herdman, T. H., & Kamitsuru, S. (Eds.). (2014). *NANDA International nursing diagnoses: Definitions and classification, 2015–2017*. Oxford, United Kingdom: Wiley-Blackwell.

SELECTED BIBLIOGRAPHY

Asconapé, J. J. (2014). Use of antiepileptic drugs in hepatic and renal disease. *Handbook of Clinical Neurology, 119*, 417–432. doi:10.1016/B978-0-7020-4086-3.00027-8

Borthen, I., & Gilhus, N. E. (2012). Pregnancy complications in patients with epilepsy. *Current Opinion in Obstetrics and Gynecology, 24*, 78–83. doi:10.1097/GCO.0b013e32834feb6a

Centers for Disease Control and Prevention. (2016). *Sudden unexpected death in epilepsy (SUDEP)*. Retrieved from http://www.cdc.gov/epilepsy/basics/sudep

Citizens United for Research in Epilepsy. (n.d.). *Epilepsy facts*. Retrieved from http://www.cureepilepsy.org/aboutepilepsy/facts.asp

Dalkara, S., & Karakurt, A. (2012). Recent progress in anticonvulsant drug research: Strategies for anticonvulsant drug development and applications of antiepileptic drugs for non-epileptic central nervous system disorders. *Current Topics in Medicinal Chemistry, 12*, 1033–1071. doi:10.2174/156802612800229215

DiFilippo, T., Parisi, L., & Roccella, M. (2012). Evaluation of creative thinking in children with idiopathic epilepsy (absence epilepsy). *Minerva Pediatrica, 64*(1), 7–14.

Faught, E. (2011). Ezogabine: A new angle on potassium gates, *Epilepsy Currents, 11*, 75–78. doi:10.5698/1535-7511-11.3.75

Foreman, B., & Hirsch, L. J. (2012). Epilepsy emergencies: Diagnosis and management. *Neurologic Clinics, 30*, 11–41. doi:10.1016/j.ncl.2011.09.005

Hirsch, L. J. (2012). Intramuscular versus intravenous benzodiazepines for prehospital treatment of status epilepticus. *New England Journal of Medicine, 366*, 659–660. doi:10.1056/NEJMe1114206

Levy, R. G., Cooper, P. N., Giri, P., & Weston, J. (2012). Ketogenic diet and other dietary treatments for epilepsy. *Cochrane Database of Systematic Reviews, 3*, Art. No.: CD001903. doi:10.1002/14651858.CD001903.pub2

National Institute of Neurologic Disorders and Stroke. (2015). *Febrile seizures fact sheet.* Retrieved at http://www.ninds.nih.gov/disorders/febrile_seizures/detail_febrile_seizures.htm

Oja, S. S., & Saransaari, P. (2013). Taurine and epilepsy. *Epilepsy Research, 104*, 187–194. doi:10.1016/j.eplepsyres

Pizzol, A. D., Martin, K. C., Mattiello, C. M., de Souza, A. C., Torres, C. M., Bragatti, J. A., & Bianchin, M. M. (2012). Impact of the chronic use of benzodiazepines prescribed for seizure control on the anxiety levels of patients with epilepsy. *Epilepsy and Behavior, 23*, 373–376. doi:10.1016/j.yebeh.2011.12.009

Schachter, S. C., Kossoff, E., & Sirven, J. (2013). *Ketogenic diet*. Retrieved from http://www.epilepsy.com/learn/treating-seizures-and-epilepsy/dietary-therapies/ketogenic-diet

Shafer, P. O., & Sirven, J. I. (2014). *Facts about seizures and epilepsy*. Retrieved from http://www.epilepsy.com/learn/epilepsy-101/facts-about-seizures-and-epilepsy

Veiby, G., Daltveit, A. K., Schjølberg, S., Stoltenberg, C., Øyen A., Vollset, S. E. . . . Gilhus, N. E. (2013). Exposure to antiepileptic drugs in utero and child development:A prospective population-based study. *Epilepsia, 54*, 1462–1472. doi:10.1111/epi.12226

Wang, H. R., Woo, Y. S., & Bahk, W. M. (2014). Anticonvulsants to treat post-traumatic stress disorder. *Human Psychopharmacology, 29*, 427–433. doi:10.1002/hup.2425

Chapter 15

Drugs for Pain Management

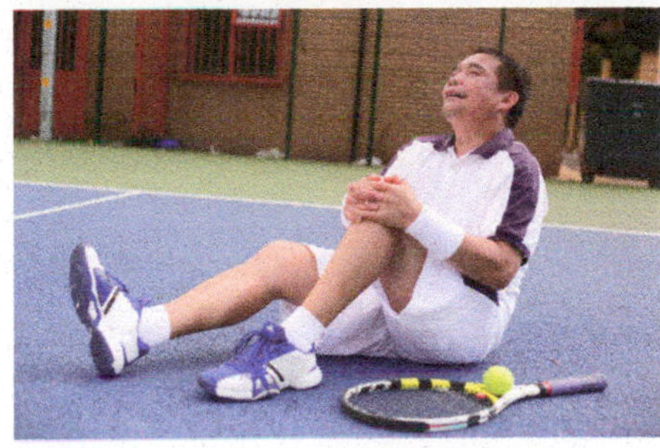

"I was playing tennis and it just popped. How many more months is this going to hurt?"

Mr. Aki Kimura

Core Concepts

15.1 **Pain assessment is the first step to pain management.**

15.2 **Pain transmission processes allow several major targets for pharmacologic intervention.**

15.3 **Nonpharmacologic techniques and adjuvant analgesics assist in providing adequate pain relief.**

15.4 **Opioid analgesic medications exert their effects by interacting with specific receptors.**

15.5 **Opioids have multiple therapeutic effects, including relief of severe pain.**

15.6 **Nonsteroidal anti-inflammatory drugs (NSAIDs) are the preferred nonopioid analgesics for inflammation and less severe pain.**

15.7 **Migraines can be effectively treated with a variety of drug classes.**

Drug Snapshot

The following drugs are discussed in this chapter:

Drug Classes	Prototype Drugs
Opioid Analgesics for Severe Pain	
Opioid agonists	Pr morphine (Astramorph PF, Duramorph, others)
Opioid antagonists	Pr naloxone (Evzio, Narcan)
Opioids with mixed agonist–antagonist activity	
Nonopioid Analgesics for Moderate Pain	
Nonsteroidal anti-inflammatory drugs (NSAIDs)	
Aspirin and other salicylates	Pr aspirin (acetylsalicylic acid, ASA)
Ibuprofen and similar drugs	
Selective COX-2 inhibitors	
Centrally acting drugs	
Antimigraine and Tension Headache Drugs	
Triptans	Pr sumatriptan (Imitrex)
Ergot alkaloids	
Other drugs	

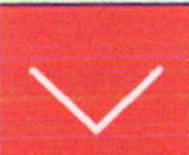

Learning Outcomes

After reading this chapter, the student should be able to:

1. Relate the importance of pain assessment to effective pharmacotherapy.
2. Explain the neural mechanism for pain processing, including the involvement of spinal neurotransmitters.

3. Describe the supportive roles of nonpharmacologic therapies and adjuvant analgesics in pain management.
4. Compare and contrast the types of opioid receptors and their importance to pharmacotherapy.
5. Explain the role of opioids in the management of severe pain, and describe the treatment of acute opioid toxicity as well as the long-term treatment of opioid dependence.
6. Identify representative drugs used in the management of less severe pain and explain their mechanisms of drug action, primary actions, and important adverse effects.
7. Discuss the pharmacotherapeutic approaches to preventing and aborting migraines

Key Terms

Aδ fibers
adjuvant analgesics (ADD-jeh-vent an- ul-JEE-ziks)
analgesics
auras (AUR-uhs)
bradykinin (bray-dee-KYE-nin)
C fibers
cyclooxygenase (COX) (sye-klo-OK-sah-jen-ays)
endogenous opioids (en-DAHJ-en-nuss O-pee-oyds)
migraine (MYE-grayne)
narcotic (nar-KOT-ik)
nociceptor (no-si-SEPP-ter)
opiates (OH-pee-ahts)
opioid (OH-pee-oyd)
patient-controlled analgesia (PCA) (an-ul-JEE-ziah)
prostaglandins (pros-tah-GLAN-dins)
substance P
tension headache

Pain is a physiological and emotional experience characterized by unpleasant feelings, usually associated with a medical procedure, trauma, or disease. On a basic level, pain has always been described as a defense mechanism that helps the body avoid a potentially dangerous situation. Pain is a natural reaction prompting patients to seek medical help. Although the neural and chemical mechanisms for pain are well characterized, psychological and emotional processes can alter pain perception. Anxiety, fatigue, and depression can increase the perception of pain; positive attitudes and support from caregivers can reduce the perception of pain. Patients are more likely to tolerate their pain if they know its source and the course of medical treatment necessary to manage it.

ACUTE OR CHRONIC PAIN

The purpose of pain assessment is to guide the appropriate course of medical treatment. Pain can be characterized as acute or chronic. Acute pain is an intense pain occurring over a brief time, usually from the time of injury until tissue repair. This may happen over several weeks. Chronic pain is longer lasting pain that may persist for 6 months or more. Chronic pain can interfere with activities of daily living (ADLs) and contribute to feelings of helplessness or hopelessness.

Core Concept 15.1 ▶

Pain assessment is the first step to pain management.

noci = *pain or injury*
ceptor = *receiver*

somatic = *referring to the body*

visceral = *deeper organ*

The psychological reaction to pain is a subjective experience. The same degree and type of pain may be described as excruciating and unbearable by one patient and not even be mentioned by another patient. Often the healthcare provider will simply ask, "How does your pain feel on a scale of zero to ten, ten being the most intense pain you have ever experienced?" Successful pain management depends on an accurate assessment of both the degree and the source of pain experienced by the patient. Pain assessment scales are important diagnostic tools for assessing the initial severity and quality of pain experienced by patients. Examples of pain assessment scales for adults are the Visual Analog Scale for Pain (VAS Pain), the Numeric Rating Scale for Pain (NRS Pain), and the McGill Pain Questionnaire (MPQ). Other scales assess pain in children, and there are even tools to assess pain in patients with dementia or other debilitating conditions. Numeric scales and survey instruments further help healthcare providers measure the progress of pain management.

Besides being termed *acute* or *chronic*, pain can also be described by its source. Injury to *tissues* produces *nociceptor pain*. This type of pain may be further subdivided into *somatic pain*, which produces sharp, localized sensations in the body, or *visceral pain*, which produces generalized dull and internal throbbing or aching pain. The term **nociceptor** refers to activation of receptor nerve endings that receive and transmit pain signals to the central nervous system (CNS). *Neuropathic pain* is caused by direct injury to the nerves. Whereas *nociceptor* pain responds quite well to conventional pain relief medications, *neuropathic* pain responds less successfully. Common types of neuropathic pain are shown in Table 15.1.

neur(o) = *nerve-related*
algia = *pain*
path(y) = *damage or disease state*
ic = *related to*

trigeminal = *fifth cranial nerve (tri = three branches; geminal = matching face)*

Table 15.1 Common Types of Neuropathic Pain

Examples	Description
Carpal tunnel syndrome	pain due to nerve compression in the wrist, thumb, and fingers
Central pain syndrome	general pain caused by damage of nerves in the CNS—that is, due to stroke or multiple sclerosis
Degenerative disk disease	back pain due to damage of nerves entering or exiting the spinal cord
Diabetic neuropathy	burning or stabbing pain in the hands and feet of patients suffering from diabetes
Intractable cancer pain	pain due to progressive or metastatic spread of cancer
Phantom limb pain	pain occurring in some patients after a limb is amputated
Postherpetic neuralgia	pain brought on by herpes and herpes-related viruses or the outbreak of shingles
Postsurgical pain	pain after a surgical procedure
Sciatica	leg pain due to compression or irritation of the sciatic nerve
Trigeminal neuralgia	shooting pain in the upper neck and jaw

CONCEPT REVIEW 15.1

- What questions would you ask to identify a patient's type of pain? How would you distinguish between acute pain and chronic pain? Which is the more difficult type of pain to treat?

Pain transmission processes allow several major targets for pharmacologic intervention.

◀ **Core Concept 15.2**

The process of pain transmission begins when nociceptors are stimulated. Nociceptors are free nerve endings located throughout the entire body. The nerve impulse signaling the pain is sent to the spinal cord along two types of sensory neurons, called Aδ and C fibers. **Aδ fibers** are sensory neurons that are thinly wrapped in myelin, a fatty substance that speeds up nerve transmission and signals sharp, well-defined pain. **C fibers** are *unmyelinated* fibers; thus, they carry nerve impulses more slowly and conduct dull, poorly localized pain.

Fast Facts **Pain**

- Pain is a common symptom.
- Approximately 52.5 million people experience debilitating symptoms associated with chronic arthritis, lupus, and fibromyalgia.
- At least 31 million adults report low back pain, with 19 million people experiencing this on a chronic basis.
- Over 40% of adults experience muscle pain each year.
- Greater than 50% of people with cancer have reported moderate to severe pain. Cancer pain is often undertreated.
- About 38 million Americans suffer from headaches and migraines.
- Use of drug therapy and other measures controls 95% of migraines.
- After puberty, women have four to eight times more migraines than men.
- Before puberty, more boys have migraines than girls.
- Headaches and migraines occur mostly among people ages 20 to 40.
- Persons with a family history of headache or migraine have a greater chance of developing these disorders.

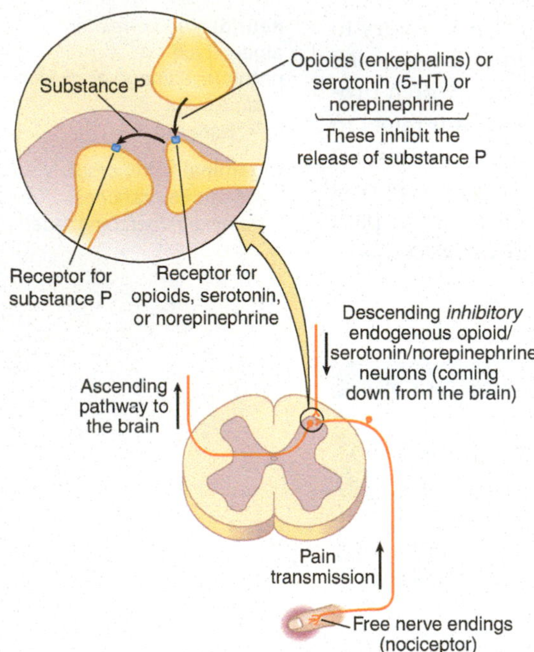

FIGURE 15.1 Neural pathways for pain.

endo = *within*
genous = *coming from*

Once pain impulses reach the spinal cord, neurotransmitters pass the message along to the next neuron. Here, a neurotransmitter called **substance P** is thought to be responsible for continuing the pain message, although other neurotransmitter candidates have been proposed. Spinal substance P is critical because it controls whether pain signals will continue to the brain. The activity of substance P may be affected by other neurotransmitters released from neurons in the CNS. One group of these neurotransmitters, called **endogenous opioids**, includes endorphins, dynorphins, and enkephalins. Figure 15.1 shows one point of contact where endogenous opioids modify sensory information at the level of the spinal cord. If pain impulses reach the brain, many possible actions may occur, ranging from immediate reaction to the stimulus, persistent aching and suffering, or thoughts of mental depression if the pain signal is repetitive and long-lasting.

Because pain signals begin at nociceptors located within peripheral body tissues and then proceed throughout the CNS, there are several targets where medications can work to stop pain transmission. In general, two major classes of drugs are employed to manage pain: opioid analgesics and nonopioid analgesics such as the nonsteroidal anti-inflammatory drugs (NSAIDs). Opioids act within the CNS, whereas NSAIDs act at the nociceptor level. There are multiple sites throughout the CNS where centrally acting drugs can produce their effects, and there are many peripheral targets as well, depending on the approach to drug therapy.

CONCEPT REVIEW 15.2

- What is a nociceptor? Consider substance P and endogenous opioids, and describe the approaches of pain management.

Core Concept 15.3 ▶

Nonpharmacologic techniques and adjuvant analgesics assist in providing adequate pain relief.

somno = *drowsiness or sleepiness*
lence = *state of*

Although drugs are quite effective at relieving pain in most patients, they can have significant adverse effects. For example, at high doses, opioids can cause nausea, constipation, loss of appetite, and profound somnolence, and aspirin can cause gastrointestinal (GI) bleeding.

To help patients obtain adequate pain relief, nonpharmacologic techniques are often used as an essential form of adjunctive therapy. Rarely will nonpharmacologic techniques be used in place of pharmacotherapy, but when used together with medication, they allow doses to be lowered. Lowered doses typically mean fewer drug-related adverse effects. Some nonpharmacologic techniques employed for reducing pain include the following:

- Physical therapy
- Massage
- Biofeedback therapy
- Heat or cold packs
- Meditation or prayer
- Counseling
- Relaxation therapy
- Art or music therapy
- Imagery
- Chiropractic manipulation
- Hypnosis
- Therapeutic touch
- Transcutaneous electrical nerve stimulation (TENS)
- Energy therapies such as reiki and qigong
- Acupuncture.

Nonpharmacologic techniques can help improve the patient's mood, reduce anxiety, and provide the patient with a sense of control. They often relax muscles, strengthen coping abilities, and generally improve the patient's quality of life. There are many determinants of successful therapy depending on the type, duration, and severity of pain. Success will also vary from patient to patient and will depend on many factors, including the patient's age, attitude, tolerance, and level of compliance with overall therapy. The patient's coping skills, capabilities, and commitment will play a role in both pain management and recovery. Costs of healthcare, availability of support from family members, and support from members within the surrounding community are extremely important.

Patients with challenging or *intractable* (not easy to relieve) pain may require additional therapy. In this case, **adjuvant analgesics** or *co-analgesics* may be used. Antiseizure drugs (Chapter 14) and local anesthetics (Chapter 16) are examples of drug categories approved by the U.S. Food and Drug Administrtion (FDA) for successful management of pain. Carbamazepine (Tegretol) is approved for treatment of pain due to trigeminal neuralgia. Valproic acid (Depakene) and derivatives are approved for the treatment of pain due to migraines. Gabapentin (Neurontin) is prescribed for the management of postherpetic neuralgia. Pregabalin (Lyrica) is approved for treatment of fibromyalgia, postherpetic neuralgia, pain due to peripheral diabetic neuropathy, and chronic pain syndrome. All these drugs were originally developed to treat conditions other than pain, but now have found useful application in pain management. Anesthetic nerve blocking drugs are another type of adjuvant analgesic used for the management of acute and chronic pain, and are administered in a variety of ways for different purposes. Lidoderm, for example, is a local anesthetic patch with 5% lidocaine applied to intact skin in order to reduce difficult pain. It is also used for postsurgical and postherpatic neuralgia pain (Chapter 16). Corticosteroids reduce inflammation and can also control certain types of inflammatory pain (Chapter 25). Topical capsaicin treats neuralgia by promoting temporary neurolysis (disruption of signal transmission due to the destruction of pain nerve fibers). Following cessation of drug therapy, reinnervation (reconnection of the nerve supply) occurs within several weeks.

in = *opposite of*
tractable = *control*

neuro = *nerve*
lysis = *disruption (breaking apart)*

re = *again*
in = *incoming*
nervation = *nerve supply*

Many medications are appropriately used for pain management, even though the FDA has not specifically approved them for a particular use. Some well-established *off-label medications* for pain management are the tricyclic antidepressants (TCAs) (Chapter 11). Examples are amitriptyline, desipramine, imipramine, and nortriptyline, which have been used to suppress a variety of pain impulses characterized as chronic and neuropathic. Neuropathic pain impulses are even slowed by dysrhythmic drugs when TCAs are not effective. Thus, cardiovascular drugs have also found a place in pain management. Examples are mexiletine and flecainide (Chapter 23).

Opioid analgesic medications exert their effects by interacting with specific receptors.

◄ **Core Concept 15.4**

Analgesics are medications used to relieve pain. The two basic categories of analgesics are the opioids (narcotics) and the nonopioids. Terminology for the narcotic analgesics may be confusing. Several of these drugs are obtained from opium, a milky extract from the unripe seeds of the poppy plant, which contains more than 20 different chemicals having pharmacologic activity. Opium consists of 9% to 14% morphine and 0.8% to 2.5% codeine. These natural substances are called **opiates**. In a search for safer analgesics, chemists have created several dozen synthetic drugs with activity similar to that of the opiates. For example, morphine is a natural narcotic; meperidine is a synthetic narcotic. **Opioid** is a general term referring to any of these substances, natural or synthetic, and is often used interchangeably with the term *opiate*. An opioid analgesic is a natural or synthetic morphine-like substance responsible for reducing moderate to severe pain. Opioids are narcotic substances, meaning that they produce numbness or stupor-like symptoms.

an = *without*
algesia = *pain*

narc = *numbness or stupor*
otic = *like*

opi = *opium*
oid = *shape or form*

Narcotic is a general term often used to describe opioid drugs that produce analgesia and CNS depression. In common usage, a narcotic analgesic is the same as an opioid, and the terms are often used interchangeably. In the context of law enforcement, however, the term *narcotic* describes a much broader range of abused drugs such as hallucinogens, heroin, amphetamines, and marijuana. This is an important fact to remember when discussing use of opioids with members of law enforcement.

Table 15.2 Responses Produced by Activation of Specific Opioid Receptors

Response	Mu Receptor	Kappa Receptor
Analgesia	✓	✓
Decreased GI motility	✓	✓
Euphoria (elated feelings)	✓	
Miosis (constricted pupils)		✓
Physical dependence	✓	
Respiratory depression	✓	
Sedation	✓	✓

eu = *well (true)*
phoria = *bearing (carrying of self)*

affective = *expressive*

Opioids exert their actions by interacting with at least four major types of receptors: mu, kappa, delta, and an opioid-like receptor called nociceptin or orphanin FQ peptide. For pain management, the *mu receptors* and *kappa receptors* have been the ones traditionally targeted. Delta receptors also have a role in analgesia; they are connected with the emotional and affective components of the pain experience and as such have become recent targets for drug development.

Body responses produced by activation of mu and kappa receptors are listed in Table 15.2. Some opioids, such as morphine, activate both mu and kappa receptors. Opioid blockers such as naloxone (Narcan) inhibit both the mu and kappa receptors. Other opioids, such as pentazocine (Talwin), exert mixed effects by activating the kappa receptors and blocking the mu receptors. Having a variety of receptor subtypes is the body's way of providing a diverse set of responses to substances circulating in the bloodstream. Figure 15.2 illustrates actions resulting from stimulation of mu and kappa receptors.

CONCEPT REVIEW 15.3

- Distinguish between the following terms: opioid, opiate, and narcotic. Name four classes of opioid receptors, and identify those that are connected with analgesia.

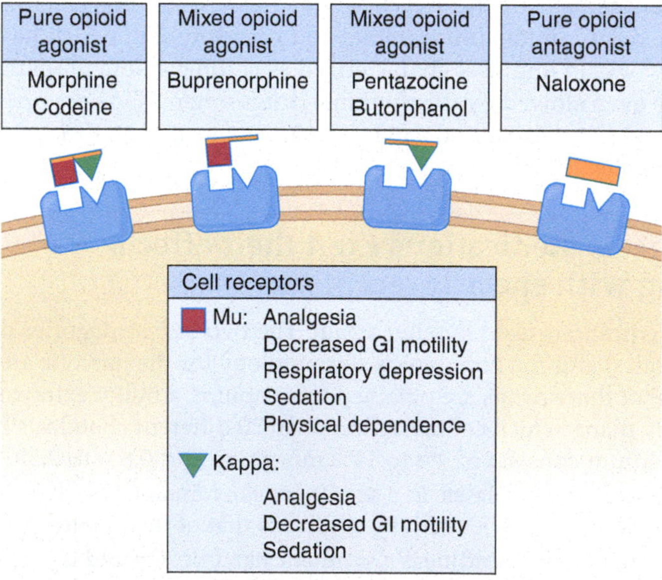

FIGURE 15.2 Opioid receptors.

OPIOID ANALGESICS FOR SEVERE PAIN

Core Concept 15.5 ▶

Opioids have multiple therapeutic effects, including relief of severe pain.

Opioids are drugs for moderate to severe pain that cannot be controlled with other classes of analgesics. Narcotic opioids bind to opioid receptors and produce multiple responses throughout the body. As powerful CNS depressants, opioid narcotics cause sedation, which may be a therapeutic effect or an adverse effect, depending on the patient's condition. Some

Table 15.3 Opioids for Pain Management

Drug	Route and Adult Dose	Remarks
OPIOID AGONISTS WITH HIGH EFFECTIVENESS		
fentanyl (Abstral, Actiq, Duragesic, Fentora, Lazanda, Onsolis, Others)	IM: 0.05–0.1 mg Transdermal: 25–100 mcg every 72 hours	Used with anesthesia for surgery and other procedures; also available by the buccal, sublingual, and nasal spray routes.
hydromorphone (Dilaudid, Exalgo)	PO: 1–4 mg every 4–6 hours prn	Also for cough; available by IM, IV, subcutaneous, and rectal routes.
levorphanol (Levo-Dromoran)	PO: 2–3 mg tid to qid prn	Also available by subcutaneous route.
meperidine (Demerol)	PO: 50–150 mg every 3–4 hours prn	For preoperative medication or obstetric analgesia; available by IM, IV, and subcutaneous routes.
methadone (Dolophine)	PO: 2.5–10 mg every 3–4 hours prn	For detoxification treatment of opioid dependency; available by IM and IV routes.
Pr morphine (Astramorph PF, Duramorph, others)	PO: 10–30 mg every 4 hours prn	Available in IM, IV, subcutaneous, intrathecal, epidural, and rectal forms.
oxymorphone (Opana)	Subcutaneous/IM: 1–1.5 mg every 4–6 hours prn; 5 mg every 4–6 hours prn	Also available by IV and rectal routes.
OPIOID AGONISTS WITH MODERATE EFFECTIVENESS		
codeine	PO: 15–60 mg qid	Also for cough; available by IM and subcutaneous routes; combination drug with aspirin is Empirin codeine; combination drug with acetaminophen is Tylenol with codeine.
hydrocodone (Hycodan)	PO: 5–10 mg every 4–6 hours prn (max: 15 mg/dose)	Also for cough; combination drug with acetaminophen is Vicodin.
oxycodone (OxyContin, Oxecta); oxycodone terephthalate (Percocet-5, Roxicet, others)	PO: 5–10 mg qid prn Controlled release; 10–20 mg every 12 hours	Combination drug with acetaminophen is Percocet or Roxicet; combination with aspirin is Percodan.
OPIOID ANTAGONISTS		
Pr naloxone (Evzio, Narcan)	IV: 0.4–2 mg, may be repeated every 2–3 min up to 10 mg if necessary Intranasal: one spray in each nostril	For opioid overdose and postoperative opioid depression.
naltrexone (ReVia, Vivatrol)	PO: 25 mg followed by another 25 mg in 1 hour if no withdrawal response (max: 800 mg/day)	For management of opiate or alcohol dependence; longer lasting effect than naloxone.
OPIOIDS WITH MIXED AGONIST–ANTAGONIST EFFECTS		
buprenorphine (Buprenex, Butrans, Suboxone)	IM/IV: 0.3 mg every 6 hours (max: 0.6 mg every 4 hours)	For moderate to severe pain; also available by subcutaneous, sublingual, epidural, and rectal routes.
butorphanol (Stadol)	IM: 1–4 mg every 3–4 hours prn (max: 4 mg/dose)	For obstetrical analgesia during labor, cancer pain, renal colic, and burns; available by IV and intranasal routes.
nalbuphine (Nubain)	Subcutaneous/IM/IV: 10–20 mg every 3–6 hours prn (max: 160 mg/day)	For moderate to severe pain.
pentazocine (Talwin Nx, Talwin)	PO: 50–100 mg every 3–4 hours (max: 600 mg/day); subcutaneous/IM/IV: 30 mg every 3–4 hours (max: 360 mg/day)	For moderate to severe pain (much lower dose for women in labor).

patients experience euphoria and intense relaxation, which are reasons why opiates are sometimes abused. There are many adverse effects, including respiratory depression, sedation, nausea, constipation, and vomiting. More than 20 different opioids are available as medications, and they can be classified by similarities in their chemical structures, by their mechanisms of action, or by their effectiveness. The most useful method is by effectiveness, which places opiates into categories of high or moderate narcotic activity (Table 15.3).

Opioid Agonists

Drugs that stimulate a particular opioid receptor are called *opioid agonists*. Morphine is the prototype opioid agonist used to treat severe pain. It is usually the standard by which the effectiveness of other opioids is compared.

All of the opioid agonists have the potential to cause physical and psychological dependence, as discussed in Chapter 8. Over the years, healthcare providers have been hesitant to administer the proper amount of opioid analgesic for fear of causing patient dependence or of producing serious adverse effects such as sedation or respiratory depression. Because of this tendency, some patients have not received complete pain relief.

When used according to accepted medical practice, patients can, and indeed should, receive the pain relief they need without fear of addiction or adverse effects. One method available to accomplish this is **patient-controlled analgesia (PCA)**. Patients are allowed to self-administer opiate medication by pressing a button on an infusion pump. The nurse programs the infusion pump so that the prescribed dose is available to the patient. If the patient attempts to self-administer the drug too often, this will not be possible due to settings established by the nurse.

The fentanyl transdermal system (Duragesic patch) is another strong prescription medication used for the control of moderate to severe chronic pain. The patch enables longer-lasting relief from persistent pain. Fentanyl (Lazanda) nasal spray is available for quick delivery across nasal mucous membranes. Fentanyl is also administered as a lozenge (Oralet, Actiq), as a tablet (Fentora, Onsolis), or in a sublingual (Abstral) form. Patients should be cautioned not to chew oral medications. They are designed to dissolve slowly in the mouth and absorb across mucous membranes of the digestive tract. Buccal fentanyl is indicated for the management of difficult pain in adult patients who are already receiving and who might already be tolerant of traditional opioid therapy. Transmucosal opioid medications should be monitored closely as they may cause serious harm or death if ingested accidentally by a child or by an adult who does not have a high level of tolerance to opioids. Respiratory depression and fatal overdose are risks.

Alfentanil (Alfenta), remifentanil (Ultiva), and sufentanil (Sufenta) are used to provide continuous pain relief during and after surgery or during the induction and maintenance of general anesthesia; these are discussed further in Chapter 16.

Prototype Drug: Pr *Morphine (Astramorph PF, Duramorph, Others)*

Therapeutic Class: Opioid analgesic **Pharmacologic Class:** Opioid agonist receptor drug

Actions and Uses: Morphine binds with both mu and kappa receptor sites to produce strong analgesia. It causes euphoria, constriction of the pupils, and stimulation of cardiac muscle. It is used for relief of serious acute and chronic pain after nonnarcotic analgesics have failed, as preanesthetic medication, to relieve shortness of breath associated with heart failure and pulmonary edema, and for acute chest pain connected with myocardial infarction (MI).

Adverse Effects and Interactions: Morphine may cause hypotension, dysphoria (restlessness, depression, and anxiety), hallucinations, nausea, constipation, dizziness, and an itching sensation. Overdose may result in severe respiratory depression or cardiac arrest. Tolerance develops to the analgesic, sedative, and euphoric effects of the drug. Cross-tolerance also develops between morphine and other opioids such as heroin, methadone, and meperidine. Physical and psychological dependence develop when high doses are taken for prolonged periods. Morphine may intensify or mask the pain of gallbladder disease.

Morphine interacts with many drugs. For example, use with CNS depressants, such as alcohol, other opioids, general anesthetics, sedatives, and antidepressants such as monoamine oxidase inhibitors (MAOIs) and TCAs, increases the action of opiates and thereby raises the risk of severe respiratory depression and death.

Use with caution with herbal supplements, such as yohimbine, which may increase the effect of morphine.

BLACK BOX WARNING:
When morphine is administered as an epidural drug, due to the risk of adverse effects, patients must be observed in a fully equipped and staffed environment for at least 24 hours. Preparations for epidural administration must be preservative free. Morphine administered as extended-release tablets has an abuse liability similar to other opioid analgesics. It is a Schedule II controlled substance and should be taken according to dispensing instructions (i.e., tabletsand capsules should be taken whole and not broken, chewed, dissolved, or crushed). Alcohol should be avoided with morphine products (e.g., Avinza). Failure to follow these warnings could result in fatal respiratory depression.

syn = *together*
erg = *work*
istically = *ability to*

In the pharmacologic management of pain, it is common practice to combine opioids and nonnarcotic analgesics into a single tablet or capsule (Core Concept 15.6). The two classes of analgesics work *synergistically* to relieve pain, and the dose of narcotic can be kept small to avoid dependence and opioid-related adverse effects. Examples of combination analgesics are as follows:

- Vicodin (hydrocodone, 5 mg; acetaminophen, 300 mg)
- Percocet (oxycodone HCl, 2.5 mg or 5 mg or 7 mg; acetaminophen, 325 mg)
- Percodan (oxycodone HCl, 4.5 mg; oxycodone terephthalate, 0.38 mg; aspirin, 325 mg)
- Empirin with Codeine No. 2 (codeine phosphate, 15 mg; aspirin, 325 mg)
- Ascomp with Codeine or Fiorinal (codeine phosphate, 30 mg; aspirin, 325 mg; caffeine, 40 mg; butalbital, 50 mg)

- Fioricet with Codeine (codeine phosphate, 30 mg; acetaminophen, 325 mg; caffeine, 40 mg; butalbital, 50 mg)
- Tylenol with Codeine (single dose may contain from 15 to 60 mg of codeine phosphate and from 300 to 325 mg of acetaminophen).

Some opioids are used primarily for conditions other than pain relief. Codeine is often prescribed as a cough suppressant and is covered in Chapter 30. Opiates used to treat diarrhea are presented in Chapter 31.

Opioid Antagonists

Drugs that block an opioid receptor are called *opioid antagonists*. Opioid antagonists are substances that prevent the effects of opioid agonists. These drugs are considered *competitive antagonists* because they compete with opioid agonists for access to the opioid receptor site.

Opioid overdose can occur as a result of overly aggressive pain therapy or substance abuse. Any opioid may be abused for its psychoactive effects; however, morphine, meperidine, and heroin are sometimes preferred because of their potency. Although heroin is currently available as a legal analgesic in many countries, it is considered by the FDA to be too dangerous for therapeutic use and is a major drug of abuse. Once injected or inhaled, heroin rapidly crosses the blood–brain barrier to enter the brain, where it is metabolized to morphine. Thus, the effects and symptoms of heroin use are actually caused by the activation of mu and kappa receptors by morphine. The initial effect is an intense euphoria, called a *rush*, followed by several hours of deep relaxation.

Opioid antagonists are often used to reverse the symptoms of opioid toxicity or overdose. Symptoms of overdose include sedation or respiratory distress. Acute opioid intoxication is a medical emergency, with respiratory depression being the most serious problem. Infusion with the opioid antagonist naloxone (Evzio, Narcan) may be used to reverse respiratory depression and other acute symptoms. Narcan is administered via subcutaneous, intravenous, or intramuscular injection and by the intranasal route. Naltrexone mixed with morphine (Embeda ER) is used for chronic severe pain control when a continuous, round-the-clock opioid analgesic is needed for an extended period. Embeda ER is administered by the oral route. In cases in which the patient is unconscious or unclear as to which drug has been taken, opioid antagonists may be given to diagnose the overdose. If the opioid antagonist fails to quickly reverse the acute symptoms, the overdose may be attributed to a nonopioid substance.

Prototype Drug: Pr *Naloxone (Evzio, Narcan)*

Therapeutic Class: Drug for treatment of acute opioid overdose and misuse **Pharmacologic Class: Opioid receptor blocker**

Actions and Uses: Naloxone is a pure opioid antagonist, blocking both mu and kappa receptors. It is used for complete or partial reversal of opioid effects in emergency situations when acute opioid overdose is suspected. Given intravenously, it begins to reverse opioid-initiated CNS and respiratory depression within minutes. It will immediately cause opioid withdrawal symptoms in patients physically dependent on opioids. It is also used to treat postoperative opioid depression (after-effect of the opioid therapy applied during surgery). In 2014 the FDA approved Evzio, which is a hand-held autoinjector containing naloxone. The device is to be used by caregivers or family members when an opioid overdose is suspected. Since reversal of opioid effects in the body is often short-lived, naloxone may need to be readministered. Naloxone is pregnancy category B.

Adverse Effects and Interactions: Naloxone itself has minimal toxicity. However, in reversing the effects of opioids, the patient may experience rapid loss of analgesia (immediate return of pain), increased blood pressure, tremors, hyperventilation, nausea, vomiting, and drowsiness.

Drug interactions include a reversal of the analgesic effects of narcotic agonists and agonist–antagonists. Any drug in the opioid family should not be taken with naloxone. Do not take naloxone with yohimbine; tremors, nervousness, and anxiety may result. Naloxone reverses the central depressant effects of ethyl alcohol.

BLACK BOX WARNING:
None; however, naltrexone, a similar opioid receptor antagonist, has the capacity to produce hepatic injury when taken in excessive doses or if taken by patients with hepatic injury or acute liver disease.

Opioids with Mixed Agonist–Antagonist Effects

Narcotic opioids stimulate the opioid receptor; thus, they cause analgesia. *Tolerance* develops relatively quickly to the euphoric and pain-relieving effects of opioids; therefore, users tend to request increased doses or take the drugs more frequently. Tolerance means the patient's reaction to the drug is reduced, requiring higher doses to achieve the same effect. Opioid agonists also have a greater risk for *dependence* than most of the other classes of medications. Dependence is an adaptive state that develops from repeated drug administration. (Concepts of *tolerance* and *dependence* were introduced in Chapter 8.) When the patient stops takings opioids or if the dose is suddenly reduced, *withdrawal symptoms* may develop, including chills, sweating, nausea, vomiting, diarrhea, restlessness, joint and muscle pain, and insomnia. Recall that withdrawal symptoms are a sign of *physical dependence*. Beyond this, the intense craving that characterizes *psychological dependence* may occur in patients for many months, even years, following discontinuation of opioids. Withdrawal symptoms with mixed agonist–antagonists are not as intense due to partial activation of the different receptor subtypes. Thus, prescribing mixed agonist–antagonists has been one method of decreasing opiate use in opioid dependent patients.

The well-known approach for treating opioid dependence has been to switch the patient from IV and inhalation forms of opioid drugs to oral methadone (Dolophine). Although oral methadone is an opioid, it does not cause the euphoria of the injectable opioids. Methadone also does not cause relief of dependency, and the patient must continue taking the drug to avoid withdrawal symptoms. This therapy, called *methadone maintenance*, may continue for many months or years, until the patient decides to enter a total withdrawal treatment program. Methadone maintenance allows the patient to return to productive work and social relationships without the physical, emotional, or criminal risks of inappropriate drug use. One caution is that methadone overdose can cause respiratory depression or death.

An alternative treatment approach is to administer buprenorphine (Buprenex, Butrans, Suboxone), a mixed opioid agonist–antagonist, by the sublingual or transdermal route. Buprenorphine is used early in opioid abuse therapy to prevent opioid withdrawal symptoms. Suboxone contains both buprenorphine and naloxone and is used later in the maintenance of opioid addiction.

Healthcare providers should always be aware that when administering mixed agonist–antagonists with opioid agonists, their pain-blocking properties are reduced. Thus, there may be a tendency to overprescribe mixed opioids, promoting drug misuse. This is true even though in most cases mixed agonist–antagonists drugs are prescribed to reduce opioid dependency.

Nursing Process Focus Patients Receiving Opioids

ASSESSMENT	POTENTIAL NURSING DIAGNOSES*
Prior to administration: • Obtain a complete health history including cardiovascular, respiratory, neurological, renal and liver conditions, allergies, drug history, likelihood of drug dependency, and possible drug interactions. • Evaluate complaints of pain (quality, intensity, location, duration). • Acquire the results of a complete physical examination including vital signs and electrocardiogram (ECG). • Evaluate laboratory blood findings: complete blood count (CBC), chemistry, renal and liver function studies, and drug screening. • Determine neurological status (level of consciousness [LOC], mental status, and identification of recent mood and behavior patterns).	• *Deficient Knowledge* related to a lack of information about drug therapy • *Acute or Chronic Pain* related to injury, disease process, surgical procedure, or inadequate medication • *Ineffective Breathing Pattern* related to adverse effects of drug therapy • *Constipation* related to adverse effect of drug therapy • *Risk for Injury* related to adverse effects of drug therapy

PLANNING: PATIENT GOALS AND EXPECTED OUTCOMES

The patient will:
- Experience therapeutic effects (report of pain relief or a reduction in pain intensity).
- Be free from or experience minimal adverse effects from drug therapy.
- Verbalize an understanding of the drug's use, adverse effects, and required precautions.

IMPLEMENTATION

Interventions and (Rationales)	Patient Education/Discharge Planning
• Monitor the use of opioids. (Opioids are Schedule II controlled substances and can produce both physical and psychological dependence.)	• Inform the patient and caregivers to take necessary steps to safeguard drug supply and to avoid sharing medications with others.

Interventions and (Rationales)	Patient Education/Discharge Planning
• Administer medication correctly and evaluate the patient knowledge of proper administration. (Depending on the drug, they may be administered PO, subcutaneously, IM, IV, or epidural. Combining opioids with some medications or food items may be contraindicated.)	Instruct the patient: • That oral *capsules* may be opened and mixed with cool foods; extended-release *tablets*, however, may not be chewed, crushed, or broken. • That the oral solution for taking sublingually may be more concentrated than the solution for swallowing. • To not use opioids concurrently with other medications (including herbal therapies) without consulting the healthcare provider.
• Monitor laboratory liver function studies. (Opioids are metabolized in the liver. Hepatic disease can increase blood levels of opioids to toxic levels.)	Instruct the patient to: • Report to healthcare provider the following symptoms: nausea; vomiting; diarrhea; rash; jaundice; abdominal pain, tenderness, or distention; or change in color of stool. • Comply with the laboratory testing regimen for liver function as ordered by the healthcare provider.
• Monitor vital signs, especially depth and rate of respirations and pulse oximetry. Withhold the drug if the patient's respiratory rate is below 12, and notify the healthcare provider. Keep resuscitative equipment and a narcotic antagonist such as naloxone (Narcan) accessible. (Opioid antagonists may reverse respiratory depression, increase LOC, and reverse other symptoms of narcotic overdose.)	Instruct the patient to: • Monitor vital signs regularly, particularly respirations. • Withhold medication for any difficulty in breathing or respirations below 12 breaths per minute; report symptoms immediately to the healthcare provider.
• Perform neurologic checks regularly. Especially monitor for changes in LOC or seizure activity. (Decreased LOC and sluggish pupillary response may occur with high doses, and the drug may increase intracranial pressure.)	Instruct the patient to: • Report headache or any significant change in sensorium, such as an aura or other visual effects that may indicate an impending seizure to the healthcare provider. • Recognize seizures and methods to ensure personal safety during a seizure. • Report any seizure activity immediately.
• If ordered prn, administer the medication upon the patient's request or when nursing observations indicate expressions of pain by the patient.	Instruct the patient to: • Alert the nurse immediately upon the return or increase of pain. • Notify the healthcare provider regarding the drug's effectiveness.
• Monitor renal status and urinary output. (Opioids may cause urinary retention, which may exacerbate existing symptoms of benign prostatic hypertrophy.)	Instruct the patient to: • Measure and monitor fluid intake and output. • Report symptoms of dysuria (hesitancy, pain, diminished stream), changes in urine quality, or scanty urine output to the healthcare provider. • Report fever or flank pain that may be indicative of a urinary tract infection.
• Monitor for other adverse effects such as restlessness, dizziness, anxiety, depression, hallucinations, nausea, and vomiting. (Hives or itching may indicate an allergic reaction due to the production of histamine. Depression, anxiety, and hallucinations may indicate overdose.)	Instruct the patient to: • Recognize adverse effects and symptoms of an allergic or anaphylactic reaction. • Immediately report to the healthcare provider any shortness of breath, tight feeling in the throat, itching, hives or other rash, feelings of dysphoria, nausea, or vomiting. • Avoid the use of sleep-inducing over-the-counter (OTC) antihistamines without first consulting the healthcare provider.
• Monitor for constipation. (Drug slows peristalsis.)	Instruct the patient to: • Maintain adequate fluid and fiber intake to facilitate stool passage. • Use a stool softener or laxative as recommended by the healthcare provider.
• Ensure patient safety. Monitor ambulation until response to the drug is known. (Drug can cause sedation and dizziness.)	Instruct the patient to: • Request assistance when getting out of bed. • Avoid driving or performing hazardous activities until effect of the drug is known.

(*Continued*)

Nursing Process Focus (*continued*)

Interventions and (Rationales)	Patient Education/Discharge Planning
• Monitor frequency of requests and stated effectiveness of narcotic administered. (Opioids cause tolerance and dependence.)	Instruct the patient: • Regarding cross-tolerance issues. • To monitor medication supply and observe for hoarding, which may signal an impending suicide attempt. • Who is suffering from a terminal illness about the issue of drug dependence as related to reduced life expectancy.

EVALUATION OF OUTCOME CRITERIA

Evaluate the effectiveness of drug therapy by confirming that patient goals and expected outcomes have been met (see "Planning"). *See Table 15.3 for a list of drugs to which these nursing actions apply.*

NONOPIOID ANALGESICS FOR MODERATE PAIN

Core Concept 15.6 ▶ **Nonsteroidal anti-inflammatory drugs (NSAIDs) are the preferred nonopioid analgesics for inflammation and less severe pain.**

The nonopioid analgesics include NSAIDs and a few centrally acting drugs, including acetaminophen. The role of the NSAIDs in the treatment of inflammation and fever is discussed more thoroughly in Chapter 25. Therefore, there is only brief mention here. Table 15.4 highlights the more common nonopioid analgesics.

Table 15.4 Nonopioid Analgesics

Drug	Route and Adult Dose	Remarks
NSAIDS: ASPIRIN AND OTHER SALICYLATES		
Pr aspirin (acetylsalicylic acid, ASA)	PO: 350–650 mg every four hours (max: 4 g/day)	Also for fever, inflammation, and thromboembolic disorders, prevention of transient ischemic attacks and heart attacks; rectal form available
salsalate (Disalcid)	PO: 325–3000 mg daily in divided doses (max: 4 g/day)	Also for fever, inflammation
NSAIDS: IBUPROFEN AND SIMILAR DRUGS		
diclofenac (Cambia, Cataflam, Voltaren XR, Zipsor)	PO: 50 mg bid to qid (max: 200 mg/day)	Also for inflammation
diflunisal	PO: 1000 mg followed by 500 mg bid to tid	Also for inflammation
etodolac	PO: 200–400 mg tid to qid	Also for inflammation
fenoprofen (Nalfon)	PO: 200 mg tid to qid (max 3200 mg/day)	Also for inflammation
flurbiprofen (Ansaid, Ocufen)	PO: 50–100 mg tid to qid (max: 300 mg/day)	Similar to ibuprofen
ibuprofen (Advil, Motrin, others)	PO: 400 mg tid to qid (max: 1200 mg/day)	Also for fever and inflammation
indomethacin (Indocin, Tivorbex)	PO: 25–50 mg bid or tid (max: 200 mg/day) or 75 mg sustained release one to two times/day	Also for moderate to severe rheumatoid arthritis and acute gouty arthritis
ketoprofen	PO: 12.5–50 mg tid to qid	Also for inflammation
ketorolac (Acular, Sprix, Toradol)	PO: 10 mg qid prn (max: 40 mg/day)	Also for allergic conjunctivitis, available by IM/IV and nasal spray routes
mefenamic acid (Ponstel)	PO: Loading dose 500 mg, maintenance dose 250 mg every 6 hours prn	Used for short-term relief of mild to moderate pain, including menstrual cramps
meloxicam (Mobic)	PO: 7.5 mg daily (max: 15 mg/day)	Used for osteoarthritis
nabumetone (Relafen)	PO: 1000 mg daily (max: 2000 mg/day)	Inhibits COX-2 more than COX-1
naproxen (Naprosyn, Naprelan)	PO: 500 mg followed by 200–250 mg tid to qid (max: 1000 mg/day)	Also for inflammation
naproxen sodium (Aleve, Anaprox, others)	PO: 250–500 mg bid (max: 1000 mg/day naproxen)	Also for dysmenorrhea
oxaprozin (Daypro)	PO: 600–1200 mg daily (max: 1800 mg/day)	Similar to naproxen; once-a-day dosage
piroxicam (Feldene)	PO: 10–20 mg daily to bid (max: 20 mg/day)	Has prolonged half-life

Drug	Route and Adult Dose	Remarks
sulindac (Clinoril)	PO: 150–200 mg bid (max: 400 mg/day)	Also for inflammation
tolmetin (Tolectin)	PO: 400 mg tid (max: 2 g/day)	Also for inflammation
NSAIDS: SELECTIVE COX-2 INHIBITORS		
celecoxib (Celebrex)	PO: 100–200 mg bid or 200 mg/daily	Also for inflammation
CENTRALLY ACTING DRUGS		
acetaminophen (Tylenol) (see the Prototype Drug box in Core Concept 25.6)	PO: 325–650 mg every 4–6 hours (max: 3000 mg/day)	Also for fever; available in rectal form; centrally acting COX inhibitor
tramadol (Ultram)	PO: 50–100 mg every 4–6 hours prn (max: 400 mg/day), may start with 25 mg/day and increase by 25 mg every 3 days up to 200 mg/day	Causes less respiratory depression than morphine
ziconotide (Prialt)	Intrathecal; 0.1 mcg/h via infusion, may increase by 0.1 mcg/h every 2–3 days (max: 0.8 mcg/h)	Also for muscle spasticity

Nonsteroidal Anti-Inflammatory Drugs (NSAIDs)

NSAIDs are drugs for mild to moderate pain, especially for pain associated with inflammation. NSAIDs inhibit **cyclooxygenase**, an enzyme responsible for the formation of **prostaglandins**. When cyclooxygenase is inhibited, inflammation and pain are reduced. These drugs have many advantages over the opioids because they have antipyretic, anti-inflammatory, and analgesic properties.

The NSAIDs act by inhibiting pain mediators at the nociceptor level. When tissue is damaged, local chemical mediators are released: histamine, potassium ion, hydrogen ion, bradykinin, and prostaglandins. **Bradykinin** is associated with sensory impulses of pain. Prostaglandins prompt pain through the formation of free radicals.

mediators = *middle drugs*

brady = *slow*
kinin = *movement*

syn = *together*
thesis = *put*

Popular NSAIDs available OTC are aspirin and ibuprofen. Ibuprofen and related medications are available in many different formulations, including those designed for children. Most are safe and well tolerated by patients when used at low to moderate doses. Higher and more prolonged doses produce hepatoxicity, which is a major concern with these classes of drugs (Chapter 25). High-dosage use of ibuprofen in particular can result in chronic kidney disease and chronic interstitial nephritis. Patients with pre-existing conditions should speak with their healthcare provider prior to use.

After tissue damage, prostaglandins are formed with the help of two enzymes called *cyclooxygenase type 1 (COX-1)* and *cyclooxygenase typ. 2 (COX-2)*. Aspirin and ibuprofen-related drugs inhibit both COX-1 and COX-2. Thus, *nonselective COX inhibition* is the basis of NSAID therapy. COX inhibition is also responsible for many of the side effects associated with NSAIDs related to kidney disease, bleeding, and ulcers. They have been linked with higher risk for cardiovascular events. Patients who have had recent cardiovascular surgery should not take NSAIDs.

Because the COX-2 enzyme is more specific for the synthesis of inflammatory prostaglandins, *selective COX-2 inhibition* provides a more focused peripheral pain relief. Celecoxib (Celebrex) is one of the COX-2 inhibitors still available in the United States; others been discontinued. Figure 15.3 illustrates the mechanism of pain transmission at the nociceptor level.

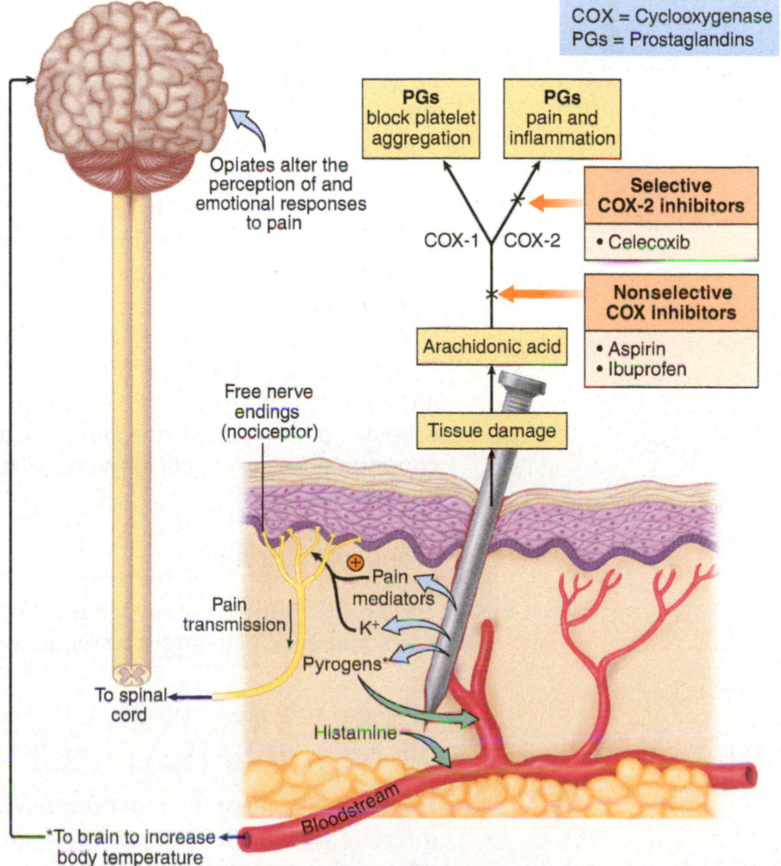

FIGURE 15.3 Mechanisms of pain at the nociceptor level.

Prototype Drug: Pr Aspirin (Acetylsalicylic Acid, ASA)

Therapeutic Class: Nonopioid analgesic, nonsteroidal anti-inflammatory drug (NSAID), antipyretic drug for myocardial infarction prophylaxis and transient ischemia **Pharmacologic Class:** Salicylate, cyclooxygenase (COX) inhibitor, prostaglandin synthesis inhibitor, platelet aggregation inhibitor

Actions and Uses: Aspirin inhibits prostaglandin synthesis involved in the processes of pain and inflammation and produces mild to moderate relief of fever. It has limited effects on peripheral blood vessels, causing vasodilation and sweating. Aspirin has significant anticoagulant activity, and this property is responsible for its ability to reduce the risk of mortality following MI and to reduce the incidence of strokes. Aspirin has also been found to reduce the risk of colorectal cancer, although the mechanism by which it affords this protective effect is unknown.

Adverse Effects and Interactions: At high doses, such as those used to treat severe inflammatory disorders, aspirin may cause gastric discomfort and bleeding because of its antiplatelet effects. Hepatotoxicity, is also a concern, especially in patients with pre-existing liver disease. Enteric-coated tablets and buffered preparations are available for patients who experience GI adverse effects.

Because aspirin increases bleeding time, it should not be given to patients receiving anticoagulant therapy such as warfarin, heparin, and plicamycin. ASA may increase the action of oral hypoglycemic drugs. Effects of NSAIDs, uricosuric drugs such as probenecid, beta blockers, spironolactone, and sulfa drugs may be decreased when combined with ASA.

Use with phenobarbital, antacids, and glucocorticoids may decrease ASA effects. Insulin, methotrexate, phenytoin, sulfonamides, and penicillin may increase effects. When taken with alcohol, pyrazolone derivatives, steroids, or other NSAIDs, there is an increased risk for gastric ulcers.

Use with caution with herbal supplements, such as feverfew, which may increase the risk of bleeding.

Centrally Acting Drugs

Centrally acting drugs are drugs that exert effects directly within the brain and spinal cord. Any analgesic drug that has a *central effect* bypasses the nociceptor level. Acetaminophen is a centrally acting nonopioid analgesic. Acetaminophen reduces fever by direct action at the level of the hypothalamus and causes dilation of peripheral blood vessels, enabling sweating and dissipation of heat. It is the primary alternative to NSAIDs when patients cannot take aspirin or ibuprofen. Acetaminophen does not produce GI bleeding or ulcers and it does not exhibit cardiotoxicity. In January 2011, the FDA announced that it was asking manufacturers of oral prescription acetaminophen combination products to limit the maximum amount of acetaminophen products to 325 mg per tablet, capsule, or other dosage unit, with the exception of IV injection. The FDA believed this would reduce the risk of severe liver injury from acetaminophen overdosing, an adverse event that can lead to liver failure, liver transplant, and death.

The safety profile of acetaminophen is excellent when administered in proper therapeutic doses. Aspirin and acetaminophen have similar efficacies in relieving pain and reducing fever. Acetaminophen is featured as a prototype drug for the treatment of fever in Chapter 25.

Tramadol (Ultram) and ziconotide (Prialt) are additional centrally acting analgesics. Of the two drugs, tramadol is the more widely prescribed. Tramadol has weak opioid activity, although it is not thought to relieve pain by this mechanism. Its main action is to inhibit reuptake of norepinephrine and serotonin in spinal neurons. Tramadol is well tolerated, but common adverse effects are vertigo, dizziness, headache, nausea, vomiting, constipation, and lethargy.

CONCEPT REVIEW 15.4

- Think about cyclooxygenase inhibitors (NSAIDs) and prostaglandins, and then describe how pain might be regulated at the nociceptor.

TENSION HEADACHES AND MIGRAINES

Headache is one of the most common complaints of patients. Living with headaches can interfere with ADLs and can cause great distress. Pain and difficulty may result in work-related absences and neglect of home and family life. When headaches are persistent, or as migraines occur, drug therapy is needed.

New Drug Focus

CGRP DRUGS TREAT MIGRAINE ATTACKS.

A new class of experimental drugs designed specifically for migraine attacks is aimed at a compound called calcitonin gene-related peptide (CGRP). CGRP is a natural neurotransmitter found within axon terminals located throughout the nervous system. It has potent vasodilator properties. When migraine attacks start, CGRP levels increase at nerve endings in areas such as the jaw and in the saliva. CGRP monoclonal antibodies bind to CGRP and prevent sensitization of nerves innervating the jaw and scalp region. Thus, this new treatment is different from the triptans and ergotamines that many migraine sufferers rely upon today. Administered as once-monthly injections, monoclonal antibodies block vasodilation, without having any vasoconstrictive properties. Since it is not known how blocking CGRP affects other organ functions in the longer term, this new class of drugs is still under Phase III clinical investigation.

Of the many types of headaches, the most common is the **tension headache**. It occurs when muscles of the head and neck tighten in response to stress. The tightness causes a steady and lingering pain. Although quite painful, tension headaches usually end when the stress is resolved. They are generally considered an annoyance rather than a medical emergency. Tension headaches are effectively treated with OTC analgesics such as aspirin, acetaminophen, or ibuprofen. More intense tension headaches may be treated with additional classes of drugs.

The most painful type of headache is the **migraine**, which is characterized by throbbing or pulsating pain, sometimes preceded by an aura similar to those that warn of a seizure (see Chapter 14). The **auras** of migraines are sensory cues, such as seeing jagged lines or flashing lights, or smelling, tasting, or hearing something strange. They let the patient know that a migraine attack is coming soon. Most patients with migraines also have nausea and vomiting. Triggers for migraines include nitrates and monosodium glutamate (MSG) found in many Asian foods, red wine, perfumes, food additives, cheese, chocolate, and aspartame (a sugar substitute). By avoiding these substances, some patients can prevent the onset of a migraine attack. Weather changes and missed medications can also prompt migraine attacks.

ANTIMIGRAINE AND TENSION HEADACHE DRUGS

Migraines can be effectively treated with a variety of drug classes.

◀ **Core Concept 15.7**

There are two primary goals for the pharmacologic management of migraines. The first is to prevent migraines from occurring (*prophylaxis*), and the second is to stop migraines in progress (*abortive therapy*). For the most part, the drugs used to stop migraines are different than those used for prophylaxis; nevertheless, drug therapy is most effective if begun before a migraine has reached a severe level. It is not unusual for pharmacotherapy for mild migraines to begin with acetaminophen or NSAIDs. If OTC analgesics are unable to stop the migraine, then more specific drugs will be necessary.

pro = *before*
phylaxis = *guarding*

The two major drug classes used to terminate migraines are the triptans and the ergot alkaloids; both stimulate receptors to serotonin also called *5-hydroxytryptamine* (5-HT). A variety of other drugs classes are also used to treat migraines. Antimigraine drugs are listed in Table 15.5.

Triptans

Triptans were introduced in the 1990s and are considered first line therapy for moderate to severe migraines. As possible agonists to the 5-HT receptor, these drugs constrict blood vessels in the brain. They are effective in stopping migraines with or without auras. The first of the triptans marketed in the United States was sumatriptan (Imitrex). Since 1993, more triptans were developed. Although oral forms of the triptans are the most convenient, patients

Table 15.5 Antimigraine Drugs

Drug	Route and Adult Dose	Remarks
TRIPTANS		
almotriptan (Axert)	PO: 6.25–12.5 mg, may repeat in 2 hours if necessary (max: two tablets/day)	May cause heart palpitations and rapid heartbeat
eletriptan (Relpax)	PO: 20–40 mg, may repeat in 2 hours if necessary (max: 80 mg/day)	May cause hypotension in older adult patients
frovatriptan (Frova)	PO: 2.5 mg, may repeat in 2 hours if necessary (max: 7.5 mg/day)	May cause chest pains and heart palpitations
naratriptan (Amerge)	PO: 1–2.5 mg, may repeat in 4 hours if necessary (max: 5 mg/day)	For termination of migraine; serotonin stimulator
rizatriptan (Maxalt)	PO: 5–10 mg, may repeat in 2 hours if necessary (max: 30 mg/day); 5 mg with concurrent propranolol (max: 15 mg/day)	May cause MI
Pr sumatriptan (Imitrex)	PO: 25 mg for one dose (max: 100 mg)	For termination of migraine; serotonin stimulator; subcutaneous and intranasal forms available
zolmitriptan (Zomig)	PO: 2.5–5 mg, may repeat in 2 hours if necessary (max: 10 mg/day)	For termination of migraine; serotonin stimulator
ERGOT ALKALOIDS		
dihydroergotamine mesylate (D.H.E. 45, Migranal)	IM: 1 mg, may be repeated at 1-hour intervals to a total of 3 mg (max: 6 mg/week)	For termination of migraine; also available as nasal spray; pregnancy category X; may be used in combination with low-dose heparin to prevent postoperative deep vein thrombosis
ergotamine tartrate (Ergostat), ergotamine with caffeine (Cafergot, Ercaf, others)	PO: 1–2 mg followed by 1–2 mg every 30 minutes until headache stops (max: 6 mg/day or 10 mg/week)	For termination of migraine; also available in sublingual, inhalant, or rectal forms; may cause physical dependence; pregnancy category X
ANTISEIZURE DRUGS		
topiramate (Topamax)	PO: Start with 25 mg/day, increase by 25 mg/week to effectiveness (max: 1600 mg/day)	Also for partial seizures; sugar-like chemical molecule; enhances the action of GABA
valproic acid (Depakene) (see the Prototype Drug box in Core Concept 14.7)	PO: 250 mg bid (max: 100 mg/day)	Also for absence seizures and mixed generalized types of seizures and mania
BETA-ADRENERGIC BLOCKERS		
atenolol (Tenormin) (see the Prototype Drug box in Core Concept 21.6)	PO: 25–50 mg daily (max: 100 mg/day)	Also for hypertension and angina
metoprolol (Lopressor)	PO: 50–100 mg daily bid (max: 450 mg/day)	Also for angina and MI; sustained-release and IV forms available
propranolol (Inderal, InnoPran XL) (see the Prototype Drug box in Core Concept 23.7)	PO: 80–240 mg/day in divided doses, may need 160–240 mg/day	Beta-adrenergic blocker for migraine prevention
timolol (Betimol, Timoptic, others) (see the Prototype Drug box in Core Concept 38.5)	PO: 10 mg bid, may increase to 60 mg/day in two divided doses	Also for hypertension, angina, and glaucoma
CALCIUM CHANNEL BLOCKERS		
nifedipine (Adalat CC, Procardia XL) (see the Prototype Drug box in Core Concept 19.9)	PO: 10–20 mg tid (max: 180 mg/day)	Also for hypertension and angina; selective for calcium channels in blood vessels; decreases peripheral vascular resistance and increases cardiac output; sustained-release form available
nimodipine (Nimotop)	PO: 60 mg every 4 hours for 21 days; start therapy within 96 hours of subarachnoid hemorrhage	Off-label use for migraines; primary use is for improvement of neurologic symptoms following a stroke
verapamil (Calan, Isoptin SR, others) (see the Prototype Drug box in Core Concept 23.9)	PO: 40–80 mg tid	Off-label use for migraine prevention
TRICYCLIC ANTIDEPRESSANTS		
amitriptyline (Elavil)	PO: 75–100 mg/day	Off-label use for migraine prevention
imipramine (Tofranil) (see the Prototype Drug box in Core Concept 11.3)	PO: 75–100 mg/day (max: 300 mg/day)	Also for alcohol or cocaine dependence; may cause cardiac dysfunction and abnormal blood cell count; may control bedwetting in children; available IM
protriptyline (Vivactil)	PO: 15–40 mg/day in three to four divided doses (max: 60 mg/day)	For symptoms of depression; few sedative qualities; causes increased heart rate

Drug	Route and Adult Dose	Remarks
MISCELLANEOUS DRUGS		
onabotulinumtoxin A (Botox)	IM: 155 units administered to muscles of the head and neck area	Direct-acting antispasmodic drug for muscle spasms and spasticity
methysergide (Sansert)	PO: 4–8 mg/day in divided doses	Similar to ergotamine; for migraine prevention
riboflavin (vitamin B_2)	PO: as a supplement: 5–10 mg/day; for deficiency: 5–30 mg/day in divided doses	Deficiency caused by chronic diarrhea, liver disease, alcoholism, or inadequate consumption of milk or animal products

who experience unpleasant symptoms during a migraine, such as nausea and vomiting, may require an alternate dosage form. Intranasal formulation and prefilled syringes of triptans are available for patients who are able to self-administer.

Ergot Alkaloids

For patients who are unresponsive to triptans, the ergot alkaloids have been used to terminate migraines. The actions of the ergot alkaloids have been known for a long time. The first purified alkaloid, ergotamine (Ergostat), was isolated from the ergot fungus in 1920. Ergotamine is an inexpensive drug that is available in oral, sublingual, and suppository forms. Modification of the original molecule has produced another useful drug, dihydroergotamine (Migranal). Dihydroergotamine is given parenterally and as a nasal spray. Because the ergot alkaloids interact with adrenergic and dopaminergic receptors as well as serotonin receptors, they produce multiple actions and adverse effects such as tachycardia or bradycardia, nausea, vomiting, muscle pain and stiffness, peripheral constriction (leg weakness, numbness or tingling), lack of urination, and hypertension. Many ergot alkaloids are pregnancy category X drugs.

Other Antimigraine and Tension Headache Drugs

Drugs for migraine prophylaxis include various classes of drugs that are discussed in other chapters of this textbook. These include antiseizure drugs (Chapter 14), beta-adrenergic blockers (Chapter 23), calcium channel blockers (Chapter 19), antidepressants (Chapter 11), neuromuscular blockers (Chapter 13), and even a little caffeine found in some OTC products (Chapter 8). Because all these drugs have the potential to produce side effects, prophylaxis is initiated only if the incidence of migraines is high and the patient is unresponsive to the drugs used to abort migraines. Of the various drugs, the beta blocker propranolol (Inderal) is one of the most commonly prescribed. Amitriptyline, an antidepressant, is often prescribed for patients who suffer from insomnia in addition to migraines. In 2010, onabotulinumtoxinA (Botox) was approved for the treatment of chronic migraines when other medications were not successful. Botox inhibits neuromuscular transmission by blocking the release of acetylcholine from axon terminals innervating skeletal muscle. With this approach, IM injections are divided across specific muscles of the head and neck. When muscles are blocked, headaches due to intense muscle tension subside for a period of up to 3 months. More indications for Botox therapy are discussed in Chapter 13.

Prototype Drug: Pr *Sumatriptan (Imitrex)*

Therapeutic Class: Antimigraine drug **Pharmacologic Class:** Triptan, 5-HT (serotonin) receptor drug, vasoconstrictor of intracranial arteries

Actions and Uses: Sumatriptan, a triptan, belongs to a relatively new group of antimigraine drugs known as the triptans. The triptans act by causing vasoconstriction of cranial arteries; this vasoconstriction is moderately selective and does not usually affect overall blood pressure. This medication is available in oral, intranasal, and subcutaneous forms. Subcutaneous administration ends migraine attacks in 10 to 20 minutes; the dose may be repeated 60 minutes after the first injection to a maximum of two doses per day. If taken orally, sumatriptan should be administered as soon as possible after the migraine is suspected or has begun.

Adverse Effects and Interactions: Some dizziness, drowsiness, or a warming sensation may be experienced after taking sumatriptan; however, these effects are not normally severe enough to warrant stopping therapy. Because of its vasconstricting action, the drug can cause chest pressure and should be used cautiously, if at all, in patients with recent MI, or with a history of angina pectoris, hypertension, or diabetes.

Sumatriptan interacts with several drugs. For example, an increased effect may occur when taken with MAOIs and selective serotonin reuptake inhibitors (SSRIs). Further vasoconstriction can occur when taken with ergot alkaloids and other triptans.

Patients Need to Know

Patients taking pain medication need to know the following facts and recommendations:

In General

1. Carefully describe the type, duration, and extent of your pain to the healthcare provider so that the analgesic medication being taken is suited to the complaint.
2. Report any OTC medication taken for pain to your healthcare provider to minimize adverse effects and interactions.
3. Aspirin has many undesirable adverse effects mainly related to gastric upset and bleeding.
4. Follow instructions carefully and watch for drug interactions or contraindications.
5. Do not drink alcohol when taking acetaminophen because this may cause liver damage.

Regarding Opiates

6. Avoid combining pain medications with alcohol and other CNS depressants (especially opioids).
7. Vital signs should be monitored with all opioid medications because of their CNS depressant effects.
8. Get up slowly from seated positions because certain pain medications cause lightheadedness.
9. Avoid operating machinery or driving a car if taking opioids because dizziness, blurred vision, and drowsiness can occur.
10. Do not abruptly stop taking opioids; this could result in withdrawal. Signs include chills, abdominal and muscle cramps, severe itching, sweating, restlessness, anxiety, yawning, and drug-seeking behavior.

Chapter Review

Core Concepts Summary

15.1 Pain assessment is the first step to pain management.

Pain is a subjective experience in which many patients describe discomfort differently. Pain may be classified as acute (from injury to recovery) or chronic (longer than 6 months). Pain may be classified as nociceptor pain and further divided into somatic or visceral pain and neuropathic pain.

15.2 Pain transmission processes allow several major targets for pharmacologic intervention.

Pain signals involve nerve impulses along two types of sensory neurons, Aδ and C fibers. Once impulses reach the spinal cord, substance P is thought to transmit pain at the spinal level. The release of substance P is controlled by ganglia that release neurotransmitters called *endogenous opioids*. If not blocked, the impulse travels to the brain, where pain information is sensed and a response to the sensation is initiated. Opioids act at the level of the central nervous system (CNS); nonsteroidal anti-inflammatory drugs (NSAIDs) act at the level of the peripheral nervous system (PNS).

15.3 Nonpharmacologic techniques and adjuvant analgesics assist in providing adequate pain relief.

Nonpharmacologic techniques may be used in place of drugs or as adjunctive to drug therapy. When used along with medication, nonpharmacologic techniques may allow lower doses to be given with possibly fewer drug-related adverse effects. Other adjunctive approaches include FDA-approved antiseizure drugs, local anesthetics, and corticosteroids, which reduce inflammation and suppress pain in some cases. Off-label drug categories include TCAs and drugs for dysrhythmia.

15.4 Opioid analgesic medications exert their effects by interacting with specific receptors.

Different types of receptors mediate analgesia (pain relief)—mu receptors and kappa receptors are the most commonly targeted. Both are opioid receptors that respond to natural or synthetic morphine-like substances. Natural substances extracted from unripe seeds of the poppy plant are called *opiates*. *Narcotic* is a general term referring to morphine-like drugs. In the context of drug enforcement, the term *narcotic* includes a much broader classification of abused drugs.

15.5 Opioids have multiple therapeutic effects, including relief of severe pain.

Opioids produce many effects, including analgesia for intense pain, cough suppression, suppression of GI motility in diarrhea treatment, sedation, and euphoria. It is common practice to place opioids and nonnarcotic analgesics in a single tablet or capsule. Acute opioid intoxication is treated with the opioid antagonist naloxone. All of the narcotic analgesics have the potential to cause physical and psychological dependence. The opioids have a greater risk of dependency than most of the other classes of medications.

15.6 Nonsteroidal anti-inflammatory drugs (NSAIDs) are the preferred nonopioid analgesics for inflammation and less severe pain.

NSAIDs are nonopioid analgesics used to treat less severe pain associated with inflammation. NSAIDs have antifever and pain-reducing properties. These effects are achieved by inhibition of enzymes called cyclooxygenase type one (COX-1) and cyclooxygenase type two (COX-2). When cyclooxygenase (COX) is inhibited, prostaglandin synthesis is prevented. Only one medication is selective for the COX-2 receptor. Another nonopioid analgesic is acetaminophen, a centrally acting drug that treats fever.

15.7 Migraines can be effectively treated with a variety of drug classes.

Two categories of headaches—tension headaches and migraines—are the most common complaints of patients. The two primary goals of migraine therapy are migraine termination and migraine prevention. The two major classes of antimigraine drugs are ergot alkaloids and triptans. Drugs for migraine prophylaxis include beta-adrenergic blockers, calcium channel blockers, antidepressants, antiseizure drugs, and drugs for muscle tension.

REVIEW Questions

Answer the following questions to assess your knowledge of the chapter material, and go back and review any material that is not clear to you.

1. The patient has osteoarthritis. Which of the following drugs would the nurse anticipate being ordered for both pain and inflammation?
   1. Sumatriptan (Imitrex)
   2. Acetaminophen (Tylenol)
   3. Fentanyl (Sublimaze)
   4. Meloxicam (Mobic)

2. The patient is starting on sumatriptan (Imitrex) for migraines. For which of the following should the nurse instruct the patient to notify his or her healthcare provider immediately?
   1. Chest pressure
   2. Gastrointestinal upset
   3. Bleeding
   4. Lethargy

3. A patient is receiving an NSAID, so the nurse monitors the patient for:
   1. Gastrointestinal upset and bleeding.
   2. Urinary retention.
   3. Blurred vision.
   4. Anorexia.

4. The patient is experiencing opioid dependency. The nurse would expect which drug to be used to treat this condition?
   1. Oxycodone (OxyContin)
   2. Tramadol (Ultram)
   3. Hydromorphone (Dilaudid)
   4. Methadone (Dolophine)

5. When planning care for a patient in pain, the nurse understands that pain signals begin at the ______ and proceed through the central nervous system.
   1. Spinal cord
   2. Viscera
   3. Nociceptors
   4. Substance P

6. Prior to administering pain medication, the nurse obtained which of the following information about the patient's pain? (Select all that apply.)
   1. The patient's medical diagnosis
   2. The location of the pain
   3. When the patient last had a meal
   4. The severity of the pain
   5. A description of the pain such as dull or throbbing.

7. The patient has been receiving morphine for pain control. An evaluation of the patient reveals a decreased level of consciousness and shallow respirations at a rate of 8 per minute. The nurse anticipates what opioid antagonist being ordered?
   1. Butorphanol (Stadol)
   2. Hydrocodone (Hycodan)
   3. Naloxone (Narcan)
   4. Oxycodone (OxyContin)

8. Because a patient is allergic to aspirin, the nurse administers what drug as an alternative for relief of mild pain?
   1. Acetaminophen
   2. Morphine
   3. Etodolac
   4. Fentanyl

9. The nurse monitors for which of the following adverse effects of ergotamine (Ergostate)? (Select all that apply.)
   1. Tachycardia
   2. Nausea and vomiting
   3. Peripheral dilation
   4. Peripheral constriction
   5. Physical dependence

10. The healthcare provider orders ibuprofen 400 mg, PO, three times a day. The pharmacy sends ibuprofen suspension 200 mg/5 mL. How many milliliters should the patient receive in each dose?
    1. 2 mL
    2. 15 mL
    3. 5 mL
    4. 10 mL

CASE STUDY Questions

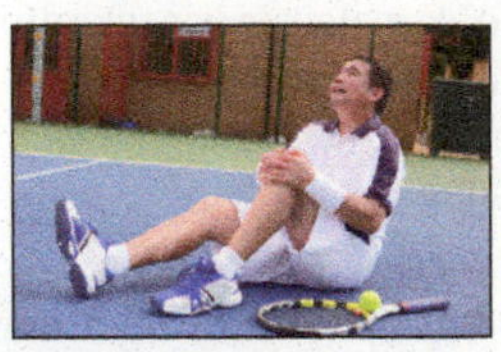

Remember Mr. Kimura, who was introduced at the beginning of the chapter? Now read the remainder of the case study. Based on the information you have learned in this chapter, answer the questions that follow.

Mr. Aki Kimura, age 48, sustained a knee injury 3 years ago, which responded well to treatment with NSAID medication. Over the last 6 months, Mr. Kimura has been seeing his healthcare provider again with complaints of "sharp painful sensations along the outer part of left knee" when he plays tennis or takes long walks. It appears that Mr. Kimura's pain is no longer responding to anti-inflammatory medication. His healthcare provider prescribes a narcotic analgesic (moderate effectiveness) with acetaminophen, hoping it might provide relief. Following three physical therapy sessions, and the new medication, Mr. Kimura reports that he is feeling better.

1. The nurse understands that when Mr. Kimura was given NSAIDs 3 years ago, the purpose was to: (Select all that apply.)
   1. Reduce pain.
   2. Reduce inflammation.
   3. Act within the CNS.
   4. Inhibit pain mediators at the nociceptors.

2. Which of the following narcotic analgesics would the nurse expect to give to Mr. Kimura?
   1. Percocet
   2. Talwin
   3. Dilaudid
   4. Demerol

3. Mr. Kimura asks the nurse why the healthcare provider put him on a narcotic that also contains acetaminophen. The nurse replies: (Select all that apply.)
   1. "The two medications work well together to decrease pain."
   2. "A lower dose of the narcotic can be used when combined with acetaminophen."
   3. "Because narcotics can have serious adverse effects, using a low dose of a narcotic can help minimize these effects."
   4. "Combining the two medication helps to lower the cost."

4. While providing Mr. Kimura with information about the use of narcotics, the nurse informs him to report which of the following adverse effects to his healthcare provider?
   1. Diarrhea
   2. Hallucinations
   3. Sedation
   4. Insomnia

Answers and complete rationales for the Review and Case Study Questions appear in Appendix A.

REFERENCE

Herdman, T. H., & Kamitsuru, S. (Eds.). (2014). *NANDA International nursing diagnoses: Definitions and classification, 2015–2017*. Oxford, United Kingdom: Wiley-Blackwell.

SELECTED BIBLIOGRAPHY

Agius, A. M., Jones, N. S., & Muscat, R. (2013). A randomized controlled trial comparing the efficacy of low-dose amitriptyline, amitriptyline with pindolol and surrogate placebo in the treatment of chronic tension-type facial pain. *Rhinology, 51*, 143–153.

American Chiropractic Association. (n.d.). *Back pain and statistics*. Retrieved from http://www.acatoday.org/Patients/Health-Wellness-Information/Back-Pain-Facts-and-Statistics

Burch, R. C., Loder, S., Loder, E., & Smitherman, T. A. (2015). The prevalence and burden of migraine and severe headache in the United States: Updated statistics from government health surveillance studies. *Headache: The Journal of Head and Face Pain, 55*, 21–34. doi:10.1111/head.12482

The Burden of Musculoskeletal Diseases in the United States. (2016). *Musculoskeletal diseases and the burden they cause in the United States*. Retrieved from http://www.boneandjointburden.org

Centers for Disease Control and Prevention. (2016). *Arthritis-related statistics*. Retrieved from http://www.cdc.gov/arthritis/data_statistics/arthritis-related-stats.htm

Finnerup, N. B., Attal, N., Haroutounian, S., McNicol, E., Baron, R., Dworkin, R. H.,... Wallace, M. (2015). Pharmacotherapy for neuropathic pain in adults: A systematic review and meta-analysis. *Lancet Neurology, 14*, 162–173. doi:10.1016/S1474-4422(14)70251-0

Fornasari, D. (2012). Pain mechanisms in patients with chronic pain. *Clinical Drug Investigation, 32*(Suppl. 1), 45–52. doi:10.2165/11630070-000000000-00000

Govenden, D., & Serpell, M. (2014). Improving outcomes for chronic pain in primary care. *The Practitioner, 258*(1774), 13–17.

Gunstein, H. B., & Akil, H. (2006). Opioid analgesics. In L. L. Brunton, J. S. Lazo, and K. L. Parker (Eds.), *The pharmacological basis of therapeutics* (11th ed., pp. 547–590). New York, NY: McGraw-Hill.

Holland, L. N. & Goldstein, B. D. (1994). Examination of tonic nociceptive behavior using a method of substance P receptor desensitization in the dorsal horn. *Pain, 56*, 339–346.

Migraine Research Foundation. (n.d.). *Migraine facts*. Retrieved from https://migraineresearchfoundation.org/about-migraine/migraine-facts

Molton, I. R., & Terrill, A. L. (2014). Overview of persistent pain in older adults. *American Psychologist, 69*(2), 197–207. doi:10.1037/a0035794

Nahin, R. L. (2015). Estimates of pain prevalence and severity in adults: United States. *Journal of Pain, 16*,769–780. doi:10.1016/j.jpain.2015.05.002

National Headache Foundation. (n.d.). *Headache fact sheets*. Retrieved from http://www.headaches.org/headache-fact-sheets/

NIH Pain Consortium. (2016). *Pain information brochure*. Retrieved from http://painconsortium.nih.gov/News_Other_Resources/pain_index.html#Anchor-Bac-14817

Penprase, B., Brunetto, E., Dahmani, E., Forthoffer, J. J., & Kapoor, S. (2015). The efficacy of preemptive analgesia for postoperative pain control: A systematic review of the literature. *AORN Journal, 101*, 94–105.e8. doi:10.1016/j.aorn.2014.01.030

Reddy, D. S. (2013). The pathophysiological and pharmacological basis of current drug treatment of migraine headache. *Expert Review of Clinical Pharmacology, 6*, 271–288. doi:10.1586/ecp.13.14

Silberstein, S. D. (2014). *Migraine*. Retrieved from http://www.merckmanuals.com/professional/neurologic_disorders/headache/migraine

Torpy, J. M., & Livingston, E. H. (2013). JAMA patient page. Aspirin therapy. *Journal of the American Medical Association, 309*, 1645. doi:10.1001/jama.2013.3866

van den Beuken-van Everdingen, M. H., de Rijke, J. M., Kessels, A. G., Schouten, H. C., van Kleef, M., & Patijn, J. (2007). Prevalence of pain in patients with cancer: A systematic review of the past 40 years. *Annals of Oncology, 18*,1437–1449. doi:10.1093/annonc/mdm056

Chapter 16

Drugs for Anesthesia

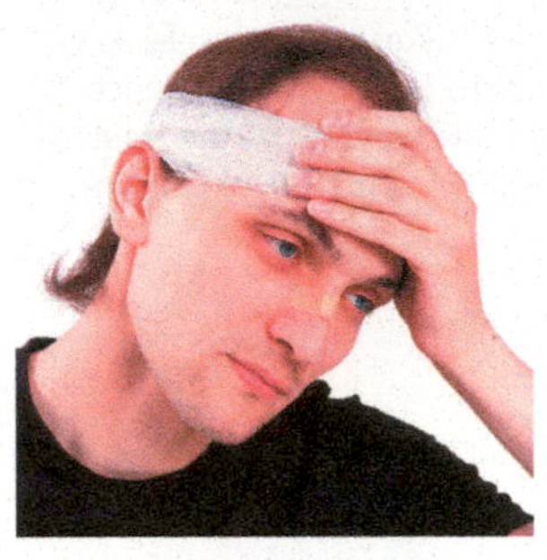

"That needle burned, but then I could only feel a little tug with the stitches."
Mr. Jeffery Wayland

Core Concepts

16.1 **Local anesthesia causes a rapid loss of sensation to a limited part of the body.**

16.2 **Local anesthetics produce their therapeutic effect by blocking the entry of sodium ions into neurons.**

16.3 **Local anesthetics are classified by their chemical structures.**

16.4 **General anesthesia induces rapid loss of consciousness, accompanied by loss of sensation occurring throughout the entire body.**

16.5 **General anesthetics are usually administered by the IV or inhalation routes.**

16.6 **Adjunctive medications complement the goals of general anesthesia.**

Drug Snapshot

The following drugs are discussed in this chapter:

Drug Classes	Prototype Drugs
Local Anesthetics	
Esters	
Amides	Pr lidocaine (Xylocaine)
Miscellaneous drugs	
General Anesthetics	
Intravenous anesthetics	Pr propofol (Diprivan)
Inhaled anesthetics	
Nitrous oxide	Pr nitrous oxide
Volatile liquids	Pr isoflurane (Forane)
Adjuncts to Anesthesia	
Neuromuscular blockers	Pr succinylcholine (Anectine)

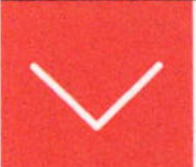

Learning Outcomes

After reading this chapter, the student should be able to:

1. Compare and contrast the five major routes for administering local anesthetics.
2. Explain the mechanism of action of local anesthetics, and explain why additives are sometimes included in the anesthetic solution.
3. Describe differences between the two major chemical classes of local anesthetics and explain their adverse effects.
4. Identify the primary actions of general anesthetics within the central nervous system, and identify the four stages of general anesthesia.

5. Explain how general anesthesia is achieved, and categorize drugs for general anesthesia based on their classifications and actions in the body.
6. For each of the adjunctive drug classes, identify representative drugs and explain their roles before, during, and after surgery.

Key Terms

amides (AM-ides)
anesthesia (ANN-ess-THEE-zee-uh)
balanced anesthesia
esters (ES-turs)
general anesthesia
local anesthesia
neuroleptanalgesia (new-row-lept-an-ul-JEE-zee-ah)
neuromuscular blockers

Anesthesia is a medical procedure performed by administering drugs that cause a loss of sensation. **Local anesthesia** occurs when sensation is lost to a limited part of the body without loss of consciousness. **General anesthesia** causes gradual loss of consciousness accompanied by loss of sensation to the entire body. This chapter examines drugs used for both local and general anesthesia, including selected drugs used before, during, and after surgical procedures.

an = *without*
esthesia = *sensation*

LOCAL ANESTHESIA

Local anesthesia is loss of sensation to a relatively small part of the body without loss of consciousness to the patient. This technique may be necessary when a relatively brief surgical, medical, or dental procedure is performed.

Local anesthesia causes a rapid loss of sensation to a limited part of the body.

◀ **Core Concept 16.1**

Although local anesthesia often causes a loss of sensation to a small, limited area, it sometimes affects relatively large portions of the body, such as an entire limb. Because of this action, some local anesthetic treatments are more accurately called *surface anesthesia* or *regional anesthesia*, depending on how the drugs are administered and the results they produce.

The five major routes (Figure 16.1) for applying local anesthetics are the following:

- Topical
- Infiltration
- Nerve block
- Spinal
- Epidural.

The methods used depend on the location and amount of anesthesia that is needed, as well as the specific procedures being performed. For example, some local anesthetics are applied topically before a needlestick or minor skin surgery. Others are used to block sensations to large areas such as limbs or the lower abdomen. The different methods of local and regional anesthesia are summarized in Table 16.1.

CONCEPT REVIEW 16.1

- What is local anesthesia? Name the five general routes for local and regional anesthesia.

Local anesthetics produce their therapeutic effect by blocking the entry of sodium ions into neurons.

◀ **Core Concept 16.2**

The mechanism of action of local anesthetics is well known. The concentration of sodium is normally higher outside the neurons compared to the inside. A rapid influx of sodium ions into the cell is necessary for neurons to fire.

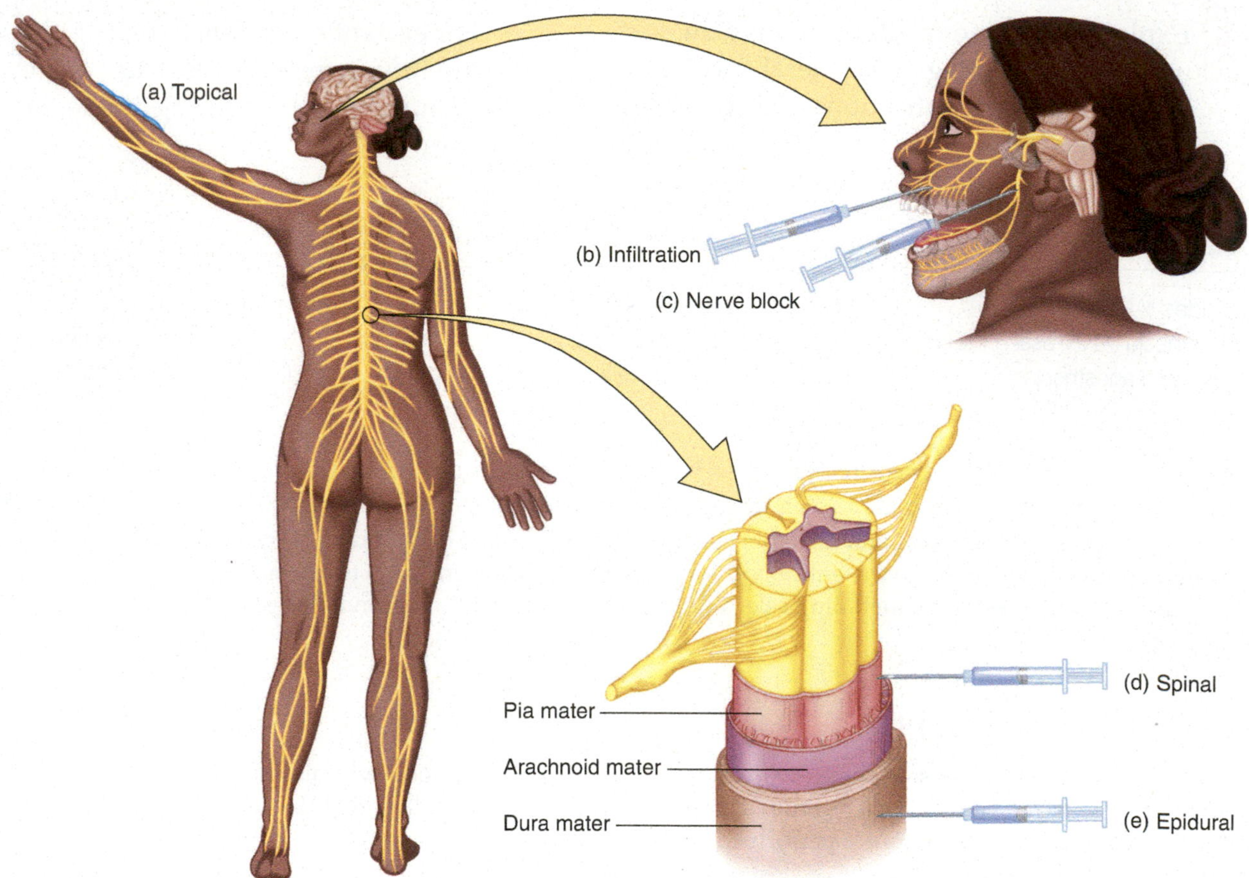

FIGURE 16.1 Routes for applying local anesthesia include (a) topical, (b) infiltration, (c) nerve block, (d) spinal, and (e) epidural.

Table 16.1 Methods of Local and Regional Anesthesia

Route	Formulation/Method	Description
Topical (surface) anesthesia	Creams, sprays, suppositories, drops, and lozenges.	Applied to mucous membranes, including the eyes, lips, gums, nasal membranes, and throat; very safe unless absorbed.
Infiltration (field block) anesthesia	Direct injection into tissue immediate to the surgical site.	Drug diffuses into tissue to block a specific group of nerves in a small area very close to the area to be operated on.
Nerve block anesthesia	Direct injection into tissue that may be distant from the operation site.	Drug affects the bundle of nerves serving the area to be operated on; used to block sensation in a limb or large area of the face.
Spinal anesthesia	Injection into the cerebrospinal fluid.	Drug affects large, regional area such as the lower abdomen and legs.
Epidural anesthesia	Injection into the epidural space (the area between the vertebrae and the spinal cord).	Drug causes numbness, without paralysis, of the areas below the injection site. A small catheter is often placed into the epidural space to allow for multiple injections.

Local anesthetics act by blocking sodium channels, as illustrated in Figure 16.2. The blocking of sodium channels is nonselective; therefore, both sensory and motor impulses are affected. The goal is to provide enough anesthetic so that sensory impulses are blocked while motor impulses remain relatively intact. Sensation and muscle activity in the treated area will be decreased temporarily. Because of their mechanism of action, local anesthetics are called *sodium channel blockers*.

During a medical or surgical procedure, it is essential for the anesthetic to last long enough to complete the procedure. Small amounts of epinephrine are sometimes added to the anesthetic solution in order to constrict blood vessels in the immediate area where the local anesthetic is applied. This keeps the drug active at the injected site and extends its duration of action while reducing bleeding. The addition of epinephrine to lidocaine (Xylocaine), for example, increases the anesthetic effect from about 20 minutes to 60 minutes. This is important for surgical and dental procedures that take longer than 20 minutes; otherwise, a second injection would be necessary.

(a)
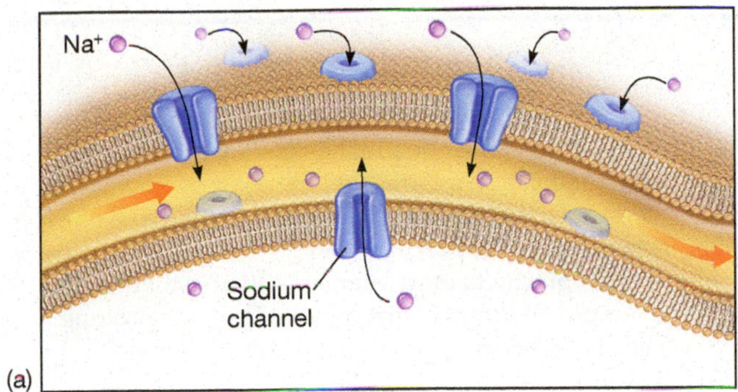

(b)
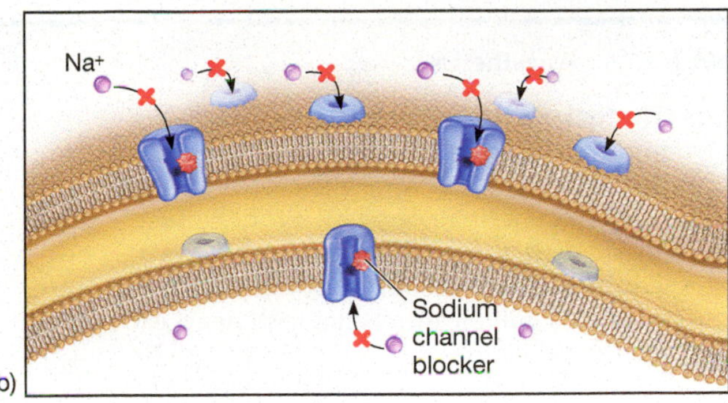

FIGURE 16.2 (a) In normal nerve conduction, sodium ions (Na^+) enter the sodium channels along a neuron and allow the neuron to fire (set off an action potential) and conduct an impulse. (b) Local anesthetics (represented by the red x) block the sodium channels. Sodium ions are not able to enter the neuronal membrane through the sodium channels. Therefore, no action potential can be conducted along the nerve.

Alkaline additives are included in some anesthetic solutions in order to increase local anesthesia in regions that have infections or abscesses. Bacteria tend to acidify an infected site, and local anesthetics are often less effective in this type of environment. Adding an alkaline solution such as sodium bicarbonate neutralizes the infected area and allows the anesthetic to work better. Methylparaben is another additive that may be included in the anesthetic solution to retard bacterial growth.

Local anesthetics are classified by their chemical structures.

◀ Core Concept 16.3

The two major classes of local anesthetics are **esters** and **amides** (Table 16.2). The terms *ester* and *amide* refer to types of chemical linkages found within the anesthetic molecules, as illustrated in Figure 16.3. A small number of miscellaneous drugs are neither esters nor amides.

Table 16.2 Selected Local Anesthetics

Drug	Clinical Uses	Remarks
ESTERS		
benzocaine (Americaine, Anbesol, Solarcaine, others) (see the Prototype Drug box in Core Concept 37.4)	Topical anesthesia	For sunburn, sore throat, earache, hemorrhoids, and other minor skins conditions
chloroprocaine (Nesacaine)	Infiltration, nerve block, and epidural anesthesia	Short duration
procaine (Novocain)	Infiltration, nerve block, epidural, and spinal anesthesia	Short duration
proparacaine (Alcaine, Ophthetic)	To numb the eye before surgery, certain tests, or procedures	Short duration
tetracaine (Pontocaine)	Topical and spinal anesthesia	Longer duration
AMIDES		
articaine (Septocaine, Zorcaine)	Infiltration and nerve block anesthesia	Longer duration
bupivicaine (Marcaine, Sensorcaine)	Infiltration and epidural anesthesia	Longer duration
dibucaine (Nupercainal)	Topical or spinal anesthesia	Longer duration
Pr lidocaine (Anestacon, Dilocaine, Xylocaine, others)	Topical anesthesia, infiltration, nerve block, epidural, and spinal anesthesia	May be combined as a mixture of lidocaine and prilocaine (EMLA cream) for topical application
mepivacaine (Carbocaine, Isocaine, Polocaine)	Infiltration, nerve block, and epidural anesthesia	Intermediate duration
Prilocaine	Infiltration, nerve block, and epidural anesthesia	Intermediate duration
ropivacaine (Naropin)	Infiltration, nerve block, and epidural anesthesia	Longer duration
MISCELLANEOUS DRUGS		
dyclonine (Dyclone)	Topical anesthesia	For ear, nose, and throat procedures
ethyl chloride or chloroethane	Topical anesthesia	For minor medical procedures
pramoxine (Tronothane)	Topical anesthesia	For minor medical procedures

Fast Facts Anesthetics

- The first medical applications of anesthetics involved ether (in 1842) and nitrous oxide (in 1846).
- About half of the general anesthetics in medical practice are administered by certified nurse anesthetists.
- Certified nurse anesthetists administer approximately 40 million anesthetics to patients each year in the United States.
- The general public often associates use of local anesthetic drugs with the practice of dentistry or topical skin applications. However, these drugs span areas of obstetrical, surgical, pain management and trauma stabilization.
- Herbal products may interact with anesthetics—for example, St. John's wort may intensify or prolong the effects of some opioids and anesthetics.

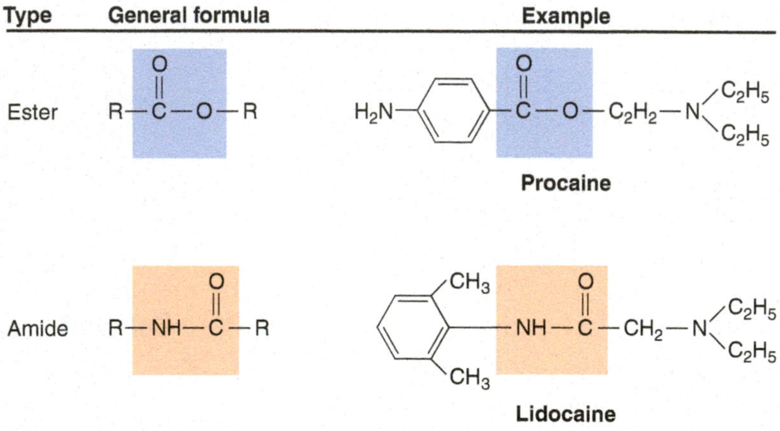

Type	General formula	Example
Ester	R—C(=O)—O—R	H_2N—C_6H_4—C(=O)—O—C_2H_2—N(C_2H_5)$_2$ **Procaine**
Amide	R—NH—C(=O)—R	(CH_3)$_2C_6H_3$—NH—C(=O)—CH_2—N(C_2H_5)$_2$ **Lidocaine**

FIGURE 16.3 The esters contain a type of chemical linkage that includes carbon and oxygen (-CO-O-). The amides contain a type of chemical linkage that includes carbon, nitrogen, and oxygen (-NH-CO-).

Esters

Cocaine, the first local anesthetic widely used for medical procedures, was used as far back as the 1880s. Cocaine is a natural ester, found in the leaves of the plant *Erythroxylon coca*, native to the Andes Mountains of Peru. Even today, cocaine is sometimes applied to the lining of the mouth, nose, and throat (mucous membranes) before biopsy, stitches, and wound cleaning. Its onset is within seconds after application. Cocaine temporarily numbs the area for about 1–2 minutes.

It constricts blood vessels, an effect that decreases bleeding and swelling during the procedure. Cocaine may be used to treat uncontrolled nose bleed. The abuse potential of cocaine is discussed in Chapter 8.

Another ester, procaine (Novocain), was the drug of choice for dental procedures from the mid-1900s to the 1960s. About that time, amide anesthetics were developed, and use of the ester anesthetics declined. One ester, benzocaine (Solarcaine, others), is used as a topical over-the-counter (OTC) drug for treating a large number of painful conditions, including sunburn, insect bites, hemorrhoids, sore throat, and minor wounds. Tetracaine is an ester that is often sprayed on the skin and mucous membranes to cause loss of feeling before and during surgery or for endoscopic procedures. For example, a topical anesthetic comprising benzocaine, butamben, and teratracaine (Cetacaine) is used in examinations of the esophagus or colon. Proparacaine (Alcaine, Ophthetic) is a drug used for short-term anesthesia in ocular procedures.

Amides

Amides have largely replaced the esters because they produce fewer adverse effects and generally have a longer duration of action. Lidocaine (Xylocaine) is the most widely used amide for short surgical procedures requiring local anesthesia. Ethyl chloride or chloroethane is a mild topical drug supplied as a liquid in a spray bottle. It is used for basic procedures such as removing splinters or small debris from the skin's surface.

Adverse effects to local anesthesia are uncommon. Allergy is rare. When it does occur, it is often due to sulfites, which are added as preservatives to prolong the shelf life of the anesthetic. Early signs of adverse effects of local anesthetics include symptoms of central nervous system (CNS) stimulation such as restlessness or anxiety. Later, drowsiness and unresponsiveness may occur due to CNS depression. Cardiovascular effects are possible, including hypotension and dysrhythmias. Patients with a history of cardiovascular disease are often given forms of local anesthetics that contain no epinephrine to reduce the possible effects of this sympathomimetic on the heart and blood pressure. CNS and cardiovascular adverse effects are rare unless the local anesthetic is absorbed rapidly or is accidentally injected directly into a blood vessel.

CONCEPT REVIEW 16.2

- How does a local anesthetic work? How does the anesthetic action of lidocaine with epinephrine differ from that of lidocaine without epinephrine?

Prototype Drug: Lidocaine (Xylocaine)

Therapeutic Class: Anesthetic (local/regional/topical), antidysrhythmic (class IB) **Pharmacologic Class:** Sodium channel blocker, amide

Actions and Uses: Lidocaine is the most frequently used injectable local anesthetic. It is available in solutions ranging from 0.5% to 2% for infiltration, nerve block, spinal, or epidural anesthesia. A topical form is also available. When given for anesthesia, its onset of action is 5 to 15 minutes. Several hours may be needed for complete sensation to reappear. Lidocaine is also given IV, IM, or subcutaneously to treat dysrhythmias, as discussed in Chapter 23. Solutions of lidocaine containing preservatives or epinephrine are used for local anesthesia only and must never be given parenterally for dysrhythmias.

Adverse Effects and Interactions: When used for anesthesia, adverse effects are uncommon. An early symptom of toxicity is excitement, leading to irritability and confusion. Serious adverse effects include convulsions, respiratory depression, and cardiac arrest. Until the effect of the anesthetic diminishes, patients may injure themselves by biting or chewing areas of the mouth that have no sensation following a dental procedure.

Barbiturates may decrease activity of lidocaine. Increased effects of lidocaine occur if taken with cimetidine, quinidine, and beta blockers. If lidocaine is used on a regular basis, its effectiveness may diminish when used with other medications.

Nursing Process Focus Patients Receiving Local Anesthesia

ASSESSMENT	POTENTIAL NURSING DIAGNOSES*
Prior to administration: • Obtain a complete health history including cardiovascular conditions, allergies (especially for amide-type drugs), drug history, and possible drug interactions. • Check for the presence of broken skin, infections, burns, and wounds where medication is to be applied. • Determine character, duration, location, and intensity of pain where medication is to be applied.	• *Deficient Knowledge* related to lack of information about drug therapy • *Acute Pain* related to administration of drug • *Risk for Injury* related to lack of sensation to a part of the body caused by the anesthetic

PLANNING: PATIENT GOALS AND EXPECTED OUTCOMES

The patient will:
- Experience therapeutic effects (no pain during surgical procedure).
- Be free from or experience minimal adverse effects from drug therapy.

IMPLEMENTATION

Interventions and (Rationales)	Patient Education/Discharge Planning
• Monitor for cardiovascular adverse effects. (These may occur if anesthetic is absorbed.)	• Instruct the patient to report any unusual heart palpitations, lightheadedness, drowsiness, or confusion. If using medication on a regular basis, instruct the patient to see the healthcare provider regularly.
• Check skin or mucous membranes for infection or inflammation. (Conditions could be worsened by the drug.)	• Instruct the patient to report any irritation or increased discomfort in areas where medication was used to the healthcare provider.
• Monitor for length of effectiveness. (Local anesthetics are effective for 1 to 3 hours.)	• Instruct the patient to report any discomfort during the procedure.
• Obtain information on and monitor the use of other medications.	• Instruct the patient to report use of any medications to the healthcare provider.
• Provide for patient safety. (There is a potential for injury related to the fact that the area being treated lacks sensation.)	• Inform the patient about having no feeling in the anesthetized area and taking extra caution to avoid heat-related and other injury.

(Continued)

Nursing Process Focus (*continued*)

Interventions and (Rationales)	Patient Education/Discharge Planning
• Monitor for gag reflex if used in the mouth or throat. (Xylocaine viscous may interfere with the swallowing reflex.)	Instruct the patient to: • Not eat within 1 hour of administration. • Not chew gum while any portion of the mouth or throat is anesthetized to prevent biting injuries.

EVALUATION OF OUTCOME CRITERIA

Evaluate the effectiveness of drug therapy by confirming that patient goals and expected outcomes have been met (see "Planning"). *See Table 16.2 for a list of drugs to which these nursing actions apply.*

CAM Therapy | Oil of Cloves for Dental Pain

One natural remedy for tooth pain is oil of cloves, a natural substance whose use dates back thousands of years in Chinese medicine. Extracted from the clove plant *Eugenia*, eugenol is the active chemical that produces a numbing effect. It works especially well for dental caries (cavities). The herb is applied by soaking a piece of cotton and packing it around the gums close to the affected tooth. Dentists sometimes recommend it for temporary relief of a toothache. Clove oil has an antiseptic effect that has been reported to kill microorganisms.

Other uses of clove oil that lack reliable scientific evidence include treatment of premature ejaculation, low libido, and fever reduction. Clove oil is very safe, with rash and gastrointestinal (GI) upset being the most common adverse effects. Clove oil may increase the risk for bleeding and should be used cautiously in patients taking anticoagulants.

GENERAL ANESTHESIA

General anesthesia involves loss of sensation to the entire body. General anesthetics are used when it is necessary for patients to remain still and without pain for a period longer than could be achieved with local anesthetics.

Core Concept 16.4 ▶

General anesthesia induces rapid loss of consciousness, accompanied by loss of sensation occurring throughout the entire body.

The goal of general anesthesia is to provide a rapid and complete loss of sensation. Signs of general anesthesia include total analgesia (no feeling of pain) and loss of consciousness, memory, and body movement. Although these signs are similar to those of sleeping, general anesthesia and sleep are not the same. General anesthetics depress most nervous activity in the brain, whereas sleeping stops activity in very specific areas. In fact, some brain activity actually increases during sleep, as described in Chapter 10.

General anesthesia is rarely achieved with a single drug. Instead, multiple medications are used to induce unconsciousness, cause muscle relaxation, and maintain deep anesthesia. This approach, called **balanced anesthesia**, allows the dose of inhalation anesthetic to be lower so that the procedure is safer for the patient.

General anesthesia is a progressive process that occurs in distinct steps, or stages. The most effective medications can quickly cause all four stages, whereas others are only able to cause stage 1 (light sedation). Most major surgery occurs in stage 3, where the patient is completely relaxed and sedated. Thus, stage 3 anesthesia is called *surgical anesthesia*. When seeking surgical anesthesia, the anesthesiologist will try to move quickly through stage 2 because this stage produces distressing symptoms. Often an IV drug will be given to calm the patient during this stage. The stages of general anesthesia are listed in Table 16.3.

Table 16.3 Stages of General Anesthesia

Stage 1	Loss of pain: the patient loses general sensation but may be awake. This stage proceeds until the patient loses consciousness.
Stage 2	Excitement and hyperactivity: the patient may be delirious and try to resist treatment. Heartbeat and breathing may become irregular, and blood pressure can increase. IV drugs are administered here to calm the patient.
Stage 3	Surgical anesthesia: skeletal muscles become paralyzed. Cardiovascular and breathing activities stabilize. Eye movements slow down and the patient becomes still.
Stage 4	Paralysis of the medulla region in the brain (responsible for controlling respiratory and cardiovascular activity): If breathing or the heart stops, death could result. This stage is usually avoided during general anesthesia.

General anesthetics are usually administered by the IV or inhalation routes.

◀ **Core Concept 16.5**

There are two primary methods of causing general anesthesia. *Intravenous drugs* are usually administered first because they act within a few seconds. After the patient loses consciousness, *inhaled drugs* are used to maintain the anesthesia. During short surgical procedures or those requiring lower stages of anesthesia, the IV drugs may be used alone.

Intravenous Anesthetics

anti = *against*
emetic = *vomiting*

IV general anesthetics, listed in Table 16.4, are important components of balanced anesthesia. Concurrent administration of IV and inhaled anesthetics allows the dose of the inhaled agent to be reduced, thus lowering the potential for serious side effects. Also, when IV and inhaled anesthetics are combined, they provide greater analgesia and greater muscle relaxation than could be provided by the inhaled anesthetic alone. If IV anesthetics are administered alone, they are generally reserved for medical procedures that take less than about 15 minutes.

Drugs employed as IV anesthetics include opioids, benzodiazepines, and miscellaneous drugs. Opioids offer the advantage of superior analgesia. Combining the opioid fentanyl (Sublimaze) with the antipsychotic agent droperidol (Inapsine) produces a state known as **neuroleptanalgesia**. In this state, patients are conscious, though insensitive to pain and

Table 16.4 Intravenous Anesthetics

Drug	Remarks
BENZODIAZEPINES	
diazepam (Valium) (see the Prototype Drug box in Core Concept 14.6)	For induction of anesthesia; prototype drug for the benzodiazepines
lorazepam (Ativan) (see the Prototype Drug box in Core Concept 10.7)	For induction of anesthesia and to produce conscious sedation; for short medical procedures or surgery
midazolam (Versed)	For induction of anesthesia and to produce conscious sedation; for short diagnostic procedures
OPIOIDS	
alfentanil (Alfenta)	For induction of anesthesia; rapid onset and short duration of action; used as a supplement to other anesthetic drugs
fentanyl (Sublimaze, others)	Used to supplement both general and regional anesthesia; short-acting analgesic used during the operative and perioperative period
remifentanil (Ultiva)	For induction and maintenance of anesthesia; approximately 7 times more potent than fentanyl; onset and duration of action more rapid than fentanyl
sufentanil (Sufenta)	For induction and maintenance of anesthesia; approximately 7 times more potent than fentanyl; onset and duration of action more rapid than fentanyl
MISCELLANEOUS IV DRUGS	
etomidate (Amidate)	For induction of anesthesia; for short medical procedures
ketamine (Ketalar)	For sedation, amnesia, and analgesia; for short diagnostic, therapeutic, or surgical procedures; most often used in children; provides dissociative anesthesia
Pr propofol (Diprivan)	For induction and maintenance of general anesthesia; for short medical procedures

amnestic = *loss of memory*

unconnected with surroundings. The premixed combination of these two agents is marketed as Innovar. A similar conscious, dissociated state is produced with the amnestic drug ketamine (Ketalar).

Prototype Drug: Pr *Propofol (Diprivan)*

Therapeutic Class: General anesthetic **Pharmacologic Class: Intravenous induction drug, N-methyl-D-aspartate (NMDA) receptor agonist**

Actions and Uses: Propofol is indicated for the induction and maintenance of general anesthesia. It has almost an immediate onset of action and is used effectively for conscious sedation. Emergence is rapid and few adverse effects occur during recovery. Propofol has an antiemetic effect that can prevent postoperative or post chemotherapy nausea and vomiting.

Adverse Effects and Interactions: Propofol is contraindicated in patients who have a known hypersensitivity reaction to the medication or its emulsion, which contains soybean and egg products. Diprivan injectable emulsion is not recommended for obstetrics, including cesarean section deliveries, or for use in nursing mothers. The drug should be used with caution in patients with cardiac or respiratory impairment.

The dose of propofol should be reduced in patients receiving preanesthetic medications such as benzodiazepines or opioids. Use with other CNS depressants can cause additive CNS and respiratory depression as well as bradycardia and hypotension.

CONCEPT REVIEW 16.3

- What is the role of IV anesthetics in surgical anesthesia? Why are these drugs often used in combination with inhaled anesthetics?

Inhaled Anesthetics

Inhaled general anesthetics, listed in Table 16.5, are gases or volatile liquids. These drugs produce their effects by preventing the flow of sodium into neurons in the CNS, thus delaying nerve impulses and producing a dramatic reduction in neural activity. The exact mechanism for how this occurs is not known, although it is likely that gamma-aminobutyric acid (GABA) receptors in the brain are activated. It is not the same mechanism as is known for local anesthetics. There is some inconclusive evidence suggesting that the mechanism may be related to some of the antiseizure drugs. There is no specific receptor that binds to general anesthetics, and they do not seem to affect neurotransmitter release.

NITROUS OXIDE

The only gas used routinely for anesthesia is nitrous oxide, commonly called *laughing gas*. Nitrous oxide is used for brief obstetric and surgical procedures and for dental procedures. It may also be used in conjunction with other general anesthetics, making it possible to decrease other dosages with high effectiveness.

Nitrous oxide should be used cautiously in patients with myasthenia gravis, because it may cause respiratory depression and prolonged hypnotic effects. Patients with cardiovascular disease, especially those with increased intracranial pressure, should be monitored carefully, because hypnotic drug effects may be prolonged or potentiated.

Table 16.5 Inhaled General Anesthetics

Drug	Remarks
GASES	
Pr nitrous oxide	Used in dental and obstetric precedures and other short medical procedures; used in combination with more potent inhaled anesthetics
VOLATILE LIQUIDS	
desflurane (Suprane)	Rapid induction and maintenance of general anesthesia, quick recovery, lower lipid and blood solubility
enflurane (Ethrane)	Induction and maintenance of general anesthesia
Pr isoflurane (Forane)	Rapid induction and maintenance of general anesthesia, quick recovery
sevoflurane (Ultane)	Rapid induction and maintenance of general anesthesia, quick recovery, lower lipid and blood solubility

Prototype Drug: Nitrous Oxide

Therapeutic Class: General anesthetic **Pharmacologic Class:** Inhalation gaseous drug

Actions and Uses: The main action of nitrous oxide is analgesia caused by suppression of pain mechanisms in the CNS. This drug has a low potency and does not produce complete loss of consciousness or extreme relaxation of skeletal muscle. Because nitrous oxide does not cause surgical anesthesia (stage 3), it is commonly combined with other surgical anesthetic drugs. Nitrous oxide is ideal for dental procedures because the patient remains conscious and can follow instruction while experiencing full analgesia.

Adverse Effects and Interactions: When used in low to moderate doses, nitrous oxide produces few adverse effects. At higher doses, patients exhibit some adverse signs of stage 2 anesthesia, such as anxiety, excitement, and combativeness. Lowering the inhaled dose will quickly reverse these adverse effects. As nitrous oxide is exhaled the patient may temporarily have some difficulty breathing at the end of a procedure. Nausea and vomiting following the procedure are more common with nitrous oxide than with other inhalation anesthetics.

VOLATILE LIQUIDS

Volatile anesthetics are liquid at room temperature but are converted into a vapor and inhaled to produce their anesthetic effects as well as skeletal muscle relaxation. Commonly administered volatile agents are desflurane (Suprane) and sevoflurane (Ultane). Some general anesthetics enhance the sensitivity of the heart to drugs such as epinephrine, norepinephrine, dopamine, and serotonin. Volatile liquids have been associated with dysrhythmias, some of which may be fatal. Isoflurane (Forane) is featured as the prototype drug in this category. Adverse reactions encountered in the administration of general anesthetics have been respiratory depression, hepatic dysfunction, hypotension, and dysrhythmias. Shivering, nausea, vomiting, and obstructive gastrointestinal signs have been observed in the postoperative period. Transient elevations in white blood count have been observed even in the absence of surgical stress. Malignant hyperthermia and elevated carboxyhemoglobin levels are common adverse reactions. The volatile liquids are excreted almost entirely by the lungs through exhalation.

hyper = *elevated*
thermia = *body temperature*

Prototype Drug: Isoflurane (Forane)

Therapeutic Class: General anesthetic **Pharmacologic Class:** Inhalation volatile liquid, GABA, and glutamate receptor agonist

Actions and Uses: Isoflurane produces a potent level of surgical anesthesia that is rapid in onset. It provides the patient with smooth induction with a low degree of metabolism required by the body. This drug provides excellent muscle relaxation and may be used off-label as adjuvant therapy in the treatment of status asthmaticus. Isoflurane with oxygen or with an oxygen and nitrous oxide mixture may be used.

Adverse Effects and Interactions: Mild nausea, vomiting, and tremor are common adverse effects. The drug produces a dose-dependent respiratory depression and a reduction in blood pressure. Malignant hyperthermia with elevated temperature has been reported. Patients with a known history of genetic predisposition to malignant hyperthermia should not use isoflurane. Caution should be used when treating patients with head trauma or brain neoplasms due to possible increases in intracranial pressure. Older adult patients are more susceptible to hypotension caused by the drug. Hypokalemia and cardiac dysrhythmias are possible.

When isoflurane is used concurrently with nitrous oxide, coughing, breath holding, and laryngospasms may occur. If isoflurane is administered with systemic polymyxin and aminoglycosides, skeletal muscle weakness, respiratory depression, or apnea may occur. Additive effects may occur with isoflurane if administered with other skeletal muscle relaxants. Additive hypotension may result if used concurrently with antihypertensive medications such as beta blockers. Epinephrine, norepinephrine, dopamine, and other adrenergic agonists should be administered with caution due to the possibility of dysrhythmias. Other drugs may cause dysrhythmias, including amiodarone, ibutilide, droperidol, and phenothiazines. Levodopa should be discontinued 6 to 8 hours before isoflurane administration. St. John's wort should be discontinued 2 to 3 weeks prior to administration due to the possible risk of hypotension.

ADJUNCTS TO ANESTHESIA

Many drugs are used either to complement the effects of general anesthetics or to treat anticipated side effects of the anesthesia. These drugs are called *adjuncts* to anesthesia.

Core Concept 16.6 ▶

Adjunctive medications complement the goals of general anesthesia.

Selected adjuncts to general anesthesia are listed in Table 16.6. They may be given prior to, during, or after surgery.

pre = *before*
operative = *surgery*
sedative = *drowsy*
hypnotic = *sleep*

Preoperative drugs are given to relieve anxiety and to provide mild sedation. Anticholinergics such as atropine may be administered to dry secretions and to suppress the bradycardia caused by some anesthetics. Sedative–hypnotic drugs (benzodiazepines) help reduce fear, anxiety, or pain associated with the surgery. Opioids such as morphine may be given to counteract pain experienced by the patient.

Neuromuscular Blockers

neuro = *nerve*
muscular = *muscle*

During surgery, the primary adjuncts are the **neuromuscular blockers** (see Chapter 13). Neuromuscular blockers cause paralysis without loss of consciousness, which means that without a general anesthetic, patients would be awake and without the ability to move. It is important to note that breathing muscles are skeletal muscle. This is why patients require intubation and mechanical ventilation. Administration of these drugs also allows a reduced amount of general anesthetic.

Neuromuscular blocking agents are classified as *depolarizing blockers* and *nondepolarizing* blockers. The only depolarizing blocker is succinylcholine (Anectine), which works by binding to acetylcholine (ACh) receptors at neuromuscular junctions to cause total skeletal

Table 16.6 Selected Adjuncts to General Anesthesia

Chemical Classification	Drug	Remarks
PREOPERATIVE		
Anticholinergic	atropine	For general anesthesia as a premedication; in emergency situations or during surgery to increase heart rate and to reverse the effects of some cholinergic drugs
Benzodiazepine	midazolam (Versed)	Generally used before other IV agents for induction of anesthesia
Dopamine blocker	droperidol (Inapsine)	For nausea and vomiting caused by opioids; reduces anxiety and relaxes muscles
Opioids	alfentanil (Alfenta)	For induction of anesthesia when endotracheal or mechanical ventilation is needed; short duration; provides analgesia
	fentanyl (Actiq, Duragesic, Sublimaze, others) fentanyl/droperidol (Innovar)	For analgesia during or after anesthesia
	morphine	For analgesia during or after anesthesia
	remifentanil (Ultiva)	For analgesia during or after anesthesia; shorter duration of action than fentanyl
	sufentanil (Sufenta)	For primary anesthesia (providing initial lack of feeling before unconsciousness) or to provide analgesia during or after anesthesia
DURING SURGERY		
Neuromuscular blockers	mivacurium (Mivacron)	For short duration muscle paralysis; nondepolarizing type muscle relaxation
	rocuronium (Zemuron)	For intermediate duration muscle paralysis; nondepolarizing type muscle relaxation
	Pr succinylcholine (Anectine, Quelicin)	For short duration muscle paralysis; depolarizing type muscle relaxation
	tubocurarine	For long duration muscle paralysis; nondepolarizing type muscle relaxation
	vercuronium (Norcuron)	For long duration muscle paralysis; non-depolarizing type muscle relaxation
POSTOPERATIVE		
Cholinergic	bethanechol (Urecholine)	For relief of constipation and urinary retention caused by opioids; stimulates GI motility
Phenothiazine	promethazine (Phenergan, others)	For nausea and vomiting caused by obstetric sedation and anesthesia
Serotonin blocker	ondansetron (Zofran)	For nausea and vomiting caused by cancer chemotherapy, radiation therapy, and surgery

muscle paralysis. Succinylcholine is used in surgery for ease of tracheal intubation. Mivacurium (Mivacron) is the shortest acting of the nondepolarizing blockers, whereas tubocurarine is a longer-acting neuromuscular blocker. The nondepolarizing blockers cause muscle paralysis by competing with ACh for cholinergic receptors at neuromuscular junctions. Once attached to the receptor, the nonpolarizing blockers prevent muscle contraction. Neuromuscular blocking agents need to be used cautiously in patients with myasthenia gravis.

Postoperative drugs include analgesics for pain and antiemetics, such as ondansetron (Zofran, Zuplenz) for the nausea and vomiting that sometimes occur during recovery from the anesthetic. Occasionally, following surgery, a parasympathomimetic such as bethanechol (Urecholine) is administered to stimulate the urinary tract and the smooth muscle of the bowel (see Chapter 9).

post = *after*
operative = *surgery*

Prototype Drug: *Succinylcholine (Anectine)*

Therapeutic Class: Skeletal muscle paralytic, neuromuscular blocker **Pharmacologic Class: Depolarizing blocker, acetylcholine receptor blocking drug**

Actions and Uses: Like the natural neurotransmitter ACh, succinylcholine acts on cholinergic receptor sites at neuromuscular junctions. At first, depolarization occurs, and skeletal muscles contract. After repeated contractions, however, the membrane is unable to repolarize as long as the drug stays on the receptor. Effects are first noted as muscle weakness and muscle spasms. Eventually paralysis occurs. Succinylcholine is rapidly broken down by the enzyme pseudocholinesterase; when the IV infusion is stopped, the duration of action is only a few minutes. Use of succinylcholine reduces the amount of general anesthetic needed for procedures.

Adverse Effects and Interactions: Succinylcholine can cause complete paralysis of the diaphragm and intercostal muscles; thus, mechanical ventilation is necessary during surgery. Bradycardia and respiratory depression are expected adverse effects. If doses are high, tachycardia, hypotension, and urinary retention may occur. Patients with certain genetic defects may experience rapid onset of extremely high fever with muscle rigidity—a serious condition known as malignant hyperthermia.

Additive skeletal muscle blockade will occur if succinylcholine is given concurrently with clindamycin, aminoglycosides, furosemide, lithium, quinidine, or lidocaine.

Increased effect of succinylcholine may occur if given with phenothiazines, oxytocin, promazine, tacrine, or thiazide diuretics. Decreased effect of succinylcholine occurs if given with diazepam.

If this drug is given with nitrous oxide, an increased risk of bradycardia, dysrhythmias, sinus arrest, apnea, and malignant hyperthermia exists. If succinylcholine is given with cardiac glycosides, there is increased risk of cardiac dysrhythmias. If narcotics are given with succinylcholine, there is increased risk of bradycardia and sinus arrest. Some patients report postoperative muscle pain.

BLACK BOX WARNING:
Succinylcholine should be administered in a facility with trained personnel to monitor, assist, and control respiration. Cardiac arrest has been reported resulting from hyperkalemic rhabdomyolysis most frequently in infants or children with undiagnosed skeletal muscle myopathy or Duchenne's muscular dystrophy. This drug is used in children only in cases of emergency intubation or in instances when immediate securing of airway is necessary.

Patients Need to Know

Patients treated with local anesthetic medications need to know the following:

1. When using topical anesthetics for skin conditions, avoid touching the eyes.
2. Never apply topical medications to large patches of skin or to areas where there is an open lesion or cut unless instructed to do so by the healthcare provider.
3. Notify the dentist or healthcare providers of any previous adverse reactions to local anesthesia before being given anesthetic medications.
4. After receiving local anesthetic solutions in the mouth, do not consume food and drink until it is clear that the anesthetic has worn off.
5. While the area is still numb, do not chew or pick at the area where a dental procedure has been performed.
6. Be careful not to inhale anesthetic sprays used for topical application.
7. Get immediate assistance if drowsiness, confusion, or blurred vision has occurred after receiving a local anesthetic. Other signs and symptoms include lightheadedness, an irregular heartbeat, or feeling faint.
8. Report all medications and conditions to the healthcare provider before receiving anesthetics.
9. For outpatient dental or medical procedures involving anesthesia, someone should be available to assist with activities such as transportation.
10. Follow post-procedure instructions carefully after anesthesia.
11. Have sufficient pain medication readily available so that post-procedure pain can be managed after the effects of the anesthesia are no longer felt.

hyper = *elevated*
kal = *kalium (potassium)*
emia = *blood levels*

rhabdo = *rod (cell shape)*
myo = *skeletal muscle*
lysis = *breakdown*

Chapter Review

Core Concepts Summary

16.1 Local anesthesia causes a rapid loss of sensation to a limited part of the body.

Local anesthesia is loss of sensation to a relatively small part of the body without causing loss of consciousness. Sometimes local anesthesia is applied to an entire limb. In these cases, it is more accurately called *surface anesthesia* or *regional anesthesia*, depending on how the drugs are administered and the results they produce.

16.2 Local anesthetics produce their therapeutic effect by blocking the entry of sodium ions into neurons.

Blocking sodium entry into neurons prevents transmission of the electrical impulse along the nerve. Epinephrine is sometimes added to anesthetic solutions to increase the duration of anesthetic action. Other additives may include alkaline substances to counter infected tissues or preservatives to increase shelf life.

16.3 Local anesthetics are classified by their chemical structures.

The two major classes of local anesthetics are esters and amides. Benzocaine (Solarcaine, others) is the most commonly used ester; lidocaine (Xylocaine) is the most used amide. A few local anesthetics are neither esters nor amides.

16.4 General anesthesia induces rapid loss of consciousness, accompanied by loss of sensation occurring throughout the entire body.

General anesthesia proceeds in stages from light sedation to total loss of consciousness. The less potent anesthetics cause stage 1 anesthesia, whereas more potent drugs cause surgical anesthesia (stage 3).

16.5 General anesthetics are usually administered by the IV or inhalation routes.

Two primary methods for producing rapid unconsciousness and total analgesia are IV drugs and inhaled general anesthetics. IV anesthetics are important supplements to inhaled general anesthetics and include benzodiazepines, opioids, and miscellaneous drugs. The only inhaled gaseous drug is nitrous oxide. Other inhaled drugs are volatile liquids.

16.6 Adjunctive medications complement the goals of general anesthesia.

Drugs are given prior to surgery to relieve anxiety, provide mild sedation, counteract pain, and dry secretions. Neuromuscular blockers, given during surgery, relax skeletal muscle and maintain a proper heart rate. Drugs after surgery include treatment for postoperative pain or nausea and vomiting, and some drugs stimulate bowel movements and urination.

REVIEW Questions

Answer the following questions to assess your knowledge of the chapter material, and go back and review any material that is not clear to you.

1. Which of the following herbal products may prolong or intensify the effects of anesthesia?
   1. Kava kava
   2. Oil of cloves
   3. Anise
   4. St. John's wort

2. While administering lidocaine, the nurse monitors for toxicity, which is manifested by: (Select all that apply.)
   1. Excitement.
   2. Irritability.
   3. Tachypnea.
   4. Confusion.
   5. Hypotension.

3. A patient in labor is advised that she can have epidural anesthesia to help relieve her pain. When she asks the nurse what will happen, the nurse tells her:
   1. "An anesthetic drug will be injected directly into the area where the pain is occurring, affecting the nerves and blocking any sensations."
   2. "A small tube (catheter) will be placed in the space between the vertebrae and the spinal cord, and an anesthetic drug will be injected through the tube. The medication will cause numbness in the areas below the injection site, but you will still be able to move your legs."
   3. "You will receive an injection of an anesthetic drug in your back, directly into the cerebrospinal spinal fluid, which will numb the lower half of your body."
   4. "An anesthetic cream will be applied to the skin in the areas causing your pain. This cream will numb those areas."

4. Before administering propofol, the nurse checks a patient's record for allergies. After reviewing the records and talking to the patient, the nurse notifies the healthcare provider and the order is discontinued because the patient is allergic to:
   1. Peanuts.
   2. Shellfish.
   3. Egg products.
   4. Milk.
5. A patient is to receive nitrous oxide during surgery. The nurse understands that he or she will need to monitor the patient for which adverse effect?
   1. Restlessness
   2. Dysrhythmia
   3. Hypertension
   4. Mania
6. The patient being prepared for surgery asks the nurse why he or she is receiving morphine and atropine prior to surgery. The nurse's best response is:
   1. "You will need to speak with your healthcare provider."
   2. "The morphine will help to provide some pain relief before surgery, and the atropine will help to decrease secretions."
   3. "The morphine and atropine will help your anesthetic work more effectively."
   4. "These medications are routinely used before we send a patient to surgery."
7. In reviewing a patient's preoperative paperwork, the nurse notes that the patient has a history of cardiovascular disease and therefore should not receive epinephrine along with the anesthetics because it can cause:
   1. Tachycardia and hypertension.
   2. Bradycardia and hypotension.
   3. Tachycardia and hypotension.
   4. Bradycardia and hypertension.
8. The nurse explains to the patient that he or she will receive both propofol (Diprivan) and nitrous oxide:
   1. Because using these anesthetics together decreases muscle relaxation.
   2. Because using both of these anesthetics together allows for the dose of the nitrous oxide to be reduced.
   3. Because isoflurane is not effective when used alone.
   4. Because nitrous oxide should not be used alone.
9. The anesthesiologist orders atropine, 1 mg IM for a patient in the recovery room. Available is 0.8 mg/mL. How many milliliters will be given?
   1. 1 mL
   2. 1.15 mL
   3. 1.2 mL
   4. 1.25 mL
10. The patient is experiencing nausea in the recovery room. The nurse anticipates which medication being ordered?
    1. Meperidine
    2. Bethanechol
    3. Ondansetron
    4. Succinylcholine

CASE STUDY Questions

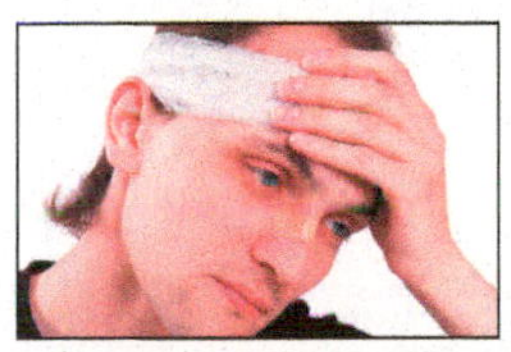

Remember Mr. Wayland, the patient introduced at the beginning of the chapter? Now read the remainder of the case study. Based on the information you have learned in this chapter, answer the questions that follow.

Mr. Jeffery Wayland, age 28, has a history of cardiovascular disease. He has collapsed and sustained an injury to his scalp. The wound is substantial, and Mr. Wayland is bleeding across his right forehead. The patient is rushed to the emergency department by his girlfriend. The girlfriend reports that Mr. Wayland felt a little dizzy and fell, hitting his head on the pavement. The doctor wants to inject the tissue surrounding the wound with 1% lidocaine with epinephrine for local anesthesia prior to suturing the laceration and asks the nurse to prepare the medication.

1. Because he is anxious, Mr. Wayland asks the nurse, "Is the doctor going to numb the area before he begins to put stitches in my head?" The nurse replies:
   1. "Yes, the doctor will apply a topical anesthetic medication to numb the area."
   2. "Yes, the doctor will inject an anesthetic medication directly around the area, or field, of the wound to help prevent pain."
   3. "Yes, the doctor will inject an anesthetic medication that will block a bundle of nerve endings."
   4. "Yes, the doctor will provide an anesthetic medication by injecting it into your epidural space."
2. The nurse understands that the addition of epinephrine to the lidocaine is to:
   1. Prevent infection.
   2. Prevent an allergic reaction.
   3. Increase the duration of the anesthetic.
   4. Decrease pain after the procedure.
3. Soon after administering the lidocaine, the nurse monitors Mr. Wayland for:
   1. Constriction of airways.
   2. Anxiety.
   3. Tachycardia.
   4. Unresponsiveness.

4. Would it be advisable to give Mr. Wayland a barbiturate to help calm his fear of pain from the suturing?
   1. No, a barbiturate might increase toxicity symptoms if Mr. Wayland is allergic to lidocaine.
   2. Yes, a barbiturate might increase the effectiveness of lidocaine in this situation and help the patient calm down.
   3. No, a barbiturate might decrease the effectiveness of lidocaine in this situation and make the patient more irritable.
   4. No, a barbiturate might decrease the effectiveness of lidocaine in this situation, although the medication would normally have a calming effect.

Answers and complete rationales for the Review and Case Study Questions appear in Appendix A.

REFERENCE

Herdman, T. H., & Kamitsuru, S. (Eds.). (2014). *NANDA International nursing diagnoses: Definitions and classification, 2015–2017*. Oxford, United Kingdom: Wiley-Blackwell.

SELECTED BIBLIOGRAPHY

American Association of Nurse Anesthetists. (2016). *Certified Registered Nurse Anesthetist fact sheet*. Retrieved from http://www.aana.com/ceandeducation/becomeacrna/Pages/Nurse-Anesthetists-at-a-Glance.aspx

American Society of Anesthesthetists. (n.d.). *Herbal products and your anesthesia.* Retrieved from https://www.aana.com/forpatients/Documents/herbal_english.pdf

Brown, E. N., Purdon, P. L., & Van Dort, C. J. (2011). General anesthesia and altered states of arousal: A systems neuroscience analysis. *Annual Review of Neuroscience, 34*, 601–628. doi:10.1146/annurevneuro-060909-153200

History of Anesthaesia Society. (n.d.). *Timeline of important dates and events in the development of anaesthesia.* Retrieved from http://www.histansoc.org.uk/timeline.html

Kye, Y. C., Rhee, J. E., Kim, K., Kim, T., Jo, Y. H., Jeong, J. H., & Lee, J. H. (2012). Clinical effects of adjunctive atropine during ketamine sedation in pediatric emergency patients. *The American Journal of Emergency Medicine, 30*, 1981–1985. doi:10.1016/j.ajem.2012.04.030

Okamoto, S., Matsuura, N., & Ichinohe, T. (2015). Effects of volatile anesthetics on oral tissue blood flow in rabbits: A comparison among isoflurane, sevoflurane, and desflurane. *Journal of Oral and Maxillofacial Surgery, 73*(9), 1714.e1-8. doi:10.1016/j.joms.2015.03.047

Persson, J. (2013). Ketamine in pain management. *CNS Neuroscience & Therapeutics, 19*, 396–402. doi:10.1111/cns.12111

Reed, K. L., Malamed, S. F., & Fonner, A. M. (2012). Local anesthesia part 2: Technical considerations. *Anesthesia Progress, 59*, 127–137. doi:10.2344/0003-3006-59.3.127

Theanesthesiaconsultant Blog. (2015). *The obese patient and anesthesia.* Retrieved from http://theanesthesiaconsultant.com/2013/03/07/anesthesia-facts-for-non-medical-people-obesity-and-anesthesia/

To, D., Kossintseva, I., & de Gannes, G. (2014). Lidocaine contact allergy is becoming more prevalent. *Dermatologic Surgery, 40*, 1367–1372. doi:10.1097/DSS.0000000000000190

Unit 3

The Cardiovascular and Urinary Systems

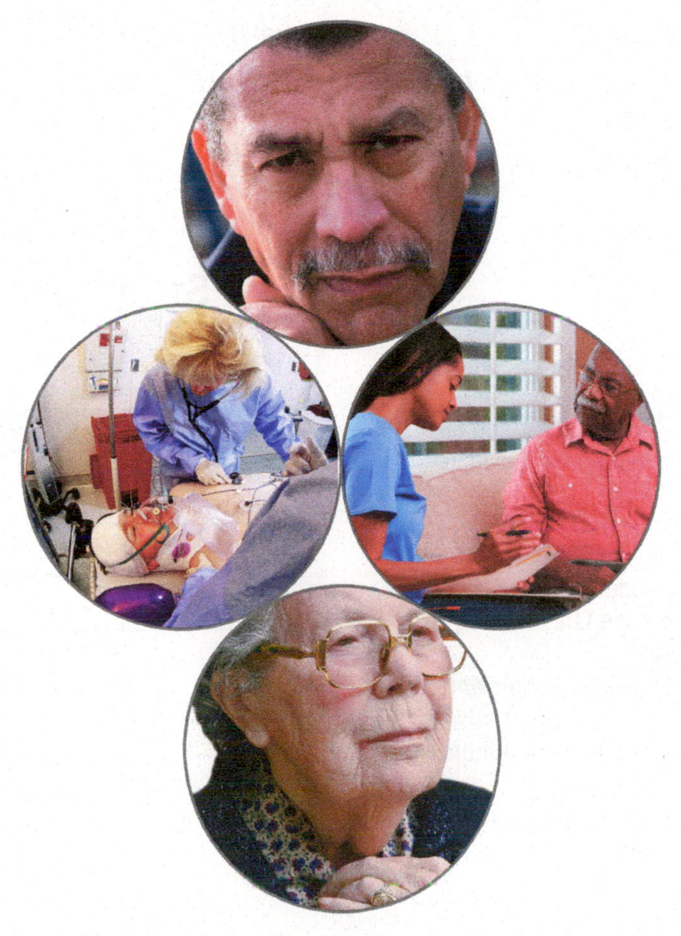

Unit Contents

Chapter 17

Drugs for Lipid Disorders

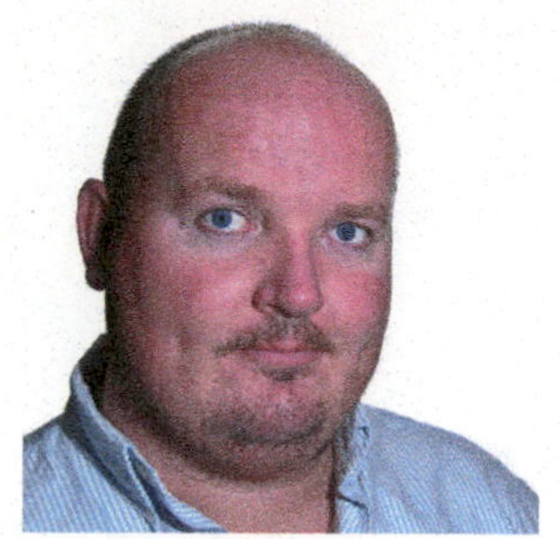

"I've lived too long to change my eating habits now. I've had bad blood tests for years and nothing has happened to me. Besides, I'm too busy to deal with one more problem in my life."

Mr. Edward Long

Core Concepts

17.1 Lipids serve essential roles in the body, but too much dietary fat can lead to disease.

17.2 Lipoproteins transport lipids through the blood for utilization by tissues, storage in adipose tissue, or excretion by the liver.

17.3 Elevated lipid levels can often be prevented or controlled through therapeutic lifestyle changes.

17.4 Statins are preferred drugs for reducing blood lipid levels.

17.5 Bile acid binding drugs can reduce LDL levels by increasing cholesterol excretion.

17.6 Niacin can reduce triglyceride and LDL-cholesterol levels.

17.7 Fibric acid drugs lower triglyceride levels, but have little effect on LDLs.

17.8 Several miscellaneous drugs and drug combinations are available to treat dyslipidemias.

Drug Snapshot

The following drugs are discussed in this chapter:

Drug Classes	Prototype Drugs
HMG-CoA reductase inhibitors (statins)	Pr atorvastatin (Lipitor)
Bile acid binding drugs	Pr cholestyramine (Questran)
Fibric acid drugs (fibrates)	Pr gemfibrozil (Lopid)

Learning Outcomes

After reading this chapter, the student should be able to:

1. Summarize the roles that fats play in human nutrition, and describe the potential consequences of excessively high lipid levels.
2. Explain the different types of lipids and how they are transported through the body.
3. Give examples of how blood lipid levels can be controlled through therapeutic lifestyle changes.
4. Explain the role of statins in the treatment of lipid disorders.
5. Explain the role of bile acid binding drugs in the treatment of lipid disorders.
6. Explain the role of niacin in the treatment of lipid disorders.
7. Explain the role of fibric acid drugs in the treatment of lipid disorders.
8. Explain the role of omega-3 fatty acids and other miscellaneous drugs in the treatment of lipid disorders.

Key Terms

atherosclerosis (ath-ur-oh-skler- OH-sis)
bile acids (BEYE-ul)
dyslipidemia (dys-lip-i-DEEM-ee-uh)
high-density lipoprotein (HDL)
HMG-CoA reductase (ree-DUCK-tase)
hypercholesterolemia (HEYE-purr-koh-LESS-tur-ol-EEM-ee-uh)
hyperlipidemia (HEYE-purr-LIP-i- DEEM-ee-uh)
hypertriglyceridemia (HEYE-purr-tri-gliss-ur-i-DEEM-ee-uh)
lipoproteins (LIP-oh-PROH-teen)
low-density lipoprotein (LDL)
plaque (PLAK)
therapeutic lifestyle changes
triglycerides (tri-GLISS-ur-ide)
very low-density lipoprotein (VLDL)

Research has brought about a nutritional revolution as new knowledge about lipids and their relationship to obesity and cardiovascular disease has allowed people to make more responsible lifestyle choices. Advances in the diagnosis of lipid disorders have helped to identify those patients at greatest risk for cardiovascular disease, and those most likely to benefit from pharmacologic intervention. Safe, effective drugs for lowering lipid levels are now available that decrease the risk of cardiovascular diseases. As a result of this knowledge and from advancements in pharmacology, the incidence of death due to most cardiovascular diseases has been declining, although they are still the leading cause of death in the United States.

Lipids serve essential roles in the body, but too much dietary fat can lead to disease.

◀ **Core Concept 17.1**

Lipids, or fats, are organic compounds that are essential for good health. Lipid tissue provides cushioning and protection of organs and insulates the body to maintain core temperature. Phospholipid is the major component of all cell membranes in the body.

The most common lipids, the **triglycerides**, are the major storage form of fat in the body and the only type of lipid that serves as an important energy source. They account for 90% of the total lipids in the body.

Cholesterol is a lipid that is a major component of cell membranes and which serves as a building block for other lipid-based biochemicals such as vitamin D, bile salts, cortisol, estrogen, and testosterone. Its negative role in promoting **atherosclerosis** or plaque on the walls of arteries is well known. Fatty **plaque** deposits narrow arteries, thereby contributing to angina, myocardial infarction (MI), and stroke, as discussed in Chapter 21. Because the body needs only small amounts of cholesterol daily, it is not necessary to ingest excess amounts of cholesterol in the diet. Dietary cholesterol is obtained solely from animal food products; humans do not absorb the sterols produced by plants.

athero = *fatty*
sclera = *hard*
osis = *condition of*

Research is still uncovering the important roles of lipids in the diet. While it is clear that too much of certain types of dietary fat are associated with disease, some types actually promote wellness. For example, evidence is strong that intake of saturated fats and trans fats should be limited because they are associated with obesity, cardiovascular disease, and possibly cancer. However, omega-3 fatty acids, which are found in abundance in deep, cold-water fish such as salmon, tuna, and herring, may have health benefits. The richest plant source of omega-3 fatty acids is flaxseed, which has become a popular dietary supplement.

Several terms are used to describe lipid disorders. **Dyslipidemia** is a general term meaning an abnormal amount of lipid in the blood. **Hyperlipidemia** is a similar term that

hyper = *above*
lipid = *fat*
emia = *blood*

Fast Facts High Blood Cholesterol

- Almost 74 million Americans (about 32% of U.S. adults) have high blood cholesterol LDL levels.
- Less than half of those with high blood cholesterol are getting treated for the condition.
- Cholesterol levels vary by race, with Mexican-American men having the highest incidence.
- People with high cholesterol levels have double the risk for heart disease compared to those with normal levels.
- The percentage of people treated for high blood LDL cholesterol increased from 28% in the year 2000, to 48% in 2008.

Source: Data from *High Cholesterol Facts*, Centers for Disease Control and Prevention, 2015.

refers to high levels of lipids in the blood. Some patients have only one specific type of lipid that is elevated. Elevated blood cholesterol, or **hypercholesterolemia**, is the type of dyslipidemia that is most familiar to the general public. **Hypertriglyceridemia**, elevated triglycerides, is a less common disorder.

Core Concept 17.2 ▶ Lipoproteins transport lipids through the blood for utilization by tissues, storage in adipose tissue, or excretion by the liver.

Knowledge of cholesterol metabolism is important to understanding cardiovascular disease and the pharmacotherapy of lipid disorders. In simplest terms, the greater the amount of cholesterol circulating in the blood, the greater the risk of cardiovascular disease. This is because the circulating cholesterol binds to vessel walls, increasing plaque buildup as years pass.

Because they are not soluble in the blood, cholesterol and other lipids are packaged as lipoprotein complexes by the liver. **Lipoproteins** contain an inner core of lipid surrounded by an outer shell of carrier protein, which makes them water soluble and able to be transported freely through the blood. The three most common lipoproteins are named based on their weight or density, which comes primarily from the amount of protein present in the complex. Figure 17.1 illustrates the three basic lipoproteins and their composition. Each type of lipoprotein serves a different function in transporting lipids to their final destination.

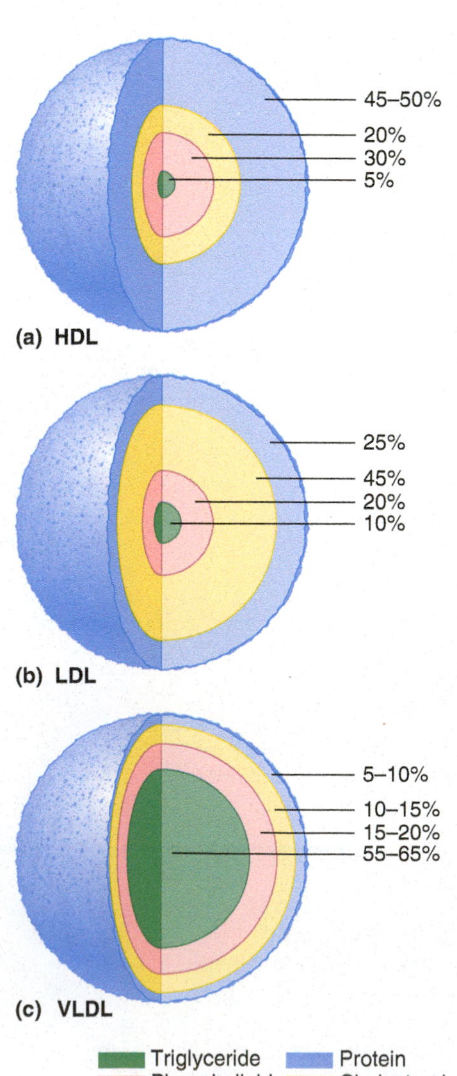

FIGURE 17.1 Composition of lipoproteins: (a) HDL; (b) LDL; (c) VLDL.

Although cholesterol is packaged in all lipoproteins, **low-density lipoprotein (LDL)** has the greatest amount: Almost 50% of LDL consists of cholesterol. The liver makes LDL, which is then transported to tissues and organs, where it is used to build plasma membranes or to synthesize other steroids. Once in the tissues, cholesterol can also be stored for later use. Storage of cholesterol in the lining of blood vessels, however, contributes to plaque buildup and atherosclerosis. LDL is often called "bad" cholesterol because it contributes significantly to plaque deposits and coronary artery disease.

Under normal circumstances, the body makes all the cholesterol it needs to construct cell membranes and other vital functions. When cholesterol is ingested, the body simply makes less to compensate for the increased amounts in the diet. If a person includes too much cholesterol in the diet, however, this feedback loop fails and LDL-cholesterol builds, increasing the risk for health problems.

The body has a remarkable method for keeping blood cholesterol levels in check. A second type of lipoprotein, **high-density lipoprotein (HDL)**, picks up cholesterol in the blood and other tissues and returns it to the liver. Once in the liver, the cholesterol is used to make bile, which is essential for digestion of lipids. The cholesterol component of bile is then excreted in the feces, although some is reabsorbed back into the circulation. Excretion via bile is the only route the body uses to remove cholesterol. Thus HDL may be thought of as a "cholesterol scavenger" that picks up cholesterol in blood and tissues and transports it for removal from the body. Because HDL transports cholesterol for destruction and removes it from the body, it is considered "good" cholesterol.

Of course, cholesterol is not the only type of lipid that can lead to cardiovascular disease. Triglycerides must also be monitored and maintained within normal levels. **Very low-density lipoprotein (VLDL)** is the primary carrier of triglycerides in the blood. VLDL is made in the liver and converted to LDL as it travels through the bloodstream as most of the triglycerides in VLDL are transported to adipose tissue for storage. The health consequences of high blood levels of VLDL are not as clear as for LDL levels. It has been demonstrated, however, that high levels of VLDL are associated with an increased risk of pancreatitis.

Elevated lipid levels can often be prevented or controlled through therapeutic lifestyle changes.

◀ **Core Concept 17.3**

Most patients with dyslipidemias are asymptomatic, and many do not seek medical intervention until cardiovascular disease has progressed, resulting in hypertension or symptoms such as chest pain. For most patients, lipid disorders are the result of a combination of genetic and environmental (lifestyle) factors. Table 17.1 gives the desirable, borderline, and high laboratory values for each of the major lipids and lipoproteins.

When a patient is found to have high LDL-cholesterol levels, most healthcare providers will recommend the initiation of pharmacotherapy. Although the drugs used to control lipid levels have certain side effects, it is clear that lowering cholesterol levels can significantly reduce the risk of heart disease or stroke.

Rather than starting pharmacotherapy immediately after diagnosis, some healthcare providers suggest that the patient try to manage their high cholesterol levels through **therapeutic lifestyle changes**. Many patients with borderline laboratory values can control their hyperlipidemia entirely through nonpharmacologic means. Even in patients with high risk for whom drug therapy is indicated, using these changes is important for reducing cholesterol levels. Following are the features of therapeutic lifestyle changes:

- Increase physical activity, which raises HDL levels and lowers triglycerides.
- Maintain weight within a normal range.
- Implement a medically supervised exercise plan.
- Reduce dietary saturated fat intake to 7% of total caloric intake.
- Reduce cholesterol intake to less than 200 mg/day.
- Increase intake of whole grains, vegetables, and fruits so that total dietary fiber is 10 to 25 g/day.
- Eliminate tobacco use.

In 2013, major revisions were made to hyperlipidemia treatment guidelines by the American College of Cardiology (ACC) and the American Heart Association (AHA) (Psaty & Weiss, 2014). The 2013 ACC/AHA guidelines no longer stress specific target goals for LDL levels. Four treatment categories were established, with three of the categories (2-4 below) for prevention of coronary heart disease. The new recommendation calls for a discussion of risks, benefits, and patient preferences before starting drug therapy for those groups.

1. Adults with preexisting cardiovascular disease
2. Adults with diabetes, aged 40 to 75 years with LDL levels between 70 and 189 mg/dL
3. Adults with LDL cholesterol levels of 190 mg/dL or higher
4. Adults aged 40 through 75 years who have LDL levels 70 through 189 mg/dL and 7.5% or greater 10-year risk of atherosclerotic cardiovascular disease.

Table 17.1 Standard Laboratory Lipid Profiles

Type of Lipid	Laboratory Value (mg/dl)	Standard
Total cholesterol	Less than 200 200–240 Greater than 240	Desirable Borderline high risk High risk
LDL cholesterol	Less than 100 100–129 130–159 160–189 Greater than 190	Optimal Near or above optimal Borderline high risk High risk Very high risk
HDL cholesterol	Less than 40 (men) or 50 (women) Greater than 60	Low risk Desirable
Triglycerides	Less than 150 150–199 200–499 Greater than 500	Normal Borderline high risk High risk Very high risk

Source: "Executive Summary of the Third Report of the National Cholesterol Education Program (NCEP) Expert Panel on Detection, Evaluation, and Treatment of High Blood Cholesterol in Adults (Adult Treatment Panel III), by Expert Panel on Detection, Evaluation, and Treatment of High Blood Cholesterol in Adults" 2001, *JAMA*, *285*, pp. 2486–2497.

Based on the results of hundreds of clinical trials, the ACC/AHA guidelines specifically recommend statins as first-line therapy for all categories. Follow-up measures of LDL are recommended to determine compliance with the drug regimen.

CAM Therapy | Red Yeast Rice and Cholesterol

Red yeast rice is a supplement that is produced when rice is fermented with the yeast *Monascus purpureus*. The product is sometimes reduced to a powder and used as a coloring or flavoring. Red yeast rice has been used for centuries in Chinese medicine to treat various digestive and liver complaints. More recently it has been used as a supplement to manage high blood cholesterol.

Red yeast rice clearly is effective at lowering blood cholesterol levels. This is likely because the product contains a chemical called monacolin, which is identical to the prescription drug lovastatin. In 2007, the U.S. Food and Drug Administration (FDA) decided that red yeast rice should be regulated as a prescription drug. Some supplement manufacturers remarketed the product after removing monacolin from the red yeast rice. It is unclear whether the "monacolin-removed" product has any ability to lower blood cholesterol. Other manufacturers kept monacolin but avoided FDA action by removing any claims about reducing cholesterol levels from the label. Patients should discuss this supplement with their healthcare provider before beginning therapy.

CONCEPT REVIEW 17.1

- Why is the cholesterol in high-density lipoproteins considered to be "good" cholesterol?

Core Concept 17.4 ▶ Statins are preferred drugs for reducing blood lipid levels.

In the late 1970s, compounds were isolated from various species of fungi that were found to inhibit cholesterol production in human cells in the laboratory. This class of drugs, known as the *statins*, has since revolutionized the treatment of lipid disorders. Statins can dramatically reduce LDL-cholesterol levels. In addition to decreasing LDL-cholesterol levels in the blood, statins can also lower triglyceride levels, lower VLDL levels, and raise "good" HDL-cholesterol levels. Research has confirmed that statins clearly reduce the incidence of serious cardiovascular related events. Statins are now first-line drugs in the treatment of dyslipidemias and are among the most widely prescribed drugs in the United States.

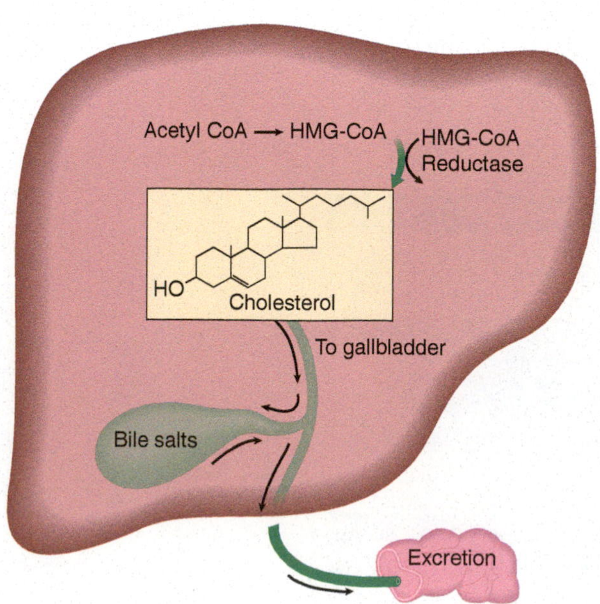

FIGURE 17.2 Cholesterol biosynthesis and excretion.

Cholesterol is made in the liver by a series of more than 25 metabolic steps. Of the many enzymes involved in this complex pathway, **HMG-CoA reductase** (hydroxymethylglutaryl-CoenzymeA reductase) serves as the primary regulator of cholesterol biosynthesis. Under normal conditions, this enzyme is controlled through negative feedback: High levels of LDL cholesterol in the blood will shut down production of HMG-CoA reductase, thus turning off the cholesterol pathway. Figure 17.2 illustrates some of the steps in cholesterol biosynthesis and the importance of HMG-CoA reductase.

The statins act by inhibiting HMG-CoA reductase. As the liver makes less cholesterol, the body responds by making more LDL receptors in order to scavenge more LDL from the blood, thus reducing blood levels of LDL. The drop in lipid levels is not permanent, however. Patients need to remain on these drugs during the remainder of their lives or until their hyperlipidemia can be controlled through lifestyle changes. The reduction in

Table 17.2 Drugs for Dyslipidemias

Drug	Route and Adult Dose	Remarks
HMG-CoA REDUCTASE INHIBITORS		
Pr atorvastatin (Lipitor)	PO: 10–80 mg/day	May be taken with or without food at any time of the day
fluvastatin (Lescol)	PO: 20 mg/day	May be taken with or without food in the evening
lovastatin (Altoprev, Mevacor)	PO: 10–80 mg daily (immediate release); 20–60 mg daily (extended release)	Should be taken with food in the evening
pitavastatin (Livalo)	PO: 1–4 mg/day	May be taken with or without food at any time of the day
pravastatin (Pravachol)	PO: 10–40 mg/day	May be taken with or without food in the evening
rosuvastatin (Crestor)	PO: 5–40 mg/day	May be taken with or without food at any time of the day
simvastatin (Zocor)	PO: 5–40 mg/day	May be taken with or without food in the evening
BILE ACID BINDING DRUGS		
Pr cholestyramine (Questran)	PO: 4–8 g bid–qid	Take with large amounts of fluid; take other drugs 1 hour before or 4 hours after
colesevelam (Welchol)	PO: 1.9 g bid	Take with meals and with at least 8 oz of fluid
colestipol (Colestid)	PO: 5–20 g/day in divided doses	Take with large amounts of fluid; take other drugs 1 hour before or 4 hours after
FIBRIC ACID DRUGS		
fenofibrate (Lofibra, Tricor, others)	PO: 54 mg daily (max: 200 mg/day)	Take with or without food. Do not take with warfarin
fenofibric acid (Fibricor, Trilipix)	PO (regular release): 35–105 mg once daily	Take with or without food. Do not take with warfarin. This is the active metabolite of fenofibrate
Pr gemfibrozil (Lopid)	PO: 600 mg bid (max: 1500 mg/day)	Take 30 minutes before morning and evening meals
OTHER DRUGS FOR DYSLIPIDEMIAS		
alirocumab (Praluent)	Subcutaneous: 75–150 mg every 2 weeks	Newer antihyperlipidemic for inherited hypercholesterolemia. Self-administer using pre-filled syringe
evolocumab (Repatha)	Subcutaneous: 140 mg every 2 weeks	Newer antihyperlipidemic for inherited hypercholesterolemia. Self-administer using pre-filled syringe
ezetimibe (Zetia)	PO: 10 mg/day	Inhibits cholesterol absorption
icosapent (Vascepa)	PO: 4 g/day	Do not open or crush capsules
lomitapide (Juxtapid)	PO: 5–60 mg once daily	For inherited hypercholesterolemia
mipomersan (Kynamro)	Subcutaneous: 200 mg once weekly	For LDL and total cholesterol
niacin (Niaspan)	PO: 1.5–3 g/day (max: 6 g/day)	Also used to treat niacin deficiency (10–20 mg/day). Take with food
omega-3-acid ethyl esters (Epanova, Lovaza)	PO: 2-4 g/day	Do not open or crush capsules; for hypertriglyceridemia

adverse cardiovascular events from the statins is especially high in those patients who have diabetes as a comorbid condition with hyperlipidemia. Doses of the HMG-CoA reductase inhibitors are shown in Table 17.2.

All statins are given orally and have very similar actions and adverse effects. Some statins should be administered in the evening because cholesterol biosynthesis in the body is higher at night.

The statins are generally safe drugs, having a low incidence of adverse effects. Gastrointestinal (GI) disturbances such as indigestion, flatulence, cramping, and constipation are usually mild and disappear with continued use. Statins can cause muscle injury, resulting in symptoms such as weakness, soreness, and pain. Muscle-related side effects are dose related and tend to occur more often in older patients. Patients should be carefully monitored for these symptoms because muscle injury may progress to more serious conditions, such as rhabdomyolysis. Rhabdomyolysis is a medical condition in which muscle tissue, including cardiac muscle, becomes extremely inflamed, resulting in breakdown of muscle. Patients reporting muscular soreness or weakness may have their statin dosage reduced, or they may be switched to a drug of a different class.

Prototype Drug: Atorvastatin (Lipitor)

Therapeutic Class: Antihyperlipidemic drug **Pharmacologic Class:** HMG-CoA reductase inhibitor (statin)

Actions and Uses: Atorvastatin slows the biosynthesis of cholesterol by blocking the rate-limiting enzyme, HMG-CoA reductase. The primary indication for atorvastatin is hypercholesterolemia. Although lovastatin (Mevacor) was the first HMG-CoA reductase inhibitor approved for use in the United States, atorvastatin has a long half-life and may be administered without regard to food or time of day. Maximum effects from atorvastatin are seen in 4–8 weeks. Effectiveness is measured by decreases in LDL, total cholesterol, and triglycerides, and an increase in HDL. Patients receiving this drug should be placed on a cholesterol-lowering diet, because this will enhance the drug's therapeutic effects. The primary goal in atorvastatin therapy is to reduce the risk of MI and stroke.

Adverse Effects and Interactions: Adverse effects of atorvastatin are rarely severe enough to cause discontinuation of therapy and include GI complaints such as intestinal cramping, diarrhea, and constipation. A small percentage of patients experience liver damage; thus, liver function is usually monitored periodically during therapy. The most serious adverse effect is rhabdomyolysis. Like other statins, atorvastatin is a pregnancy category X drug. Pregnancy testing should be conducted prior to treatment in women of childbearing years, and the patient should be advised to take precautions to prevent pregnancy during therapy.

Atorvastatin interacts with many drugs. For example, it may increase digoxin levels by 20%, as well as increase levels of oral contraceptives. Erythromycin may increase atorvastatin levels by 40%. Azole antifungals, HIV protease inhibitors, and telaprevir are contraindicated due to an increased risk for myopathy.

Grapefruit juice inhibits the metabolism of statins, allowing them to reach toxic levels. Because HMG-CoA reductase inhibitors also decrease the synthesis of coenzyme Q10 (CoQ10), patients may benefit from CoQ10 supplements.

Nursing Process Focus Patients Receiving Drug Therapy with HMG-CoA Reductase Inhibitors (Statins)

ASSESSMENT	POTENTIAL NURSING DIAGNOSES*
Prior to administration: • Obtain a complete health history including cardiovascular, musculoskeletal, gastrointestinal, renal and liver conditions, diet, allergies, drug history, and possible drug interactions. • Evaluate laboratory blood findings: complete blood count (CBC), electrolytes, lipid panel, renal and liver function studies, glucose and pregnancy testing for women of childbearing age. • Acquire the results of a complete physical examination, including vital signs, height, and weight.	• *Deficient Knowledge* related to a need for an altered lifestyle and lack of information about drug therapy • *Noncompliance* related to difficulty adhering to dietary and drug regimen • *Chronic Pain* related to drug-induced myopathy • *Ineffective Health Maintenance* related to insufficient knowledge of seriousness of disease and drug therapy regimen

PLANNING: PATIENT GOALS AND EXPECTED OUTCOMES

The patient will:
- Experience therapeutic effects (lowered cholesterol and triglyceride levels).
- Be free from or experience minimal adverse effects from drug therapy.
- Verbalize an understanding of the drug's use, adverse effects, and required precautions.

IMPLEMENTATION

Interventions and (Rationales)	Patient Education/Discharge Planning
• Monitor blood cholesterol and triglyceride levels at intervals during therapy. (Monitoring these levels will help to determine the effectiveness of therapy.)	• Advise the patient of the importance of keeping appointments for laboratory testing.
• Monitor liver function tests after 12 weeks and every 6 months thereafter. (Liver toxicity can occur.)	Advise patients: • To notify the healthcare provider if anorexia, vomiting, nausea, or jaundice occurs. • That it is important to keep all appointments for laboratory testing.
• Monitor patient compliance with the dietary regimen. (Maintenance of controlled saturated fat diet is essential to the effectiveness of medications.)	• Ensure that patient and family understand that drug therapy is used in addition to diet therapy. Provide the patient with information needed to maintain a low-saturated fat, low-cholesterol diet.
• Monitor the patient for alcohol abuse. (Excessive alcohol intake may result in liver damage and interfere with drug effectiveness.)	• Instruct the patient to avoid or limit alcohol use.

Interventions and (Rationales)	Patient Education/Discharge Planning
• Monitor the patient for adverse effects of drug therapy, e.g., GI effects, muscle soreness or joint pain unrelated to usual activity. (May indicate muscle inflammation related to medication.)	• Instruct the patient to report symptoms of GI effects such as cramping and diarrhea; unexplained muscle tenderness and pain, tingling of extremities, or effects that hinder normal activities of daily living to the healthcare provider.
• If complaints of increasing muscle soreness, monitor creatine phosphokinase (CPK) level. (Elevated CPK may be indicative of myopathy.)	• Instruct the patient to see healthcare provider immediately if having increased muscle pain and weakness.
• Obtain the patient's smoking history. (Smoking increases risk of cardiovascular disease and may decrease HDL levels.)	• Encourage smoking cessation. Provide information about medications and smoking cessation programs.
• Monitor patient's pregnancy status. (Statins are classified as pregnancy category X.)	• Advise the patient of childbearing age of the dangers of using statins while pregnant, and to report any prospects of pregnancy or possible side effects or symptoms.
• Administer medication correctly and evaluate the patient's knowledge of proper administration. (Some medications interact with statins, and grapefruit juice inhibits metabolism and can lead to dangerously high statin levels.)	Instruct the patient: • Not to take medication with grapefruit juice. • To notify the healthcare provider when taking oral contraceptives, erythromycin, and some cardiac medication such as digoxin, diltiazem, and verapamil.

EVALUATION OF OUTCOME CRITERIA

Evaluate the effectiveness of drug therapy by confirming that patient goals and expected outcomes have been met (see "Planning"). *See Table 17.2 for a list of drugs to which these nursing actions apply.*

*Herdman, T.H. & Kamitsuru, S. (Eds.), *Nursing Diagnoses: Definitions & Classification* 2015–2017. Copyright © 2014, 1994–2014 NANDA International. Used by arrangement by John Wiley & Sons, Inc. Companion website: www.wiley.com/go/nursingdiagnoses.

Bile acid binding drugs can reduce LDL levels by increasing cholesterol excretion.

◄ **Core Concept 17.5**

Prior to the discovery of the statins, the primary means of lowering blood cholesterol was through use of bile acid binding drugs. **Bile acids** contain a high concentration of cholesterol and are secreted by the liver to aid in the digestion of fats in the small intestine. Once bound in the intestine, the cholesterol in the bile acids is eliminated in the feces. Although they are no longer considered first-line drugs for dyslipidemias, they are sometimes combined with statins for patients who are unable to achieve sufficient response from the statins alone. Doses of these drugs are listed in Table 17.2. Bile acid binding drugs are also called bile acid resins and bile acid sequestrants. The prototype drug for this drug class is cholestyramine (Questran).

Although effective at producing a 20% decrease in LDL-cholesterol levels, the bile acid binding drugs tend to cause more frequent adverse effects than do the statins. Taken orally, bile acid binding drugs are not absorbed into the circulation; therefore, their adverse effects are limited to the GI tract. A high percentage of patients, however, experience constipation, bloating, nausea, or indigestion. Also of concern is that bile acid binding drugs can prevent the absorption of other medications and vitamins that may be taken at the same time. This can be avoided by teaching the patient to take these drugs 1 hour before, or 4 hours after, other medications. Bile-acid binding drugs are sometimes combined with statins to produce

Prototype Drug: Pr *Cholestyramine (Questran)*

Therapeutic Class: Antihyperlipidemic drug **Pharmacologic Class:** Bile acid binding drug

Actions and Uses: Cholestyramine is used to treat elevated levels of cholesterol and LDLs. The drug is formulated as a powder that is mixed with fluid before being taken once or twice daily. It is not absorbed or metabolized once it enters the intestine; thus, it does not produce systemic effects. It may take 30 days or longer to produce its maximum effect. Cholestyramine is sometimes combined with other cholesterol-lowering drugs, such as the statins or niacin, to produce additive effects.

Adverse Effects and Interactions: Although cholestyramine rarely produces serious adverse effects, patients may experience constipation, bloating, gas, and nausea that may limit its use. Cholestyramine has the ability to bind to other drugs and interfere with their absorption. Examples include binding to vitamin K, thiazide diuretics, and penicillins. To prevent potential interactions, other medications should be taken 1 hour before or 4 hours after administration of cholestyramine. The drug is contraindicated in patients with biliary obstruction, biliary cirrhosis, or GI obstruction.

additional reductions in lipid levels, or they may be prescribed as monotherapy for patients who have contraindications to the use of statins. All three of the bile-acid binding drugs have similar effectiveness and side effects.

Core Concept 17.6 ▶

Niacin can reduce triglyceride and LDL-cholesterol levels.

Niacin, also called nicotinic acid, is a water-soluble B-complex vitamin whose primary pharmacologic action is to decrease VLDL levels. When VLDL is diminished, the patient also experiences a reduction in LDL-cholesterol and triglyceride levels. Niacin also has the desirable effect of increasing HDL levels. Thus, niacin is unique in that it can improve multiple types of dyslipidemias. As with other lipid-lowering drugs, maximum therapeutic effects may take a month or longer to achieve.

Niacin may also be used to treat pellagra, a condition resulting from chronic dietary niacin deficiency. The doses used for correcting niacin deficiency are only 14-18 mg/day, whereas the doses for decreasing cholesterol are about 2000 mg/day.

Although effective at reducing LDL cholesterol, niacin produces more adverse effects than the statins. Flushing and hot flashes occur in almost every patient, although taking one aspirin tablet 30 minutes prior to niacin administration can reduce flushing in many patients. Uncomfortable GI effects such as nausea, excess gas, and diarrhea are frequently reported. Although uncommon, more serious adverse effects such as liver toxicity and gout are possible. Because of these adverse effects, niacin is most often used in lower doses in combination with a statin or bile acid binding drug because the beneficial effects of these drugs are additive. Several fixed-dose combination drugs are available, including Advicor (niacin with lovastatin) and Simcor (niacin with simvastatin). Extended-release niacin, which is taken once daily, causes less flushing and fewer GI adverse effects.

As a dietary supplement, niacin is available without a prescription. However, patients should be instructed not to attempt self-medication to lower cholesterol with this drug. One form of niacin, available over the counter as a vitamin supplement called *nicotinamide*, has no lipid-lowering effects. Patients should be informed that if niacin is used to lower cholesterol, it should be done under medical supervision.

CONCEPT REVIEW 17.2

- How does the mechanism of the statins differ from that of niacin?

CAM Therapy | Coenzyme Q10 for Heart Disease

Coenzyme Q10 (CoQ10) is a vitamin-like substance found in most animal cells. It is an essential component in the mitochondria of cells, which produce energy or adenosine triphosphate (ATP). Because the heart requires high levels of ATP, a sufficient level of CoQ10 is essential to that organ. Foods richest in this substance are pork, sardines, beef, salmon, broccoli, spinach, and nuts. Older adults appear to have an increased need for CoQ10.

Reports of the benefits of CoQ10 for treating heart disease began to emerge in the mid-1960s. Subsequent reports have claimed that CoQ10 may be beneficial in angina pectoris, dysrhythmias, periodontal disease, immune disorders, neurologic disease, obesity, diabetes mellitus, and certain cancers. Considerable research has been conducted on this antioxidant.

The statins decrease CoQ10 levels. Indeed, many of the adverse effects of statins may be due to the decrease in CoQ10 levels, including muscle weakness and rhabdomyolysis. Supplementation with CoQ10 may diminish myopathy symptoms. In addition, there is scientific evidence to suggest that CoQ10 causes a small decrease in blood pressure in patients with hypertension. Evidence to support the use of CoQ10 in treating patients with heart disease, neurologic disorders, or cancer is weak. As for most dietary supplements, controlled research studies are often lacking and give conflicting results.

Core Concept 17.7 ▶

Fibric acid drugs lower triglyceride levels, but have little effect on LDLs.

The fibric acid drugs, or fibrates, are older medications that have been largely replaced by the statins. They are sometimes used in combination with the statins to produce an enhanced lipid-lowering effect. Fenofibrate (Lofibra, Tricor), fenofibric acid (Fibricor, Trilipix), and gemfibrozil (Lopid) are sometimes indicated for patients with excessive triglyceride and VLDL levels. They are preferred drugs for treating severe hypertriglyceridemia. Unfortunately, these drugs have little effect on LDL-cholesterol levels. Doses of the fibrates are listed in Table 17.2.

Fibrates cause few serious adverse effects. Flushing, dizziness, fatigue, rashes, and GI complaints are the most common adverse effects. Like the statins, some patients experience muscle pain or weakness; therefore, patients receiving concurrent therapy with both statins and fibrates should be monitored carefully. The mechanisms of action of the fibrates and other drugs for dyslipidemias are shown in Figure 17.3. Dosages of these drugs are listed in Table 17.2.

Prototype Drug: *Gemfibrozil (Lopid)*

Therapeutic Class: Antihyperlipidemic drug **Pharmacologic Class:** Fibric acid drug

Actions and Uses: Gemfibrozil can cause up to a significant reduction in VLDL with a moderate increase in HDL. Because it is less effective than the statins, it is not a drug of first choice for reducing LDL-cholesterol levels. However, it is useful for patients with high triglyceride levels who have not responded favorably to diet modification and those at risk for pancreatitis.

Adverse Effects and Interactions: The most common adverse effects of gemfibrozil are related to the GI system: diarrhea, nausea, and abdominal cramping. The drug produces few serious adverse effects, but it may increase the likelihood of gallstones and occasionally affect liver function.

Using gemfibrozil with oral anticoagulants may increase the risk of bleeding. Concurrent use with statins should be avoided because this increases the risk of myopathy and rhabdomyolysis.

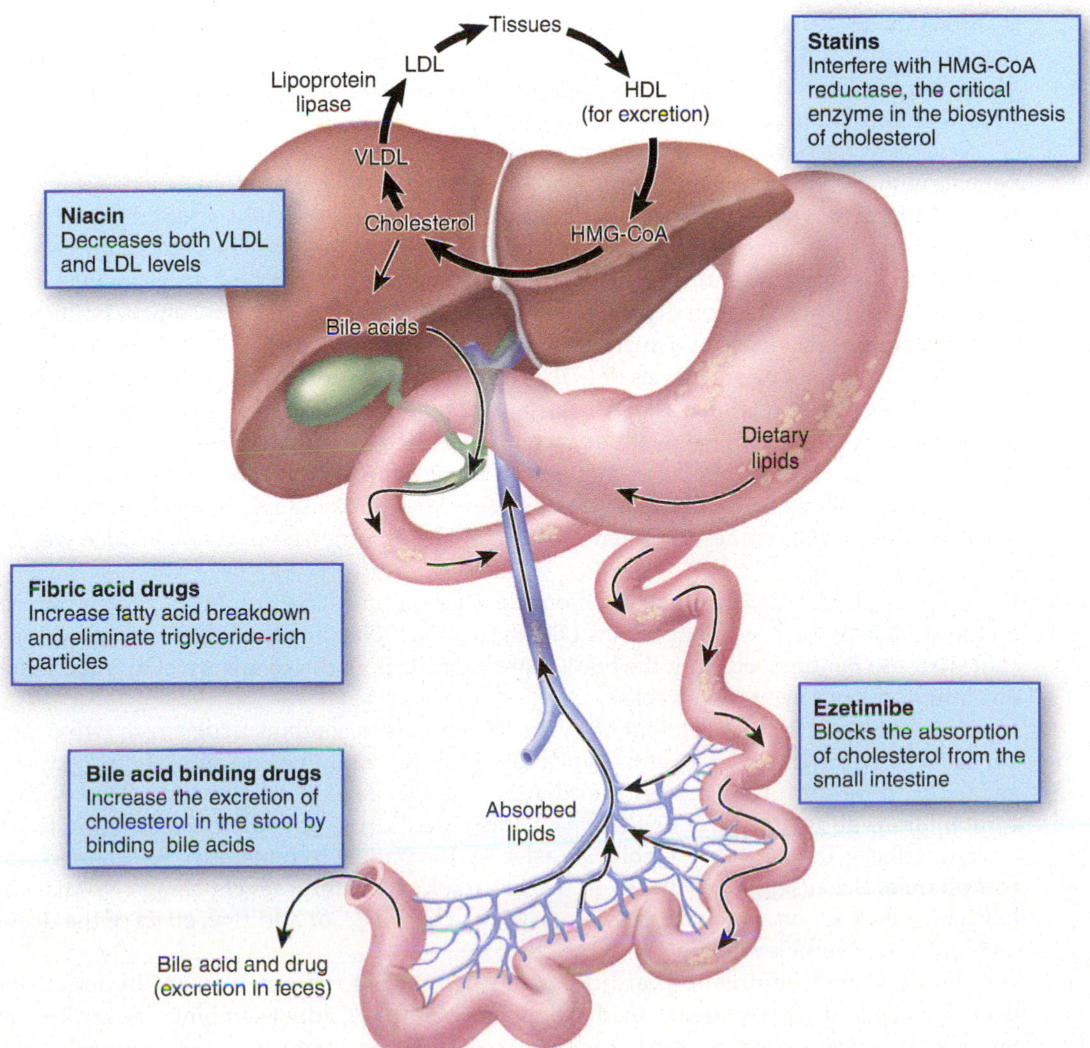

FIGURE 17.3 Mechanisms of action of lipid-lowering drugs.

New Drug Focus

TREATMENT OF FAMILIAL HYPERCHOLESTEROLEMIA

While most cases of high blood cholesterol are believed to be caused by lifestyle factors, research has identified genetic causes for the disease, called familial hypercholesterolemia (FH). In these patients, a genetic mutation renders the liver unable to remove cholesterol, which then builds to high lipid levels early in life. Children who receive the mutation from both parents (homozygous FH) inherit an especially aggressive form of the condition. Affecting enzymes in the pathway for cholesterol metabolism, three drugs have recently been approved for FH: mipomersen (Kynamaro), lomitapide (Lojuxta), and evolocumab (Repatha). These drugs are used concurrently with statins and dietary modifications. They represent a significant breakthrough for patients with FH.

Core Concept 17.8 ▶

Several miscellaneous drugs and drug combinations are available to treat dyslipidemias.

Several newer approaches for treating high blood cholesterol levels have emerged in recent years. Ezetimibe (Zetia) blocks the absorption of cholesterol in the small intestine. LDL-cholesterol and triglyceride levels are reduced, with a slight increase in HDL. It is used as monotherapy or combined with statins. Adverse effects from ezetimibe are uncommon and include abdominal pain, back pain, diarrhea, and arthralgia. The dose for ezetimibe is listed in Table 17.2.

Omega-3-acid ethyl esters (Epanova, Lovaza) and icosapent (Vascepa) are prescription forms of omega-3 fatty acids found in fish oil. Fish oil has long been a natural therapy for the treatment of high blood lipid levels. Both drugs are approved as an adjunct to diet in the treatment of severe hypertriglyceridemia. Most adverse effects are minor and include burping, fishy taste, and dyspepsia (indigestion). Those patients allergic to seafood may be allergic to fish oil. High doses of omega-3 fatty acids may prolong clotting time and should be used with caution in patients taking anticoagulants.

Several drugs have been recently approved for a very narrow indication: lowering LDL in patients with homozygous familial hypercholesterolemia (HoFH). HoFH is a genetic disorder in which the body has such high levels of cholesterol and LDL that cardiovascular disease begins in childhood and results in death by the mid thirties. Many of these patients have a diminished response to therapy with statins and other antihyperlipidemics. The new drugs include lomitapide (Juxtapid), mipomersen (Kynamro), evolocumab (Repatha), and alirocumab (Praluent).

Lomitapide is classified as a microsomal triglyceride transfer protein (MTP) inhibitor. Inhibition of MTP lowers plasma levels of LDL. The drug is given orally and is indicated only for HoFH. GI adverse effects such as diarrhea, nausea, vomiting, dyspepsia, and abdominal pain occur in almost all patients. Lomitamide is contraindicated during pregnancy (category X).

Mipomersan is classified as an inhibitor of Apolipoprotein B (apo B) synthesis, the primary protein that makes up LDL particles. By preventing the synthesis of apo B, mipomersen is able to lower LDL values in patients with HoFH. Mipomersen is given as once weekly subcutaneous injection.

Evolocumab and alirocumab are monoclonal antibodies that inhibit PCSK9, a protein on the surface of liver cells that retains LDL in the body. Blocking the PCSK9 protein allows cholesterol to be removed from the body more rapidly. Both drugs are given by subcutaneous injection, once every two weeks.

A recent trend in the treatment of hyperlipidemia is to combine drugs from two different classes in a single tablet. Examples include Vytorin (ezetimibe and simvastatin), Liptruzet (ezetimibe and atorvastatin), and Advicor (lovastatin and niacin). Fixed-dose combinations allow for lower doses of each individual drug, potentially resulting in fewer adverse effects. Taking a single tablet is easier for the patient to remember, which increases compliance. Because the combination drugs attack cholesterol levels using two distinct mechanisms of action, it may be possible to get a synergistic, or additive, effect of the drugs on blood cholesterol levels.

A second trend in treating cardiovascular disease is to combine an antihypertensive drug with an antihyperlipidemic medication. For example, Caduet combines the antihypertensive amlodipine with atorvastatin. These combination agents are targeted for the millions of patients who have both hypertension and elevated blood cholesterol levels.

Patients Need to Know

Patients treated for lipid disorders need to know the following:

In General

1. Because high cholesterol and triglyceride levels in the blood increase the risk for heart disease and stroke, follow the healthcare provider's instructions even when feeling well.
2. Continuation of a low-fat, low-cholesterol diet while taking lipid-lowering drugs will provide the best results.

Regarding Statin Medications

3. Atorvastatin and rosuvastatin are effective regardless of the time of day they are taken. Taking other statin drugs in the evening makes them available to work on the higher amount of cholesterol that the body makes at night.
4. The healthcare provider may prescribe a fibric acid drug to lower triglycerides and another drug to lower cholesterol. One drug should not be stopped when the second drug is ordered, except by advice of the provider.

Regarding Bile Acid Binding Drugs

5. Self-medication with high doses of niacin can cause gout and liver damage. It will not lower cholesterol at low doses. Supervision by a healthcare provider supports safe and effective use of this drug.
6. If prescribed bile acid resins, such as psyllium (Metamucil), cholestyramine (Questran), or colestipol (Colestid), take 1 hour after or 4 hours before other drugs to avoid counteracting drug effectiveness. Dissolving the bile acid resin in water and keeping fluid intake high helps to avoid irritation of the mouth and constipation.

Chapter Review

Core Concepts Summary

17.1 Lipids serve essential roles in the body, but too much dietary fat can lead to disease

Lipids, or fats, have important roles in human physiology. Excessive dietary triglyceride or cholesterol can cause dyslipidemias, an abnormal amount of lipid in the blood. Dyslipidemias are major risk factors for cardiovascular disease.

17.2 Lipoproteins transport lipids through the blood for utilization by tissues, storage in adipose tissue, or excretion by the liver.

Lipids are packaged for travel through the blood in lipoprotein complexes. High VLDL and LDL are associated with an increased incidence of cardiovascular disease, whereas HDL provides a protective effect.

17.3 Elevated lipid levels can often be prevented or controlled through therapeutic lifestyle changes.

Before starting pharmacotherapy for hyperlipidemia, patients are usually advised to manage the condition through lifestyle changes, such as restriction of dietary saturated fats and cholesterol, increased exercise, and smoking cessation.

17.4 Statins are preferred drugs for reducing blood lipid levels.

Drugs in the statin class inhibit HMG-CoA reductase, a critical enzyme in the biosynthesis of cholesterol. They are safe and effective at lowering LDL cholesterol and are the most widely prescribed class of drugs for hyperlipidemias.

17.5 Bile acid binding drugs can reduce LDL levels by increasing cholesterol excretion.

The bile acid binding drugs are effective at lowering LDL cholesterol, although they produce more adverse effects than the statins. They should be taken separately from other medications because they can interfere with drug absorption.

17.6 Niacin can reduce triglyceride and LDL-cholesterol levels.

Niacin, or nicotinic acid, can be effective at lowering LDL cholesterol and triglycerides when given in large amounts. It is not usually a first-choice drug but is sometimes combined in smaller doses with statins.

17.7 Fibric acid drugs lower triglyceride levels, but have little effect on LDLs.

Fibric acids such as gemfibrozil are effective at lowering triglycerides but less effective than the statins at lowering LDLs. Their use is limited because of frequent adverse effects. However, they are sometimes combined with statins to produce an additive effect.

17.8 Several miscellaneous drugs and drug combinations are available to treat dyslipidemias.

Ezetimibe lowers LDL levels by blocking the absorption of cholesterol from the intestine. Omega-3 fatty acids are available by prescription to lower LDL cholesterol. Combination drugs such as Advicor and Vytorin attack high blood cholesterol levels using two different mechanisms. Lomitapide, mipomersen, evolocumab, and alirocumab are newer medications used to treat HoFH.

REVIEW Questions

Answer the following questions to assess your knowledge of the chapter material, and go back and review any material that is not clear to you.

1. This lipoprotein is responsible for transporting cholesterol from the blood to the liver.
   1. LDL
   2. VLDL
   3. HDL
   4. Triglycerides

2. Which of the following HMG-CoA reductase inhibitors should be taken with meals?
   1. Atorvastatin (Lipitor)
   2. Simvastatin (Zocor)
   3. Lovastatin (Mevacor)
   4. Rosuvastatin (Crestor)

3. The nurse is instructing a patient on how to take statin drugs. The patient is informed that statin drugs are most effective when taken:
   1. In the morning.
   2. In the evening.
   3. With other medications.
   4. On an empty stomach.

4. The healthcare provider orders lovastatin (Mevacor) 20 mg at bedtime. The supply is 10-mg tablets. How many tablets will the nurse give?
   1. 1 tablet
   2. 1½ tablets
   3. 2 tablets
   4. 2½ tablets

5. Which of the following patient complaints would be considered to be an adverse reaction to a bile acid resin?
   1. Constipation
   2. Headache
   3. Anxiety
   4. Double vision

6. When administering colestipol (Colestid), the nurse administers the drug:
   1. With large amounts of fluid to prevent gastrointestinal upset.
   2. 30 minutes prior to meals.
   3. At least 1 hour before or 4 hours after meals.
   4. At bedtime.

7. A patient is interested in taking niacin to help reduce cholesterol. When the patient asks the nurse about possible adverse effects, the nurse informs that niacin can cause: (Select all that apply.)
   1. Flushing.
   2. Excess gas.
   3. Constipation.
   4. Diarrhea.
   5. Headaches.

8. On assessment, the patient is found to have a total cholesterol level of 326 mg/dL and prehypertension. When assisting the RN in the development of a care plan, the LPN or LVN recognizes that the best treatment for this patient would be a low-fat diet and:
   1. An exercise program only.
   2. Cholesterol-lowering medication.
   3. Over-the-counter supplements.
   4. An antihypertensive.

9. After a review of a patient's chart, the nurse notices that the patient has developed gallstones and elevated liver enzymes. Which of the following cholesterol-lowering medications could have caused this?
   1. Cholestyramine (Questran)
   2. Niacin (Nicotinic acid)
   3. Gemfibrozil (Lopid)
   4. Lovastatin (Mevacor)

10. A patient hears that taking fish oil helps reduce triglyceride levels. He asks for information concerning this form of treatment. The nurse would explain that: (Select all that apply.)
    1. A minor adverse effect of this drug is dyspepsia.
    2. Some people who are allergic to seafood may be allergic to fish oil.
    3. Omega-3 fatty acids are the beneficial component found in fish oil.
    4. No matter what the dose, omega-3-fatty acids may decrease the ability of the blood to clot.
    5. It commonly causes constipation.

CASE STUDY Questions

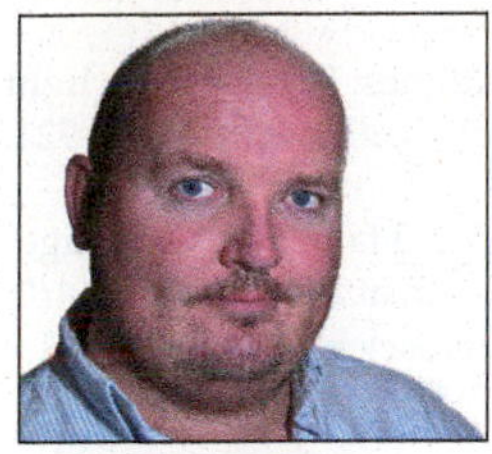

Remember Mr. Long, the patient introduced at the beginning of the chapter? Now read the remainder of the case study. Based on the information you have learned in this chapter, answer the questions that follow.

Mr. Edward Long is a 50-year-old office worker who has gained 50 pounds over the past 5 years. His blood pressure has consistently been high, but he has declined to take medication for the condition. His LDL-cholesterol level has been above 210 mg/dL on his last three office visits. He claims to have no chronic diseases and is at the office seeking assistance concerning his weight gain. While there, his healthcare provider speaks to him about his cholesterol level.

1. The healthcare provider ordered cholestyramine for Mr. Long. You inform Mr. Long that this drug acts by:
   1. Inhibiting enzymes that make cholesterol.
   2. Binding bile acids in the intestine, which increases cholesterol excretion.
   3. Increasing the breakdown of cholesterol in the liver.
   4. Making more bile acids, which bind cholesterol.
2. After 2 months of therapy, the healthcare provider switched the prescription to lovastatin (Mevacor). Mr. Long asks what makes this drug different from the other one he was on. You reply that this drug acts by:
   1. Inhibiting enzymes that make cholesterol.
   2. Binding bile acids in the intestine, which increase cholesterol excretion.
   3. Increasing the breakdown of cholesterol in the liver.
   4. Making more bile acids, which bind cholesterol.
3. After several weeks of lovastatin therapy, Mr. Long returns to the office for follow-up. What question should you ask to determine if he may be suffering from a very serious adverse effect of the statins?
   1. "Do you have bloody diarrhea more than once a week?"
   2. "Have you felt confused, lethargic, or drowsy since starting the drug?"
   3. "Have you experienced excessive muscle weakness or pain?"
   4. "Have you experienced acid indigestion or nausea?"
4. You are checking the results of Mr. Long's laboratory work. Which of the following therapeutic results would you expect to see now that he has been taking lovastatin?
   1. Higher LDL level
   2. Higher VLDL level
   3. Lower HDL level
   4. Higher HDL level

Answers and complete rationales for Review and Case Study Questions appear in Appendix A.

REFERENCES

Centers for Disease Control and Prevention. (2015). *High cholesterol facts*. Retrieved from http://www.cdc.gov/cholesterol/facts.htm

Expert Panel on Detection, Evaluation, and Treatment of High Blood Cholesterol in Adults. (2001). Executive Summary of the Third Report of the National Cholesterol Education Program (NCEP) Expert Panel on Detection, Evaluation, and Treatment of High Blood Cholesterol in Adults (Adult Treatment Panel III). *JAMA 285*, 2486–2497. doi:10.1001/jama.285.19.2486

Herdman, T. H., & Kamitsuru, S. (Eds.). (2014). *NANDA International nursing diagnoses: Definitions and classification, 2015–2017*. Oxford, United Kingdom: Wiley-Blackwell.

Psaty, B. M., & Weiss, N. S. (2014). 2013 ACC/AHA guideline on the treatment of blood cholesterol: A fresh interpretation of old evidence. *JAMA, 311*, 461–462. doi:10.1001/jama.2013.284203

SELECTED BIBLIOGRAPHY

Ahn, C. H., & Choi, S. H. (2015). New drugs for treating dyslipidemia: Beyond statins. *Diabetes and Metabolism Journal, 39*, 87–94. doi:10.4093/dmj.2015.39.2.87

Anderson, T. J., Grégoire, J., Hegele, R. A., Couture, P., Mancini, G. B., McPherson, R., . . . Ur, E. (2013). 2012 update of the Canadian Cardiovascular Society guidelines for the diagnosis and treatment of dyslipidemia for the prevention of cardiovascular disease in the adult. *Canadian Journal of Cardiology, 29*, 151–167. doi:10.1016/j.cjca.2012.11.032

Bamba, V. (2014). Update on screening, etiology, and treatment of dyslipidemia in children. *The Journal of Clinical Endocrinology & Metabolism, 99*, 3093–3102. doi:10.1210/jc.2013-3860

Citkowitz, E. (2015). *Familial hypercholesterolemia*. Retrieved from http://emedicine.medscape.com/article/121298-overview

Lefler, L. L., Hadley, M., Tackett, J., & Thomason, A. P. (2016). New cardiovascular guidelines: Clinical practice evidence for the nurse practitioner. *Journal of the American Association of Nurse Practitioners, 28*, 241–248. doi:10.1002/2327-6924.12262

National Center for Complementary and Integrative Health. (2015). *Coenzyme Q10 (CoQ10): In depth*. Retrieved from https://nccih.nih.gov/health/supplements/coq10

Smith, R. J., & Hiatt, W. R. (2013). Two new drugs for homozygous familial hypercholesterolemia: Managing benefits and risks in a rare disorder. *JAMA Internal Medicine, 173*, 1491–1492. doi:10.1001/jamainternmed.2013.6624

Stone, N. J., Robinson, J. G., Lichtenstein, A. H., Merz, C. N. B., Blum, C. B., Eckel, R. H., . . . Wilson, P. W. F. (2014). 2013 ACC/AHA guideline on the treatment of blood cholesterol to reduce atherosclerotic cardiovascular risk in adults: A report of the American College of Cardiology/American Heart Association Task Force on Practice Guidelines. *Journal of the American College of Cardiology, 63*(25_PA), 2889-2934. doi:10.1016/j.jacc.2013.11.002

Vogel, R. A. (2014). The new cholesterol guidelines: Finally more light than heat. *Journal of the American College of Cardiology, 64*, 920–921. doi:10.1016/j.jacc.2014.06.1168

Weintraub, H. (2013). Update on marine omega-3 fatty acids: Management of dyslipidemia and current omega-3 treatment options. *Atherosclerosis, 230*, 381–389. doi:10.1016/j.atherosclerosis.2013.07.041

Chapter 18

Drugs for Electrolyte and Acid–Base Imbalances

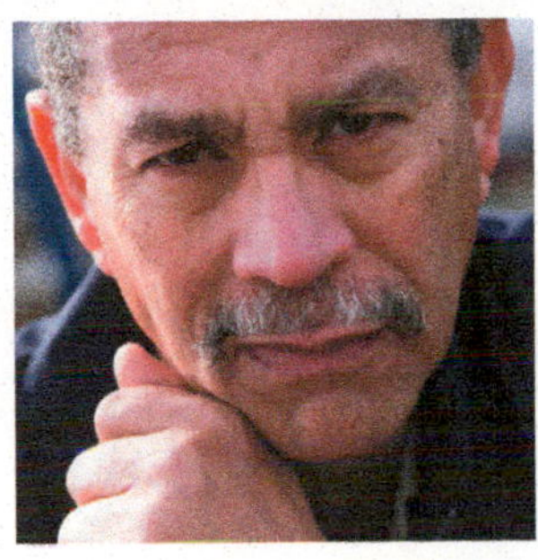

"I did everything the nurse told me to do. Why is my blood pressure so high when I've been taking all my medications?"
Mr. Joseph Grant

Core Concepts

18.1 **The kidneys regulate fluid volume, electrolytes, acids, and bases.**
18.2 **The composition of filtrate changes dramatically as a result of the processes of reabsorption and secretion.**
18.3 **Renal failure significantly impacts pharmacotherapy.**
18.4 **Diuretics are used to treat hypertension, heart failure, and fluid retention disorders.**
18.5 **The most effective diuretics are those that affect the loop of Henle.**
18.6 **The thiazides are the most widely prescribed class of diuretics.**
18.7 **Although less effective than the loop diuretics, potassium-sparing diuretics may help prevent hypokalemia.**
18.8 **Several less commonly prescribed diuretics have specific indications.**
18.9 **Electrolytes are charged substances that play important roles in maintaining homeostasis.**
18.10 **Acidic and basic drugs can be administered to correct pH imbalances.**

Drug Snapshot

The following drugs are discussed in this chapter:

Drug Classes	Prototype Drugs
Loop (high-ceiling) diuretics	Pr furosemide (Lasix)
Thiazide diuretics	Pr hydrochlorothiazide (Microzide)
Potassium-sparing diuretics	Pr spironolactone (Aldactone)
Miscellaneous diuretics	
Electrolytes	Pr potassium chloride (KCl)
Acid–base agents	Pr sodium bicarbonate ($NaHCO_3$)

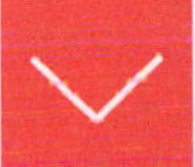

Learning Outcomes

After reading this chapter, the student should be able to:

1. Explain the role of the kidneys in maintaining fluid, electrolyte, and acid–base balance.
2. Explain how the processes of reabsorption and secretion can affect the composition of the filtrate.

3. Describe how pharmacotherapy is modified for patients with renal failure.
4. Identify indications and general uses for diuretics.
5. Explain the role of loop diuretics in the treatment of fluid volume disorders.
6. Explain the role of thiazide diuretics in the treatment of fluid volume disorders.
7. Explain the role of potassium-sparing diuretics in the treatment of fluid volume disorders.
8. Explain the role of miscellaneous diuretics in the treatment of fluid volume disorders.
9. Explain the importance of electrolytes in maintaining homeostasis.
10. Identify common causes of acidosis and alkalosis and the drugs used to treat these conditions.

Key Terms

acidosis (ah-sid-OH-sis)
aldosterone (al-DOH-stair-own)
alkalosis (al-kah-LOH-sis)
carbonic anhydrase (kar-BON-ik an-HY-drase)
diuretic (dye-your-ET-ik)
electrolytes (ee-LEK-troh-lites)
end-stage renal disease (ESRD)
erythropoietin (ee-rith-ro-po-EE-tin)
filtrate (FIL-trate)
hyperkalemia (heye-purr-kah-LEE-mee-ah)
hypernatremia (heye-purr-nuh-TREE-mee-ah)
hypokalemia (heye-poh-kah-LEE-mee-uh)
hyponatremia (hy-po-nay-TREE-mee-uh)
nephrons (NEF-ron)
pH
reabsorption
renal failure
secretion

The volume and composition of fluids in the body must be maintained within narrow limits. Excess fluid volume can lead to hypertension (HTN) or heart failure (HF), whereas depletion may result in dehydration or shock. Body fluids must also contain specific amounts of essential ions or electrolytes and be maintained at specific pH values. The kidneys serve a remarkable role in keeping the volume and composition of body fluids within normal limits. This chapter examines diuretics and drugs used to reverse electrolyte and acid–base imbalances.

Core Concept 18.1 ▶

The kidneys regulate fluid volume, electrolytes, acids, and bases.

When most people think of the kidneys, they think of excretion. Although this is certainly one of their roles, the kidneys have many other essential functions. The kidneys are the primary organs for regulating fluid volume, electrolyte composition, and the acid–base balance of body fluids. They also secrete the enzyme renin, which helps to regulate blood pressure (see Chapter 19), and the hormone erythropoietin, which stimulates red blood cell production. In addition, the kidneys are responsible for the production of calcitriol, the active form of vitamin D, which helps maintain bone homeostasis (see Chapter 36). It is not surprising that overall wellness is strongly dependent on proper functioning of the kidneys.

The urinary system consists of two kidneys, two ureters, a urinary bladder, and a urethra. These structures are shown in Figure 18.1. Each kidney contains more than 2 million **nephrons**, the functional units of the kidney. As blood enters a nephron, it is filtered through a porous capillary known as the glomerulus. Once in the nephron, the fluid is called **filtrate**. Water and other small molecules readily pass through and enter the Bowman's capsule, the first section of the renal tubule. After leaving the Bowman's capsule, the filtrate travels through the proximal tubule, the loop of Henle, and, subsequently, the distal tubule. Nephrons empty their filtrate into tubes called common collecting ducts, and then into larger and larger collecting structures inside the kidney. Fluid leaving the collecting ducts and entering subsequent portions of the kidney is called urine. The parts of the nephron are illustrated in Figure 18.2.

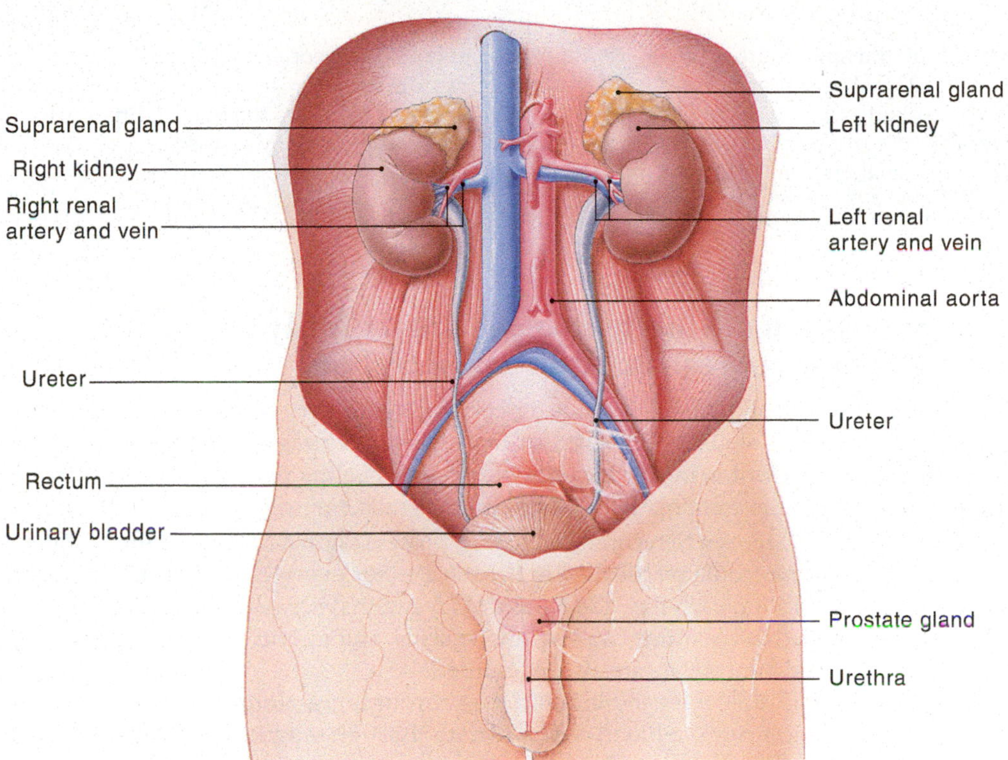

FIGURE 18.1 The urinary system.

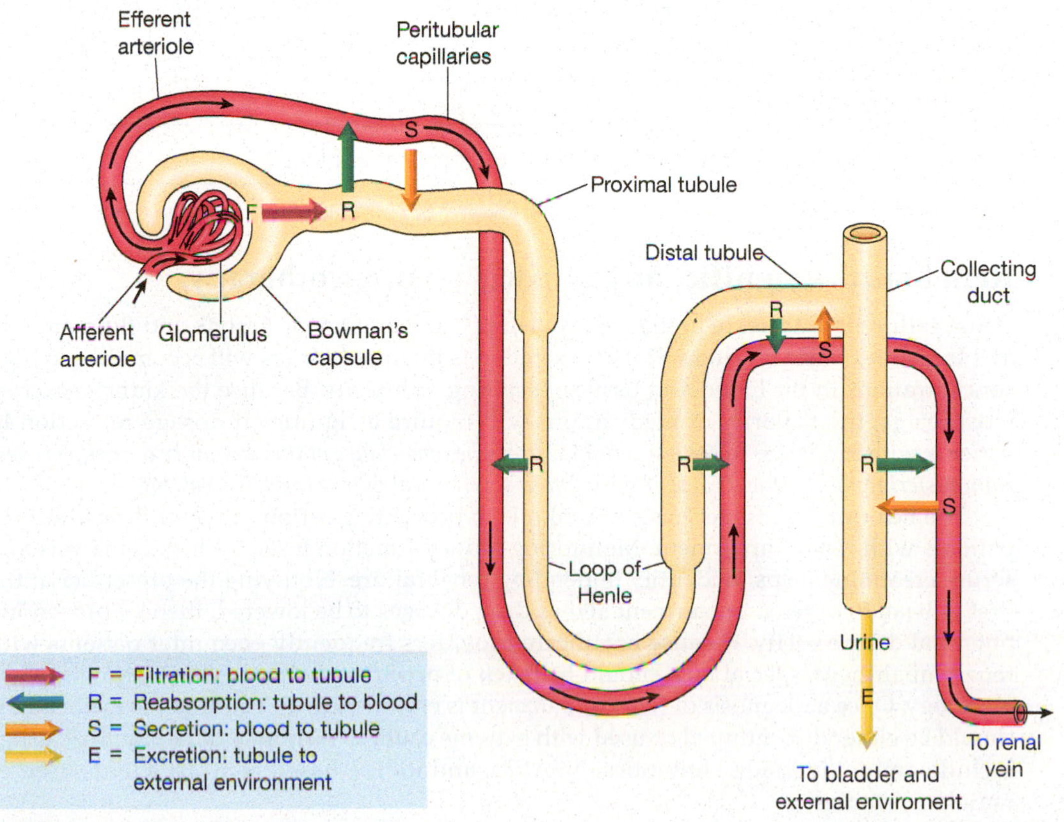

FIGURE 18.2 The nephron.

Fast Facts Renal Disorders

- Although more than 17,000 kidney transplants are performed annually, more than 120,000 people are on a waiting list for kidney transplants.
- Approximately 47,000 Americans die from kidney disease annually; this is more deaths than from prostate cancer or breast cancer.
- Approximately 24% of people over age 60 have chronic kidney disease,.
- Type 2 diabetes and HTN are the two leading causes of new cases of chronic kidney disease.

Core Concept 18.2 ▶

The composition of filtrate changes dramatically as a result of the processes of reabsorption and secretion.

When filtrate enters the Bowman's capsule, its composition is very similar to that of plasma. Plasma proteins such as albumin, however, are too large to have passed through the glomerulus and will not be present in the filtrate or in the urine of healthy patients. As filtrate travels through the nephron, its composition changes dramatically. Some substances in the filtrate cross the walls of the nephron to reenter the blood, a process known as **reabsorption**. Water is the most important molecule reabsorbed in the tubule. For every 180 liters (47 gallons) of water entering the filtrate each day, 178.5 liters (45.5 gallons) are reabsorbed, leaving only 1.5 liters to be excreted in the urine. Glucose, amino acids, and essential ions such as sodium, chloride, calcium, and bicarbonate are also reabsorbed.

Certain ions and molecules too large to pass through the glomerulus can still enter the urine by crossing from the blood to the filtrate through a process known as tubular **secretion**. Potassium, phosphate, hydrogen, and ammonium ions enter the filtrate through secretion. Examples of drugs secreted in the proximal tubule include penicillin G, ampicillin, nonsteroidal anti-inflammatory drugs (NSAIDs), furosemide, epinephrine, and trimethoprim.

Reabsorption and secretion are critical to the pharmacokinetics of many drugs. Some drugs are reabsorbed, whereas others are secreted into the filtrate. For example, approximately 90% of a dose of penicillin G enters the urine through secretion. When the kidney is damaged, reabsorption and secretion mechanisms are impaired, and serum drug levels may be dramatically affected. The processes of reabsorption and secretion are depicted in Figure 18.2.

CONCEPT REVIEW 18.1

- How does the composition of filtrate differ from that of blood?

Core Concept 18.3 ▶

Renal failure significantly impacts pharmacotherapy.

Renal failure is a decrease in the kidneys' ability to maintain electrolyte and fluid balance and to excrete waste products. If renal excretion is impaired, drugs will accumulate to high concentrations in the blood and tissues, resulting in toxicity. Because the kidneys excrete most drugs, the majority of medications will require a significant dosage reduction in patients with moderate to severe renal failure. *The importance of this cannot be overemphasized: Administering the "average" dose to a patient in severe renal failure can kill a patient.*

The healthcare provider has a critical role in preventing serious adverse drug effects in patients with renal impairment. Monitoring kidney function tests, such as urinalysis and serum creatinine helps to identify impending renal failure. Notifying the prescriber at the first indication of renal impairment allows drug dosages to be lowered, thereby preventing potential drug toxicity. Because healthcare providers frequently encounter patients with renal impairment, special note should be taken of nephrotoxic drugs when learning pharmacology. Once a diagnosis of renal impairment is established, all nephrotoxic medications should be either discontinued or used with extreme caution. Examples of nephrotoxic drugs include aminoglycoside antibiotics, NSAIDs, and iodine-based contrast agents used in radiologic studies.

Renal failure is classified as acute or chronic, depending on its onset. Acute renal failure requires immediate treatment because accumulation of waste products, such as urea and creatinine, can result in death if untreated. The cause of acute renal failure must be quickly identified and corrected. The most common cause of acute renal failure is lack of sufficient blood flow through the kidneys due to underlying conditions such as HF, dysrhythmias, hemorrhage, or dehydration.

Chronic renal failure occurs over a period of months or years. Over half of patients with chronic renal failure have a medical history of longstanding HTN or diabetes mellitus. Because of its long, gradual development and nonspecific symptoms, chronic renal failure may go undiagnosed for many years until the impairment becomes irreversible. When the kidneys are no longer able to function at a level necessary for day-to-day living, the patient has **end-stage renal disease (ESRD)**, and dialysis and kidney transplantation become treatment alternatives.

Pharmacotherapy of renal impairment includes administering diuretics, which can increase urine output. In addition, cardiovascular drugs are commonly administered to treat underlying HTN or HF. Dietary management, such as protein restriction and reduction of sodium, potassium, phosphorus, and magnesium intake, is often necessary to prevent worsening of renal impairment.

Many patients with chronic renal failure will also have a deficiency of **erythropoietin**, a hormone secreted by the kidney. Erythropoietin serves as a primary signal to increase red blood cell production in the bone marrow. A synthetic form of erythropoietin, epoetin alfa (Epogen, Procrit) is effective in treating several disorders caused by a deficiency in red blood cells. Epoetin is sometimes given to patients undergoing cancer chemotherapy to counteract the anemia caused by antineoplastic drugs (see Chapter 29). It is occasionally prescribed for patients prior to blood transfusions or surgery and to treat anemia in HIV-infected patients. Epoetin alfa is usually administered three times per week until an increase in the number of red blood cells is achieved.

CAM Therapy | Cranberry for Urinary System Health

Nearly everyone is familiar with the bright red cranberries that are eaten during holiday times. Native Americans used the colorful, ripe berries to treat wounds and to cure anorexia and for other digestive complaints. In the 1900s, it was noted that the acidity of the urine increases after eating cranberries; thus began the belief that cranberry juice is a natural cure for urinary tract infections.

Cranberry juice or berries contain a significant amount of vitamin C and other antioxidants that can promote health. They contain a substance that can prevent bacteria from sticking to the walls of the bladder. Research suggests that cranberries can prevent symptomatic urinary tract infections in some patients, especially in women who have recurrent infections.

Cranberry is a safe supplement, although large amounts may cause gastrointestinal (GI) upset and diarrhea. The juice should be 100% cranberry and not "cocktail" juice because that contains sugar, which enhances bacteria growth and may be contraindicated in patients with diabetes. Some individuals may prefer to take cranberry capsules, which are available at most pharmacies.

Diuretics are used to treat hypertension, heart failure, and fluid retention disorders.

◀ **Core Concept 18.4**

A **diuretic** is a drug that increases urine output. The goal of most diuretic therapy is to reverse abnormal fluid retention by the body. Excretion of excess body fluid is important in managing the following conditions:

dia = *thoroughly*
uretic = *to urinate*

- Hypertension
- Heart failure

- Kidney failure
- Pulmonary edema
- Liver failure or cirrhosis.

The most common mechanism by which diuretics act is by blocking sodium ion (Na^+) reabsorption in the nephron, thus sending more Na^+ to the urine. Chloride ion (Cl^-) follows Na^+. Because water molecules travel with sodium, blocking the reabsorption of Na^+ will increase the volume of urination, or diuresis. Some drugs, such as furosemide (Lasix), act by preventing the reabsorption of Na^+ in the loop of Henle, and thus they are called loop diuretics. Because of the abundance of Na^+ in the loop of Henle, furosemide is capable of producing large increases in urine output. Other drugs, such as the thiazides, act on the distal tubule. Because most Na^+ has already been reabsorbed from the filtrate by the time it reaches this point in the nephron, the thiazides produce less diuresis than does furosemide. The sites at which the various diuretics act are shown in Figure 18.3.

Core Concept 18.5 ▶

The most effective diuretics are those that affect the loop of Henle.

The most effective diuretics are the loop or high-ceiling diuretics. Drugs in this class act by blocking the reabsorption of Na^+ and Cl^- in the loop of Henle. When given by IV route, they have the ability to cause large amounts of fluid to be excreted by the kidney in a very short time. Loop diuretics are used to reduce the fluid accumulation associated with HF, hepatic cirrhosis, or chronic renal failure. Furosemide (Lasix) and torsemide (Demadex) are also approved for HTN.

Furosemide is the most frequently prescribed loop diuretic. Unlike the thiazide diuretics, furosemide is able to increase urine output even when blood flow to the kidneys is

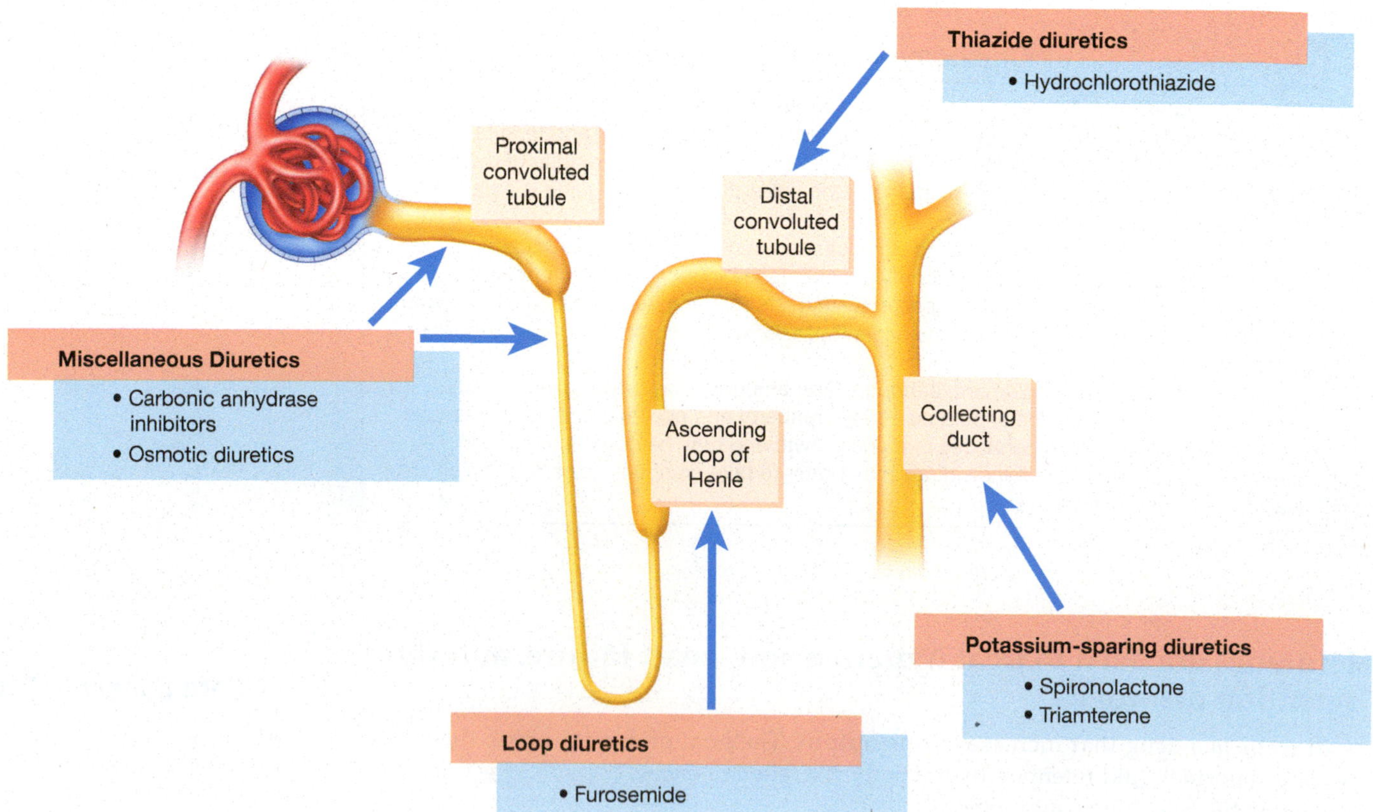

FIGURE 18.3 Sites of action of diuretics.

diminished. Torsemide (Demadex) has a longer half-life than furosemide, which offers the advantage of once-a-day dosing. Bumetanide (Bumex) is 40 times more potent than furosemide but has a shorter duration of action.

The rapid excretion of large amounts of water caused by loop diuretics may produce adverse effects such as dehydration and electrolyte imbalances. Signs of dehydration include thirst, dry mouth, weight loss, and headache. Hypotension, dizziness, and even fainting can result from the rapid fluid loss. When urine flow increases, potassium ion (K^+) is lost from the body. Potassium depletion, or **hypokalemia**, may cause abnormal heart rhythms called *dysrhythmias*, and thus potassium supplements may be indicated during loop diuretic therapy. Potassium loss is of particular concern to patients who are also taking digoxin (Lanoxin). Although rare, impairment of hearing or balance (ototoxicity) is possible. Because of the potential for serious adverse effects, the loop diuretics are normally reserved for patients with moderate to severe fluid retention, or when other diuretics have failed to achieve therapeutic goals. Information on the loop diuretics is given in Table 18.1.

de = *not/without*
hydration = *water*

hypo = *low or below normal*
kal = *potassium*
emia = *blood condition*

CONCEPT REVIEW 18.2

- Why are drugs that block Na^+ reabsorption at the loop of Henle more effective than those that act on the distal tubule?

Prototype Drug: Pr *Furosemide (Lasix)*

Therapeutic Class: Drug for heart failure, edema, and hypertension **Pharmacologic Class:** Diuretic (loop type)

Actions and Uses: Furosemide is used for conditions in which the patient is retaining fluid. In the treatment of acute HF furosemide has the ability to remove large amounts of edema fluid from the patient in a short time. Patients often receive quick relief from their distressing symptoms. Compared to other diuretics, furosemide is particularly beneficial when cardiac output and renal flow are severely diminished.

Furosemide acts by preventing the reabsorption of sodium and chloride in the loop of Henle. By blocking sodium chloride (NaCl) reabsorption, furosemide interferes with water reabsorption. When water reabsorption is blocked, increased urination results.

Adverse Effects and Interactions: Adverse effects of furosemide, like those of most diuretics, include electrolyte imbalances, the most important of which is hypokalemia. Because hypokalemia may cause dysrhythmias in patients taking digoxin, combination therapy with furosemide and digoxin must be carefully monitored. When furosemide is given with corticosteroids and amphotericin B, it can increase the risk for hypokalemia. When given with sulfonylureas and insulin, furosemide may diminish their hypoglycemic effects. Because furosemide is such a potent drug, fluid loss must be carefully monitored to prevent possible dehydration and hypotension.

Furosemide should be monitored carefully in patients receiving aminoglycoside antibiotics because additive ototoxicity may result. Patients allergic to sulfur or sulfonamide antibiotics should not receive furosemide because of potential allergic response.

BACK BOX WARNING:
Furosemide is a potent diuretic that, if given in excessive amounts, may lead to profound diuresis with water and electrolyte depletion. Careful medical supervision is required.

Table 18.1 Loop Diuretics

Drug	Route and Adult Dose	Remarks
bumetanide (Bumex)	PO: 0.5–2 mg daily (max: 10 mg/day)	IV form available; this drug is 40 times more potent than furosemide
ethacrynic acid (Edecrin)	PO: 50–100 mg once or twice per day (max: 400 mg/day)	IV form available; exhibits the most ototoxicity of the drugs in this class
Pr furosemide (Lasix)	PO: 20–80 mg daily (max: 600 mg/day) IV/IM: 20–40 mg in one or more divided doses (max: 600 mg/day)	Should be used with great caution in premature infants, neonates, and older adults
torsemide (Demadex)	PO: 4–20 mg daily (max: 200 mg/day)	IV form available; exhibits the lowest risk of ototoxicity of the drugs in this class

Core Concept 18.6 ▶ The thiazides are the most widely prescribed class of diuretics.

The thiazides comprise the largest, most frequently prescribed class of diuretics. These drugs act on the distal tubule to block sodium reabsorption and increase water excretion. Their primary use is for the treatment of mild to moderate HTN. They are less effective at producing diuresis than the loop diuretics, and they are ineffective in patients with severe renal disease. All the thiazide diuretics are available by the oral route and have equivalent efficacy and safety profiles. Three drugs—chlorthalidone (Hygroton), indapamide (Lozol), and metolazone (Zaroxolyn)—are not true thiazides, although they are included with this drug class because they have similar mechanisms of action and adverse effects. The thiazide and thiazide-like diuretics are listed in Table 18.2.

The frequency of adverse effects with the thiazides is lower than that of the loop diuretics. As is true with other diuretics, dehydration is possible because of excessive or rapid fluid loss, and patients may experience dizziness due to hypotension when moving from a supine or sitting to an upright position. Electrolyte levels are monitored periodically to prevent hypokalemia. To avoid adverse effects from the drug, patients taking thiazides should be advised to drink plenty of water and beverages containing electrolytes and to eat a balanced diet. Diabetic patients should be aware that thiazide diuretics sometimes raise blood glucose levels.

Prototype Drug: Pr *Hydrochlorothiazide (Microzide)*

Therapeutic Class: Drug for hypertension and edema **Pharmacologic Class:** Thiazide diuretic

Actions and Uses: Hydrochlorothiazide is the most widely prescribed diuretic, belonging to a class of drugs known as the thiazides. Hydrochlorothiazide is approved to treat ascites, edema, HF, and HTN. Like many diuretics, it produces few serious adverse effects and is effective at producing a 10–20 mmHg reduction in blood pressure. Patients with severe HTN require the addition of a second drug from a different class to control the disease.

Hydrochlorothiazide acts on the kidney tubule to decrease the reabsorption of Na^+. When hydrochlorothiazide blocks this reabsorption, more Na^+ and water are sent into the urine, thus reducing blood volume and decreasing blood pressure. The volume of urine produced is directly proportional to the amount of Na^+ reabsorption blocked by the diuretic.

Adverse Effects and Interactions: The most common adverse effects of hydrochlorothiazide include possible electrolyte imbalances, especially loss of excessive K^+ and Na^+. Because potassium deficiency may cause cardiac conduction abnormalities, patients are usually asked to increase their intake of dietary potassium as a precaution.

Hydrochlorothiazide increases the action of antihypertensives and skeletal muscle relaxants. It may reduce the effectiveness of anticoagulants, antigout drugs, and antidiabetic drugs, including insulin.

Central nervous system (CNS) depressants such as alcohol, barbiturates, and opioids may increase the orthostatic hypotension caused by hydrochlorothiazide. Steroids or amphotericin B increase K^+ loss when given in conjunction with hydrochlorothiazide, leading to hypokalemia.

Hydrochlorothiazide increases the risk of serum toxicity of the following drugs: digoxin, lithium, allopurinol, anesthetics, and antineoplastics. It also alters vitamin D metabolism and calcium conservation; use of calcium supplements may cause hypercalcemia. It should be used with caution with ginkgo biloba, which may cause an increase in blood pressure.

Hydrochlorothiazide is often combined with drugs from other classes for the pharmacotherapy of HTN. The combination of hydrochlorothiazide with another antihypertensive allows for lower doses of each individual drug, thus decreasing the incidence of side effects. In addition, a combination drug can sometimes cause a greater reduction in blood pressure than using a single drug. Examples of combination drugs include Lopressor HCT (hydrochlorothiazide with metoprolol, a beta adrenergic blocker) and Zestoretic (hydrochlorothiazide with lisinopril, an ACE inhibitor)

Table 18.2 Thiazide and Thiazide-Like Diuretics

Drug	Route and Adult Dose	Remarks
bendroflumethiazide and nadolol (Corzide)	PO: 1 tablet/day (40–80 mg nadolol/5 mg bendroflumethiazide)	Intermediate acting
chlorothiazide (Diuril)	PO: 250–500 mg one or two times/day	IV form available; short acting
chlorthalidone (Hygroton)	PO: 50–100 mg/day	Thiazide-like; long acting
Pr hydrochlorothiazide (Microzide)	PO: 25–100 mg/day	Short acting
indapamide (Lozol)	PO: 1.25–2.5 mg once daily	Thiazide-like; long acting
methyclothiazide (Aquatensen, Enduron)	PO: 2.5–10 mg/day	Long acting
metolazone (Zaroxolyn)	PO: 2.5–10 mg once daily	Thiazide-like; intermediate acting

Although less effective than the loop diuretics, potassium-sparing diuretics may help prevent hypokalemia.

◀ **Core Concept 18.7**

Potassium depletion is a potentially serious adverse effect of the thiazide and loop diuretics. The therapeutic advantage of the potassium-sparing diuretics is that they are able to increase diuresis without adversely affecting blood potassium levels. These diuretics are shown in Table 18.3.

Table 18.3 Potassium-Sparing Diuretics

Drug	Route and Adult Dose	Remarks
amiloride (Midamor)	PO: 5 mg/day (max: 20 mg/day)	Moduretic is a fixed-dose combination of amiloride and hydrochlorothiazide.
Pr spironolactone (Aldactone)	PO: 25–100 mg one or two times/day	Used in combination with other antihypertensives to increase diuresis; monitor serum potassium level carefully
eplerenone (Inspra)	PO: 25–50 mg once daily	Newer drug in class; actions very similar to spironolactone
triamterene (Dyrenium)	PO: 50–100 mg bid	Dyazide is a fixed-dose combination of triamterene and hydrochlorothiazide.

Normally, Na^+ and K^+ are exchanged in the distal tubule; Na^+ is reabsorbed into the bloodstream and K^+ is secreted into the tubule. Potassium-sparing diuretics block this exchange, causing sodium to stay in the tubule and ultimately leave through the urine. When Na^+ is blocked, the body retains more K^+. Because most of the Na^+ has already been removed by the time the filtrate reaches the distal tubule, potassium-sparing diuretics produce only a mild diuresis. Their primary use is in combination with thiazide or loop diuretics to minimize K^+ loss.

Spironolactone and eplerenone (Inspra) are potassium-sparing diuretics that act by blocking the actions of the hormone aldosterone; thus they are commonly called aldosterone antagonists. Secreted by the adrenal cortex, **aldosterone** is a hormone that promotes the retention of Na^+ by increasing its reabsorption by the kidney. Although it produces only a mild diuresis, spironolactone has been found to significantly reduce mortality in patients with HF.

Unlike the loop and thiazide diuretics, patients taking potassium-sparing diuretics should not take potassium supplements and should not add potassium-rich foods to their diet. Intake of excess potassium when taking these medications may lead to **hyperkalemia**, which is dangerously high K^+ levels in the blood. Coadministration of these diuretics with angiotensin converting enzyme (ACE) inhibitors such as lisinopril increases the risk for hyperkalemia, especially in older adults or those with renal impairment.

Prototype Drug: Pr *Spironolactone (Aldactone)*

Therapeutic Class: Antihypertensive, drug for reducing edema **Pharmacologic Class:** Potassium-sparing diuretic, aldosterone antagonist

Actions and Uses: Spironolactone, the most frequently prescribed potassium-sparing diuretic, is primarily used to treat mild HTN, often in combination with other antihypertensives. It may also be used to reduce edema associated with kidney or liver disease, and it is effective in slowing the progression of HF.

Spironolactone blocks sodium reabsorption in the distal tubule by inhibiting aldosterone. Aldosterone is a hormone secreted by the adrenal cortex that is responsible for increasing the renal reabsorption of Na^+ in exchange for K^+, thus causing water retention. When blocked by spironolactone, sodium and water excretion is increased, and the body retains more potassium.

Adverse Effects and Interactions: Spironolactone does such an efficient job of retaining potassium that hyperkalemia may develop. The risk of hyperkalemia is increased if the patient takes potassium supplements or is also taking angiotensin-converting enzyme (ACE) inhibitors. Signs and symptoms of hyperkalemia include muscle weakness, fatigue, and bradycardia. When potassium levels are monitored carefully and maintained within normal values, adverse effects from spironolactone are uncommon. Spironolactone is contraindicated during pregnancy and lactation.

When spironolactone is combined with ammonium chloride, acidosis may occur. Aspirin and other salicylates may decrease the diuretic effect of the medication. Use of spironolactone with digoxin may decrease the effects of digoxin.

BLACK BOX WARNING:

Because spironolactone has been found to cause tumors in animals in clinical studies, it should be used only for specified indications.

Table 18.4 Miscellaneous Diuretics

Drug	Route and Adult Dose	Remarks
acetazolamide (Diamox)	PO: 250–375 mg/day in a.m.	Carbonic anhydrase inhibitor; IV form available
glycerin	PO: 1–1.8 g/kg, 1–2 hours before ocular surgery	Osmotic type; also used to treat constipation and acute glaucoma
mannitol (Osmitrol)	IV: 100 g infused over 2–6 hours	Osmotic type
methazolamide (Neptazane)	PO: 50–100 mg bid or tid	Carbonic anhydrase inhibitor

Core Concept 18.8 ▶ Several less commonly prescribed diuretics have specific indications.

intra = *within*
ocular = *eye*

A few miscellaneous diuretics have very limited and specific indications. Two of these drugs inhibit **carbonic anhydrase**, an enzyme involved with acid–base balance. Acetazolamide (Diamox) is a carbonic anhydrase inhibitor used to decrease intraocular pressure in patients with glaucoma (see Chapter 38). Unrelated to its diuretic effect, acetazolamide is also used to treat acute mountain sickness in patients at very high altitudes. The carbonic anhydrase inhibitors are not commonly used as diuretics, because they produce a very weak diuresis and have a higher incidence of adverse effects than other diuretics.

The osmotic diuretics also have very specific applications. Mannitol (Osmitrol) is used to maintain urine flow in patients with acute renal failure during prolonged surgery. Mannitol is also used to reduce swelling in the brain (increased intracranial pressure) and lower intraocular pressure in certain types of glaucoma. It is a very potent diuretic that is only given by the IV route. Osmotic diuretics are rarely drugs of first choice due to their potential toxicity. Table 18.4 lists some of the miscellaneous diuretics.

Nursing Process Focus Patients Receiving Diuretic Therapy

ASSESSMENT

Prior to administration:
- Obtain a complete health history including cardiovascular disease, renal and liver conditions, diabetes, pregnancy, allergies, diet, and data on recent surgeries or trauma.
- Acquire the results of a complete physical examination, including vital signs, height, and weight.
- Obtain the patient's medication history, including cardiac medications, nicotine and alcohol consumption, and use of over-the-counter and herbal supplements or alternative therapies. Determine possible drug allergies or interactions.
- Evaluate laboratory blood findings: complete blood count (CBC), electrolytes, renal and liver function studies.

POTENTIAL NURSING DIAGNOSES*

- *Deficient Fluid Volume* related to effects of drug therapy
- *Impaired Urinary Elimination* related to diuretic use
- *Deficient Knowledge* related to a lack of information about drug therapy
- *Noncompliance* related to adverse effects of medications
- *Risk for Electrolyte Imbalance* related to diuretic use

PLANNING: PATIENT GOALS AND EXPECTED OUTCOMES

The patient will:
- Experience therapeutic effects (normal fluid balance and maintenance of normal electrolyte levels).
- Be free from or experience minimal adverse effects from drug therapy.
- Verbalize an understanding of the drug's use, adverse effects, and required precautions.

IMPLEMENTATION

Interventions and (Rationales)	Patient Education/Discharge Planning
• Monitor for fluid overload by measuring intake, output, and daily weights. (Intake, output, and daily body weight can be indications of the effectiveness of diuretic therapy.)	Instruct the patient to: • Immediately report any severe shortness of breath, frothy sputum, profound fatigue, edema in extremities, potential signs of HF, or pulmonary edema. • Accurately measure fluid intake, fluid output, and body weight, and report decrease in output or weight gain of 2 lb (1 kg) or more within 2 days. • Avoid excessive heat, which contributes to fluid loss through perspiration. • Consume adequate amounts of plain water.

Interventions and (Rationales)	Patient Education/Discharge Planning
• Monitor laboratory findings, especially potassium and sodium. (Diuretics can cause electrolyte imbalances.)	• Advise the patient of the importance of keeping appointments for laboratory testing. • Instruct the patient to inform laboratory personnel of diuretic therapy when providing blood or urine samples.
• Monitor vital signs, especially blood pressure. (Diuretics reduce blood volume, resulting in lowered blood pressure.)	Instruct the patient to: • Monitor blood pressure as specified by the healthcare provider and ensure proper use of home equipment. • Stop medication if severe hypotension exists, as specified by the healthcare provider (e.g., "hold for blood pressure levels below 88/50 mmHg").
• Observe for changes in level of consciousness, dizziness, fatigue, and orthostatic hypotension. (Reduction in blood volume due to diuretic therapy may produce changes in level of consciousness or syncope.)	Instruct the patient to: • Immediately report any change in consciousness, especially feeling faint. • Change positions slowly. • Obtain blood pressure readings in sitting, standing, and lying positions.
• Monitor nutritional status, especially intake of foods with sodium and potassium. (These electrolytes can become depleted with thiazide or loop diuretics. Potassium sparing diuretics may cause sodium loss but potassium increase.)	Instruct patients: • Receiving *loop or thiazide diuretics* to eat foods high in potassium. • Receiving *potassium-sparing diuretics* to avoid foods high in potassium. • To consult with a healthcare provider before using vitamin or mineral supplements or electrolyte-fortified sports drinks. Combining potassium supplements with a high potassium diet may lead to hyperkalemia.
• Observe for signs of hypersensitivity reaction. (Allergic responses may be life threatening.)	Instruct the patient or caregiver to report: • Difficulty breathing, throat tightness, hives, rash, or bleeding. • Flu-like symptoms such as shortness of breath, fever, sore throat, malaise, joint pain, profound fatigue.
• Monitor hearing and vision. (Loop diuretics are ototoxic. Thiazide diuretics increase serum digoxin levels and may cause digoxin toxicity, which can produce visual changes.)	• Instruct the patient to report any changes in hearing or vision such as ringing or buzzing in the ears, becoming "hard of hearing," or experiencing dimness of sight, seeing halos, or having "yellow vision."
• Monitor reactivity to light exposure. (Some diuretics cause photosensitivity.)	Instruct the patient to: • Limit exposure to the sun. • Wear dark glasses and light-colored loose-fitting clothes when outdoors. • Always use high SPF sunscreen lotion when outdoors.
• Administer medication correctly, and evaluate the patient's knowledge of proper administration. (Some medications interact with other medications.)	Instruct the patient: • About the appropriate dosing and administration of the specific diuretic being taken. • To take diuretic in the morning instead of at night to avoid interruption of sleep.

EVALUATION OF OUTCOME CRITERIA

Evaluate the effectiveness of drug therapy by confirming that patient goals and expected outcomes have been met (see "Planning"). *See Tables 18.1 through 18.4 for lists of drugs to which these nursing actions apply.*

*Herdman, T.H. & Kamitsuru, S. (Eds.), *Nursing Diagnoses: Definitions & Classification* 2015–2017. Copyright © 2014, 1994–2014 NANDA International. Used by arrangement by John Wiley & Sons, Inc. Companion website: www.wiley.com/go/nursingdiagnoses.

Core Concept 18.9 ▶

Electrolytes are charged substances that play important roles in maintaining homeostasis.

Minerals are inorganic substances needed in very small amounts by the body (see Chapter 32). When placed in water, some of these minerals become ions and possess a positive or negative charge. Small, inorganic molecules possessing a positive or negative charge are called **electrolytes**. Electrolytes are essential to many body functions, including nerve conduction, muscle contraction, and bone growth and remodeling. Too little or too much of an electrolyte may result in serious disease and must be quickly corrected.

electro = *conducts electricity*
lyte = *solution*

Levels of electrolytes in body fluids are maintained within very narrow ranges, primarily by the kidney and GI tract. As electrolytes are lost due to normal excretory functions, they must be replaced by adequate fluid intake; otherwise, electrolyte imbalances can result. Although imbalances can occur in any ion, sodium, potassium, and calcium are of greatest importance. Calcium homeostasis is presented in vitamins, minerals, and nutritional supplements because it is associated with the pharmacotherapy of bone disorders. Sodium and potassium are discussed in the following paragraphs. The major electrolyte imbalances and their treatments are described in Table 18.5.

An electrolyte imbalance is a sign of an underlying medical condition that needs attention. The most common cause is renal impairment. In some cases, drug therapy itself can cause the electrolyte imbalance. For example, aggressive therapy with loop diuretics such as furosemide (Lasix) can rapidly deplete the body of Na^+ and K^+. Treatment includes correcting the electrolyte imbalance as well as treating the underlying medical condition. Treatments for electrolyte imbalances range from simple changes in dietary intake for mild imbalances to rapid electrolyte infusions in severe cases.

Sodium Imbalances

Because Na^+ is the major electrolyte in extracellular fluid, imbalances of this ion can have serious consequences. Sodium excess, or **hypernatremia**, is most commonly caused by kidney disease; Na^+ accumulates in the blood due to decreased excretion. Another cause of hypernatremia is high net water losses, such as occur from inadequate water intake, watery diarrhea, fever, or burns. A high serum Na^+ level can cause cellular dehydration with symptoms such as thirst, fatigue, weakness, muscle twitching, convulsions, and a decreased level of consciousness. For minor hypernatremia, a salt-restricted diet may be effective in returning serum Na^+ to normal levels. In patients with acute hypernatremia, however, IV fluids such as 5% dextrose in water or diuretics may be administered to quickly remove sodium from the body.

hyper = *high or above normal*
natri = *sodium*
emia = *blood condition*

Table 18.5 Electrolyte Imbalances

Ion	Condition	Abnormal Serum Value (mEq/L)	Supportive Treatment*
Calcium	Hypercalcemia	Greater than 11	Hypotonic fluid or calcitonin
	Hypocalcemia	Less than 4	Calcium supplements or vitamin D
Chloride	Hyperchloremia	Greater than 112	Hypotonic fluid
	Hypochloremia	Less than 95	Hypertonic salt solution
Magnesium	Hypermagnesemia	Greater than 4	Hypotonic fluid
	Hypomagnesemia	Less than 0.8	Magnesium supplements
Phosphate	Hyperphosphatemia	Greater than 6	Dietary phosphate restriction
	Hypophosphatemia	Less than 1	Phosphate supplements
Potassium	Hyperkalemia	Greater than 5	Hypotonic fluid, buffers, or dietary potassium restriction
	Hypokalemia	Less than 3.5	Potassium supplements
Sodium	Hypernatremia	Greater than 145	Hypotonic fluid or dietary sodium restriction
	Hyponatremia	Less than 135	Hypertonic salt solution or sodium supplement

**For all electrolyte imbalances, the primary therapeutic goal is to identify and correct the cause of the imbalance.*

Sodium deficiency, or **hyponatremia**, may occur when Na^+ is lost because of serious skin burns, vomiting, diarrhea, kidney disease, and with conditions associated with excessive sweating or prolonged fever. Symptoms of hyponatremia include nausea, vomiting, anorexia, abdominal cramping, confusion, lethargy, convulsions, coma, and muscle twitching or tremors. Hyponatremia is usually treated with solutions of NaCl or with IV fluids containing salt, such as normal saline or lactated Ringer's solution. Tolvaptan (Samsca) is a newer drug administered to raise sodium levels in hospitalized patients with serious hyponatremia.

Potassium Imbalances

Potassium levels must be carefully balanced between adequate dietary intake and renal excretion. Levels of K^+ in the blood must be maintained within narrow limits because too little or too much of this electrolyte is associated with fatal cardiac dysrhythmias and serious neuromuscular disorders.

Hyperkalemia may be caused by high consumption of potassium-rich foods or dietary supplements, particularly when patients are taking potassium-sparing diuretics such as spironolactone. Excess potassium may also accumulate when renal excretion is diminished due to kidney pathology. The most serious consequences of hyperkalemia are cardiac dysrhythmias.

In mild cases of hyperkalemia, K^+ levels may be returned to normal by restricting major dietary sources of potassium, such as bananas, dried fruits, peanut butter, broccoli, and green leafy vegetables. If the patient is taking a potassium-sparing diuretic, the dose is lowered or an alternate drug is considered. In acute cases, administration of furosemide (Lasix) can increase potassium excretion within minutes. Serum K^+ levels may also be lowered by administering sodium polystyrene sulfate (Kayexalate), a resin that removes K^+ by exchanging it for Na^+ in the large intestine. This drug is given concurrently with a laxative to promote rapid evacuation of the potassium. Sodium polystyrene sulfate is available in oral and enema formulations. An additional method of treating hyperkalemia is to administer glucose and insulin, which causes K+ to leave the extracellular fluid and enter cells.

Prototype Drug: Pr *Potassium Chloride (KCl)*

Therapeutic Class: Potassium supplement **Pharmacologic Class:** Electrolyte

Actions and Uses: Potassium is one of the most important electrolytes in body fluids, and levels must be maintained within a narrow range of values between 3.5 and 5.5 mEq/L. Too much or too little K^+ may lead to serious consequences and must be immediately corrected. Neurons and muscle fibers are most sensitive to potassium loss. Muscle weakness, dysrhythmias, and cardiac arrest are possible consequences. KCl is also used to treat mild forms of alkalosis.

KCl is the preferred drug for treating or preventing hypokalemia. Therapy with loop or thiazide diuretics is the most common cause of excessive potassium loss. Patients taking thiazide or loop diuretics are usually instructed to take oral potassium supplements to prevent hypokalemia. Oral forms include tablets, powders, and liquids, usually heavily flavored because of the unpleasant taste of the drug. IV forms may be given in critical care situations.

Adverse Effects and Interactions: KCl irritates the GI mucosa; therefore, nausea and vomiting are common. The drug may be taken with meals or antacids to lessen the gastric distress. Taking too much KCl can cause hyperkalemia, especially when it is combined with a diet that contains potassium-rich foods.

Hyperkalemia may occur if potassium supplements are given concurrently with potassium-sparing diuretics or ACE inhibitors. If patients are taking these drugs, the healthcare provider should warn them not to take OTC potassium supplements.

Hypokalemia is a relatively common adverse effect resulting from high doses of loop diuretics such as furosemide. Strenuous muscular activity and severe vomiting or diarrhea can also result in significant potassium loss. Mild hypokalemia is treated by increasing the dietary intake of potassium-rich foods. More severe deficiencies require oral or parenteral potassium supplements. KCl is available in IV and a wide variety of oral formulations to increase blood potassium levels.

Core Concept 18.10 ▶ Acidic and basic drugs can be administered to correct pH imbalances.

One of the most important homeostatic functions of the blood is to neutralize strong acids and bases. Much of the food we eat is either more acidic or more alkaline than body fluids. Furthermore, during the breakdown of food, the body generates significant amounts of acid. If body fluids become too acidic or too alkaline, enzymes will not function efficiently and cells may be injured.

The degree of acidity or alkalinity of a solution is measured by its **pH**. A pH of 7 is defined as neutral, above 7 as basic or alkaline, and below 7 as acidic. To maintain homeostasis, the pH of plasma and most body fluids must be kept within the very narrow range of 7.35 to 7.45. At pH values above 7.45, **alkalosis** develops, and symptoms of CNS stimulation occur that include nervousness and convulsions. **Acidosis** occurs below a pH of 7.35, and symptoms of CNS depression may result in coma. In either alkalosis or acidosis, death may result if large changes in pH are not corrected immediately.

alkal = *basic*
osis = *condition*

Acidosis and alkalosis are not diseases; they are symptoms of underlying disorders. Primary treatment of acid–base disorders is always targeted to correct the underlying cause. Drugs are administered to support the patient's vital functions while the disease is being treated. Common causes of alkalosis and acidosis are listed in Table 18.6.

Treatment of alkalosis is directed toward addressing the underlying condition that is causing the excess bases to be retained. In mild cases, alkalosis may be corrected by administering NaCl concurrently with KCl. This combination increases the renal excretion of bicarbonate ion (a base), which indirectly increases the acidity of the blood. For acute patients, acidifying agents may be used. Hydrochloric acid and ammonium chloride are two drugs that can quickly lower the pH in patients with severe alkalosis.

Prototype Drug: Pr *Sodium Bicarbonate ($NaHCO_3$)*

Therapeutic Class: Agent to treat acidosis or bicarbonate deficiency **Pharmacologic Class:** Electrolyte

Actions and Uses: Acidosis is a more common event than alkalosis, occurring during shock or cardiac arrest, or with diabetes mellitus. Sodium bicarbonate is the drug of choice for correcting acidosis: The bicarbonate ion (HCO_3^-) directly raises the pH of body fluids. Sodium bicarbonate may be given orally if acidosis is mild, or IV in cases of acute disease. Although sodium bicarbonate neutralizes gastric acid, it is rarely used to treat peptic ulcers because of its tendency to cause gas and gastric distention.

Sodium bicarbonate may also be used to make the urine more basic. An alkaline urine will speed the excretion of acidic drugs, such as barbiturates and aspirin.

Adverse Effects and Interactions: Most of the adverse effects of sodium bicarbonate therapy are the result of alkalosis caused by *too much* HCO_3^-. Symptoms may include confusion, irritability, slow respiration rate, and vomiting. Simply discontinuing the sodium bicarbonate infusion often reverses these symptoms; however, KCl or ammonium chloride may be administered to reverse the alkalosis.

Sodium bicarbonate may decrease the absorption of ketoconazole and may decrease elimination of dextroamphetamine, ephedrine, pseudoephedrine, and quinidine. Sodium bicarbonate may increase the elimination of salicylates and tetracyclines. Chronic use of sodium bicarbonate with milk or calcium supplements may cause milk–alkali syndrome, a condition characterized by very high serum calcium levels and possible kidney failure.

Table 18.6 Causes of Acidosis and Alkalosis

Acidosis	Alkalosis
RESPIRATORY ORIGINS OF ACIDOSIS	RESPIRATORY ORIGIN OF ALKALOSIS
• Hypoventilation or shallow breathing • Airway constriction • Damage to respiratory center in medulla	• Hyperventilation due to asthma, anxiety, or high altitude
METABOLIC ORIGINS OF ACIDOSIS	METABOLIC ORIGINS OF ALKALOSIS
• Severe diarrhea • Kidney failure • Diabetes mellitus • Excess alcohol ingestion • Starvation	• Constipation for prolonged periods • Ingestion of excess sodium bicarbonate • Diuretics that cause potassium depletion • Severe vomiting

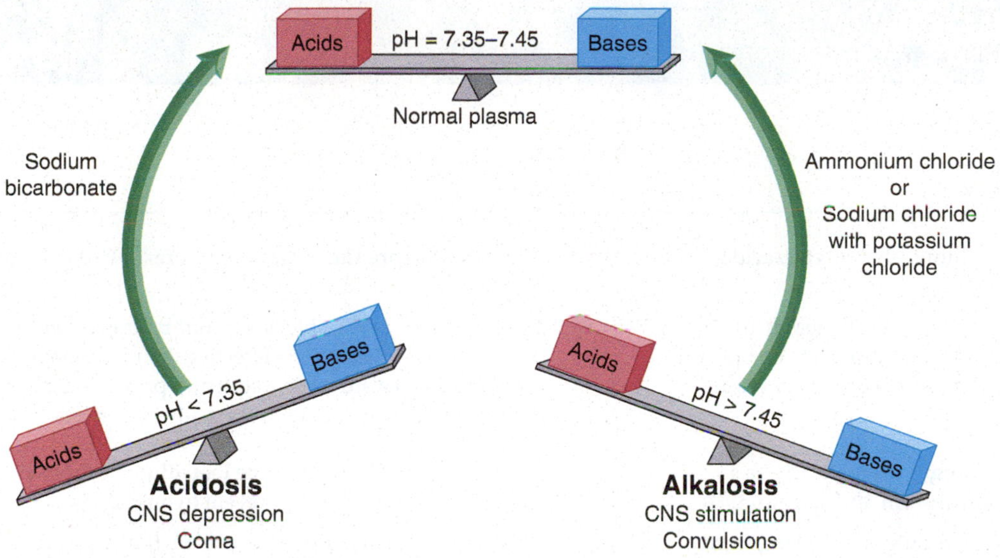

FIGURE 18.4 Correction of acid–base imbalances.

In patients with acidosis, the goal is to quickly reverse the level of acids in the blood. A preferred treatment for acute acidosis is to administer infusions of sodium bicarbonate. Bicarbonate ion acts as a base to quickly neutralize acids in the blood and other body fluids. The patient must be carefully monitored during infusions because this drug can "over-correct" the acidosis, causing blood pH to turn alkaline. The correction of acid–base imbalances is illustrated in Figure 18.4.

Patients Need to Know

Patients treated for urinary, acid–base, and fluid disorders need to know the following:

Regarding Diuretics

1. See the healthcare provider regularly and have serum electrolytes, CBC, and glucose levels monitored as instructed.
2. When taking diuretics, drink plenty of water if dry mouth or thirst develops, unless otherwise directed by a healthcare provider.
3. Take diuretics in the morning or at least 2 hours before bedtime to avoid nighttime diuresis.
4. If diabetes is present, monitor blood sugar levels very closely when taking thiazide diuretics because these drugs may elevate blood glucose levels.
5. Do not take thiazide diuretics during pregnancy or when breastfeeding.
6. When taking loop or thiazide diuretics, increase dietary sources of potassium-rich foods such as dark leafy vegetables, nuts, citrus fruits, bananas, and potatoes unless prescribed a potassium supplement or otherwise instructed by the healthcare provider. If taking a potassium-sparing diuretic, avoid these foods unless otherwise instructed by a healthcare provider.
7. Avoid caffeinated beverages when taking diuretics. The diuretic effect of the caffeine combined with the effects of these medications may cause dehydration.

Regarding Potassium Supplements

8. Because KCl tablets are irritating to the GI mucosa, they should be taken with food. Do not crush or suck the tablets. If nausea or heartburn occurs, take antacids along with the KCl.

Chapter Review

Core Concepts Summary

18.1 The kidneys regulate fluid volume, electrolytes, acids, and bases.

The kidneys are essential to the overall health of the patient, and to control fluid volume, electrolyte composition, and acid–base balance. The functional unit of the kidney is the nephron.

18.2 The composition of filtrate changes dramatically as a result of the processes of reabsorption and secretion.

Filtrate entering the proximal tubule resembles plasma without proteins. Through the processes of reabsorption and secretion, the filtrate composition changes, producing urine.

18.3 Renal failure significantly impacts pharmacotherapy.

Because the kidneys excrete most drugs, a large number of medications require a significant dosage reduction in patients with moderate to severe renal failure. Renal failure is classified as acute or chronic. Pharmacotherapy of renal failure attempts to cure the cause of the dysfunction. Diuretics may be used to maintain urine output. Epoetin alfa is a form of erythropoietin used to treat anemia in which there is a deficiency in red blood cell production.

18.4 Diuretics are used to treat hypertension, heart failure, and fluid retention disorders.

Diuretics are drugs that increase urine output, usually by blocking sodium reabsorption. Indications for diuretics include HTN, HF, kidney failure, and liver disease.

18.5 The most effective diuretics are those that affect the loop of Henle.

The high-ceiling or loop diuretics such as furosemide act by blocking sodium reabsorption in the loop of Henle. They are the most effective diuretics but are more likely to cause dehydration and electrolyte loss.

18.6 The thiazides are the most widely prescribed class of diuretics.

The thiazide diuretics block sodium reabsorption in the distal tubule. Although less effective than the loop diuretics, the thiazides are more frequently prescribed because of their lower incidence of serious adverse effects.

18.7 Although less effective than the loop diuretics, potassium-sparing diuretics may help prevent hypokalemia.

Potassium-sparing diuretics act on the distal tubule, although they are less effective than the loop diuretics. Their primary advantage is that they do not cause potassium loss.

18.8 Several less commonly prescribed diuretics have specific indications.

Carbonic anhydrase inhibitors and osmotic diuretics are not commonly prescribed. They have specific applications, such as decreasing intraocular pressure and maintaining urine flow during renal failure.

18.9 Electrolytes are charged substances that play important roles in maintaining homeostasis.

Electrolyte imbalances can cause significant signs and symptoms. Hypokalemia is a serious potential adverse effect of drug therapy with certain diuretics. Oral or IV KCl can reverse symptoms of hypokalemia. Although less common, hyperkalemia may be just as serious and may be reversed by administration of glucose or insulin.

18.10 Acidic and basic drugs can be administered to correct pH imbalances.

NaCl with KCl may be administered to reverse mild to moderate alkalosis. Hydrochloric acid or ammonium chloride may be administered for acute alkalosis. Sodium bicarbonate is used to reverse acidosis.

REVIEW Questions

Answer the following questions to assess your knowledge of the chapter material, and go back and review any material that is not clear to you.

1. Which of the following is not a function of the kidneys?
   1. Acid–base balance
   2. Secretion of renin
   3. Production of white blood cells
   4. Production of calcitriol

2. While collecting data on a patient suspected of being dehydrated, the nurse is looking for:
   1. Headache and increased urinary output.
   2. Weight gain and edema.
   3. Hypertension and decreased urinary output.
   4. Hypotension, headache, and dry mouth.

3. A patient, newly diagnosed with hypertension, was just seen by the healthcare provider. The office nurse was asked to give the patient samples of the most commonly prescribed diuretic used for this condition. The nurse gives the patient which of the following diuretics?
   1. Ethacrynic acid (Edecrin)
   2. Chlorothiazide (Diuril)
   3. Spironolactone (Aldactone)
   4. Mannitol (Osmitrol)

4. A female patient, recently started on diuretic therapy, is taught that she should:
   1. Take medication at night.
   2. Rise slowly from a sitting position.
   3. Increase sodium intake.
   4. Decrease fluid intake.

5. A patient is receiving intravenous sodium bicarbonate for treatment of metabolic acidosis. During this infusion, how will the nurse monitor for therapeutic effect?
   1. Liver function tests
   2. White blood cell count
   3. Serum pH
   4. Glucose levels

6. The nurse is monitoring a patient for which of the following common adverse effects of oral potassium chloride?
   1. Drowsiness
   2. Nausea and vomiting
   3. Hypoglycemia
   4. Muscle weakness

7. When instructing a patient about taking potassium-sparing diuretics, the nurse teaches the patient to:
   1. Take potassium supplements.
   2. Not take potassium supplements.
   3. Add potassium rich foods to the diet.
   4. Have their magnesium levels monitored regularly.

8. The patient is receiving IV normal saline because of hyponatremia. On assessment, the nurse determines that the hyponatremia may have been caused by: (Select all that apply.)
   1. Constipation.
   2. Severe diarrhea and vomiting.
   3. Prolonged fever and sweating.
   4. Hemorrhage.
   5. Mild skin burns.

9. When taking diuretics, the patient is instructed to decrease or avoid the intake of:
   1. Dark green, leafy vegetables.
   2. Nuts.
   3. Fruits.
   4. Caffeine.

10. The healthcare provider orders 1000 mL of 0.9% NaCl to infuse intravenously over 8 hours. How many mL should the nurse expect to infuse in 1 hour?
    1. 100 mL
    2. 125 mL
    3. 135 mL
    4. 150 mL

CASE STUDY Questions

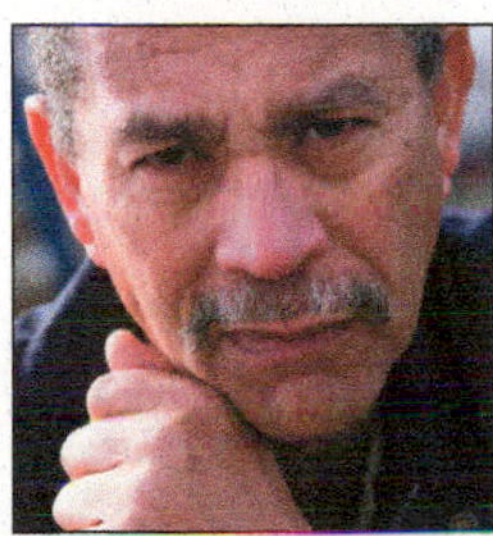

Remember Mr. Grant, the patient introduced at the beginning of the chapter? Now read the remainder of the case study. Based on the information you have learned in this chapter, answer the questions that follow.

Mr. Joseph Grant has been placed on hydrochlorothiazide (Microzide) for high blood pressure, and potassium chloride as a dietary supplement. His wife tells him to eat lots of bananas because she read that this was necessary when taking diuretics. After a few weeks, Mr. Grant becomes weak and feels as if his heart is skipping beats. His blood pressure remains high, despite the diuretic.

1. When providing education on his medications, which of the following should have been explained to Mr. Grant?
   1. Never eat bananas when taking Microzide.
   2. Eat lots of bananas when taking Microzide.
   3. Limit potassium-rich foods when taking potassium supplements.
   4. Never eat bananas and take Microzide at the same meal.

2. Given the previous information, the nurse believes it is quite possible that Mr. Grant's cardiac symptoms and weakness were caused by:
   1. Hyperkalemia.
   2. Hypokalemia.
   3. Hypernatremia.
   4. Hyponatremia.

3. The healthcare provider examines Mr. Grant and decides to administer a dose of sodium polystyrene sulfonate (Kayexalate). The reason for administering this drug is to:
   1. Increase fluid volume.
   2. Decrease fluid volume.
   3. Increase serum potassium levels.
   4. Decrease serum potassium levels.

4. After Mr. Grant's condition stabilized, the healthcare provider decided to select furosemide (Lasix), a more effective diuretic to treat hypertension. Which of the following information should the nurse provide to Mr. Grant?
   1. Never eat bananas when taking Lasix.
   2. Eat lots of bananas when taking Lasix.
   3. Limit potassium-rich foods when taking potassium supplements.
   4. Never eat bananas and take Lasix at the same meal.

Answers and complete rationales for the Review Questions appear in Appendix A.

REFERENCE

Herdman, T. H., & Kamitsuru, S. (Eds.). (2014). *NANDA International nursing diagnoses: Definitions and classification, 2015–2017*. Oxford, United Kingdom: Wiley-Blackwell.

SELECTED BIBLIOGRAPHY

Armstrong, A. (2013). Practical tips for prescribing in renal impairment. *Nurse Prescribing, 11*, 222–227. doi:10.12968/npre.2013.11.5.222

de Groot, M. H., van Campen, J. P., Moek, M. A., Tulner, L. R., Beijnen, J. H., & Lamoth, C. J. (2013). The effects of fall-risk-increasing drugs on postural control: A literature review. *Drugs & Aging, 30*, 901–920. doi:10.1007/s40266-013-0113-9

Gardner, J., Mooney, J., & Forester, A. (2013). HEAL: A strategy for advanced practitioner assessment of reduced urine output in hospital inpatients. *Journal of Clinical Nursing, 23*, 1562–1572. doi:10.1111/jocn.12254

National Institute of Diabetes and Digestive and Kidney Diseases. (n.d.). *Kidney disease statistics for the United States*. Retrieved from http://www.niddk.nih.gov/health-information/health-statistics/Pages/kidney-disease-statistics-united-states.aspx

National Kidney Foundation. (2016). *Organ donation and transplant statistics*. Retrieved from https://www.kidney.org/news/newsroom/factsheets/Organ-Donation-and-Transplantation-Stats

Saccomano, S. J., & DeLuca, D. A. (2012). Living with chronic kidney disease: Related issues and treatment. *The Nurse Practitioner, 37*(8), 32–38. doi:10.1097/01.NPR.0000415873.61843.68.

Tamargo, J., Segura, J., & Ruilope, L. M. (2014). Diuretics in the treatment of hypertension. Part 1: Thiazide and thiazide-like diuretics. *Expert Opinion on Pharmacotherapy, 15*, 527–547. doi:10.1517/14656566.2014.879118

Tamargo, J., Segura, J., & Ruilope, L. M. (2014). Diuretics in the treatment of hypertension. Part 2: Loop diuretics and potassium-sparing agents. *Expert Opinion on Pharmacotherapy, 15*, 605–621. doi:10.1517/14656566.2014.879117

von Lueder, T. G., Atar, D., & Krum, H. (2013). Diuretic use in heart failure and outcomes. *Clinical Pharmacology & Therapeutics, 94*, 490–498. doi:10.1038/clpt.2013.140

Wang, P. (2013). The effectiveness of cranberry products to reduce urinary tract infections in females: A literature review. *Urologic Nursing, 33*(1), 38.

Williams, H. (2013). An update on hypertension for nurse prescribers. *Nurse Prescribing, 11*. 70–75. doi:10.12968/npre.2013.11.2.70

Williams, T., Szekendi, M., & Thomas, S. (2014). An analysis of patient falls and fall prevention programs across academic medical centers. *Journal of Nursing Care Quality, 29*, 19–29. doi:10.1097/NCQ.0b013e3182a0cd19

Chapter 19

Drugs for Hypertension

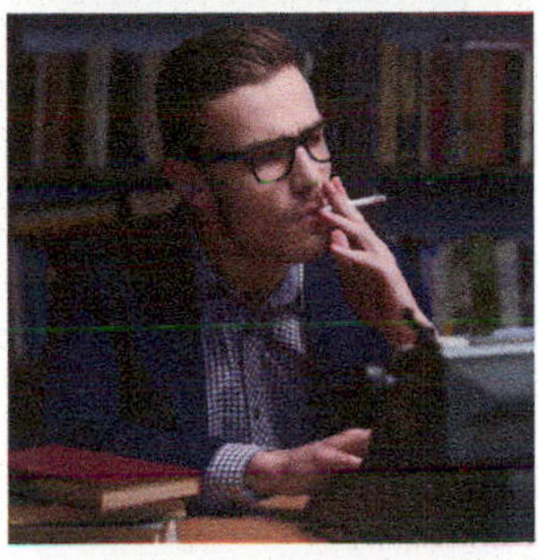

"I have all these reports to finish by Friday. I just don't have time to deal with high blood pressure."

Mr. Paul Rodriguez

Core Concepts

19.1 **Failure to treat chronic hypertension can lead to stroke, heart failure, or myocardial infarction.**

19.2 **Blood pressure is caused by the pumping action of the heart.**

19.3 **The primary factors responsible for blood pressure are cardiac output, the resistance of the small arteries, and blood volume.**

19.4 **Many nervous and hormonal factors help to keep blood pressure within normal limits.**

19.5 **Positive lifestyle changes can reduce blood pressure and lessen the need for medications.**

19.6 **The goal in treating hypertension is to reduce the long-term morbidity and mortality associated with the disease.**

19.7 **Diuretics are sometimes preferred drugs for treating mild to moderate hypertension.**

19.8 **Blocking the renin-angiotensin-aldosterone system leads to a decrease in blood pressure.**

19.9 **Calcium channel blockers have emerged as important drugs in the treatment of hypertension.**

19.10 **Adrenergic blockers are used to treat a wide variety of cardiovascular disorders, including hypertension.**

19.11 **Vasodilators lower blood pressure by relaxing arteriolar smooth muscle.**

Drug Snapshot

The following drugs are discussed in this chapter:

Drug Classes	Prototype Drugs
Diuretics	
Renin-angiotensin-aldosterone modifiers	Pr enalapril (Vasotec)
Calcium channel blockers	Pr nifedipine (Adalat CC, Procardia XL, Others)
Adrenergic blockers	Pr doxazosin (Cardura)
Direct-acting vasodilators	Pr hydralazine (Apresoline)

Learning Outcomes

After reading this chapter, the student should be able to:

1. Identify the long-term consequences of untreated hypertension.
2. Describe how the pumping action of the heart creates blood pressure.
3. Explain the effects of cardiac output, peripheral resistance, and blood volume on blood pressure.

4. Discuss nervous and hormonal factors that influence blood pressure.
5. Discuss the role of positive lifestyle changes in the management of hypertension.
6. Describe the goals in using pharmacotherapy to treat hypertension.
7. Explain the role of diuretics in the management of hypertension.
8. Explain the role of calcium channel blockers in the management of hypertension.
9. Explain the role of renin-angiotensin-aldosterone modifiers in the management of hypertension.
10. Explain the role of adrenergic blockers in the management of hypertension.
11. Explain the role of direct vasodilators in the management of hypertension.

Key Terms

angiotensin II (AN-geo-TEN-sin)
angiotensin-converting enzyme (ACE)
antidiuretic hormone (ADH) (ANT-eye-deye-your-ET-ik)
baroreceptors (BARE-oh-ree-sep-tours)
bradycardia (bray-dee-KAR-DEE-ah)
calcium channel blockers (CCBs)
cardiac output
diastolic pressure (DEYE-ah-stall-ik)
false neurotransmitter (NYUR-oh-TRANS-mitt-ur)
hypertension (HTN) (heye-purr-TEN-shun)
lumen (LOO-men)
orthostatic (postural) hypotension (or-tho-STAT-ik)
peripheral resistance (per-IF-ur-ul)
reflex tachycardia (ta-kee-CAR-dee-ah)
renin-angiotensin-aldosterone system (RAAS) (REN-in–an-geo-TEN-sin-al-DOS-ter-own)
systolic pressure (SIS-tol-ik)
vasomotor center (VAZO-mo-tor)

Diseases affecting the heart and blood vessels are the most common causes of death in the United States. Hypertension (HTN), or high blood pressure, is the most common of the cardiovascular diseases. Because healthcare providers encounter numerous patients with this disease, a firm grasp of the underlying principles of antihypertensive therapy is critical. By improving public awareness of HTN and teaching the importance of early intervention, the healthcare provider can contribute significantly to reducing cardiovascular mortality.

Core Concept 19.1 ▶

Failure to treat chronic hypertension can lead to stroke, heart failure, or myocardial infarction.

hyper = *high*
tension = *pressure*

Hypertension is defined as the consistent elevation of arterial blood pressure. A patient is said to have chronic HTN if he or she presents with a sustained systolic blood pressure of greater than 140 mmHg or diastolic pressure of greater than 90 to 99 mmHg after multiple measurements are made over several clinic visits.

HTN results from a combination of genetic and environmental factors. In 90% of the patients with HTN, no specific cause for the elevated blood pressure can be identified. This type of HTN is called *primary* or *essential*. Although the actual cause of primary HTN may not be known, many conditions or risk factors are associated with the disease. Advanced age and weight gain, particularly around the hips and thighs, tends to be associated with HTN. The disease is most prevalent in African Americans and least prevalent in Mexican Americans. Men in all ethnic groups experience more HTN compared to women. The disease also has a hereditary component, with family members of patients with HTN having greater risk of acquiring the disease than nonfamily members. Other factors, such as tobacco use and high-fat diets, clearly contribute to the disease.

In 10% of patients, a specific cause of the HTN *can* be identified. This is called *secondary* hypertension. Certain diseases, such as Cushing's syndrome, hyperthyroidism, and chronic renal disease, cause elevated blood pressure. Certain drugs are also associated with HTN, including corticosteroids, oral contraceptives, and epoetin alfa (Epogen). The therapeutic goal for secondary HTN is to treat or remove the underlying condition that is causing the blood pressure elevation. In many cases, correcting this underlying condition will cure the associated HTN.

Because chronic HTN may produce no symptoms for as long as 10 to 20 years, many people are not aware of their condition. Convincing patients to control their diets, spend money on medication, and take drugs on a regular basis when they are feeling healthy is a difficult task for the healthcare provider. Failure to control HTN, however, can lead to accelerated narrowing of the arteries, resulting in strokes, kidney failure, and cardiac arrest. One of the most serious consequences of chronic HTN is that the heart must work harder to pump blood to organs and tissues. This excessive workload can cause the heart to fail and the lungs to fill with fluid, a condition known as heart failure (HF). Drug therapy for HF is covered in Chapter 20.

The death rate from cardiovascular-related diseases has dropped significantly over the past 30 years because of the improved diagnosis and treatment of HTN, as well as the acceptance of healthier lifestyle habits. Early treatment, however, is essential; the long-term cardiovascular damage caused by HTN is irreversible if the disease is allowed to progress unchecked.

Fast Facts Hypertension

- High blood pressure affects more than 77 million adults, or approximately one in three Americans.
- Among people with HTN, more about one in 5 do not realize they have the condition.
- African American men have the highest rate of HTN, which is more than double the rate for white males
- Approximately 47% of Americans diagnosed with HTN do not have their condition under adequate control.
- HTN is the most common complication of pregnancy.
- Approximately 348,000 Americans die of HTN and HTN-related causes each per year.

Source: Norman Holland, Michael Adams and Jeanine Brice, Core Concepts in Pharmacology, 5e, 9780134514161, © 2018.

Blood pressure is caused by the pumping action of the heart.

◀ Core Concept 19.2

Although pressure can be measured in nearly any vessel in the body, the term *blood pressure* commonly refers to the pressure in the large arteries. Because the pumping action of the heart is the source of blood pressure, those arteries closest to the heart, such as the aorta, have the highest pressure. Pressure decreases gradually as the blood travels farther from the heart, until it falls close to zero in the largest veins. This is illustrated in Figure 19.1.

When the ventricles of the heart contract and eject blood, the pressure created in the arteries is called **systolic pressure**. When the ventricles relax and the heart temporarily stops ejecting blood, pressure in the arteries will fall, and this results in **diastolic pressure**. Blood pressure is measured in units of millimeters of mercury, abbreviated as mmHg. (Hg is the chemical symbol for the element mercury.) The average normal systolic pressure in a healthy adult is considered to be less than 120 mmHg, whereas the average normal diastolic pressure is less than 80 mmHg. The systolic and diastolic pressures are usually measured and reported together, with the systolic given first. For example, average normal blood pressure is said to be less than 120/80 mmHg. Figure 19.2 illustrates how the pumping action of the heart determines systolic and diastolic blood pressure.

The primary factors responsible for blood pressure are cardiac output, the resistance of the small arteries, and blood volume.

◀ Core Concept 19.3

In order to understand how drugs affect blood pressure, students must know cardiovascular physiology. Investing time to understand the details of how this system functions will reap great rewards later when studying the cardiovascular and respiratory drugs.

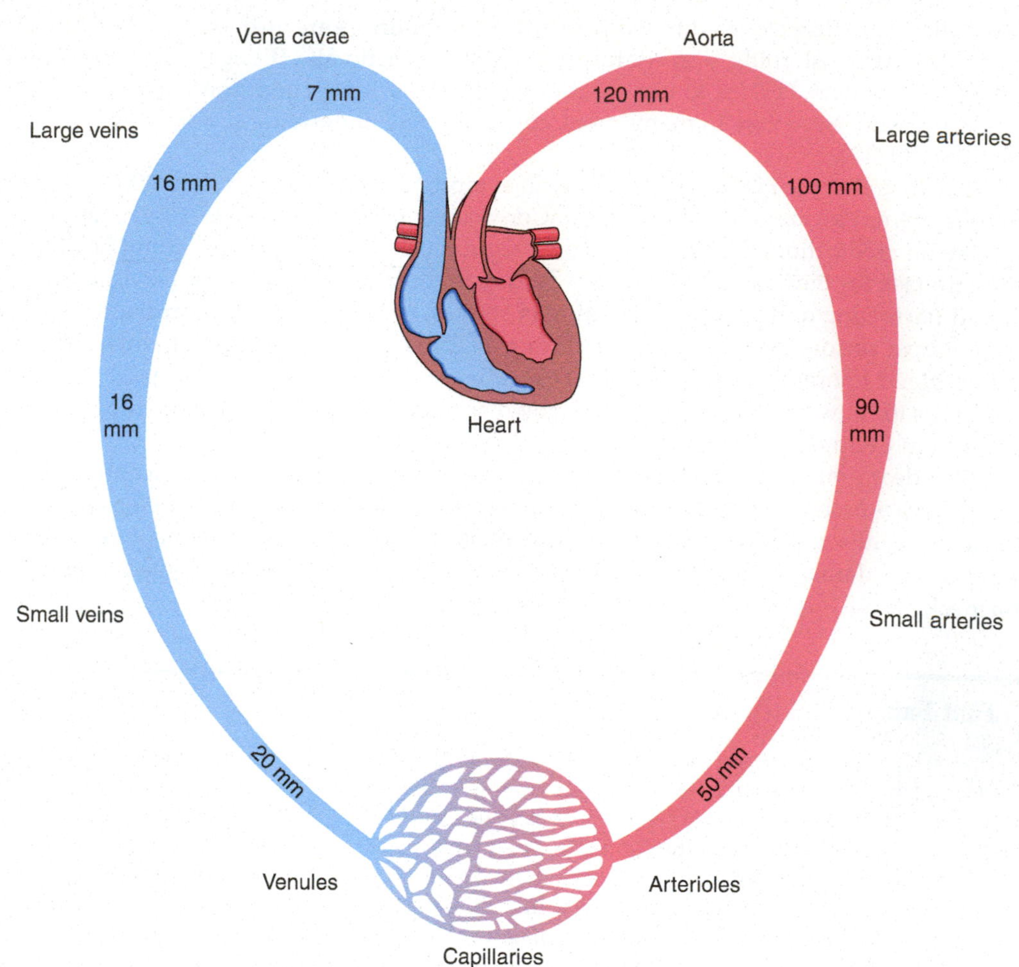

FIGURE 19.1 Blood pressure changes throughout the circulation.

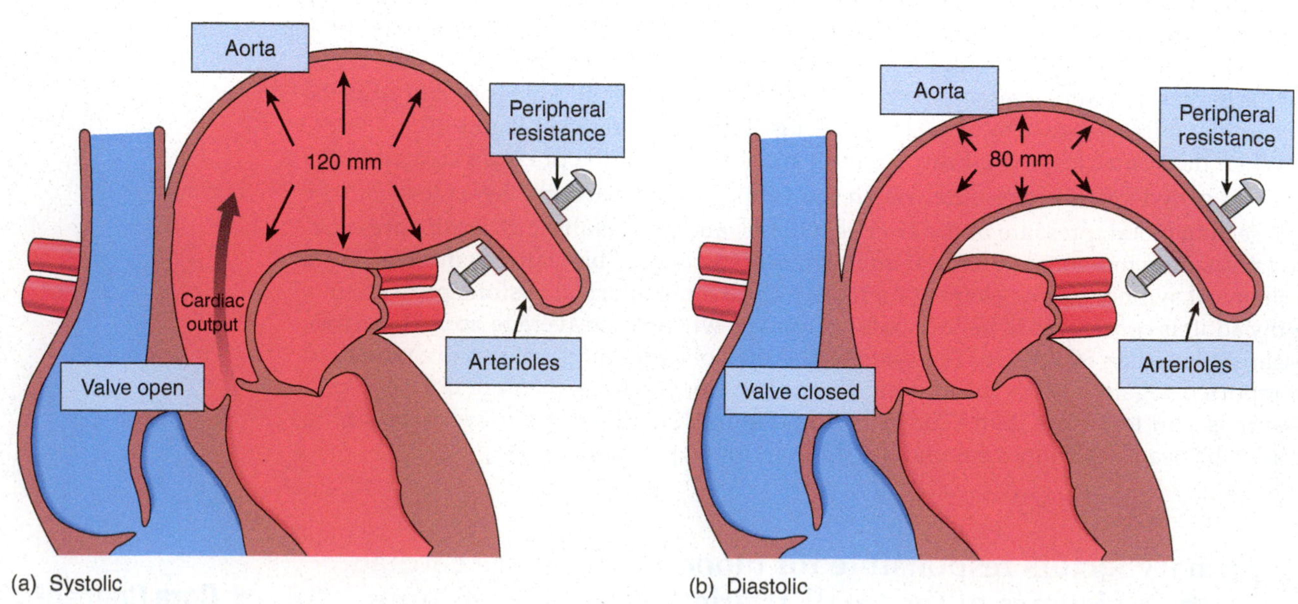

FIGURE 19.2 (a) Systolic pressure occurs when the heart ejects blood, creating high pressure in the arteries. (b) Diastolic pressure occurs when the heart relaxes, resulting in less pressure in the arteries.

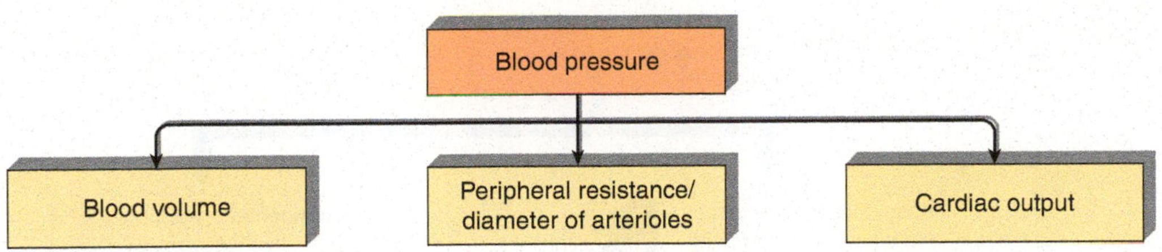

FIGURE 19.3 Primary factors affecting blood pressure.

Although many factors can influence blood pressure, three factors are truly responsible for determining the pressure. The three primary factors—cardiac output, peripheral resistance, and blood volume—are shown in Figure 19.3.

The volume of blood pumped per minute is called the **cardiac output**. Although resting cardiac output is approximately 5 liters per minute (L/min), strenuous exercise can increase this output to as much as 35 L/min. This is important to pharmacology because drugs that change the cardiac output have the potential to influence a patient's blood pressure. It is important to remember that the higher the cardiac output, the higher the blood pressure.

As blood flows at high speeds through the vascular system, it bumps and drags across the walls of the vessels. Although the vessel walls are extremely smooth, this friction reduces the velocity of the blood. This dragging or friction in the arteries is called **peripheral resistance**. Arteries have smooth muscle in their walls that, when constricted, will cause the inside diameter or **lumen** to become smaller, thus creating more resistance and higher pressure. This is how the body controls normal minute-by-minute changes in blood pressure. This is also important to pharmacology because a number of drugs affect vascular smooth muscle, causing vessels to constrict, thus raising blood pressure. Other drugs cause the smooth muscle to relax, thereby opening the lumen and lowering blood pressure. These drugs are among those used to treat HTN. The role of the autonomic nervous system in controlling peripheral resistance is presented in Chapter 9.

The third factor responsible for blood pressure is the total amount of blood in the vascular system, or blood volume. Although the average person maintains a relatively constant blood volume of approximately 5 L, this can change as a result of certain regulatory factors and with certain disease states. More blood in the vascular system will exert additional pressure on the walls of the arteries and raise blood pressure. For example, high sodium diets cause water to be retained by the body, thus increasing blood volume and raising blood pressure. On the other hand, drugs called diuretics can cause fluid loss by enhancing urination, thus decreasing blood volume and lowering blood pressure. Diuretics are discussed later in this chapter.

Many nervous and hormonal factors help to keep blood pressure within normal limits.

◀ Core Concept 19.4

It is critical that the body maintains a normal range of blood pressure and that it has the ability to safely and rapidly change pressure as it proceeds through daily activities, such as sleep and exercise. Too little blood pressure can cause dizziness and lack of urine formation, whereas too much pressure can cause vessels to rupture. A diagram explaining how the body maintains homeostasis during periods of blood pressure change is shown in Figure 19.4.

Blood pressure is regulated on a minute-to-minute basis by a cluster of neurons in the medulla oblongata called the **vasomotor center**. Nerves travel from the vasomotor center to the arteries, where the smooth muscle is directed to either constrict (raise blood pressure) or relax (lower blood pressure).

Receptors in the aorta and the carotid artery act as sensors to provide the vasomotor center with vital information on current conditions in the vascular system. Some of these neurons, called **baroreceptors**, have the ability to sense blood pressure within these large vessels. The baroreceptors are important to the pharmacotherapy of HTN. When a drug is given to lower blood pressure, the baroreceptors respond by trying to return pressure to its original (high) level. The baroreceptor response includes an immediate increase in heart

baro = *pressure*
receptor = *sensor*

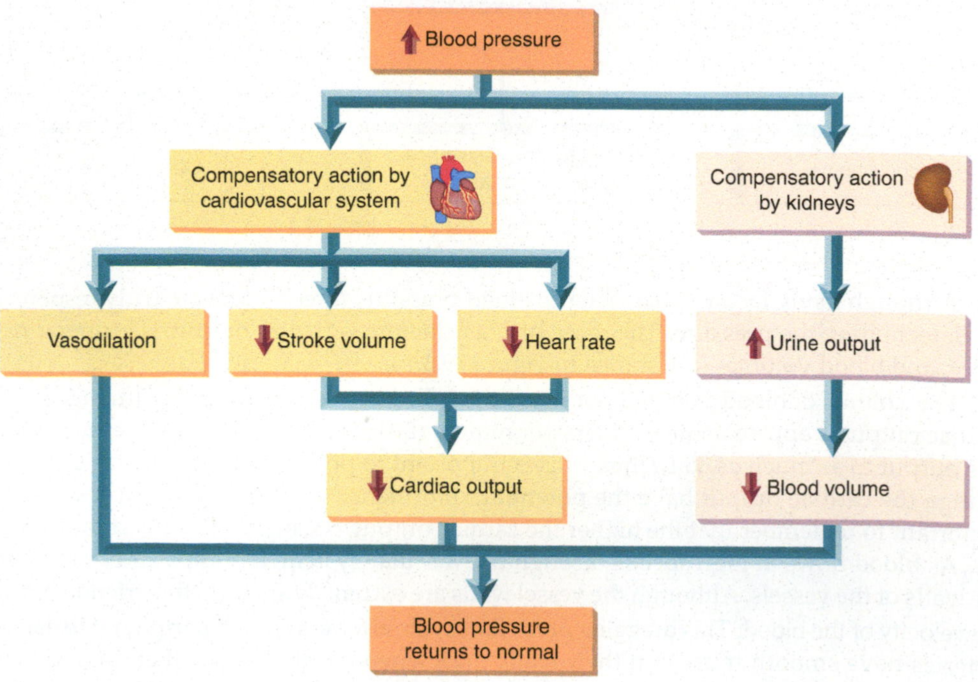

FIGURE 19.4 Blood pressure is controlled by the actions of the cardiovascular system and kidneys.

tachy = *rapid*
cardia = *heart*

rate, known as **reflex tachycardia**. In time, the body will recognize the lower blood pressure as normal, "reset" the baroreceptors, and reflex tachycardia will diminish. If reflex tachycardia does not decrease, a patient may be administered a beta-adrenergic blocker to prevent heart rate increase.

Emotions can also have a profound effect on blood pressure. Anger and stress can cause blood pressure to rise, whereas mental depression and lethargy may cause it to fall. Strong emotions, if present for a long time, may be important contributors to chronic HTN.

anti = *against*
diuretic = *urination*

A number of hormones and other agents affect blood pressure on a daily basis. When given as medications, some of these agents may have a profound effect on blood pressure. For example, an injection of epinephrine or norepinephrine will immediately raise blood pressure. **Antidiuretic hormone (ADH)** is a strong vasoconstrictor that can increase blood pressure by raising blood volume. The renin-angiotensin-aldosterone system is particularly important in the pharmacotherapy of HTN and is discussed in Core Concept 19.8. A summary of the various nervous and hormonal factors influencing blood pressure is shown in Figure 19.5.

CONCEPT REVIEW 19.1

- Because hypertension may cause no symptoms, how would you convince a patient to take his or her medication regularly?

Core Concept 19.5 ▶

Positive lifestyle changes can reduce blood pressure and lessen the need for medications.

When a patient is first diagnosed with HTN, the healthcare provider obtains a comprehensive medical history to determine if the disease can be controlled without medications. Positive lifestyle changes should be recommended for most patients with HTN. Of great importance is maintaining optimal weight, because obesity is closely associated with blood lipid elevation and HTN.

For many patients, implementing positive lifestyle changes may eliminate the need for pharmacotherapy altogether. Even if pharmacotherapy is required, it is important that the patients continue these lifestyle modifications so that dosages can be minimized. Because all blood pressure medications have potential adverse effects, it is important that patients

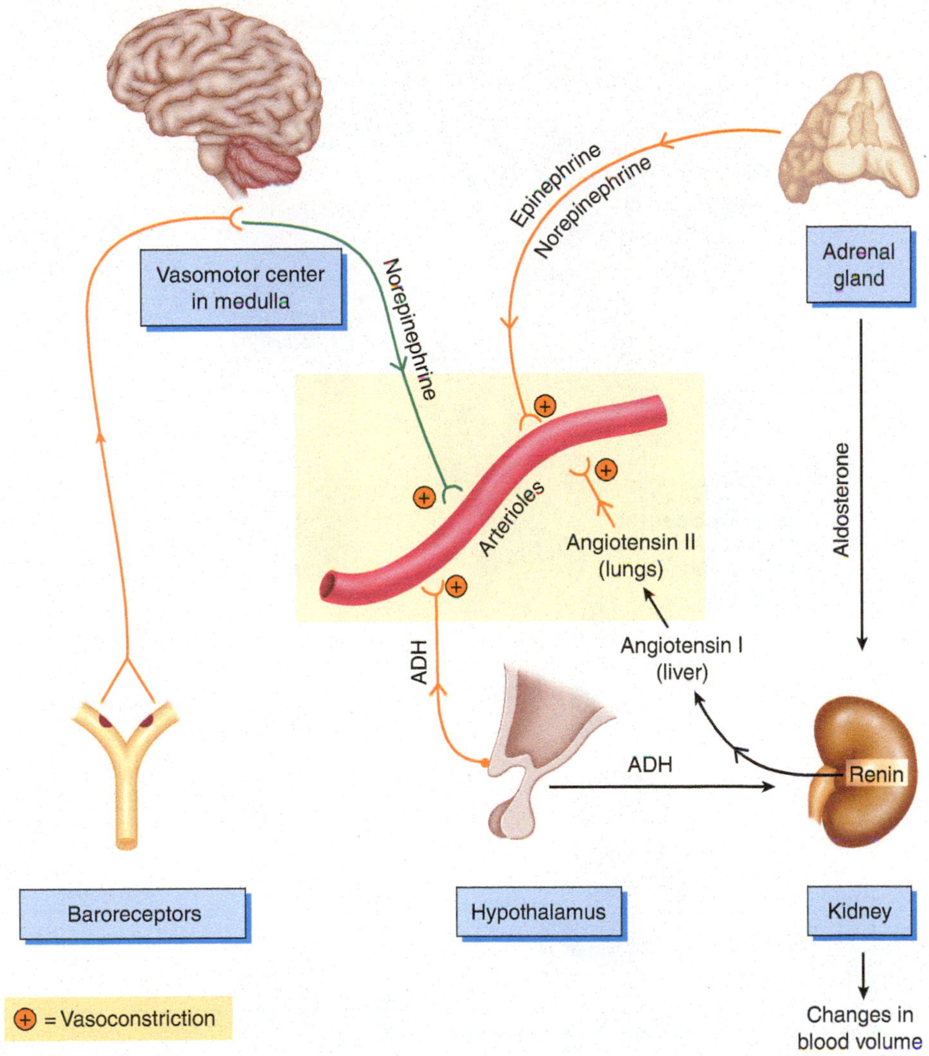

FIGURE 19.5 Hormonal and nervous factors influencing blood pressure.

attempt to control their disease through nonpharmacologic means to the greatest extent possible. Important nonpharmacologic methods for controlling HTN are as follows:

- Implement a medically supervised, safe weight-reduction plan, if 20% or more over normal body weight.
- Stop using tobacco.
- Restrict salt (sodium) intake and eat foods rich in potassium and magnesium.
- Limit alcohol consumption.
- Implement a medically supervised aerobic exercise plan.
- Reduce sources of stress and learn to implement coping strategies.

▶ Lifespan and Diversity

Control of blood pressure is particularly important in older adults. Age often causes blood vessels to be less elastic, thus impairing their ability to dilate or constrict with activities of daily living. Healthcare providers should emphasize to their older adult patients the importance of blood pressure monitoring and control.

The goal in treating hypertension is to reduce the long-term morbidity and mortality associated with the disease.

◀ **Core Concept 19.6**

Keeping blood pressure within optimal limits has been shown to reduce the risk of HTN-related diseases, such as stroke and HF. The pharmacotherapeutic strategies used to achieve this goal are summarized in Figure 19.6.

Practice guidelines for the management of HTN are periodically revised to reflect ongoing research. Late in 2013, the Eighth Joint National Committee (JNC-8) significantly revised the HTN guidelines, based on newer research (James et al., 2014). The JNC-8 committee kept the previously accepted definition of HTN: 140/90 mmHg. The primary difference is

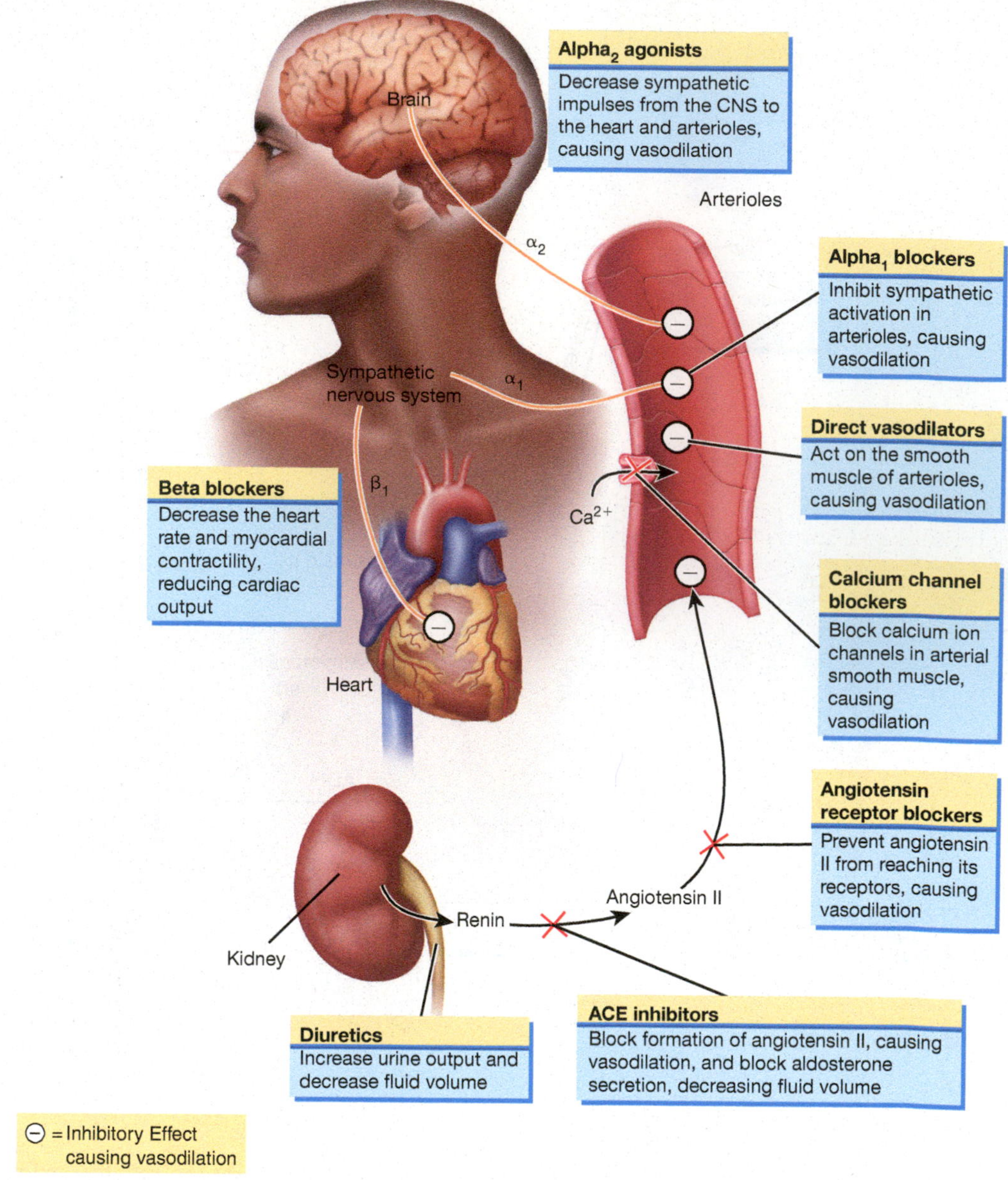

FIGURE 19.6 Mechanism of action of antihypertensive drugs.

that research has shown that not all people with a blood pressure higher than 140/90 mmHg need pharmacotherapy. For example, patients over age 60 who do not have chronic kidney disease or diabetes do not need pharmacotherapy until the 150/90 mmHg threshold. Furthermore, the classes of medications recommended as first-line therapy changed: Beta-adrenergic blockers are no longer considered first-line drugs.

Patient responses to antihypertensive medications vary because of the many complex genetic and environmental factors affecting blood pressure. A large number of antihypertensive drugs are available. Medications recommended as first-line drugs by the JNC-8 are the most effective and provide the lowest incidence of adverse effects for most patients. Second-line drugs are used if additional medications are necessary to achieve blood pressure goals. The drug classes are summarized in Table 19.1.

Pharmacotherapy usually begins with low doses of a single antihypertensive medication. The patient is reevaluated after an appropriate time interval. If necessary, the healthcare provider may increase the dose of the initial drug or substitute another antihypertensive drug from a different class. Prescribing two antihypertensives from different drug classes results in a greater reduction in blood pressure, allows for lower doses of each drug to be used, and is common practice when managing resistant HTN.

Table 19.1 Drug Classes for Hypertension

Type	Class
First-line drugs	Angiotensin-converting enzyme (ACE) inhibitors
	Angiotensin receptor blockers (ARBs)
	Calcium channel blockers (CCBs)
	Thiazide diuretics
Second-line drugs	Adrenergic blockers
	Centrally acting drugs
	Direct-acting vasodilators
	Direct renin inhibitors

For convenience, drug manufacturers often combine two drugs into a single pill or capsule. The diuretic hydrochlorothiazide (Microzide) is the most common drug used in combination antihypertensive products. Examples of antihypertensive combination drugs include Diovan HCT (hydrochlorothiazide and valsartan), Zestoretic (hydrochlorothiazide and lisinopril), and Lotrel (benazepril and amlodipine).

Diuretics are sometimes preferred drugs for treating mild to moderate hypertension.

◀ **Core Concept 19.7**

Diuretics act by increasing the amount of urine produced by the kidneys. They are widely used in the treatment of HTN, HF, and fluid balance disorders. Diuretics were presented in detail in Chapter 18, and prototype drug features for hydrochlorothiazide (Microzide), furosemide (Lasix), and spironolactone (Aldactone) are included in that chapter. This section focuses on the role of diuretics in treating HTN. Table 19.2 lists diuretics commonly used to treat HTN.

Diuretics were the first widely prescribed class of drugs used to treat HTN in the 1950s. Despite many advances in drug therapy since then, diuretics are still considered first-line drugs because they produce few adverse effects and are very effective at controlling mild to moderate HTN. For resistant HTN, they are prescribed in combination with medications from other antihypertensive classes.

Table 19.2 Diuretics for Hypertension

Drug	Route and Adult Dose	Remarks
amiloride (Midamor)	PO: 5–10 mg/day (max: 20 mg/day)	Potassium-sparing type
bumetanide (Bumex)	PO: 0.25–2 mg once daily (max: 10 mg/day)	Loop diuretic type; decreases blood potassium levels; IV and IM forms available
chlorothiazide (Diuril)	PO/IV: 250 mg–1 g/day in one or two divided doses (max: 2 g/day)	Thiazide type; decreases blood potassium levels
chlorthalidone (Thalitone)	PO: 12.5–25 mg daily (max: 50 mg/day)	Thiazide type; decreases blood potassium levels
eplerenone (Inspra)	PO: 25–50 mg once daily (max: 100 mg/day)	Potassium-sparing type
furosemide (Lasix) (see the Prototype Drug box in Core Concept 18.5)	PO: 20–80 mg/day (max: 600 mg/day)	Loop diuretic type; decreases blood potassium levels; IV and IM forms available
hydrochlorothiazide (Microzide) (see the Prototype Drug box in Core Concept 18.6)	PO: 25–100 mg in one to two divided doses (max: 200 mg/day)	Thiazide type; decreases blood potassium levels
indapamide (Lozol)	PO: 2.5–5 mg daily (max: 5 mg/day)	Similar to thiazide type; decreases blood potassium levels
spironolactone (Aldactone) (see the Prototype Drug box in Core Concept 18.7)	PO: 25–100 mg 1–2 times/day (max: 400 mg/day)	Potassium-sparing type
torsemide (Demadex)	PO/IV: 10–20 mg/day (max: 200 mg/day)	Loop diuretic type; decreases blood potassium levels
triamterene (Dyrenium)	PO: 50–100 mg bid (max: 300 mg/day)	Potassium sparing type

Although many different diuretics are available for HTN, all produce a similar outcome: the reduction of blood volume through the urinary excretion of water and electrolytes. Electrolytes are inorganic ions such as sodium (Na^+), calcium (Ca^{2+}), chloride (Cl^-), and potassium (K^+) that possess a positive or negative charge. The mechanisms by which diuretics reduce blood volume differ among the various diuretics. Differences among the diuretic classes are presented in Chapter 18.

de = *without or absence of*
hydra = *water*
tion = *condition*

A common adverse effect of diuretic therapy is dehydration, the excessive loss of water from the body. Early signs of dehydration include thirst, dry mouth, dizziness, lethargy, and a fall in blood pressure.

▶ Lifespan and Diversity

Older adults are especially at risk for dehydration and must be carefully monitored during the initial stages of diuretic therapy.

Electrolyte imbalances of potassium, sodium, and magnesium ions are additional adverse effects of diuretic therapy. Depletion of K^+, or hypokalemia, is of particular concern because it can lead to serious abnormalities in cardiac rhythm. When taking thiazide or loop diuretics, patients should be encouraged to include a potassium supplement or to eat foods rich in potassium content, such as bananas, oranges, tomatoes, milk, salmon, and beef.

hyper = *high*
hypo = *low*
ka = *potassium*
emia = *blood*

Certain diuretics, such as spironolactone (Aldactone), have fewer tendencies to cause K^+ depletion, and, for this reason, are called *potassium-sparing diuretics*. Taking potassium supplements with potassium-sparing diuretics may lead to dangerously high K^+ levels in the blood, or hyperkalemia, which can cause cardiac conduction abnormalities.

CONCEPT REVIEW 19.2

- State the major reasons why patients should continue lifestyle changes even though their antihypertensive drugs appear to be effective.

Core Concept 19.8 ▶

Blocking the renin-angiotensin-aldosterone system leads to a decrease in blood pressure.

The **renin-angiotensin-aldosterone system (RAAS)** is one of the primary homeostatic mechanisms controlling blood pressure and fluid balance in the body. Drugs that modify the RAAS decrease blood pressure and increase urine output. They are widely used in the treatment of HTN, HF, and MI. Some of the ACE inhibitors are also used to slow the progress of diabetic nephropathy, a type of kidney damage found in patients with diabetes. Table 19.3 lists the RAAS modifiers commonly used to treat HTN.

angio = *vessels*
tensin = *pressure*

Renin is an enzyme secreted by specialized cells in the kidneys when blood pressure falls or when there is a decrease in Na^+ flowing through the kidney tubules. In a series of enzymatic steps, **angiotensin II**, one of the most potent natural vasoconstrictors known, is formed. The enzyme responsible for the final step of this pathway is called **angiotensin-converting enzyme (ACE)**. The intense vasoconstriction of arterioles caused by angiotensin II raises blood pressure by increasing peripheral resistance.

A second, equally important effect of angiotensin II is stimulation of the secretion of aldosterone, a hormone from the adrenal gland that increases Na^+ reabsorption in the kidney. The enhanced Na^+ reabsorption causes the body to retain water, which raises blood volume and increases blood pressure. Drugs that inhibit the RAAS block the effects of angiotensin II, thus decreasing blood pressure through *two* mechanisms: dilating arteries and decreasing blood volume.

First detected in the venom of pit vipers in the 1960s, drugs that inhibit ACE have been approved for HTN since the 1980s. Since then, the ACE inhibitors have become first-line drugs in the treatment of HTN. ACE inhibitors are preferred drugs for patients with both diabetes and HTN because they have been shown to reduce the progression of kidney failure that often occurs in patients with diabetes. Because of cardiovascular changes associated with diabetes, these patients often require therapy with at least two antihypertensive drugs. Adverse effects of ACE inhibitors are relatively minor and include persistent dry cough and hypotension following the first dose of the drug. As with many other antihypertensive drugs, patients may experience **orthostatic (postural) hypotension**, a condition in which they become dizzy, lightheaded, or faint when moving rapidly from a recumbent to a sitting

Table 19.3 ACE Inhibitors and Angiotensin-Receptor Blockers for Hypertension

Drug	Route and Adult dose	Remarks
ACE INHIBITORS		
benazepril (Lotensin)	PO: 10–40 mg in one to two divided doses (max: 40 mg/day)	Approved for HTN only
captopril (Capoten)	PO: 6.25–25 mg tid (max: 450 mg/day)	Also for HF and diabetic nephropathy
Pr enalapril (Vasotec)	PO: 5–40 mg in 1–2 divided doses (max: 40 mg/day)	Also for HF and asymptomatic left ventricular dysfunction; IV form available
fosinopril (Monopril)	PO: 5–40 mg daily (max: 80 mg/day)	Also for HF
lisinopril (Prinivil, Zestril) (see the Prototype Drug box in Core Concept 20.5)	PO: 10 mg daily (max: 80 mg/day)	Also for HF and post-MI therapy
moexipril (Univasc)	PO: 7.5–30 mg daily (max: 30 mg/day)	Approved for HTN only
perindopril (Aceon)	PO: 4 mg once daily (max: 16 mg/day)	Also for HF, stable angina, and post MI therapy
quinapril (Accupril)	PO: 10–20 mg daily (max: 80 mg/day)	Also for HF
ramipril (Altace)	PO: 2.5–5 mg daily (max: 20 mg/day)	Also for HF, stroke prophylaxis, and post-MI therapy
trandolapril (Mavik)	PO: 1–4 mg daily (max: 8 mg/day)	Also for post-MI therapy
ANGIOTENSIN-RECEPTOR BLOCKERS (ARBs)		
azilsartan (Edarbi)	PO: 40–80 mg once daily	Approved for HTN only. Newer drug in this class
candesartan (Atacand)	PO: start at 16 mg/day (max: 32 mg/day)	Also for HF
eprosartan (Teveten)	PO: 600 mg/day or 400 mg qid–bid (max: 800 mg/day)	Approved for HTN only
irbesartan (Avapro)	PO: 150–300 mg/day (max: 300 mg/day)	Approved for HTN only; maximum effect may take 6–12 weeks
losartan (Cozaar)	PO: 25–50 mg in one to two divided doses (max: 100 mg/day)	Approved for HTN only
olmesartan (Benicar)	PO: 20–40 mg/day (max: 40 mg/day)	Approved for HTN only
telmisartan (Micardis)	PO: 40–80 mg/day (max: 80 mg/day	Approved for HTN only
valsartan (Diovan)	PO: 80 mg/day (max: 320 mg/day)	Also for HF

or standing position. Though rare, the most serious adverse effect of ACE inhibitors is the development of angioedema, an intense swelling around the lips, eyes, throat, and other body regions. In advanced cases, angioedema may lead to airway closure due to serious swelling in the neck. When angioedema does occur, it most often develops within hours or days after beginning ACE inhibitor therapy.

A second method of modifying the RAAS is blocking the action of angiotensin II *after* it is formed. This class of drugs is called the angiotensin-receptor blockers (ARBs). These drugs, which include irbesartan (Avapro), losartan (Cozaar), and valsartan (Diovan), block the receptors for angiotensin II in arteriolar smooth muscle and in the adrenal gland, thus causing blood pressure to fall. Their actions of arteriolar dilation and increased renal Na^+ excretion are quite similar to those of the ACE inhibitors. ARBs have relatively minor adverse effects, such as headache, dizziness, and facial flushing. Unlike the ACE inhibitors, they do not cause cough, and angioedema is rare. Drugs in this class are usually combined with drugs from other classes; for example, the drug Hyzaar combines losartan with the diuretic hydrochlorothiazide.

The newest method of modifying the RAAS is to inhibit the effects of renin itself. The direct renin inhibitors prevent the formation of angiotensin I and II. Aliskiren (Tekturna) was the first drug marketed in this class of antihypertensives. Pharmaceutical companies were quick to add aliskiren to other drugs to create fixed-dose combinations containing hydrochlorothiazide (Tekturna HCT) and amlodipine (Amturnide, Tekamlo). The most common adverse effects of aliskiren are diarrhea, cough, flu-like symptoms, and rash.

All drugs affecting the RAAS contain a black box warning that the drug should be discontinued as soon as possible when pregnancy is detected because it may result in fetal injury or death.

Prototype Drug: Pr *Enalapril (Vasotec)*

Therapeutic Class: Drug for hypertension and heart failure **Pharmacologic Class: ACE inhibitor**

Actions and Uses: Enalapril is one of the most common ACE inhibitors prescribed for HTN. Unlike captopril, the first ACE inhibitor to be marketed, enalapril has a prolonged half-life, which permits administration once or twice daily. Enalapril acts by reducing angiotensin II and aldosterone levels to produce a significant reduction in blood pressure, with few adverse effects. Enalapril has effectiveness comparable to the thiazide diuretics and the beta-adrenergic blockers. It may be used by itself or in combination with other antihypertensives. Vaseretic is a fixed-dose combination of enalapril and hydrochlorothiazide.

Adverse Effects and Interactions: Unlike diuretics, ACE inhibitors such as enalapril have little effect on electrolyte balance, and unlike beta-adrenergic blockers, they cause few cardiac adverse effects. Like other antihypertensive drugs, enalapril may cause orthostatic hypotension, especially in older adults. Care must be taken because a rapid fall in blood pressure may occur following the first dose. Most drugs in this class cause a persistent, dry cough. Other adverse effects include headache and dizziness.

Thiazide diuretics increase the risk of excessive potassium loss when used with enalapril. On the other hand, potassium-sparing diuretics increase the risk of hyperkalemia when used with ACE inhibitors.

Enalapril may induce lithium toxicity by reducing renal clearance of lithium. Nonsteroidal anti-inflammatory drugs (NSAIDs) may reduce the effectiveness of ACE inhibitors.

BLACK BOX WARNING:
Fetal injury and death may occur when ACE inhibitors or ARBs are taken during pregnancy. When pregnancy is detected, they should be discontinued as soon as possible.

Nursing Process Focus Patients Receiving ACE Inhibitor Therapy

ASSESSMENT

Prior to administration:
- Obtain a complete health history including cardiovascular conditions, neurological status, incidence of angioedema, allergies, drug history, and possible drug interactions.
- Acquire the results of a complete physical examination, including vital signs, height, weight, and electrocardiogram (ECG), and compare to previous baseline values.
- Evaluate laboratory blood findings: complete blood count (CBC), electrolytes, lipid panel, and renal and liver function studies.

POTENTIAL NURSING DIAGNOSES*

- *Deficient Knowledge* related to lack of information about drug therapy
- *Risk for Decreased Cardiac Tissue Perfusion* related to hypertension
- *Noncompliance* related to adverse effects of medications
- *Risk for Injury* related to orthostatic hypotension

PLANNING: PATIENT GOALS AND EXPECTED OUTCOMES

The patient will:
- Experience therapeutic effects (a reduction in systolic/diastolic blood pressure and normal electrolyte levels).
- Be free from or experience minimal adverse effects from drug therapy.
- Verbalize an understanding of the drug's use, adverse effects, and required precautions.

IMPLEMENTATION

Interventions and (Rationales)	Patient Education/Discharge Planning
• Monitor for first-dose phenomenon of profound hypotension. (First-dose phenomenon includes the relatively minor adverse effects of dry cough and hypotension.)	• Warn the patient about the first-dose phenomenon; reassure that this effect diminishes with continued therapy.
• Monitor vital signs, especially blood pressure. (ACE inhibitors can cause hypotension.)	Instruct the patient: • To monitor blood pressure as specified by the healthcare provider and ensure proper use of home equipment. • That changes in consciousness may occur due to rapid reduction in blood pressure and to immediately report feelings of syncope. • That the drug takes effect in approximately 1 hour and peaks in 3 to 4 hours. • To rest in the supine position beginning 1 hour after administration and for 3 hours after the first dose. • To always rise slowly, avoiding sudden postural changes.

Interventions and (Rationales)	Patient Education/Discharge Planning
• Monitor for changes in level of consciousness, dizziness, drowsiness, or lightheadedness. (Signs of decreased blood flow to the brain are due to the drug's hypotensive action. Sudden fainting episodes are possible.)	Instruct the patient to: • Report dizziness or syncope that persists beyond the first dose as well as unusual sensations (e.g., numbness and tingling) or other changes in the face or limbs to the healthcare provider. • Contact the healthcare provider before the next scheduled dose of the drug if syncope occurs.
• Ensure patient safety. (Orthostatic hypotension may cause dizziness, affecting the ability to perform normal activities.)	Instruct the patient to: • Obtain help prior to getting out of bed or attempting to walk alone. • Avoid driving or other activities that require mental alertness or physical coordination until effects of the drug are known.
• Observe for hypersensitivity reaction, particularly angioedema. (Angioedema may arise at any time during ACE inhibitor therapy, but it is generally expected shortly after initiation of therapy.)	Instruct the patient: • To immediately report any difficulty breathing, throat tightness, muscle cramps, hives, rash, or tremors to the healthcare provider. (These symptoms can occur as early as the first dose or much later as a delayed reaction.) • That angioedema can be life threatening and to call emergency medical services if severe dyspnea or hoarseness is accompanied by swelling of the face or mouth.
• Monitor for persistent dry cough, a possible adverse effect of the drug. Monitor changes in cough pattern. (This may indicate another disease process.)	Instruct the patient to: • Expect persistent dry cough. • Report any change in the character or frequency of cough. (Any cough accompanied by shortness of breath, fever, or chest pain should be reported *immediately* to the healthcare provider because it may indicate MI.) • Sleep with the head elevated if cough becomes troublesome when in the supine position. • Use nonmedicated sugar-free lozenges or hard candies to relieve cough.
• Monitor for dehydration or fluid overload. (Dehydration causes low circulating blood volume and will exacerbate hypotension. Severe dehydration may cause fainting.)	Instruct the patient to: • Observe for signs of dehydration, such as oliguria, dry lips and mucous membranes, or poor skin turgor. • Report any bodily swelling that leaves sunken marks on the skin when pressed to the healthcare provider. • Measure and monitor fluid intake and output, and weigh daily. • Monitor increased need for fluids caused by vomiting, diarrhea, or excessive sweating. • Avoid excessive heat that contributes to sweating and fluid loss. • Consume adequate amounts of *plain* water.
• Monitor for high potassium levels. (Hyperkalemia is a potentially life-threatening complication. Patients on ACE inhibitors should regularly have blood tests to measure potassium levels.)	Instruct the patient to: • Immediately report any signs of hyperkalemia to the healthcare provider: nausea, irregular heartbeat, profound fatigue, muscle weakness, and slow or faint pulse. • Avoid consuming electrolyte-fortified snacks or sports drinks that may contain potassium. • Avoid using salt substitute (KCl) to flavor foods. • Consult the healthcare provider before taking any nutritional supplements containing potassium.
• Monitor for liver and kidney function. (ACE inhibitors are metabolized by the liver and excreted by the kidneys.)	Instruct the patient to: • Report signs of liver toxicity such as nausea; vomiting; anorexia; diarrhea; rash; jaundice; abdominal pain, tenderness, or distension; or change in the color or character of stools to the healthcare provider. • Discontinue the drug immediately and contact the healthcare provider if jaundice occurs. • Adhere to laboratory testing regimen as ordered by the healthcare provider.

(Continued)

Nursing Process Focus (*continued*)

Interventions and (Rationales)	Patient Education/Discharge Planning
• Administer the medication correctly and evaluate the patient's knowledge level of proper administration. (Some medications interact with other medications.)	Instruct the patient: • That taking other antihypertensive drugs may increase the risk for hypotension. • Not to take the medication with grapefruit juice. • To consult a healthcare provider before taking potassium supplements or potassium-sparing diuretics. • That NSAIDs may reduce the actions of ACE inhibitors.

EVALUATION OF OUTCOME CRITERIA

- Evaluate the effectiveness of drug therapy by confirming that patient goals and expected outcomes have been met (see "Planning"). *See Table 19.5 for a list of drugs to which these nursing actions apply.*

*Herdman, T.H. & Kamitsuru, S. (Eds.), *Nursing Diagnoses: Definitions & Classification* 2015–2017. Copyright © 2014, 1994–2014 NANDA International. Used by arrangement by John Wiley & Sons, Inc. Companion website: www.wiley.com/go/nursingdiagnoses.

Core Concept 19.9 ▶ Calcium channel blockers have emerged as important drugs in the treatment of hypertension.

Calcium channel blockers (CCBs) comprise a group of drugs that are used to treat a number of cardiovascular diseases, including angina pectoris, cardiac dysrhythmias, and HTN. When CCBs were first approved for the treatment of angina in the early 1980s, it was quickly noted that a "side effect" of the drugs was the lowering of blood pressure in patients with HTN. Although not usually prescribed as monotherapy for chronic HTN, CCBs are useful in treating patients who are unresponsive to other antihypertensive classes, such as older and African American patients. Table 19.4 lists CCBs that are used to treat HTN.

Contraction of a muscle is regulated by the amount of calcium ions inside the muscle cell. Muscular contraction occurs when Ca^{2+} enters the cell through channels in the plasma membrane. CCBs block these channels and prevent Ca^{2+} from entering the cell, thus inhibiting muscular contraction. At low doses, CCBs cause vasodilation in arterioles, thus decreasing blood pressure. Some CCBs, such as nifedipine (Adalat CC, Procardia XL, others), are selective for calcium channels in arterioles, whereas others, such as verapamil (Calan, Isoptin, others), affect channels in both arterioles and cardiac muscle. CCBs vary in their potency and in the frequency and types of adverse effects produced. The use of CCBs in the treatment of dysrhythmias and angina is discussed in Chapters 23 and 21, respectively.

Table 19.4 Calcium Channel Blockers for Hypertension

Drug	Route And Adult Dose	Remarks
amlodipine (Norvasc)	PO: 5–10 mg once daily (max: 10 mg/day)	Selective for calcium channels in blood vessels; also for angina
diltiazem (Cardizem, Cartia XT, Dilacor XR, others) (see the Prototype Drug box in Core Concept 21.7)	PO (extended release): 120–240 mg daily or 20–120 mg bid	Dilates coronary arteries; affects calcium channels in both heart and blood vessels; IV form available; also for angina and dysrhythmias
felodipine (Plendil)	PO: 2.5–10 mg/day (max: 20 mg/day)	Selective for calcium channels in blood vessels; may be used off-label for angina and HF
isradipine (DynaCirc)	PO: 2.5 mg bid (max: 20 mg/day)	Selective for calcium channels in blood vessels; may be used off-label for angina
nicardipine (Cardene SR)	PO: 30–60 mg bid	Selective for calcium channels in blood vessels; also for angina; IV form is available
Pr nifedipine (Adalat CC, Procardia XL, others)	PO: 30–60 mg once daily	Selective for calcium channels in blood vessels; also for angina
nisoldipine (Sular)	PO: 17 mg once daily (max: 34 mg/day)	Selective for calcium channels in blood vessels; may be used off-label for angina
verapamil (Calan, Isoptin SR, others) (see the Prototype Drug box in Core Concept 23.9)	PO: 80–120 mg tid (max: 480 mg/day) PO (extended release): 1080 mg once daily	Affects calcium channels in both heart and blood vessels; IV form available for specific dysrhythmias; also for angina

Two CCBs, clevidipine (Cleviprex) and nicardipine (Cardene), are important drugs for treating patients with serious, life-threatening HTN. Clevidipine has an ultrashort half-life of 1 minute and is only available by the IV route for hypertensive emergencies.

The high safety profile of CCBs has contributed to their popularity in treating HTN. Common adverse effects related to their vasodilation action include headache, facial flushing, and dizziness. The CCBs that affect the heart should be used cautiously in patients with preexisting cardiac disease.

Prototype Drug: Pr *Nifedipine (Adalat CC, Procardia XL, Others)*

Therapeutic Class: Drug for hypertension and angina **Pharmacologic Class:** Calcium channel blocker

Actions and Uses: Nifedipine is a CCB prescribed for angina as well as for HTN. Nifedipine selectively blocks calcium channels in myocardial and vascular smooth muscle, including that in the coronary arteries. This results in reduced oxygen demands by the heart, an increase in cardiac output, and a fall in blood pressure. The immediate-release capsules are indicated for angina, and the extended-release tablets (XL) are indicated for HTN.

Adverse Effects and Interactions: Adverse effects of nifedipine are generally minor and related to vasodilation, such as headache, dizziness, and flushing. Fast-acting forms of nifedipine can cause significant reflex tachycardia. To avoid rebound hypotension, discontinuation of drug therapy should occur gradually.

Nifedipine may increase serum levels of digoxin, cimetidine, and ranitidine, and increase the effects of warfarin, resulting in increased partial thromboplastin time (PTT). It may also increase the effects of fentanyl anesthesia, resulting in severe hypotension and an increased need for fluids. Grapefruit juice may enhance the absorption of nifedipine.

Alcohol increases the vasodilating action of nifedipine and can lead to a severe drop in blood pressure. Nicotine causes vasoconstriction, countering the desired effect of nifedipine. Use with melatonin may increase blood pressure and heart rate.

Nursing Process Focus Patients Receiving Calcium Channel Blocker Therapy

ASSESSMENT

Prior to administration:

- Obtain a complete health history including cardiovascular, respiratory, neurological, renal and liver conditions, allergies, drug history, and possible drug interactions.
- Evaluate laboratory blood findings: CBC, electrolytes, lipid panel, and renal and liver function studies.
- Acquire the results of a complete physical examination, including vital signs, height, weight, ECG, neurologic status, and signs of edema.

POTENTIAL NURSING DIAGNOSES*

- *Ineffective Health Maintenance* related to insufficient knowledge of seriousness of disease and drug therapy regimen
- *Deficient Knowledge* related to a lack of information about drug therapy unfamiliarity with medication information
- *Decreased Cardiac Output* related to effects of drug therapy
- *Noncompliance* related to adverse effects of medications
- *Risk for Injury* related to possible orthostatic hypotension

PLANNING: PATIENT GOALS AND EXPECTED OUTCOMES

The patient will:

- Experience therapeutic effects (reduction in systolic/diastolic blood pressure).
- Be free from or experience minimal adverse effects from drug therapy.
- Verbalize an understanding of the drug's use, adverse effects, and required precautions.

IMPLEMENTATION

Interventions and (Rationales)	Patient Education/Discharge Planning
• Monitor vital signs and ECG. Obtain blood pressure readings in sitting, standing, and supine positions to monitor fluctuations in blood pressure. (CCBs dilate the arteries, reducing blood pressure and possibly causing hypotension.)	Instruct the patient to: • Monitor vital signs as specified by the nurse, particularly the blood pressure, ensuring proper use of home equipment. • Withhold medication for severe hypotensive readings as specified by the nurse (e.g., "hold for levels below 88/50 mmHg"). • Immediately report palpitations or rapid heartbeat.

(Continued)

Nursing Process Focus *(continued)*

Interventions and (Rationales)	Patient Education/Discharge Planning
• Observe for changes in level of consciousness, dizziness, fatigue, orthostatic hypotension. (These adverse effects can be caused by vasodilation.) • Observe for paradoxical increase in chest pain, angina symptoms, or increase in heart rate. (These complaints may be related to severe hypotension.)	Instruct the patient to: • Report dizziness or lightheadedness to the healthcare provider. • Rise slowly from prolonged periods of sitting or lying down. • Report chest pain or other angina-like symptoms immediately to the healthcare provider.
• Monitor for signs of HF. (CCBs can decrease myocardial contractility, increasing the risk of HF.)	• Instruct the patient to immediately report any severe shortness of breath, frothy sputum, profound fatigue, and swelling to the healthcare provider. These may be signs of HF or fluid accumulation in the lungs.
• Monitor for fluid accumulation. Measure intake and output and daily weights. (Edema is an adverse effect of some CCBs.)	Instruct the patient to: • Avoid excessive heat, which contributes to excessive sweating and fluid loss. • Measure and monitor fluid intake and output, and weigh daily. • Consume enough *plain* water to remain adequately, but not overly, hydrated.
• Observe for hypersensitivity reaction. (Allergic responses may be life threatening.)	• Instruct the patient to immediately report difficulty breathing, throat tightness, hives, rash, muscle cramps, or tremors to the healthcare provider.
• Monitor liver and kidney function. (CCBs are metabolized in the liver and excreted by the kidneys.)	Instruct the patient to: • Report signs of liver toxicity to the healthcare provider: nausea, vomiting, anorexia, bleeding, severe upper abdominal pain, heartburn, jaundice, or a change in the color or character of stools. • Report signs of renal toxicity to the healthcare provider: fever, flank pain, changes in urine output, color, or character (cloudy, with sediment). • Adhere to laboratory testing regimens as ordered by the healthcare provider.
• Observe for constipation. May need to increase dietary fiber or administer laxatives. (CCBs may cause constipation.)	Advise the patient to: • Maintain adequate fluid and fiber intake to facilitate stool passage. • Use a bulk laxative or stool softener, as recommended by the healthcare provider.
• Ensure patient safety. Monitor ambulation until response to the drug is known. (Some CCBs may cause drowsiness.)	• Instruct the patient to avoid driving or other activities that require mental alertness or physical coordination until the effects of the drug are known.
• Administer medication correctly and evaluate the patient's knowledge level of proper administration. (Some medications interact with other medications.)	Instruct the patient: • That taking other antihypertensive drugs may increase risk for hypotension. • To avoid rebound hypotension, this drug should be discontinued gradually. • Not to take nifedipine with grapefruit juice because it may enhance absorption. • That alcohol potentiates vasodilating action of nifedipine

EVALUATION OF OUTCOME CRITERIA

Evaluate the effectiveness of drug therapy by confirming that patient goals and expected outcomes have been met (see "Planning"). *See Table 19.4 for a list of drugs to which these nursing actions apply.*

*Herdman, T.H. & Kamitsuru, S. (Eds.), *Nursing Diagnoses: Definitions & Classification* 2015–2017. Copyright © 2014, 1994–2014 NANDA International. Used by arrangement by John Wiley & Sons, Inc. Companion website: www.wiley.com/go/nursingdiagnoses.

CAM Therapy | Grape Seed Extract for Hypertension

Grapes and grape seeds have been used to enhance wellness for thousands of years. Their primary use has been for cardiovascular conditions such as HTN, high blood cholesterol, and atherosclerosis, and to improve circulation. Some claim that grape seed extract improves wound healing, prevents cancer, and lowers the risk for the long-term consequences of diabetes.

The grape seeds, usually obtained from winemaking, are crushed and placed into tablet, capsule, or liquid forms. Grape seed extract has antioxidant properties. In general, antioxidants improve wound healing and repair cellular injury. Some evidence suggests that it may have some benefit in repairing blood vessel damage that sometimes leads to atherosclerosis and HTN. Controlled, long-term studies on the effects of grape seed extract on HTN have not been conducted. It has few adverse effects, but caution should be used if taking anticoagulant drugs because increased bleeding may result. Overall, the benefits of grape seed extract are no different than those of a diet balanced with natural antioxidants and an occasional glass of red wine.

Adrenergic blockers are used to treat a wide variety of cardiovascular disorders, including hypertension.

◀ **Core Concept 19.10**

Stimulation of the sympathetic division of the autonomic nervous system causes "fight-or-flight" responses such as faster heart rate, an increase in blood pressure, and bronchodilation. By blocking the sympathetic fight-or-flight responses, adrenergic drugs can cause the heart rate to slow, blood pressure to decline, and the bronchi to dilate. Adrenergic antagonists (or blockers) that are important in managing HTN are listed in Table 19.5.

Because of their beneficial effects on the heart and vessels, adrenergic blockers are used for a wide variety of cardiovascular disorders. Although no longer recommended as first-line drugs for HTN, they are still frequently prescribed for this condition. These drugs can block the effects of the sympathetic division through a number of different mechanisms, although they all have in common the effect of lowering blood pressure. These mechanisms include the following:

- Blockade of alpha$_1$-receptors in the arterioles
- Blockade of beta$_1$-receptors in the heart
- Nonselective blockade of both beta$_1$- and beta$_2$-receptors
- Stimulation of alpha$_2$-adrenergic receptors in the brainstem (centrally acting).

Prototype Drug: Pr *Doxazosin (Cardura)*

Therapeutic Class: Drug for hypertension and benign prostatic hyperplasia **Pharmacologic Class:** Alpha$_1$-adrenergic blocker

Actions and Uses: Doxazosin is an adrenergic blocker available only in oral form. Because it is selective for blocking alpha$_1$-receptors in vascular smooth muscle, it has few adverse effects on other autonomic organs and is sometimes preferred over nonselective beta blockers such as propranolol. Doxazosin dilates both arteries and veins and is capable of causing a rapid, profound fall in blood pressure.

Doxazosin and several other alpha blockers also relax smooth muscle around the prostate gland. Patients who have difficulty urinating due to an enlarged prostate, a condition known as benign prostatic hyperplasia (BPH), sometimes receive these drugs to relieve symptoms of this disease, as discussed in Chapter 35. The immediate release form is indicated for HTN and BPH. The extended-release form (Cardura XL) is only indicated for BPH.

Adverse Effects and Interactions: When starting doxazosin therapy, some patients experience orthostatic hypotension, although tolerance normally develops to this adverse effect after a few doses. Dizziness and headache are also common adverse effects, although they are rarely severe enough to cause discontinuation of therapy. Oral cimetidine may cause a mild increase (10%) in the half-life of doxazosin. Concurrent administration of doxazosin with phosphodiesterase–5 inhibitors, such as sildenafil (Viagra), can result in extreme hypotension.

Table 19.5 Adrenergic Blockers and Central-Acting Drugs for Hypertension

Drug	Route and Adult Dose	Remarks
acebutolol (Sectral)	PO: 400–800 mg/day (max: 1200 mg/day)	Selective $beta_1$-blocker; also for premature ventricular beats
atenolol (Tenormin) (see the Prototype Drug box in Core Concept 21.6)	PO: 25–50 mg/day (max: 100 mg/day)	Selective $beta_1$-blocker; IV form available for MI; monitor apical pulse prior to administration
betaxolol (Kerlone)	PO: 10–40 mg/day (max: 40 mg/day)	Selective $beta_1$-blocker; approved for HTN only; discontinue drug gradually to avoid rebound HTN
bisoprolol (Zebeta)	PO: 2.5–5 mg daily (max: 20 mg/day)	Selective $beta_1$-blocker; also for angina; discontinue the drug gradually to avoid rebound HTN
carvedilol (Coreg) (see the Prototype Drug box in Core Concept 20.8)	PO: 6.25 mg bid (max: 50 mg/day)	Blocks both alpha and beta receptors; also for HF
clonidine (Catapres)	PO: 0.1 mg bid–tid (max: 0.8 mg/day)	Central-acting $alpha_2$-adrenergic drug; transdermal patch available; epidural infusion form available for management of cancer pain
Pr doxazosin (Cardura)	PO: 1 mg; may increase to 16 mg/day in one to two divided doses (max: 16 mg/day)	Selective $alpha_1$-blocker; also for benign prostatic hyperplasia (BPH)
methyldopa (Aldomet)	PO: 250 mg bid or tid (max: 3 g/day)	Central-acting $alpha_2$-adrenergic drug; IV form available; lowers standing and supine blood pressure
metoprolol (Lopressor, Toprol)	PO: 50–100 mg daily or bid (max: 450 mg/day)	Selective $beta_1$-blocker; sustained-release and IV forms available; also for angina and MI
nadolol (Corgard)	PO: 40 mg/day (max: 320 mg/day)	Nonselective beta blocker; also for angina
pindolol (Visken)	PO: 5 mg bid (max: 60 mg/day)	Nonselective $beta_1$- and $beta_2$-blocker; for HTN only
prazosin (Minipress) (see the Prototype Drug box in Core Concept 9.9)	PO: 1 mg; may increase to 1 mg bid–tid (max: 20 mg/day)	Selective $alpha_1$-blocker; also for BPH, Raynaud's disease, and pheochromocytoma
propranolol (Inderal, InnoPran XL) (see the Prototype Drug box in Core Concept 23.7)	PO: 40 mg bid but may be increased to 160–480 mg/day in divided doses (max: 480 mg/day)	Nonselective $beta_1$- and $beta_2$-blocker; also for angina, MI, dysrhythmias, and migraine prophylaxis; IV form available
terazosin (Hytrin)	PO: 1 mg; may increase 1–5 mg/day (max: 20 mg/day)	Selective $alpha_1$-blocker; also for BPH
timolol (Betimol, Timoptic, others) (see the Prototype Drug box in Core Concept 38.5)	PO: 10 mg bid (max: 60 mg/day)	Nonselective $beta_1$- and $beta_2$-blocker; also for MI and migraine prophylaxis and for glaucoma

Some drugs, such as epinephrine, affect both beta- and alpha-adrenergic receptors and can cause serious adverse effects. Drugs that affect only one receptor subtype produce fewer adverse effects. Prazosin (Minipress), for example, is specific to $alpha_1$-receptors and thus has less effect on the heart, which contains $beta_1$-receptors. On the other hand, atenolol (Tenormin) and metoprolol (Lopressor, Toprol) are selective for $beta_1$-receptors and thus have little effect on the bronchi, which have $beta_2$-receptors. Of the adrenergic antagonists, only the beta-blockers are widely used for the pharmacotherapy of HTN.

The adverse effects of adrenergic antagonists are predictable because they are extensions that would be expected from blocking the fight-or-flight response. The $alpha_1$-blockers tend to cause orthostatic hypotension, nausea, **bradycardia** (slow heart rate), and dry mouth. Less common, though sometimes a major cause of noncompliance, is their adverse effect on male sexual function (impotence). Because nonselective beta blockers slow the heart rate and cause bronchoconstriction, they should be used with caution in patients with asthma or HF.

ortho = *straight*
static = *causing to stand*
brady = *slow*
cardia = *heart*

Some adrenergic blockers affect the production of neurotransmitters in the *central* nervous system rather than affecting the *peripheral* nervous system. For example, methyldopa (Aldomet) is converted to a **false neurotransmitter** in the brainstem, thus causing a shortage of the "real" neurotransmitter and inhibition of the sympathetic nervous system. Clonidine (Catapres), an $alpha_2$ blocker, affects alpha-adrenergic receptors in the cardiovascular control centers in the brainstem. The central acting drugs have a tendency to produce sedation and are infrequently prescribed.

CONCEPT REVIEW 19.3

- Why is it important for patients to weigh themselves on a regular basis when taking antihypertensive drugs?

Vasodilators lower blood pressure by relaxing arteriolar smooth muscle.

◀ **Core Concept 19.11**

Many of the antihypertensive drugs discussed thus far lower blood pressure through *indirect* means by affecting enzymes (ACE inhibitors), autonomic nerves (alpha and beta blockers), or fluid volume (diuretics). It would seem that a more efficient way to reduce blood pressure would be to cause a direct relaxation of arteriolar smooth muscle. Indeed, drugs that directly affect vascular smooth muscle are highly effective at lowering blood pressure, but they produce too many adverse effects to be first-line drugs. The direct-acting vasodilators used for HTN are listed in Table 19.6.

Table 19.6 Direct-Acting Vasodilators for Hypertension

Drug	Route and Adult Dose	Remarks
Pr hydralazine (Apresoline)	PO: 10–50 mg qid (max: 300 mg/day)	Diastolic response usually greater than systolic; IV and IM forms available
minoxidil (Loniten)	PO: 5–40 mg/day (max: 100 mg/day)	Reserved for severe HTN; topical form used to promote hair growth
nitroprusside (Nitropress)	IV: 0.5–10 mcg/kg/min	For hypertensive crisis; produces both arteriolar and venous dilation; infusion not to exceed 10 min

Direct vasodilators produce reflex tachycardia, a normal physiologic response to the sudden decrease in blood pressure caused by the drug. Reflex tachycardia forces the heart to work harder, and blood pressure increases, counteracting the effect of the antihypertensive drug. Patients with coronary artery disease could experience an acute angina attack. Fortunately, reflex tachycardia can be prevented by the concurrent administration of a beta blocker, such as propranolol.

A second potentially serious adverse effect of direct vasodilator therapy is sodium and water retention. As the kidney retains more sodium and water, blood volume increases, thus raising blood pressure and canceling the antihypertensive action of the vasodilator. A diuretic may be administered concurrently with a direct vasodilator to prevent fluid retention.

One direct-acting vasodilator, nitroprusside (Nitropress), is the traditional drug of choice for hypertensive emergency, a condition in which diastolic pressure is greater than 120 mmHg and there is evidence of organ damage, usually to the heart, kidney, or brain. This potentially life-threatening condition must be controlled quickly. Nitroprusside has the ability to lower blood pressure almost instantaneously on IV administration. Care must be taken not to decrease blood pressure too quickly because this can result in hypotension and severe restriction of blood flow to the cerebral, coronary, or renal capillaries.

Prototype Drug: Pr *Hydralazine (Apresoline)*

Therapeutic Class: Drug for hypertension and heart failure **Pharmacologic Class:** Direct-acting vasodilator

Actions and Uses: Hydralazine was one of the first oral antihypertensive drugs marketed in the United States. Therapy is generally begun with low doses, which are gradually increased until the desired therapeutic response is obtained. After several months of therapy, tolerance to the drug develops, and a dosage increase may be necessary. Although it produces an effective reduction in blood pressure, drugs in other antihypertensive classes have largely replaced hydralazine because of its many adverse effects. However, this may change due to the approval of BiDil, a fixed-dose combination of isosorbide dinitrate and hydralazine that appears to be effective at lowering blood pressure in African Americans.

Adverse Effects and Interactions: Headache, reflex tachycardia, palpitations, flushing, nausea, and diarrhea are common but may resolve as therapy progresses. Patients taking hydralazine often receive a beta blocker to counteract reflex tachycardia. The drug may produce a lupus-like syndrome with extended use. Sodium and fluid retention is another potentially serious adverse effect. The use of hydralazine is mostly limited to patients whose HTN cannot be controlled with safer medications.

Administering hydralazine with other antihypertensives or monoamine oxidase inhibitors (MAOIs) may cause severe hypotension. This includes all drug classes used as antihypertensives. NSAIDs may decrease the antihypertensive response of hydralazine.

Patients Need to Know

Patients treated for HTN need to know the following:

1. Take medications as prescribed.
2. Never discontinue the medication without approval from a healthcare provider.
3. To control HTN, incorporate lifestyle changes such as diet and exercise, even if blood pressure is brought into normal limits by the medication.
4. Check blood pressure on a regular basis and report significant changes to the healthcare provider.
5. Get out of bed slowly to avoid dizziness.
6. If taking loop or thiazide diuretics, potassium supplements or an increased intake of potassium-rich foods such as bananas, dried fruits, and orange juice may be necessary.
7. Take weight measurements regularly and report abnormal weight gains or losses.
8. Do not take any over-the-counter (OTC) medications for colds, flu, or allergies without first checking with a healthcare provider.
9. If taking an ACE inhibitor or ARB for HTN, immediately notify your healthcare provider if you suspect you are pregnant.

Safety Alert Drug-Food Interactions

Certain drug-food interactions can be very dangerous. For example, the combination of grapefruit juice and certain blood pressure-lowering drugs or some cholesterol-lowering drugs can cause toxic levels of the drug in the blood. It is advisable for patients to keep medications in their original, labeled containers so that instructions are readily available. The nurse should ensure that patients are fully informed about how to take their drugs by providing both oral and written instructions.

Chapter Review

Core Concepts Summary

19.1 Failure to treat chronic hypertension can lead to stroke, heart failure, or myocardial infarction.

HTN is one of the most common cardiovascular diseases. Uncontrolled HTN can cause chronic and debilitating disorders such as stroke, heart attack, and HF.

19.2 Blood pressure is caused by the pumping action of the heart.

As the heart pumps, it creates pressure that is greatest in the arteries closest to the heart. The pressure created by the heart's contraction is called systolic pressure, and that present during the heart's relaxation is called diastolic pressure.

19.3 The primary factors responsible for blood pressure are cardiac output, the resistance of the small arteries, and blood volume.

As blood leaves the heart, its pressure depends on how much blood is present in the vessels (blood volume), how much is ejected per minute, and how much resistance it encounters from the small arteries (peripheral resistance). These are considered the primary factors controlling blood pressure.

19.4 Many nervous and hormonal factors help to keep blood pressure within normal limits.

Clusters of neurons in the medulla known as the vasomotor center regulate blood pressure. Feedback is provided to the vasomotor center by baroreceptors in the aorta and carotid arteries. Hormones such as epinephrine or ADH may have profound effects on blood pressure.

19.5 Positive lifestyle changes can reduce blood pressure and lessen the need for medications.

Because antihypertensive drugs may have uncomfortable adverse effects, lifestyle changes such as proper diet and exercise are often implemented prior to and during drug therapy to enable lower drug doses.

19.6 The goal in treating hypertension is to reduce the long-term morbidity and mortality associated with the disease.

Keeping blood pressure within normal limits can reduce the incidence of long-term consequences of HTN such as stoke and HF. Drug therapy of HTN often begins with low doses of a single drug. If ineffective, a second drug from a different class may be added to the regimen. Multidrug therapy is common.

19.7 Diuretics are sometimes preferred drugs for treating mild to moderate hypertension.

Diuretics are first-line drugs for HTN because they have few adverse effects and can control minor to moderate HTN. Electrolytes should be carefully monitored in patients taking diuretics.

19.8 Blocking the renin-angiotensin-aldosterone system leads to a decrease in blood pressure.

Blocking angiotensin-converting enzyme (ACE) or the angiotensin II receptor can prevent the intense vasoconstriction caused by angiotensin. These drugs also decrease blood volume, which aids in producing their antihypertensive effect.

19.9 Calcium channel blockers have emerged as important drugs in the treatment of hypertension.

CCBs block calcium ions from entering smooth muscle cells, causing arterioles to relax, thus reducing blood pressure. Some CCBs are also used to treat angina, HF, and dysrhythmias.

19.10 Adrenergic blockers are used to treat a wide variety of cardiovascular disorders, including hypertension.

Autonomic drugs that block $alpha_1$-receptors, block $beta_1$- or $beta_2$-receptors, or stimulate $alpha_2$-receptors in the brainstem (centrally acting) to lower blood pressure are available. Although acting by different mechanisms, these drugs all lower blood pressure.

19.11 Vasodilators lower blood pressure by relaxing arteriolar smooth muscle.

A few drugs lower blood pressure by directly relaxing arteriolar smooth muscle. Other than their use in treating hypertensive crisis, drugs in this class are not widely used because of their numerous adverse effects.

REVIEW Questions

Answer the following questions to assess your knowledge of the chapter material, and go back and review any material that is not clear to you.

1. Which of the following is not a first-line drug class used for hypertension?
   1. Angiotensin-converting enzyme (ACE) inhibitors
   2. Calcium channel blockers (CCBs)
   3. Adrenergic blockers
   4. Thiazide diuretics

2. Prior to starting antihypertensive therapy, the nurse obtains an ECG and the baseline heart rate of a patient. This was done because the patient will be taking medication that affects heart function and rate. What medication will the patient most likely be taking?
   1. Cardizem
   2. Micardis
   3. Diuril
   4. Nitropress

3. The patient is on two antihypertensive drugs. The advantage of multidrug treatment is:
   1. Blood pressure decreases faster.
   2. Adverse effects are always fewer.
   3. Doses of the two drugs can be lower.
   4. Multidrug therapy treats the patient's other medical conditions.

4. The patient is taking furosemide (Lasix) 40 mg bid. The nurse monitors the patient's laboratory report for:
   1. Hyperkalemia.
   2. Hypokalemia.
   3. Hypernatremia.
   4. Hypercalcemia.

5. The patient has been taking losartan (Cozaar) for hypertension. The healthcare provider has determined that the current medication regimen is not effective. Which of the following drugs may be added to the treatment plan?
   1. Felodipine (Plendil)
   2. Methyldopa (Aldomet)
   3. Atenolol (Tenormin)
   4. Hydrochlorothiazide (Microzide)

6. The patient has been started on antihypertensives and will be monitored for:
   1. Nausea and vomiting.
   2. Diarrhea.
   3. Dizziness.
   4. Tetany.

7. A patient with hypertension has a medication order for diltiazem HCL 60 mg PO twice a day. How many tablet(s) will the nurse administer in a day if the medication comes only as 120 mg per tablet?
   1. Half tablet in the morning
   2. Half tablet, once in the morning and once in the evening
   3. One tablet in the morning
   4. One tablet in the morning and one in the evening

8. The nurse is helping to develop a presentation on the different types of medications used for hypertension. One type of antihypertensive medication that will be included affects the renin-angiotensin-aldosterone system to increase urine. This medication is a(n):
   1. Calcium channel blocker.
   2. Adrenergic blocker.
   3. Angiotensin-converting enzyme inhibitor.
   4. Direct-acting vasodilator.

9. To make sure the patient understands how a direct-acting vasodilator medication works, the nurse includes what information in the teaching plan?
   1. They block calcium from entering smooth muscle, causing arterioles to relax.
   2. They block receptors in the brainstem to lower blood pressure.
   3. They block the angiotensin-converting enzyme to prevent vessel constriction.
   4. They relax smooth muscles in the blood vessels to decrease peripheral resistance.

10. The patient is on an angiotensin-converting enzyme inhibitor. As a result of this therapy, the nurse checks for:
    1. Hypokalemia.
    2. Hyperkalemia.
    3. Hypernatremia.
    4. Hyperglycemia.

CASE STUDY Questions

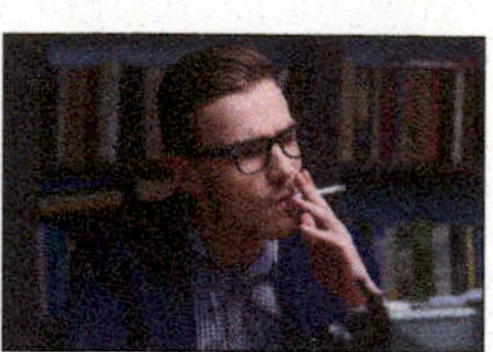

Remember Mr. Rodriguez, the patient introduced at the beginning of the chapter? Now read the remainder of the case study. Based on the information you have learned in this chapter, answer the questions that follow.

Mr. Paul Rodriguez was admitted to the emergency department unconscious with a nose bleed that wouldn't stop. His blood pressure was measured as 210/120 mmHg, and the healthcare provider ordered that he be immediately placed on nitroprusside (Nitropress). He stayed in the hospital for 2 days and was discharged with a blood pressure of 135/88 mmHg. On discharge, Mr. Rodriguez was given a prescription for Hyzaar with information about how it works, possible adverse effects, and guidelines for taking the medication.

1. Why was nitroprusside, rather than Hyzaar, used in the emergency department?
   1. Nitroprusside is safer.
   2. Nitroprusside has a longer duration of action.
   3. Nitroprusside has a faster onset of action.
   4. Mr. Rodriguez is allergic to Hyzaar.
2. What two drug classes are contained in Hyzaar?
   1. Thiazide diuretic and angiotensin-receptor blocker
   2. Thiazide diuretic and potassium-sparing diuretic
   3. Angiotensin-converting enzyme inhibitor and potassium-sparing diuretic
   4. Alpha-adrenergic blocker and angiotensin-converting enzyme inhibitor
3. What instructions did the nurse provide to Mr. Rodriguez about Hyzaar?
   1. Always rise slowly and avoid sudden changes in posture.
   2. Take a daily potassium supplement.
   3. Eat plenty of calcium-rich foods such as yogurt.
   4. Do not exercise regularly because exercise may interfere with blood pressure regulation.
4. After 8 months on Hyzaar, the healthcare provider switched Mr. Rodriguez to nifedipine (Procardia). The patient then reported to the nurse that he stopped taking the Procardia because it made him dizzy, and he felt his heart was racing. The nurse explained that these common adverse effects were probably due to:
   1. Electrolyte imbalance.
   2. Underdosing of nifedipine.
   3. Excessive vasodilation of arteries.
   4. Reflex tachycardia.

Answers and complete rationales for the Review and Case Study Questions appear in Appendix A.

REFERENCE

James, P. A., Oparil, S., Carter, B. L., Cushman, W. C., Dennison-Himmelfarb, C., Handler, J., . . . Ortiz, E. (2014). 2014 Evidence based guideline for the management of high blood pressure in adults: Report from the panel members appointed to the Eighth Joint National Committee (JNC 8). *JAMA: The Journal of the American Medical Association, 311*, 507–520. doi:10.1001/jama.2013.284427

SELECTED BIBLIOGRAPHY

American Heart Association. (2013). *High blood pressure, 2013 statistical fact sheet*. Retrieved from http://www.heart.org/idc/groups/heart-public/@wcm/@sop/@smd/documents/downloadable/ucm_319587.pdf

Carson, M.P. (2016). *Hypertension and pregnancy*. Retrieved from http://emedicine.medscape.com/article/261435-overview

Centers for Disease Control and Prevention. (2015). *High blood pressure facts*. Retrieved from http://www.cdc.gov/bloodpressure/facts.htm

De Simoni, A., Hardeman, W., Mant, J., Farmer, A. J., & Kinmonth, A. L. (2013). Trials to improve blood pressure through adherence to antihypertensives in stroke/TIA: A systematic review and metaanalysis. *Journal of the American Heart Association, 2*, e000251. doi:10.1161/JAHA.113.000251

Hopkins, C. (2015). *Hypertensive emergencies.* Retrieved from http://emedicine.medscape.com/article/1952052-overview

Krakoff, L. R., Gillespie, R. L., Ferdinand, K. C., Fergus, I. V., Akinboboye, O., Williams, K. A., ... Pepine, C. J. (2014). 2014 hypertension recommendations from the Eighth Joint National Committee Panel Members raise concerns for elderly black and female populations. *Journal of the American College of Cardiology, 64*, 394–402. doi:10.1016/j.jacc.2014.06.014

Madhur, M. S. (2014). *Hypertension: Practice essentials.* Retrieved from http://emedicine.medscape.com/article/241381-overview

National Center for Complementary and Integrative Health. (2012). *Grape Seed Extract.* Retrieved at http://nccam.nih.gov/health/grapeseed/ataglance.htm

Ramos, A. P., & Varon, J. (2014). Current and newer agents for hypertensive emergencies. *Current Hypertension Reports, 16*, 450. doi:10.1007/s11906-014-0450-z

Turgut, F., Yesil, Y., Balogun, R. A., & Abdel-Rahman, E. M. (2013). Hypertension in the elderly: Unique challenges and management. *Clinics in Geriatric Medicine, 29*, 593–609. doi:10.1016/j.cger.2013.05.002

Williams, H. (2013). An update on hypertension for nurse prescribers. *Nurse Prescribing, 11*, 70–75. doi:10.12968/npre.2013.11.2.70

University of Maryland Medical Center. (2015). *Grape seed.* Retrieved from http://www.umm.edu/altmed/articles/grape-seed-000254.htm

Chapter 20

Drugs for Heart Failure

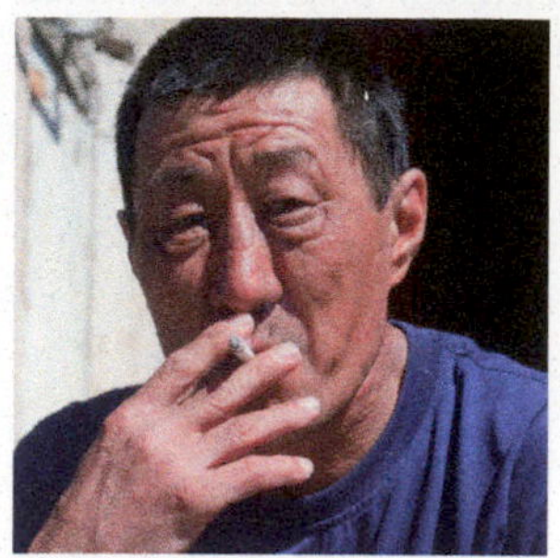

"My parents and grandparents smoked their whole lives and lived to be in their 90s. I just can't believe smoking has damaged my heart. I knew about possible lung damage. . .but my heart?"

Mr. Lei Chen

Core Concepts

20.1 **Heart failure is closely associated with disorders such as chronic hypertension, coronary artery disease, and diabetes.**

20.2 **The central cause of heart failure is weakened heart muscle.**

20.3 **The three primary characteristics of heart function are force of contraction, heart rate, and speed of impulse conduction.**

20.4 **The specific therapy for heart failure depends on the severity of the disease.**

20.5 **Angiotensin-converting enzyme (ACE) inhibitors are the preferred drugs for heart failure.**

20.6 **Diuretics relieve symptoms of heart failure by reducing fluid overload and decreasing blood pressure.**

20.7 **Cardiac glycosides increase the force of myocardial contraction and were once the traditional drugs of choice for heart failure.**

20.8 **Beta-adrenergic blockers are used in combination with other drugs to slow the progression of heart failure.**

20.9 **Vasodilators reduce symptoms of heart failure by decreasing cardiac workload.**

20.10 **Phosphodiesterase inhibitors are used for short-term therapy of advanced heart failure.**

Drug Snapshot

The following drugs are discussed in this chapter:

Drug Classes	Prototype Drugs
Angiotensin-converting enzyme (ACE) inhibitors	Pr lisinopril (Prinivil, Zestril)
Diuretics	
Cardiac glycosides	Pr digoxin (Lanoxin, Lanoxicaps)
Beta-adrenergic blockers	Pr carvedilol (Coreg)
Vasodilators	
Phosphodiesterase inhibitors	Pr milrinone (Primacor)

Learning Outcomes

After reading this chapter, the student should be able to:

1. Identify the major risk factors associated with the progression to heart failure.
2. Relate how the symptoms associated with heart failure may be caused by weakened heart muscle.

3. Describe the three fundamental characteristics of cardiac function.
4. Identify drug classes that are used as first-line and second-line choices for the pharmacotherapy of heart failure.
5. Categorize heart failure drugs based on their classifications and mechanisms of action.
6. For each of the classes listed in the Drug Snapshot, identify representative drugs and explain their mechanisms of drug action, primary actions, and important adverse effects.

Key Terms

afterload
contractility (kon-trak-TILL-eh-tee)
heart failure (HF)
inotropic effect (in-oh-TRO-pik)
natriuretic peptide (hBNP) (na-tree-ur-ET-ik)
peripheral edema (purr-IF-ur-ul eh-DEE-mah)
phosphodiesterase (fos-fo-die-ES-tur-ase)
preload

Heart failure (HF) is one of the most common and fatal cardiovascular diseases, and its incidence is expected to increase as the population ages. Improved treatment of myocardial infarction (MI) and hypertension (HTN) has led to declines in mortality due to HF: Deaths due to HF have declined an average of 12% per decade over the past 50 years. However, approximately one in five patients dies within 1 year of being diagnosed with HF, and 50% die within 5 years.

Heart failure is closely associated with disorders such as chronic hypertension, coronary artery disease, and diabetes.

◀ **Core Concept 20.1**

Heart failure (HF) is the inability of the ventricles to pump enough blood to meet the body's metabolic demands. HF can be caused by any disorder that affects the heart's ability to receive or eject blood. Although weakening of cardiac muscle is a natural consequence of aging, the process can be accelerated by a number of diseases associated with HF that are shown in Table 20.1. There is no cure for HF; however, effective drug therapy can relieve many of the distressing symptoms of HF and may prolong the lives of patients.

For many patients, HF is considered a preventable condition; controlling associated diseases will greatly reduce the risk of eventual HF. For example, controlling lipid levels and keeping blood pressure within normal limits will reduce the incidence of MI. Maintaining blood glucose within normal values can reduce the cardiovascular consequences of uncontrolled diabetes. Therefore, the therapy of HF is no longer just focused on end stages of the disorder. Pharmacotherapy is now targeted at prevention and slowing the progression of HF. This change in emphasis has led to significant improvements in survival and quality of life for patients with HF.

Table 20.1 Disorders Commonly Associated with Heart Failure

Disease	Description
Chronic hypertension	Sustained high systemic blood pressure
Coronary artery disease	Atherosclerosis of the coronary arteries
Diabetes	Lack of insulin or inability to tolerate carbohydrates
Mitral stenosis	Inability of the mitral valve to open fully
Myocardial infarction	Heart muscle death due to coronary artery obstruction

Fast Facts **Heart Failure**

- About 550,000 new cases of HF are diagnosed in the United States every year.
- More than 287,000 people die of HF or HF-related illnesses each year.
- African Americans are 1.5 times more likely to develop HF than Caucasians.
- HF occurs equally frequent in men and women.
- HF occurs in people of all age groups: About 1.4 million persons with HF are under age 60.

Source: Based on *Heart Failure Statistics*, Emory Healthcare, n.d.

Core Concept 20.2 ▶ The central cause of heart failure is weakened heart muscle.

Although a number of diseases can lead to HF, the end result is the same: The heart is unable to pump out the volume of blood required to meet the needs of the other organs. To understand how drugs act on the weakened heart muscle, it is essential to understand the underlying cardiac physiology.

The right side of the heart receives blood from the venous system and sends it to the lungs, where the blood receives oxygen and gives up its carbon dioxide. The blood returns to the left side of the heart, which sends it out to the rest of the body through the aorta. The amount of blood received by the right side should exactly equal that sent out by the left side. If this does not happen, HF may occur. The amount of blood pumped by each ventricle per minute is the cardiac output. The relationship between cardiac output and blood pressure is explained in Chapter 19.

Although many variables affect cardiac output, the two most important factors are preload and afterload. Just before the chambers of the heart contract (systole), they are filled to their maximum capacity with blood. The degree to which the cardiac muscle fibers are stretched just prior to contraction is **preload**. The more these fibers are stretched, the more forcefully they will contract. This is somewhat analogous to a rubber band: The more it is stretched, the more forcefully it will snap back. This strength of contraction of the heart is called **contractility**.

The second important factor affecting cardiac output is afterload. For the left ventricle to pump blood out of the heart, it must overcome a fairly substantial pressure in the aorta. The **afterload** is the amount of pressure in the aorta that must be overcome for blood to be ejected from the left ventricle. The greater afterload that occurs with chronic HTN creates a constant increased workload for the heart. This explains why patients with chronic HTN are more likely to experience HF. Lowering blood pressure results in less workload for the heart.

In HF, the myocardium becomes weakened, and the heart cannot eject all the blood it receives. This weakening may occur on the left side, the right side, or both sides of the heart. If it occurs on the left side, excess blood accumulates in the left ventricle. The wall of the left ventricle thickens and enlarges (*hypertrophy*) in an attempt to compensate for the increased workload. Because the left ventricle has limits to its ability to compensate, blood "backs up" into the lungs, resulting in the classic symptoms of cough and shortness of breath, particularly when the patient is lying down. Left HF is sometimes called *congestive* HF.

Although left-sided HF is more common, the right side of the heart can also become weak, either simultaneously with the left side or independently from the left side. In right HF, the blood "backs up" into the peripheral veins. This results in swelling of the feet and ankles, a condition known as **peripheral edema**, and engorgement of organs such as the liver. Figure 20.1 illustrates the underlying pathophysiology of HF. Figure 20.2 illustrates the signs and symptoms of the patient in HF.

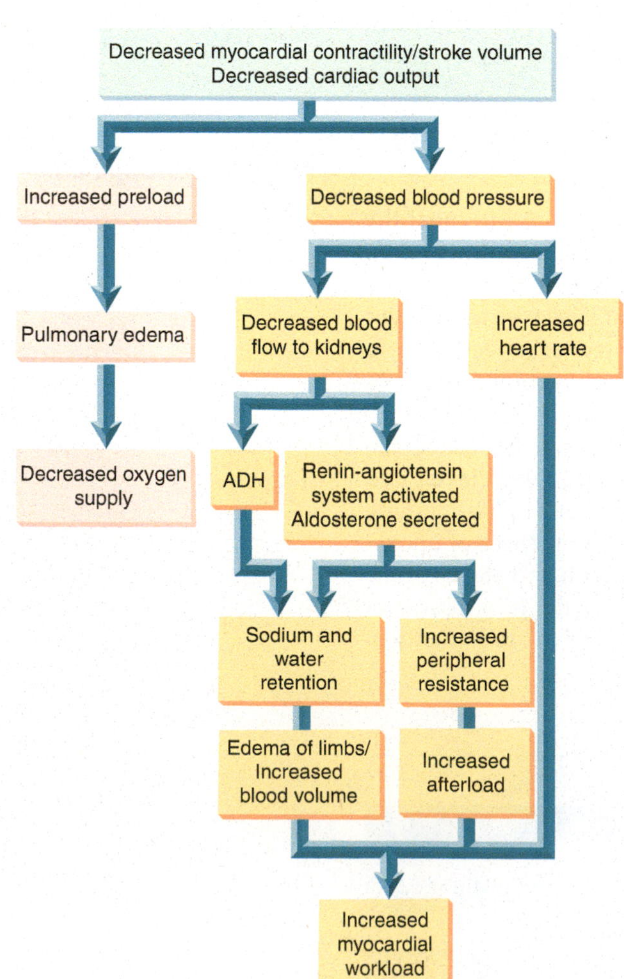

FIGURE 20.1 Pathophysiology of heart failure.

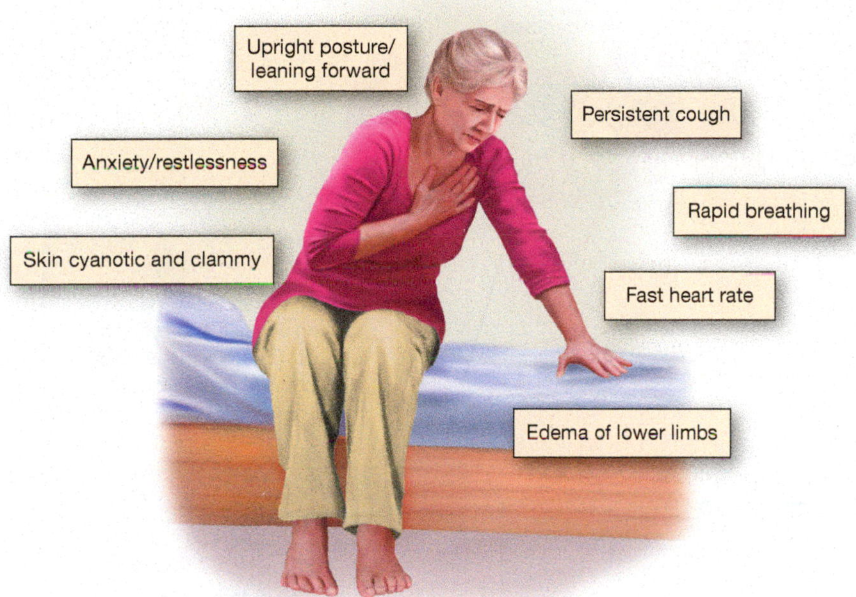

FIGURE 20.2 Signs and symptoms of heart failure.

The three primary characteristics of heart function are force of contraction, heart rate, and speed of impulse conduction.

◀ **Core Concept 20.3**

Cardiac physiology is quite complex, particularly when the heart is challenged with a chronic disease such as HF. A simplified method for understanding cardiac function, and one that is quite useful for understanding drug therapy, is to visualize the heart as having three fundamental characteristics:

1. It contracts with a specific force or strength (contractility).
2. It beats at a certain rate (beats per minute).
3. It conducts electrical impulses at a particular speed.

The ability to change the force of contraction, or contractility, is of particular interest to the pharmacotherapy of HF. Because the fundamental cause of HF is a weak myocardium, causing the muscle to beat more forcefully seems to be an ideal solution. The ability to increase the strength of contraction is called a positive **inotropic effect** and is a fundamental characteristic of the class of drugs known as the cardiac glycosides.

ino = *fiber*
tropic = *to influence*

The ability of the heart to speed up or slow down is a second characteristic important to pharmacology. A faster heart works harder but not necessarily more efficiently. A slower heart has a longer time to rest between beats, thus decreasing the workload on the heart.

A third fundamental characteristic of cardiac physiology is the electrical conduction through the heart. Some cardiovascular drugs influence the speed of this conduction. Slowing the conduction speed through the heart will cause the heart to beat slower, thus lessening cardiac workload.

These primary characteristics of cardiac function can be modified through pharmacotherapy to assist the heart in meeting the body's metabolic demands. The mechanisms by which HF medications accomplish this are shown in Figure 20.3.

The specific therapy for heart failure depends on the severity of the disease.

◀ **Core Concept 20.4**

Although HF can be acute and require immediate treatment, it is often considered a progressive, chronic disorder. In its early stages, many of its symptoms can be improved through nonpharmacologic interventions. Through certain lifestyle changes, the patient can experience a higher quality of life either without drug therapy or with lower drug doses

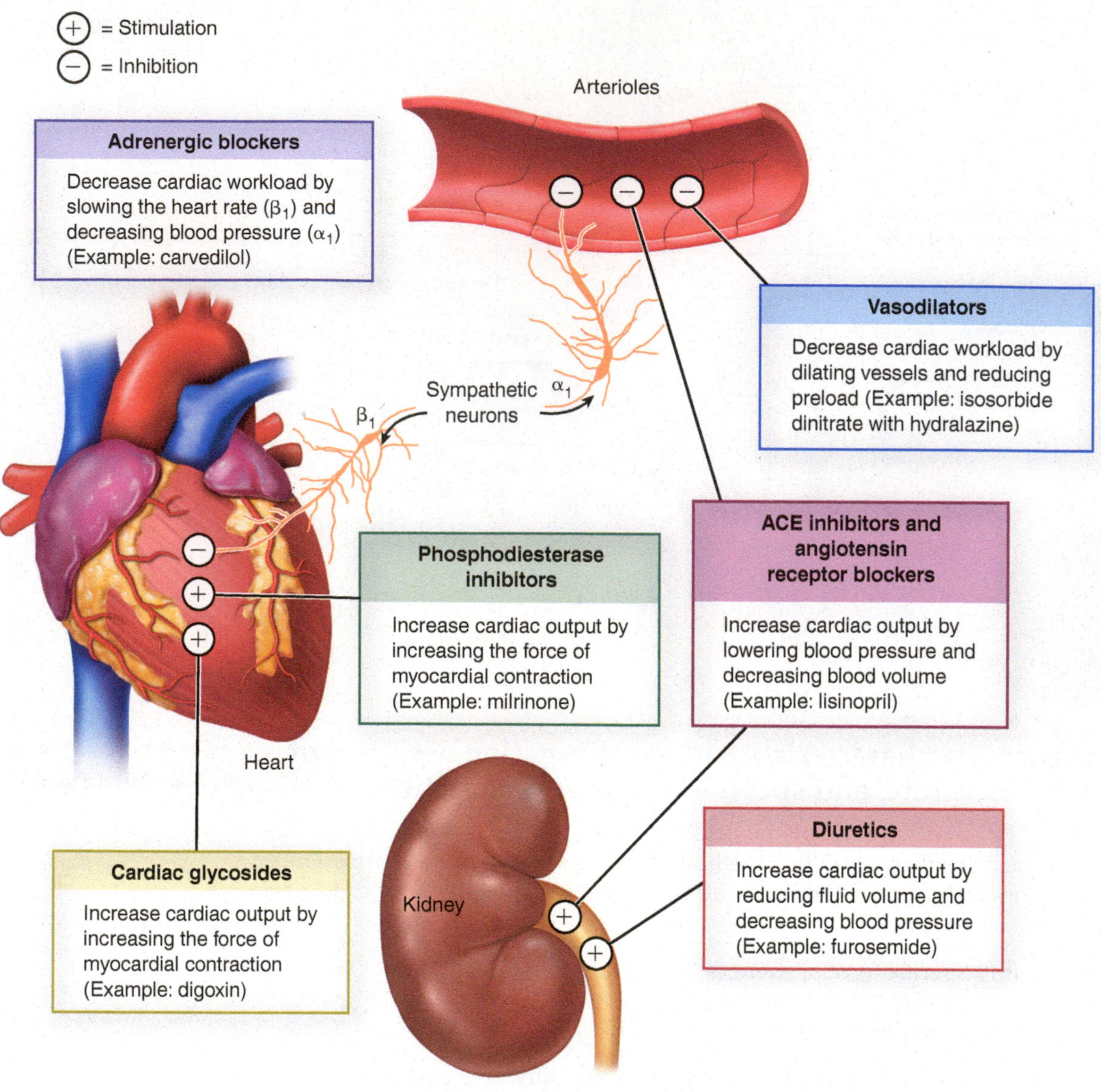

FIGURE 20.3 Mechanisms of action of drugs used to treat heart failure.

that have less risk for adverse effects. It should be noted that the following nonpharmacologic methods for controlling HF are the same strategies also used to manage HTN.

- Stop using tobacco.
- Restrict salt (sodium) intake, and be sure to eat foods rich in potassium and magnesium.
- Limit alcohol consumption.
- Implement a medically supervised aerobic exercise plan.
- Reduce sources of stress and learn to implement coping strategies.
- Maintain optimal weight.
- Limit caffeine consumption.

Once heart disease progresses such that it significantly affects activities of daily living, drug therapy is indicated. Drugs for HF may be classified as first-line or second-line drugs. If first-line drugs are not effective, then second-line drugs will be tried or added to the regimen. The first-line drugs are the angiotensin-converting enzyme (ACE) inhibitors and diuretics. These medications relieve most symptoms of mild to moderate HF and produce the fewest number of adverse effects. Sometimes considered first-line drugs, the cardiac glycosides are effective but have the potential for more serious adverse effects. Drugs of second choice are those used in acute HF, or when the ACE inhibitors and diuretics prove ineffective. Second-line drugs include the phosphodiesterase inhibitors, vasodilators, and beta-adrenergic blockers. The use of multiple drugs is common in the pharmacotherapy of HF.

Angiotensin-converting enzyme (ACE) inhibitors are the preferred drugs for heart failure.

◀ **Core Concept 20.5**

Drugs affecting the renin-angiotensin-aldosterone system reduce the workload on the heart by lowering blood pressure. They are drugs of choice for the treatment of HF. Table 20.2 lists the ACE inhibitors approved to treat HF.

The basic pharmacology of the ACE inhibitors and their effects on the renin-angiotensin-aldosterone pathway are discussed in Chapter 19. Approved for the treatment of HTN since the 1980s, ACE inhibitors have been shown to slow the progression of HF and reduce deaths from this disease. They have replaced digoxin as the preferred drugs for the treatment of chronic HF.

Prototype Drug: *Lisinopril (Prinivil, Zestril)*

Therapeutic Class: Drug for HF, HTN, and MI prevention **Pharmacologic Class:** ACE inhibitor

Actions and Uses: Lisinopril is one of the most frequently prescribed drugs for HTN and HF. An additional indication for this medication is to improve survival in patients when given within 24 hours of an acute MI.

Lisinopril lowers blood pressure by blocking ACE. Like other ACE inhibitors, doses of lisinopril may require 2 to 3 weeks of therapy for optimal effectiveness, and several months of therapy may be needed for a patient's cardiac function to return to normal. Because of their combined hypotensive action, concurrent therapy with lisinopril and diuretics should be carefully monitored to avoid the development of hypotension.

Adverse Effects and Interactions: Lisinopril exhibits few serious adverse effects. The most common adverse effects are cough, headache, dizziness, orthostatic hypotension, and rash. Because high potassium levels may occur during therapy, use of potassium supplements or potassium-sparing diuretics should be avoided. Thus, electrolyte levels are usually monitored periodically. Angioedema is a rare, though potentially serious, adverse effect.

Lisinopril interacts with nonsteroidal anti-inflammatory drugs (NSAIDs) to cause decreased antihypertensive activity. Lisinopril may increase lithium levels and toxicity.

BLACK BOX WARNING:
Fetal injury and death may occur when ACE inhibitors are taken during pregnancy. When pregnancy is detected, they should be discontinued as soon as possible.

CAM Therapy | Carnitine and Heart Disease

Carnitine is a natural substance structurally similar to amino acids. Its primary function in metabolism is to move fatty acids from the bloodstream into cells, where carnitine assists in the breakdown of lipids and the production of energy. The best food sources of carnitine are organ meat, fish, muscle meats, and milk products. Carnitine is available as a supplement in several forms, including L-carnitine, D-carnitine, and actetyl-L-carnitine. D-carnitine is associated with potential adverse effects and thus should be avoided.

L-carnitine has been claimed to enhance energy and sports performance, heart health, memory, immune function, and male fertility. It is also being marketed as a "fat burner" for weight reduction.

L-carnitine has been extensively studied. There is solid evidence to support supplementation in patients who are deficient in carnitine. Certain patients, such as vegetarians or those with heart disease, may need additional amounts. L-carnitine supplementation has been shown to improve exercise tolerance in patients with angina. The use of carnitine may prevent the occurrence of dysrhythmias in the early stages of heart disease. L-carnitine has also been shown to decrease triglyceride levels while increasing high-density lipoprotein (HDL) serum levels, thus helping to minimize one of the major risk factors associated with heart disease. Research has not shown L-carnitine supplementation to be of significant benefit in enhancing sports performance or weight loss.

dys = *difficult or bad*
rhythmia = *rhythm*

Table 20.2 First-Line Drugs for Heart Failure

Drug	Route and Adult Dose	Remarks
ACE INHIBITORS AND ANGIOTENSIN RECEPTOR BLOCKERS		
candesartan (Atacand)	PO: 4 mg once daily, may increase to a dose of 32 mg	Also for HTN
captopril (Capoten)	PO: 6.25-12.5 mg tid (max: 450 mg/day)	Also for HTN, post MI therapy, and diabetic nephropathy
enalapril (Vasotec) (see the Prototype Drug box in Core Concept 19.8)	PO: 2.5 mg bid-qid (max: 40 mg/day)	IV form available; also for HTN and asymptomatic left ventricular dysfunction
fosinopril (Monopril)	PO: 5–10 mg daily (max: 40 mg/day)	Also for HTN
Pr lisinopril (Prinivil, Zestril)	PO: 5–10 mg daily (max: 40 mg/day)	Therapy should not begin until 2 to 3 days after diuretics are stopped; also for HTN and post MI therapy.
quinapril (Accupril)	PO: 5 mg bid (max: 40 mg/day)	Also for HTN; may be used off-label for diabetic nephropathy
ramipril (Altace)	PO: 2.5–5 mg bid (max: 10 mg/day)	Also for HTN, stroke prophylaxis, and post-MI therapy
valsartan (Diovan)	PO: 40 mg bid (max: 160 mg bid	Also for HTN and post-MI therapy
SELECTED DIURETICS		
bumetanide (Burinex, Bumex)	PO: 0.5–2 mg daily (max: 10 mg/day)	Diuretic activity is 40 times greater and duration of action is shorter than furosemide; IM and IV forms available.
eplerenone (Inspra)	PO: 50 mg once daily (max: 100 mg/day)	Also for HTN; potassium-sparing diuretic
furosemide (Lasix) (see the Prototype Drug box in Core Concept 18.5)	PO: 20–80 mg in one or more divided doses (max: 600 mg/day)	Monitor for hypokalemia; also for HTN; IV and IM forms available; loop diuretic.
hydrochlorothiazide (Microzide) (see the Prototype Drug box in Core Concept 18.6)	PO: 25–200 mg in one to three divided doses (max: 200 mg/day)	May bring on diabetes in patients with prediabetes; also for HTN; thiazide diuretic
spironolactone (Aldactone) (see the Prototype Drug box in Core Concept 18.7)	PO: 5–200 mg in divided doses (max: 200 mg/day)	Used for edema associated with HF; also for HTN; potassium-sparing diuretic
torsemide (Demadex)	PO: 10–20 mg/day (max: 200 mg/day)	Also for HTN; IV form available; loop diuretic

The ACE inhibitors produce their effects by blocking ACE, thus preventing the formation of angiotensin, an extremely potent vasoconstrictor. The primary actions of the ACE inhibitors are to lower blood pressure and reduce blood volume by enhancing the excretion of sodium and water. The resultant reduction of arterial blood pressure increases cardiac output. An additional effect of the ACE inhibitors is dilation of the veins returning blood to the heart. This action decreases preload and reduces pulmonary congestion and peripheral edema. The combined actions of ACE inhibitors substantially decrease the workload on the heart and allow it to work more efficiently. ACE inhibitors have been shown to reduce mortality following acute MI when therapy is started soon after the onset of symptoms (see Chapter 21).

A related group of drugs act by blocking the effects of angiotensin *after* it is formed. The angiotensin-receptor blockers (ARBs) have similar effectiveness to the ACE inhibitors. Although the ARBs are usually prescribed for HTN, valsartan (Diovan) and candesartan (Atacand) are also approved for HF. Because research has not yet demonstrated a clear advantage of ARBs over other medications, their use in the treatment of HF is usually reserved for patients unable to tolerate the adverse effects of ACE inhibitors. Both the ARBs and the ACE inhibitors are contraindicated during pregnancy because they may cause fetal injury or death.

Core Concept 20.6 ▶

Diuretics relieve symptoms of heart failure by reducing fluid overload and decreasing blood pressure.

Diuretics are commonly used for the symptomatic treatment of HF. They produce few adverse effects and are effective at increasing urine flow, lowering blood volume, and reducing edema and congestion. When diuretics reduce fluid overload and lower blood pressure, the workload on the heart is reduced and cardiac output increases. They are widely used in the treatment of cardiovascular disease in patients with fluid overload. When used to treat HF in patients who have edema, diuretics are usually prescribed in combination with ACE inhibitors and other HF medications.

The most common adverse effects from diuretic therapy are electrolyte imbalances. Of greatest concern are the effects of diuretics on potassium levels, because too little or too much potassium can greatly affect a failing heart. This can be especially important in patients taking cardiac glycosides; patients with potassium or magnesium deficiencies are at greater risk for toxicity from digoxin. Potassium or magnesium supplements may be prescribed to prevent this adverse effect. Frequent laboratory testing may be necessary to monitor electrolyte levels in patients with HF.

The mechanisms by which diuretics reduce blood volume, specifically where and how the nephron of the kidney is affected among the various drugs, are discussed in Chapter 18. A Nursing Process Focus chart for diuretics, and prototype features for furosemide (Lasix), hydrochlorothiazide (Microzide), and spironolactone (Aldactone), are also included in Chapter 18.

Cardiac glycosides increase the force of myocardial contraction and were once the preferred drugs for heart failure.

◀ **Core Concept 20.7**

The value of the cardiac glycosides in treating heart disorders has been known for over 2000 years. They have been used as arrow poisons by African tribes and as medicines by the ancient Egyptians and Romans.

Extracted from the common plants *Digitalis purpura* (purple foxglove) and *Digitalis lanata* (white foxglove), drugs from this class are sometimes called *digitalis glycosides.* Until the discovery of the ACE inhibitors, the cardiac glycosides were the mainstay of HF treatment. Digoxin (Lanoxin) is the only drug in this class available in the United States. The routes and dose for digoxin are listed in Table 20.3.

The primary action of digoxin is an increase in the force of myocardial contraction. This action, a positive inotropic effect, allows the weakened heart to eject more blood per beat, thus increasing cardiac output. The increased cardiac output helps the heart to meet the metabolic demands of the tissues.

A second important action of digoxin is its ability to slow electrical conduction through the heart. This results in fewer beats per minute. The reduced heart rate, combined with more forceful contractions, allows for much greater efficiency of the heart.

Table 20.3 Second-Line Drugs for Heart Failure

Drug	Route and Adult Dose	Remarks
CARDIAC GLYCOSIDE		
Pr digoxin (Lanoxin, Lanoxicaps)	PO: 0.125–0.5 mg/day (max: 0.5 mg/day)	Increases cardiac output; larger dose may be given to initiate therapy; IV form available; also used for dysrhythmias
BETA-ADRENERGIC BLOCKERS		
Pr carvedilol (Coreg)	PO: 3.125 mg bid for 2 weeks, then gradually increase to 25 mg bid (max: 25 mg bid)	Reduces cardiac workload; dose must be increased slowly; also for HTN and left ventricular dysfunction
metoprolol (Toprol XL)	PO: 25 mg/day for 2 weeks, then gradually increase dose (max: 200 mg/day)	Also for HTN, angina, and post-MI therapy
DIRECT-ACTING VASODILATORS		
hydralazine with isosorbide dinitrate (BiDil)	PO: 1–2 tablets tid (each tablet contains 20 mg isosorbide dinitrate and 37.5 mg hydralazine) (max: 2 tablets/day)	Increases heart rate and cardiac output; decreases myocardial oxygen consumption; hydralazine also for HTN and isosorbide dinitrate for angina
nesiritide (Natrecor)	IV: 2 mcg/kg bolus followed by continuous infusion at 0.01 mcg/kg/min	Also called atrial natriuretic peptide; only for acute HF
PHOSPHODIESTERASE INHIBITORS		
inamrinone (Inocor)	IV: 0.75 mg/kg bolus given slowly over 2–3 min; then 5–10 mcg/kg/min (max: 10 mg/kg/day)	Larger dose is given to initiate therapy; peak effect reached in 10 min.
Pr milrinone (Primacor)	IV: 50 mcg/kg over 10 min; then 0.375–0.75 mcg/kg/min	Larger dose is given to initiate therapy; peak effect reached in 2 min.

Unfortunately, digoxin has the potential to cause serious adverse effects at high doses and in certain patients. The margin of safety between a beneficial dose and a toxic dose is very small; thus, therapy should be closely monitored to prevent severe adverse effects. Serum digoxin levels above 1.8 mg/mL are considered toxic. Initial adverse effects are gastrointestinal related and include loss of appetite, vomiting, and diarrhea. Headache, drowsiness, confusion, and blurred vision may occur. Excessive slowing of the heart rate and other cardiac abnormalities can be fatal if not corrected. Because of these adverse effects, digitalis is usually used only in the late stages of HF.

The antidote for digoxin toxicity is administration of digoxin immune fab (Ovine). This drug binds digoxin, preventing it from reaching the tissues. Onset of action is rapid—less than 1 minute after the IV infusion is begun.

CONCEPT REVIEW 20.1

- If cardiac glycosides are so effective at increasing myocardial contraction, why are they no longer first-line drugs for HF?

Prototype Drug: Pr *Digoxin (Lanoxin, Lanoxicaps)*

Therapeutic Class: Drug for heart failure **Pharmacologic Class:** Cardiac glycoside

Actions and Uses: The primary benefit of digoxin is its ability to increase the strength of cardiac contraction (positive inotropic effect). Digoxin accomplishes this by inhibiting Na^+–K^+ ATPase, an enzyme in myocardial cells.

By increasing myocardial contractility, digoxin directly increases cardiac output, thus alleviating symptoms of HF and improving exercise tolerance. The increased cardiac output also results in increased urine production and a desirable reduction in blood volume, thus relieving the distressing symptoms of lung congestion and peripheral edema.

In addition to its positive inotropic effect, digoxin also has the ability to suppress the sinoatrial (SA) node (the pacemaker of the heart) and slow electrical conduction through the atrioventricular (AV) node. Because of these actions, digoxin is sometimes used to treat cardiac rhythm abnormalities known as dysrhythmias, which is discussed in Chapter 23. Pulse rate should be monitored daily, and values less than 60 beats per minute or greater than 100 beats per minute should be reported to the healthcare provider.

Adverse Effects and Interactions: The most dangerous adverse effect of digoxin is its ability to create dysrhythmias, particularly in patients who have hypokalemia. Because diuretics can cause hypokalemia and are also often used to treat HF, use of digoxin and diuretics together must be carefully monitored. Levels of potassium, magnesium, calcium, blood urea nitrogen (BUN), and creatinine should be monitored frequently (hypokalemia predisposes the patient to digoxin toxicity). Other adverse effects of digoxin therapy include nausea, vomiting, anorexia, and abnormalities of the nervous system such as blurred vision. Periodic serum levels are checked to determine if the digoxin level is within the therapeutic range, and the dosage may be adjusted based on the laboratory results. Digoxin also interacts with many other medications. Concurrent use with beta blockers may result in additive bradycardia. Because small changes in digoxin levels can produce serious adverse effects, the healthcare provider must constantly be alert for drug–drug interactions.

Core Concept 20.8 ▶

Beta-adrenergic blockers are used in combination with other drugs to slow the progression of heart failure.

Drugs that produce a positive inotropic effect, such as the cardiac glycosides and phosphodiesterase inhibitors, play important roles in treating the diminished contractility that is the hallmark of HF. It may seem somewhat surprising then to find medications that exhibit a *negative* inotropic effect prescribed for this disease. Yet such is the case with the beta-adrenergic blockers. Beta blockers have been shown to dramatically reduce the number of hospitalizations and deaths associated with HF.

Beta-adrenergic antagonists block the cardiac actions of the sympathetic nervous system, thus slowing the heart rate and reducing blood pressure. Workload on the heart is decreased. Carvedilol (Coreg) and metoprolol (Toprol XL) are the two beta blockers approved to treat HF. Patients with HF must be carefully monitored when taking beta blockers because these drugs have the potential to worsen HF. They are always used in combination with other agents, usually ACE inhibitors. The basic pharmacology of the beta blockers is presented in Chapter 9. Other indications, routes, and dosages of the beta-adrenergic blockers are discussed elsewhere in this text: HTN in Chapter 19, dysrhythmias in Chapter 23, and angina and myocardial infarction in Chapter 21.

In 2015, a new drug was introduced for patients who do not achieve a therapeutic response with beta blockers. Ivabradine (Corlanor) acts by a unique mechanism that slows ion currents through the SA node. The drug reduces cardiac workload by slowing the heart. Bradycardia is the most common adverse effect.

Prototype Drug: Pr *Carvedilol (Coreg)*

Therapeutic Class: Drug for heart failure and HTN **Pharmacologic Class:** Beta-adrenergic blocker

Actions and Uses: Carvedilol has been found to reduce symptoms of HF, slow the progression of the disease, and increase exercise tolerance when combined with other drugs for HF, such as ACE inhibitors. Unlike many drugs in this class, carvedilol blocks $beta_1$- and $beta_2$- as well as $alpha_1$-adrenergic receptors. The primary therapeutic effects relevant to HF are a reduction in heart rate and a drop in blood pressure. The lower blood pressure reduces the workload on the heart. The drug is also approved to treat HTN and for reducing cardiac complications following an MI.

Adverse Effects and Interactions: The most frequent adverse effects of carvedilol include back pain, bradycardia, dizziness, shortness of breath, fatigue, orthostatic hypotension, and weight gain. It should be used with caution in patients with asthma or cardiac dysrhythmias.

Carvedilol's effect in decreasing heart rate and contractility has the potential to worsen HF; therefore, dosage must be carefully monitored. Because of the potential for adverse cardiac effects, beta-adrenergic blockers such as carvedilol are usually given concurrently with other drugs in the treatment of HF.

Carvedilol interacts with many drugs. For example, levels of carvedilol are significantly increased when the drug is taken with rifampin. Monoamine oxidase inhibitors (MAOIs), clonidine, and reserpine can cause hypotension or bradycardia when given with carvedilol. When given with digoxin, carvedilol may increase digoxin levels. It may also enhance the hypoglycemic effects of insulin and oral hypoglycemic agents.

Vasodilators reduce symptoms of heart failure by decreasing cardiac workload.

◀ Core Concept 20.9

The two direct-acting vasodilators, hydralazine (Apresoline) and isosorbide dinitrate (Isordil), act directly on vascular smooth muscle to relax blood vessels and lower blood pressure. Hydralazine acts on arterioles, whereas isosorbide dinitrate acts on veins. Because the two drugs act synergistically, isosorbide dinitrate is combined with hydralazine in the treatment of HF. BiDil is a fixed-dose combination of 20 mg of isosorbide dinitrate with 37.5 mg of hydralazine. Dosing for the drug is shown in Table 20.2.

Because of a high incidence of reflex tachycardia and orthostatic hypotension, vasodilators play a minor role in the drug therapy of HF. They are generally reserved for patients with more severe disease, or those who cannot tolerate ACE inhibitors. BiDil appears to be especially effective in treating HF in African American patients, who often exhibit resistance to standard therapies. Hydralazine is featured as a prototype drug for direct vasodilators in the treatment of HTN in Chapter 19. Isosorbide dinitrate belongs to a class of drugs called organic nitrates that are widely used in the treatment of angina pectoris (see Chapter 21).

A third vasodilator used for HF is very different from hydralazine or isosorbide dinitrate. Nesiritide (Natrecor) is a small peptide hormone that is structurally identical to a hormone known as human beta-type **natriuretic peptide (hBNP)**, which is secreted by the heart when the heart begins to fail. Nesiritide reduces both preload and afterload, improving cardiac efficiency in patients with HF. Nesiritide has limited uses because of its ability to cause severe hypotension. The medication is given only by IV infusion, and patients require continuous monitoring. It is approved for patients with severe HF.

natri = *sodium*
uretic = *urinary excretion*

CONCEPT REVIEW 20.2

- Why are the ACE inhibitors preferred over both the nitrates and the diuretics in the treatment of HF?

New Drug Focus

NEW APPROACH FOR TREATING HEART FAILURE

A new class of drugs, the neprilysin inhibitors, is able to slow the progression of HF with minimal side effects. Neprilysin is an enzyme normally present in the body that breaks down natriuretic peptides (see Section 20.9) and other substances that affect fluid balance. By blocking neprilysin, the concentration of natriuretic peptides in the blood increases and cardiac efficiency improves. The new drug is Entresto, a combination of sacubitril (a neprilysin inhibitor) and valsartan (an angiotensin-receptor blocker). The nepilysin inhibitors may lead to the discovery of other new approaches to treating angina, HTN, and HF.

Core Concept 20.10 ▶ Phosphodiesterase inhibitors are used for short-term therapy of advanced heart failure.

Phosphodiesterase inhibitors are drugs with a very brief half-life that are occasionally used for the short-term control of acute HF. The doses of phosphodiesterase inhibitors are given in Table 20.3.

The two drugs in this class block the enzyme **phosphodiesterase** in cardiac and smooth muscle. Blocking phosphodiesterase has the effect of increasing the amount of calcium available for myocardial contraction. The inhibition results in two main actions that benefit patients with HF: an increased force of contraction (positive inotropic response) and vasodilation. Because of their toxicity, however, phosphodiesterase inhibitors are reserved for patients who have not responded to ACE inhibitors or cardiac glycosides, and they are generally used for 2 to 3 days only.

Prototype Drug: Pr *Milrinone (Primacor)*

Therapeutic Class: Drug for severe heart failure **Pharmacologic Class:** Phosphodiesterase inhibitor

Actions and Uses: Of the two phosphodiesterase inhibitors available, milrinone is generally preferred because it has a shorter half-life and fewer adverse effects. It is given IV only and is primarily used for the short-term support of advanced HF. Peak effects occur in two minutes. Immediate effects of milrinone include an increased force of contraction and an increase in cardiac output.

Adverse Effects and Interactions: The most serious adverse effect of milrinone is ventricular dysrhythmia, which can occur in more than 1 of every 10 patients taking the drug. The patient's electrocardiogram (ECG) should be monitored continuously during the infusion of the drug. Less serious adverse effects include headache, nausea, and vomiting.

Use with disopyramide may cause excessive hypotension. Caution should be used when administering milrinone with digoxin, dobutamine, or other inotropic drugs because their positive inotropic effects on the heart may be additive.

Patients Need to Know

Patients treated for HF need to know the following:

In General

1. Take blood pressure regularly because many drugs for HF affect blood pressure. Report any persistent changes.
2. Take weight measurements regularly, and report abnormal weight gains or losses.
3. Salt intake should be limited.

Regarding ACE Inhibitors

4. Avoid sudden position changes because these can cause lightheadedness.

Regarding Cardiac Glycosides

5. Check pulse rate before taking digoxin. If the rate is less than 60 beats per minute or the rate designated by a healthcare provider, the drug should not be taken.
6. Many drugs interact with digoxin to increase or decrease its effects on the heart. For this reason, it is important to consult with a healthcare provider before taking any other medication.
7. Report visual disturbances (seeing halos or a yellow-green tinge, blurring), nausea, headaches, or irregular heartbeat without delay because they are signs and symptoms of digoxin toxicity.

Regarding Diuretics

8. Limit salt intake as directed by the healthcare provider.
9. Drink at least six to eight glasses of water daily.
10. Report any of the following adverse effects: abdominal pain, jaundice, dark urine, flu-like symptoms.
11. To prevent dizziness, avoid sudden position changes.
12. An increased intake of potassium-rich foods, such as bananas, dried fruits, and orange juice, or a potassium supplement may be necessary if certain diuretics are taken. Taking potassium supplements with food reduces stomach irritation.

Chapter Review

Core Concepts Summary

20.1 Heart failure is closely associated with disorders such as chronic hypertension, coronary artery disease, and diabetes.

Heart failure (HF) is not considered a distinct disease in itself. Instead, a number of diseases that affect the heart, such as chronic HTN, coronary artery disease, and diabetes, lead to the collection of symptoms known as HF.

20.2 The central cause of heart failure is weakened heart muscle.

HF occurs when the heart cannot pump enough blood to meet the demands of the tissues. This usually occurs when the heart muscle cannot contract with sufficient force. HF may occur on the right side, left side, or both sides of the heart, producing symptoms such as shortness of breath, coughing, and peripheral edema.

20.3 The three primary characteristics of heart function are force of contraction, heart rate, and speed of impulse conduction.

The ability of the heart to effectively pump blood depends on the strength of contraction of the myocardial fibers. Heart rate and the speed of the impulse conduction across the myocardium also directly affect the ability of the heart to pump blood.

20.4 The specific therapy for heart failure depends on the severity of the disease.

Mild HF can be improved through lifestyle changes such as tobacco cessation and maintaining optimal weight. As HF progresses, pharmacotherapy with preferred drugs, such as ACE inhibitors or diuretics, is indicated. More advanced disease may require therapy with cardiac glycosides, phosphodiesterase inhibitors, beta blockers, or vasodilators.

20.5 Angiotensin-converting enzyme (ACE) inhibitors are the preferred drugs for heart failure.

ACE inhibitors improve HF by reducing peripheral edema and increasing cardiac output. Because of their effectiveness and their relatively low potential for serious adverse effects, they have become preferred drugs in the treatment of HF.

20.6 Diuretics relieve symptoms of heart failure by reducing fluid overload and decreasing blood pressure.

Diuretics produce few serious adverse effects and are often used in combination with other HF drugs to reduce patients' symptoms. Potent diuretics such as furosemide are particularly valuable in treating acute HF.

20.7 Cardiac glycosides increase the force of myocardial contraction and were once the preferred drugs for heart failure.

Cardiac glycosides, long the mainstay for pharmacotherapy of HF, increase myocardial contractility and are effective. The large number of drug–drug interactions and the potential for serious adverse effects such as dysrhythmias limit their use.

20.8 Beta-adrenergic blockers are used in combination with other drugs to slow the progression of heart failure.

Although beta blockers decrease myocardial contractility, they also lower heart rate and blood pressure, which is beneficial in reducing the symptoms of HF. When administered to treat patients with HF, they are nearly always used in combination with other drugs.

20.9 Vasodilators reduce symptoms of heart failure by decreasing cardiac workload.

Direct vasodilators are effective at relaxing blood vessels, thus reducing myocardial oxygen demand on the heart. BiDil is a combination of two vasodilators: isosorbide dinitrate and hydralazine. Their use is limited by their high incidence of adverse effects. Nesiritide (Natrecor) is a small peptide hormone that is approved only for severe HF because of its potentially serious adverse effects.

20.10 Phosphodiesterase inhibitors are used for short-term therapy of advanced heart failure.

Phosphodiesterase inhibitors are a relatively new class of drugs used for the short-term treatment of HF. Although effective, they are given IV only and can produce potentially serious adverse effects.

REVIEW Questions

Answer the following questions to assess your knowledge of the chapter material, and go back and review any material that is not clear to you.

1. The patient has developed a cough and shortness of breath when lying down. After thoroughly collecting data on the patient, the nurse suspects:
   1. Right heart failure.
   2. Left heart failure.
   3. Liver engorgement.
   4. Peripheral edema.

2. The patient has been started on digoxin (Lanoxin) therapy. Which of the following should be monitored carefully?
   1. Phosphate levels
   2. Amylase levels
   3. Sodium levels
   4. Potassium levels

3. The nurse is teaching a patient about beta blockers. The patient states that he or she is already taking another kind of medication for heart failure. The nurse tells the patient that this is not uncommon. What other drug is usually given with beta blockers?
   1. Cardiac glycosides
   2. Diuretics
   3. Phosphodiesterase inhibitors
   4. Angiotensin-converting enzyme (ACE) inhibitors

4. A patient who is taking hydralazine for heart failure is also experiencing angina. Which of the following drugs would be used in combination with hydralazine to help relieve this patient's symptoms?
   1. Isosorbide dinitrate (Isordil)
   2. Carvedilol (Coreg)
   3. Chlorothiazide (Diuril)
   4. Milrinone (Primacor)

5. The patient is admitted with heart failure. The healthcare provider orders IV milrinone (Primacor). The most serious adverse effect of this drug is:
   1. Headache.
   2. Dysrhythmias.
   3. Confusion.
   4. Drowsiness.

6. Which of the following should be included in the education provided to a patient on lisinopril (Prinivil)? (Select all that apply.)
   1. "It may take several weeks for your blood pressure to return to normal."
   2. "You must have your potassium monitored from time to time."
   3. "This medication may change your vision from time to time."
   4. "It interacts with nonsteroidal anti-inflammatory drugs (NSAIDs) to cause decreased antihypertensive activity."
   5. "You must have an ECG done on a regular basis."

7. In addition to decreasing cardiac contractility, beta blockers:
   1. Lower heart rate and blood pressure.
   2. Increase heart rate and afterload.
   3. Produce systemic vasoconstriction.
   4. Increase the force of myocardial contraction.

8. A patient is taking digoxin. Just in case the patient develops digoxin toxicity, which drug would you expect to be ordered for this patient?
   1. Digoxin immune fab
   2. Milrinone (Primacor)
   3. Inamrinone (Inocor)
   4. Flecainide (Tambocor)

9. A patient is receiving digoxin and furosemide (Lasix). Which of the following electrolyte levels should the nurse most carefully monitor?
   1. Potassium
   2. Creatinine
   3. Sodium
   4. Calcium

10. The healthcare provider orders a patient to have 0.5 mg of digoxin. On hand, you have a bottle labeled digoxin 0.25 mg per tablet. How many tablet(s) will you give?
    1. One tablet
    2. One and one-half tablets
    3. Two tablets
    4. Half tablet

CASE STUDY Questions

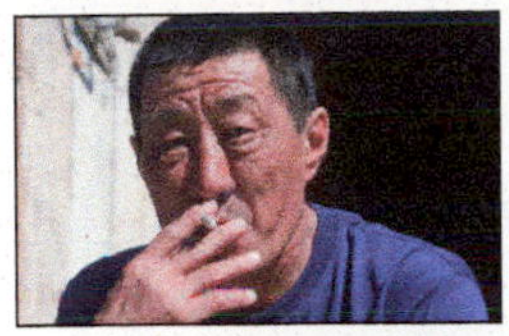

Remember Mr. Chen, the patient introduced at the beginning of the chapter? Now read the remainder of the case study. Based on the information you have learned in this chapter, answer the questions that follow.

Mr. Lei Chen, age 60, has smoked since age 18. He recently has had trouble breathing when mowing the lawn, and he coughs when he lies down to sleep at night. The healthcare provider has diagnosed Mr. Chen with early HF and is planning to start him on some medication to help his heart function more effectively, in addition to providing information on a smoking cessation program.

1. Which of the following drugs would *most* likely be prescribed for Mr. Chen?
   1. Isosorbide dinitrate (Isordil)
   2. Enalapril (Vasotec)
   3. Milrinone (Primacor)
   4. Digoxin (Lanoxin)
2. Which of the following actions would be most desirable for a drug used to treat heart failure in Mr. Chen?
   1. Increase the heart rate.
   2. Increase cardiac output.
   3. Increase arterial blood pressure.
   4. Increase blood volume by retaining water.
3. After a year, Mr. Chen enters the emergency department with acute shortness of breath and severe congestion in both lungs. The nurse understands that the plan of care for a patient with these symptoms will most likely include which medication?
   1. Inamrinone (Inocor)
   2. Captopril (Capoten)
   3. Carvedilol (Coreg)
   4. Spironolactone (Aldactone)
4. Mr. Chen is eventually placed on digoxin and furosemide. Which of the following adverse effects of furosemide should the nurse tell the patient about because it could lead to dysrhythmias and other cardiac disease while taking digoxin?
   1. Hypotension
   2. Bradycardia
   3. Hypokalemia
   4. Hyperkalemia

Answers and complete rationales for the Review and Case Study Questions appear in Appendix A.

REFERENCE

Emory Healthcare. (n.d.). *Heart failure statistics*. Retrieved from http://www.emoryhealthcare.org/heart-failure/learn-about-heart-failure/statistics.html

SELECTED BIBLIOGRAPHY

Allen, L. A., Stevenson, L. W., Grady, K. L., Goldstein, N. E., Matlock, D. D., Arnold, R. M., . . . Spertus, J. A. (2012). Decision making in advanced heart failure: A scientific statement from the American Heart Association. *Circulation, 125*, 1928–1952. doi:10.1161/CIR.0b013e31824f2173

Corotto, P. S., McCarey, M. M., Adams, S., Khazanie, P., & Whellan, D. J. (2013). Heart failure patient adherence: Epidemiology, cause, and treatment. *Heart Failure Clinics, 9*, 49–58. doi:10.1016/j.hfc.2012.09.004

Dumitru, I. (2016). *Heart failure*. Retrieved from http://emedicine.medscape.com/article/163062-overview

Go, A. S., Mozaffarian, D., Roger, V. L., Benjamin, E. J., Berry, J. D., Blaha, M. J., . . . Turner, M. B. (2014). Executive summary: Heart disease and stroke statistics—2014 update: A report from the American Heart Association. *Circulation, 129*, 399–410. doi:10.1161/01.cir.0000442015.53336.12

Rossano, J. W., & Shaddy, R. E. (2014). Heart failure in children: Etiology and treatment. *The Journal of Pediatrics, 165*, 228–233. doi:10.1016/j.jpeds. 2014.04.055

van Deursen, V. M., Damman, K., van der Meer, P., Wijkstra, P. J., Luijckx, G. J., van Beek, A., . . . Voors, A. A. (2014). Co-morbidities in heart failure. *Heart failure reviews, 19*, 163–172. doi:10.1007/s10741-012-9370-7

Yancy, C. W., Jessup, M., Bozkurt, B., Butler, J., Casey, D. E., Drazner, M. H., . . . & Wilkoff, B. L. (2013). 2013 ACCF/AHA guideline for the management of heart failure: A report of the American College of Cardiology Foundation/American Heart Association Task Force on Practice Guidelines. *Journal of the American College of Cardiology, 62*(16), e147–e239. doi:10.1016/j.jacc.2013.05.019

Chapter 21

Drugs for Angina Pectoris, Myocardial Infarction, and Stroke

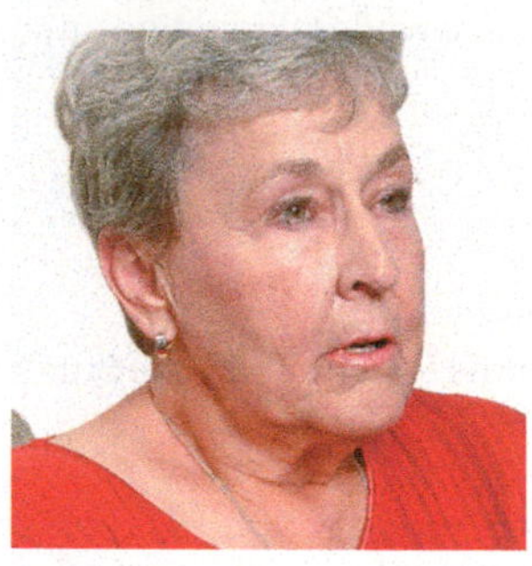

"Every time I mow the lawn it happens. The pain is so crushing, it takes my breath away."
Ms. Shirley Bush

Core Concepts

21.1 **Coronary artery disease can lead to serious cardiac impairment.**
21.2 **Angina pectoris is characterized by severe chest pain caused by lack of sufficient oxygen flow to cardiac muscle.**
21.3 **Angina pain can often be controlled through positive lifestyle changes, medications, and surgical procedures.**
21.4 **The pharmacologic management of angina is achieved by reducing cardiac workload.**
21.5 **The organic nitrates relieve angina pain by dilating veins and the coronary arteries.**
21.6 **Beta-adrenergic blockers are sometimes preferred drugs for reducing the frequency of angina attacks.**
21.7 **Calcium channel blockers relieve angina pain by reducing the cardiac workload.**
21.8 **The early diagnosis and treatment of myocardial infarction increases chances of survival.**
21.9 **Thrombolytics dissolve clots blocking the coronary arteries.**
21.10 **Drugs are used to treat the symptoms and complications of acute myocardial infarction.**
21.11 **Aggressive treatment of stroke can increase survival.**

Drug Snapshot

The following drugs are discussed in this chapter:

Drug Classes	Prototype Drugs
Organic nitrates	Pr nitroglycerin (Nitrostat, Nitro-Bid, Nitro-Dur, others)
Beta-adrenergic blockers	Pr atenolol (Tenormin)
Calcium channel blockers	Pr diltiazem (Cardizem, Cartia XT, Dilacor XR, others)
Thrombolytics	Pr reteplase (Retavase)

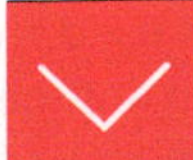

Learning Outcomes

After reading this chapter, the student should be able to:

1. Describe how the myocardium receives its oxygen and nutrient supply.
2. Explain the pathophysiology of angina pectoris.
3. Identify positive lifestyle changes that may be implemented to manage symptoms of angina.
4. Explain the pharmacologic treatment of MI.
5. Describe the pharmacologic treatment of stroke.
6. Categorize drugs used to treat angina, MI, and stroke based on their classification and mechanisms of action.
7. For each of the classes listed in the Drug Snapshot, identify representative drugs and explain their mechanisms of drug action, primary actions, and important adverse effects as they relate to the treatment of angina, MI, or stroke.

Key Terms

angina pectoris (an-JEYE-nuh PEK-tore-us)
atherosclerosis (ath-ur-oh-skler-OH-sis)
coronary arteries (KOR-un-air-ee AR-tur-ees)
hemorrhagic stroke (hee-moh-RAJ-ik)
myocardial infarction (MI) (meye-oh-KAR-dee-ul in-FARK-shun)
myocardial ischemia (meye-oh-KAR-dee-ul is-KEE-mee-uh)
percutaneous coronary intervention (PCI) (per-cue-TAIN-ee-us)
plaque (plak)
stable angina
stroke
thrombotic stroke (throm-BOT-ik)
unstable angina
vasospastic (Prinzmetal's) angina

All tissues in the body are dependent on a continuous supply of oxygen and vital nutrients to support life and health. The heart and brain are especially demanding. Should the blood supply to cardiac (heart) muscle become compromised, cardiovascular function may become impaired, resulting in angina pectoris, myocardial infarction (MI), and, possibly, death. Interruption of blood supply to the brain can cause fainting or stroke. This chapter focuses on the pharmacologic interventions related to angina pectoris, MI, and stroke (also called cerebrovascular accident or CVA).

cerebro = *head or brain*
vascular = *vessels*

Coronary artery disease can lead to serious cardiac impairment.

◄ **Core Concept 21.1**

The heart is the hardest working organ in the body. Whereas the activity of most organs slows considerably during rest and sleep, the heart must continue pumping so that the tissues can receive the nutrients they need and dispose of the wastes they have accumulated. Because it is such a vital organ, the cardiac muscle (myocardium) must receive a continuous supply of oxygen and nutrients. Any disturbance in blood flow to the vital organs or to the myocardium itself—even for brief episodes—can result in life-threatening consequences.

myo = *muscle*
cardium = *heart*

Because the heart chambers fill with blood more than 60 times per minute, one would think that the myocardium would have an ample supply of oxygen and nutrients. The myocardium, however, receives essentially no nutrients from the blood traveling through the heart's chambers. Instead, cardiac muscle receives its nutrients from the first two arteries branching off the aorta, the right and left **coronary arteries**. As these arteries branch, they circle the heart, bringing cardiac muscle a continuous supply of oxygen and nutrients.

Coronary artery disease (CAD), also called coronary heart disease, is the term used to describe restricted blood flow in the coronary arteries. Moderate restriction leads to angina pectoris. Severe impairment or complete loss of blood flow causes MI and a high risk of sudden death. CAD can also cause dysrhythmias and lead to heart failure.

ANGINA PECTORIS

Angina pectoris is acute chest pain caused by insufficient oxygen to a portion of the myocardium. Angina is characterized by chest pain on physical exertion or emotional stress. Although it produces many of the same symptoms as a heart attack, its pharmacologic treatment is quite different.

Core Concept 21.2 ▶ Angina pectoris is characterized by severe chest pain caused by lack of sufficient oxygen flow to cardiac muscle.

athero = *fatty*
sclera = *hard*
osis = *abnormal condition*

The most common cause of angina is **atherosclerosis**: a buildup of fatty, fibrous material called **plaque** in the walls of arteries. Although plaque may take as long as 40 to 50 years to accumulate to a level that would cause symptoms, plaque deposition actually begins very early in life. If plaque accumulates in a coronary artery, the myocardium downstream from the affected artery begins to receive less oxygen than it needs to perform its metabolic functions. This condition of having a reduced blood supply to cardiac muscle cells is called **myocardial ischemia**. Figure 21.1 illustrates the progressive accumulation of plaque that is characteristic of atherosclerosis.

The classic presentation of angina pectoris is intense pain in the chest, often radiating to the left side of the neck and lower jaw and down the left arm. Angina pain is usually preceded by physical exertion or emotional excitement—events associated with *increased myocardial oxygen demand*. The plaque-filled coronary artery is unable to supply the amount of nutrients needed by the stressed myocardium. With rest and effective pharmacotherapy, angina pain usually diminishes in less than 15 minutes.

There are several types of angina. Angina pectoris that is predictable in its frequency, intensity, and duration is called **stable angina**. If angina episodes become more frequent or severe and occur during periods of rest, the condition is called **unstable angina**. Unstable angina requires more aggressive medical intervention. It is sometimes considered a medical emergency because it is associated with an increased risk of MI. A third type of angina is known as **vasospastic** or **Prinzmetal's angina**. This type is caused by *spasms* of the coronary arteries, which may or may not contain plaque. Vasospastic angina pain occurs most often during periods of rest.

Angina pain may closely mimic that of an MI. It is necessary for the healthcare provider to distinguish quickly between the two diseases because the pharmacologic treatment of angina is much different than that of MI. Angina is rarely fatal. In contrast, MI has a high mortality rate if treatment is delayed, so drug therapy must begin immediately.

Chest pain is a common complaint of patients seeking care in healthcare providers' offices and emergency departments. It is also one of the most frightening symptoms for patients, who often equate their pain to having MI with a real risk of sudden death. The pain experienced by the patient, however, is only a symptom of an underlying disorder. A number of diverse diseases can produce chest pain, and some of these are unrelated to the heart. A major goal of the healthcare provider is to quickly determine the cause of the pain so that the proper treatment can be administered. Table 21.1 lists some of the common diseases that can produce chest pain as a symptom.

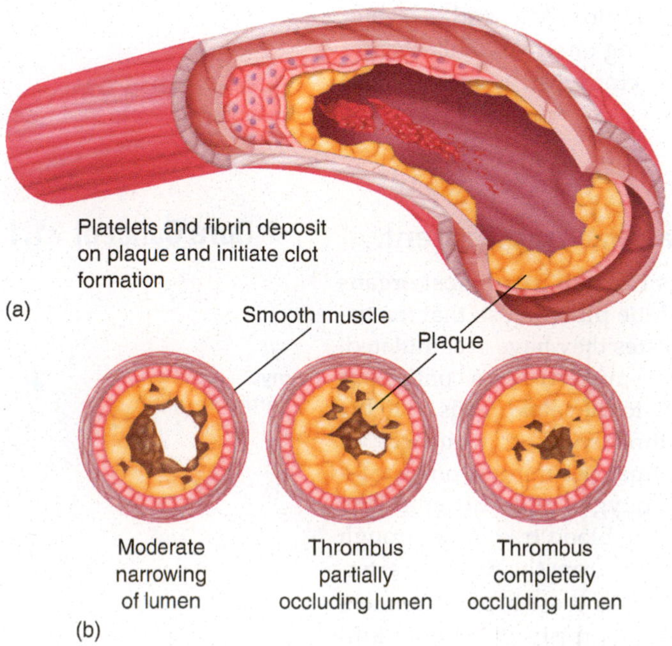

(a) Platelets and fibrin deposit on plaque and initiate clot formation
Smooth muscle
Plaque
(b) Moderate narrowing of lumen | Thrombus partially occluding lumen | Thrombus completely occluding lumen

FIGURE 21.1 Plaque and thrombus formation in the coronary artery.

Table 21.1 Examples of Disorders That May Produce Chest Pain

Name of Disease	Description
Coronary artery disease	Atherosclerosis of the coronary arteries
Diabetes	Lack of insulin or lack of insulin receptors
Gastric reflux	Backflow of stomach contents into the esophagus
Hypertension	High systemic blood pressure
Mitral stenosis	Inability of the mitral valve to fully open
Myocardial infarction	Cardiac muscle tissue death due to clots in coronary arteries
Peptic ulcer disease	Erosion of the mucosa of the stomach or small intestine

Fast Facts Angina Pectoris

- Almost 10 million Americans have angina pectoris; 500,000 new cases occur each year.
- Angina is the presenting symptom for CAD much more often in women than men.
- Among ethnic groups, the incidence of angina is highest among African Americans.
- Angina occurs more frequently in women than men; African American women have approximately twice the risk of African American men.

Source: Data from *Angina Pectoris*, by J. Alaeddini, 2015, Medscape News and Perspective.

Angina pain can often be controlled through positive lifestyle changes and surgical procedures.

◄ **Core Concept 21.3**

A combination of variables influences the development and progression of CAD, including dietary patterns and lifestyle choices. The healthcare provider should help the patient control the frequency of angina episodes by advising him or her to implement some or all of the following lifestyle changes:

- Limit alcohol consumption to small amounts.
- Eliminate foods high in cholesterol or saturated fats.
- Keep blood cholesterol and other lipid indicators within the normal ranges.
- Do not use tobacco.
- Keep blood pressure within the normal range.
- Exercise regularly and maintain optimal weight.
- Keep blood glucose levels within normal range.
- Limit salt (sodium) intake.
- Reduce stress levels as much as possible.

When the coronary arteries are significantly obstructed, surgical intervention may be necessary. **Percutaneous coronary intervention (PCI)** is a procedure in which a severely narrowed coronary artery is opened during cardiac catheterization. The occluded area may be opened by using a balloon catheter or a laser, or by removal of plaque (atherectomy). PCI sometimes involves placing a stent in the narrowed area to keep the vessel open.

per = *through procedure*
cutaneous = *skin*

CONCEPT REVIEW 21.1

- How can a healthcare provider distinguish between stable angina and unstable angina?

The pharmacologic management of angina is achieved by reducing cardiac workload.

◄ **Core Concept 21.4**

The treatment goals for a patient with angina are twofold: to *reduce the frequency* of angina episodes and to *terminate* acute angina pain in progress. Long-term goals include extending the patient's lifespan by preventing serious consequences of ischemic heart disease, such as dysrhythmias, heart failure, and MI. The primary means by which antianginal drugs act is by reducing the myocardial demand for oxygen. This reduced demand can be accomplished by at least four mechanisms:

- Slowing the heart rate
- Dilating veins so that the heart receives less blood (reduced *preload*)
- Causing the heart to contract with less force (reduced *contractility*)
- Lowering blood pressure, thus offering the heart less resistance when ejecting blood from the ventricles (reduced *afterload*).

Three classes of drugs—organic nitrates, beta-adrenergic blockers, and calcium channel blockers—are used to treat angina. Rapid-acting organic nitrates are preferred drugs for *terminating* acute angina pain. Beta-adrenergic blockers are considered first-line drugs for *preventing* angina pain. Calcium channel blockers are used when beta blockers or long-acting organic nitrates are not tolerated well by a patient. It is important to understand that the antianginal medications relieve symptoms but do not cure the underlying disorder. A summary of the drugs used to prevent and treat CAD is shown in Figure 21.2.

Patients with angina will also likely be taking several secondary medications. Daily low-dose aspirin reduces the risk of serious cardiovascular events. Aggressive therapy with statins to lower blood cholesterol levels has been found to reduce the number of cardiac events and mortality associated with angina. Ranolazine (Ranexa) is a newer drug for angina that is approved for chronic angina that has not responded to other agents.

Core Concept 21.5 ▶

The organic nitrates relieve angina pain by dilating veins and the coronary arteries.

All drugs in this chemical class possess at least one nitrate (NO_2) group. The vasodilation effect of these agents is a result of the conversion of nitrate to its active form, nitric oxide (NO). Another nitrogen containing drug, nitrous oxide (N_2O), is used in anesthesia (see Chapter 16). Organic nitrates used to treat angina are listed in Table 21.2.

FIGURE 21.2 Mechanisms of action of drugs used to treat angina pectoris.

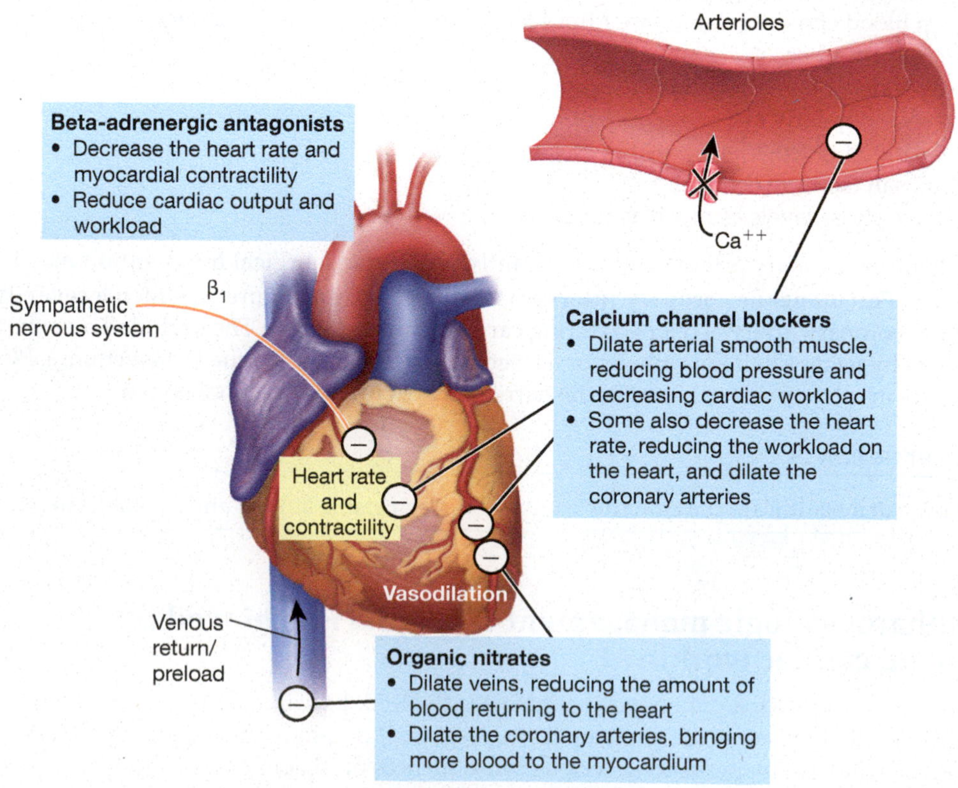

Table 21.2 Selected Drugs for Angina and Myocardial Infarction

Drug	Route and Adult Dose	Remarks
ORGANIC NITRATES		
isosorbide dinitrate (Dilatrate SR, Isordil)	PO (sustained release): 40 mg 2–4 times/day	For both acute attacks and long-term management; sublingual and chewable forms; smaller dose is given to initiate therapy
isosorbide mononitrate (Imdur, Ismo, Monoket)	PO (regular release): 20 mg bid; PO (sustained release): 30–60 mg once daily	For prevention of angina; smaller dose is given to initiate therapy; give in morning, if taking once daily
Pr nitroglycerin (Nitrostat, Nitro-Bid, Nitro-Dur, others)	Sublingual: 1 tablet (0.3–0.6 mg) or 1 spray (0.4–0.8 mg) every 3–5 minutes (max: three doses in 15 minutes)	Dilates both arteries and veins; extended-release form available
BETA-ADRENERGIC BLOCKERS		
acebutolol (Sectral)	PO: 400–800 mg/day in 1–2 divided doses (max: 1200 mg/day)	Cardioselective $beta_1$-blocker; decreases cardiac output; also for hypertension (HTN) and dysrhythmias
Pr atenolol (Tenormin)	PO: 25–50 mg daily (max: 100 mg/day)	Cardioselective $beta_1$-blocker; also for dysrhythmias, MI, and HTN
metoprolol (Lopressor, Toprol XL)	For angina: PO: 100 mg bid (max: 400 mg/day) For MI: IV: 5 mg every 2 minutes for three doses followed by PO doses	Cardioselective $beta_1$-blocker; also for MI and HTN
nadolol (Corgard)	PO: 40 mg once daily (max: 240 mg/day)	Nonselective $beta_1$- and $beta_2$-blocker; also for HTN
propranolol (Inderal, InnoPran XL) (see the Prototype Drug box in Core Concept 23.7)	PO: 10–80 mg bid–tid (max: 320 mg/day)	Nonselective $beta_1$- and $beta_2$-blocker; IV form available; also for HTN, dysrhythmias, MI, and migraine prophylaxis
CALCIUM CHANNEL BLOCKERS		
amlodipine (Norvasc)	PO: 5–10 mg daily (max: 10 mg/day)	Also for HTN
Pr diltiazem (Cardizem, Cartia XT, Dilacor XR, others)	PO (regular release): 30 mg tid-qid (max: 480 mg/day) PO (extended release): 20–240 mg bid (max: 540 mg/day)	Dilates coronary arteries and decreases coronary artery spasm; also for HTN; IV form available for dysrhythmias
nicardipine (Cardene)	PO: 20–40 mg tid or 30–60 mg PO (sustained release): bid (max: 120 mg/day)	Also for HTN; IV form available
nifedipine (Adalat CC, Procardia XL, others) (see the Prototype Drug box in Core Concept 19.9)	PO (regular release): 10–20 mg tid (max: 180 mg/day) PO (extended release): 30–90 mg once daily	Used in the treatment of vasospastic angina; also for HTN
verapamil (Calan, Isoptin SR, others) (see the Prototype Drug box in Core Concept 23.9)	PO (regular release): 80 mg tid–qid (max: 480 mg/day) PO (sustained release): 180 mg once daily	Dilates coronary arteries and inhibits coronary artery spasm; also for HTN; IV form available for dysrhythmias
MISCELLANEOUS DRUG		
ranolazine (Ranexa)	PO: 500–1000 mg bid (max: 1000 mg bid)	Acts by shifting myocardial metabolism from fatty acids to glucose, which decreases the oxygen demands of the heart

Since the discovery of their medicinal properties in 1879, the organic nitrates have been the mainstay for the treatment of angina. The primary therapeutic action of these agents is their ability to relax both arterial and venous smooth muscle. Dilation of veins reduces the amount of blood returning to the heart (preload), so the chambers contain a smaller volume. With less blood for the ventricles to pump, the workload on the heart is decreased, thereby lowering myocardial oxygen demand. The therapeutic outcome is that chest pain is terminated and episodes of angina become less frequent.

Organic nitrates also have the ability to dilate coronary arteries, and this was once thought to be their primary mechanism of action. It seems logical that dilating a partially occluded coronary vessel would allow more oxygen to reach ischemic myocardial tissue. Although this effect does indeed occur, it is not believed to be the primary mechanism of nitrate action in stable angina. This action, however, is important in treating the less common form of angina known as vasospastic angina. The organic nitrates can relax these spasms and stop the pain.

Organic nitrates are of two types: short acting and long acting. The short-acting agents, such as nitroglycerin, are taken sublingually to quickly stop an acute angina attack in

trans = *across or through*
dermis = *skin*

progress. Long-acting nitrates, such as isosorbide dinitrate (Dilatrate SR, Isordil), are taken orally or delivered through a transdermal patch to decrease the frequency and severity of angina episodes. Long-acting nitrates are also useful in reducing the symptoms of heart failure (see Chapter 20).

Prototype Drug: Pr *Nitroglycerin (Nitrostat, Nitro-Bid, Nitro-Dur, Others)*

Therapeutic Class: Antianginal drug **Pharmacologic Class:** Organic nitrate, vasodilator

Actions and Uses: Nitroglycerin, the oldest and most widely used of the organic nitrates, can be delivered by a number of different routes, including sublingual, lingual spray, oral, IV, transmucosal, transdermal, topical, and extended-release forms. It is normally taken while an acute angina episode is in progress or just prior to physical activity. When given sublingually, it reaches peak plasma levels in only 4 minutes and thus can stop angina pain rapidly. Chest pain that does not respond quickly to sublingual nitroglycerin may indicate MI. The transdermal and oral sustained-release forms are for prophylaxis only, because they have a relatively slow onset of action.

Adverse Effects and Interactions: Adverse effects of nitroglycerin are usually cardiovascular and rarely life threatening. Because nitroglycerin can dilate vessels in the head, headache is common and may be persistent and severe. Occasionally, the venodilation created by nitroglycerin causes *reflex tachycardia.* Many adverse effects of nitroglycerin diminish after a few doses.

Using with sildenafil (Viagra) may cause life-threatening hypotension and cardiovascular collapse. Nitrates should not be taken 24 hours before or after taking Viagra.

tachy = *rapid*
cardia = *heart*

Although nitrates are safe drugs that have few serious adverse effects, some adverse effects may be troublesome to patients. Dilation of veins can reduce blood pressure and cause patients to become dizzy when moving from a recumbent or sitting to a standing position (orthostatic hypotension). This fall in blood pressure can result in reflex tachycardia, causing patients to feel as if their heart is having palpitations or skipping a beat. A beta-adrenergic blocker may be prescribed to diminish this undesirable increase in heart rate. Dilation of cerebral vessels may cause headache, which can sometimes be severe. Flushing of the skin is common. Most of these effects are temporary and rarely cause discontinuation of drug therapy.

Tolerance commonly occurs with the long-acting organic nitrates when they are taken for extended periods. The magnitude of the tolerance depends on the dosage and the frequency of drug administration. Patients are often instructed to remove the transdermal patch for 6–12 hours each day or withhold the nighttime dose of the oral organic nitrate to delay the development of tolerance.

Nursing Process Focus Patients Receiving Organic Nitrate Therapy

ASSESSMENT	POTENTIAL NURSING DIAGNOSES*
Prior to administration: • Obtain a complete health history including cardiovascular conditions, allergies, drug history, and possible drug interactions. • Acquire the results of a complete physical examination, including vital signs, height, weight, and electrocardiogram (ECG). • Evaluate laboratory blood findings: complete blood count (CBC), electrolytes, cardiac enzymes, lipid panel, and renal and liver function studies. • Obtain information regarding medications such as sildenafil (Viagra), vardenafil (Levitra), or tadalafil (Cialis) used within the past 24 hours.	• *Acute Pain* (headache) related to adverse effects of drug • *Deficient Knowledge* related to lack of information about drug therapy • *Ineffective Health Maintenance* related to lack of knowledge about seriousness of disease and drug therapy regimen • *Risk for Injury* (dizziness or fainting) related to hypotension from drug therapy

PLANNING: PATIENT GOALS AND EXPECTED OUTCOMES

The patient will:

- Experience therapeutic effects (relief or prevention of chest pain).
- Be free from or experience minimal adverse effects from drug therapy.
- Verbalize an understanding of the drug's use, adverse effects, and required precautions.

IMPLEMENTATION

Interventions and (Rationales)	Patient Education/Discharge Planning
• In cases of chest pain, administer medication, and evaluate the patient's knowledge of correct administration. Ask the patient to describe and rate pain prior to and throughout drug administration for documentation of angina episode. (Location and quality of pain will determine need for medication; patients at risk for angina or MI will need to carry drug in case of emergencies.)	In case of chest pain, instruct the patient to: • Place one tablet under the tongue every 5 minutes during an attack, up to three times, or until pain is relieved. • If using medication in spray form, spray under the tongue once every 5 minutes during an attack, up to three times, or until pain is relieved. Be sure not to inhale. • Call emergency medical services (EMS) if chest pain is not relieved after two or three doses.
• Obtain a 12-lead ECG to differentiate between angina and infarction. (Pharmacotherapy depends on which disorder is presenting.)	• Explain to the patient the reason for and importance of conducting an ECG.
• Monitor vital signs, especially blood pressure and pulse. Do not administer drug if the patient is hypotensive. (Drug will further reduce blood pressure.)	Instruct the patient to: • Monitor blood pressure as specified by the healthcare provider, and ensure proper use of home equipment. • Sit or lie down before taking medication and to avoid abrupt changes in position. • Explain to the patient the reason for and importance of monitoring blood levels that indicate cardiac function.
• Monitor laboratory findings, especially cardiac enzymes, CBC, blood urea nitrogen (BUN), creatinine, and liver function test. (Monitoring blood levels supplies valuable information on patient's status.)	• Advise the patient of the importance of keeping appointments for laboratory testing.
• Monitor alcohol use. (Use of alcohol with nitrates may cause extremely low blood pressure.)	• Emphasize the importance of avoiding alcohol while taking nitroglycerin.
• Monitor for headache in response to use of nitrates. (Nitrates cause vasodilation, including vessels in the head, which may cause pain.)	Instruct the patient that: • Headache is a common adverse effect that usually decreases over time. • Over-the-counter (OTC) medicines usually relieve the headache. • Their healthcare provider must be notified if headaches continue.
• Monitor for use of erectile dysfunction drugs (e.g., sildenafil) concurrently with nitrates. (Life-threatening hypotension may result with concurrent use of these drugs.)	Instruct the patient to: • Not take erectile dysfunction drugs within 24 hours after taking nitrates. • Wait at least 24 hours after taking erectile dysfunction drugs to resume nitrate therapy.
• For use of prophylactic nitrates, administer medication correctly and evaluate the patient's knowledge of proper administration. (Some patients may need the vasodilation effect of nitrates on a continuous basis.)	Instruct the patient: • In the appropriate dosing and administration of the specific nitrate being taken. • To take medication prior to a stressful event or physical activity to prevent angina. • To store nitrates according to recommendations; tablets are to be kept in a tightly closed dark glass container. All nitrates should be kept away from sources of heat and discarded at expiration date.

EVALUATION OF OUTCOME CRITERIA

Evaluate the effectiveness of drug therapy by confirming that patient goals and expected outcomes have been met (see Planning). *See Table 21.2 for a list of drugs to which these nursing actions apply.*

Core Concept 21.6 ▶ Beta-adrenergic blockers are sometimes the preferred drugs for reducing the frequency of angina attacks.

Beta-adrenergic blockers reduce the workload on the heart and are used for angina prophylaxis. Drugs for angina include cardioselective $beta_1$-blockers and mixed $beta_1$-$beta_2$-blockers. The beta-adrenergic blockers of importance in treating angina are listed in Table 21.2. The non-selective beta blockers are not used to treat vasospastic angina because they may worsen this condition.

The pharmacology of the beta-adrenergic blockers, including a Nursing Process Focus, was presented in Chapter 9. Beta blockers are widely used in medicine, including for the treatment of hypertension (see Chapter 19), heart failure (see Chapter 20), and dysrhythmias (see Chapter 23). Because of their ability to reduce oxygen consumption of the heart by slowing heart rate and reducing contractility, several beta blockers are used to decrease the frequency and severity of angina attacks caused by exertion.

Beta-adrenergic blockers are well tolerated by most patients. In some patients, fatigue, lethargy, and depression occur. Because beta blockers slow the heart rate, they are contraindicated in patients with bradycardia and heart block. Heart rate should be closely monitored so that it does not fall below 60 beats per minute (bpm) at rest or 100 bpm during exercise. Patients with diabetes should be aware that blood glucose levels should be monitored more frequently and that insulin doses may need to be adjusted accordingly. Patients should be advised against abruptly stopping beta-blocker therapy because this may result in a sudden increase in workload on the heart and acute angina symptoms. Patients should also be advised to make position changes slowly to prevent dizziness and possible fainting due to orthostatic hypotension.

Prototype Drug: Pr *Atenolol (Tenormin)*

Therapeutic Class: Drug for angina, hypertension, or MI **Pharmacologic Class:** Beta-adrenergic blocker

Actions and Uses: Atenolol is one of the most frequently prescribed drugs in the United States due to its relative safety and effectiveness in treating a number of chronic disorders, including heart failure, hypertension, stable angina, and MI. Atenolol selectively blocks $beta_1$ receptors in the heart. Its effectiveness in angina is attributed to its ability to slow heart rate and reduce contractility (negative inotropic effect), both of which lower myocardial oxygen demand. Because of its long half-life, it may be taken once a day.

Adverse Effects and Interactions: As a cardioselective $beta_1$-blocker, atenolol has few adverse effects on the lungs and is useful for patients experiencing bronchospasm. Like other beta blockers, therapy generally begins with low doses, which are gradually increased until the therapeutic effect is achieved. The most frequent adverse effects of atenolol include fatigue, weakness, dizziness, and hypotension.

Using atenolol together with CCBs may cause excessive cardiac suppression. Using atenolol together with digoxin may cause slowed atrioventricular conduction, leading to heart block. Patients should avoid using this drug with nicotine or caffeine because their vasoconstriction action will diminish the beneficial effects of atenolol.

BLACK BOX WARNING:
Abrupt discontinuation of atenolol should be avoided in patients with ischemic heart disease because this can cause acute angina pain; doses should be reduced over a 1- to 2-week period.

Core Concept 21.7 ▶ Calcium channel blockers relieve angina pain by reducing the cardiac workload.

Several calcium channel blockers (CCBs) reduce myocardial oxygen demand by lowering blood pressure and slowing the heart rate. They are widely used in the treatment of cardiovascular diseases. The first approved use of CCBs was for the treatment of angina. CCBs that are important to the pharmacotherapy of angina are listed in Table 21.2.

Blockade of calcium ion channels has a number of effects on the heart, most of which are similar to those of beta-adrenergic blockers. Like beta blockers, actions of the CCBs are presented in several chapters in this text for the treatment of hypertension (see Chapter 19) and dysrhythmias (see Chapter 23). A Nursing Process Focus for this drug class is included in Chapter 19.

CCBs cause arteriolar smooth muscle to relax, thus lowering peripheral resistance and reducing blood pressure. This decreases the myocardial oxygen demand, thus reducing the frequency of angina pain. Some CCBs are selective for arterioles. Others, such as verapamil and diltiazem, have an additional beneficial effect of slowing the heart rate (negative chronotropic effect). An additional effect of the CCBs is their ability to dilate the coronary arteries, bringing more oxygen to the myocardium. This is especially important in patients with vasospastic angina. Because they are able to relieve the acute spasms of vasospastic angina, CCBs are considered preferred drugs for this condition.

Most adverse effects of CCBs are related to vasodilation, such as headache, dizziness, and edema of the ankles and feet. CCBs should be used with caution in patients taking other cardiovascular medications that slow conduction through the atrioventricular (AV) node, particularly digoxin or beta-adrenergic blockers. The combined effects of these drugs may cause partial or complete AV heart block, heart failure, or dysrhythmias.

Prototype Drug: Pr *Diltiazem (Cardizem, Cartia XT, Dilacor XR, Others)*

Therapeutic Class: Drug for angina and hypertension **Pharmacologic Class:** Calcium channel blocker

Actions and Uses: Diltiazem inhibits the transport of calcium ions into myocardial cells and has the ability to relax both coronary and peripheral blood vessels. It is useful in the treatment of atrial dysrhythmias and hypertension as well as angina. When given as sustained-release capsules, it may be administered once daily.

Adverse Effects and Interactions: Adverse effects of diltiazem are generally not serious and are related to vasodilation such as headache, dizziness, and edema of the ankles and feet. Although diltiazem produces few adverse effects on the heart or vessels, it should be used with caution in patients taking other cardiovascular medications, particularly digoxin or beta-adrenergic blockers; the combined effects of these drugs may cause heart failure or dysrhythmias.

Diltiazem increases the levels of digoxin or quinidine if taken together. It should be used cautiously with ginger because this combination may interfere with blood clotting.

CONCEPT REVIEW 21.2

- How does decreasing the workload on the heart result in reduction in angina pain?

MYOCARDIAL INFARCTION

A **myocardial infarction (MI)** is the result of a sudden occlusion of a coronary artery. Immediate pharmacologic treatment may reduce patient mortality.

The early diagnosis and treatment of myocardial infarction increases chances of survival.

◀ **Core Concept 21.8**

MIs are responsible for a substantial number of deaths each year. Some patients die before reaching a medical facility for treatment, and many others die within 48 hours after the initial MI. Clearly, MI is a serious and frightening disease and is responsible for a large percentage of sudden deaths.

The primary cause of MI is advanced CAD. Plaque buildup can severely narrow one or more branches of the coronary arteries. Pieces of plaque may break off and lodge in a small vessel that serves a portion of the myocardium. Deprived of its oxygen supply, the affected area of the myocardium becomes ischemic and cardiac muscle cells begin to die unless the blood supply is quickly restored. Figure 21.3 illustrates this blockage and the resulting reperfusion process.

Goals for the pharmacologic treatment of acute MI include the following:

- Restore blood supply (reperfusion) to the damaged myocardium as quickly as possible through the use of thrombolytics or PCI.
- Reduce myocardial oxygen demand with organic nitrates, beta blockers, CCBs, or angiotensin-converting enzyme (ACE) inhibitors to prevent another MI.
- Control or prevent MI-associated dysrhythmias with beta blockers or other antidysrhythmics.
- Reduce post-MI mortality with aspirin, beta blockers, and ACE inhibitors.
- Manage severe chest pain and associated anxiety with analgesics.
- Prevent enlargement of the clot with anticoagulants and antiplatelet drugs. (NSAIDS should not be used due to the risk for bleeding.)

Fast Facts **Myocardial Infarction**

- About 1.5 million Americans experience a new or recurrent MI each year.
- About one third of patients experiencing an MI will die; half the deaths occur prior to arrival at the hospital.
- About 60% of patients who died suddenly of MI had no previous symptoms of the disease.
- Mortality from MI is three times higher in men than in women.
- More than 20% of men and 40% of women will die from an MI within 1 year of being diagnosed.

Source: Data from *Myocardial Infarction*, by A. M. Zafari, 2016, Medscape News and Reference.

Core Concept 21.9 ▶ Thrombolytics dissolve clots blocking the coronary arteries.

Thrombolytics are medications that are administered to dissolve an existing blood clot. In the treatment of MI, the goal of thrombolytic therapy is to dissolve clots that are obstructing the coronary arteries and restore circulation to the myocardium as quickly as possible. Thrombolytics are most effective when administered from 20 minutes to 12 hours after the onset of MI symptoms. Quick restoration of cardiac circulation has been found to prevent permanent damage to the myocardium, thereby reducing mortality and the incidence of heart failure from the MI. After the clot is successfully dissolved, anticoagulant or antiplatelet therapy is initiated to prevent the formation of additional thrombi.

Thrombolytics have a narrow margin of safety and the primary risk is excessive bleeding from interference in the clotting process. Older adults have an increased risk of serious bleeding and intracranial hemorrhage. Patients with recent trauma or surgery should not receive these drugs. Vital signs must be monitored continuously, and any signs of bleeding generally call for discontinuation of therapy. Because these medications are rapidly destroyed in the blood, stopping the infusion normally results in the rapid termination of any adverse effects.

Since the discovery of streptokinase, the first thrombolytic, there have been a number of generations of thrombolytics. The more recent drugs such as tenecteplase (TNKase) have a more rapid onset and a longer duration and may produce fewer adverse effects than older drugs in this class. Table 21.3 lists the major thrombolytics.

Prototype Drug: Pr *Reteplase (Retavase)*

Therapeutic Class: Drug for dissolving clots **Pharmacologic Class:** Thrombolytic

Actions and Uses: Reteplase is indicated for dissolving clots associated with acute MI. Like other drugs in this class, reteplase is most effective if given within 30 minutes but not later than 12 hours of the onset of MI symptoms. It usually acts within 20 minutes. A second bolus may be delivered 30 minutes after the first, if necessary. After the clot has been dissolved, therapy with heparin or another anticoagulant is started to prevent additional clots from forming.

Adverse Effects and Interactions: The major adverse effect of reteplase is hemorrhage. Healthcare providers must be vigilant in recognizing and reporting any abnormal bleeding that may occur during thrombolytic therapy. The drug is contraindicated in patients with active bleeding.

Drug interactions with anticoagulants and platelet aggregation inhibitors will produce an additive effect and increase the risk of bleeding.

Table 21.3 Thrombolytics

Drug	Route and Adult Dose	Remarks
alteplase (Activase) (see the Prototype Drug box in Core Concept 24.6)	IV: 60 mg initially, then 20 mg/h over the second hour and 20 mg/h over the third hour	Naturally occurring tissue plasminogen activator; must be given within 6 hours of start of MI or 3 hours of thrombotic stroke
Pr reteplase (Retavase)	IV: 10 units over two minutes; repeat dose in 30 minutes	Given during an acute MI to decrease the risk of heart failure and death
streptokinase (Kabikinase)	IV: 250,000–1.5 million units over 60 minutes	For acute deep vein thrombosis, pulmonary embolism, and MI
tenecteplase (TNKase)	IV: 30–50 mg infused over five seconds	Newer thrombolytic with longer half-life

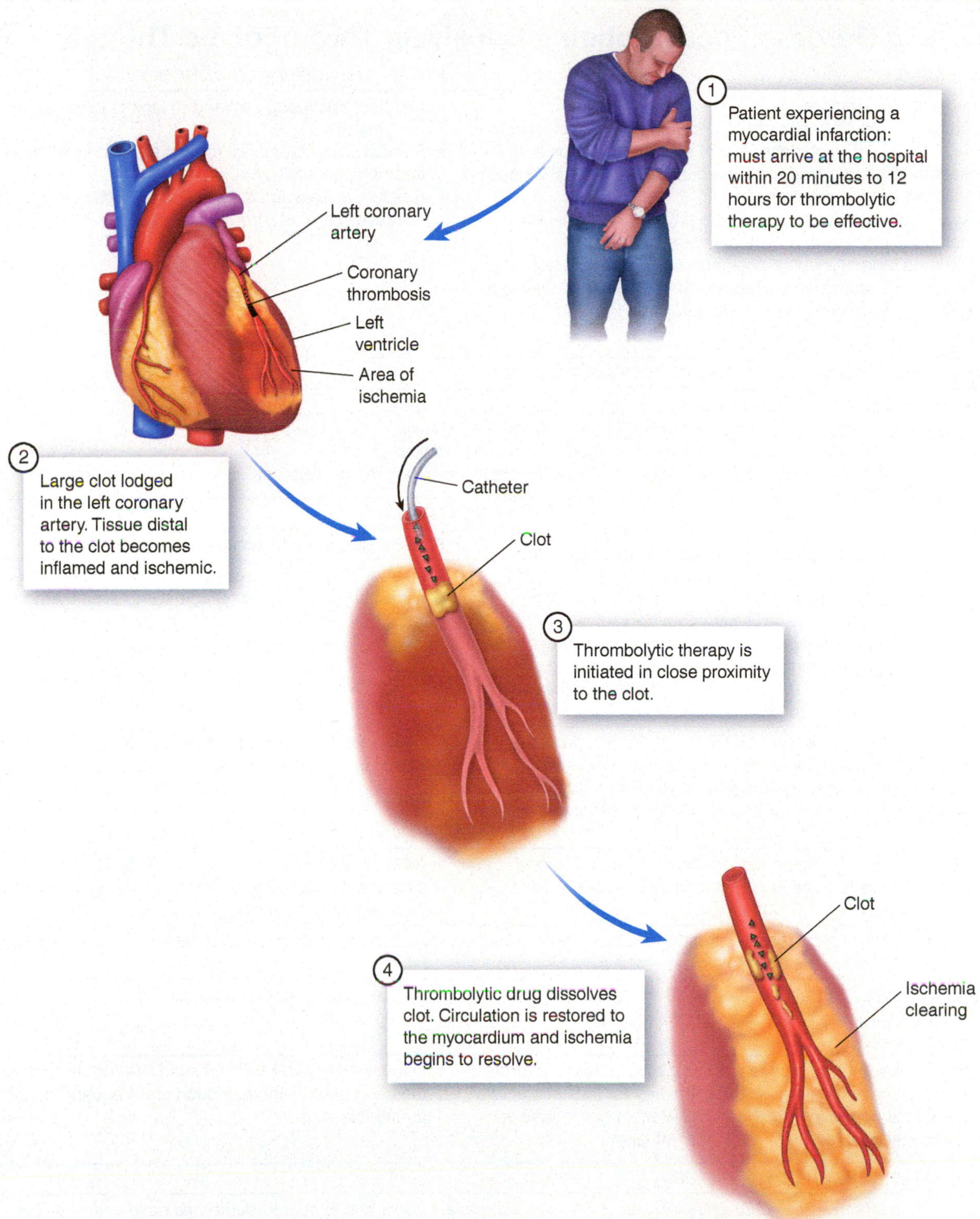

FIGURE 21.3 Blockade and reperfusion following myocardial infarction (MI): (1) blockage of left coronary artery with myocardial ischemia, (2) infusion of thrombolytics, (3) blood supply returning to myocardium, and (4) thrombus dissolving and ischemia clearing.

Nursing Process Focus Patients Receiving Thrombolytic Therapy

ASSESSMENT	POTENTIAL NURSING DIAGNOSES*
Prior to administration: • Obtain complete health history including cardiovascular, renal, and liver conditions; recent surgeries or trauma; allergies; drug history (especially cardiovascular and OTC); and possible drug interactions. • Acquire the results of a complete physical examination, including vital signs, height, and weight. • Evaluate laboratory blood findings: CBC, electrolytes, clotting factors (activated partial thromboplastin time, thromboplastin time, platelet count), and renal and liver function studies.	• *Deficient Knowledge* related to lack of information about drug therapy • *Risk for Injury* (bleeding) related to adverse effects of thrombolytic therapy • *Risk for Decreased Cardiac Tissue Perfusion* related to increase in size of thrombus and altered blood flow

PLANNING: PATIENT GOALS AND EXPECTED OUTCOMES

The patient will:
- Experience therapeutic effects (dissolving of preexisting blood clot(s)).
- Be free from or experience minimal adverse effects from drug therapy.
- Verbalize an understanding of the drug's use, adverse effects, and required precautions.

IMPLEMENTATION

Interventions and Rationales	Patient Education/Discharge Planning
• Administer medication correctly; have IV lines initiated or Foley catheter inserted *prior* to beginning therapy. (The placement of IV lines and urinary catheters allows for the ability to monitor the patient's condition, but, because they are invasive procedures, they must be done prior to the start of thrombolytic therapy to prevent the increased risk for bleeding associated with these drugs.)	• Instruct the patient about procedures and why they are necessary prior to beginning thrombolytic therapy.
• Monitor vital signs every 15 minutes during the first hour of infusion, then every 30 minutes during the remainder of infusion. (A change in vital signs may indicate indication excessive bleeding, a major adverse effect of thrombolytic therapy.)	• Advise the patient on the need for frequent monitoring of vital signs.
• Patient should be moved as little as possible during the infusion. (This is done to prevent internal injury.)	• Advise the patient that activity will be limited during infusion and that a pressure dressing may be needed to prevent any active bleeding.
• If given for thrombotic stroke, monitor neurologic status frequently. (Changes in LOC can indicate excessive bleeding.)	• Advise the patient about assessments and why they are necessary.
• Have cardiac rhythm monitored while medication is infusing. (Dysrhythmias may occur with reperfusion of myocardium.)	• Advise the patient that cardiac rhythm will be monitored during therapy.
• Monitor laboratory findings (CBC, clotting factors and arterial blood gases) during and after therapy for indications of blood loss due to internal bleeding. (Patient has increased risk of bleeding for 2 to 4 days post infusion.)	• Instruct the patient on increased risk for bleeding and on the need for activity restriction and frequent monitoring during this time.

EVALUATION OF OUTCOME CRITERIA

Evaluate the effectiveness of drug therapy by confirming that patient goals and expected outcomes have been met (see "Planning"). *See Table 21.3 for a list of drugs to which these nursing actions apply.*

*Herdman, T.H. & Kamitsuru, S. (Eds.), *Nursing Diagnoses: Definitions & Classification* 2015–2017. Copyright © 2014, 1994–2014 NANDA International. Used by arrangement by John Wiley & Sons, Inc. Companion website: www.wiley.com/go/nursingdiagnoses.

Core Concept 21.10 ▶ Drugs are used to treat the symptoms and complications of acute myocardial infarction.

The most immediate needs of the patient with MI are to ensure that the heart continues functioning and that permanent damage from the infarction is minimized. Drugs from several classes are administered soon after the onset of symptoms to prevent reinfarction and, ultimately, to reduce mortality from the episode.

Beta-Adrenergic Blockers

Beta blockers are used for MI, as they are for angina, to reduce the cardiac workload. Beta blockers have the ability to slow the heart rate, decrease contractility, and reduce blood pressure. These three actions reduce the cardiac oxygen demand, which is beneficial for those who have experienced a recent MI. In addition, the ability of beta blockers to slow impulse conduction through the heart tends to suppress dysrhythmias, which are serious and sometimes fatal complications that occur following an MI. Their use has been found to reduce mortality if given within 8 hours of an MI.

Antiplatelet and Anticoagulant Drugs

Aspirin has been found to dramatically reduce mortality, as much as 50%, in the weeks following an acute MI. Unless contraindicated, 160–324 mg of aspirin is given as soon as possible following a suspected MI. Clopidogrel (Plavix) is another effective antiplatelet agent that has been shown to reduce mortality associated with thrombi formation following an MI. Patients at high risk for thrombi formation may receive anticoagulants such as heparin, low-molecular weight heparin, or warfarin (Coumadin) following an MI. Some patients may remain on anticoagulant therapy on a continual basis after hospital discharge. The various coagulation modifiers are presented in Chapter 24.

Angiotensin-Converting Enzyme (ACE) Inhibitors

The ACE inhibitors captopril (Capoten) and lisinopril (Prinivil, Zestril) have also been found to reduce mortality following MI. These drugs are most effective when therapy is started within 1 or 2 days of the onset of symptoms. Oral therapy with the ACE inhibitors normally begins after thrombolytic therapy has been completed and the patient's condition has stabilized. The pharmacology of the ACE inhibitors is presented in Chapter 19.

Pain Management

Pain control is essential following acute MI to ensure the patient's comfort and reduce stress. Opioids such as morphine are sometimes given to ease the severe pain associated with acute MI and to sedate the anxious patient. Details on the pharmacology of the opioids were presented in Chapter 15.

CONCEPT REVIEW 21.3

- Why is it important to treat an MI within the first 24 hours after symptoms have begun? What classes of drugs are used for this purpose?

STROKE

A stroke is caused by a thrombus within or bleeding from a vessel serving the brain. Stroke is the third leading cause of death, behind heart disease and cancer. Although drug therapy is limited, immediate treatment may reduce the degree of permanent disability resulting from a stroke.

Aggressive treatment of stroke can increase survival.

◀ **Core Concept 21.11**

Stroke is a major cause of permanent disability caused by blockage of blood to the brain or rupture of a blood vessel in the brain. The majority of strokes are caused by a thrombus in a vessel serving the brain (**thrombotic stroke**). Areas downstream from the clot lose their oxygen supply, and neural tissue will begin to die unless circulation is quickly restored. A smaller percentage of strokes, about 20%, are caused by rupture of a cerebral vessel and its associated bleeding into neural tissue (**hemorrhagic stroke**). Symptoms are the same for the two types of stroke, and a computerized tomography (CT) scan is usually performed to distinguish the type of stroke before treatment is initiated. Specific symptoms of stroke vary widely depending on the affected area of the brain and may include blindness, paralysis, speech problems, coma, and even dementia. Mortality from stroke is very high: As many as 40% of patients die within the first year of a stroke.

Drug therapy of thrombotic stroke focuses on two main goals: prevention of strokes through the use of anticoagulants and antihypertensive agents, and restoration of blood supply to the affected portion of the brain as quickly as possible after an acute stroke through the use of thrombolytics.

Treatment for hemorrhage strokes depends on the cause and severity of the bleeding. Drugs used in the treatment of acute hemorrhagic stroke may include anticonvulsants to prevent seizure activity, antihypertensive agents to reduce blood pressure, and osmotic diuretics to decrease intracranial pressure. Thrombolytic therapy is contraindicated in hemorrhagic strokes because its use would prolong bleeding into the intracranial space and cause further damage.

As discussed in Chapter 19, sustained, chronic hypertension is closely associated with stroke. Antihypertensive therapy with beta-adrenergic blockers, CCBs, diuretics, and ACE inhibitors can help manage blood pressure and reduce the probability of stroke.

In very low doses, aspirin reduces the incidence of stroke by discouraging the formation of thrombi by inhibiting platelet aggregation. Patients are often placed on low-dose aspirin therapy on a continual basis following their first stroke. Clopidogrel (Plavix) is an antiplatelet drug that may be used to provide antiplatelet activity in patients who cannot tolerate aspirin. Other anticoagulants such as warfarin may be given to prevent stroke in high-risk patients such as those with prosthetic heart valves.

The single most important breakthrough in the treatment of stroke was development of the thrombolytic agents. Prior to the discovery of these drugs, the treatment of thrombotic stroke was largely a passive, wait-and-see strategy. Now stroke is aggressively treated with thrombolytics as soon as the patient arrives at the hospital: These agents are most effective if administered within 3 hours of the attack. Use of aggressive thrombolytic therapy can completely restore brain function in a significant number of patients with stroke.

CAM Therapy | Ginseng and Cardiovascular Disease

Ginseng is one of the oldest known herbal remedies. *Panax ginseng* is distributed throughout China, Korea, and Siberia, whereas *Panax quinquefolius* is native to Canada and the United States. American ginseng is not considered equivalent to Siberian ginseng.

Ginseng has been used for centuries to promote general wellness, boost immune function, and reduce fatigue. There are some claims that the herb lowers blood glucose and can help in the management of hypertension.

Ginseng is thought to have calcium channel blocking actions. The herb appears to improve blood flow to the heart in times of low oxygen supply, such as with myocardial ischemia. Some research has shown that ginseng lowers blood sugar levels in patients with type 2 diabetes. In addition, some studies have found ginseng to boost the immune system. The healthcare provider should caution patients who take ginseng, because herb–drug interactions are possible with CCBs, oral hypoglycemics, warfarin, and loop diuretics.

Patients Need to Know

Patients treated for chest pain need to know the following:

Regarding Drugs for Angina

1. Dissolve one nitroglycerin tablet under the tongue as soon as angina pain is felt. If pain is not relieved in 5 minutes, use another. Many healthcare providers recommend a third nitroglycerin tablet for pain not relieved 5 minutes after the second dose. If chest pain or pressure is not relieved by two or three doses of nitroglycerin, call EMS.
2. Rotate the application site of transdermal patches, and do not apply a new patch until after the old patch has been removed.

3. Change positions slowly. Orthostatic hypotension may cause dizziness and even fainting.
4. Monitor blood pressure regularly, and report any consistent changes to a healthcare provider.
5. Abrupt discontinuation of atenolol should be avoided with ischemic heart disease because acute angina pain may occur.
6. Report to the healthcare provider if any of the following symptoms occur: headache, dizziness, or edema of ankles and feet.

Regarding Drugs for MI or Stroke

7. A variety of drugs are used in the treatment of MI and stroke. It is important to understand and comply with the drug therapy regimen prescribed by the healthcare provider.

Chapter Review

Core Concepts Summary

21.1 Coronary artery disease can lead to serious cardiac impairment.

The high metabolic rate of the heart requires that a continuous supply of oxygen be maintained in the coronary arteries. Restriction of flow caused by coronary artery disease can lead to angina pectoris or MI.

21.2 Angina pectoris is characterized by severe chest pain caused by lack of sufficient oxygen flow to cardiac muscle.

The coronary arteries can become partially occluded with plaque, resulting in ischemia. Lack of sufficient oxygen to the myocardium upon emotional or physical exertion causes sharp chest pain, the characteristic symptom of angina.

21.3 Angina pain can often be controlled through positive lifestyle changes and surgical procedures.

A number of lifestyle changes can reduce the deposition of plaque in the coronary arteries and help prevent coronary heart disease. These include stopping tobacco use, limiting alcohol consumption, and getting adequate exercise. Surgical procedures may be necessary to correct severe angina.

21.4 The pharmacologic management of angina is achieved by reducing cardiac workload.

Reducing the workload on the heart can relieve angina pain. This can be accomplished by slowing the heart rate, dilating the vessels, reducing the force of myocardial contraction, or reducing blood pressure.

21.5 The organic nitrates relieve angina pain by dilating veins and the coronary arteries.

Fast-acting organic nitrates can quickly terminate angina pain by causing venodilation, which reduces the workload on the heart. They also dilate the coronary arteries, bringing more oxygen to the myocardium. Long-acting nitrates can prevent acute angina episodes, but the patient may become tolerant to their protective effect.

21.6 Beta-adrenergic blockers are sometimes preferred drugs for reducing the frequency of angina attacks.

Beta blockers lower blood pressure, slow the heart rate, and reduce the force of contraction, thus reducing the workload on the myocardium. They are prescribed to reduce the frequency of acute angina episodes.

21.7 Calcium channel blockers relieve angina pain by reducing the cardiac workload.

CCBs are effective at lowering blood pressure, thus reducing the workload on the heart. They are prescribed to reduce the frequency of acute angina attacks.

21.8 The early diagnosis and treatment of myocardial infarction increases chances of survival.

MI is caused by a thrombus in a coronary artery and is responsible for a substantial number of sudden deaths. Fast, effective diagnosis and treatment can reduce mortality.

21.9 Thrombolytics dissolve clots blocking the coronary arteries.

When used within hours of the onset of an MI, thrombolytics can dissolve clots and restore circulation to the myocardium.

21.10 Drugs are used to treat the symptoms and complications of acute myocardial infarction.

Beta blockers can slow the heart rate and reduce blood pressure, and have been shown to reduce mortality when given soon after MI symptoms appear. Aspirin and ACE inhibitors have been shown to reduce mortality when given soon after the onset of MI. Narcotic analgesics are sometimes given to reduce the pain and anxiety associated with an MI.

21.11 Aggressive treatment of stroke can increase survival.

Stroke is now viewed as an emergency condition requiring immediate treatment to improve survival. Thrombolytics, when given quickly after the onset of thrombotic strokes, can restore some or all brain function. Some degree of stroke prevention can be achieved by using anticoagulants and by controlling blood pressure.

REVIEW Questions

Answer the following questions to assess your knowledge of the chapter material, and go back and review any material that is not clear to you.

1. The patient is being discharged with nitroglycerin (Nitrostat) tablets. Patient education would include instructions to:
   1. "Swallow three tablets immediately for pain, and call 911."
   2. "For chest pain, place one tablet under your tongue every 5 minutes; taking no more than a total of three tablets."
   3. "Call your healthcare provider when you have chest pain. The provider will tell you how many tablets to take."
   4. "Place three tablets under your tongue, and call 911."

2. What is the most common adverse effect of nitroglycerin for which the patient is monitored?
   1. Headache
   2. Hypertension
   3. Diuresis
   4. Bradycardia

3. Which of the following classes of medication decreases heart rate, contractility, and blood pressure, and is used to increase survival rates in post-myocardial infarction patients?
   1. ACE inhibitors
   2. Beta blockers
   3. Vasodilators
   4. Diuretics

4. The most common adverse effect of reteplase (Retavase) is:
   1. Dehydration.
   2. Bleeding.
   3. Confusion.
   4. Increased clotting times.

5. The healthcare provider should be vigilant in observing for which of the following adverse effects during a reteplase infusion?
   1. An increase in blood pressure
   2. An increase in heart rate
   3. Abnormal bleeding
   4. Vomiting or diarrhea

6. A patient in the emergency department at the local hospital has been diagnosed with a hemorrhagic stroke. All of the following drug classes may be used in treatment *except*:
   1. Anticonvulsants.
   2. Thrombolytics.
   3. Antihypertensives.
   4. Osmotic diuretics.

7. The healthcare provider ordered an IV drip of D5W at 150 mL/hr. The tubing has a drip factor of 15 drops/mL. The IV drip rate is maintained at how many drops per minute?
   1. 25 drops/minute
   2. 28 drops/minute
   3. 35 drops/minute
   4. 38 drops/minute

8. In the treatment of angina, the mechanism of action of a beta-adrenergic blocker is:
   1. Slowed heart rate and decreased contractility of the heart.
   2. Relaxation of arterial and venous smooth muscle.
   3. Increased contractility and heart rate.
   4. Decreased peripheral resistance.

9. The patient is instructed when taking calcium channel blockers to use extreme caution when taking which of the following medications?
   1. Acetaminophen (Tylenol)
   2. Ibuprofen (Motrin)
   3. Digoxin (Lanoxin)
   4. Ranitidine (Zantac)

10. The patient is complaining of a viselike pain in the chest and has been diagnosed with a myocardial infarction. The nurse anticipates that he may be given which of the following medications? (Select all that apply.)
   1. Aspirin
   2. A beta blocker
   3. Thrombolytics
   4. An ACE inhibitor
   5. A potassium-sparing diuretic

CASE STUDY Questions

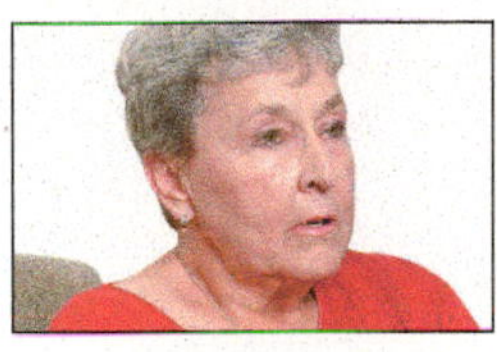

Remember Ms. Bush, the patient introduced at the beginning of the chapter? Now read the remainder of the case study. Based on the information you have learned in this chapter, answer the questions that follow.

Ms. Shirley Bush, a 65-year-old woman, arrives in your office with a complaint of chest pain when she does strenuous activity such as mowing the grass. Subsequent tests show a 10% occlusion of two coronary arteries. Her blood pressure is 126/78 mmHg. The healthcare provider prescribes one aspirin per day, sublingual nitroglycerin, and metoprolol.

1. The purpose of the nitroglycerin is to:
   1. Prevent acute angina attacks.
   2. End an angina attack in progress.
   3. Prevent MI or stroke.
   4. Relieve epigastric pain.

2. What instructions should be given to Ms. Bush about taking sublingual nitroglycerin?
   1. Take before exercising.
   2. Take on first indication of chest pain.
   3. Take three or four times per day to prevent chest pain.
   4. Take before bedtime and when rising.

3. Ms. Bush says, "What about the metoprolol?" The nurse tells her that she has been prescribed metoprolol to:
   1. Prevent acute angina attacks.
   2. End an angina attack in progress.
   3. Prevent MI or stroke.
   4. Lower blood pressure.

Ms. Bush discontinues her drugs without notifying her healthcare provider. Three months later, she arrives in the emergency department with a thrombotic stroke. Her blood pressure is 186/100 mmHg. The provider orders a reteplase infusion.

4. As the infusion is started, Ms. Bush asks, "What is this drug for?" She is told that the function of reteplase is to:
   1. Dissolve existing blood clots.
   2. Prevent possible formation of blood clots.
   3. Stabilize blood pressure.
   4. Reduce workload on the heart.

Answers and complete rationales for the Review and Case Study Questions appear in Appendix A.

REFERENCE

Herdman, T. H., & Kamitsuru, S. (Eds.). (2014). *NANDA International nursing diagnoses: Definitions and classification, 2015–2017*. Oxford, United Kingdom: Wiley-Blackwell.

SELECTED BIBLIOGRAPHY

Alaeddini, J. (2015). *Angina Pectoris*. Retrieved from http://emedicine.medscape.com/article/150215-overview

Cucherat, M., & Borer, J. S. (2012). Reduction of resting heart rate with antianginal drugs: Review and meta-analysis. *American Journal of Therapeutics, 19*, 269–280. doi:10.1097/MJT.0b013e3182246a49

Gupta, A. K., Winchester, D., & Pepine, C. J. (2013). Antagonist molecules in the treatment of angina. *Expert Opinion on Pharmacotherapy, 14*, 2323–2342. doi:10.1517/14656566.2013.834329

Jones, D. A., Timmis, A., & Wragg, A. (2013). Novel drugs for treating angina. *BMJ, 347*, f4726. doi:10.1136/bmj.f4726

Parker, J. D., & Parker, J. O. (2012). Stable angina pectoris: The medical management of symptomatic myocardial ischemia. *Canadian Journal of Cardiology, 28*(2 Suppl.), S70–S80. doi.org/10.1016/j.cjca.2011.11.002

Pedrinelli, R., Ballo, P., Fiorentini, C., Galderisi, M., Ganau, A., Germanò, G., & Zacà, V. (2013). Hypertension and stable coronary artery disease: An overview. *Journal of Cardiovascular Medicine, 14*, 545–552. doi:10.2459/JCM.0b013e3283609332

Potts, K. (2012). Preventing thromboembolic events and stroke. *Nursing & Residential Care, 14*, 179–183. doi:10.12968/nrec.2012.14.4.179

Sharma, V., Bell, R. M., & Yellon, D. M. (2012). Targeting reperfusion injury in acute myocardial infarction: A review of reperfusion injury pharmacotherapy. *Expert Opinion on Pharmacotherapy, 13*, 1153–1175. doi:10.1517/14656566.2012.685163

Tallantyre, E. C., & Robertson, N. P. (2015). Acute stroke management. *Journal of neurology, 262*, 239–242. doi:10.1007/s00415-014-7607-1

Valgimigli, M., & Biscaglia, S. (2014). Stable Angina Pectoris. *Current Atherosclerosis Reports, 16*(7), 422. doi:10.1007/s11883-014-0422-4

Winchester, D. E., & Pepine, C. J. (2015). Angina treatments and prevention of cardiac events: An appraisal of the evidence. *European Heart Journal Supplements, 17*(Suppl. G), G10–G18. doi:10.1093/eurheartj/suv054

Wood, J., & Gordon, P. (2012). Preventing CVD in women: The NP's role. *The Nurse Practitioner, 37*(2), 26–33. doi:10.1097/01.NPR.0000410275.21998.b5

Young, J. W., & Melander, S. (2013). Evaluating symptoms to improve quality of life in patients with chronic stable angina. *Nursing Research and Practice, Article ID 504915*. doi:10.1155/2013/504915

Zafari, A. M. (2016). *Myocardial Infarction*. Retrieved from http://emedicine.medscape.com/article/155919-overview

Zellweger, M. J. (2015). Management of stable coronary artery disease. *Cardiovascular Medicine, 18*, 16–19.

Chapter 22

Drugs for Shock and Anaphylaxis

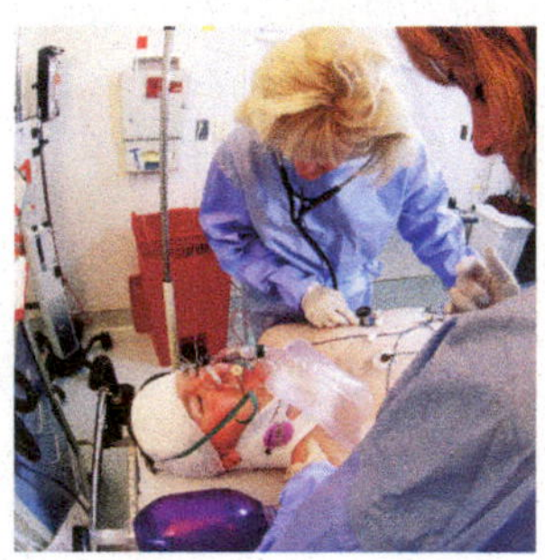

"Where am I? What happened? I really hurt."
Mr. Joshua Hanks

Core Concepts

22.1 **Shock is a syndrome characterized by the collapse of the circulatory system.**
22.2 **The initial treatment of shock includes basic life support and identification of the underlying cause.**
22.3 **Intravenous fluid replacement drugs are given to replace fluids lost during shock.**
22.4 **Vasoconstrictors are administered during shock to raise and maintain blood pressure.**
22.5 **Inotropic drugs are useful in reversing the decreased cardiac output that occurs during shock.**
22.6 **Anaphylaxis is a type of shock caused by a hyper-response of body defense mechanisms.**

Drug Snapshot

The following drugs are discussed in this chapter:

Drug Classes	Prototype Drugs
Fluid replacement drugs	Pr normal serum albumin (Albuminar, Plasbumin, others)
Vasoconstrictors	Pr norepinephrine (Levophed)
Inotropic drugs	Pr dopamine (Intropin)
Drug for anaphylaxis	Pr epinephrine (Adrenalin)

Learning Outcomes

After reading this chapter, the student should be able to:

1. Compare and contrast the different types of shock.
2. Explain the initial treatment of a patient with shock.
3. Compare and contrast the use of blood products, colloids, and crystalloids in the pharmacotherapy of shock.
4. Identify the rationale for administering vasoconstrictors to patients experiencing shock.
5. Identify the rationale for administering inotropic drugs to patients experiencing shock.
6. Identify drugs used in the pharmacotherapy of anaphylaxis.

Key Terms

anaphylactic (ann-ah-fuh-LAK-tick) shock
antigen (ANN-tuh-jen)
cardiogenic shock (kar-dee-oh-JEN-ik)
colloids (KO-loyds)
crystalloids (KRIS-tuh-loyds)
hypovolemic shock (high-poh voh-LEEM-ik)
inotropic drug (eye-noh-TROW-pik)
neurogenic shock (nyoor-oh-JEN-ik)
septic shock (SEP-tik)
shock

Shock is a condition in which vital organs are not receiving enough blood to function properly. Without an adequate supply of oxygen and other nutrients, cells cannot carry on normal metabolism. Shock is a medical emergency; failure to reverse the causes and symptoms of shock may lead to irreversible organ damage and death. This chapter examines how drugs are used to aid in the treatment of different types of shock.

SHOCK

Shock is a syndrome characterized by the collapse of the circulatory system.

◀ Core Concept 22.1

There are several types of shock, each having different causes. A simple method for classifying shock is by naming the underlying pathologic process or organ system causing the condition. Table 22.1 describes the different types of shock and their primary causes. This chapter focuses on the pharmacologic therapy of three common types of shock: hypovolemic, cardiogenic, and anaphylactic.

Shock is a collection of signs and symptoms, many of which are nonspecific. Although symptoms vary among the different kinds of shock, there are some similarities. The patient may appear pale and claim to feel sick or weak without reporting any specific symptoms. Behavioral changes are often some of the earliest symptoms and may include restlessness, anxiety, confusion, depression, and lack of interest. Thirst is a common complaint. The skin may feel cold or clammy.

Assessing the patient's cardiovascular status may provide important clues for a diagnosis of shock. Blood pressure is usually low, with a diminished cardiac output. Heart rate may be rapid, with a weak pulse. Breathing is rapid and shallow. Figure 22.1 illustrates some of the common symptoms of a patient in shock.

Diagnosis of shock is rarely based on such nonspecific symptoms. A careful medical history, however, will provide the healthcare provider with valuable clues as to what type of shock may be present. For example, obvious trauma or bleeding combined with the symptoms mentioned previously would suggest **hypovolemic shock**. If trauma to the brain or spinal cord is evident, **neurogenic shock** may be suspected. A history of heart disease would suggest **cardiogenic shock**, whereas a recent infection may indicate **septic shock**. A history of allergy with a sudden onset of symptoms following food or drug intake suggests **anaphylactic shock**.

hypo = *below*
vol = *volume*
emic = *pertaining to the blood*

neuro = *nervous system*
genic = *origin*

cardio = *heart*
genic = *origin*

Table 22.1 Classification of Shock

Type of Shock	Definition	Underlying Pathology
Anaphylactic	Acute allergic reaction	Severe reaction to allergens such as penicillin, nuts, shellfish, or animal proteins
Cardiogenic	Failure of the heart to pump sufficient blood to tissues	Left heart failure, myocardial ischemia, myocardial infarction (MI), dysrhythmias, pulmonary embolism, and myocardial or pericardial infection
Hypovolemic	Loss of blood volume	Hemorrhage, burns, profuse sweating, excessive urination, vomiting, or diarrhea
Neurogenic	Vasodilation due to overstimulation of the parasympathetic nervous system or understimulation of the sympathetic nervous system	Trauma to the spinal cord or medulla, severe emotional stress or pain, drugs that depress the central nervous system
Septic	Multiple organ dysfunction as a result of pathogenic organisms in the blood	Widespread inflammatory response to bacterial, fungal, or parasitic infection

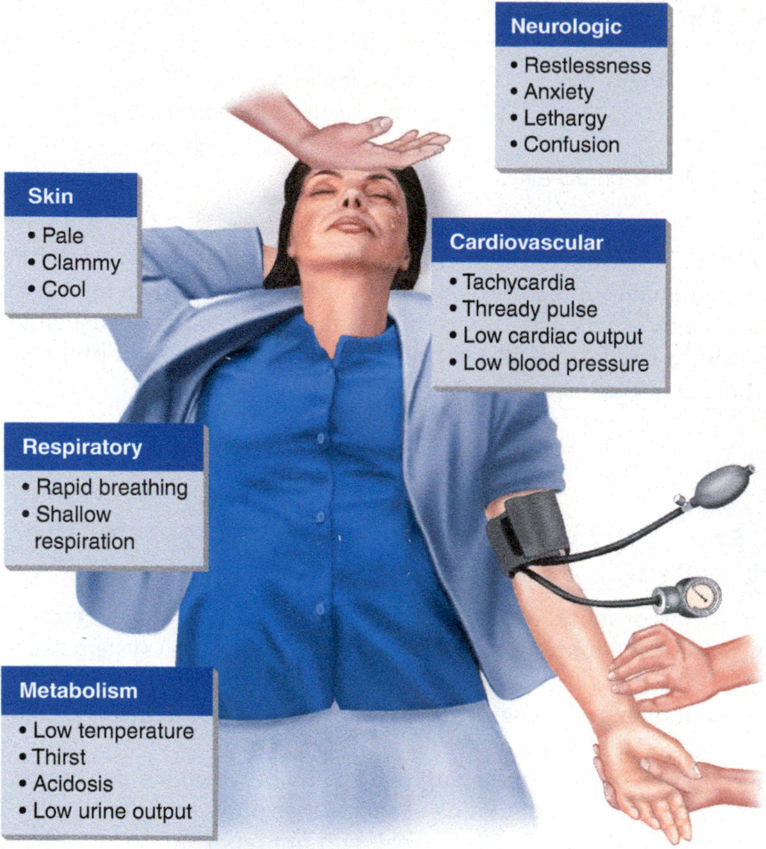

FIGURE 22.1 Symptoms of a patient in shock.

The brain and heart are affected early in the progression of shock. Lack of blood to the brain may result in fainting, whereas disruption of blood supply to the myocardium can result in permanent damage to the heart. Immediate treatment is necessary to prevent failure of other organ systems, including respiratory collapse or renal failure.

Core Concept 22.2 ▶

The initial treatment of shock includes basic life support and identification of the underlying cause.

Acute shock is treated as a medical emergency, and the first goal is to provide basic life support. Rapid identification of the underlying cause is essential because the patient's condition may deteriorate rapidly without specific, emergency measures. Keeping the patient quiet and warm until specific therapy can be initiated is important. Maintaining the CABs of life support—chest compression, airway, and breathing—is critical. Once basic life support is established, the healthcare provider can begin more specific treatment of the underlying causes of the shock.

The remaining therapies for shock depend on the specific cause of the condition. The two primary pharmacotherapeutic goals are to restore normal fluid volume and composition and to maintain adequate blood pressure. Unless contraindicated, oxygen is administered. For anaphylaxis, an additional therapeutic goal is to prevent or stop the hypersensitive inflammatory response. Specific pharmacotherapies are illustrated in Figure 22.2.

CONCEPT REVIEW 22.1

- What signs or symptoms might help a paramedic arriving on the scene of a motorcycle accident determine the cause of the patient's shock?

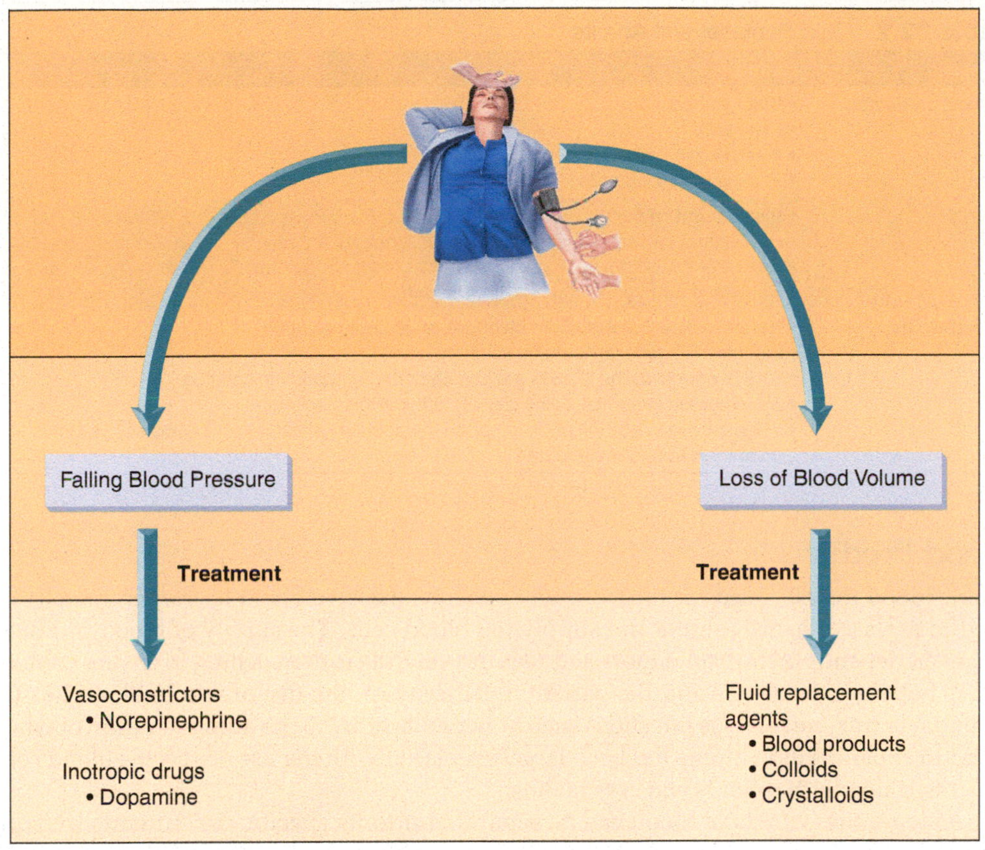

FIGURE 22.2 Physiologic changes occurring during shock and their pharmacologic interventions.

Fast Facts Shock

- Cardiogenic shock occurs in about 5–10% of the patients suffering from an acute MI.
- Cardiogenic shock is the leading cause of death in patients hospitalized with acute MI.
- The mortality rate for patients with sepsis who develop septic shock is 20–50%.
- The estimated death rate for anaphylaxis is 0.65–2% of all patients who experience the condition.
- Fewer than 100 fatal cases of anaphylaxis caused from insect stings occur annually in the United States.

Source: Based on Kalil, A. (2015). Septic shock. Retrieved from http://emedicine.medscape.com/article/168402-overview; Mustafa, S. S. (2015). Anaphylaxis. Retrieved from http://emedicine.medscape.com/article/135065-overview; Ren, Xiushui, (2015). Cardiogenic shock. Retrieved from http://emedicine.medscape.com/article/152191-overview.

Intravenous fluid replacement drugs are given to replace fluids lost during shock.

◀ **Core Concept 22.3**

When a patient loses significant amounts of blood or other body fluids, immediate treatment with fluid replacement drugs is essential. Fluid loss can occur due to hemorrhage, extensive burns, severe dehydration, persistent vomiting or diarrhea, or aggressive diuretic therapy. Death can result if a major fluid imbalance is not corrected. Fluid replacement drugs are sometimes referred to as *fluid expanders*.

The immediate goal in treating hypovolemic shock is to replace the lost fluid. In mild cases, this may be accomplished by drinking extra water or beverages containing electrolytes. In acute situations, therapy with intravenous (IV) infusions can immediately replace lost fluids. Regardless of how fluids are administered, careful attention must be paid to restoring normal levels of electrolytes as well as fluid volume.

Fluid replacement agents may be categorized as blood products, colloids, or crystalloids. Colloid and crystalloid infusions are often used when up to one-third of an adult's blood volume is lost. Examples of fluid replacement agents are listed in Table 22.2.

Table 22.2 Fluid Replacement Agents

Drug	Examples
Blood products	• Whole blood • Platelets • Fresh frozen plasma • Packed red blood cells
Colloids	• Plasma protein fraction (Plasmanate, Plasma-Plex, Plasmatein, PPF, Protenate) • Pr Normal serum albumin (Albuminar, Plasbumin, others) • Dextran 40 (Gentran 40, Hyskon, Rheomacrodex) or dextran 70 (Macrodex) • Hetastarch or hydroxyethyl starch (Hespan)
Crystalloids	• Normal saline (0.9% sodium chloride), an isotonic solution • Lactated Ringer's, an isotonic solution • 0.45% normal saline (0.45% sodium chloride), a hypotonic solution • 5% dextrose in normal saline (D5NS), a hypertonic solution • 5% dextrose in water (D5W), although the solution is isotonic, it becomes hypotonic once infused and metabolized

Blood Products

Whole blood may be used for the treatment of acute, massive blood loss when there is the need to replace plasma volume and supply red blood cells. The supply of blood products, however, depends on human donors and requires careful cross-matching to ensure compatibility between the donor and the patient. Furthermore, the use of whole blood has the potential to transmit serious infections such as hepatitis or HIV. The administration of whole blood to expand fluid volume has been largely replaced with the use of specific blood components, along with colloids and crystalloids.

A single unit of whole blood can be separated into its specific constituents (red and white blood cells, platelets, fresh frozen plasma, and immunoglobulins). This allows a single blood donation to be used to treat more than one patient.

Colloids

Colloids are proteins or other large molecules that stay suspended in the blood for a long period and draw water molecules from the body's cells and tissues into the blood vessels. Colloids include normal human serum albumin, dextran, and hetastarch or hydroxyethyl starch (Hespan). These drugs are administered to provide life-sustaining support following massive hemorrhage and to treat shock, burns, acute liver failure, and neonatal hemolytic disease.

Crystalloids

Crystalloids are IV solutions that contain electrolytes in amounts resembling those of natural plasma. Unlike colloids, crystalloid solutions can readily leave the blood and enter the cells or tissues. They are used to replace fluids that have been lost and to increase urine

Prototype Drug: Pr *Normal Serum Albumin (Albuminar, Plasbumin, Others)*

Therapeutic Class: Fluid replacement drug **Pharmacologic Class:** Blood product, colloid

Actions and Uses: Normal serum albumin is a protein extracted from whole blood or plasma. Because of this, it may be classified as both a blood product and a colloid. Its functions are to maintain plasma osmotic pressure and to shuttle certain substances through the blood, including a substantial number of drug molecules. After extraction from blood or plasma, albumin is sterilized to remove possible contamination by the hepatitis viruses or HIV.

Administered IV, albumin is used to restore plasma volume during hypovolemic shock or to restore blood proteins in patients with hypoproteinemia. It may also be administered to patients who have below normal serum protein levels due to nutritional deficiency. It has an immediate onset of action and is available in concentrations of 5% and 25%.

Adverse Effects and Interactions: Because albumin is a natural blood product, the patient may have antibodies to the donor's albumin, and allergic reactions are possible. Signs of allergy include fever, chills, rash, dyspnea, and possibly hypotension. Circulatory overload and edema may occur if excessive albumin is infused, due to fluid being moved into the vascular system.

No clinically significant drug interactions have been identified.

output. Crystalloid solutions are classified by their tonicity in relation to plasma. Tonicity refers to the concentration of dissolved molecules (solutes) within the solution. These solutions are classified as either *isotonic* (having the same concentration of solutes as plasma), *hypertonic* (having a greater concentration of solutes than plasma), or *hypotonic* (having a lesser concentration of solutes than plasma). The most common crystalloids used for the treatment of shock are isotonic solutions; they are primarily used to replace the loss of fluid volume.

Nursing Process Focus **Patients Receiving Intravenous Fluid Therapy**

ASSESSMENT	POTENTIAL NURSING DIAGNOSES*
Prior to administration: • Obtain a complete health history including cardiovascular, respiratory, neurological, renal and skin conditions, allergies, drug history, and possible drug interactions. • Acquire the results of a complete physical examination, including vital signs, height, weight, presence of burns, lung sounds, loss of consciousness, and urinary and cardiac output. • Evaluate laboratory blood findings: complete blood count, electrolytes, arterial blood gas, clotting factors, total protein/albumin, lipid panel, and renal and liver function studies.	• *Deficient Fluid Volume* related to injury • *Ineffective Tissue Perfusion* related to decreased blood volume • *Deficient Knowledge* related to a lack of information about drug therapy • *Risk for Injury* related to loss of blood or adverse effect of drug therapy • *Risk for Electrolyte Imbalance* related to fluid loss • *Risk for Imbalanced Fluid Volume* related to drug therapy • *Risk for Infection* related to broken skin, invasion of pathogenic organisms

PLANNING: PATIENT GOALS AND EXPECTED OUTCOMES

The patient will:
- Experience therapeutic effects (urinary output of at least 30 mL/h and systolic blood pressure greater than 90 mmHg).
- Be free from or experience minimal adverse effects from drug therapy.
- Verbalize an understanding of the drug's use, adverse effects, and required precautions.

IMPLEMENTATION

Interventions and (Rationales)	Patient Education/Discharge Planning
• Administer IV fluids correctly, checking type of fluid and frequently monitoring flow rate and IV site. (Frequently monitoring the infusion of IV fluids will help prevent adverse effects.)	• Inform the patient about the need for IV fluids and the reason for frequent monitoring.
• Monitor respiratory status: respirations, effort, O_2 saturation, and lung sounds. Report any signs of distress immediately to the healthcare provider. (Effects of drugs and rapid infusion may result in fluid overload.)	Instruct the patient to report to the healthcare provider: • Any signs of respiratory distress such as shortness of breath. • Changes in sensorium such as lightheadedness, drowsiness, or dizziness.
• Monitor cardiac function: blood pressure, pulse, heart rate/rhythm, cardiac output, electrocardiogram, and laboratory blood tests. (Effects of drugs and rapid infusion may result in fluid overload and put stress on the circulatory system.)	• Instruct the patient about the rationale for monitoring cardiac function and to immediately report any palpitations, chest pain, or headache.
• Monitor renal function: Intake/output, urine color, BUN, creatinine, presence of edema, or dehydration. (Renal function changes with an increase or decrease in fluid volume. A decrease is usually seen with shock.)	• Instruct the patient about the rationale for monitoring fluid intake and output, laboratory tests, and possible need for a Foley catheter.
• Weigh the patient daily. (Daily weight is an accurate measure of fluid status.)	• Teach the patient the rationale for monitoring weight and to report any evidence of weight gain.
• Monitor electrolytes. (Crystalloid drugs may cause hypernatremia and the resulting fluid retention.)	• Instruct the patient to report any evidence of edema.
• Observe the patient for signs of allergic reactions. (Administration of blood and blood products could cause allergic reactions.)	Instruct the patient: • To report itching, rash, chills, and difficulty breathing to the healthcare provider.

EVALUATION OF OUTCOME CRITERIA

Evaluate the effectiveness of drug therapy by confirming that patient goals and expected outcomes have been met (see Planning).

*Herdman, T.H. & Kamitsuru, S. (Eds.), *Nursing Diagnoses: Definitions & Classification* 2015–2017. Copyright © 2014, 1994–2014 NANDA International. Used by arrangement by John Wiley & Sons, Inc. Companion website: www.wiley.com/go/nursingdiagnoses.

Core Concept 22.4 ▶ Vasoconstrictors are administered during shock to maintain blood pressure.

In the early stages of shock, the body compensates for the rapid fall in blood pressure by activating the sympathetic nervous system. This sympathetic activity causes vasoconstriction, which raises blood pressure and increases the heart rate and force of myocardial contractions. These compensatory measures help to maintain blood flow to vital organs such as the heart and brain and to decrease the flow to "less essential" organs such as the kidneys and liver.

The body's ability to compensate is limited, however, and profound hypotension may develop as shock progresses. In severe cases, vasoconstrictors, also called vasopressors, may be needed to help stabilize blood pressure. Because of the potential for serious adverse effects and potential organ damage due to the rapid and intense vasoconstriction, vasopressors are used only after fluid infusions have failed to raise blood pressure. Patients receiving these drugs must be monitored continuously during the infusion to avoid hypertension. Vasoconstrictor therapy is discontinued as soon as the patient's condition stabilizes. Discontinuation is always gradual, due to the possibility of rebound hypotension and undesirable cardiac effects.

Vasoconstrictors used to treat shock include dopamine (Intropin), norepinephrine (Levophed), phenylephrine (Neo-Synephrine), and epinephrine. Because dopamine also affects the strength of myocardial contraction, it is considered both a vasopressor and an inotropic drug (see Concept Section 22.5). Epinephrine is usually associated with the treatment of anaphylaxis (Section 22.6). The basic pharmacology of the sympathomimetic drugs is presented in Chapter 9. Table 22.3 gives the dosages for these drugs.

Table 22.3 Vasoconstrictors and Inotropic Drugs for Shock

Drug	Rate and Adult Dose	Remarks
digoxin (Lanoxin, Lanoxicaps) (see the Prototype Drug box in Core Concept 20.7)	IV: digitalizing dose 2.5–5 mcg every 6 hours for 24 hours; maintenance dose 0.125–0.5 mg/day	Doses are highly individualized for each patient; also for dysrhythmias and heart failure
dobutamine (Dobutrex)	IV: infused at a rate of 0.5–15 mcg/kg/min (max: 40 mcg/kg/min)	Selective to $beta_1$-adrenergic receptors; for cardiac decompensation
Pr dopamine (Intropin)	IV: 2–5 mcg/kg/min initial dose; may be increased to 20–50 mcg/kg/min	May activate dopaminergic, $beta_1$- or $alpha_1$-adrenergic receptors, depending on dose
Pr epinephrine (Adrenalin)	Subcutaneous: 0.1–0.5 mL of 1:100 every 10–15 min; IV: 0.1–0.25 mL of 1:1000 every 10–15 min	Nonselective adrenergic drug; available by other routes for cardiac arrest and asthma and as an adjunct to local anesthesia
isoproterenol (Isuprel)	IV: 0.02-0.06 mg bolus followed by 5mcg/min infusion	Nonselective beta-adrenergic drug; also to reverse acute bronchospasm caused by anesthesia
Pr norepinephrine (Levophed)	IV: Initial 0.5–1 mcg/min, titrate to response; usual range 8–30 mcg/min	Activates alpha- and $beta_1$-adrenergic receptors; also for cardiac arrest
phenylephrine (Neo-Synephrine) (see the Prototype Drug box in Core Concept 9.8)	IV: 0.1–0.18 mg/min until pressure stabilizes, then 0.04–0.06 mg/min for maintenance	Selective to $alpha_1$-receptors; used to maintain blood pressure during general anesthesia; also for certain dysrhythmias, nasal congestion, and glaucoma, and to dilate the pupil during eye exams; subcutaneous, IM, ophthalmic, and intranasal forms available

Prototype Drug: Pr *Norepinephrine (Levophed)*

Therapeutic Class: Drug for shock **Pharmacologic Class:** Sympathomimetic, vasoconstrictor

Actions and Uses: Norepinephrine is indicated for acute hypotension, septic shock, and cardiac arrest. It acts directly on alpha-adrenergic receptors in the smooth muscle of blood vessels to immediately raise blood pressure. Its stimulation of $beta_1$-receptors in the heart increases the force of contraction and increases cardiac output. It is given by the IV route and has a duration of only 1 to 2 minutes after the infusion is terminated.

Adverse Effects and Interactions: Norepinephrine is a powerful vasoconstrictor; thus, continuous monitoring of blood pressure is required to prevent the development of hypertension. When first administered, reflex bradycardia is sometimes experienced. It also has the ability to produce various types of dysrhythmias. Because of its potent effects on the cardiovascular system, it should be used with great caution in patients with heart disease.

Norepinephrine interacts with many drugs, including alpha and beta blockers, which may decrease its effects on blood pressure. Conversely, ergot alkaloids and tricyclic antidepressants may increase vasopressor effects.

BLACK BOX WARNING:
Following extravasation, the affected area should be infiltrated immediately with 5–10 mg of phentolamine, an adrenergic blocker.

Inotropic drugs are useful in reversing the decreased cardiac output that occurs during shock.

◀ **Core Concept 22.5**

As shock progresses, the heart begins to fail and cardiac output declines. This lowers the amount of blood reaching vital tissues and deepens the degree of shock. **Inotropic drugs**, also called *cardiotonic drugs*, have the potential to reverse the cardiac symptoms of shock by increasing the force of myocardial contraction. The role of the inotropic drug digoxin (Lanoxin) in treating patients with heart failure was presented in Chapter 20. Digoxin increases myocardial contractility and cardiac output, thus rapidly bringing tissues their needed oxygen. Chapter 20 should be reviewed because drugs prescribed for heart failure are sometimes used for the treatment of shock.

Dopamine is often a preferred drug for increasing the cardiac output in acute situations because it has both inotropic and vasoconstriction actions. Dobutamine (Dobutrex) is a beta$_1$-adrenergic agent that has value in the short-term treatment of certain types of shock because of its ability to cause the heart to beat more forcefully without significantly increasing heart rate. The resulting increase in cardiac output assists in maintaining blood flow to vital organs. Although very effective, dobutamine has a half-life of only 2 minutes, and therapy is limited to 72 hours.

Prototype Drug: Pr *Dopamine (Intropin)*

Therapeutic Class: Drug for shock **Pharmacologic Class:** Nonselective adrenergic agonist, inotropic drug

Actions and Uses: Dopamine is the immediate metabolic precursor to norepinephrine. Although classified as a sympathomimetic, the mechanism of dopamine's action is dependent on the dose. At low doses, dopamine selectively increases blood flow through the kidneys. This makes dopamine of particular value in treating hypovolemic and cardiogenic shock. At higher doses, dopamine stimulates beta$_1$-adrenergic receptors, causing the heart to beat with more force and increasing cardiac output. Another beneficial effect of dopamine when given in higher doses is its ability to stimulate alpha-adrenergic receptors, thus causing vasoconstriction and raising blood pressure.

Adverse Effects and Interactions: Because of its intense effects on the cardiovascular system, patients receiving dopamine are continuously monitored for signs of dysrhythmias and hypotension. Adverse effects are normally self-limiting because of the short half-life of the drug.

Dopamine interacts with many other drugs. For example, administering it with monoamine oxidase inhibitors (MAOIs) and ergot alkaloids increases alpha-adrenergic effects. Phenytoin may decrease dopamine action. Beta blockers may block the cardiac effects of dopamine. Alpha blockers decrease peripheral vasoconstriction. Halothane increases the risk of hypertension and ventricular dysrhythmias.

BLACK BOX WARNING:
Following extravasation, the affected area should be infiltrated immediately with 5 mg to 10 mg of phentolamine, an adrenergic blocker.

ANAPHYLAXIS

Anaphylaxis is a type of shock caused by a hyper-response of body defense mechanisms.

◀ **Core Concept 22.6**

an = *without or against*
phylaxis = *protection*

Anaphylaxis is a condition in which the natural body defenses produce a hyper-response to an antigen. An **antigen** is anything that is recognized as foreign by the body. Certain foods, industrial chemicals, drugs, pollen, animal proteins, and even latex gloves can be antigens. A more detailed discussion of the immune system and the pharmacotherapy of immune disorders are included in Chapter 25.

Following the exposure to an antigen, the body normally responds with actions such as inflammation, antibody production, and activation of lymphocytes that rid the body of the foreign substance. During anaphylaxis, however, the body responds quickly—usually within minutes after exposure to the antigen—by releasing massive amounts of histamine and other inflammatory mediators. The patient may experience itching, hives, and a tightness in the throat or chest. Swelling occurs around the larynx, causing a hoarse voice and a nonproductive cough. As anaphylaxis progresses, the patient experiences a rapid fall in blood pressure and difficulty breathing due to

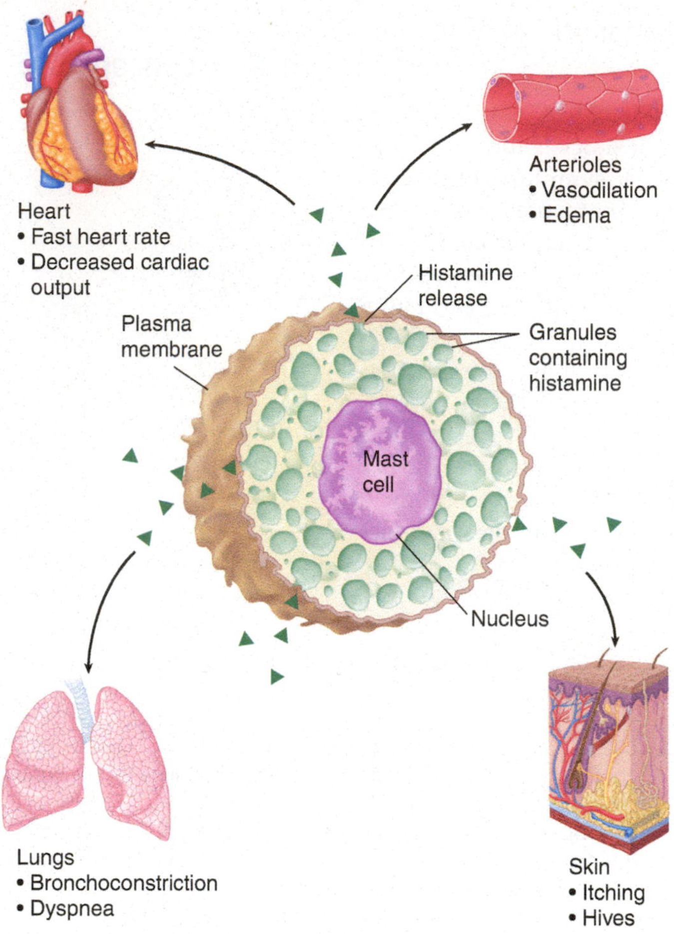

FIGURE 22.3 Symptoms of anaphylaxis.

bronchoconstriction. The fall in blood pressure causes *reflex tachycardia*, a rebound speeding up of the heart. Untreated anaphylactic shock may result in death. Figure 22.3 illustrates the signs and symptoms of anaphylaxis.

It is always easier to *prevent* anaphylaxis than it is to *treat* it. Patients should be strongly advised to avoid substances that might trigger acute allergic reactions. This includes carefully reading all food and cosmetic labels to avoid exposure to known allergens. Individuals with known allergies to insect stings or food should carry a portable form of epinephrine, such as an EpiPen. The healthcare provider should always obtain a comprehensive drug allergy history before administering medications. Common allergens include the penicillin antibiotics and iodine-based contrast media used for radiologic exams. The patient should be observed in the outpatient setting for 20 to 60 minutes after a drug injection because delayed anaphylactic reactions are possible.

The pharmacotherapy of anaphylaxis involves supporting the cardiovascular system and preventing further hyper-response by body defenses. Various medications are used to treat the symptoms of anaphylaxis, depending on the severity of the symptoms.

At the first suspicion of anaphylaxis, epinephrine is administered and IV fluid infusions are begun. Epinephrine is an initial drug for acute shock because it causes vasoconstriction and can rapidly relieve symptoms of bronchoconstriction. It may be necessary to use other vasoconstrictors (see Table 22.3) to overcome severe hypotension. Infusion of large amounts of fluids may be needed to overcome circulatory shock. These may include blood products, colloids, or crystalloids. Fluid infusions continue until systolic blood pressure reaches at least 90 mmHg and is stable.

Prototype Drug: Epinephrine (Adrenalin)

Therapeutic Class: Drug for anaphylaxis and shock **Pharmacologic Class:** Sympathomimetic, vasoconstrictor

Actions and Uses: Subcutaneous or IV epinephrine is a preferred drug for treating acute anaphylactic shock because it can reverse many of the distressing symptoms within minutes. Epinephrine is nonselective and activates both alpha- and beta-adrenergic receptors. Immediately after injection, blood pressure rises due to the stimulation of $alpha_1$-receptors. Activation of $beta_2$-receptors in the bronchi opens the airways to relieve shortness of breath. Cardiac output increases due to stimulation of $beta_1$-receptors in the heart. Epinephrine can also be administered topically, by inhalation, or by the intracardiac route.

Adverse Effects and Interactions: The most common adverse effects of epinephrine are nervousness, tremors, palpitations, dizziness, headache, and stinging or burning at the site of application. When administered parenterally, hypertension and dysrhythmias may occur rapidly; therefore, the patient is monitored continuously following IV or subcutaneous injections.

Epinephrine interacts with many drugs. For example, it may increase hypotension with phenothiazines and oxytocin. There may be additive toxicities with other sympathomimetics. MAOIs, tricyclic antidepressants, and alpha- and beta-adrenergic drugs inhibit the actions of epinephrine.

A number of other drugs are useful in treating symptoms of anaphylaxis. Oxygen is usually administered immediately. Antihistamines such as diphenhydramine (Benadryl) may be given intramuscularly or intravenously to prevent additional release of histamine. A bronchodilator such as albuterol (Ventolin, Proventil) is sometimes administered by inhalation to relieve the acute shortness of breath caused by histamine release. Corticosteroids such as hydrocortisone may be administered to dampen the acute inflammatory response that occurs during anaphylaxis. Corticosteroids may be administered for 24 hours or longer to prevent the possibility of delayed anaphylactic reactions. Additional effects of antihistamines are discussed in Chapter 25, bronchodilators in Chapter 30, and corticosteroids in Chapter 33, respectively.

CONCEPT REVIEW 22.2

- How can inotropic drugs reduce the symptoms of shock without causing vasoconstriction?

Patients Need to Know

Patients treated for shock need to know the following:

1. Seek emergency medical assistance immediately if signs or symptoms of shock are being experienced.
2. While waiting for medical assistance, keep warm by using blankets.
3. Have a caregiver, if present, monitor temperature, pulse, and blood pressure until emergency medical assistance arrives.
4. Do not move around. Lie down and elevate the feet.
5. Report any changes in mental status, such as depression, confusion, or anxiety, to the healthcare provider immediately.
6. Take medications for shock (such as epinephrine) exactly as prescribed.

Patients using epinephrine injectable pens need to know the following:

7. Learn how to use the pen prior to actually needing to use it.
8. Carry medication at all times in case of allergy exposure. Inform others of any allergies, where medication is kept, and how to administer it.
9. Report to the healthcare provider if any of the following occurs after using epinephrine pen: difficulty in breathing, severe headache, blurred vision, ringing in the ears, irregular heartbeat.
10. Seek emergency medical attention immediately after using the pen. Drug effects may wear off after 10-20 minutes.

Chapter Review

Core Concepts Summary

22.1 Shock is a syndrome characterized by the collapse of the circulatory system.

Basic types of shock include cardiogenic, hypovolemic, neurogenic, septic, and anaphylactic shock. Nonspecific symptoms of shock include hypotension, cold or clammy skin, reduced cardiac output, and behavioral changes such as confusion, apathy, or disorientation.

22.2 The initial treatment of shock includes basic life support and identification of the underlying cause.

Shock may be life threatening if allowed to proceed without medical intervention. Immediate therapy is targeted at restoring or maintaining vital processes such as respiratory function, blood pressure, and cardiac output. Immediate drug therapy includes vasoconstrictors, inotropic drugs, and IV fluid agents.

22.3 Intravenous fluid replacement drugs are given to replace fluids lost during shock.

IV fluid replacement agents include blood products, colloids, and crystalloids. These drugs help to maintain circulation and raise blood pressure.

22.4 Vasoconstrictors are administered during shock to maintain blood pressure.

An immediate concern for the patient in shock is a fall in blood pressure. A variety of adrenergic drugs, both selective and nonselective, are used to maintain blood pressure and cardiac function.

22.5 Inotropic drugs are useful in reversing the decreased cardiac output that occurs during shock.

Circulatory failure can occur during shock if the cardiac output falls below a critical level. A number of inotropic drugs are used to strengthen myocardial function and to improve cardiac output.

22.6 Anaphylaxis is a type of shock caused by a hyper-response of body defense mechanisms.

When the body mounts a hyper-response to an antigen, anaphylactic shock may result. Epinephrine is a preferred drug for immediately reversing the cardiovascular symptoms. IV fluid infusion agents, antihistamines, and corticosteroids also serve roles in treating this form of shock.

REVIEW Questions

Answer the following questions to assess your knowledge of the chapter material, and go back and review any material that is not clear to you.

1. The patient with severe burns has just been admitted to the hospital. The nurse will monitor for signs and symptoms of:
1. Cardiogenic shock.
2. Hypovolemic shock.
3. Septic shock.
4. Anaphylactic shock.

2. In the plan of care, the *most* important intervention for a patient experiencing shock is assessing:
1. Temperature.
2. Heart rate.
3. Respirations rate.
4. Blood pressure.

3. Which intravenous solution would be most appropriate for a patient in hypovolemic shock?
1. 0.45% NS
2. Normal serum albumin
3. 0.33% NS
4. D5W

4. The patient's family is asking questions about the medications used in the treatment for shock. The nurse explains that dopamine is one of the drugs being used and that it works: (Select all that apply.)
1. At low doses, to cause increased blood flow to the kidneys.
2. At high doses, to increase cardiac output.
3. To cause vasoconstriction and increases blood pressure.
4. At high doses, to treat anaphylaxis.
5. At low doses, to treat anaphylaxis.

5. The patient is experiencing anaphylaxis. Which drug would be administered to increase blood pressure and treat bronchospasm related to anaphylaxis?
1. Epinephrine
2. Dobutamine (Dobutrex)
3. Digoxin (Lanoxin)
4. Dopamine

6. In reviewing a plan of care for a patient exhibiting the symptoms of anaphylaxis, which of the following medications would be avoided?
1. Antihistamines
2. Corticosteroids
3. Bronchodilators
4. Vasodilators

7. After administering an inotropic medication to a patient in shock, the nurse monitors the patient for signs of:
1. Decreased cardiac output.
2. Increased cardiac output.
3. Slowing of the heart rate.
4. Increased afterload.

8. When administering norepinephrine (Levophed), the nurse monitors the patient for:
1. Bradycardia.
2. Hypotension.
3. Hypertension.
4. Liver failure.

9. Dobutamine (Dobutrex) is used to treat shock because:
1. It increases myocardial contractility and heart rate.
2. It increases myocardial contractility without significantly increasing heart rate.
3. It decreases cardiac output.
4. It is a powerful vasoconstrictor.

10. The healthcare provider has ordered 1000 mL of 0.9% sodium chloride to be administered intravenously over 5 hours. The drop factor on the tubing is 15 drops/mL. How many milliliters per hour will you administer and how many drops per minute?
    1. 250 mL/hr and 50 drops/min
    2. 200 mL/hr and 50 drops/min
    3. 200 mL/hr and 45 drops/min
    4. 250 mL/hr and 45 drops/min

CASE STUDY Questions

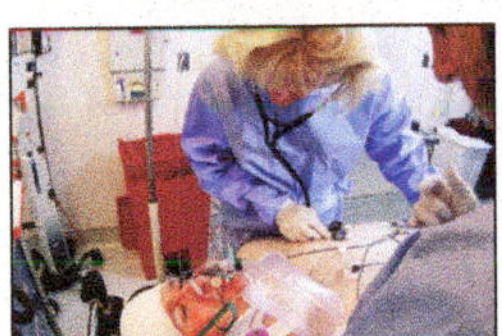

Remember Mr. Hanks from the beginning of the chapter? Now read the remainder of the case study. Based on the information you have learned in this chapter, answer the questions that follow.

Mr. Joshua Hanks arrives in the emergency department having lost a considerable amount of blood in an automobile crash. His blood pressure is 60/30 mmHg. His skin is clammy, and he is going in and out of consciousness. He is gasping for breath. The healthcare provider orders an infusion of 0.9% sodium chloride, IV dobutamine, IM hydrocortisone, and subcutaneous epinephrine.

1. The nurse notices that Mr. Hanks's breathing is labored and he appears anxious. The nurse administers which of the prescribed medications to help reduce Mr. Hanks's bronchospasm?
    1. 0.9% sodium chloride
    2. Dobutamine
    3. Hydrocortisone
    4. Epinephrine
2. Which drug was given to replace the fluids lost during Mr. Hanks's accident?
    1. 0.9% sodium chloride
    2. Dobutamine
    3. Hydrocortisone
    4. Epinephrine
3. Within 2 minutes, Mr. Hanks's blood pressure increases to 100/60 mmHg. Which drug most likely caused this effect?
    1. 0.9% sodium chloride
    2. Dobutamine
    3. Hydrocortisone
    4. Epinephrine
4. After 4 hours, Mr. Hanks has stabilized, but he still has some difficulty breathing. As ordered by the healthcare provider, which of the following drugs would the nurse most likely be administering to help Mr. Hanks with his breathing difficulties?
    1. Diphenhydramine (Benadryl)
    2. Hydrocortisone
    3. Phenylephrine (Neo-Synephrine)
    4. Albuterol (Ventolin)

Answers and complete rationales for the Review and Case Study Questions appear in Appendix A.

REFERENCE

Herdman, T. H., & Kamitsuru, S. (Eds.). (2014). *NANDA International nursing diagnoses: Definitions and classification, 2015–2017*. Oxford, United Kingdom: Wiley-Blackwell.

SELECTED BIBLIOGRAPHY

American Heart Association. (2015). *Highlights of the 2015 American Heart Association Guidelines Update for CPR and ECC*. Retrieved from http://eccguidelines.heart.org/wp-content/uploads/2015/10/2015-AHA-Guidelines-Highlights-English.pdf

Asfar, P., Meziani, F., Hamel, J. F., Grelon, F., Megarbane, B., Anguel, N., . . . Radermacher, P. (2014). High versus low blood-pressure target in patients with septic shock. *The New England Journal of Medicine, 370*, 1583–1593. doi:10.1056/NEJMoa1312173

Avni, T., Lador, A., Lev, S., Leibovici, L., Paul, M., & Grossman, A. (2015). Vasopressors for the treatment of septic shock: Systematic review and meta-analysis. *PloS ONE, 10*(8), e0129305. doi:10.1371/journal.pone.0129305

Crawford, A., & Harris, H. (2015). Anaphylaxis: Rapid recognition and treatment. *Nursing2015 Critical Care, 10*(4), 32–37. doi:10.1097/01.CCN.0000466766.77929.1a

Fawzy, A., Evans, S. R., & Walkey, A. J. (2015). Practice patterns and outcomes associated with choice of initial vasopressor therapy for septic shock. *Critical Care Medicine, 43*(10), 2141–2146. doi: 10.1097/CCM.0000000000001149

Kalil, A. (2015). *Septic shock*. Retrieved from http://emedicine.medscape.com/article/168402-overview

Mustafa, S. S. (2015). *Anaphylaxis*. Retrieved from http://emedicine.medscape.com/article/135065-overview

Nagendran, M., Maruthappu, M., Gordon, A. C., & Gurusamy, K. S. (2016). Comparative safety and efficacy of vasopressors for mortality in septic shock: A network meta-analysis. *Journal of the Intensive Care Society, 17*(2), 136–145 doi:10.1177/1751143715620203

Pierce, J. D., Shen, Q., & Thimmesch, A. (2016). The ongoing controversy: Crystalloids versus colloids. *Journal of Infusion Nursing*, 39 40–44. doi:10.1097/NAN.0000000000000149

Rance, K., & Goldberg, P. (2015). Anaphylaxis overview: Addressing unmet patient needs. *The Journal for Nurse Practitioners, 11*(3), 352–359. doi:10.1016/j.nurpra.2014.09.006

Ren, Xiushui, (2015). *Cardiogenic shock*. Retrieved from http://emedicine.medscape.com/article/152191-overview

Thibeault, S. (2015). Massive transfusion for hemorrhagic shock: What every critical care nurse needs to know. *Critical Care Nursing Clinics of North America, 27*, 47–53. doi:10.1016/j.cnc.2014.10.008

Chapter 23

Drugs for Dysrhythmias

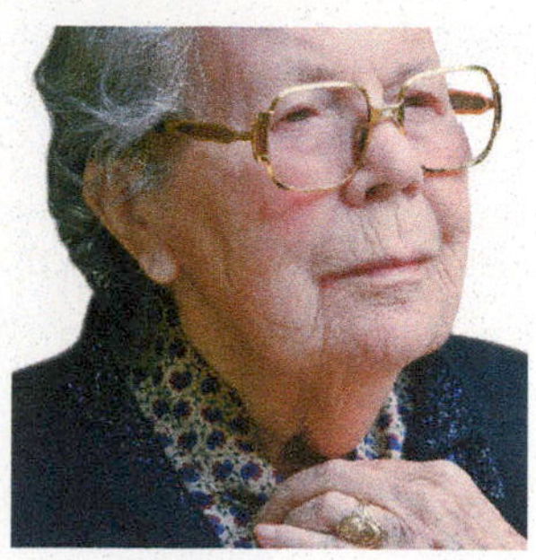

"I've never had anything happen like this. I was watching TV, and all of a sudden, my heart started racing."

Mrs. Margaret Duncan

Core Concepts

23.1 **Some types of dysrhythmias produce no patient symptoms, whereas others may be life threatening.**

23.2 **Dysrhythmias are classified by the type of rhythm abnormality produced and its location.**

23.3 **The electrical conduction pathway in the myocardium keeps the heart beating in a synchronized manner.**

23.4 **Most antidysrhythmic drugs act by blocking ion channels in myocardial cells.**

23.5 **Antidysrhythmic drugs are classified by their mechanisms of action.**

23.6 **Sodium channel blockers slow the rate of impulse conduction through the heart.**

23.7 **Beta-adrenergic blockers reduce automaticity and slow conduction velocity in the heart.**

23.8 **Potassium channel blockers prolong the refractory period of the heart.**

23.9 **Calcium channel blockers are available to treat supraventricular dysrhythmias.**

23.10 **Digoxin and adenosine are used for specific dysrhythmias but do not act by blocking ion channels.**

Drug Snapshot

The following drugs are discussed in this chapter:

Drug Classes	Prototype Drugs
Sodium channel blockers	Pr procainamide
Beta-adrenergic blockers	Pr propranolol (Inderal, InnoPran XL)
Potassium channel blockers	Pr amiodarone (Cordarone)
Calcium channel blockers	Pr verapamil (Calan, Isoptin SR, others)
Miscellaneous drugs	

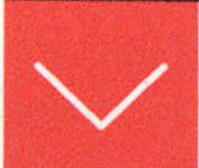

Learning Outcomes

After reading this chapter, the student should be able to:

1. Identify patient symptoms associated with cardiac dysrhythmias.
2. Classify dysrhythmias based on their location and type of conduction abnormality.
3. Illustrate the flow of electrical impulses through the normal heart.
4. Explain the importance of ion channels to cardiac function and the pharmacotherapy of dysrhythmias.

5. Explain the basic mechanisms by which antidysrhythmic drugs act.
6. Explain the role of sodium channel blockers in treating dysrhythmias.
7. Explain the role of beta-adrenergic blockers in treating dysrhythmias.
8. Explain the role of potassium channel blockers in treating dysrhythmias.
9. Explain the role of calcium channel blockers in treating dysrhythmias.
10. Explain the role of digoxin and adenosine in treating dysrhythmias.

Key Terms

atrioventricular (AV) node (ay-tree-oh-ven-TRIK-you-lur noad)
atrioventricular bundle (ay-tree-oh-ven-TRIK-you-lur BUN-dul)
automaticity (aw-toh-muh-TISS-uh-tee)
bundle branches (BUN-dul BRAN-chez)
calcium ion channels (KAL-see-um)
depolarization (dee-po-lur-eye-ZAY-shun)
dysrhythmias (diss-RITH-mee-uh)
ectopic foci/pacemakers (ek-TOP-ik FO-si)
electrocardiogram (ECG) (e-lek-tro-KAR-dee-oh-gram)
fibrillation (fi-bruh-LAY-shun)
polarized (POLE-uh-rized)
potassium ion channels (po-TASS-ee-um)
Purkinje fibers (purr-KEN-gee FI-burrs)
refractory period (ree-FRAK-tor-ee)
sinoatrial (SA) node (si-no-AYE-tree-ul noad)
sodium ion channels (SO-dee-um)

Dysrhythmias are abnormalities of electrical conduction or rhythm in the heart. Sometimes called arrhythmias, they encompass a number of different disorders that range from harmless to life threatening. Diagnosis is often difficult because patients usually must be connected to an electrocardiogram (ECG) and be experiencing symptoms to determine the exact type of rhythm disorder. Accurate diagnosis and optimum pharmacologic treatment can significantly reduce the frequency of serious dysrhythmias and their consequences.

dys = *difficult or bad*
rhythm = *rhythm*
ia = *condition*

Some types of dysrhythmias produce no patient symptoms, whereas others may be life threatening.

◀ **Core Concept 23.1**

Whereas some dysrhythmias produce no symptoms and have negligible effects on heart function, others are life threatening and require immediate treatment. Typical symptoms of a dysrhythmia include dizziness, weakness, decreased exercise tolerance, shortness of breath, and fainting. Many patients report palpitations or a sensation that their heart has skipped a beat. Persistent dysrhythmias are associated with increased risk of stroke and heart failure. Severe dysrhythmias may cause sudden death. Because asymptomatic patients may not seek medical attention, it is difficult to estimate the frequency of the disease.

a = *no or not*
symptomat = *symptoms*
ic = *pertaining to*

Dysrhythmias are classified by the type of rhythm abnormality produced and its location.

◀ **Core Concept 23.2**

There are many types of dysrhythmias, and they may be classified by a number of different methods. The simplest method is to name dysrhythmias according to the type of rhythm abnormality produced and their locations. A summary of the different dysrhythmias along with a brief description of each type is given in Table 23.1. Dysrhythmias that originate in the atria are sometimes referred to as supraventricular. Those that originate in the ventricles are generally more serious because they are more likely to interfere with the normal function of the heart. Although obtaining a correct diagnosis of the type of dysrhythmia is sometimes difficult, it is essential for effective treatment. Atrial **fibrillation (commonly called A-fib)** is the most common type of dysrhythmia.

supra = *above*
ventricular = *cardiac ventricle*

Table 23.1 Types of Dysrhythmias

Name of Dysrhythmia	Description
Atrial or ventricular flutter or fibrillation	Very rapid, uncoordinated beats; atrial may require treatment but is not usually fatal; ventricular flutter or fibrillation requires immediate treatment
Atrial or ventricular tachycardia	Rapid heartbeat greater than 100 beats per minute in adults; ventricular tachycardia is more serious than atrial tachycardia
Heart block	Area of nonconduction in the myocardium; may be partial or complete; classified as first, second, or third degree
Premature atrial or premature ventricular contractions (PVCs)	An extra beat often originating from a source other than the sinoatrial (SA) node; not normally serious unless it occurs frequently
Sinus bradycardia	Slow heartbeat, less than 60 beats per minute; may require a pacemaker
Torsades de pointes	Serious type of ventricular tachycardia that often occurs in patients with a long QT interval; may occur as a side effect of certain drugs such as amiodarone, fluoroquinolones, and amphetamine

Fast Facts Dysrhythmias

- Atrial fibrillation is much more common in men than in women.
- The incidence of atrial fibrillation increases with age. They affect:
  - About 0.1% of those younger than age 55
  - About 3.8% of those over age 60
  - About 10% of those over age 80
- The risk of stroke is between two and seven times above normal in patients with atrial fibrillation.
- Up to a third of sudden cardiac deaths are believed to be caused by ventricular dysrhythmias.
- Ventricular fibrillation is responsible for 5% of all deaths in the pediatric and adolescent age groups.

Source: Based on Rosenthal, L. (2016) *Atrial fibrillation*. Retrieved from http://emedicine.medscape.com/article/151066-overview

Dysrhythmias can occur in both healthy and diseased hearts. Although the actual cause of most dysrhythmias is elusive, dysrhythmias are often associated with certain conditions, primarily heart disease and myocardial infarction (MI). Following are some conditions associated with dysrhythmias:

- Hypertension (HTN)
- Cardiac valve disease, such as mitral stenosis
- Coronary artery disease
- Medications such as digoxin
- Low potassium levels in the blood
- Myocardial infarction
- Adverse effect from antidysrhythmic medication
- Stroke
- Diabetes mellitus
- Congestive heart failure.

Core Concept 23.3 ▶

The electrical conduction pathway in the myocardium keeps the heart beating in a synchronized manner.

Although there are many different types of dysrhythmias, all have in common a defect in the formation or conduction of electrical impulses across the myocardium. These electrical impulses carry the signal for cardiac muscle cells to contract and must be coordinated precisely for the chambers to beat in a synchronized manner. For the heart to function properly, the atria must contract simultaneously, sending their blood into the ventricles. Following atrial contraction, the right and left ventricles then must contract simultaneously. Lack of synchronization of the atria and ventricles or of the right and left sides of the heart may have serious consequences. The normal conduction pathway in the heart is illustrated in Figure 23.1.

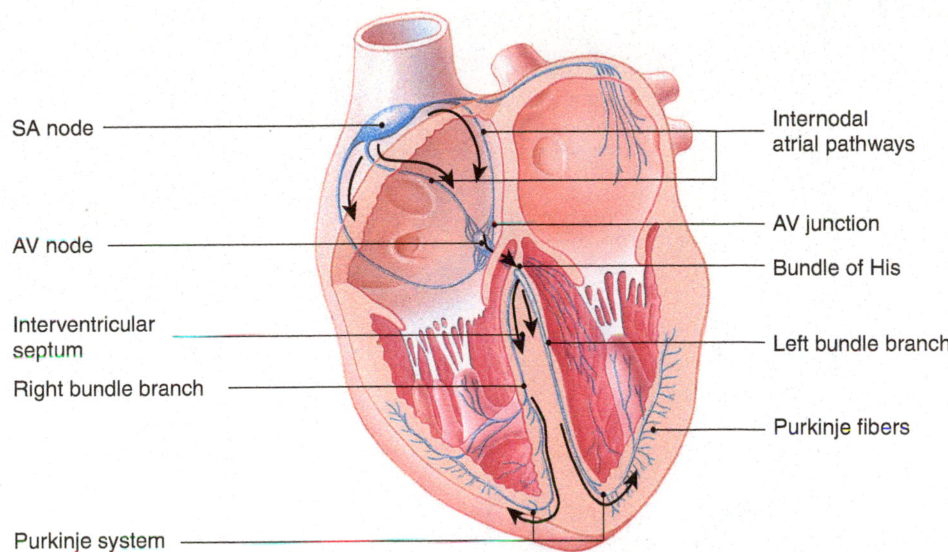

FIGURE 23.1 Normal conduction pathway in the heart.

Control of this synchronization begins in a small area of tissue in the wall of the right atrium called the **sinoatrial (SA) node**. The SA node or pacemaker of the heart has a property called **automaticity**, the ability of certain cells to spontaneously generate an electrical impulse known as an *action potential*, without instructions from the nervous system. The SA node generates a new action potential approximately 75 times every minute under resting conditions.

On leaving the SA node, the action potential travels quickly across both atria to the **atrioventricular (AV) node**, a small area of specialized fibers that lies in the wall separating the two atria. The AV node also has the property of automaticity, although less than the SA node. If the SA node malfunctions, the AV node has the ability to spontaneously generate action potentials and continue the heart's contraction.

As the action potential leaves the AV node, it travels rapidly to the **atrioventricular bundle** or bundle of His, which is responsible for carrying the electrical signal from the atria to the ventricles. The impulse is then conducted down the right and left **bundle branches** (tissue that carries electrical signal impulse from the AV bundle to the Purkinje fibers). The **Purkinje fibers** carry the electrical impulse to all regions of the ventricles almost simultaneously.

The wave of electrical activity across the myocardium can be measured by an **electrocardiogram (ECG)**. The total time for the electrical impulse to be generated by the SA node and travel across the heart is about 0.22 second. A normal ECG and its relationship to impulse conduction in the heart are shown in Figure 23.2.

Although action potentials normally begin at the SA node and spread across the myocardium in a coordinated manner, other regions of the heart may begin to initiate beats. These areas, known as **ectopic foci** or **ectopic pacemakers**, may send impulses across the myocardium that compete with those from the normal conduction system. Although healthy hearts often experience an extra beat without incident, ectopic foci in diseased hearts have the potential to cause many of the types of dysrhythmias noted in Table 23.1.

ec = *outside*
top = *place*
ic = *pertaining to*

It is important to understand that the underlying purpose of this conduction system is to keep the heart beating in a regular, synchronized manner so that cardiac output can be maintained. Some dysrhythmias occur sporadically, produce no symptoms, and cause little or no effect on cardiac output. These types of abnormalities may go unnoticed by the patient and rarely require treatment. Some dysrhythmias, however, seriously affect cardiac output, producing patient symptoms and resulting in potentially serious, if not mortal, consequences. It is these types of dysrhythmias that require pharmacotherapy.

CONCEPT REVIEW 23.1

- Trace the flow of electrical conduction across the heart. What would happen if the impulse never reached the AV node?

FIGURE 23.2 Relationship of the electrocardiogram to electrical conduction in the heart.

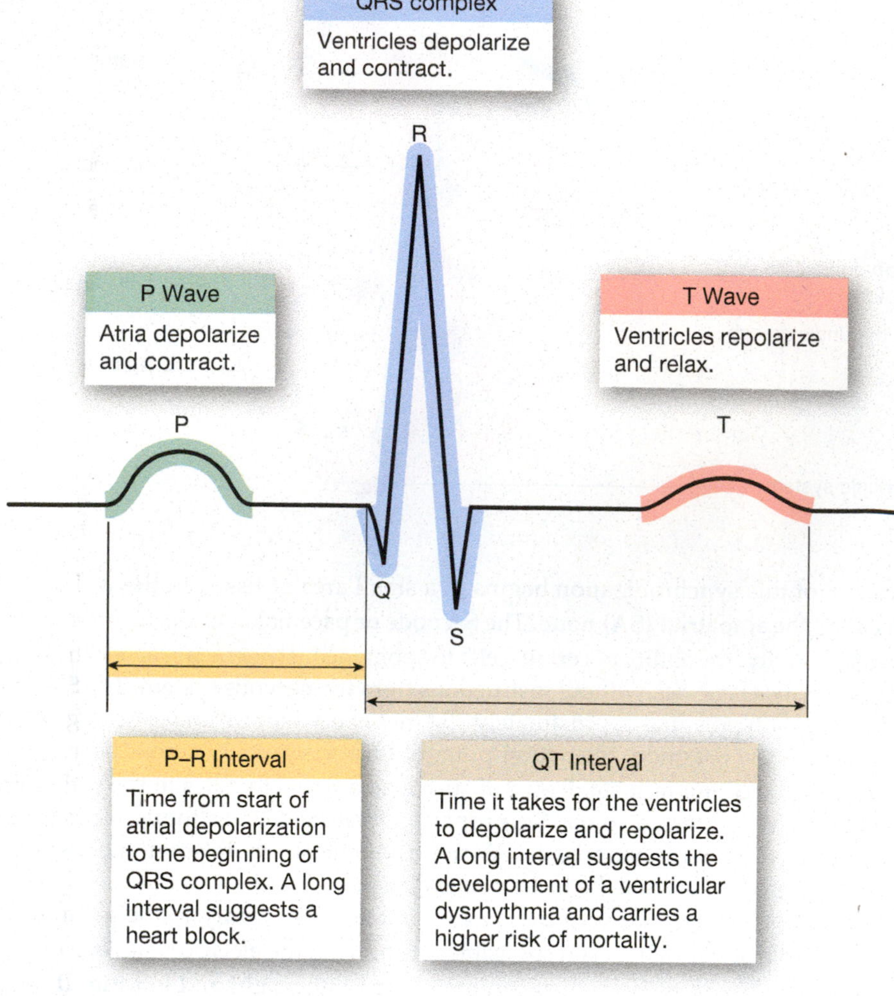

Core Concept 23.4 ▶

Most antidysrhythmic drugs act by blocking ion channels in myocardial cells.

Because most antidysrhythmic drugs act by interfering with the cardiac action potential, a firm grasp of this phenomenon is necessary for understanding drug mechanisms. Action potentials occur in both neurons and cardiac muscle cells due to differences in the concentration of certain ions found inside and outside the cell. Under resting conditions, sodium ions (Na^+) and calcium ions (Ca^{2+}) are found in higher concentrations *outside* the myocardial cells, whereas potassium ions (K^+) are found in higher concentrations *inside* these cells. These imbalances are, in part, responsible for the inside of a myocardial cell membrane being slightly negatively charged relative to the outside of the membrane. A cell having this negative membrane potential is said to be **polarized**.

An action potential begins when **sodium ion channels** located in the plasma membrane open and Na^+ rushes into the cell, producing a rapid **depolarization**, or loss of membrane potential. During this period, Ca^{2+} also enters the cell through **calcium ion channels**. It is this influx of Ca^{2+} that is responsible for the contraction of cardiac muscle. The cell returns to its polarized state by the removal of Na^+ from the cell via the sodium pump and movement of K^+ back into the cell through **potassium ion channels**. In cells located in the SA and AV nodes, it is the influx of Ca^{2+}, rather than Na^+, that generates the rapid depolarization of the membrane.

Although it may seem complicated to learn the different ions involved in an action potential, this knowledge is vital to understanding cardiac pharmacology. Blocking

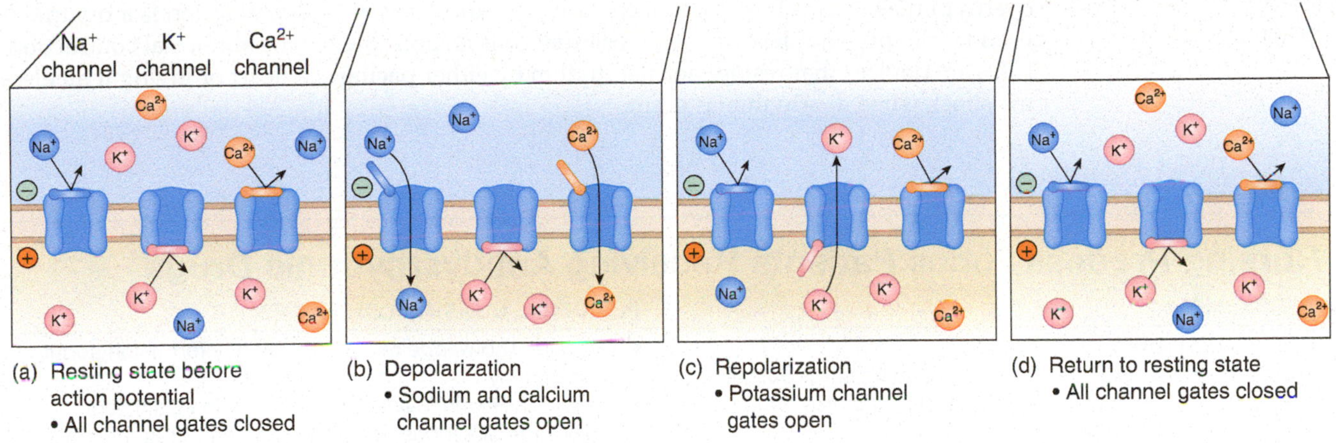

FIGURE 23.3 The flow of ions through ion channels in myocardial cells.

potassium, sodium, or calcium ion channels is the primary pharmacologic strategy used to prevent or terminate dysrhythmias. Figure 23.3 illustrates the flow of ions during the action potential.

The pumping action of the heart requires alternating periods of contraction and relaxation. There is a brief period following depolarization when the cell cannot initiate another action potential. This time, known as the **refractory period**, ensures that the myocardial cell finishes contracting before a second action potential begins. Some antidysrhythmic drugs produce their effects by prolonging the refractory period.

Antidysrhythmic drugs are classified by their mechanisms of action.

◀ **Core Concept 23.5**

The therapeutic goal of antidysrhythmic pharmacotherapy is to prevent or terminate dysrhythmias to reduce the risk for sudden death, stroke, or other complications resulting from the disease. All antidysrhythmic drugs have the potential to profoundly affect the heart's conduction system. Because they can cause serious adverse effects, antidysrhythmic drugs are normally reserved for patients experiencing symptoms of dysrhythmia or for those whose condition cannot be controlled by other means. Treating asymptomatic dysrhythmias with medications provides little or no benefit to the patient.

Antidysrhythmic drugs are grouped by the stage at which they affect the action potential. These drugs fall into four primary classes and a miscellaneous group that does not act by one of the first four mechanisms. Classes of antidysrhythmics include the following:

- Sodium channel blockers (Class I)
- Beta-adrenergic blockers (Class II)
- Potassium channel blockers (Class III)
- Calcium channel blockers (Class IV)
- Miscellaneous antidysrhythmic drugs.

The use of antidysrhythmic drugs has significantly declined in the past 20 years. Research has determined that the use of antidysrhythmic medications for prophylaxis can actually *increase* mortality in some patients. This is because there is a narrow margin between a therapeutic effect and a toxic effect with drugs that affect cardiac rhythm. They have the ability not only to *correct* dysrhythmias but also to worsen or even *create* new dysrhythmias. The healthcare provider must carefully monitor patients taking antidysrhythmic drugs. Often, the patient is hospitalized during the initial stages of therapy so that the optimum dose can be accurately determined.

Another reason for the decline in antidysrhythmic drug use is the success of nonpharmacologic techniques. Research has demonstrated that catheter ablation and implantable cardioverter defibrillators (ICDs) are more successful in managing certain types of dysrhythmias than is the prophylactic use of medications. Catheter ablation is a treatment used to identify and destroy the myocardial cells responsible for the abnormal conduction. ICDs are devices that restore normal rhythm by either pacing the heart or giving it an electric shock when dysrhythmias occur.

Nursing Process Focus Patients Receiving Antidysrhythmic Drugs

ASSESSMENT	POTENTIAL NURSING DIAGNOSES*
Prior to administration: • Obtain a complete health history including cardiovascular, neurological, renal and liver conditions, allergies, drug history, and possible drug interactions. • Evaluate laboratory blood findings: complete blood count (CBC), electrolytes, lipid panel, and renal and liver function studies. • Acquire the results of a complete physical examination, including vital signs, height, weight, ECG, level of consciousness (LOC), and urinary output.	• *Deficient Knowledge* related to lack of information about drug therapy • *Ineffective Health Maintenance* related to insufficient knowledge of seriousness of disease and drug therapy regimen • *Risk for Ineffective Tissue Perfusion* related to cardiac conduction abnormality • *Risk for Injury* related to adverse effects of drug therapy

PLANNING: PATIENT GOALS AND EXPECTED OUTCOMES

The patient will:

- Experience therapeutic effects (stabilization of heart rate, heart rhythm, sensorium, urinary output, and vital signs).
- Be free from or experience minimal adverse effects from drug therapy.
- Verbalize an understanding of the drug's use, adverse effects, and required precautions.

IMPLEMENTATION

Interventions and (Rationales)	Patient Education/Discharge Planning
• Administer medication correctly, and evaluate the patient's knowledge of proper administration. (Proper use of medication ensures that the patient will receive intended results and minimize adverse effects.)	Instruct the patient to: • Never discontinue the drug abruptly. • Take the drug exactly as prescribed, even if feeling well. • Take the pulse prior to taking the drug (may need to demonstrate technique). • Immediately notify the healthcare provider for further instructions if pulse is below the "reportable" pulse rate, usually 60 beats per minute. • Take blood pressure frequently if taking an antidysrhythmic medication that also lowers blood pressure.
• Ensure cardiac rate and rhythm are monitored continuously if administering the drug IV and regularly if administered orally. (The IV route is used when rapid therapeutic effects are needed. Monitoring is needed to detect any potential serious dysrhythmias. Immediately report any changes in heart sounds or rhythm.)	• Explain to the patient the need for continuous ECG monitoring when administering the medication intravenously. • For patients taking oral medications, explain the need to follow up with intermittent cardiac/holter monitoring as prescribed by the healthcare provider.
• Monitor the IV site, and administer all IV medications via an infusion pump. (Administering IV cardiac medications via an infusion pump helps to ensure safety and accuracy.)	• Instruct the patient to report any burning or stinging pain, swelling, warmth, redness, or tenderness at the IV insertion site.
• Obtain information regarding possible causes of the dysrhythmia. (Electrolyte imbalances, hypoxia, pain, anxiety, caffeine ingestion, and tobacco use can contribute to dysrhythmias.)	Instruct the patient to: • Maintain a diet low in sodium and fat with sufficient potassium. • Report to the healthcare provider symptoms such as vomiting, diarrhea, and dehydration because they may enhance the development of an electrolyte imbalance, an adverse effect associated with some antidysrhythmic drugs. • Avoid the use of caffeine and tobacco products.
• Observe for adverse effects specific to the antidysrhythmic used. (These drugs affect heart function and can cause serious adverse effects. Continuing or worsening cardiac symptoms may indicate inadequate drug therapy.)	Instruct the patient to report to the healthcare provider: • Any adverse effects specific to the prescribed antidysrhythmic, such as visual disturbances or skin rashes caused by potassium channel blockers. • Any cardiac-related symptoms such as dizziness, hypotension, palpitations, chest pain, dyspnea, unusual fatigue, and weakness.

Interventions and (Rationales)	Patient Education/Discharge Planning
• Check for edema, noting location and character. Weigh patient daily, and report a weight gain or loss of 2 lb (1 kg) or more in a 24-hour period. (Daily weight is an accurate measure of fluid status; weight gain or edema may indicate adverse drug effect or worsening cardiac disease.)	Have the patient: • Weigh and record their weight daily, ideally at the same time of day. • Report to healthcare provider a weight loss or gain of more than 2 lb (1 kg) in a 24-hour period.
• Monitor ongoing laboratory results of electrolytes, especially potassium and magnesium; renal function, and drug levels. (Hypokalemia or hypomagnesemia increases the risk of dysrhythmias. Inadequate or high drug levels may lead to increased dysrhythmias.)	Instruct the patient on the need to: • Return periodically for laboratory work. • Carry a wallet ID card or wear medical alert jewelry indicating antidysrhythmia medication.
• Monitor lung sounds. Immediately report if patient is experiencing worsening dyspnea, crackles, or pink, frothy pink-tinged sputum. (New or worsening dysrhythmias may cause lung congestion and possible heart failure.)	• Instruct the patient to immediately report to the healthcare provider any severe shortness of breath, frothy sputum, profound fatigue, or swelling of extremities.
EVALUATION OF OUTCOME CRITERIA	
Evaluate the effectiveness of drug therapy by confirming that patient goals and expected outcomes have been met (see "Planning"). *See Tables 23.2 through 23.5 for lists of drugs to which these nursing actions apply.*	

*Herdman, T.H. & Kamitsuru, S. (Eds.), *Nursing Diagnoses: Definitions & Classification* 2015–2017. Copyright © 2014, 1994–2014 NANDA International. Used by arrangement by John Wiley & Sons, Inc. Companion website: www.wiley.com/go/nursingdiagnoses.

Sodium channel blockers slow the rate of impulse conduction through the heart.

◄ **Core Concept 23.6**

The first medical uses of the sodium channel blockers were recorded in the 18th century. Quinidine, the oldest antidysrhythmic drug, was originally obtained as a natural substance from the bark of the South American *Cinchona* tree. Although a prototype for many decades, quinidine (Quinidex, others) is rarely used today owing to the availability of safer antidysrhythmics. Sodium channel blockers used as antidysrhythmics are listed in Table 23.2.

Sodium channel blockers, the Class I drugs, are the largest group of antidysrhythmics. They are divided into three subgroups—IA, IB, and IC—based on subtle differences in their mechanisms of action. Because the action potential is dependent on the opening of sodium ion channels, a blockade of these channels will slow the spread of impulse conduction across the myocardium. This slowing of conduction will suppress ectopic pacemaker activity.

The chemical structures and actions of the sodium channel blockers are similar to those of the local anesthetics. In fact, the antidysrhythmic drug lidocaine is a prototype local anesthetic in Chapter 16. This anesthetic-like action slows impulse conduction across the heart.

Table 23.2 Sodium Channel Blockers (Class I)

Drug	Rate and Adult Dose	Remarks
disopyramide (Norpace)	PO (immediate release): 100–200 mg q6h PO (controlled release): 300 mg bid	Class 1A; usually reserved for serious ventricular dysrhythmias
flecainide (Tambocor)	PO: 100 mg bid (max: 300-400 mg/day)	Class 1C; usually reserved for serious ventricular dysrhythmias
lidocaine (Xylocaine) (see the Prototype Drug box in Core Concept 16.3)	IV: 1–4 mg/min infusion rate (max: 3 mg/kg per 5–10 min)	Class 1B; usually reserved for rapid control of ventricular dysrhythmias; IM, subcutaneous, and topical forms available; also widely used as a local anesthetic
mexiletine (Mexitil)	PO: 200–300 mg tid (max: 1200 mg/day)	Class 1B; usually reserved for serious ventricular dysrhythmias
Pr procainamide	IV: 100 mg q5min at a rate of 25-50 mg/min (max: 1 g)	Class 1A; IM, IV, and sustained-release forms available; for both atrial and ventricular dysrhythmias
propafenone (Rythmol)	PO: (immediate release) 150-300 mg bid PO (sustained release): 225-425 mg bid	Class 1C; usually reserved for serious ventricular dysrhythmias
quinidine sulfate	PO: 200–400 mg tid or qid (max: 3–4 g/day)	Class 1A; gluconate salt is also available in IM and IV forms; sustained-release forms available for the sulfate and gluconate salts

A few, such as quinidine and procainamide, are effective against many different types of dysrhythmias. The remaining Class I drugs are more specific and indicated only for life-threatening ventricular dysrhythmias.

All the sodium channel blockers have the potential to cause new dysrhythmias or worsen existing ones; thus, frequent ECGs should be obtained. The reduced heart rate caused by the drugs can result in hypotension, dizziness, and fainting. Some Class I drugs have significant anticholinergic adverse effects such as dry mouth, constipation, and urinary retention.

CONCEPT REVIEW 23.2

- Why does slowing the speed of the electrical impulse across the myocardium sometimes correct a dysrhythmia?

Prototype Drug: Pr *Procainamide*

Therapeutic Class: Antidysrhythmic (Class 1A) **Pharmacologic Class: Sodium channel blocker**

Actions and Uses: Procainamide is an older drug, approved in 1950, that is chemically related to the local anesthetic procaine. Procainamide blocks sodium ion channels in myocardial cells, thus slowing conduction of the action potential across the myocardium. This slight delay in conduction velocity prolongs the refractory period and can suppress dysrhythmias. Procainamide has the ability to correct many different types of dysrhythmias. The most common dosage form is the extended-release tablet; however, procainamide is also available in IV and IM formulations for emergency conditions.

Adverse Effects and Interactions: Procainamide has a narrow margin of safety, and dosage must be monitored carefully to avoid serious adverse effects. Nausea, vomiting, abdominal pain, and headache are common during therapy. The drug can cause fever accompanied by anorexia, weakness, nausea, and vomiting. High doses may produce central nervous system (CNS) effects such as confusion or psychosis. Procainamide should be reserved for life-threatening dysrhythmias because it has the ability to produce new dysrhythmias or worsen existing ones.

Additive cardiac depressant effects may occur if procainamide is administered with other antidysrhythmics. Additive anticholinergic adverse effects will occur if procainamide is used concurrently with other medications that have anticholinergic effects.

BLACK BOX WARNING:
Chronic administration may result in a lupus-like syndrome. The drug may increase the risk of mortality in certain patients. Due to an increased risk for blood dyscrasias, complete blood counts should be monitored frequently and the drug discontinued at the first sign of potential blood abnormalities.

Core Concept 23.7 ▶

Beta-adrenergic blockers reduce automaticity and slow conduction velocity in the heart.

Beta-adrenergic blockers are used to treat a large number of cardiovascular diseases, including HTN, MI, heart failure, and dysrhythmias. Their ability to slow the heart rate and conduction velocity can suppress several types of dysrhythmias. Beta blockers of importance to dysrhythmias are listed in Table 23.3.

The basic pharmacology of beta-adrenergic blockers is explained in Chapter 9. Although the effects of beta blockers on the heart are complex, their basic actions are to slow the heart rate and decrease conduction velocity through the AV node. Myocardial automaticity is

Table 23.3 Beta-Adrenergic Blockers Used for Dysrhythmias (Class II)

Drug	Rate and Adult Dose	Remarks
acebutolol (Sectral)	PO: 200–600 mg bid (max: 1200 mg/day)	Cardioselective $beta_1$ blocker; usually reserved for ventricular dysrhythmias; also for HTN and angina
esmolol (Brevibloc)	IV: 50 mcg/kg/min maintenance dose (max: 200 mcg/kg/min)	Cardioselective $beta_1$ blocker; usually reserved for immediate control of severe atrial dysrhythmias; very short half-life of 9 minutes
Pr propranolol (Inderal, InnoPran XL)	PO: 10–30 mg tid or qid (max: 480 mg/day) IV: 1–3 mg every 4 hours	Sustained-release forms available; also for HTN, prevention of MI, angina, and migraines

reduced, and many types of dysrhythmias are stabilized. The main value of beta blockers as antidysrhythmic drugs is to treat atrial dysrhythmias that are associated with heart failure.

Only a few beta blockers are approved for dysrhythmias because of the potential for adverse effects. Blockade of beta receptors in the heart may result in bradycardia, and hypotension may cause dizziness and possible fainting. Beta blockers that affect beta$_2$-receptors will also affect the lungs, increasing the risk for bronchospasm. This is of particular concern in patients with asthma and in older patients with chronic obstructive pulmonary disease (COPD).

▶ Lifespan and Diversity

Special attention should be given to older adults because anticholinergic adverse effects may worsen urinary hesitancy in patients with prostate enlargement.

Prototype Drug: Pr *Propranolol (Inderal, InnoPran XL)*

Therapeutic Class: Antidysrhythmic (Class II) **Pharmacologic Class:** Beta-adrenergic blocker

Actions and Uses: Propranolol is a nonselective beta-adrenergic blocker, affecting both beta$_1$-receptors in the heart and beta$_2$-receptors in the lungs. Propranolol reduces heart rate, slows conduction velocity, and lowers blood pressure. Propranolol is most effective in treating tachycardia. It is approved to treat a wide variety of disorders, including HTN, angina, and migraine headaches, and to prevent MI.

Adverse Effects and Interactions: Frequent adverse effects of propranolol include hypotension and bradycardia. Because of its ability to slow the heart rate, patients with serious cardiac disorders such as heart failure must be carefully monitored. Patients with diabetes should be monitored carefully because beta blockers can affect blood glucose levels. Adverse effects such as diminished sex drive and impotence may result in noncompliance.

Propranolol interacts with many other drugs, including phenothiazines, which have additive hypotensive effects. Propranolol should not be given within 2 weeks of a monoamine oxidase inhibitor (MAOI). Beta-adrenergic drugs such as albuterol block the actions of propranolol.

BLACK BOX WARNING:

Abrupt withdrawal is not advised in patients with angina or heart disease. Dosage should gradually be reduced over 1 to 2 weeks, and the drug should be restarted if angina symptoms develop during this period.

CONCEPT REVIEW 23.3

- Why are selective alpha-adrenergic blockers such as doxazosin (Cardura) of no value in treating dysrhythmias?

Potassium channel blockers prolong the refractory period of the heart.

◀ Core Concept 23.8

Although a small class of drugs, the potassium channel blockers (Class III) have important applications to the treatment of dysrhythmias. Potassium channel blockers used as antidysrhythmics are listed in Table 23.4.

The drugs in Class III exert their actions by blocking potassium ion channels in myocardial cells. After the action potential has passed and the myocardial cell is in a depolarized state, repolarization depends on removal of potassium from the cell. The Class III drugs

Table 23.4 Potassium Channel Blockers (Class III)

Drug	Rate and Adult Dose	Remarks
Pr amiodarone (Cordarone, Pacerone)	PO: 400–600 mg/day maintenance dose	IV form available; usually reserved for serious ventricular dysrhythmias
dofetilide (Tikosyn)	PO: 125–500 mcg bid based on creatinine clearance	Usually for atrial dysrhythmias; must be hospitalized for first 3 days of therapy to monitor for possible drug-induced dysrhythmias
dronedarone (Multaq)	PO: 400 mg bid	Newer drug; given to reduce the risk of cardiovascular hospitalization in patients with atrial dysrhythmias
ibutilide (Corvert)	IV: 1 mg infused over 10 minutes	Usually reserved for atrial flutter or fibrillation
sotalol (Betapace, Betapace AF, Sorine)	PO: 80 mg bid and increase gradually to 240-320 mg/day (max: 320 mg/day)	Usually reserved for serious ventricular dysrhythmias; also a nonselective beta-adrenergic blocker

prolong the duration of the action potential by lengthening the refractory period (resting stage), which tends to stabilize dysrhythmias.

Potassium channel blockers are reserved for serious dysrhythmias because of potentially serious adverse effects. Like other antidysrhythmics, potassium channel blockers slow the heart rate, resulting in bradycardia and possible hypotension. These adverse effects occur in a significant number of patients. These medications can worsen dysrhythmias, especially following the first few doses. Older adults with preexisting heart failure must be carefully monitored because they are particularly at risk for adverse cardiac effects of potassium channel blockers.

Prototype Drug: Pr *Amiodarone (Cordarone)*

Therapeutic Class: Antidysrhythmic (Class III) **Pharmacologic Class:** Potassium channel blocker

Actions and Uses: Amiodarone is approved for the treatment of resistant ventricular tachycardia that may prove life threatening. It is also a preferred drug for treating atrial dysrhythmias in patients with heart failure. In addition to blocking potassium ion channels, some of amiodarone's actions on the heart relate to its blockade of sodium ion channels. Amiodarone is available as oral tablets and as an IV infusion. IV infusions are limited to short-term therapy, normally only 2 to 4 days. Its onset of action may take several weeks when the drug is given orally. Its effects, however, can last 4 to 8 weeks after the drug is discontinued because it has an extended half-life that may exceed 50 days.

Adverse Effects and Interactions: Amiodarone may cause blurred vision, rashes, photosensitivity, nausea, vomiting, anorexia, fatigue, dizziness, and hypotension. Because this medication is concentrated by certain tissues and has a prolonged half-life, adverse effects may be slow to resolve. As with other antidysrhythmics, patients must be closely monitored to avoid serious toxicity. Amiodarone is a pregnancy category D drug.

Amiodarone interacts with many other drugs. For example, it increases digoxin levels in the blood and enhances the actions of anticoagulants. If used together with beta blockers, sinus bradycardia may increase, and sinus arrest and atrioventricular block may occur. Protease inhibitors such as ritonavir and indinavir increase the levels of amiodarone, and the combinations should not be used.

Use cautiously with herbal supplements such as echinacea, which may cause increased liver toxicity. Aloe may increase the effect of amiodarone.

BLACK BOX WARNING:

(Oral form only): Amiodarone causes a pneumonia-like syndrome in the lungs. Because the pulmonary toxicity may be fatal, baseline and periodic assessment of lung function is essential. Amiodarone has prodysrhythmic action and may cause bradycardia, cardiogenic shock, or AV block. Mild liver injury is frequent with amiodarone.

Core Concept 23.9 ▶

Calcium channel blockers are available to treat supraventricular dysrhythmias.

Like the beta blockers, the calcium channel blockers (Class IV) are widely prescribed for various cardiovascular disorders. By slowing conduction velocity, they are able to stabilize certain dysrhythmias. Although about 10 calcium channel blockers (CCBs) are available to treat cardiovascular diseases, only a limited number have been approved for dysrhythmias. Doses for the CCBs used for treating dysrhythmias are listed in Table 23.5. The basic pharmacology of this drug class is presented in Chapter 19. Diltiazem is featured as a prototype drug in Chapter 21.

Table 23.5 Calcium Channel Blockers (Class IV) and Miscellaneous Drugs for Dysrhythmias

Drug	Rate and Adult Dose	Remarks
diltiazem (Cardizem, Cartia XT, Dilacor XR, others) (see the Prototype Drug box in Core Concept 21.7)	IV: 0.25 mg/kg bolus over 2 min then 5-10 mg/h continuous infusion (max: 15 mg/h)	Oral and sustained-release forms available for HTN and angina
Pr verapamil (Calan, Isoptin SR, others)	PO (immediate release): 240–480 mg/day IV: 2.5-5 mg over 2 minutes: then give 5-10 mg every 15–30 minutes if needed	Sustained-release and IV forms available; also for HTN, angina, and migraines
MISCELLANEOUS DRUGS		
adenosine (Adenocard, Adenoscan)	IV: 6–12 mg given as a bolus injection for 3 doses (max: 12 mg/dose)	Usually reserved for atrial dysrhythmias; half-life is only 10 seconds
digoxin (Lanoxin) (see the Prototype Drug box in Core Concept 20.7)	PO: 0.1–0.375 mg/day maintenance dose; dose is individualized for each patient	Usually reserved for atrial dysrhythmias; IV and IM forms available; also for heart failure

Blockade of calcium ion channels produces effects on the heart that are similar to those of beta-adrenergic blockers. Effects include reduced automaticity in the SA node and slowed impulse conduction through the AV node. This prolongs the refractory period and stabilizes many types of dysrhythmias. CCBs are only effective against atrial dysrhythmias.

Prototype Drug: *Verapamil (Calan, Isoptin SR, Others)*

Therapeutic Class: Antidysrhythmic (Class IV) **Pharmacologic Class:** Calcium channel blocker

Actions and Uses: Verapamil was the first CCB approved by the U.S. Food and Drug Administration (FDA). The drug acts by inhibiting the flow of Ca^{2+} into myocardial cells and in vascular smooth muscle. In the heart, this action slows conduction velocity and stabilizes dysrhythmias. In the vessels, calcium ion channel inhibition lowers blood pressure. Verapamil also dilates the coronary arteries, an action that is important when the drug is used to treat angina (see Chapter 21).

Adverse Effects and Interactions: Adverse effects are generally minor and may include headache, constipation, and hypotension. Because verapamil can cause bradycardia, patients with heart failure should be carefully monitored. Like many other antidysrhythmics, it has the ability to elevate blood levels of digoxin. Because both digoxin and verapamil have the effect of slowing conduction through the AV node, their concurrent use must be carefully monitored.

Grapefruit juice may increase verapamil levels. The drug should be used cautiously with hawthorn, which may have additive hypotensive effects.

CCBs are well tolerated by most patients. As with other antidysrhythmics, patients should be carefully monitored for bradycardia and hypotension. Because their cardiac effects are almost identical to those of beta-adrenergic blockers, patients concurrently taking drugs from both classes are especially at risk for bradycardia and possible heart failure. Because older patients often have multiple cardiovascular disorders, such as HTN, heart failure, and dysrhythmias, it is not unusual for them to be taking drugs from multiple classes.

▶ Lifespan and Diversity

The healthcare provider should carefully monitor older adults with preexisting heart failure because these patients are particularly at risk from the cardiac effects of potassium channel blockers.

CONCEPT REVIEW 23.4

- Remembering the effects of digoxin on the heart from Chapter 20, explain why most antidysrhythmic drugs have the potential to cause serious adverse effects in patients taking cardiac glycosides.

Digoxin and adenosine are used for specific dysrhythmias but do not act by blocking ion channels.

◀ Core Concept 23.10

Two other drugs, adenosine and digoxin, are used to treat specific dysrhythmias, but they do not act by the mechanisms described previously. These drugs are summarized in Table 23.5.

Adenosine (Adenocard, Adenoscan) is given as a 1- to 2-second bolus IV injection to terminate serious atrial tachycardia by slowing conduction through the AV node and decreasing automaticity of the SA node. Its primary indication is a specific dysrhythmia known as paroxysmal supraventricular tachycardia (PSVT), for which it is a preferred drug. Although dyspnea is common, adverse effects are generally brief, because of its 10-second half-life.

Although digoxin (Lanoxin) is primarily used to treat heart failure, it is also prescribed for certain types of atrial dysrhythmias because it decreases automaticity of the SA node and slows conduction through the AV node. Excessive levels of digoxin can produce serious dysrhythmias, and interactions with other medications are common; therefore, patients must be carefully monitored during therapy. The adverse effects of digoxin are described in Chapter 20.

Patients Need to Know

Patients treated for dysrhythmias need to know the following recommendations:

In General

1. Monitor blood pressure regularly during treatment.
2. Monitor for a decreased heart rate and changes in rhythm while taking antidysrhythmic drugs. Report changes to a healthcare provider.
3. Do not discontinue the medication suddenly. It should be stopped gradually under the supervision of a healthcare provider.

Regarding CCBs

4. Notify the healthcare provider if a very slow heart rate (less than 60 beats per minute), dizziness when standing up quickly, headache, or constipation is experienced.
5. Inform a healthcare provider if systolic blood pressure is less than 90 mmHg, and do not take the next dose of the CCB until instructed to do so.

Regarding Beta Blockers

6. Notify the healthcare provider if experiencing a very slow heart rate (less than 60 beats per minute), systolic pressure less than 90 mmHg, dizziness when standing up quickly, or headache.
7. Notify dentists, surgeons, and eye doctors if taking propranolol (Inderal, InnoPran XL). This drug lowers intraocular pressure.
8. For those with diabetes, check blood glucose regularly while taking beta blockers. These medications can change how the body uses sugars and starches.

Regarding Potassium Channel Blockers

9. Notify the healthcare provider immediately if difficulty in breathing or chest discomfort occurs.

Chapter Review

Core Concepts Summary

23.1 Some types of dysrhythmias produce no patient symptoms, whereas others may be life threatening.

Some dysrhythmias produce no symptoms and are harmless, whereas others are life threatening. The frequency of dysrhythmias is difficult to ascertain, although they are thought to be quite common, particularly in the geriatric population.

23.2 Dysrhythmias are classified by the type of rhythm abnormality produced and its location.

Dysrhythmias are classified by their site of origin, either atrial or ventricular, and by the type of rhythm abnormality produced, such as tachycardia, flutter, or fibrillation. Dysrhythmias are associated with diseases such as HTN, MI, and heart failure.

23.3 The electrical conduction pathway in the myocardium keeps the heart beating in a synchronized manner.

The normal rhythm of the heart is established by the SA node, which ensures that the chambers beat in a synchronized manner. The central problem with dysrhythmias is their potential to affect the function of the heart, reduce cardiac output, and cause certain consequences such as stroke or heart failure.

23.4 Most antidysrhythmic drugs act by blocking ion channels in myocardial cells.

Antidysrhythmic drugs affect the action potential in myocardial cells. They act by blocking sodium, potassium, or calcium channels in the cell membrane.

23.5 Antidysrhythmic drugs are classified by their mechanisms of action.

All antidysrhythmic drugs have the ability to cause rhythm abnormalities or worsen existing ones. Most antidysrhythmic medications are placed into one of five classes, based on their mechanisms of action. Class I drugs are further subdivided into IA, IB, and IC. Nonpharmacologic treatments such as cardioversion or catheter ablation are sometimes preferred over drug therapy.

23.6 Sodium channel blockers slow the rate of impulse conduction through the heart.

Sodium channel blockers stabilize dysrhythmias by slowing the spread of impulse conduction across the myocardium. Quinidine, a Class IA drug, is the oldest antidysrhythmic drug.

23.7 Beta-adrenergic blockers reduce automaticity and slow conduction velocity in the heart.

Beta blockers such as propranolol stabilize dysrhythmias by slowing the heart rate and decreasing the conduction velocity through the AV node.

23.8 Potassium channel blockers prolong the refractory period of the heart.

Potassium channel blockers such as amiodarone stabilize dysrhythmias by prolonging the duration of the action potential and extending the refractory period.

23.9 Calcium channel blockers are available to treat supraventricular dysrhythmias.

Calcium channel blockers such as verapamil have effects similar to those of beta-adrenergic blockers. These include reduced automaticity in the SA node, slowed impulse conduction through the AV node, and a prolonged refractory period.

23.10 Digoxin and adenosine are used for specific dysrhythmias but do not act by blocking ion channels.

Digoxin and adenosine are used for specific dysrhythmias but do not act by the mechanisms of Class I, II, III, or IV drugs. Adenosine is used for short-term, rapid termination of dysrhythmias.

REVIEW Questions

Answer the following questions to assess your knowledge of the chapter material, and go back and review any material that is not clear to you.

1. The nurse is monitoring the electrolytes and electrocardiogram of a patient with a cardiac dysthymia because which of the following electrolytes produces depolarization when it rushes into cardiac cells?
   1. Potassium
   2. Magnesium
   3. Sodium
   4. Chloride
2. A patient has been ordered a sodium channel blocker. This class of drug works by:
   1. Increasing automaticity.
   2. Slowing impulse conduction.
   3. Prolonging the refractory period.
   4. Increasing impulse conduction.
3. The healthcare provider has ordered propranolol, 15 mg by mouth (PO), three times a day. The pharmacy has propranolol in 30-mg tablets. How many tablets will be given per dose, and how many milligrams will the patient receive in a day?
   1. One-half tablet per dose, 30 mg per day
   2. One-half tablet per dose, 45 mg per day
   3. One and one-half tablets per dose, 45 mg per day
   4. One and one-half tablets per dose, 35 mg per day
4. The patient is on amiodarone (Cordarone). What changes will the nurse expect to see to the patient's digoxin order?
   1. Discontinued
   2. Increased
   3. Decreased
   4. Doubled
5. The nurse is monitoring a patient taking an antidysrhythmic drug. What outcome would be expected?
   1. Decreased heart rate
   2. Increased heart rate
   3. Increased renal insufficiency
   4. Increased hepatic insufficiency
6. The patient taking an antidysrhythmic is instructed to notify the healthcare provider if:
   1. Constipation occurs.
   2. The heart rate is less than 60 beats per minute.
   3. The heart rate is greater than 90 beats per minute.
   4. Blood pressure does not decrease.
7. A group of patients is being taught about the common adverse effects of antidysrhythmic medications. Some of the adverse effects include: (Select all that apply.)
   1. Dizziness.
   2. Hypotension.
   3. Weakness.
   4. Anorexia.
   5. Insomnia.
8. Which of the following would be included in the teaching plan for a patient taking an antidysrhythmic medication?
   1. "Take the drug only when you are feeling excessively tired."
   2. "Take your pulse prior to taking your medication."
   3. "Do not drink alcohol unless you have spoken with your healthcare provider."
   4. "You will need to increase your sodium and potassium intake."

9. A patient taking an antidysrhythmic medication learns in a patient education session that sometimes this medication is also used to treat angina. What medication is being discussed?
1. Digoxin (Lanoxin)
2. Verapamil (Calan)
3. Adenosine (Adenocard)
4. Quinidine sulfate

10. Which of the following antidysrhythmics is used to treat hypertension and angina?
1. Diltiazem (Cardizem)
2. Digoxin (Lanoxin)
3. Adenosine (Adenocard)
4. Quinidine sulfate

CASE STUDY Questions

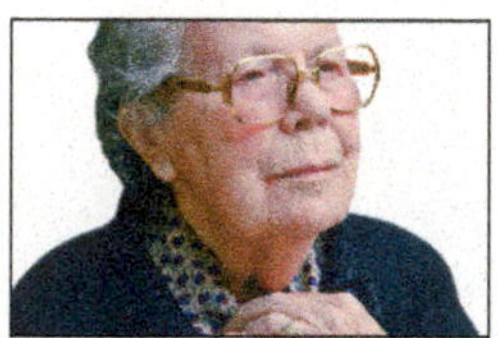

Remember Mrs. Duncan, the patient introduced at the beginning of the chapter? Now read the remainder of the case study. Based on the information you have learned in this chapter, answer the questions that follow.

Mrs. Margaret Duncan, age 72, who has a history of HTN, has arrived in the emergency department with a life-threatening ventricular dysrhythmia. She is frightened and is wondering what is happening. The healthcare provider has ordered that an IV lidocaine infusion be started on Mrs. Duncan.

1. The nurse explains to Mrs. Duncan that lidocaine would be expected to terminate her dysrhythmia primarily by which of the following mechanisms?
1. Speeding up the heart rate
2. Lowering blood pressure
3. Increasing the strength of myocardial contractions
4. Slowing the speed of electrical conduction across the myocardium

2. When Mrs. Duncan is discharged from the hospital, she is placed on propranolol. The nurse informs the patient that this drug should:
1. Raise her blood pressure.
2. Lower her blood pressure.
3. Have no effect on her hypertension.
4. First raise her blood pressure, then lower it.

3. The healthcare provider lowers the dose of propranolol and adds amiodarone (Cordarone) to the drug regimen. Mrs. Duncan begins to experience dizziness and fatigue. This is most likely caused by which of the following?
1. Mrs. Duncan is not eating enough potassium-rich foods.
2. The drug combination is causing bradycardia or hypertension.
3. The drug combination is causing respiratory depression.
4. Mrs. Duncan's hypertension is out of control.

4. When taking these medications, Mrs. Duncan is instructed to:
1. Check her pulse rate prior to taking her medication.
2. Keep a log of weight gain or loss.
3. Eat plenty of foods containing potassium.
4. Avoid taking aspirin, unless instructed to do so by the healthcare provider.

Answers and complete rationales for the Review and Case Study Questions appear in Appendix A.

REFERENCES

Herdman, T. H., & Kamitsuru, S. (Eds.). (2014). *NANDA International nursing diagnoses: Definitions and classification, 2015–2017*. Oxford, United Kingdom: Wiley-Blackwell.

Rosenthal, L. (2016) *Atrial fibrillation*. Retrieved from http://emedicine.medscape.com/article/151066-overview

SELECTED BIBLIOGRAPHY

Charneski, L., & Hollands, J. M. (2014). Recent changes in practice guidelines for atrial fibrillation management. *Pharmacotherapy: The Journal of Human Pharmacology and Drug Therapy, 34*, 1118–1120. doi:10.1002/phar.1498

Goyal, S. K. (2014). *Ventricular fibrillation*. Retrieved from http://emedicine.medscape.com/article/158712-overview

Ismail, H., & Lewin, R. J. (2013). The role of a new arrhythmia specialist nurse in providing support to patients and caregivers. *European Journal of Cardiovascular Nursing, 12*, 177–183. doi:10.1177/1474515112442446

National Heart, Lung, and Blood Institute. (2011). *What is long QT syndrome?* Retrieved from http://www.nhlbi.nih.gov/health/dci/Diseases/qt/qt_whatis.html

National Heart, Lung, and Blood Institute. (2015). *What is sudden cardiac arrest?* Retrieved from http://www.nhlbi.nih.gov/health/health-topics/topics/scda/

Piccini, J. P., Zhao, Y., Steinberg, B. A., He, X., Mathew, J. P., Fullerton, D. A., . . . Peterson, E. D. (2013). Comparative effectiveness of pharmacotherapies for prevention of atrial fibrillation following coronary artery bypass surgery. *The American Journal of Cardiology, 112,* 954–960. doi:10.1016/j.amjcard.2013.05.029

Sullivan, S. D., Orme, M. E., Morais, E., & Mitchell, S. A. (2013). Interventions for the treatment of atrial fibrillation: A systematic literature review and meta-analysis. *International Journal of Cardiology, 165,* 229–236. doi:10.1016/j.ijcard.2012.03.070

Chapter 24

Drugs for Coagulation and Hematologic Disorders

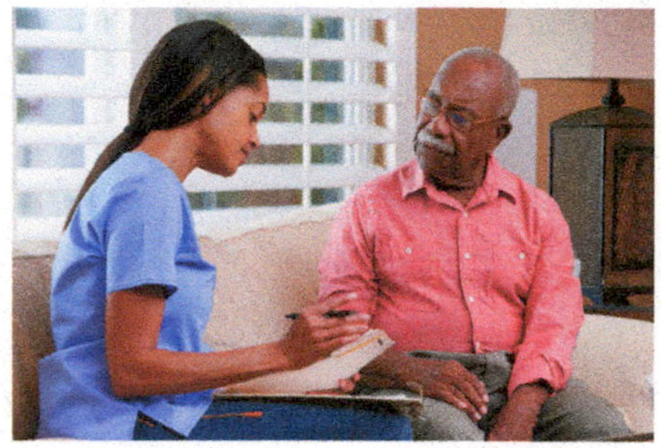

"Let me see if I understand this . . . I need to go to the lab and get stuck every other day for the next 2 weeks?"

Mr. Thomas Hawkins

Core Concepts

24.1 **Hemostasis is a complex process involving multiple steps and many clotting factors.**

24.2 **Removing a blood clot is essential to restoring normal circulation.**

24.3 **Drugs are used to modify the coagulation process.**

24.4 **Anticoagulants prevent the formation and enlargement of clots.**

24.5 **Antiplatelet drugs prolong bleeding time by interfering with platelet aggregation.**

24.6 **Thrombolytics are used to dissolve existing clots.**

24.7 **Hemostatics are used to promote the formation of clots.**

24.8 **Hematopoietic growth factors are administered to boost blood cell production.**

Drug Snapshot

The following drugs are discussed in this chapter:

Drug Classes	Prototype Drugs
Anticoagulants	Pr heparin Pr warfarin (Coumadin)
Antiplatelet drugs	Pr clopidogrel (Plavix)
Thrombolytics	Pr alteplase (Activase)
Hemostatics	Pr aminocaproic acid (Amicar)
Hematopoietic growth factors	Pr epoetin alfa (Epogen, Procrit)

Learning Outcomes

After reading this chapter, the student should be able to:

1. Explain the importance of hemostasis.
2. Identify the importance of removing blood clots to the restoration of blood circulation.
3. Construct a diagram that illustrates how drugs are used to modify the coagulation process.

4. Explain the primary mechanism by which anticoagulants act.
5. Explain the primary mechanism by which antiplatelet drugs act.
6. Describe indications for the administration of thrombolytics.
7. Describe indications for the administration of hemostatics.
8. Explain reasons for administering hematopoietic growth factors.

Key Terms

activated partial thromboplastin time (aPTT) (throm-bow-PLAS-tin)
anticoagulants (ANT-eye-co-AG-you lents)
antiplatelet drugs (ant-eye-PLAY-tuh let)
clotting factors
coagulation (co-ag-you-LAY-shun)
coagulation cascade (cass-KADE)
deep vein thrombosis (DVT)
embolus (EM-boh-luss)
fibrin (FEYE-brin)
fibrinogen (feye-BRIN-oh-jen)
fibrinolysis (feye-brin-OL-oh-sis)
glycoprotein IIb/IIIa (GLEYE-koh-proh-teen)
hematopoiesis (hee-mato-po-EE-sis)
hemostasis (hee-moh-STAY-sis)
hemostatics (hee-moh-STAT-iks)
international normalized ratio (INR)
low molecular weight heparins (LMWHs)
plasmin (PLAZ-min)
plasminogen (plaz-MIN-oh-jen)
prothrombin (PRO-throm-bin)
prothrombin time (PT)
thrombin (THROM-bin)
thromboembolic disorder (THROM-bow-EM-bow-lik)
thrombolytics (throm-bow-LIT-iks)
thrombus (THROM-bus)
tissue plasminogen activator (tPA)

The blood serves all cells in the body and is the only fluid tissue. Because of this, disorders of the blood can affect a large number of organ systems. For example, lack of adequate numbers of blood cells or blood cofactors can cause excessive bleeding or decreased effectiveness of the immune system. This chapter examines how drugs are used to manage two important homeostatic mechanisms: control of coagulation and blood growth factors.

Many diseases and conditions affect hemostasis. Some common disorders that often require pharmacotherapy with coagulation modifiers are described in Table 24.1.

Hemostasis is a complex process involving multiple steps and many clotting factors.

◀ **Core Concept 24.1**

hemo = *blood*
stasis = *stopping*

Hemostasis, or the stopping of blood flow, is an essential mechanism protecting the body from both external and internal injury. Without efficient hemostasis, bleeding from wounds would lead to shock and perhaps death. Too much clotting, however, can be just as deadly as too little. Thus, hemostasis must maintain a delicate balance between blood fluidity and coagulation.

Table 24.1 Disorders Commonly Treated with Coagulation Modifier Drugs

Disorder/Condition	Description
Angina	Pain due to narrowing of the coronary vessels that interferes with blood flow to cardiac muscle
Deep vein thrombosis (DVT)	Clot within a vein in the legs
Indwelling devices	Mechanical heart valves, stents
Myocardial infarction	Death of cardiac muscle tissue due to blockage of a coronary artery
Postoperative hemorrhage	Bleeding following a surgical procedure
Pulmonary embolus	Clot within a pulmonary artery that blocks blood flow to the lungs
Kidney dialysis	Procedure used to filter waste products or excess fluid or ions from the blood
Stroke (cerebrovascular accident)	Clot within an artery that blocks blood flow to the brain
Valvular heart disease	Disease of heart valves or replacement of a heart valve

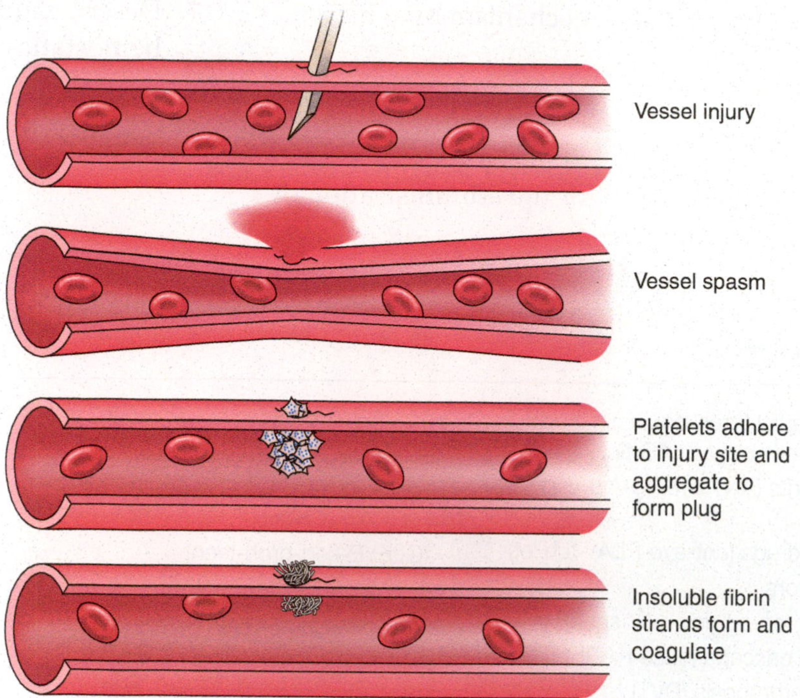

FIGURE 24.1 Basic steps in hemostasis.

Hemostasis is complex and involves a number of substances called **clotting factors**. The clotting factors are activated in a series of sequential steps, sometimes referred to as a *cascade*. Drugs can be used to modify several of these steps.

When an injury occurs, cells lining damaged blood vessels release chemicals that begin the process of hemostasis. The vessel immediately spasms, which limits blood flow to the injured area. Platelets become sticky, adhere to the injured area, and aggregate or clump to plug the damaged vessel. Blood flow is further slowed, resulting in **coagulation**, the formation of an insoluble clot. The basic steps of hemostasis are shown in Figure 24.1.

pro = *before*
thrombin = *clot*

The **coagulation cascade** is a complex series of steps that begins when the injured cells release a chemical called *prothrombin activator* or prothrombinase. Prothrombin activator converts the clotting factor **prothrombin** to an enzyme called **thrombin**. Thrombin then converts **fibrinogen**, a plasma protein, to long strands of **fibrin**. Thus two of the factors essential to clotting, thrombin and fibrin, are only formed *after* injury to the vessels. The fibrin strands form an insoluble web over the injured area to stop blood loss. Normal blood clotting occurs in about 6 minutes. The primary steps in the coagulation cascade are illustrated in Figure 24.2.

thrombo = *clot*
plastin = *to form*

It is important to note that several clotting factors, including thromboplastin and fibrinogen, are proteins made by the liver that are constantly circulating through the blood in an *inactive* form. Vitamin K is required for the liver to make four of the clotting factors. Because the liver supplies many of the clotting factors, patients with serious hepatic impairment usually exhibit abnormal coagulation.

Fast Facts Clotting Disorders

- Many patients with DVT (60-80%) also have pulmonary emboli, although they may be asymptomatic.
- Von Willebrand's disease is a hereditary platelet disorder; the average time from symptoms to diagnosis is often prolonged (about 16 years).
- Hemophilia A, or classic hemophilia, is a hereditary condition in which a person lacks clotting factor VIII.
- More than 20,000 people in the United States have hemophilia; the median age at diagnosis is about 36 months.

Source: Based on Ouellette, D. R. (2015). Pulmonary embolism. Retrieved from http://emedicine.medscape.com/article/300901-overview#a6.

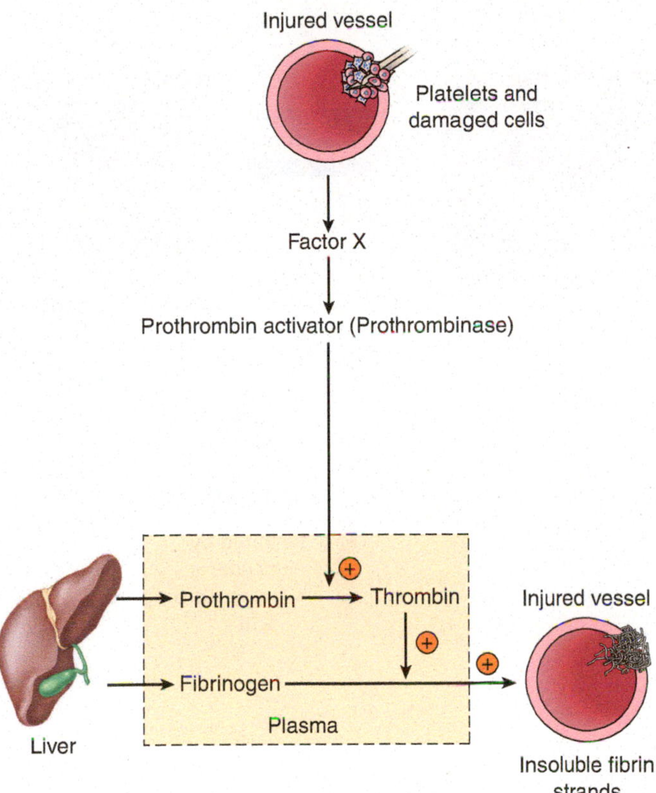

FIGURE 24.2 Major steps in the coagulation cascade.

Removing a blood clot is essential to restoring normal circulation.

◀ **Core Concept 24.2**

The goal of hemostasis has been achieved once a blood clot is formed, and the body is protected from excessive hemorrhage. Large clots, however, may prevent adequate blood flow to the affected area; circulation must eventually be restored so that the tissue can resume normal activities. The process of clot removal is called **fibrinolysis**.

fibrin = *fiber*
lysis = *break apart*

Fibrinolysis also involves several sequential steps. When the fibrin clot is formed, nearby blood vessel cells secrete **tissue plasminogen activator (tPA)**. tPA converts the inactive protein **plasminogen**, which is present in the fibrin clot, to its active form called **plasmin**. Plasmin then digests the fibrin strands to remove the clot. The body normally regulates fibrinolysis such that *unwanted* fibrin clots are removed, whereas fibrin present in wounds is left to maintain hemostasis. The steps of fibrinolysis are shown in Figure 24.3.

Drugs are used to modify the coagulation process.

◀ **Core Concept 24.3**

There are many types of disorders in which abnormal coagulation might occur. The term **thromboembolic disorder** is used to describe conditions in which the body forms undesirable clots. Thromboembolic disorders may occur in either veins or arteries and can place patients in extreme danger. Once a stationary clot, or **thrombus**, forms in a vessel, it often grows larger as more fibrin is added. Thrombi in the venous system usually form in the veins of the legs due to sluggish blood flow, a condition called **deep vein thrombosis (DVT)**. Pieces of a thrombus may break off and travel in the bloodstream to lodge in other vessels. A traveling clot is called an **embolus**. When thrombi or emboli form, or when a patient is at very high risk for thrombus formation, drug therapy is indicated.

Drugs can be used to modify hemostasis in a number of ways. **Anticoagulants** are drugs used to prevent excessive clotting, usually by interfering with some aspect of the coagulation cascade. The **antiplatelet drugs**, also frequently prescribed to modify hemostasis, act by diminishing the clotting action of platelets. Regardless of the mechanism, all anticoagulant and antiplatelet drugs will increase the time the body takes to form clots. These

anti = *against*
coagulation = *clotting*

FIGURE 24.3 Primary steps in fibrinolysis.

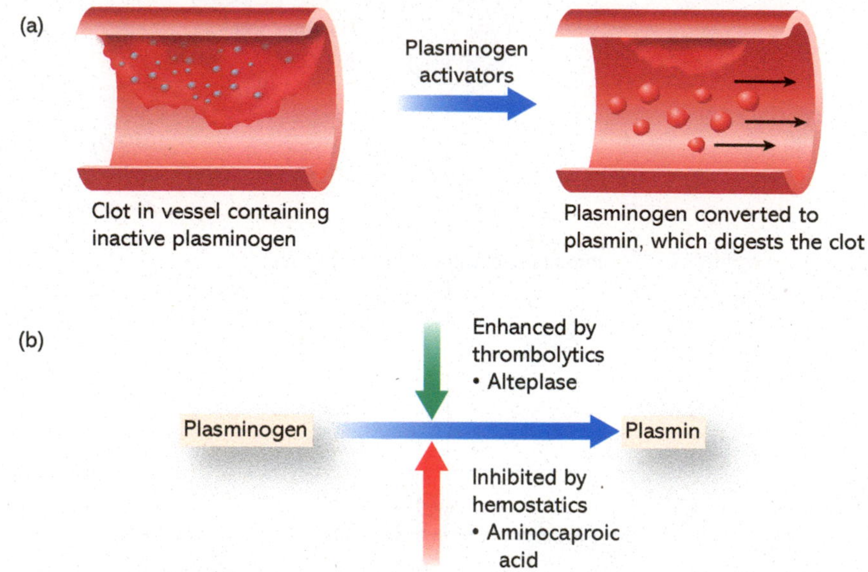

drugs are often referred to as *blood thinners*, which is an incorrect term, because they do not change the thickness of the blood. Disorders commonly treated with coagulation modifiers are shown in Table 24.1.

thrombo = *clot*
lytic = *remove/destroy*

Once an abnormal clot has formed, it may be critical to quickly remove it in order to restore normal function. This is particularly important for blood vessels serving the heart, lungs, and brain. A specific class of drugs, the **thrombolytics**, is used to dissolve such life-threatening clots.

hemo = *blood*
static = *halting or stopping*

In some cases, the blood may not clot quickly enough—for example, following surgery. In this case, it is sometimes desirable to administer medications that make the blood clot more quickly in order to prevent excessive bleeding. These drugs, called **hemostatics**, inhibit the normal removal of fibrin, thus keeping the clot in place for a longer period. Hemostatics are used to speed clot formation, thereby limiting bleeding from a surgical site (see Figure 24.3).

CONCEPT REVIEW 24.1

- Which clotting factors are always circulating in the blood? Which are formed only once coagulation is underway?

Core Concept 24.4 ▶ Anticoagulants prevent the formation and enlargement of clots.

Anticoagulants are drugs used to prolong bleeding time and prevent thrombi from forming or growing larger. Because thromboembolic disease can be life threatening, therapy is often begun by administering anticoagulants intravenously or subcutaneously to achieve a rapid onset of action. As the disease stabilizes, the patient is switched to oral anticoagulants. Anticoagulants act by a number of different mechanisms, which are illustrated in Figure 24.4. Table 24.2 lists the primary anticoagulants.

The most frequent, and potentially serious, adverse effect of anticoagulant and antiplatelet drugs is bleeding. The patient must be observed for signs of hemorrhage, such as bruising, bleeding gums, and blood in the urine or stools. Patients who have recently experienced a traumatic injury or recent surgery are especially at risk. Any symptoms of bleeding must be immediately reported to the healthcare provider. Specific blockers may be administered to reverse the anticoagulant effects: Protamine sulfate is used for heparin, and vitamin K is administered for warfarin.

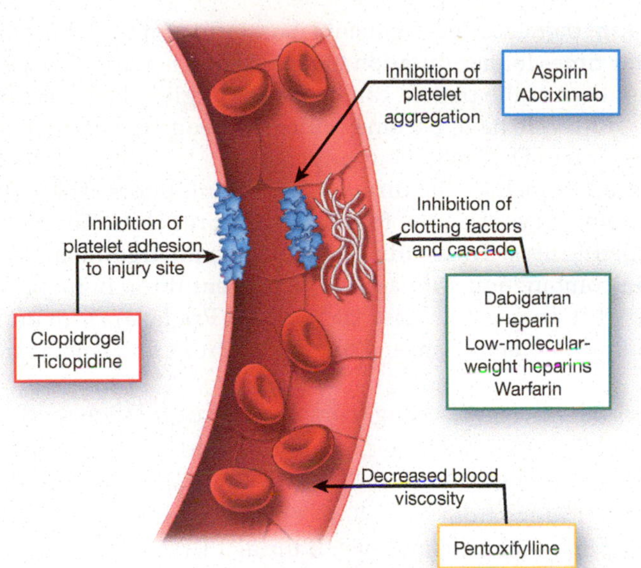

FIGURE 24.4 Mechanism of action of coagulation modifiers.

Table 24.2 Anticoagulants

Drug	Route and Adult Dose	Remarks
antithrombin, recombinant (ATryn)	IV: Dose is individualized based on the patient's pretreatment antithrombin level and body weight	Thrombin inhibitor; for prevention of perioperative and peripartum thromboembolic events in hereditary antithrombin deficient patients
apixaban (Eliquis)	PO: 2.5–10 mg bid	Factor Xa inhibitor; for prevention of DVT, stroke, and pulmonary embolism
argatroban (Acova, Novastan)	IV: 2–10 mcg/kg/min	Thrombin inhibitor; for prevention of clots in patients with heparin-induced thrombocytopenia
bivalirudin (Angiomax)	IV: 0.75 mg/kg initial bolus followed by 1.75 mg/kg/h for the duration of the procedure	Thrombin inhibitor; used with aspirin to prevent clots during percutaneous coronary intervention (PCI)
dabigatran (Pradaxa)	PO: 75–150 mg bid	Thrombin inhibitor; for prevention of DVT, stroke, and systemic embolism in patients with atrial fibrillation
desirudin (Iprivask)	Subcutaneous: 15 mg bid for 9–12 days	Thrombin inhibitor; for DVT prophylaxis in patients undergoing hip replacement surgery
edoxaban (Savaysa)	PO: 30–60 mg once daily	Factor Xa inhibitor; for prevention of DVT, stroke, and pulmonary embolism
fondaparinux (Arixtra)	Subcutaneous: 2.5–10 mg/daily	For prevention of DVT and pulmonary embolism
Pr heparin	IV infusion: 5000–40,000 units/day Subcutaneous: 5000–20,000 units/bid	For prevention and treatment of DVT and pulmonary edema; therapy begins with a higher dose, which is gradually reduced
pentoxifylline (Trental)	PO: 400 mg tid	Reduces blood viscosity and increases the flexibility of red blood cells; for intermittent claudication (pain in legs while walking or exercising)
rivaroxaban (Xarelto)	PO: 10–20 mg once daily	Factor Xa inhibitor; for prevention of DVT, stroke, and pulmonary embolism
Pr warfarin (Coumadin)	PO: 2–10 mg/day	Same use as heparin but effect is more prolonged; IV form is available
Low Molecular Weight Heparins (LMWHs)		
dalteparin (Fragmin)	Subcutaneous: 2500–10,000 units/day	For prevention and treatment of DVT following knee or hip replacement or abdominal surgery, unstable angina, or acute coronary syndromes
enoxaparin (Lovenox)	Subcutaneous: 30–40 mg bid for 7–10 days	
tinzaparin (Innohep)	Subcutaneous: 175 units/kg daily for at least 6 days	

Parenteral Anticoagulants

The traditional drug of choice for rapid anticoagulation is heparin. Heparin inactivates thrombin and several other clotting factors within minutes after it is given by the IV route. In recent years, the heparin molecule was shortened and modified to create **low molecular weight heparins (LMWHs)**, parenteral drugs that possess the same anticoagulant activity as heparin but have several advantages. They produce a more predictable anticoagulant response than heparin; therefore, less frequent laboratory monitoring is required. They also exhibit a two to four times longer duration of action than heparin that permits once daily dosing. Family members or the patient can be taught to give the necessary subcutaneous injections at home. LMWHs have become preferred drugs for many clotting disorders, including the prevention of DVT following surgery.

Other anticoagulants include the direct thrombin inhibitors. These drugs bind to the active site of thrombin, preventing the formation of fibrin clots. The thrombin inhibitors have limited therapeutic uses. Bivalirudin (Angiomax) and argatraban (Acova, Novastan) are administered in combination with aspirin to prevent thrombi in patients undergoing angioplasty. The newest drug in this class, dabigatran (Pradaxa), is an oral drug approved to treat DVT and pulmonary embolism and to prevent stroke and embolism in patients with atrial fibrillation.

To avoid serious adverse effects, drug therapy with coagulation modifier drugs is individualized to each patient and must be carefully monitored. For heparin, the **activated partial thromboplastin time (aPTT)** test is used to monitor the extent of anticoagulation. Baseline values of aPTT range from 25 to 40 seconds. During heparin therapy, the aPTT is maintained at 1.5 to 2 times the baseline level. If the aPTT rises above 80 seconds, the heparin dosage should be reduced. During the first few days of heparin therapy, aPTT is measured every 4 to 6 hours to avoid abnormal bleeding.

Prototype Drug: Pr *Heparin*

Therapeutic Class: Anticoagulant **Pharmacologic Class:** Indirect thrombin inhibitor

Actions and Uses: Heparin is a natural substance found in the lining of blood vessels. Its normal function is to prevent excessive clotting within blood vessels. When given as a drug, heparin provides immediate anticoagulant activity. The binding of heparin to a substance called antithrombin III results in an inactivation of some of the clotting factors and an inhibition of thrombin activity. Heparin must be given either subcutaneously or through IV infusion. The onset of action for IV heparin is immediate, whereas subcutaneous heparin may take up to an hour for maximum therapeutic effect.

Adverse Effects and Interactions: Abnormal bleeding is common during heparin therapy. If aPTT becomes prolonged or toxicity is observed, stopping the heparin infusion will result in loss of anticoagulant activity within hours. If serious hemorrhage occurs, a specific blocker, protamine sulfate, may be administered to neutralize the anticoagulant activity of heparin. Protamine sulfate has an onset time of 5 minutes and is also a blocker of the LMWHs.

Heparin-induced thrombocytopenia (HIT) is a serious complication that occurs in up to 30% of patients taking the drug. The patient may experience serious and even life-threatening thrombosis. Although the half-life of heparin is short, it may take a week after the drug is discontinued for platelets to completely recover.

Oral anticoagulants, including warfarin, increase the action of heparin. Ibuprofen, ASA, and other drugs that inhibit platelet aggregation may induce bleeding. Nicotine, digoxin, tetracyclines, or antihistamines may inhibit anticoagulation. Herbal supplements that may affect coagulation, such as ginger, garlic, green tea, feverfew, or ginkgo, should be avoided because they may increase the risk of bleeding.

BLACK BOX WARNING:
Epidural or spinal hematomas may occur when heparin or LMWHs are used in patients receiving spinal anesthesia or lumbar puncture. Because these can result in long-term or permanent paralysis, frequent monitoring for neurologic impairment is essential.

Oral Anticoagulants

The most frequently prescribed oral anticoagulant is warfarin (Coumadin). Often, patients begin anticoagulation therapy with heparin and are switched to warfarin when their condition stabilizes. When transitioning, the two drugs are administered concurrently for 2 to 3 days because warfarin takes several days of therapy before it achieves optimal anticoagulation effects.

Warfarin inhibits two enzymes involved in the formation of activated vitamin K, which is required for the synthesis of several clotting factors. Warfarin inhibits the synthesis of *new* clotting factors but does not affect clotting factors that are already circulating in the blood. The result is slowed clot formation and increased bleeding time.

Although not a true anticoagulant, pentoxifylline (Trental) reduces the viscosity of red blood cells and increases their flexibility. It is given to increase the microcirculation in patients with intermittent claudication. A newer class of drugs, the Factor X inhibitors, have emerged as significant alternatives to warfarin. Apixaban (Eliquis), edoxaban (Savaysa), and rivaroxaban directly inhibit Factor X in the clotting cascade. These drugs are indicated for the prophylaxis of DVT in patients undergoing knee or hip replacement surgery and to reduce the incidence of stroke and pulmonary embolism in patients with atrial fibrillation. Patients with atrial fibrillation are at increased risk for thrombus formation. The Factor X inhibitors are given orally and do not require international normalized ratio monitoring.

The laboratory test used during therapy with the oral anticoagulants is **prothrombin time (PT)**. Although the normal range for PT is 12 to 15 seconds, this value becomes prolonged with anticoagulant treatment. Daily PT tests may be conducted at the start of pharmacotherapy to ensure optimal dose levels. The frequency of PT tests is decreased to weekly or monthly as therapy progresses and the patient's condition stabilizes. Because the method of performing PT tests varies from laboratory to laboratory, clotting time is sometimes reported as an **international normalized ratio (INR)**, which is the PT multiplied by a correction factor. Recommended post-treatment INR values range from 2 to 4.

▶ Lifespan and Diversity

Bleeding complications are more likely to occur in older adults. Prescribed doses of anticoagulants are generally lower for older patients, and this group receives more frequent assessments and laboratory testing to avoid serious complications.

Prototype Drug: Pr *Warfarin (Coumadin)*

Therapeutic Class: Anticoagulant **Pharmacologic Class:** Vitamin K antagonist

Actions and Uses: Warfarin is used to prevent thrombi and emboli formation. Thus it is administered to patients at high risk for stroke, myocardial infarction (MI), DVT, and pulmonary embolism. This includes patients undergoing hip or knee surgery, those with long-term indwelling central venous catheters or prosthetic heart valves, and those who have experienced a recent MI.

Unlike heparin, the anticoagulant activity of warfarin can take several days to reach its maximum effect. This explains why heparin and warfarin therapy are overlapped. Warfarin inhibits the action of vitamin K that is essential for the synthesis of several clotting factors. Because these clotting factors are normally circulating in the blood, it takes several days for them to clear the plasma and for the anticoagulant effect of warfarin to appear. Another reason for the slow onset is that 99% of warfarin binds to plasma proteins and is unavailable to produce its effect. This high level of protein binding is responsible for a significant number of drug–drug interactions that may occur during warfarin therapy.

Adverse Effects and Interactions: Like all anticoagulants, the most serious adverse effect of warfarin is abnormal bleeding. On discontinuation of therapy, the activity of warfarin can take up to 10 days to diminish. If life-threatening bleeding occurs during therapy, the anticoagulant effects of warfarin can be reduced in 6 hours through the IM or subcutaneous administration of its blocker, vitamin K. For most patients, the therapeutic range of serum warfarin levels varies from 1 to 10 mcg/mL to achieve an INR value of 2–3. Warfarin is contraindicated during pregnancy, except in women with mechanical heart valves.

Extensive protein binding is responsible for numerous drug interactions, some of which occur with NSAIDs, diuretics, selective serotonin reuptake inhibitors (SSRIs) and other antidepressants, steroids, antibiotics, vaccines, and vitamins (e.g., vitamin K). Use with NSAIDs may increase bleeding risk. During warfarin therapy, the patient should not take any other prescription or over-the-counter (OTC) drugs unless approved by the healthcare provider. Use of warfarin with herbal supplements such as green tea, ginkgo, feverfew, garlic, cranberry, chamomile, and ginger may increase the risk of bleeding.

BLACK BOX WARNING:

Warfarin can cause major or fatal bleeding. Regular monitoring of INR is required. Patients should be instructed about prevention measures to minimize bleeding risk and to immediately notify healthcare providers of signs and symptoms of bleeding.

Nursing Process Focus Patients Receiving Anticoagulant and Antiplatelet Therapy

ASSESSMENT	POTENTIAL NURSING DIAGNOSES*
Prior to administration: • Obtain complete health history, including cardiovascular and renal conditions, surgeries or trauma, allergies, drug history, and possible drug interactions. • Acquire the results of a complete physical examination, including vital signs, height, and weight. • Evaluate laboratory blood findings: complete blood count (CBC), electrolytes, lipid panel, clotting factors, and renal and liver function studies.	• *Ineffective Tissue Perfusion* related to altered blood flow • *Deficient Knowledge* related to lack of information about drug therapy • *Noncompliance* related to adverse effects of medications • *Ineffective Health Maintenance* related to insufficient knowledge of seriousness of disease and drug therapy regimen • *Risk for Injury (bleeding)* related to adverse effects of anticoagulant therapy

(Continued)

Nursing Process Focus (*continued*)

PLANNING: PATIENT GOALS AND EXPECTED OUTCOMES

The patient will:
- Experience therapeutic effects (a decrease in the blood's ability to clot).
- Be free from or experience minimal adverse effects from drug therapy.
- Verbalize an understanding of the drug's use, adverse effects, and required precautions.

IMPLEMENTATION

Interventions and (Rationales)	Patient Education/Discharge Planning
• Administer the medication correctly, and evaluate the patient knowledge of proper administration. (Proper medication administration will increase effectiveness and help reduce complications and adverse effects.)	Instruct patient and caregivers that: • Correct self-administration of medication is extremely important. • Injections of heparin or LMWH should be administered in the fatty layers of the abdomen. • Skin is drawn up (pinched) and the needle is inserted at 45-90 degree angle. • Injections are done without aspirating for blood return. • Oral medications should be taken at the same time every day.
Monitor for adverse clotting reaction(s): • Observe for skin necrosis, blue or purple mottling of the feet that blanches with pressure or fades when the legs are elevated. (Patients on anticoagulant therapy remain at risk for developing emboli resulting in cerebrovascular accident or pulmonary embolism. Coumadin may cause cholesterol microemboli, which result in gangrene, localized vasculitis, or "purple toes syndrome." Heparin can cause thrombus formation with thrombocytopenia, or "white clot syndrome.")	Instruct the patient to: • Immediately report to the healthcare provider any sudden dyspnea or chest pain, and if temperature or color change occurs in the hands, arms, legs, and feet. (Gangrene may occur between days 3 and 8 of warfarin therapy. Purple toes syndrome usually occurs within weeks 3–10 or later.) • Feel pedal pulses daily to check circulation. • Protect feet from injury by wearing loose-fitting socks; avoid going barefoot.
• Use with caution in patients with GI, renal, or liver disease, alcoholism, diabetes, hypertension, hyperlipidemia, and in older adult patients and premenopausal women. (Patients with coronary artery disease risk factors are at increased risk of developing cholesterol microemboli.)	• Advise older adult patients; menstruating women; and those with peptic ulcer disease, alcoholism, or kidney or liver disease that they have an increased risk of bleeding. • Advise patients with diabetes and those with high blood pressure or high cholesterol that they are at risk of developing microscopic clots, despite anticoagulant therapy.
• Monitor for signs of bleeding: flu-like symptoms, excessive bruising, pallor, epistaxis, hemoptysis, hematemesis, menorrhagia, hematuria, melena, frank rectal bleeding, or excessive bleeding from wounds or in the mouth. (Bleeding is a sign of anticoagulant overdose.)	Instruct the patient to: • Immediately report to the healthcare provider flu-like symptoms (dizziness, chills, weakness, pale skin); blood coming from a cough, the nose, mouth, or rectum; menstrual "flooding," "coffee grounds" vomit; tarry stools, excessive bruising; bleeding from wounds that cannot be stopped within 10 minutes, and all physical injuries. • Avoid all contact sports and amusement park rides that cause intense or violent bumping or jostling. • Use a soft toothbrush and electric shaver. • Keep a "pad count" during menstrual periods to estimate blood losses.
• Monitor vital signs. (Increase in heart rate accompanied by low blood pressure or subnormal temperature may signal bleeding.)	• Instruct the patient to immediately report palpitations, fatigue, or feeling faint, which may signal low blood pressure related to bleeding.
• Monitor laboratory values: CBC, especially in premenopausal women; liver function studies, platelets, aPTT, PT, or INR for therapeutic values. (The aPTT and PT are usually 1.5–2.5 the normal control values. The value for INR is usually 2–4. Values below normal indicate below-therapeutic levels. Values above the norm indicate a high potential for bleeding. CBC and platelet levels should remain within normal limits. Heparin may also cause significant elevations of liver function tests because the drug is metabolized by the liver.)	Instruct the patient: • About the importance and need for regular laboratory testing. • To always inform laboratory and dental personnel of anticoagulant therapy when providing samples. • To carry a wallet card or wear medical ID jewelry indicating anticoagulant therapy.

IMPLEMENTATION	
• Monitor the use of other medications or herbal supplements.	• Instruct the patient to consult a healthcare provider before taking any other drugs, including OTC or herbal supplements. Many drugs decrease the action of anticoagulants.
• Maintain a normal diet, avoiding alcohol and increases in vitamin-K rich foods. (Vitamin K is used in the formation of clots; therefore, ingesting high amounts may decrease the effectiveness of warfarin. Alcohol may also alter the effectiveness of anticoagulants.)	• Inform the patient to avoid alcohol and increases in vitamin K-rich foods such as broccoli, cabbage, dark leafy greens, and asparagus.

EVALUATION OF OUTCOME CRITERIA

Evaluate the effectiveness of drug therapy by confirming that patient goals and expected outcomes have been met (see "Planning"). *See Tables 24.2 and 24.3 for a list of drugs to which these nursing actions apply.*

Antiplatelet drugs prolong bleeding time by interfering with platelet aggregation.

◀ **Core Concept 24.5**

Antiplatelet medications produce an anticoagulant effect by interfering with platelet aggregation. Unlike the anticoagulants, which are used primarily to prevent thrombosis in *veins,* antiplatelet drugs are used to prevent clot formation in *arteries*. Doses for antiplatelet medications are listed in Table 24.3.

Platelets are a key component of hemostasis. Too few platelets or diminished platelet function can profoundly increase bleeding time. The three primary classes of antiplatelet drugs include the following:

- Aspirin
- Adenosine diphosphate (ADP) receptor blockers
- Glycoprotein IIb/IIIa receptor blockers

Table 24.3 Antiplatelet Drugs

Drug	Route and Adult Dose	Remarks
anagrelide (Agrylin)	PO: 0.5 mg qid or 1 mg bid (max: 10 mg/day)	For essential thrombocythemia (production of too many platelets)
aspirin (acetylsalicylic acid, ASA) (see the Prototype Drug box in Core Concept 15.6)	PO: 80 mg/day–650 mg bid	Available without a prescription; higher doses are used to treat inflammation or pain
cilostazol (Pletal)	PO: 100 mg bid	For intermittent claudication
dipyridamole (Persantine)	PO: 75–100 mg qid	Used to prevent thromboembolism in cardiac valve replacement; usually used with warfarin
vorapaxar (Zontivity)	PO: 2.08 mg/day	For prevention of thrombotic events in patients with history of MI
ADP RECEPTOR BLOCKERS		
Pr clopidogrel (Plavix)	PO: 75 mg daily (300 mg loading dose for patients with acute coronary syndrome)	For prevention of MI and stroke; often used with a daily dose of aspirin
prasugrel (Effient)	PO: 60 mg loading dose followed by 10 mg/day	For prevention of thrombotic events in patients undergoing PCI
ticagrelor (Brilinta)	PO: 90 mg bid	For prevention of thrombotic events and to reduce the rate of stent thrombosis; used with daily dose of aspirin
ticlopidine (Ticlid)	PO: 250 mg bid	For stroke prevention and to reduce the rate of stent thrombosis
GLYCOPROTEIN IIB/IIIA BLOCKERS		
abciximab (ReoPro)	IV: 0.25 mg/kg initial bolus; then 10 mcg/min for 12–4 hours	For prevention of cardiac events during PCI or in patients with unstable angina
eptifibatide (Integrilin)	IV: 180 mcg/kg initial bolus; then 2 mcg/kg/min for 24–72 hours	
tirofiban (Aggrastat)	IV: 0.4 mcg/kg/min for 30 minutes; then 0.1 mcg/kg/min for 12–18 hours	

Aspirin deserves special mention as an antiplatelet drug. Because it is available OTC, patients may not consider aspirin a strong medication. However, its anticoagulant activity is well documented. Aspirin acts by inhibiting thromboxane A_2, a powerful inducer of platelet aggregation. The anticoagulant effect of a single dose of aspirin may last for as long as a week. Use of aspirin with other coagulation modifiers should be avoided unless approved by the prescriber. The primary actions and adverse effects of aspirin are described in a Prototype Drug feature in Chapter 15.

The ADP receptor blockers are a small group of drugs that irreversibly alter the plasma membrane of platelets, preventing them from aggregating. Both ticlopidine (Ticlid) and clopidogrel (Plavix) are given orally to prevent thrombi formation in patients who have experienced a recent thromboembolic event such as a stroke or MI. Clopidogrel is considerably safer and much more widely prescribed, having adverse effects comparable to those of aspirin. Prasugrel (Effient) and ticagrelor (Brilinta) are newer drugs in this class, approved to reduce thrombotic events in patients undergoing PCI.

CAM Therapy | Garlic for Cardiovascular Health

Garlic (*Allium sativum*) is one of the best-studied herbs. Several substances have been isolated from garlic and shown to have pharmacologic activity. Dosage forms include eating prepared garlic oil or the fresh bulbs from the plant.

Modern claims for garlic uses have focused on the cardiovascular system: treatment of high blood lipid levels, atherosclerosis, and hypertension. Other modern claims are that garlic reduces blood glucose levels and has antibacterial and antineoplastic activity.

Like many other supplements, garlic likely has some health benefits, but controlled, scientific studies are often lacking and the results are mixed. Garlic has been shown to decrease the aggregation or "stickiness" of platelets, thus producing an anticoagulant effect. There is some research to show that the herb has a small effect on lowering blood cholesterol, although the effects seem to be short term.

Garlic is safe for consumption in moderate amounts. Patients taking anticoagulant medications should limit their intake of garlic to avoid bleeding complications. Patients with diabetes should monitor their blood glucose levels closely if taking high doses of garlic.

Prototype Drug: Pr *Clopidogrel (Plavix)*

Therapeutic Class: Antiplatelet drug **Pharmacologic Class:** ADP receptor blocker

Actions and Uses: Clopidogrel is an oral drug that prolongs bleeding time by inhibiting platelet aggregation. It is approved to reduce the risk of thrombotic events in patients with a recent history of stroke, MI, or unstable angina. It is sometimes used off-label to prevent blockage of coronary stents. Because it is expensive, it is usually prescribed for patients who are unable to tolerate aspirin, which has similar anticoagulant activity. Ticlopidine (Ticlid) acts by the same mechanism as clopidogrel but causes more adverse effects.

Adverse Effects and Interactions: Clopidogrel has approximately the same tolerability as aspirin. The incidence of gastrointestinal bleeding is less than that for aspirin. Frequent adverse effects include a flu-like syndrome, headache, diarrhea, dizziness, bruising, upper respiratory tract infection, and rash or pruritus. Excessive bleeding is a potential adverse effect, although it only occurs in about 1% of patients. The other drug in this class, ticlopidine, can cause an acute blood disorder known as thrombotic thrombocytopenia purpura, which can be fatal in up to 30% of patients who develop the disorder.

Use with anticoagulants, other antiplatelet drugs, thrombolytics, or NSAIDS, including aspirin, will increase the risk of bleeding. Proton pump inhibitors, rifampin, or carbamazepine may increase the anticoagulant activity of clopidogrel. The azole antifungals, protease inhibitors, erythromycin, verapamil, or zafirlukast may diminish the antiplatelet actions of clopidogrel.

BLACK BOX WARNING:
Because the effectiveness of clopidogrel is dependent on its metabolic activation by hepatic enzymes, poor metabolizers will exhibit less therapeutic effect and more adverse cardiovascular events.

Glycoprotein IIb/IIIa inhibitors are relatively new additions to the treatment of thromboembolic disease. **Glycoprotein IIb/IIIa** is a receptor on the surface of platelets that is necessary for platelet aggregation. Blocking this receptor has the effect of preventing thrombus formation in patients experiencing a recent MI, stroke, or PCI. These drugs are expensive and administered only by the IV route.

Thrombolytics are used to dissolve existing clots.

◀ **Core Concept 24.6**

It is often mistakenly believed that the purpose of anticoagulants such as heparin and warfarin is to digest and remove preexisting clots. This is not the case: A totally different type of drug is needed for this purpose. These drugs, called thrombolytics, are administered quite differently than the anticoagulants and produce their effects by different mechanisms. Thrombolytics are prescribed for situations in which a clot has already formed, including the following:

- Acute MI
- Pulmonary embolism
- Stroke
- DVT
- Arterial or coronary thrombosis
- Clearing thrombi in arteriovenous cannulas and blocked IV catheters.

The goal of thrombolytic therapy is to restore blood flow quickly to essential tissues served by the blocked vessel. Delays in reestablishing circulation may result in permanent tissue damage. The therapeutic effect of thrombolytics is greater when they are administered as soon as possible after clot formation occurs, preferably within 4 hours. The role of the thrombolytics in treating MI, and a Nursing Process Focus for this drug class, are presented in Chapter 21.

Thrombolytics have a narrow margin of safety between dissolving normal and abnormal clots. Vital signs must be monitored continuously, and signs of bleeding usually call for discontinuation of therapy. Because these medications are rapidly destroyed in the bloodstream, discontinuation normally results in the immediate end of thrombolytic activity. After the clot is successfully removed by the thrombolytic medication, coagulation modifier therapy is initiated to prevent the reformation of clots.

Prototype Drug: Pr *Alteplase (Activase)*

Therapeutic Class: Drug for dissolving clots **Pharmacologic Class:** Thrombolytic

Actions and Uses: Produced through recombinant DNA technology, alteplase is identical to the enzyme human tPA. Like other thrombolytics, the primary action of alteplase is to convert plasminogen to plasmin, which then dissolves clots. Alteplase should be given within 6 hours of the onset of symptoms of MI and within 3 hours of thrombotic stroke to be effective. Peak effect occurs in 5–10 minutes. Alteplase is a preferred drug for the treatment of acute MI and thrombotic stroke. It is occasionally used to reopen occluded IV catheters.

Adverse Effects and Interactions: Thrombolytics such as alteplase are contraindicated in patients with active bleeding or with a history of recent trauma. The patient must be monitored carefully for signs of bleeding every 15 minutes for the first hour of therapy and every 30 minutes thereafter. Signs of bleeding such as bruising, hematomas, or nosebleeds should be reported to the healthcare provider immediately.

Concurrent use with anticoagulants, antiplatelet drugs, or NSAIDs, including aspirin, may increase the risk of bleeding. Use with supplements that affect coagulation, such as feverfew, green tea, ginkgo, fish oil, ginger, or garlic, should be avoided because they may increase the risk of bleeding.

CONCEPT REVIEW 24.2

- Both warfarin and heparin are effective anticoagulants. Why would a physician choose heparin over warfarin?

Hemostatics are used to promote the formation of clots.

◀ **Core Concept 24.7**

Hemostatics, also called *antifibrinolytics*, have an action opposite to that of anticoagulants: to shorten bleeding time. The name *hemostatics* comes from their ability to slow blood flow. They are used to prevent and treat excessive bleeding following surgical procedures.

All of the hemostatics have very specific indications for use, and none are commonly prescribed. Aminocaproic acid is administered IV to prevent bleeding in patients who have systemic clotting disorders. A PO form of tranexamic acid (Lysteda) is available for the

Table 24.4 Hemostatics

Drug	Route and Adult Dose	Remarks
Pr aminocaproic acid (Amicar)	IV/PO: 4–5 g for first hour, then 1–1.25 g/h until bleeding is controlled	For control of bleeding where fibrinolysis contributes to bleeding, such as surgical complications following heart surgery
thrombin (Evithrom, Recothrom, Thrombinar)	Topical: Dose varies based on the size of the treated area	Used to prevent blood loss following cardiopulmonary bypass surgery
tranexamic acid (Cyklokapron, Lysteda)	IV: 10 mg/kg, 3–4 times daily for 2–8 days PO: Two 650 mg tablets, tid for a maximum of 5 days	Used just prior to and following dental surgery in patients with hemophilia (IV) and for heavy menstrual bleeding (PO)

treatment of heavy menstrual bleeding. Thrombin (Evithrom, Recothrom, Thrombinar) is a topical drug to prevent minor oozing and bleeding from surgical sites. Although their mechanisms differ, all drugs in this class prevent fibrin from dissolving, thus enhancing the stability of the clot. The hemostatics are listed in Table 24.4.

Prototype Drug: Pr *Aminocaproic Acid (Amicar)*

Therapeutic Class: Clot stabilizer **Pharmacologic Class:** Hemostatic/Antifibrinolytic

Actions and Uses: Aminocaproic acid is prescribed in situations in which there is excessive bleeding as a result of clots being dissolved prematurely. The drug acts by inactivating plasminogen, the precursor of the enzyme plasmin, which dissolves the fibrin clot. During acute hemorrhages, it can be given IV to reduce bleeding in 1 to 2 hours. It is most commonly prescribed following surgery to reduce postoperative bleeding.

Adverse Effects and Interactions: Because aminocaproic acid tends to stabilize clots, it should be used cautiously in patients with a history of thromboembolic disease. Adverse effects are generally mild. The therapeutic serum level is 100–400 mcg/mL.

Drug interactions include hypercoagulation when used with estrogens and oral contraceptives.

Patients Need to Know

Patients treated for coagulation disorders need to know the following:

1. Keep all scheduled laboratory appointments for PT, aPTT, and INR testing. Test results are used in making decisions about drug dose adjustments.
2. Report unusual bruising or bleeding, such as nosebleeds, bleeding gums, black or red stool, heavy menstrual periods, or spitting up blood, to healthcare providers.
3. Inform dental hygienists and dentists about the use of anticoagulant medication.
4. Use caution when engaged in activities that can cause bleeding, such as shaving, brushing teeth, trimming nails, and using kitchen knives. A soft toothbrush and an electric razor are safe choices. Contact sports, with their high risk for injury, should be avoided.
5. Take medications on time and as directed. Do not skip a dose, double up on doses, or discontinue taking medication without guidance from a healthcare provider.
6. Do not eat large or inconsistent amounts of foods high in vitamin K when taking warfarin because it interferes with clotting time.
7. Speak with the healthcare provider before taking any other drugs, including OTC drugs or herbal supplements. Many drugs increase or decrease the action of anticoagulants.

Patients being treated for hematopoietic disorders need to know the following:

8. Keep all laboratory appointments for CBC and other blood-related testing. Test results are used to determine effectiveness of medication and in making decisions about drug dosing.
9. Rest when fatigued, and allow enough time between activities throughout the day to allow for adequate rest periods.
10. Take blood pressure and pulse as recommended by the healthcare provider, using the monitoring equipment properly.
11. Consult with a dietitian, and follow dietary recommendations to ensure nutritional needs are being met.
12. Drink water when thirsty instead of heavily concentrated drinks in order to maintain adequate fluid levels in the blood.
13. Notify the healthcare provider if experiencing pain, especially chest and bone pain.

Safety Alert: Medication Label Confusion: Heparin

Medication errors have occurred because of a nurse's failure to read the information provided on medication labels properly, such as when the strength of heparin was labeled only on a per-milliliter basis, and the volume of the vial was stated in another location. To help prevent these types of errors, the U.S. Food and Drug Administration (FDA) requires that heparin labels express the strength of the entire container and milliliters together. However, nurses should not rely on safety organizations alone to prevent medication errors. It is ultimately the responsibility of the nurse to read and understand the entire label before preparing and administering any medication.

Hematopoietic growth factors are administered to boost blood cell production.

◀ **Core Concept 24.8**

Hematopoiesis is the process of blood cell production. The body controls blood cell production through natural hormones called hematopoietic growth factors (HGFs). If more of a certain type of blood cell is needed, the body secretes these hormones to bring the body back to homeostasis. Scientists have developed drugs that are either identical to, or very similar to, natural HGFs. These medications are shown in Table 24.5.

Some of the HGFs have become important adjunct medications in cancer therapy. Many of the drugs used to treat cancers are toxic to the blood forming tissues in the body and dramatic reductions in blood cells can occur. The HGFs can boost the production of red blood cells, white blood cells, or platelets in these patients.

Table 24.5 Hematopoietic Growth Factors and Enhancers

Drug	Route and Adult Dose	Remarks
RED BLOOD CELL ENHANCERS		
darbepoetin alfa (Aranesp)	Subcutaneous/IV: 0.45 mcg/kg once per week	For disorders associated with a deficiency of red blood cells; therapeutic response may take 2–6 weeks
Pr epoetin alfa (Epogen, Procrit)	Subcutaneous/IV: 50–100 units/kg/dose until target hematocrit range is reached	
COLONY-STIMULATING FACTORS		
filgrastim (Granix, Neupogen)	IV/Subcutaneous: 5-10 mcg/kg/day (max: 20–30 mcg/kg/day)	For disorders associated with a deficiency of white blood cells; therapeutic response may take 1–2 days
pegfilgrastim (Neulasta)	Subcutaneous: 6 mg once per chemotherapy cycle	
sargramostim (Leukine)	IV: 250 mcg/m^2/day	
PLATELET ENHANCERS		
eltrombopag (Promacta)	PO: 50 mg once daily (max: 75 mg/day)	For disorders associated with a deficiency of platelets; therapeutic response may take 5–9 days
oprelvekin (Neumega)	Subcutaneous: 50 mcg/kg once daily	
romiplostim (Nplate)	Subcutaneous: 1 mcg/kg once weekly (max; 10 mcg/kg/week)	

Red Blood Cell Enhancers

The most frequently prescribed HGF is epoetin alfa (Epogen, Procrit), a drug that is identical to the natural hormone erythropoietin. Epoetin alfa, the prototype for the HGFs, stimulates the production of red blood cells. A second red blood cell enhancer, darbepoetin alfa (Aranesp), has the same action and effectiveness as epoetin alfa but an extended duration of action that allows it to be given once weekly or once every 2 weeks.

White Blood Cell Enhancers

Substances that stimulate the production of white blood cells are called colony-stimulating factors (CSFs). The three drugs in this group are identical to natural HGFs in the body. Drugs such as filgrastim (Granix, Neupogen) are very important for restoring white blood cell counts in patients who have suppressed immune systems due to cancer chemotherapy, tissue transplants, or debilitating infections.

Platelet Enhancers

Thrombopoietin is the hormone in the body responsible for controlling the number of platelets. A severe reduction in platelets, or thrombocytopenia, may result in excessive bleeding.

Prototype Drug: Pr *Epoetin Alfa (Epogen, Procrit)*

Therapeutic Class: Drug for anemia **Pharmacologic Class:** Hematopoietic growth factor, erythropoietin

Actions and Uses: Epoetin alfa is made through recombinant DNA technology and functions like human erythropoietin. Because of its ability to stimulate red blood cell formation, epoetin alfa is effective in treating specific disorders caused by a deficiency in the number of red blood cells. Patients with chronic renal failure often cannot secrete enough erythropoietin and thus will benefit from epoetin administration. Epoetin is sometimes given to patients undergoing cancer chemotherapy to counteract the anemia caused by antineoplastic drugs. It is occasionally prescribed for patients prior to blood transfusions or surgery and to treat anemia in patients infected with HIV. Epoetin alfa is usually administered three times per week until a therapeutic response is achieved.

Adverse Effects and Interactions: Epoetin alfa has some serious adverse effects, which are described in the black box warning. The most common adverse effect of epoetin alfa is hypertension, which may occur in as many as 30% of patients receiving the drug. Blood pressure should be monitored during therapy, and an antihypertensive drug may be indicated.

The effectiveness of epoetin alfa will be greatly reduced in patients with iron deficiency or other vitamin-depleted states because erythropoiesis cannot be enhanced without these vital nutrients. There are no clinically significant drug interactions with epoetin alfa.

BLACK BOX WARNING:
The risk of serious cardiovascular events is increased with epoetin alfa therapy. Transient ischemic attacks (TIAs), MIs, and strokes have occurred in patients who are on dialysis and being treated with epoetin alfa. Epoetin increased the rate of DVT in patients not receiving concurrent anticoagulation. The lowest dose possible should be used in patients with cancer because the drug can promote tumor progression and shorten overall survival in some patients.

Oprelvekin (Neumega) is equivalent to thrombopoietin and is commonly prescribed to prevent or reverse the platelet reduction caused by intensive cancer chemotherapy. Romiplostim (Nplate) and eltrombopag (Promacta) have more limited applications in treating a disorder called chronic immune (idiopathic) thrombocytopenic purpura (ITP), in which patients have increased destruction of platelets.

Chapter Review

Core Concepts Summary

24.1 Hemostasis is a complex process involving multiple steps and many clotting factors.

Hemostasis is an essential mechanism protecting the body from both external and internal injury; it occurs in a sequential series of steps known as the coagulation cascade. The final result of coagulation is the formation of a fibrin clot that protects the body from excessive blood loss.

24.2 Removing a blood clot is essential to restoring normal circulation.

Blood clots are removed by fibrinolysis. Plasmin digests the fibrin strands, thus restoring circulation to the injured area.

24.3 Drugs are used to modify the coagulation process.

Anticoagulants prevent the formation of clots, thrombolytics dissolve existing clots, and hemostatics promote the formation of clots. Coagulation is always carefully monitored through the use of PT or aPTT laboratory tests.

24.4 Anticoagulants prevent the formation and enlargement of clots.

Anticoagulants prolong coagulation time by inhibiting platelets or a specific clotting factor in the coagulation cascade. Heparin is given IV or subcutaneously to provide immediate anticoagulation activity, and warfarin is given orally to offer more prolonged action. Protamine sulfate can reverse the anticoagulant activity of heparin, and vitamin K can reverse the effects of warfarin.

24.5 Antiplatelet drugs prolong bleeding time by interfering with platelet aggregation.

Aspirin, ADP receptor blockers, and glycoprotein IIb/IIIa receptor blockers prolong bleeding time by interfering with platelet function. They are used to prevent thrombus formation in arteries.

24.6 Thrombolytics are used to dissolve existing clots.

By dissolving existing clots, thrombolytics restore circulation to an injured area. For maximum effectiveness, they should be given as soon as possible after the thrombus is diagnosed.

24.7 Hemostatics are used to promote the formation of clots.

Hemostatics inhibit fibrin in a clot from dissolving and are used primarily to prevent excessive bleeding from surgical sites.

24.8 Hematopoietic growth factors are administered to boost blood cell production.

HGFs are natural hormones secreted by the body to control blood cell production. Drugs have been developed that mimic the actions of HGFs to boost the production of red blood cells, white blood cells, and platelets.

REVIEW Questions

Answer the following questions to assess your knowledge of the chapter material, and go back and review any material that is not clear to you.

1. A patient has started taking clopidogrel (Plavix) after experiencing a transient ischemic attack. What adverse effects are associated with this drug? (Select all that apply)
   1. Headache
   2. Diarrhea
   3. Constipation
   4. Bruising
   5. Rash

2. The patient has been started on warfarin (Coumadin) for deep vein thrombosis. The patient asks when the medication will break up the clots. The nurse's best response would be:
   1. "It will take 7 to 10 days for the clot to break down."
   2. "This medication will not break down clots but will make it less likely that the clot will get larger."
   3. "It will break down the clot within 8 to 12 hours of administration."
   4. "You will need to be on this medication for a long time before it will break down the clot."

3. The patient has been started on oprelvekin (Neumega). The patient asks when the medication will begin to create new platelets. The nurse's best response would be:
   1. "It will take 5 to 9 days to see any results from the medication."
   2. "We should see an immediate increase in the number of platelets."
   3. "Oprelvekin does not help create new platelets."
   4. "We should see an immediate increase in the number of white blood cells."

4. The patient is receiving enoxaparin (Lovenox) subcutaneously every 12 hours following knee replacement surgery. The patient is monitored for:
   1. Gingival hyperplasia.
   2. Signs and symptoms of bruising and bleeding.
   3. Clotting at the incision site.
   4. Increased pain.

5. The healthcare provider prescribes clopidogrel (Plavix) for a patient at risk for a myocardial infarction. While instructing the patient about the adverse effects and precautions associated with this drug, the nurse tells him that the following drugs should not be used while on clopidogrel unless the doctor is consulted. (Select all that apply.)
   1. Coumadin
   2. Ibuprofen
   3. Diltiazem
   4. Aspirin
   5. Tissue plasminogen activator

6. The nurse is conducting an informational session with patients being prescribed *epoetin alfa*. The nurse knows that the patients understand what they must do while taking this medication when they say: (Select all that apply)
   1. "We will avoid eating raw vegetables."
   2. "We will avoid direct sunlight."
   3. "We will take frequent rest periods to avoid excessive fatigue."
   4. "We will monitor our blood pressure and pulse."
   5. "We will protect our eyes from bright light."

7. The healthcare provider has ordered that a patient be placed on a hemostatic drug to control postoperative bleeding. Which of the following medications will most likely be given in this situation?
   1. Aminocaproic acid (Amicar)
   2. Aspirin
   3. Trombin (Evithrom)
   4. Tranexamic acid (Cyklokapron)

8. The patient on intermittent heparin is found to have hematuria and bleeding from old intravenous sites. The nurse anticipates what being ordered?
   1. Protamine sulfate
   2. Vitamin K
   3. Pentoxifylline (Trental)
   4. Ardeparin (Normiflo)

9. The healthcare provider orders 35,000 units of heparin to be given subcutaneously daily after the patient's aPTT has been checked. The label on the vial states 10,000 units/mL. How many units should the patient receive daily should the aPTT be in the recommended range?
   1. 3.2 mL
   2. 3.3 mL
   3. 3 mL
   4. 3.5 mL

10. A patient is receiving alteplase (Activase), a thrombolytic drug. The nurse monitors the patient for which of the following possible adverse effects?
    1. Temperature of 100.8°F (38.2°C)
    2. Bruising and epistaxis
    3. Skin rash with urticaria
    4. Wheezing with labored breathing

CASE STUDY Questions

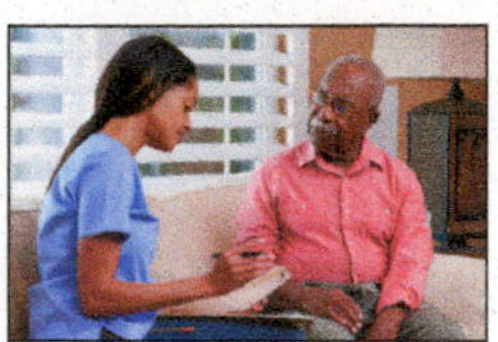

Remember Mr. Hawkins, the patient introduced at the beginning of the chapter? Now read the remainder of the case study. Based on the information you have learned in this chapter, answer the questions that follow.

Mr. Thomas Hawkins was recently admitted to the hospital with chest pain and a suspected pulmonary embolism. He was immediately placed on heparin for 2 days and then switched to warfarin. He is now leaving the hospital with instructions to have laboratory testing every other day for the next 2 weeks.

1. The goal of initially placing Mr. Hawkins on heparin was to:
    1. Dissolve pulmonary emboli.
    2. Prevent excessive bleeding.
    3. Reduce blood viscosity.
    4. Prevent additional thrombi from forming.
2. Mr. Hawkins is taught that the most common adverse effect of heparin therapy is:
    1. Nausea and vomiting
    2. Myocardial infarction
    3. Bleeding
    4. Sedation
3. In planning for Mr. Hawkins's discharge from the hospital, he was switched from heparin to warfarin. When he inquired why his drug was switched, the nurse informed him that:
    1. Warfarin is more effective.
    2. Warfarin is given orally.
    3. Warfarin causes less risk of hemorrhage.
    4. Warfarin is less expensive.
4. As part of the discharge instructions, Mr. Hawkins is told that he will need to have blood drawn and which of the following laboratory tests performed during the 2 weeks after his discharge?
    1. Prothrombin time/international normalized ratio (PT/INR)
    2. Complete blood count (CBC)
    3. Activated partial thromboplastin time (aPTT)
    4. White blood cell count

Answers and complete rationales for the Review and Case Study Questions appear in Appendix A.

REFERENCE

Herdman, T. H., & Kamitsuru, S. (Eds.). (2014). *NANDA International nursing diagnoses: Definitions and classification, 2015–2017*. Oxford, United Kingdom: Wiley-Blackwell.

SELECTED BIBLIOGRAPHY

Angiolillo, D. J., & Ferreiro, J. L. (2013). Antiplatelet and anticoagulant therapy for atherothrombotic disease: The role of current and emerging agents. *American Journal of Cardiovascular Drugs, 13*, 233–250. doi:10.1007/s40256-013-0022-7

Berra, K. (2014). Antithrombotics for stroke prevention in non-valvular atrial fibrillation: An update. *European Journal of Cardiovascular Nursing, 13*, 32–40. doi:10.1177/1474515113477957

Boonyawat, K., & Crowther, M. A. (2015). Venous thromboembolism prophylaxis in critically ill patients. *Seminars in Thrombosis and Hemostasis 41*, 68–74. doi:10.1055/s-0034-1398386

Fareed, J., Hoppensteadt, D., & Jeske, W. P. (2014). An update on low molecular-weight heparins. In H. I. Saba & H. R. Roberts (Eds.), *Hemostasis and thrombosis*, (pp. 296–313). Oxford, United Kingdom: John Wiley & Sons, Ltd. doi:10.1002/9781118833391.ch31

Patel, K. (2015). *Deep venous thrombosis*. Retrieved from http://emedicine.medscape.com/article/1911303-overview

Centers for Disease Control (2015). *Hemophilia: Data and statistics in the United States*. Retrieved from http://www.cdc.gov/ncbddd/hemophilia/data.html

Centers for Disease Control (2015). *Venous thromboembolism (blood clots) data and statistics*. Retrieved from http://www.cdc.gov/ncbddd/dvt/data.html

Centers for Disease Control (2015). *Von Willebrand disease*. Retrieved from http://www.cdc.gov/ncbddd/vwd/facts.html

Hörl, W. H. (2013). Differentiating factors between erythropoiesis stimulating agents: An update to selection for anaemia of chronic kidney disease. *Drugs, 73,* 117–130. doi:10.1007/s40265012-0002-2

Lissiman, E., Bhasale, A. L., & Cohen, M. (2012). Garlic for the common cold. *Cochrane Database of Systematic Reviews, 3,* Art. No.: CD006206. doi:10.1002/14651858.CD006206.pub3

National Center for Complementary and Integrative Health. (2016). *Garlic.* Retrieved from https://nccih.nih.gov/health/garlic/ataglance.htm

Ouellette, D. R. (2015). *Pulmonary emobolism.* Retrieved from http://emedicine.medscape.com/article/300901-overview#a6

Pollack, C. V. (2013). Current and future options for anticoagulant therapy in the acute management of ACS. *Current Treatment Options in Cardiovascular Medicine, 15,* 21–32. doi:10.1007/s11936-012-0216-3

Schulman, S. (2015). Treatment of venous thromboembolism with new oral anticoagulants according to patient risk. *Seminars in Thrombosis and Hemostasis, 41,* 160–165. doi:10.1055/s-0035-1544157

Unit 4

The Immune System

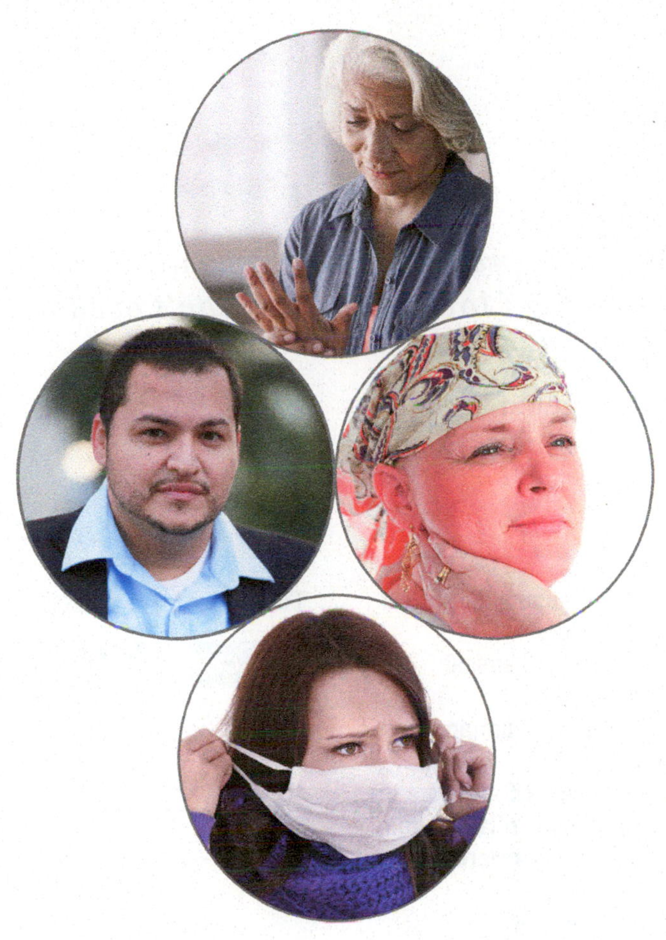

Unit Contents

Chapter 25

Drugs for Inflammation and Fever

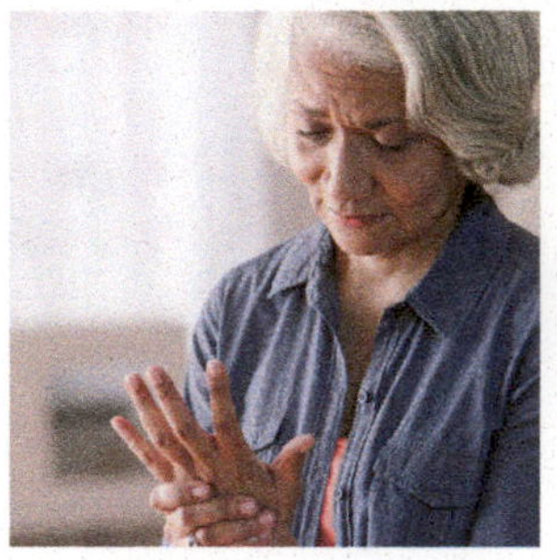

"It's so depressing. My hands are swollen all the time; and the gardening I love so much, I can't even do anymore. It's just too painful."

Mrs. Eugenia Ford

Core Concepts

25.1 Inflammation is a body defense that limits the spread of invading microorganisms and injury.

25.2 The body reacts to injury by releasing chemical mediators that cause inflammation.

25.3 Inflammation may be treated with nonpharmacologic and pharmacologic therapies.

25.4 Nonsteroidal anti-inflammatory drugs (NSAIDs) are the primary drugs for the treatment of mild inflammation.

25.5 Corticosteroids are effective in treating severe inflammation.

25.6 Antipyretics are drugs used to reduce fever.

Drug Snapshot

The following drugs are discussed in this chapter:

Drug Classes	Prototype Drugs
NSAIDs	Pr naproxen (Naprosyn) and naproxen sodium (Aleve, Anaprox)
Corticosteroids	Pr prednisone
Antipyretics	Pr acetaminophen (Tylenol)

Learning Outcomes

After reading this chapter, the student should be able to:

1. Identify the functions of inflammation as part of the body's normal defenses.
2. Explain the role of chemical mediators in inflammation.
3. Outline the general strategies for treating inflammation.
4. Explain why NSAIDs are the primary pharmacotherapy for mild to moderate inflammation.
5. Identify the advantages and disadvantages of using corticosteroids to treat inflammation.
6. Explain the pharmacotherapy of fever.

Key Terms

alternate-day therapy
anaphylaxis (ANN-ah-fah-LAX-iss)
antipyretics
Cushing syndrome (KUSH-ing)
cyclooxygenase (COX) (SYE-klo-OK-sah-jen-ays)
histamine (HISS-tuh-meen)
inflammation (IN-flah-MAY-shun)
mast cells
salicylism (sal-IH-sill-izm)

The pain and redness of inflammation following minor abrasions and cuts is something everyone has experienced. Although there may be discomfort from such scrapes, inflammation is a normal and expected part of our body's defense against injury. For some diseases, however, inflammation can rage out of control, producing severe pain, fever, and other distressing symptoms. The purpose of this chapter is to examine these sorts of inflammatory conditions for which drug therapy may be needed.

Fast Facts Inflammatory Disorders

- Osteoarthritis affects about 27 million people and is the leading cause of disability in the United States.
- About 1.3 million Americans are afflicted with rheumatoid arthritis, which has an average onset between the ages of 30 and 60.
- In the United States, approximately 70 million NSAID prescriptions are written, and 30 billion over-the-counter (OTC) nonsteroidal anti-inflammatory drug (NSAID) tablets are sold each year.
- Over 50,000 accidental poisonings occur with NSAIDs each year in American children.
- It is estimated that NSAIDs cause about 16,000 deaths in the United States annually, largely as a result of gastrointestinal (GI) complications.

INFLAMMATION

Inflammation is a body defense that limits the spread of invading microorganisms and injury.

◀ Core Concept 25.1

The human body has developed complex ways to defend itself against physical injury and invasion by microorganisms. Inflammation is one of these defense mechanisms. **Inflammation** is a nonspecific process that occurs in response to many different stimuli, including physical injury, exposure to toxic chemicals, extreme heat, invading microorganisms, or death of cells. The central purpose of inflammation is to contain the injury or destroy the microorganism. By removing cellular debris and dead cells, repair of the injured area can move at a faster pace. Inflammation proceeds the same regardless of the cause that triggered it. Signs of inflammation include swelling, pain, warmth, and redness of the affected area.

Inflammation may be classified as *acute* or *chronic*. Acute inflammation has an immediate onset and lasts 1 to 2 weeks. During acute inflammation, 8–10 days are normally needed for the symptoms to resolve and for repair to begin. If the body cannot destroy or neutralize the damaging agent, inflammation may continue for long periods and become chronic. In chronic diseases such as lupus and rheumatoid arthritis, inflammation may persist for years, with symptoms becoming progressively worse over time. Other disorders such as seasonal allergy arise at predictable times each year, and inflammation may produce only minor, annoying symptoms.

The body reacts to injury by releasing chemical mediators that cause inflammation.

◀ Core Concept 25.2

Whether the injury is due to an infection, chemicals, or physical trauma, the damaged tissue releases chemical mediators that act as "alarms" that notify the surrounding area of the injury. These chemical mediators initiate the processes and steps of inflammation. Chemical mediators include histamine, leukotrienes, bradykinin, complement, and prostaglandins. Table 25.1 describes the sources and actions of these mediators.

Table 25.1 Chemical Mediators of Inflammation

Bradykinin	Vasodilator that causes pain; effects are similar to those of histamine
C-reactive protein	Protein found in the plasma that serves as an early marker of inflammation
Complement	Series of at least 20 proteins that combine in a cascade fashion to neutralize or destroy an antigen
Histamine	Stored and released by mast cells; causes dilation of blood vessels, smooth muscle constriction, tissue swelling, and itching
Leukotrienes	Stored and released by mast cells; effects are similar to those of histamine
Prostaglandins	Present in most tissues; stored and released by mast cells; increase capillary permeability, attract white blood cells to the site of inflammation, cause pain and induce fever

Histamine is a key chemical mediator of inflammation. It is primarily stored within **mast cells** located in tissue spaces under epithelial membranes such as the skin, in the bronchial tree and digestive tract, and along blood vessels. Mast cells detect invading microorganisms or injury and respond by releasing histamine, which initiates the inflammatory response within seconds. In addition, histamine directly stimulates pain receptors.

When released at an injury site, histamine and other mediators dilate nearby blood vessels, causing the capillaries to become more permeable or leaky. Plasma and components such as complement proteins and phagocytes can then enter the area to neutralize foreign agents. The affected area may become congested with blood, which can lead to significant swelling and pain. Thrombosis or blood clotting may result. Figure 25.1 shows the basic steps in acute inflammation.

Rapid release of histamine on a larger scale throughout the body is responsible for **anaphylaxis**, a life-threatening allergic response that may result in shock and death. A number of chemicals, insect stings, foods, and some therapeutic drugs can cause this widespread release of histamine from mast cells. Drug therapy of anaphylactic shock is discussed in Chapter 22.

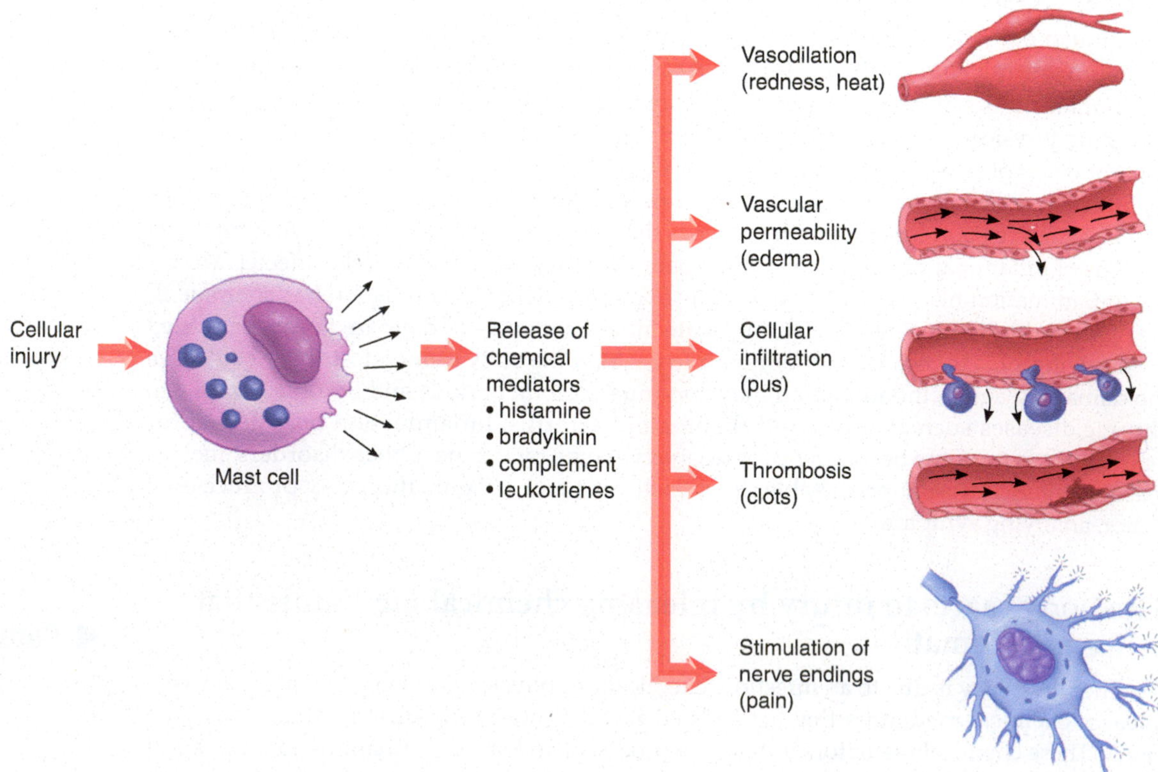

FIGURE 25.1 Steps in acute inflammation.

Inflammation may be treated with nonpharmacologic and pharmacologic therapies.

◀ **Core Concept 25.3**

Because inflammation is a nonspecific process and may be caused by such a diverse variety of causes, it may occur in nearly any tissue or organ system. When treating inflammation, the following general principles apply:

- Inflammation is not a disease but a symptom of an underlying disorder. Whenever possible, the *cause* of the inflammation is identified and treated.
- Inflammation is a natural process for ridding the body of foreign agents, and it is usually self-limiting. For mild symptoms, nonpharmacologic therapies such as ice packs, rest, and elevating the affected extremity should be used, as appropriate for the condition.
- When pharmacotherapy is necessary, topical drugs are used when applicable because they cause fewer adverse effects. Topical sprays, ointments, and creams are often the most effective drugs for treating inflammation of the skin and mucous membranes of the mouth, nose, rectum, and vagina. Many of these are available over the counter (OTC).

The goal of pharmacotherapy with anti-inflammatory drugs is to prevent or decrease the intensity of the inflammatory response and reduce fever, if present. Most anti-inflammatory medications are nonspecific; the drug will exhibit the same inhibitory actions regardless of the cause of the inflammation. Diseases that benefit from anti-inflammatory drugs include allergic rhinitis, anaphylaxis, ankylosing spondylitis, contact dermatitis, Crohn's disease, glomerulonephritis, Hashimoto's thyroiditis, peptic ulcer disease, rheumatoid arthritis, systemic lupus erythematosus, and ulcerative colitis. If the inflammation is the result of an infection, antibiotic therapy may be necessary.

rhin = *nose*
itis = *inflammation*

The two primary drug classes used for inflammation are the NSAIDs and the corticosteroids (also called glucocorticoids). For mild to moderate pain and inflammation, NSAIDs are the preferred drugs. Should inflammation become severe, oral corticosteroid therapy is begun. Due to their serious long-term adverse effects, oral corticosteroids are usually used for only 1 to 3 weeks to bring inflammation under control, and then the patient is switched to NSAIDs. Topical corticosteroids are used whenever possible, because they do not exhibit the serious adverse effects of oral corticosteroids.

Nonsteroidal anti-inflammatory drugs (NSAIDs) are the primary drugs for the treatment of mild inflammation.

◀ **Core Concept 25.4**

NSAIDs such as aspirin and ibuprofen have analgesic, antipyretic, and anti-inflammatory effects. They are preferred drugs for the oral therapy of mild to moderate inflammation. Specific NSAIDs used to treat inflammation are listed in Table 25.2.

The analgesic action of NSAIDs is discussed in Chapter 15. Because many of these medications are inexpensive and available OTC, NSAIDs such as aspirin and ibuprofen are some of the most widely used drugs. Acetaminophen has no anti-inflammatory action and is thus not classified as an NSAID. It is, however, an effective analgesic and antipyretic (see Section 25.6).

Aspirin is useful in treating inflammation because it inhibits **cyclooxygenase (COX)**, a key enzyme in the pathway of prostaglandin synthesis that is found in every tissue. Aspirin causes irreversible inhibition of both forms of cyclooxygenase, COX-1 and COX-2. Because it is readily available, inexpensive, and effective, aspirin is sometimes a drug of first choice for treating mild inflammation. The basic pharmacology and a drug profile of aspirin are presented in Chapter 15.

Unfortunately, large doses of aspirin are necessary to suppress severe inflammation, and these doses result in a greater incidence of serious adverse effects. The most common adverse effects observed during high-dose therapy relate to the digestive system. By increasing gastric acid secretion and irritating the stomach lining, aspirin may cause pain, heartburn, and even bleeding due to ulceration. In some patients, even small doses may cause GI bleeding. Some aspirin formulations are buffered or given an enteric coating to minimize GI adverse effects. Because aspirin also has an antiplatelet effect (see Chapter 24), the potential for bleeding must be carefully monitored by the healthcare provider. High doses may

Table 25.2 Selected Nonsteroidal Anti-Inflammatory Drugs (NSAIDs)

Drug	Route and Adult Dose	Remarks
aspirin (acetylsalicylic acid [ASA], others) (see the Prototype Drug box in Core Concept 15.6)	PO: 350–650 mg every 4 hours (max: 4 g/day) PO: 3.6–5.4 g/day in 4–6 divided doses for arthritic conditions	Inhibits the formation of prostaglandins; also for fever, pain, and prevention of stroke and myocardial infarction (MI)
celecoxib (Celebrex)	PO: 100–400 mg bid (max: 800 mg/day)	Selective COX-2 inhibitor
diclofenac (Cataflam, Solaraze, Voltaren)	PO: 50 mg bid–qid (max: 200 mg/day)	Sustained-release and transdermal forms available
diflunisal	PO: 250–500 mg bid (max: 1500 mg/day)	Similar to ibuprofen
etodolac	PO: 200–1200 mg in divided doses (max: 3200 mg/day)	Extended-release form available
fenoprofen (Nalfon)	PO: 200–600 mg in divided doses (max: 3200 mg/day)	Similar to ibuprofen
flurbiprofen (Ansaid)	PO: 50–300 in divided doses (max: 300 mg/day)	Similar to ibuprofen
ibuprofen (Advil, Motrin, others)	PO: 400–800 mg tid–qid (max: 3200 mg/day)	Blocks prostaglandin synthesis as well as modulates T-cell function; also for dysmenorrhea
ketoprofen	PO: 25–75 mg tid (immediate release) or 200 mg/day (extended release)	Similar to ibuprofen; also for dysmenorrhea
meloxicam (Mobic)	PO: 7.5–15 mg once daily (max: 15 mg/day)	Similar to ibuprofen
nabumetone (Relafen)	PO: 1000 mg daily (max: 2000 mg/day)	Similar to ibuprofen
Pr naproxen (Naprosyn) and naproxen sodium (Aleve, Anaprox)	PO: 250–500 mg bid (max: 1000 mg/day)	Also for dysmenorrhea
oxaprozin (Daypro)	PO: 600–1200 mg daily (max: 1800 mg/day)	Similar to naproxen; once-a-day dosage
piroxicam (Feldene)	PO: 10–20 mg once or twice a day (max: 40 mg/day)	Has prolonged half-life
tolmetin (Tolectin)	PO: 200–600 mg tid (max: 1800 mg/day)	Similar to ibuprofen

produce **salicylism**, a syndrome that includes symptoms such as tinnitus (ringing in the ears), dizziness, headache, and sweating. Patients with preexisting kidney disease should be monitored carefully because aspirin and other NSAIDs may affect kidney function.

Ibuprofen and ibuprofen-like drugs such as naproxen are available as alternatives to aspirin. Like aspirin, they exhibit their effects through inhibition of COX-1 and COX-2. Because of their similar mechanisms, they all have similar pharmacologic properties and a relatively low incidence of adverse effects. The most common adverse effects of these drugs

Prototype Drug: Pr *Naproxen (Naprosyn) and Naproxen Sodium (Aleve, Anaprox)*

Therapeutic Class: Analgesic, anti-inflammatory drug, antipyretic **Pharmacologic Class:** Nonsteroidal anti-inflammatory drug (NSAID)

Actions and Uses: Naproxen is an older NSAID that is prescribed for the treatment of mild to moderate pain, fever, and inflammation. Its efficacy at relieving pain and inflammation is similar to that of aspirin. Common indications include treating the pain associated with rheumatoid arthritis and osteoarthritis, gout, and bursitis. In treating rheumatoid arthritis, the therapeutic effects may take 3 to 4 weeks to appear.

Naproxen inhibits prostaglandin synthesis through the nonselective inhibition of cyclooxygenase type-1 and type-2 enzymes. It also inhibits platelet aggregation and prolongs bleeding time.

Adverse Effects and Interactions: Adverse effects of naproxen are generally not serious and include GI upset, dizziness, and drowsiness. Administration with food will decrease the incidence of stomach upset, which is the most common adverse effect. Because naproxen can interfere with platelet action and prolong bleeding time, the drug should be administered with caution to those with bleeding disorders. Patients taking naproxen should notify their dental hygienist before dental procedures are performed.

Using naproxen concurrently with oral anticoagulants can prolong bleeding time. Lithium levels may be increased. Bleeding potential increases when used with herbal supplements such as feverfew, garlic, ginger, and ginkgo biloba.

BLACK BOX WARNING (PRESCRIPTION FORMS):
All prescription NSAIDs carry the same black box warning. NSAIDs may increase the risk of serious cardiovascular thrombotic events, MI, and stroke, which may be fatal. Patients with existing cardiovascular disease may be at greater risk. NSAIDs are contraindicated for the treatment of perioperative pain in those undergoing coronary artery bypass graft surgery. NSAIDs increase the risk of serious GI adverse events, including bleeding, ulceration, and perforation of the stomach or intestines, which can be fatal. These events occur more frequently in older adults and can occur at any time during use or without warning symptoms.

are nausea and vomiting. Although the incidence of gastric ulceration and bleeding is less than that of aspirin, this can still be a serious problem in patients with peptic ulcers who are taking high doses of these medications. Recently, the U.S. Food and Drug Administration (FDA) strengthened the warning labels on NSAIDs to include an increased risk for MI or stroke.

Selective inhibition of COX-2 produces the analgesic, anti-inflammatory, and antipyretic effects seen with the NSAIDs without causing some of the serious adverse effects of the older NSAIDs. Celecoxib (Celebrex) is the sole drug in this class. Because it has no adverse GI effects and does not affect blood coagulation, celecoxib quickly became the preferred treatment for moderate to severe inflammation.

Nursing Process Focus Patients Receiving NSAID Therapy

ASSESSMENT	POTENTIAL NURSING DIAGNOSES*
Prior to administration: • Obtain a complete health history, including musculoskeletal, GI, renal and liver conditions, infectious diseases, allergies, drug history, and possible drug interactions. • Evaluate laboratory blood findings: compete blood count (CBC), electrolytes, and renal and liver function studies. • Determine reasons for analgesic use and patterns (amount and times) of medication usage. • Acquire the results of a complete physical examination, including vital signs, height, and weight.	• *Chronic Pain* related to tissue damage • *Deficient Knowledge* related to a lack of information about drug therapy • *Ineffective Health Maintenance* related to pain and drug usage

PLANNING: PATIENT GOALS AND EXPECTED OUTCOMES

The patient will:

- Experience therapeutic effects (pain relief or a reduction in pain intensity).
- Be free from or experience minimal adverse effects from drug therapy.
- Verbalize an understanding of the drug's use, adverse effects, and required precautions.

IMPLEMENTATION

Interventions and (Rationales)	Patient Education/Discharge Planning
• Determine need for medication. Record the character, duration, location, and intensity of pain and the presence of inflammation. (NSAIDs are usually given to patients who have inflammatory conditions that cause pain. Monitoring pain and medication use helps to determine medication effectiveness.)	• Instruct the patient to report to the healthcare provider any pain or inflammation that remains unresolved.
• Administer NSAIDs correctly, and evaluate the patient's knowledge of proper administration. (May be administered PO, topical, or transdermal. Overuse may cause severe adverse effects.)	Inform the patient to: • Take only the prescribed amount of NSAIDs to decrease the potential for adverse effects. • Not cut or crush enteric-coated tablets. Regular tablets may be broken or pulverized and mixed with food. • Take liquid aspirin (ASA) products immediately after mixing because they break down rapidly. • Not take different drugs and formulations, such as ibuprofen and naproxen, concurrently. Consult the healthcare provider regarding appropriate OTC analgesics for specific types of pain. • Consult the healthcare provider regarding aspirin therapy following surgery. (ASA also has antiplatelet properties. The body needs time to manufacture new platelets to make clots that promote wound healing.) • Advise laboratory personnel of aspirin therapy when providing urine samples.
• Monitor vital signs, especially temperature. (Increased temperature may indicate infection. Increased pulse and blood pressure may indicate discomfort; if accompanied by pallor or dizziness, may indicate bleeding.)	Instruct the patient to: • Immediately report the occurrence of a rapid heartbeat, palpitations, dizziness, or pallor to the healthcare provider. • Monitor blood pressure and temperature, ensuring proper use of home equipment.

(Continued)

Nursing Process Focus (*continued*)

Interventions and (Rationales)	Patient Education/Discharge Planning
• Monitor for signs of GI bleeding, patterns of GI elimination, or hepatic toxicity. Conduct guaiac stool testing for occult blood, and monitor CBC for anemia-related blood loss. (NSAIDs can be a local irritant to the GI tract with anticoagulant action that is metabolized in the liver.)	Instruct the patient to: • Report any bleeding, abdominal pain, anorexia, heartburn, nausea, vomiting, jaundice, or change in the color or character of stools to the healthcare provider. • Know the proper method of obtaining stool samples and home testing for occult blood. • Adhere to a regimen of laboratory testing as ordered by the healthcare provider. • Take NSAIDs with food to reduce stomach upset.
• Monitor for hypersensitivity reaction.	• Advise the patient to monitor for shortness of breath, wheezing, throat tightness, itching, or hives. If these occur, stop taking ASA immediately and inform the healthcare provider.
• Monitor urinary output and edema in feet and ankles. (Medication is excreted through the kidneys. Long-term use may lead to renal dysfunction.)	• Instruct the patient to report changes in urination, flank pain, or pitting edema.
• Monitor for sensory changes indicative of drug toxicity. (Signs and symptoms of toxicity include tinnitus and blurred vision.)	• Inform the patient to immediately report any sensory changes in sight or hearing, especially blurred vision or tinnitus, to the healthcare provider.

EVALUATION OF OUTCOME CRITERIA

Evaluate the effectiveness of drug therapy by confirming that patient goals and expected outcomes have been met (see "Planning"). *See Table 25.2 for a list of drugs to which these nursing actions apply.*

Core Concept 25.5 ▶ Corticosteroids are effective in treating severe inflammation.

Corticosteroids or glucocorticoids are natural hormones released by the adrenal cortex that have powerful effects on nearly every cell in the body. One of their most useful actions is the ability to suppress severe inflammation. When used to treat inflammatory disorders, the drug doses are many times higher than those naturally present in the blood. Corticosteroids have numerous therapeutic applications, including the treatment of arthritis, dermatitis, psoriasis, asthma, inflammatory bowel disease, allergies, and cancer. The uses of these drugs in treating hormonal imbalances are presented in detail in Chapter 33. Doses of the corticosteroids used to treat severe inflammatory disease are listed in Table 25.3.

Table 25.3 Selected Corticosteroids for Severe Inflammation

Drug	Route and Adult Dose	Remarks
betamethasone (Celestone, Diprolene, others)	PO: 0.6–7.2 mg/day	Topical, intra-articular, IM, and IV forms available
cortisone	PO: 20–300 mg/day in divided doses	IM form available; also for adrenal insufficiency
dexamethasone	PO: 0.25–4 mg bid–qid	IM and IV forms available; also for adrenal insufficiency and immunosuppression
hydrocortisone (Cortef, Hydrocortone, Solu-Cortef, others) (see the Prototype Drug box in Core Concept 33.8)	Topical: 0.5% cream applied 1–4 times daily PO: 10–320 mg tid–qid	Used widely for skin inflammation; IM, rectal, and IV forms available; may be injected intra-articular
methylprednisolone (Depo-Medrol, Medrol)	PO: 4–48 mg/day in divided doses	Available in IM, IV, and rectal forms; also for neoplasia and adrenal insufficiency
prednisolone (Prelone)	PO: 5–60 mg 1–4 times daily	Available in IM and IV forms; also for neoplasia and adrenal insufficiency
Pr prednisone	PO: 5–60 mg 1–4 times daily	Available in oral form only; also for neoplasia
triamcinolone (Aristospan, Kenalog)	PO: 4–48 mg 1–4 times daily	Available in IM, subcutaneous, intradermal, intra-articular, and aerosol forms

Corticosteroids affect inflammation in multiple ways. They suppress the actions of chemical mediators of inflammation such as histamine and prostaglandins. In addition, they inhibit the immune system by suppressing certain functions of phagocytes and lymphocytes. These multiple effects have the ability to markedly reduce inflammation, making corticosteroids the most effective medications for the treatment of severe inflammatory disorders.

Unfortunately, medications in the corticosteroid class have several potentially serious adverse effects that limit their therapeutic usefulness when they are given by the oral or parenteral routes. These include suppression of the normal functions of the adrenal gland (adrenal insufficiency), elevated blood glucose, mood changes, cataracts, peptic ulcers, electrolyte imbalances, and osteoporosis. Because of their effectiveness at reducing the signs and symptoms of inflammation, corticosteroids can mask infections that may be present in the patient. This combination of masking inflammation and suppressing the immune system creates a potential for existing infections to grow rapidly and undetected. An active infection is usually a contraindication for corticosteroids therapy.

Because the appearance of these adverse effects is a function of the dose and duration of therapy, treatment with oral corticosteroids is often limited to the short-term control of acute disease. When longer therapy is indicated, doses are kept as low as possible and **alternate-day therapy** is sometimes used. The medication is taken every other day to encourage the patient's adrenal glands to function on the days when no drug is taken. During long-term therapy, the healthcare provider must be alert for signs of overtreatment, a condition called **Cushing syndrome**. Signs include bruising and a characteristic pattern of fat deposits in the cheeks (moon face), shoulders (buffalo hump), and abdomen. The body becomes accustomed to the high doses of corticosteroids, and patients must discontinue the drug gradually because abrupt withdrawal can result in lack of adrenal function.

The serious adverse effects of the corticosteroids may be prevented by giving the drugs by the intranasal, topical, or intravaginal routes. Although small amounts of the drug are absorbed across the skin and mucous membranes, the amount reaching the blood is generally small and too low to cause serious systemic effects.

Prototype Drug: Pr *Prednisone*

Therapeutic Class: Anti-inflammatory drug **Pharmacologic Class:** Corticosteroid

Actions and Uses: Prednisone is a synthetic corticosteroid. Its actions are the result of being metabolized to an active form, which is also available as a drug called prednisolone. When used for inflammation, a 4- to 10-day duration for therapy is common. Alternate-day dosing is used for long-term therapy. Prednisone is occasionally used to terminate acute bronchospasm in patients with asthma (see Chapter 30) and for patients with certain cancers such as Hodgkin's disease, acute leukemia, and lymphomas (see Chapter 29).

Adverse Effects and Interactions: When used for short-term therapy, prednisone has few adverse effects. Long-term therapy may result in Cushing syndrome, a condition that includes elevated blood glucose, fat redistribution to the shoulders and face, muscle weakness, bruising, and bones that easily fracture. Corticosteroids can raise blood glucose levels. Patients with diabetes may require an adjustment in insulin dose. Gastric ulcers may occur with long-term therapy, and an antiulcer medication may be prescribed prophylactically. Patients must report any potential infections immediately. This drug should be discontinued gradually.

Barbiturates, phenytoin, and rifampin increase the metabolism of prednisone; increased doses of prednisone may be needed. Amphotericin B and diuretics together with prednisone can increase potassium loss. Prednisone may inhibit the effectiveness of vaccines and toxoids, resulting in a serious or life-threatening infection. In patients with myasthenia gravis, use of prednisone with ambenonium, neostigmine, or pyridostigmine can cause severe muscle weakness.

FEVER

Antipyretics are drugs used to reduce fever.

◄ **Core Concept 25.6**

Like inflammation, fever is a natural defense mechanism for neutralizing foreign substances. Many species of bacteria are killed by high fever. Often, the healthcare provider must determine whether the fever needs to be treated aggressively or allowed to run its course without drug therapy. Drugs used to treat fever are called **antipyretics**.

Prototype Drug: Pr *Acetaminophen (Tylenol)*

Therapeutic Class: Antipyretic, nonopioid analgesic **Pharmacologic Class:** Centrally acting prostaglandin inhibitor

Actions and Uses: Acetaminophen reduces fever by direct action at the level of the hypothalamus and causes dilation of peripheral blood vessels, enabling sweating and dissipation of heat. Acetaminophen and aspirin have equal efficacy in relieving pain and reducing fever. Acetaminophen is administered as a substitute for aspirin when NSAIDs are contraindicated due to age, allergy, or gastric irritation. It is not linked with Reye's syndrome, as is aspirin; thus it is safe to administer to infants, children, and adolescents who have flu-like symptoms or chickenpox. Acetaminophen is sometimes combined with opioid analgesics to provide additional pain relief.

Acetaminophen has no peripheral anti-inflammatory action; therefore, it is not effective in treating arthritis or pain caused by tissue swelling following injury. Acetaminophen is pregnancy category B. It does not affect platelet aggregation, as do the NSAIDs.

Adverse Effects and Interactions: At recommended doses, acetaminophen is well tolerated. The risk for adverse effects is dose related and increases with long-term use. Acute acetaminophen poisoning is very serious, and symptoms include anorexia, nausea, vomiting, dizziness, lethargy, diaphoresis, chills, abdominal pain, and diarrhea. Excessive acetaminophen use is a major cause of acute hepatic failure in the United States. Because of this risk, doses of acetaminophen are now limited to a maximum of 325 mg per tablet or capsule.

Acetaminophen inhibits warfarin metabolism, causing warfarin to accumulate to toxic levels. High-dose or long-term acetaminophen usage may result in elevated warfarin levels and bleeding. Ingestion of this drug with alcohol is not recommended due to the possibility of liver failure from hepatic necrosis.

The patient should avoid taking herbs that have the potential for liver toxicity, including comfrey, coltsfoot, and chaparral.

BLACK BOX WARNING:
Acetaminophen has the potential to cause severe liver injury and may cause serious allergic reactions with symptoms of angioedema, difficulty breathing, itching, or rash.

In most patients, fever is more of a discomfort than a life-threatening problem. Prolonged, high fever, usually above 102°f (38.9°c), however, can become dangerous, especially in young children in whom fever can stimulate seizures. In adults, excessively high fever can break down body tissues, reduce mental acuity, and lead to delirium or coma, particularly among older patients. In rare instances, an elevated body temperature may be fatal.

The goal of antipyretic therapy is to lower body temperature while identifying and treating the underlying cause of the fever, which is often an infection. Aspirin, ibuprofen, and acetaminophen are safe, inexpensive, and effective drugs for reducing fever. Many of these antipyretics are marketed for different age groups, including special, flavored brands for infants and children. For fast delivery and effectiveness, drugs may come in various forms including gels, caplets, enteric-coated tablets, and suspensions. Aspirin and acetaminophen are also available as suppositories.

Patients Need to Know

Patients treated for inflammatory disorders or fever need to know the following:

Regarding Anti-Inflammatory Medications and Antipyretics

1. Take NSAIDs with food to decrease stomach irritation.
2. Avoid drinking alcohol when taking high doses of NSAIDs or aspirin because it increases stomach irritation.
3. If ringing in the ears (tinnitus), dizziness, headache, or signs of bleeding or bruising occur, discontinue aspirin use immediately and report the incident to the healthcare provider.
4. Take corticosteroids exactly as prescribed because improper use may lead to serious adverse effects.
5. Acetaminophen may be found in many OTC cold and flu products. Be careful not to take multiple products containing this drug, because additive toxicity may result.

Chapter Review

Core Concepts Summary

25.1 Inflammation is a body defense that limits the spread of invading microorganisms and injury.

Inflammation is a nonspecific response designed to rid the body of invading pathogens or to contain the spread of injury. Acute inflammation occurs over a period of several days, whereas chronic inflammation may continue for months or years.

25.2 The body reacts to injury by releasing chemical mediators that cause inflammation.

Inflammation is initiated by chemical mediators, the most important of which is histamine. Release of these meditators causes vasodilation, allowing capillaries to become leaky, thus causing tissue swelling. Extremely rapid release of histamine throughout the body can trigger anaphylaxis.

25.3 Inflammation may be treated with nonpharmacologic and pharmacologic therapies.

When possible, topical drugs are used because they produce fewer adverse effects than oral or parenteral drugs. The two primary drug classes used for inflammation are the NSAIDs and corticosteroids.

25.4 Nonsteroidal anti-inflammatory drugs (NSAIDs) are the primary drugs for the treatment of mild inflammation.

NSAIDs are drugs that inhibit the enzyme cyclooxygenase. Nonselective cyclooxygenase inhibitors, including aspirin, are effective at reducing inflammation and pain but cause significant GI adverse effects in some patients.

25.5 Corticosteroids are effective in treating severe inflammation.

Corticosteroids are hormones that are extremely effective at reducing inflammation. Because overtreatment with these drugs can cause Cushing syndrome, corticosteroid therapy for inflammation is generally short term.

25.6 Antipyretics are drugs used to reduce fever.

Fever is often self-limiting, but when it is elevated or prolonged, pharmacotherapy is indicated. Acetaminophen is often a preferred drug for fever, although ibuprofen is equally effective.

REVIEW Questions

Answer the following questions to assess your knowledge of the chapter material, and go back and review any material that is not clear to you.

1. The nurse and a patient who is getting ready to be discharged from the hospital are discussing the available types of over-the-counter (OTC) nonsteroidal anti-inflammatory drugs (NSAIDs). The nurse states that an OTC medication that is not classified as an NSAID is:
   1. Aspirin.
   2. Ibuprofen.
   3. Acetaminophen.
   4. Motrin.

2. The patient has been taking aspirin for several days for a headache. While collecting information, the nurse discovers that the patient is experiencing tinnitus and dizziness. The most appropriate action by the nurse is to:
   1. Question the patient about history of sinus infection.
   2. Determine if the patient has mixed the aspirin with other medications.
   3. Tell the patient to not take any more aspirin until seen by the healthcare provider.
   4. Tell the patient to take the aspirin with food or milk.

3. The nurse informs the patient that the most common adverse effect of NSAIDs is:
   1. Edema.
   2. Rash.
   3. Gastrointestinal irritation.
   4. Bleeding.
   5. Myocardial infarction

4. The patient is taking corticosteroids, so the nurse monitors for:
   1. Bleeding.
   2. Respiratory distress.
   3. Dehydration.
   4. Infection.

5. A patient with diabetes taking prednisone states that his blood sugar is higher than normal. The nurse's most appropriate response would be:
   1. "You must not be following your diet for diabetes."
   2. "Prednisone can cause blood sugar levels to increase."
   3. "You must be developing an illness."
   4. "Your diabetes must be getting worse."

6. The nurse is to administer 10 grains of aspirin by mouth. Available are 325 mg tablets. How many tablets will the nurse administer?
   1. One-half tablet
   2. One tablet
   3. One and one-half tablets
   4. Two tablets
7. While educating a patient about acetaminophen, the nurse instructs the patient to report to the healthcare provider if the following occurs: (Select all that apply.)
   1. Lethargy
   2. Anorexia
   3. Tearing of the eyes
   4. Difficulty breathing
   5. Itching and rash
8. A patient has been taking prednisone for an extended period of time. The nurse observes that the patient has a very round moon-shaped face, bruising, and shoulder hump. What does the nurse suspect based on these findings?
   1. These are normal reactions.
   2. These are probably birth defects.
   3. These are the symptoms of myasthenia gravis.
   4. These are the symptoms of adverse drug effects from prednisone.
9. A patient has been taking acetaminophen fairly regularly for headaches but has questions regarding food and beverage restrictions. The nurse informs the patient that taking this drug while regularly drinking alcohol may cause:
   1. Liver failure.
   2. Renal damage.
   3. Thrombosis.
   4. Pulmonary damage.
10. A patient has developed a skin rash on his arm and is being seen at the local clinic. The healthcare provider prescribes a topical corticosteroid instead of an oral steroid because:
    1. It is cheaper than the oral corticosteroids.
    2. The topical corticosteroids have fewer adverse effects.
    3. The rash is localized and shows signs of infection.
    4. It is easier to take than oral medications.

CASE STUDY Questions

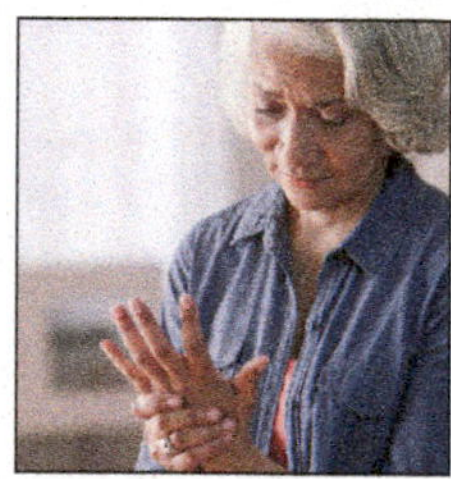

Remember Mrs. Ford, the patient introduced at the beginning of the chapter? Now read the remainder of the case study. Based on the information you have learned in this chapter, answer the questions that follow.

Mrs. Eugenia Ford, 62 years old, has been experiencing a gradual increase in pain and swelling of her hands. Her knuckles have also become red and warm to the touch. She enjoys gardening and sewing, but over the past 6 months has not been able to participate in these activities because it is "too painful." Mrs. Ford has been treating herself with NSAIDs, specifically ibuprofen and naproxen.

1. Regarding Mrs. Ford's use of NSAIDs, what question should you ask to determine potential adverse effects?
   1. "Have you experienced excessive drowsiness?"
   2. "Have you experienced gastrointestinal upset?"
   3. "Have you experienced excessive dryness or stinging sensations in your nose?"
   4. "Have you experienced any rashes or dryness of the skin?"
2. To help Mrs. Ford alleviate the adverse effects of NSAIDs, the nurse advises her:
   1. To take NSAIDs with food.
   2. To take NSAIDs on an empty stomach.
   3. To take both types of NSAIDs at the same time.
   4. That there are no adverse effects for most NSAIDs.
3. Mrs. Ford is diagnosed with rheumatoid arthritis. She experiences a flare (acute exacerbation) of her disease. Which of the following drug classes would likely be prescribed over a 10-day period?
   1. Biologic response modifiers
   2. Intranasal corticosteroids
   3. Systemic corticosteroids
   4. Sympathomimetics
4. Mrs. Ford asks why her healthcare provider has prescribed prednisone. The office nurse tells her that:
   1. "He just wanted to try something different."
   2. "Prednisone markedly reduces inflammation and is beneficial for short-term use."
   3. "Prednisone is used only for pain control."
   4. "Prednisone has very few adverse effects, even when used for long periods."

Answers and complete rationales for the Review and Case Study Questions appear in Appendix A.

REFERENCE

Herdman, T. H., & Kamitsuru, S. (Eds.). (2014). *NANDA International nursing diagnoses: Definitions and classification, 2015–2017*. Oxford, United Kingdom: Wiley-Blackwell.

SELECTED BIBLIOGRAPHY

Aminoshariae, A., Kulild, J. C., & Donaldson, M. (2016). Short-term use of nonsteroidal anti-inflammatory drugs and adverse effects: An updated systematic review. *The Journal of the American Dental Association, 147*, 98–110. doi:10.1016/j.adaj.2015.07.020

Atkinson, T. J., Fudin, J., Jahn, H. L., Kubotera, N., Rennick, A. L., & Rhorer, M. (2013). What's new in NSAID pharmacotherapy: Oral agents to injectables. *Pain Medicine, 14* (Suppl. 1), S11–S17. doi:10.1111/pme.12278

Banks, T., Paul, S. P., & Wall, M. (2013). Managing fevers in children with a single antipyretic. *Nursing Times, 109*(7), 24–25.

Farrell, S. E. (2016). *Acetaminophen toxicity*. Retrieved from http://emedicine.medscape.com/article/820200-overview#aw2aab6b2b4

Hymes, S. R. (2014). *Fever without a focus*. Retrieved from http://emedicine.medscape.com/article/970788-overview

Moore, N., Pollack, C., & Butkerait, P. (2015). Adverse drug reactions and drug–drug interactions with over-the-counter NSAIDs. *Therapeutics and Clinical Risk Management, 11*, 1061. doi:10.2147/TCRM.S79135

Niven, D. J., Stelfox, H. T., & Laupland, K. B. (2013). Antipyretic therapy in febrile critically ill adults: A systematic review and meta-analysis. *Journal of Critical Care, 28*, 303–310. doi:10.1016/j.jcrc.2012.09.009

Pavlidis, P., & Bjarnason, I. (2015). Aspirin induced adverse effects on the small and large intestine. *Current Pharmaceutical Design, 21*, 5089–5093. doi:10.2174/1381612821666150915110058

Sherman, J. M., & Sood, S. K. (2012, June). Current challenges in the diagnosis and management of fever. *Current Opinion in Pediatrics, 24*, 400–406. doi:10.1097/MOP.0b013e32835333e3

University of Rochester Medical Center. (n.d). *Arthritis and other rheumatic diseases statistics*. Retrieved from https://www.urmc.rochester.edu/encyclopedia/Content.aspx?ContentTypeID=85&ContentID=P00043

Wiegand, T. J. (2015). *Nonsteroidal anti-inflammatory agent toxicity*. Retrieved from http://emedicine.medscape.com/article/816117-overview

Chapter 26

Drugs for Immune System Modulation

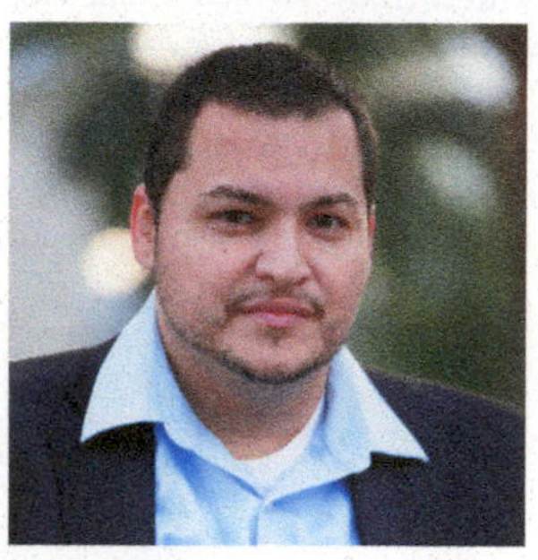

"Because of my lifestyle choices, I thought it might be a good idea to get the hepatitis B vaccine series."
Mr. Jose Martel

Core Concepts

26.1 **The human body has both innate and adaptive body defenses.**
26.2 **The immune response results from activation of the humoral and cell-mediated immune systems.**
26.3 **Vaccines are biologic agents used to prevent illness.**
26.4 **Biologic response modifiers are used to boost the immune response.**
26.5 **Immunosuppressants are used to prevent transplant rejection and to treat autoimmune disorders.**

Drug Snapshot

The following drugs are discussed in this chapter:

Drug Classes	Prototype Drugs
Vaccines	Pr hepatitis B vaccine (Energix-B, Recombivax HB)
Biologic response modifiers	Pr interferon alfa-2b (Intron a)
Immunosuppressants	Pr cyclosporine (Gengraf, Neoral, Sandimmune)

Learning Outcomes

After reading this chapter, the student should be able to:

1. Compare and contrast innate and adaptive body defenses.
2. Compare and contrast the humoral and cell-mediated immune responses.
3. Explain the types of vaccines and how they are used to prevent illness.
4. Identify indications for pharmacotherapy with biologic response modifiers.
5. Explain the need for immunosuppressant medications following organ transplants and for treating severe inflammation.

Key Terms

active immunity
adaptive body defenses
antibodies (ANN-tee-BOD-ees)
antigen (ANN-tih-jen)
B cell
biologic response modifiers
boosters
cytokines (SYE-toh-kines)
cytotoxic T cells

helper T cells
humoral immunity (HYOU-mor-ul eh-MEWN-uh-tee)
immune response
immunization (IH-mewn-ize-AYE-shun)
immunoglobulins (Ig) (ih-MEW-noh-GLOB-you-lins)
immunomodulator (ih-mew-no-MOF-you-layter)
immunosuppressants (ih-MEW-noh-suh-PRESS-ents)
innate body defenses
passive immunity
plasma cells
T cells
titer (TIE-ter)
toxoid vaccines (TOX-oid vaks-EENs)
transplant rejection
vaccination (VAK-sin-AYE-shun)
vaccines (vaks-EENs)

Our bodies come under continuous attack from a host of foreign invaders that include viruses, bacteria, fungi, and even multicellular organisms. In defending the body, our immune system is capable of mounting a rapid and effective response against many of these pathogens.

Immunomodulator is a general term referring to any drug that affects body defenses. In some patients, immunomodulators are used to *stimulate* body defenses so that microbes or cancer cells can be more effectively attacked. For example, **vaccines** (substances given to stimulate the body's defense so that disease can be prevented or controlled) are given at various times throughout the lifespan to prevent major illnesses. On other occasions, it is desirable to *suppress* body defenses to prevent a transplanted organ from being rejected by the immune system. The purpose of this chapter is to examine the pharmacotherapy of drugs that are used to modulate the body's immune response to disease.

The human body has both innate and adaptive body defenses.

◀ **Core Concept 26.1**

anti = *against*
gen = *formation*

A foreign substance that is detected by body defenses and elicits a response is called an **antigen**. Proteins such as those present on the surfaces of pollen grains, bacteria, and viruses are the strongest antigens. When normal cells become damaged, injured, or cancerous, they too can be viewed as antigens by body defenses. The human body has an elaborate set of body defenses that is able to respond to virtually any antigen it may encounter. Dozens of different cells and processes are used to battle disease and internal threats such as cancer cells. These disease-fighting cells and processes are classified into two groups: innate defenses or adaptive defenses.

The first line of protection from pathogens consists of the **innate body defenses**, which serve as general barriers to microbes or environmental hazards. The innate defenses are called *nonspecific* because they are unable to distinguish one type of threat from another; the response or protection is the same regardless of the pathogen. These defenses include physical barriers, such as the skin and the lining of the respiratory and gastrointestinal tracts, which are potential entry points for pathogens. Other innate defenses are phagocytes, natural killer (NK) cells, the complement system, inflammation, fever, and interferons. The purposes of the innate body defenses are to neutralize or destroy the antigen and to alert other components of body defenses that a threat has arrived. From a pharmacologic perspective, two of the most important of the innate defenses are inflammation and fever, which were presented in Chapter 25.

Fast Facts Vaccines and Immune Disorders

- Vaccines lowered the number of measles cases in the United States from more than 3–4 million to only a few hundred cases annually. Most cases of measles in the United States are due to importation from other countries.
- About 40% of girls aged 13–17 in the United States receive the three-dose recommended vaccine for human papillomavirus (HPV).
- Severe combined immunodeficiency disorder (SCID) is rare, occurring in less than 1 per 58,000 births annually in the United States.
- Over 23 million Americans suffer from autoimmune disorders, and the frequency is rising.
- The most common organ transplant is kidney, with about 100,000 people annually awaiting a transplant.

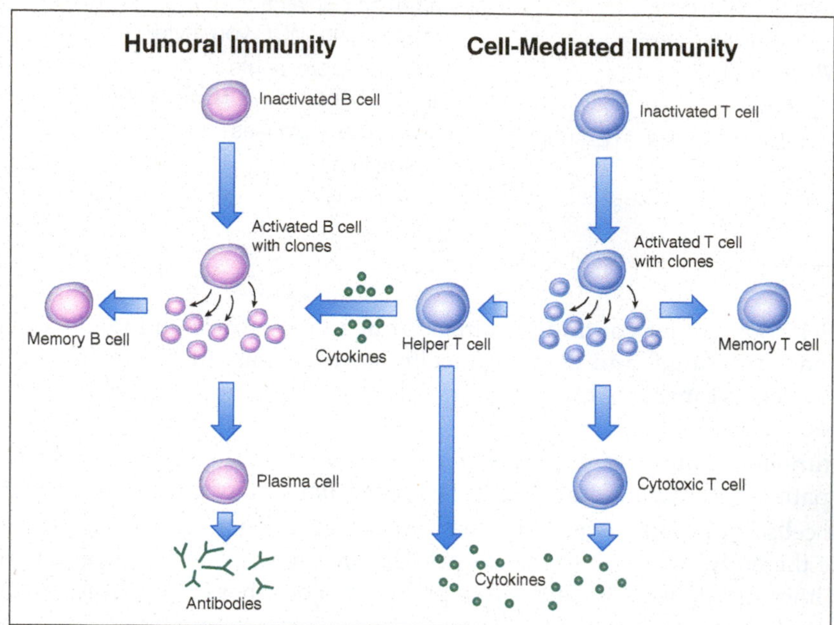

FIGURE 26.1 Steps in the humoral and cell-mediated immune responses.

The body also has the ability to mount a *second* line of defense known as **adaptive body defenses**, which are specific to particular threats. For example, a specific defense may act against only a single species of bacteria and be ineffective against all others. Adaptive body defenses are also known as the **immune response**. The primary cells that accomplish most of the functions of the immune response are the *lymphocytes*. The two primary divisions of the immune response are antibody-mediated (humoral) immunity and cell-mediated immunity. These are illustrated in Figure 26.1.

Core Concept 26.2 ▶

The immune response results from activation of the humoral and cell-mediated immune systems.

Humoral immunity is initiated when an antigen encounters a type of lymphocyte known as a **B cell**. The antigen activates the B cell, which then divides rapidly to form many copies, or clones, of itself. Most cells in this clone are called **plasma cells**. The primary function of the plasma cells is to secrete **antibodies**, also called **immunoglobulins (Ig)**, which are specific to the antigen that initiated the immune response. As they circulate through the body, antibodies physically interact with the antigens to neutralize or target them for destruction by other cells of the immune response. Peak production of antibodies occurs about 10 days after an immune response.

immuno = *body defenses or immune system*
globulin = *blood protein*

After the antigen challenge, *memory B cells* are formed that will remember the specific antigen–antibody interaction. Should the body be exposed to the same antigen in the future, the body will be able to manufacture even higher levels of antibodies in a shorter period, approximately 2 to 3 days. For some antigens, such as those for measles, mumps, or chickenpox, memory can be retained for an entire lifetime. Vaccines, discussed later in this chapter, are sometimes administered to produce these memory cells in advance of exposure to the antigen, so that when the body is exposed to the real organism it can mount a fast, effective response.

The second branch of the immune response involves lymphocytes called **T cells**. When they encounter their specific antigen, T cells become activated and rapidly form clones. Unlike B cells, however, T cells do not produce antibodies. Instead, T cells produce huge amounts of **cytokines**, which are chemicals that regulate important aspects of the immune response. Some cytokines kill foreign organisms directly, whereas others act as messengers to the immune system, stimulating T cells, B cells, and other body defenses to rid the body of the foreign agent. Specific cytokines released by activated T cells include several interleukins, interferon, colony stimulating factors, and tumor necrosis factor (TNF). Some of these

cyto = *cell*
kine(sis) = *movement*

cytokines have been developed as medications to treat certain immune disorders and cancers. This class of medications, called *biologic response modifiers*, is discussed later in this chapter.

The two major types of T cells are **helper T cells** and **cytotoxic T cells**. These cells are often named after a protein receptor on their plasma membrane; the helper T cells have a CD4 receptor, and the cytotoxic T cells have a CD8 receptor. Helper T cells are particularly important because they are responsible for activating most other immune cells, including B cells. Cytotoxic T cells travel throughout the body, secreting cytokines that directly kill bacteria, parasites, virus-infected cells, and cancer cells.

Like B cells, some of the activated T cells become memory cells. If the person encounters the same antigen in the future, the memory T cells will assist in mounting a more rapid immune response.

CAM Therapy | Echinacea for Boosting the Immune System

Echinacea purpurea, or purple coneflower, is one of the most popular medicinal botanicals. This plant is native to the midwestern United States and central Canada. Its flowers, leaves, and stems are harvested and dried. Preparations include dried powder, tinctures, fluid extracts, and teas. No single ingredient seems to be responsible for the herb's activity; many active chemicals have been identified from the extracts.

Echinacea was used by Native Americans to treat various wounds and injuries. Echinacea is claimed to boost the immune system by increasing phagocytosis and inhibiting bacterial enzymes. Some substances in echinacea appear to have antiviral activity; the herb is sometimes taken to prevent and treat the common cold and influenza, indications for which it has received official approval in Germany. A summary analysis of 24 double-blind research studies revealed some weak evidence that echinacea prevented colds, although it was not statistically significant (Karsch-Völk, Barrett, & Linde, 2015). In general, it is used as a supportive treatment for any disease involving inflammation and to enhance the immune system.

IMMUNOSTIMULANTS

Drugs that enhance the immune response are called *immunostimulants*. These types of immunomodulators include vaccines and biologic response modifiers such as interferons and interleukins.

Vaccines are biological agents used to prevent illness.

◀ Core Concept 26.3

Vaccination, or **immunization**, is the process of introducing a foreign substance (a vaccine) into the body to trigger immune activation *before* the patient is exposed to the real pathogen. As a result of the vaccination, memory B cells are formed. When later exposed to the actual infectious organism, these cells will react quickly by producing large quantities of antibodies that will help to neutralize or destroy the pathogen. Some immunizations require follow-up doses, called **boosters**, to provide sustained protection. The effectiveness of most vaccines can be assessed by measuring the amount of antibody produced after the vaccine has been administered, a quantity called **titer**. If the antibody titer falls below a specified protective level over time, a booster may be indicated.

The goal of vaccine administration is to induce long-lasting immunity to a pathogen *without* producing an illness in an otherwise healthy person. Therefore, the microorganisms and other substances used as vaccines must be able to strongly trigger the immune response but be modified to pose no significant risk of disease development. The four methods of producing safe and effective vaccines include the following:

- Attenuated (live) vaccines contain microbes that are alive but weakened so they are unable to produce disease. Some attenuated vaccines cause mild symptoms of the disease. An example of a live attenuated vaccine is the measles, mumps, and rubella (MMR) vaccine.

- Inactivated (killed) vaccines contain microbes that have been inactivated by heat or chemicals and are unable to replicate or cause disease. Examples of inactivated vaccines include the influenza and hepatitis A vaccines.
- **Toxoid vaccines** contain bacterial toxins that have been chemically modified to be incapable of causing disease. When injected, toxoid vaccines induce the formation of antibodies that are capable of neutralizing the real toxins. Examples include diphtheria and tetanus toxoids.
- Recombinant technology vaccines are those that contain partial organisms or bacterial proteins that are generated in the laboratory using biotechnology. The best example of this type is the hepatitis B vaccine.

tox = *poison*
oid = *resembling*

The widespread use of vaccines has prevented illness in millions of people, particularly children. One disease—smallpox—has been virtually eliminated from the planet through immunization, and others, such as polio, have diminished to extremely low levels. Table 26.1 identifies some common vaccines and their recommended schedules.

Common side effects of vaccine administration include redness and discomfort at the site of injection, minor aches, and fever. Although severe reactions are rare, anaphylaxis is possible. In the vast majority of cases, the benefits of disease prevention far outweigh the small risk of adverse effects from the vaccine. Vaccinations are contraindicated for patients who have a weakened immune system or who are currently experiencing symptoms such as diarrhea, vomiting, or fever. Some vaccines are pregnancy category C: These vaccinations are often postponed in pregnant patients until after delivery to avoid any potential harm to

Table 26.1 Selected Vaccines and Their Schedules

Vaccine	Schedule and Age
Adacel and Boostrix (combination of tetanus toxoid and DTaP)	IM: Single dose as an active booster after age 10 (Boostrix) or between ages 11 and 64 (Adacel)
Comvax (combination of haemophilus and hepatitis B vaccines)	IM: Three doses at 2, 4, and 2–15 months of age
Diphtheria, tetanus, and pertussis (Daptacel, DTaP, Infanrix, Tripedia)	IM: Ages 2 months, 4 months, 6 months, 15–18 months, and 4–6 years
Haemophilus influenza type B conjugate (ActHIB, Hiberix, PedvaxHIB)	IM: Ages 2 months, 4 months, 6 months, and 12–15 months
Hepatitis A (Havrix, VAQTA)	Children, IM: Age 12 months, followed by a booster 6–12 months later Adults, IM: 1 mL followed by a booster 6 to 12 months later
Pr Hepatitis B (Engerix-B, Recombivax HB)	Children and adults, IM: Three doses with the second dose 1 month after the first and the third dose 6 months after the first
Human papilloma virus (Cervarix, Gardasil)	Ages 9–26 years, IM: Three doses with the second dose 2 months after the first and the third dose 6 months after the first
Influenza vaccine (Afluria, Fluarix, FluLaval, FluMist, Fluvirin, Fluzone)	Children, IM: Two doses 1 month apart starting at age 6 months; then annual dose Adults, IM: Single annual dose or intranasal (FluMist)
Measles, mumps, and rubella (MMR II)	Subcutaneous: Single dose at age 12–15 months; second dose at age 4–6 years
Meningococcal conjugate vaccine (Menactra, Menomune, Menveo)	IM: First dose at age 11–12 years and second dose at age 16 years
Pneumococcal, polyvalent (Pneumovax 23), or 7-valent (Prevnar)	Adults (Pneumovax 23 or Pnu-Immune 23): Subcutaneous or IM: Single dose Children (Prevnar), IM: Four doses at ages 2 months, 4 months, 6 months, and 12–15 months
Poliovirus, inactivated (IPOL, poliovax)	Children, subcutaneous: Four doses at ages 2 months, 4 months, 6–18 months, and 4–6 years
Proquad (combination of MMR and varicella vaccines)	Subcutaneous: First dose at ages 12–15 months, second dose at ages 4–6 years
Rotavirus (Rotarix, RotaTeq)	PO: Three doses at ages 2 months, 4 months, and 6 months (Rotarix does not require a dose at 6 months)
Tetanus toxoid	IM, primary immunization, age 7 or older: Three doses with the second dose 4–8 weeks after the first dose and the third dose 6–12 months after the second dose
Twinrix (combination of hepatitis A and hepatitis B vaccines)	Over age 18: Three doses, with the second dose 1 month after the first, and the third dose 6 months after the first
Varicella (Varivax, Zostavax)	Subcutaneous (Varivax): Two doses at ages 12–15 months and 4–6 years; subcutaneous (Zostavax): Single dose at age 50 or older

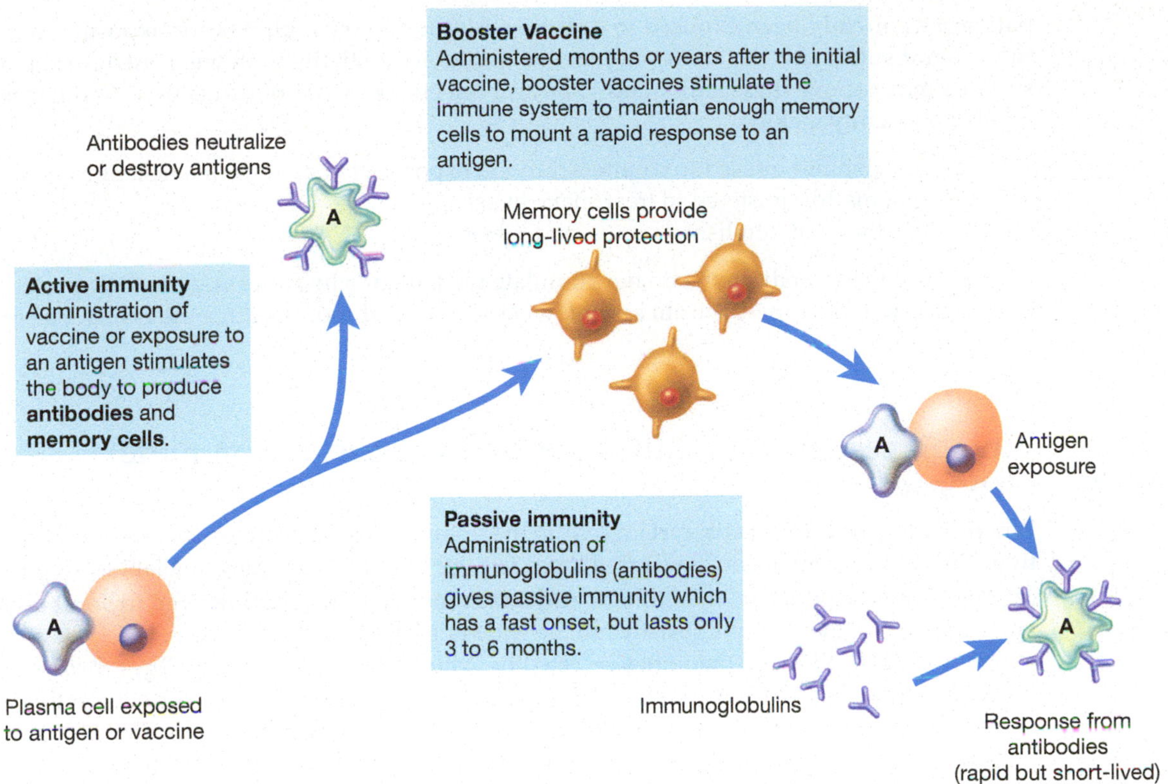

FIGURE 26.2 Mechanisms of active and passive immunity.

the fetus. Because pregnant women are at increased risk for hospitalization from influenza, routine influenza vaccination is recommended for all women who are or will likely become pregnant during influenza season.

There are two types of immunity that can be obtained through the administration of pharmacologic agents, as illustrated in Figure 26.2. The type of response induced by the real pathogen, or its vaccine, is called **active immunity**: The body produces its own antibodies in response to exposure. The active immunity induced by vaccines closely resembles that caused by natural exposure to the antigen, including the generation of memory cells.

Passive immunity occurs when preformed antibodies are transferred or "donated" from one person to another. Drugs for passive immunity are usually administered when the

Prototype Drug: Pr *Hepatitis B Vaccine (Energix-B, Recombivax HB)*

Therapeutic class: Vaccine **Pharmacologic class:** Vaccine

Actions and Uses: Hepatitis B vaccine is administered via IM injection to provide prophylaxis against exposure to the hepatitis B virus (HBV). Following injection, the body produces antibodies against the virus. It is indicated for all infants at birth, and for those at high risk for exposure to HBV-infected blood, including nurses, physicians, dentists, dental hygienists, morticians, and paramedics. Because HBV infection is extremely difficult to treat, it is prudent for all healthcare workers to receive the HBV vaccine before beginning their clinical education, unless contraindicated. The vaccine is also indicated for all persons who engage in high-risk sexual practices, such as heterosexual activity with multiple partners, prostitution, or homosexual or bisexual practices, or for persons who repeatedly contract sexually transmitted infections. The regimen involves three doses of the vaccine, usually followed by a titer to confirm that active immunity has been achieved.

Hepatitis B vaccine is sometimes given to patients *after* they have been exposed to the virus. In this case, it is often combined with hepatitis B immune globulin (HBIG), which will provide passive immunity while the body is building its own antibodies to the virus. Once a hepatitis B infection is acquired, it is difficult to eliminate; therefore, prevention is the best treatment.

Adverse Effects and Interactions: The adverse effects of hepatitis B vaccine are similar to those of other vaccines. Pain and inflammation may appear at the injection site. A fever may develop, and the patient may feel tired and lethargic. Although anaphylaxis is rare, epinephrine should be kept available. The vaccine should be given to pregnant or lactating women only if clearly needed to protect the health of the mother or child.

patient has already been exposed to a pathogen or is at very high risk for exposure, and there is not sufficient time to develop active immunity. Patients with weakened immune systems may receive these antibodies to *prevent* infections. Types of drugs used to provide passive immunity include:

- Gamma globulin infused to counteract recent exposure to hepatitis or chickenpox
- Antivenoms administered to treat snake bites
- Sera used to treat botulism, tetanus, and rabies.

Because these medications do not stimulate the patient's immune system, their protective effects will disappear within several weeks to several months after the infusions are discontinued.

Core Concept 26.4 ▶ Biologic response modifiers are used to boost the immune response.

When challenged by antigens, certain cells in the immune system secrete cytokines that help fight the invading organism. Several of these natural chemicals are now available as medications. Drugs in this class, the **biologic response modifiers**, are administered to boost certain functions of the immune system and are shown in Table 26.2.

Interferons (IFNs) are cytokines secreted by lymphocytes and macrophages that have been infected with a virus. IFNs slow the spread of viral infections and enhance the activity of existing leukocytes. In addition to antiviral properties, these drugs exhibit anticancer and anti-inflammatory actions. Alpha IFNs have the widest therapeutic application (when used as medications, the spelling is changed to *alfa*). Indications for IFN alpha therapy include cancers, such as hairy cell leukemia and AIDS-related Kaposi's sarcoma, and chronic hepatitis virus B or C infections. Interferon alfa-2b (Intron A) is one of the most common IFNs used in therapy and is featured as a prototype drug. IFN beta is primarily used for treatment of severe multiple sclerosis (see Chapter 13). Patients receiving IFN therapy must be closely monitored because drugs in this class can cause serious adverse effects, including depression, suicidal ideation, psychosis, cardiovascular disease (including myocardial infarction), pulmonary impairment, hepatic or renal failure, and a number of other life-threatening disorders.

Interleukins are another class of cytokines secreted by lymphocytes, monocytes, and macrophages. Although 30 different interleukins have been identified, only a few are available as medications. The interleukins have widespread effects on immune function, and all of them boost the activity of natural defense mechanisms. Interleukin-2 is available as aldesleukin (Proleukin), which is approved for the treatment of metastatic renal carcinoma. Interleukin-11, which is derived from bone marrow cells, is a growth factor with multiple

Table 26.2 Selected Biologic Response Modifiers

Drug	Route and Adult Dose	Remarks
aldesleukin (Proleukin): interleukin-2	IV: 600,000 units/kg (0.037 mg/kg) every 8 hours for a total of 14 doses	For metastatic renal cell carcinoma and metastatic melanoma
Bacillus Calmette–Guérin (BCG) vaccine (Tice, TheraCys)	Intradermal (Tice): 0.1 mL as vaccine Intravesical (TheraCys): Bladder instillation	For bladder cancer
INTERFERONS		
interferon alfa-2b (Intron-A)	IM/Subcutaneous: Highly variable depending upon indication	For hairy cell leukemia, malignant melanoma, follicular lymphoma, condylomata acuminata, Kaposi's sarcoma, chronic hepatitis B, and chronic hepatitis C
interferon alfa-n3 (Alferon N)	Intralesion: 0.05 mL (250,000 international units) per wart twice per week for up to 8 weeks	For treatment of genital warts
interferon beta-1a (Avonex, Rebif)	IM (Avonex): 30 mcg/wk Subcutaneous (Rebif); 44 mcg three times per week	For multiple sclerosis
interferon beta-1b (Betaseron, Extavia)	Subcutaneous: 0.25 mg (8 million units) every other day	For multiple sclerosis
peginterferon alfa-2a (Pegasys)	Subcutaneous: 180 mcg/wk for 48 weeks	For chronic hepatitis B and chronic hepatitis C

hematopoietic effects. A recombinant form of interleukin-11 is available as oprelvekin (Neumega) to stimulate platelet production in patients with weakened immune systems.

In addition to IFNs and interleukins, a few additional biologic response modifiers are available to enhance the immune system. Bacillus Calmette–Guérin (BCG) vaccine (Tice, TheraCys) is an attenuated strain of *Mycobacterium bovis* used for the pharmacotherapy of certain types of bladder cancer. Colony-stimulating factors such as filgrastim (Neupogen) and sargramostim (Leukine) promote the production of white blood cells (WBCs). These drugs are used to shorten the length of neutropenia (reduced leukocyte count) in patients with cancer and in those who have had a bone marrow transplant.

Prototype Drug: Pr *Interferon alfa-2b (Intron-A)*

Therapeutic Class: Immunostimulant **Pharmacologic Class:** Interferon, biologic response modifier

Actions and Uses: Interferon alfa-2b is a biologic response modifier that is prepared by recombinant DNA technology and is approved to treat cancers (hairy cell leukemia, melanoma, non-Hodgkin's lymphoma, AIDS-related Kaposi's sarcoma), as well as viral infections (HPV, chronic hepatitis virus B and C). It is available for IV, IM, and subcutaneous administration.

Peginterferon alfa-2b (PegIntron) has a molecule of polyethylene glycol (PEG) attached to the IFN molecule, which gives the drug an extended half-life. Peginterferon alfa-2b is approved in combination with other antiviral medications such as ribavirin to treat chronic hepatitis C virus infections.

Adverse Effects and Interactions: A flu-like syndrome of fever, chills, dizziness, and fatigue occurs in 50% of patients, although this usually diminishes as therapy progresses. Headache, nausea, vomiting, diarrhea, and anorexia are relatively common. Depression and suicidal ideation have been reported and may be severe enough to require discontinuation of the drug. With prolonged therapy, immunosuppression, and serious toxicity such as hepatotoxicity and neurotoxicity may be observed.

Use with ethanol may cause excessive drowsiness and dehydration. Zidovudine may increase hematologic toxicity.

BLACK BOX WARNING:

IFNs may cause or aggravate fatal or life-threatening neuropsychiatric, autoimmune, ischemic, or infectious disorders. Therapy should be discontinued in patients with persistently severe or worsening signs or symptoms of these conditions.

Immunosuppressants are used to prevent transplant rejection and to treat autoimmune disorders.

◀ Core Concept 26.5

The immune system is normally viewed as a lifesaver that protects us from pathogens in the environment. For those receiving organ or tissue transplants, however, the immune system is the enemy. Despite careful tissue matching and typing, donated organs and tissues always contain some antigens that trigger the recipient's immune response. This response, called **transplant rejection**, is sometimes acute, with antibodies rushing to destroy the transplanted tissue within a few days. The cell-mediated immune system reacts more slowly to the transplant, attacking it about 2 weeks following surgery. Even if the organ survives these challenges, chronic rejection of the transplant may occur months or even years after surgery.

Immunosuppressants are medications given to lessen the immune response. One or more of these drugs are administered at the time of transplantation and continued for several months following surgery. In some cases, they are continued indefinitely at low doses. Transplantation would be impossible without the use of effective immunosuppressant drugs.

In addition, these drugs may be prescribed to treat the symptoms of autoimmune disorders, conditions in which the body creates antibodies against its own cells. Over a hundred different disorders have been found to have some degree of autoimmune involvement. Examples of common autoimmune disease include diabetes mellitus (type I), psoriasis, rheumatoid arthritis, systemic lupus erythematosus (SLE), myasthenia gravis, and Hashimoto's thyroiditis. Although these disorders affect different organs, most have in common a hypersensitive immune system that causes symptoms of acute inflammation. When the disease becomes acute, immunosuppressant pharmacotherapy may be initiated. Unlike transplant recipients who may receive immunosuppressants indefinitely, patients with acute inflammation from an autoimmune disorder usually are given these drugs only for brief periods to control relapses.

Although the various immunosuppressant drugs act by different mechanisms, all suppress some aspect of lymphocyte function. Some act nonselectively by inhibiting all aspects of the immune system. Other, newer drugs suppress only a limited aspect of the immune response. The nonselective agents provide more widespread immunosuppression but carry a greater risk of adverse effects.

Nearly all the immunosuppresants are toxic to bone marrow. Because the immune system is suppressed, infections are common and the patient must be protected from situations in which exposure to pathogens is likely. Long-term survivors of transplants are also at increased risk of developing cancers, especially lymphoma, skin cancer, cervical cancer, and Kaposi's sarcoma. Doses for these drugs are listed in Table 26.3.

Drug classes that have immunosuppressant activity include corticosteroids (glucocorticoids), antimetabolites, antibodies, and calcineurin inhibitors. The corticosteroids are potent inhibitors of inflammation and are often drugs of choice in the short-term therapy of severe inflammation (see Chapter 25). Antimetabolites such as sirolimus (Rapamune) and azathioprine (Imuran) inhibit aspects of lymphocyte replication. By binding to the intracellular messenger calcineurin, cyclosporine (Gengraf, Sandimmune, Neoral), and tacrolimus (Prograf) disrupt T-cell function. The calcineurin inhibitors are of value in treating psoriasis, an inflammatory disorder of the skin (see Chapter 37).

The final group of immunosuppressants, and the most recently developed, are monoclonal antibodies (MABs). MABs have been designed to attack very specific target receptors. By binding to overactive cells in the immune system, MABs can dampen the immune response. For example, basiliximab (Simulect) and belatacept (Nulojix) are given to prevent the acute rejection of kidney transplants by host T cells. Infliximab (Remicade) is used to suppress the severe inflammation that often accompanies autoimmune disorders such as Crohn disease and rheumatoid arthritis. Belimumab (Benlysta) suppresses abnormal B cells that are a problem in people with severe SLE. Because many drugs in the MAB class are used as antineoplastics, the student should refer to Chapter 29 for additional information.

Table 26.3 Selected Immunosuppressants

Drug	Route and Adult Dose	Remarks
anakinra (Kineret)	Subcutaneous: 100 mg once daily	For rheumatoid arthritis that has not responded to safer drugs
azathioprine (Azasan, Imuran)	PO/IV: 3–5 mg/kg daily	Inhibits DNA, RNA, and protein synthesis; also for rheumatoid arthritis
basiliximab (Simulect)	IV: 20 mg times two doses (first dose 2 hours before surgery; second dose 4 days after transplant)	Monoclonal antibody against the CD25 receptor on T cells; for preventing rejection of kidney transplants
belatacept (Nulojix)	IV: 5–10 mg/kg	For preventing rejection of kidney transplants
belimumab (Benlysta)	IV: 10 mg/kg at 2-week intervals	Suppresses B cells; for severe SLE
Pr cyclosporine (Gengraf, Neoral, Sandimmune)	PO: Initial dose 14–18 mg/kg just prior to surgery; after 2 weeks, then 5–10 mg/kg/day	IV and ophthalmic forms available; inhibits T cells; also for rheumatoid arthritis, psoriasis, and other severe inflammatory disorders
infliximab (Remicade)	IV: 5 mg/kg at 0, 2, and 6 weeks, then every 8 weeks	Blocks tumor necrosis factor; for severe inflammatory disorders such as Crohn disease
lymphocyte immune globulin or antithymocyte globulin (Atgam)	IV: 10–30 mg/kg daily for 1–2 weeks	Polyclonal antibodies that suppress T cells; for preventing rejection of kidney transplants
methotrexate (Rheumatrex, Trexall) (see the Prototype Drug box in Core Concept 29.8)	PO: 15–30 mg/day for 5 days; repeat every 12 weeks for three courses	IV, IM, and intrathecal forms available; blocks metabolism of folic acid; also for neoplasia, psoriasis, and rheumatoid arthritis
mycophenolate (CellCept, Myfortic)	PO/IV: 720 mg bid	Inhibits B cells, T cells, and antibody formation; for preventing rejection of kidney, liver or heart transplants
sirolimus (Rapamune)	PO: 6 mg loading dose, then 2 mg/day	Suppresses antibody production; for preventing rejection of kidney transplants
tacrolimus (Prograf)	PO: 0.15–0.3 mg/kg/day in two divided doses every 12 hours	IV form available; inhibits T cells; for preventing rejection of kidney, liver, or heart transplants; ointment is approved to treat atopic dermatitis

CONCEPT REVIEW 26.1

- Why are oral glucocorticoids usually used concurrently with immunosuppressant drugs following a transplant operation?

Prototype Drug: Cyclosporine (Gengraf, Neoral, Sandimmune)

Therapeutic Class: Immunosuppressant **Pharmacologic Class:** Calcineurin inhibitor

Actions and Uses: Cyclosporine is a complex chemical obtained from a soil fungus that inhibits helper T cells. It is approved for the prophylaxis of kidney, heart, and liver transplant rejection, psoriasis, and xerophthalmia, an eye condition of diminished tear production caused by ocular inflammation. Cyclosporine is normally administered by the oral route but an IV form is available for severe cases of ulcerative colitis or Crohn disease. When prescribed for transplant recipients, it is usually administered in combination with high doses of corticosteroids such as prednisone.

Adverse Effects and Interactions: The primary adverse effect of cyclosporine occurs in the kidney, with up to 75% of patients experiencing reduction in urine output. Frequent laboratory tests of kidney function, such as BUN and creatinine, are necessary. Other common adverse effects are tremor, hypertension, and elevated hepatic enzyme values. Although opportunistic infections are common during cyclosporine therapy, they are fewer than with other immunosuppressants. Periodic blood counts are necessary to be certain that WBCs do not fall below 4000 or platelets below 75,000.

Because cyclosporine is extensively metabolized in the liver, many drug interactions are possible. The following drugs increase the metabolism of cyclosporine, making the drug *less effective*: phenytoin, carbamazepine, TMP–SMZ, and phenobarbital. The following drugs decrease the metabolism of cyclosporine, causing the drug to build high concentrations and become *potentially toxic*: macrolide antibiotics, azole antifungals, and amphotericin B. Because cyclosporine can damage the kidneys, other nephrotoxic drugs such as amphotericin B, NSAIDs, or aminoglycosides should be administered with great caution.

BLACK BOX WARNING:
Therapy with cyclosporine may result in serious infections and increases the risk of malignancies.

Nursing Process Focus Patients Receiving Immunosuppressants

ASSESSMENT

Prior to administration:

- Obtain a complete health history, including cardiovascular, neurological, immune, oral, renal and liver conditions, allergies, drug history, and possible drug interactions.
- Evaluate laboratory blood findings: complete blood count (CBC), electrolytes, lipid panel, and renal and liver function studies.
- Attain history or current cases of cancer, fever, or active infections (such as herpes and HIV).
- Acquire the results of a complete physical examination, including vital signs, height, and weight.

POTENTIAL NURSING DIAGNOSES*

- *Deficient Knowledge* related to lack of information about drug therapy
- *Risk for Infection* related to adverse effects of drug therapy
- *Risk for Injury* related to adverse effects of drug therapy
- *Risk for Impaired Mucous Membrane, Oral,* related to adverse effects of drug therapy

PLANNING: PATIENT GOALS AND EXPECTED OUTCOMES

The patient will:

- Experience therapeutic effects (depending on the reason the drug is being given).
- Be free from or experience minimal adverse effects from drug therapy.
- Verbalize an understanding of the drug's use, adverse effects, and required precautions.

IMPLEMENTATION

Interventions and (Rationales)	Patient Education/Discharge Planning
• Administer medications correctly and evaluate the patient's knowledge of proper administration. (Most immunosuppressants are administered either PO or IV and require specific instructions.)	Inform the patient to: • Use enclosed equipment to mix the drug. • Use glass, not paper or plastic cups unless package directions indicate they are to be used. • Mix drug with milk, chocolate milk, or orange juice, stirring well. Take additional liquid to ensure the drug is consumed.

(*Continued*)

Nursing Process Focus (*continued*)

Interventions and (Rationales)	Patient Education/Discharge Planning
• Monitor all vital signs, and observe for signs and symptoms of infection such as fever, elevated pulse, respiration, and blood pressure, fatigue, cough, white patches on mucous membranes, vaginal discharge, or itchy blister-like vesicles on skin. (Immunosuppressants increase the risk of infection, especially opportunistic infections such as herpes and yeast.)	Advise the patient to: • Immediately report any signs and symptoms of infection such as wounds with redness or drainage, increasing cough, fatigue, and fever to the healthcare provider. • Use proper hand hygiene techniques. • Avoid large crowds and people with known infections or young children who have higher risk of infection. • Cook food thoroughly, allowing others to prepare raw foods and clean up afterward.
• Monitor changes in level of consciousness, disorientation, confusion, or tremors. (Neurological changes may indicate adverse effects of drug therapy.)	• Instruct the patient to report increasing lethargy, disorientation, confusion, changes in behavior or mood, slurred speech, or tremors to the healthcare provider.
• Continue to monitor serum and urine laboratory tests, specifically noting: CBC, platelets, electrolytes, glucose, liver and renal studies, and lipid levels. (Depending on the drug, immunosuppressants may cause leukopenia, anemia, thrombocytopenia, hyperglycemia, hyperkalemia, and renal failure.)	Instruct the patient: • That it is extremely important to keep scheduled laboratory and doctor appointments. • To carry a wallet identification or wear medical ID jewelry indicating immunosuppressant therapy.
• Inspect oral mucous membrane and dental health. (Immunospressants increase the risk of oral candidiasis and gingivitis. Oral antifungal medications may be needed.)	Instruct the patient to: • Maintain excellent oral hygiene, inspecting the mouth daily. • Keep regular dental visits, and consult with dentist about frequency.
• Determine the patient's diet and consumption of grapefruit juice. (Grapefruit juice significantly increases cyclosporine levels and should be avoided while on immunosuppressant therapy.)	• Advise the patient to avoid or eliminate grapefruit and grapefruit juice from the diet while on the drug.
• Collect information about pregnancy status. (Pregnancy should be avoided for up to 4 months after discontinuing immunosuppressive therapy.)	• Explain the effects of medications on pregnancy and breastfeeding and the need to delay pregnancy. • Discuss options for family planning; alternative contraception methods may be necessary.
• Monitor for the development of hirsutism or alopecia. (Hirsutism is reversible when the drug is discontinued. Alopecia indicates significant immunosuppression.)	• Advise the patient to notify the healthcare provider of changes in hair growth or texture.

EVALUATION OF OUTCOME CRITERIA

Evaluate the effectiveness of drug therapy by confirming that patient goals and expected outcomes have been met (see "Planning"). *See Table 26.3 for a list of drugs to which these nursing actions apply.*

*Herdman, T.H. & Kamitsuru, S. (Eds.), *Nursing Diagnoses: Definitions & Classification* 2015–2017. Copyright © 2014, 1994–2014 NANDA International. Used by arrangement by John Wiley & Sons, Inc. Companion website: www.wiley.com/go/nursingdiagnoses.

Patients Need to Know

Patients treated for inflammatory or immune disorders need to know the following:

Regarding Vaccines

1. Maintain an accurate, written record of vaccinations, including the date of the vaccination, route and site of vaccination, type of vaccine (including manufacturer and lot number), and the address of the healthcare provider's office where the vaccination occurred.
2. Keep immunizations up to date to prevent illness. Because recommendations can change, seek current information from a healthcare provider periodically.
3. Vaccines may contain a number of additives, including antibiotics, formaldehyde, thimersol, and monosodium glutamate. If an allergy is known or suspected to any of these additives, notify a healthcare provider before getting a vaccination.

Regarding Biologic Response Modifiers

4. Regular laboratory testing is extremely important, especially monitoring CBC.
5. Immediately report neurological symptoms (depression, suicidal ideations) and cardiovascular effects to the healthcare provider.

Regarding Immunosuppressants

6. Never take cyclosporine with grapefruit juice; blood levels of the drug are increased by this combination.
7. Reduce risk of illness by avoiding crowds, avoiding those with colds or infections, and washing hands frequently.
8. Keep scheduled laboratory and healthcare provider appointments. Regular laboratory testing is extremely important, especially monitoring CBC, electrolytes, hormone levels, and urine studies.
9. Immediately report an elevation in temperature, sore throat, mouth ulcers, and fatigue to the healthcare provider.

Chapter Review

Core Concepts Summary

26.1 The human body has both innate and adaptive body defenses.

Innate body defenses such as the skin, inflammation, and phagocytes, are nonspecific, general barriers to disease. Adaptive body defenses, known as the immune response, involve lymphocytes and are specific to the particular threats.

26.2 The immune response results from activation of the humoral and cell-mediated immune systems.

B cells become plasma cells and secrete large quantities of antibodies. The antibodies are specific to the antigen and neutralize the foreign agent or destroy it. Some B cells remember the antigen for many years. T cells also recognize specific antigens, but instead of producing antibodies, they produce cytokines, some of which rid the body of the foreign agent. Memory B and T cells remember the antigen for many years and mount a faster immune response on subsequent exposures.

26.3 Vaccines are biologic agents used to prevent illness.

Vaccines are usually given to prevent a serious infectious disease. Vaccines may be live, attenuated, or toxoids. They are effective when taken according to schedule and rarely produce serious adverse effects.

26.4 Biologic response modifiers are used to boost the immune response.

Several drugs are available to boost a patient's immune function. Interleukins, interferons, and other agents enhance the body's natural defenses, primarily in the pharmacotherapy of cancer.

26.5 Immunosuppressants are used to prevent transplant rejection and to treat autoimmune disorders.

For an organ or tissue transplant to be successful, the patient's immune system must be suppressed following surgery. Immunosuppressants are effective in lessening the immune response but must be monitored carefully because loss of immune function can lead to infections and cancer.

REVIEW Questions

Answer the following questions to assess your knowledge of the chapter material, and go back and review any material that is not clear to you.

1. The nurse is evaluating drug effects in a patient who has been given interferon alfa-2b (Intron A) for multiple sclerosis. Which of the following are common adverse effects? (Select all that apply.)
   1. Thoughts of suicide
   2. Hepatotoxicity
   3. Hypotension
   4. Depression

2. The nurse would question an order for aldesleukin (Proleukin) if the patient had which of the following conditions? (Select all that apply.)
   1. Liver disease
   2. Metastatic lung cancer
   3. Metastatic renal cancer
   4. Metastatic melanoma
   5. Colon cancer

3. The healthcare provider has ordered oprelvekin (Neumega) for a patient who has just had chemotherapy. The patient asks the nurse why she needs this drug. The nurse responds:
   1. "You are being given this drug to suppress your immune system because you are having a hypersensitivity reaction."
   2. "You are being given this drug to help reduce any inflammation response you may develop."
   3. "You are being given this drug because it acts as an antiviral, helping to reduce infection."
   4. "You are being given this drug to stimulate platelet production."

4. While receiving filgrastim (Neupogen), the nurse should monitor for a(n):
   1. Increase in the production of white blood cells.
   2. Increase in the production of platelets.
   3. Increase in the production of red blood cells.
   4. Decrease in the production of red blood cells.

5. A patient who is pregnant with her first child is at the clinic for a checkup and an infant care class. The nurse begins to review an informational pamphlet with the patient and informs her that the DTaP vaccine should be given at ages:
   1. 1 months, 4 months, 12 months, 15–18 months, and 4–6 years.
   2. 2 months, 6 months, 15–18 months, and 4–6 years.
   3. 2 months, 4 months, 6 months, 15–18 months, and 4–6 years.
   4. 2 months, 4 months, 6 months, and 15–18 months.

6. A patient comes to the healthcare provider's office immediately after a suspected exposure to hepatitis B. He is to start the hepatitis B vaccine series and also receive the hepatitis B immune globulin (HBIG) vaccine injection. He tells the nurse that he understands how the hepatitis B vaccine series works but wants to know why he also needs to have the HBIG vaccine. The nurse responds the HIBG vaccine is given to:
   1. Enhance the ability of the hepatitis B (Engerix-B) series of vaccines to provide permanent immunity.
   2. Ensure that the hepatitis B (Engerix-B) series eliminates the virus.
   3. Provide temporary immunity while the body is building its own antibodies to the virus.
   4. Provide active immunity by causing the immune system to form antibodies.

7. The nurse evaluates the patient on immunosuppressants for:
   1. Hypotension.
   2. Infection.
   3. Hypoglycemia.
   4. Bleeding.

8. A patient is to receive tacrolimus (Prograf) 0.15 mg/kg/day to be given in two doses (every 12 hours). She weighs 100 pounds. How many milligrams will the patient receive per dose?
   1. 6.82 mg
   2. 6.60 mg
   3. 3.30 mg
   4. 3.41 mg

9. Which of the following statements by a patient taking cyclosporine (Neoral, Sandimmune) would indicate the need for more information?
   1. "I will report any reduction in urine output to my healthcare provider."
   2. "I will wash my hands frequently."
   3. "I will take my blood pressure at home every day."
   4. "I will take my cyclosporine at breakfast with a glass of grapefruit juice."

10. The nurse should monitor a transplant patient for the primary adverse effect of cyclosporine (Neoral, Sandimmune) therapy by collecting information on which of the following laboratory tests?
    1. Complete blood count
    2. BUN and creatinine
    3. Liver enzymes
    4. Electrolytes

CASE STUDY Questions

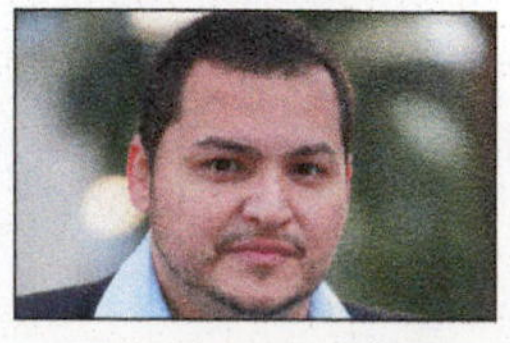

Remember Mr. Martel, the patient introduced at the beginning of the chapter? Now read the remainder of the case study. Based on the information you have learned in this chapter, answer the questions that follow.

Mr. Jose Martel, a 32-year-old night club manager, arrives at the office for his annual check-up. While being interviewed by the nurse, he says that he had called the office in advance and made arrangements to begin the hepatitis B vaccine series. He states, "Because of my lifestyle choices, I thought it might be a good idea." He has read about the vaccine on several online sites but still has some questions.

1. Mr. Martel asks how the hepatitis B vaccine works. The nurse responds that the vaccine stimulates the immune system to produce antibodies after exposure to components of the vaccine. This type of vaccine provides ______ immunity.
   1. Passive
   2. Attenuated
   3. Live
   4. Active

2. While providing information about the hepatitis B vaccine series, the nurse informs Mr. Martel that:
   1. It is a series of three shots: the first one today, the second one a month from now, and the last shot 6 months after the first shot.
   2. It is a series of two shots: the first one today and then the last one a month from now.
   3. It is a series of three shots: the first one today, the second one a month from now, and the last shot 6 months after the second shot.
   4. It is a series of four shots: the first one today, the second one a month from now, the third one 6 months after the first shot, and the last one a year after the first one.

3. The nurse and Mr. Martel are reviewing his health history. Which of the following information would cause the nurse to withhold the vaccine and check with the healthcare provider?
   1. Mr. Martel smokes cigarettes, one-half pack a day.
   2. Mr. Martel is frightened by needles and injections.
   3. Mr. Martel is allergic to yeast and yeast products.
   4. Mr. Martel drinks several glasses of wine on the weekends.

4. Just prior to administering the first injection of the series, the nurse tells Mr. Martel that he might expect which adverse effect(s) to occur? (Select all that apply.)
   1. Pain or inflammation at the injection site
   2. Nausea
   3. Fatigue
   4. Fever

Answers and complete rationales for the Review and Case Study Questions appear in Appendix A.

REFERENCES

Herdman, T. H., & Kamitsuru, S. (Eds.). (2014). *NANDA International nursing diagnoses: Definitions and classification, 2015–2017*. Oxford, United Kingdom: Wiley-Blackwell.

Karsch-Völk, M., Barrett, B., & Linde, K. (2015). Echinacea for preventing and treating the common cold. *JAMA, 313*, 618–619. doi:10.1001/jama.2014.17145

SELECTED BIBLIOGRAPHY

American Autoimmune Related Diseases Association. (n.d.). *Autoimmune statistics*. Retrieved from http://www.aarda.org/autoimmune-information/autoimmune-statistics

Bamoulid, J., Staeck, O., Halleck, F., Dürr, M., Paliege, A., Lachmann, N., . . . Budde, K. (2015). Advances in pharmacotherapy to treat kidney transplant rejection. *Expert Opinion on Pharmacotherapy, 16*, 1627–1648. doi:10.1517/14656566.2015.1056734

Centers for Disease Control and Prevention. (2014). *Guidelines for vaccinating pregnant women*. Retrieved from http://www.cdc.gov/vaccines/pubs/preg-guide.htm#flu1

Centers for Disease Control and Prevention. (2015). *ACIP vaccine recommendations*. Retrieved from http://www.cdc.gov/vaccines/hcp/acip-recs/index.html

Centers for Disease Control and Prevention. (2015). *Human papillomavirus (HPV)*. Retrieved from http://www.cdc.gov/hpv/infographics/vacc-coverage.html

Centers for Disease Control and Prevention. (2015). *Measles – Q&A about disease and vaccine*,. Retrieved from http://www.cdc.gov/vaccines/vpd-vac/measles/faqs-dis-vac-risks.htm

Centers for Disease Control and Prevention. (2015). *Parent's guide to childhood immunizations*. Retrieved from http://www.cdc.gov/vaccines/parents/tools/parents-guide/downloads/parents-guide-508.pdf

Macartney, K. K., Chiu, C., Georgousakis, M., & Brotherton, J. M. (2013). Safety of human papillomavirus vaccines: A review. *Drug Safety, 36*, 393–412. doi:10.1007/s40264-013-0039-5

Pelligrino, B. (2016). *Immunosuppression*. Retrieved from http://emedicine.medscape.com/article/432316-overview

Phillips, D. (2014). *SCID prevalence doubles previous estimates*. Retrieved from http://www.medscape.com/viewarticle/830156

U.S. Department of Health and Human Services. (2016). *Organ procurement and transplantation network: Data*. Retrieved from https://optn.transplant.hrsa.gov/data

Vichnin, M., Bonanni, P., Klein, N. P., Garland, S. M., Block, S. L., Kjaer, S. K., . . . Lievano, F. (2015). An overview of quadrivalent human papillomavirus vaccine safety: 2006 to 2015. *The Pediatric Infectious Disease Journal, 34*, 983–991. doi:10.1097/INF.0000000000000793

Chapter 27

Drugs for Bacterial Infections

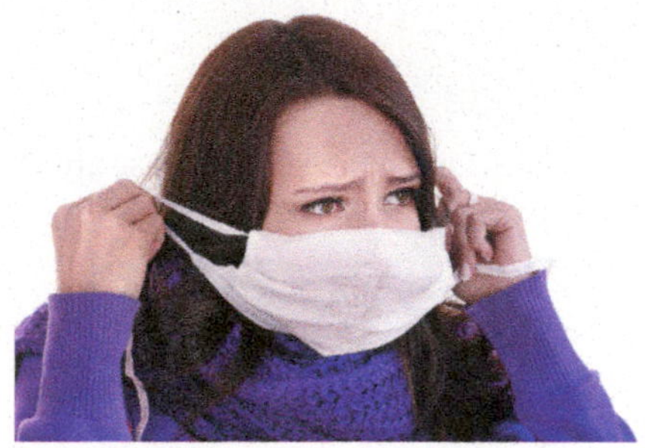

"I don't know what is going on. Ever since I had my kidney transplant, I've been experiencing repeated bacterial infections and now I have to wear this mask when I'm around people."

Ms. Shelly Jackson

Core Concepts

27.1 **Pathogens are organisms that cause disease by invading tissues or secreting toxins.**
27.2 **Anti-infective drugs are classified by their chemical structures or by their mechanisms of action.**
27.3 **Anti-infective drugs act by selectively targeting a pathogen's metabolism or life cycle.**
27.4 **Acquired resistance is a major clinical problem that is worsened by improper use of anti-infectives.**
27.5 **Careful selection of the correct antibiotic is essential for effective pharmacotherapy and to limit adverse effects.**
27.6 **The penicillins are one of the oldest and safest groups of anti-infectives.**
27.7 **The cephalosporins are similar in structure and function to the penicillins and are one of the most widely prescribed anti-infective classes.**
27.8 **The tetracyclines have broad spectrums but are preferred drugs for few diseases.**
27.9 **The macrolides are safe alternatives to penicillin for many infections.**
27.10 **The aminoglycosides are narrow-spectrum drugs that have the potential to cause serious toxicity.**
27.11 **Fluoroquinolones have wide clinical applications because of their broad spectrum of activity and relative safety.**
27.12 **Sulfonamides and urinary antiseptics are traditional drugs for urinary tract infections.**
27.13 **A number of additional anti-infectives have distinct mechanisms of action and specific indications.**
27.14 **The pharmacotherapy of tuberculosis requires special dosing regimens and schedules.**

Drug Snapshot

The following drugs are discussed in this chapter:

Drug Classes	Prototype Drugs
Penicillins	Pr penicillin G
Cephalosporins	Pr cefazolin (Ancef, Kefzol)
Tetracyclines	Pr tetracycline (Sumycin, others)
Macrolides	Pr erythromycin (E-Mycin, Erythrocin)
Aminoglycosides	Pr gentamicin (Garamycin)
Fluoroquinolones	Pr ciprofloxacin (Cipro)
Sulfonamides	Pr trimethoprim–sulfamethoxazole (Bactrim, Septra)
Miscellaneous antibacterials	Pr vancomycin (Vancocin)
Antitubercular drugs	Pr isoniazid (INH)

Learning Outcomes

After reading this chapter, the student should be able to:

1. Explain how bacteria cause disease.
2. Explain how bacteria are described and classified.
3. Describe the basic mechanisms by which antibacterial drugs act.
4. Using an example, explain how resistance can develop to an anti-infective drug.
5. Explain the importance of culture and sensitivity testing to anti-infective chemotherapy.
6. Explain the role of penicillins in treating bacterial infections.
7. Explain the role of cephalosporins in treating bacterial infections.
8. Explain the role of tetracyclines in treating bacterial infections.
9. Explain the role of macrolides in treating bacterial infections.
10. Explain the role of aminoglycosides in treating bacterial infections.
11. Explain the role of fluoroquinolones in treating bacterial infections.
12. Explain the role of sulfonamides and urinary antiseptics in treating bacterial infections.
13. Explain the role of miscellaneous antibiotics in treating bacterial infections.
14. Explain how the pharmacotherapy of tuberculosis differs from that of other infections.

Key Terms

acquired resistance
antagonism
antibiotic (ann-tie-bye-OT-ik)
anti-infective (ann-tie-in-FEK-tive)
bactericidal (bak-teer-ih-SY-dall)
bacteriostatic (bak-teer-ee-oh-STAT-ik)
beta-lactam ring (bay-tuh LAK-tam)
beta-lactamase/penicillinase (bay-tuh-LAK-tam-ace/pen-uh-SILL-in-ace)
broad-spectrum antibiotic
chemoprophylaxis (kee-moh-pro fill-AX-is)
culture and sensitivity (C&S) testing
directly observed therapy (DOT)
healthcare-associated infections (HAIs)
host flora (host FLOR-uh)
mutations (myou-TAY-shuns)
narrow-spectrum antibiotic
nephrotoxicity (NEF-row-toks ISS-ih-tee)
ototoxicity (OH-toh-toks-ISS-ih-tee)
pathogen (PATH-oh-jen)
pathogenicity (path-oh-jen ISS-ih-tee)
photosensitivity
plasmids (PLAZ-midz)
red man syndrome
superinfections
toxins (TOX-in)
tubercles (TOO-burr-kyouls)
urinary antiseptics
virulence (VEER-you-lens)

The human body has adapted quite well to living in a world teeming with microorganisms (microbes). Present in the air, water, food, and soil, microbes are an essential component to life on the planet. In some cases, microorganisms, such as those in the colon, play a beneficial role in human health. When in an unnatural environment or when present in unusually high numbers, however, microorganisms can cause a variety of ailments ranging from mildly annoying to fatal. The development of the first anti-infective drugs in the mid-1900s was a milestone in the field of medicine. In the past 60 years, pharmacologists have attempted to keep pace with microbes that rapidly become resistant to therapeutic drugs. This chapter examines two groups of anti-infectives: the antibacterial drugs and the specialized medications used to treat tuberculosis (TB).

Fast Facts Bacterial Infections

- It is estimated that over 110 million people in the United States have sexually transmitted infections (STIs), with about 70% of these being infection by human papillomavirus.
- It is estimated that about 23,000 deaths occur each year due to organisms that are resistant to antibiotics.
- Foodborne illness is responsible for 48 million illnesses, 128,000 hospitalizations, and 3000 deaths each year in the United States.
- Significant reductions in the incidence of nearly all types of healthcare-associated infections occurred from 2008–2014, the largest being a 44% reduction in central line-associated bloodstream infections.
- About half of all the antibiotics prescribed are not needed or are not optimally effective as prescribed.

Source: Data from Centers for Disease Control and Prevention.

Core Concept 27.1 ▶ Pathogens are organisms that cause disease by invading tissues or secreting toxins.

An organism that can cause disease in humans is called a **pathogen**. Human pathogens include viruses, bacteria, fungi, unicellular organisms (protozoans), and multicellular animals. Examples of these pathogens are illustrated in Figure 27.1. To infect humans, pathogens must bypass a number of elaborate body defenses, such as those described in Chapter 26. Pathogens may enter through broken skin, or by ingestion, inhalation, or contact with a mucous membrane such as the nasal, urinary, or vaginal mucosas.

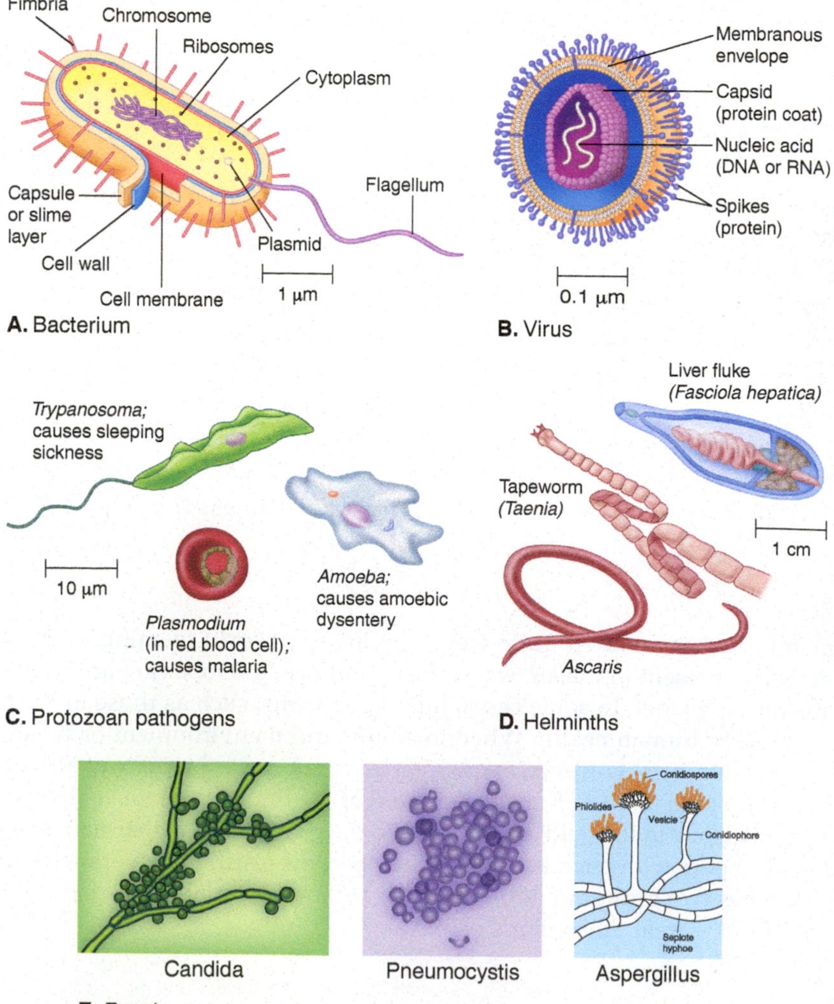

FIGURE 27.1 Types of pathogenic organisms: (a) bacterium, (b) virus, (c) protozoan pathogens, (d) multicellular parasites, and (e) fungi.

Some pathogens are extremely infectious and life threatening to humans, whereas others simply cause annoying symptoms or none at all. The ability of an organism to cause infection is called its **pathogenicity**. Pathogenicity depends on an organism's ability to bypass or overcome the body's immune system. Fortunately for us, only a few dozen pathogens commonly cause disease in humans. Some of these are listed in Table 27.1. Another common word used to describe a pathogen is **virulence**. A highly virulent organism is one that can produce disease when present in very small numbers.

patho = *disease*
gen = *producing*

After gaining entry, pathogens generally cause disease by one of two basic mechanisms. Invasiveness is the ability of a pathogen to grow extremely rapidly and damage surrounding tissues by their sheer numbers. Because a week or more may be needed to mount an immune response against the organism, this rapid growth can easily overwhelm body defenses. A second mechanism is the production of **toxins**. Even very small amounts of some bacterial toxins may disrupt normal cellular activity and, in extreme cases, result in death of the individual.

Several methods are used to describe and classify the millions of species of bacteria on the planet. The three most common methods are shown in Table 27.2. Healthcare providers must learn these organizational schemes because anti-infective drugs are often effective only for a specific type of bacteria, such as gram-positive bacilli or gram-negative anaerobes.

Table 27.1 Common Bacterial Pathogens

Name of Organism	Disease(s)	Remarks
Bacillus anthracis	Anthrax	Appears in cutaneous and respiratory forms
Borrelia burgdorferi	Lyme disease	Acquired from tick bites
Chlamydia trachomatis	Venereal disease, eye infection	Most common cause of STIs in the United States
Enterococcus	Wounds, UTI, endocarditis, bacteremia	Common opportunistic microbe; part of normal flora of the genitourinary and intestinal tracts
Escherichia coli	Traveler's diarrhea, UTI, bacteremia, meningitis in children	Part of normal flora of the intestinal tract
Haemophilus	Pneumonia, meningitis in children, bacteremia, otitis media, sinusitis	Some species are part of the normal host flora of the upper respiratory tract
Klebsiella	Pneumonia, UTI	Common opportunistic microbe
Mycobacterium tuberculosis	Tuberculosis	Incidence high in patients infected with HIV
Mycoplasma pneumoniae	Pneumonia	Most common cause of pneumonia in patients ages 5 to 35
Neisseria gonorrhoeae	Gonorrhea, endometriosis, neonatal eye infection	Common cause of STI
Neisseria meningitidis	Meningitis in children	Can be part of the normal host flora in the nasopharynx
Pneumococcus	Pneumonia, otitis media, meningitis, bacteremia, endocarditis	Part of normal flora in upper respiratory tract
Proteus mirabilis	UTI, skin infections	Part of normal flora in the gastrointestinal (GI) tract
Pseudomonas aeruginosa	UTI, skin infections, septicemia	Common opportunistic microbe
Rickettsia rickettsii	Rocky Mountain spotted fever	Acquired from tick bites
Salmonella enteritidis	Food poisoning	From infected animal products, raw eggs, or undercooked meat or chicken
Staphylococcus aureus	Pneumonia, food poisoning, impetigo, wounds, bacteremia, endocarditis, toxic shock syndrome, osteomyelitis, UTI	Can be part of the normal host flora on the skin and mucous membranes
Streptococcus	Pharyngitis, pneumonia, skin infections, septicemia, endocarditis, otitis media	Some species are part of the normal host flora of the respiratory, genital, and intestinal tracts

Table 27.2 Methods of Describing and Classifying Bacteria

Method	Description
Staining	Gram-positive or gram-negative
Shape	Bacilli (rods), cocci (spheres), and spirilla (spirals)
Ability to use O_2	Aerobic (uses O_2) or anaerobic (without O_2)

Core Concept 27.2 ▶

Anti-infective drugs are classified by their chemical structures or by their mechanisms of action.

Anti-infective is a general term that applies to any drug that is effective against pathogens. In its broadest sense, an anti-infective drug may be used to treat bacterial, fungal, viral, or parasitic infections. The most frequent term used to describe an anti-infective drug is *antibiotic*. Technically, **antibiotic** refers to a natural substance produced by bacteria that can kill other bacteria. In clinical practice, however, the terms *antibacterial, anti-infective, antimicrobial*, and *antibiotic* are often used interchangeably.

anti = *against*
bio = *life*
ic = *pertaining to*

With more than 300 anti-infective drugs available, it is helpful to group these drugs into classes that have similar properties. Two means of grouping are widely used: chemical classes and pharmacologic classes.

Chemical class names such as aminoglycosides, fluoroquinolones, and sulfonamides refer to the fundamental chemical structure of the anti-infectives. Anti-infectives belonging to the same chemical class usually share similar antibacterial properties and adverse effects. Although chemical names are often long and difficult to pronounce, placing drugs into chemical classes will assist the student in mentally organizing these drugs into distinct therapeutic groups.

Pharmacologic classes are used to group anti-infectives by their *mechanism of action*. Examples include cell wall inhibitors, protein synthesis inhibitors, folic acid inhibitors, and reverse trancriptase inhibitors. These classifications are used in this text, where appropriate.

Core Concept 27.3 ▶

Anti-infective drugs act by selectively targeting a pathogen's metabolism or life cycle.

The primary goal of antimicrobial therapy is to assist the body's defenses in eliminating a pathogen. Drugs that accomplish this goal by *killing* bacteria are called **bactericidal**. Some medications do not kill the bacteria but instead *slow their growth*, allowing the body's natural defenses to eliminate the microorganisms. These growth-slowing drugs are called **bacteriostatic**.

bacterio = *bacteria*
cidal = *killing*
static = *staying the same*

Bacterial cells are quite different from human cells. Bacteria have cell walls and contain certain enzymes that human cells lack. Antibiotics exert selective toxicity on bacterial cells by targeting these unique differences. Through this selective action, pathogens can be killed or their growth severely hampered without major effects on human cells. Of course, there are limits to this selective toxicity; therefore, adverse effects can be expected from all the anti-infectives. The basic mechanisms of action of antimicrobial drugs are shown in Figure 27.2.

Core Concept 27.4 ▶

Acquired resistance is a major clinical problem that is worsened by improper use of anti-infectives.

Microorganisms have the ability to replicate extremely rapidly. For example, under ideal conditions, *E. coli* can produce a million cells every 20 minutes. During this rapid replication, bacteria make frequent errors, or **mutations**, while duplicating their genetic code. These mutations occur spontaneously and randomly in the bacterial cell. Although most mutations are harmful to the organism, mutations occasionally result in a bacterial cell that has reproductive advantages over its neighbors. The mutated bacterium may be able to survive in harsher conditions or perhaps grow faster than surrounding cells. One such mutation of particular importance to medicine is that which confers drug resistance on a microorganism.

Antibiotics help promote the appearance of drug-resistant bacterial strains. Killing populations of bacteria that are sensitive to the drug leaves behind those microbes that possess mutations that make them *insensitive* to the effects of the antibiotic. These drug-resistant bacteria are then free to grow faster because they are no longer competing for food with neighboring bacteria that were killed by the antibiotic. Soon the patient develops an infection that is resistant to conventional antibiotics. This phenomenon, called **acquired resistance**, is illustrated in Figure 27.3. Bacteria may pass the resistance gene to other bacteria by transferring small pieces of circular DNA called **plasmids**.

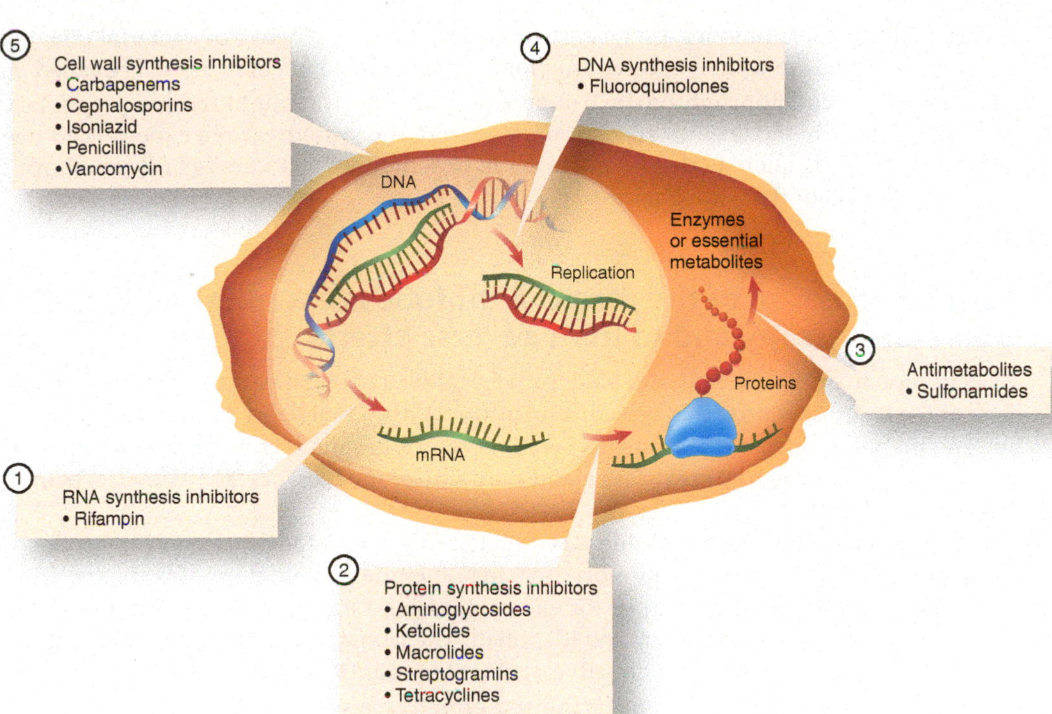

FIGURE 27.2 Mechanisms of action of antimicrobial drugs.

The widespread and sometimes inappropriate use of antibiotics has led to many resistant strains. For example, the majority of *Staphylococcus* bacteria are now resistant to penicillin, and resistant strains of other pathogenic bacteria have become major clinical problems. The longer an antibiotic is used in the population and the more often it is prescribed, the larger will be the percentage of resistant strains. Infections acquired in a hospital or other healthcare setting, called **healthcare-associated infections (HAIs)**, are often resistant to common antibiotics. Two particularly serious resistant infections are those caused by methicillin-resistant *Staphylococcus aureus* (MRSA) and vancomycin-resistant enterococci (VRE).

Healthcare providers play important roles in delaying the emergence of resistance. The following are four principles recommended by the Centers for Disease Control and Prevention (CDC):

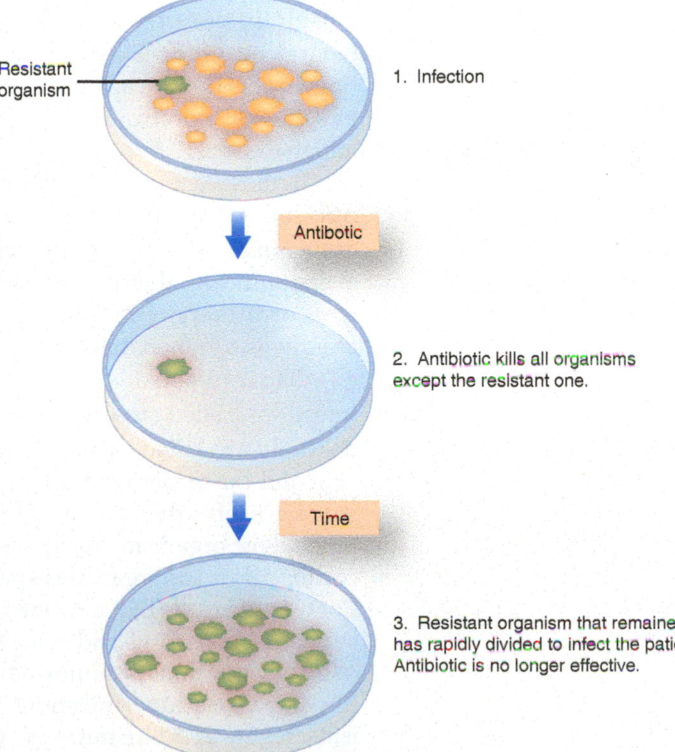

FIGURE 27.3 Acquired resistance.

- Prevent infections when possible. It is always easier to prevent an infection than to treat one. This includes teaching the patient the importance of getting immunizations against diseases such as influenza, tetanus, measles, and hepatitis B.
- Restrict the use of antibiotics to those conditions deemed medically necessary. Antibiotics should be prescribed only when there is a clear rationale for their use.
- Advise the patient to take anti-infectives for the full length of therapy, even if symptoms disappear before the regimen is finished. Prematurely stopping antibiotic therapy allows some pathogens to survive, thus promoting the development of resistant strains.
- Prevent transmission of the pathogen. This includes the use of standard infection control procedures and teaching patients the methods of proper hygiene for preventing transmission in the home and community settings.

In most cases, antibiotics are given when there is clear evidence of bacterial infection. Some patients, however, may receive antibiotics to *prevent* an infection, a practice called *prophylactic use*, or **chemoprophylaxis**. Examples of patients who might receive prophylactic antibiotics include those who have suppressed immune systems, have experienced deep puncture wounds such as dog bites, or have prosthetic heart valves and are about to undergo medical or dental procedures.

Core Concept 27.5 ▶ Careful selection of the correct antibiotic is essential for effective pharmacotherapy and to limit adverse effects.

Selection of an antibiotic that will be effective against a specific pathogen is an important task of the healthcare provider. Selecting an incorrect drug will delay proper treatment, giving the microorganisms more time to invade. Prescribing ineffective antibiotics also promotes the development of resistance and may cause unnecessary adverse effects in the patient.

Ideally, laboratory tests should be conducted to identify the organism prior to beginning anti-infective therapy. Laboratory tests may include examination of body specimens such as urine, sputum, blood, or pus for microorganisms. Organisms isolated from the specimens are grown in the laboratory and identified. The laboratory then tests several antibiotics to determine which is most effective against the identified pathogen. This process of growing the organism and identifying the effective antibiotic is called **culture and sensitivity (C&S) testing**.

Ideally, the pathogen should be identified *before* anti-infective therapy is begun. However, laboratory testing and identification may take several days and, in the case of viruses, several weeks. If the infection is severe, therapy is often begun with a **broad-spectrum antibiotic**, one that is effective against a wide variety of different microbial species. After laboratory testing is completed, the drug may be changed to a **narrow-spectrum antibiotic**, one that is effective against a smaller group of microbes or only the isolated species. In general, narrow-spectrum antibiotics have less effect on normal host flora, thus causing fewer adverse effects.

In most cases, anti-infective therapy uses a single drug, because combining two antibiotics may actually decrease each drug's effectiveness. This phenomenon is known as **antagonism**. Use of multiple antibiotics also has the potential to promote resistance. However, multidrug therapy is warranted if the patient's infection is caused by different organisms or if therapy must be started before C&S testing has been completed. Multidrug therapy is common in the treatment of TB and HIV infection.

One common adverse effect of anti-infective therapy is the appearance of secondary infections, called **superinfections**, which occur when microorganisms normally present in the body are killed by the drug. These normal microorganisms, or **host flora**, inhabit the skin and the upper respiratory, urogenital, and intestinal tracts. Some of these organisms serve a useful purpose by producing antibacterial substances and by competing with pathogenic organisms for space and nutrients. Removal of host flora by an antibiotic gives pathogenic microorganisms space to grow or allows for overgrowth of nonaffected normal flora. Appearance of a new infection while receiving anti-infective therapy is suspicious of a superinfection. Signs and symptoms of a superinfection may include diarrhea, bladder pain, painful urination, or abnormal vaginal discharges. Broad-spectrum antibiotics are more likely to cause superinfections because they kill so many different species of microorganisms. Figure 27.3 illustrates the production of a superinfection.

Core Concept 27.6 ▶ The penicillins are one of the oldest and safest groups of anti-infectives.

Although not the first anti-infective discovered, penicillin was the first *mass-produced* antibiotic. Isolated from the fungus *Penicillium* in 1941, penicillin quickly became a miracle medicine by preventing thousands of deaths from what are now considered to be minor infections. The penicillins are listed in Table 27.3.

Table 27.3 Penicillins

Drug	Route and Adult Dose	Remarks
amoxicillin (Amoxil, Trimox)	PO: 250–500 mg tid	Broad-spectrum penicillin
amoxicillin–clavulanate (Augmentin)	PO: 250–500 mg every 8–12 hours	Broad-spectrum penicillin with a beta lactamase inhibitor
ampicillin (Principen)	PO: 250–500 mg qid	Broad-spectrum penicillin; IM and IV forms available
ampicillin–sulbactam (Unasyn)	IV/IM: 1.5–3 g qid	Broad-spectrum penicillin
dicloxacillin	PO: 125–500 mg qid	Penicillinase resistant
nafcillin	IV/IM: 500 mg–1 g qid (max: 12 g/day)	Penicillinase resistant
oxacillin	IV: 250–500 mg–1 g every 4–6 hours (max: 12 g/day)	Penicillinase resistant; IM form available
penicillin G benzathine (Bicillin)	IM: 1.2 million units as a single dose	Prolonged duration of action
Pr penicillin G potassium	IV/IM: 2–24 million units divided every 4–6 hours	Ineffective against most forms of *S. aureus*
penicillin G procaine (Wycillin)	IM: 600,000–1.2 million units daily	Prolonged duration of action
penicillin V (Pen-Vee K, Veetids, others)	PO: 125–500 mg qid	Acid stable
piperacillin	IM: 2–4 g tid–qid (max: 24 g/day)	Extended-spectrum penicillin
piperacillin–tazobactam (Zosyn)	IV: 3.375–4.5 g qid over 30 minutes	Extended-spectrum penicillin with a beta lactamase inhibitor
ticarcillin–clavulanate (Timentin)	IV: 3.1 g qid	Extended-spectrum penicillin with a beta lactamase inhibitor

Penicillins kill bacteria by disrupting their cell walls. The chemical structure of penicillin that is responsible for its antibacterial activity is called the **beta-lactam ring**. However, some bacteria secrete an enzyme, called **beta-lactamase/penicillinase**, which splits the beta-lactam ring. This structural change allows these bacteria to become resistant to the effects of most penicillins. The action of penicillinase is illustrated in Figure 27.4. Since their discovery, large numbers of resistant bacterial strains that limit the therapeutic usefulness of the penicillins have emerged.

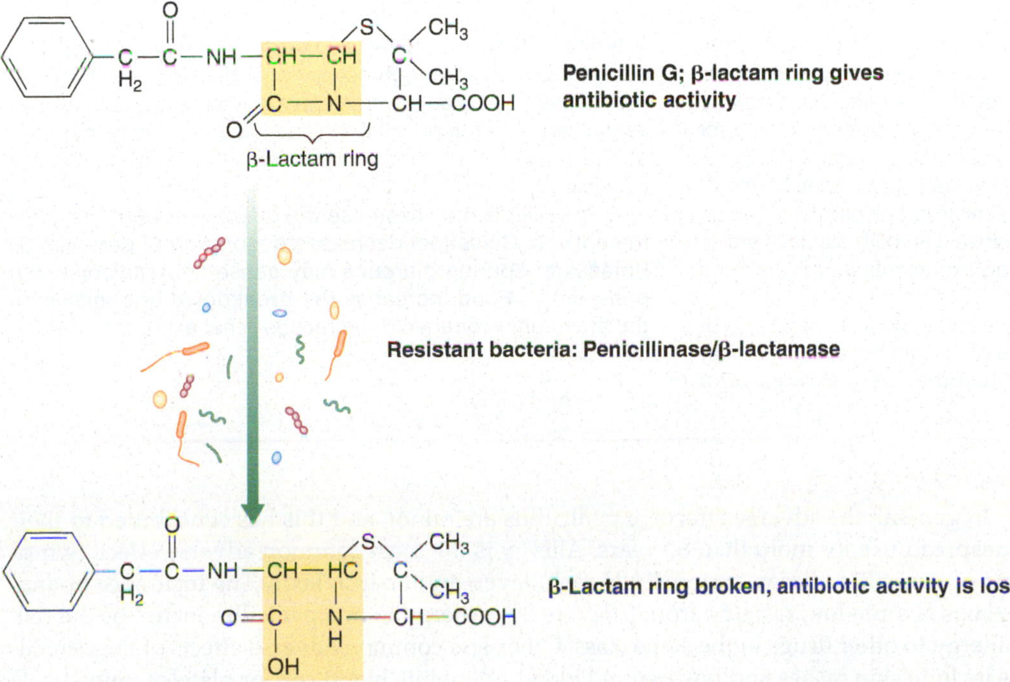

FIGURE 27.4 Action of penicillinase.

Chemical modifications to the natural penicillin molecule produced drugs offering several advantages.

- *Penicillinase-resistant penicillins* Oxacillin and dicloxacillin (Cloxapen) are examples of drugs that are effective against penicillinase-producing bacteria. These are sometimes called antistaphylococcal penicillins.
- *Broad-spectrum penicillins* Ampicillin (Principen) and amoxicillin (Amoxil, Trimox) are effective against a wide range of microorganisms and are called *broad-spectrum* penicillins. These are sometimes referred to as aminopenicillins.
- *Extended-spectrum penicillins* Ticaricillin and piperacillin are effective against even more microbial species than the aminopenicillins, including *Pseudomonas, Enterobacter, Klebsiella,* and *Bacteroides fragilis.*

Several drugs are available that inhibit the bacterial beta-lactamase enzyme. When combined with penicillin, these drugs protect the penicillin molecule from destruction, extending its spectrum of activity. The beta-lactamase inhibitors—clavulanate, sulbactam, and tazobactam—are available in fixed-dose combinations with specific penicillins. These include Augmentin (amoxicillin plus clavulanate), Timentin (ticarcillin plus clavulanate), Unasyn (ampicillin plus sulbactam), and Zosyn (piperacillin plus tazobactam).

CAM Therapy | The Antibacterial Properties of Goldenseal

Goldenseal (*Hydrastis canadensis*) was once a common plant found in woods in the eastern and midwestern United States. As word spread of its medicinal properties, the plant was harvested to near extinction. In particular, goldenseal was reported to mask the appearance of drugs in the urine of patients wanting to hide their drug abuse. This claim has been proven false.

The roots and leaves of goldenseal are dried and available as capsules, tablets, salves, and tinctures. One of the primary ingredients in goldenseal is hydrastine, which is reported to have antibacterial and antifungal properties. When used topically or locally, it is claimed to be of value in treating bacterial and fungal skin infections and oral conditions such as gingivitis and thrush. Other possible indications include hypertension, duodenal ulcers, and conjunctivitis.

Prototype Drug: Pr *Penicillin G Potassium*

Therapeutic Class: Antibacterial **Pharmacologic Class: Cell wall inhibitor, natural penicillin**

Actions and Uses: Penicillin G is sometimes a preferred drug against *streptococcal, pneumococci*, and *staphylococcal* organisms that do not produce penicillinase and are shown to be susceptible by C&S testing. It is also a preferred drug for gonorrhea and syphilis caused by susceptible strains. Because of its low oral absorption, penicillin G is usually given by the IV or IM routes. Penicillin G is very similar to penicillin V, although the latter can be given orally because it is more stable in stomach acid. Penicillinase-producing organisms inactivate both penicillin G and penicillin V.

Penicillin G is available in potassium, benzathine, and procaine salts. They have equal effectiveness; however, the benzathine and procaine salts are absorbed very slowly over a 24-hour period.

Adverse Effects and Interactions: Penicillin G has few adverse effects. Although not serious, diarrhea, nausea, and vomiting are common adverse effects. Anaphylaxis is the most serious adverse effect, although its incidence is very low. Pain at the injection site may occur, and superinfections are possible.

Penicillin G may decrease the effectiveness of oral contraceptives. Colestipol decreases absorption of penicillin G. Potassium-sparing diuretics may cause hyperkalemia with penicillin G. Food increases the breakdown of penicillin in the stomach. Probenecid decreases renal excretion of penicillin G.

In general, the adverse effects of penicillins are minor, and this has contributed to their widespread use for more than 60 years. Allergy is the most common adverse effect. Symptoms of penicillin allergy may include rash, fever, and anaphylaxis. The incidence of anaphylaxis is quite low, ranging from 0.04% to 2%. Allergy to one penicillin increases the risk of allergy to other drugs in the same class. Other less common adverse effects of the penicillins include skin rashes and lowered red blood cell, white blood cell, or platelet counts.

CONCEPT REVIEW 27.1

- Why does antibiotic resistance become more of a problem when antibiotics are prescribed too often?

The cephalosporins are similar in structure and function to the penicillins and are one of the most widely prescribed anti-infective classes.

◄ **Core Concept 27.7**

Isolated shortly after the penicillins, the four generations of cephalosporins comprise the largest antibiotic class. Like the penicillins, the cephalosporins contain a beta-lactam ring that is primarily responsible for their antimicrobial activity. The cephalosporins are bactericidal and inhibit bacterial cell wall synthesis. Table 27.4 lists the cephalosporins and their dosages.

About 20 cephalosporins are available and they have similar sounding names that can challenge even the best memory. They are classified by their "generation." The first-generation drugs contain a beta-lactam ring, and bacteria that produce beta-lactamase will normally be resistant to these medications. The second-generation cephalosporins are more potent and more resistant to beta-lactamase and exhibit a broader spectrum than the first-generation drugs. The third-generation cephalosporins generally have a longer duration of action, an even broader spectrum, and are resistant to beta-lactamases. Third-generation cephalosporins are preferred drugs against infections by *Pseudomonas, Klebsiella, Neisseria, Salmonella, Proteus,* and *Haemophilus influenzae.* Newer, fourth- and fifth-generation drugs are more effective against organisms that have developed resistance to earlier cephalosporins. There are not always clear distinctions between the generations.

In 2014 and 2015 two cephalosporin combinations were approved for the treatment of serious intra-abdominal and urinary tract infections. Zerbaxa combines ceftolozane, a new fifth generation cephalosporin, with tazobactam. Avycaz combines the third generation drug ceftazidime with avibactam, a new beta-lactamase inhibitor.

The primary therapeutic use of the cephalosporins is for gram-negative infections and for patients who cannot tolerate the less expensive penicillins. Like the penicillins, allergic reactions are the most common adverse effect. Skin rashes are a common sign of allergy and may appear several days following the initiation of therapy. GI complaints are common.

Table 27.4 Selected Cephalosporins

Drug	Route and Adult Dose	Remarks
FIRST GENERATION		
cefadroxil (Duricef)	PO: 500 mg–1 g once or twice daily (max: 2 g/day)	Bactericidal
Pr cefazolin (Ancef, Kefzol)	IM: 250 mg–2 g tid (max: 12 g/day)	IV form available
cephalexin (Keflex)	PO: 250–500 mg qid	Bactericidal; broad spectrum
SECOND GENERATION		
cefaclor (Ceclor)	PO: 250–500 mg tid	Extended-release form available; bactericidal
cefotetan (Cefotan)	IM: 1–2 g every 12 hours	IV form available
cefprozil (Cefzil)	PO: 250–500 mg once or twice daily	Bactericidal
cefuroxime (Ceftin, Zinacef)	PO: 250–500 mg bid	IM and IV forms available; bactericidal
THIRD TO FIFTH GENERATIONS		
cefdinir (Omnicef)	PO: 300 mg bid	Third generation; broad spectrum
cefditoren (Spectracef)	PO: 400 mg bid for 10 days	Third generation
cefepime (Maxipime)	IM: 0.5–1 g bid (max: 3 g/day)	Fourth generation; IV form available
cefixime (Suprax)	PO: 400 mg daily or 200 mg bid	Third generation; bactericidal
cefotaxime (Claforan)	IM: 1–2 g bid–tid (max: 12 g/day)	Third generation; bactericidal; IV form available
ceftaroline (Teflaro)	IV: 600 mg every 12 hours for 5–14 days	Fifth generation; broad spectrum effective against MRSA
ceftriaxone (Rocephin)	IM: 1–2 g once or twice daily (max: 4 g/day)	Third generation; IV form also available; bactericidal

Prototype Drug: Pr Cefazolin (Ancef, Kefzol)

Therapeutic Class: Antibacterial **Pharmacologic Class:** Cell wall inhibitor; first-generation cephalosporin

Actions and Uses: Cefazolin is a first-generation cephalosporin used for the treatment and prophylaxis of susceptible gram-positive bacterial infections. Cefazolin has been used to treat infections of the respiratory tract, urinary tract, skin structures, biliary tract, bones, and joints. It has also been useful in the pharmacotherapy of genital infections, septicemia, and endocarditis. This drug is sometimes used for infection prophylaxis in patients who are undergoing surgical procedures. Cefazolin is not effective against MRSA.

Cefazolin has a longer half-life than other first-generation cephalosporins, which allows for less frequent dosing. It is one of the most frequently prescribed parenteral antibiotics.

Adverse Effects and Interactions: The cephalosporins are well tolerated by most patients. Rash and diarrhea are the most common adverse effects, and superinfections are likely when the antibiotic is used for prolonged periods. Approximately 1% to 4% of patients will experience some kind of an allergic reaction. Severe hypersensitivity reactions are rare, though potentially fatal. Pain and phlebitis can occur at injection sites.

Cefazolin can lower the levels of estradiol in the blood, possibly leading to contraceptive failure. Cefazolin can increase the effects of anticoagulants, including both heparin and warfarin; therefore, blood coagulation should be carefully monitored.

Earlier generation cephalosporins exhibited kidney toxicity, but this is diminished with the newer drugs. The nurse must be aware that up to 10% of patients who are allergic to penicillin will also be allergic to cephalosporins. Despite this small incidence of cross allergy, cephalosporins offer a reasonable alternative for *most* patients who are unable to take penicillins. However, cephalosporins are contraindicated if the patient has previously experienced a *severe* allergic reaction to a penicillin.

Core Concept 27.8 ▶

The tetracyclines have broad spectrums but are preferred drugs for few diseases.

The first tetracyclines were extracted from *Streptomyces* soil microorganisms in 1948. Their widespread use in the 1950s and 1960s resulted in a large number of resistant bacterial strains that now limits their therapeutic usefulness. Table 27.5 lists the tetracyclines and their dosages.

Tetracyclines exert a bacteriostatic effect by inhibiting bacterial protein synthesis. They are effective against a wide range of gram-negative and gram-positive organisms and have one of the broadest spectrums of any class of antibiotics. They are preferred drugs for a few diseases, including Rocky Mountain spotted fever, typhus, cholera, Lyme disease, ulcers caused by *Helicobacter pylori*, and *Chlamydia* infections. Drugs in this class are occasionally used for the treatment of acne vulgaris, for which they are given topically or PO at low doses. Minocycline (Arestin) and doxycycline (Atridox, Periostat) are used to treat periodontal disease. A newer tetracycline, tigecycline (Tygacil) is approved to treat drug-resistant intra-abdominal infections and complicated skin infections, especially those caused by MRSA.

The tetracyclines cause few serious adverse effects. Gastric distress is relatively common, so patients tend to take tetracyclines with food. Tetracyclines bind ions such as aluminum, calcium, and iron that may significantly decrease absorption. Therefore these

Table 27.5 Tetracyclines

Drug	Route and Adult Dose	Remarks
demeclocycline (Declomycin)	PO: 150 mg every 6 hours or 300 mg bid (max: 3 g total)	Intermediate duration of action; broad spectrum
doxycycline (Vibramycin, others)	PO: 100 mg bid on day 1, then 100 mg daily (max: 200 mg/day)	Long duration of action; IV form available; subgingival form available for periodontitis
minocycline (Minocin, others)	PO: 200 mg as one dose followed by 100 mg bid	Long duration of action; IV form available; available as microsphere powder for periodontitis and as extended-release tablet for acne
Pr tetracycline (Sumycin)	PO: 250–500 mg bid–qid (max: 2 g/day)	Short acting; inhibits protein synthesis; bacteriostatic; IM and topical forms available
tigecycline (Tygacil)	IV: 100 mg, followed by 50 mg every 12 hours	Newest tetracycline; very limited indications

Prototype Drug: Pr *Tetracycline (Sumycin, Others)*

Therapeutic Class: Antibacterial **Pharmacologic Class:** Tetracycline, protein synthesis inhibitor

Actions and Uses: Tetracycline is effective against many different microorganisms, including some protozoans. Its use has increased due to its effectiveness against *H. pylori* in the treatment of peptic ulcer disease. It is given PO and has a short half-life. A topical preparation is available for treating acne. It should be administered at least 1 hour before or 2 hours after a meal to avoid drug interactions.

Adverse Effects and Interactions: As a broad-spectrum antibiotic, tetracycline has a tendency to affect vaginal, oral, and intestinal flora and cause superinfections. Diarrhea may be severe enough to cause discontinuation of therapy. Other common adverse effects include nausea, vomiting, and photosensitivity.

Tetracycline can decrease the effectiveness of oral contraceptives, and thus alternative precautions should be taken during therapy to prevent pregnancy. Pregnant patients and those who are breastfeeding should not take tetracyclines because they are pregnancy category D.

antibiotics should not be taken with milk or calcium or aluminum-based medications. Patients should be advised to avoid direct exposure to sunlight because tetracyclines can cause **photosensitivity**, which makes the skin particularly susceptible to sunburn. Unless suffering from a life-threatening infection, patients younger than 9 years are not given tetracyclines because these drugs may cause permanent yellow-brown teeth discoloration in young children. Because of their broad spectrum, the risk for superinfection is relatively high, and nurses should always be observant for signs of a secondary infection. Outdated tetracyclines may deteriorate and become nephrotoxic; therefore, unused prescriptions should be discarded promptly.

The macrolides are safe alternatives to penicillin for many infections.

◀ **Core Concept 27.9**

Erythromycin (E-Mycin, Erythrocin), the first macrolide antibiotic, was isolated from *Streptomcyes* in a soil sample in 1952. Macrolides are prescribed for infections that are resistant to penicillins. Commonly prescribed macrolides are listed in Table 27.6.

Prototype Drug: Pr *Erythromycin (E-Mycin, Erythrocin)*

Therapeutic Class: Antibacterial **Pharmacologic Class:** Macrolide protein synthesis inhibitor

Actions and Uses: Erythromycin is inactivated by stomach acid and is thus administered as coated tablets or capsules that dissolve in the small intestine. The drug's main application is for patients who are allergic to penicillins or who may have a penicillin-resistant infection. It is a preferred drug for infections by *Bordetella pertussis* (whooping cough), *Legionella pneumophila* (Legionnaire's disease), *Mycoplasma pneumoniae*, and *Corynebacterium diphtheriae*.

Adverse Effects and Interactions: The most common adverse effects from erythromycin are nausea, abdominal cramping, and vomiting, although these are rarely serious enough to cause discontinuation of therapy. Concurrent administration with food reduces these symptoms. Its spectrum of activity is similar to that of the penicillins. Due to the potential for hepatotoxicity, liver function should be monitored, especially in patients with preexisting hepatic impairment.

Concurrent use with fluconazole will increase the effects of erythromycin. Erythromycin will increase the levels of certain antiseizure drugs, such as cabamazepine, resulting in potentially serious adverse effects. This drug interacts with cyclosporine, increasing the risk for kidney toxicity. It may increase the anticoagulant effects of warfarin. The concurrent use of erythromycin with lovastatin or simvastatin is not recommended because it may increase the risk of muscle toxicity.

Table 27.6 Macrolides

Drug	Route and Adult Dose	Remarks
azithromycin (Zithromax, Zmax)	PO (Zithromax): 500 mg for one dose, then 250 mg daily for 4 days PO (Zmax): 1–2 g single dose	Inhibits protein synthesis; bacteriostatic; IV form available
clarithromycin (Biaxin)	PO: 250–500 mg bid	Inhibits protein synthesis; bacteriostatic; part of regimen for *H. pylori* infections
Pr erythromycin (E-Mycin, Erythrocin)	PO: 250–500 mg qid or 333 mg tid	Bacteriostatic or bactericidal depending on nature of organism and drug concentration; IV form available
fidaxomicin (Dificid)	PO: 200 mg bid	Newer macrolide for treatment of pseudomembranous colitis or *Clostridium difficile*–associated diarrhea

The macrolide antibiotics inhibit bacterial protein synthesis and may be either bactericidal or bacteriostatic, depending on the dose and the target organism. Macrolides are considered safe alternatives to penicillin, although they are preferred drugs for relatively few infections. Common uses of macrolides include the treatment of whooping cough, Legionnaire's disease, and infections by *Streptococcus, H. influenzae, M. pneumoniae*, and *Chlamydia*. Clarithromycin is one of several antibiotics used to treat peptic ulcer disease.

The macrolides are well tolerated by most patients. Mild GI upset, diarrhea, and abdominal pain are the most common adverse effects. Because macrolides are broad-spectrum drugs, patients should be observed for signs of superinfection. Like most of the older antibiotics, macrolide-resistant strains are becoming more common. Macrolides should be used with caution in patients with known QT prolongation due to the potential for dysrhythmias. The only major contraindication to therapy is prior allergic reactions to macrolides.

Some of the macrolides have a longer half-life and cause less GI irritation than erythromycin. For example, azithromycin (Zithromax) has such an extended half-life that it can be administered for only 5 days, rather the 10 days required for most antibiotics. Even shorter durations, often a single dose, are sometimes used when azithromycin (Zmax) is administered to treat gonorrhea, otitis media, or acute bacterial sinusitis. The shorter duration of therapy is thought to increase patient compliance.

CONCEPT REVIEW 27.2

- If penicillins are inexpensive, why might a healthcare provider prescribe a more expensive cephalosporin or macrolide antibiotic?

Core Concept 27.10 ▶ The aminoglycosides are narrow-spectrum drugs that have the potential to cause serious toxicity.

The aminoglycosides, first isolated from soil organisms in 1942, share a common chemical structure of an amino group (NH_2) and a sugar group. Although more toxic than most other antibiotic classes, they have important therapeutic applications for the treatment of a number of aerobic gram-negative bacteria, mycobacteria, and some protozoans. Table 27.7 lists the aminoglycosides and their dosages.

Aminoglycosides are bactericidal and act by inhibiting bacterial protein synthesis. They are normally reserved for serious aerobic gram-negative infections, including those caused by *E. coli, Serratia, Proteus, Klebsiella*, and *Pseudomonas*. When used for systemic bacterial infections, they are given parenterally because they are poorly absorbed from the GI tract. They are occasionally given orally to sterilize the bowel before intestinal surgery. Neomycin is available for topical infections of the skin, eyes, and ears. Paromomycin (Humatin) is given orally for the treatment of parasitic infections. The first aminoglycoside, streptomycin, was once widely prescribed, but its use is now limited to the treatment of TB due to the development of a large number of resistant strains. The student should note the differences in spelling of some of these drugs, from *mycin* to *micin*, which reflects the different organisms from which the drugs were originally isolated.

Table 27.7 Aminoglycosides

Drug	Route and Adult Dose	Remarks
amikacin (Amikin)	IM: 5–7.5 mg/kg as a loading dose, then 7.5 mg/kg bid	Broader spectrum than others in this class; usually bactericidal; IV form available
Pr gentamicin (Garamycin)	IM: 1.5–2 mg/kg as a loading dose, then 1–2 mg/kg bid–tid	IV, topical, and ophthalmic forms available
kanamycin	IM: 5–7.5 mg/kg bid–tid	Also used to sterilize the bowel prior to colon surgery; oral, inhalation, and IV forms available
neomycin	PO: 4–12 g/day in divided doses	Oral, topical, and IV forms available
paromomycin (Humatin)	PO: 7.5–12.5 mg/kg tid	For parasitic infections of the intestine; also used to treat hepatic coma
streptomycin	IM: 15 mg/kg up to 1 g as a single dose	For TB, tularemia, and plague
tobramycin	IM/IV: 3 mg/kg tid (max: 5 mg/kg/day)	Most effective aminoglycoside against *P. aeruginosa*

The clinical applications of the aminoglycosides are limited by their potential to cause serious adverse effects. The degree and types of potential toxicity are similar for all drugs in this class. Of greatest concern are their effects on the inner ear and the kidney. Damage to the inner ear, or **ototoxicity**, causes hearing impairment, dizziness, loss of balance, persistent headache, and ringing in the ears. Because permanent deafness may occur, aminoglycosides are usually discontinued when symptoms of hearing impairment first appear. Kidney damage, or **nephrotoxicity**, is recognized by abnormal urinary function tests, such as elevated serum creatinine or blood urea nitrogen (BUN). The healthcare provider should use great caution if concurrently administering other neurotoxic or nephrotoxic drugs. Serum drug levels are sometimes monitored during therapy to prevent toxic doses of these antibiotics.

oto = *ear*
toxicity = *poison*

nephron = *kidney*

Prototype Drug: Pr *Gentamicin (Garamycin)*

Therapeutic Class: Antibacterial **Pharmacologic Class:** Aminoglycoside, protein synthesis inhibitor

Actions and Uses: Gentamicin is a broad-spectrum, bactericidal antibiotic usually prescribed for serious urinary, respiratory, nervous, or GI system infections. Activity includes *Enterobacter, E. coli, Klebsiella, Citrobacter, Pseudomonas*, and *Serratia*. It is often used in combination with other antibiotics or when other antibiotics have proven ineffective. A topical formulation (Genoptic) is available for infections of the external eye.

Adverse Effects and Interactions: As with other aminoglycosides, adverse effects from gentamicin may be severe. Ototoxicity is possible and may become permanent with continued use. Ringing in the ears, dizziness, and persistent headaches are early signs of ototoxicity. Frequent hearing tests should be conducted so that gentamicin may be discontinued if early signs of ototoxicity are detected. The healthcare provider must also be alert for signs of nephrotoxicity because this may limit drug therapy with gentamicin. Renal function should be monitored during therapy.

Using this drug together with amphotericin B, cisplatin, polymyxin B, or vancomycin increases the risk of nephrotoxicity. The risk of ototoxicity increases if the patient is currently taking amphotericin B, furosemide, aspirin, bumetanide, ethacrynic acid, cisplatin, or paromomycin.

BLACK BOX WARNING:
Adverse effects from parenteral gentamicin may be severe and include neurotoxicity, neuromuscular blockade, and nephrotoxicity. The concurrent use with potent diuretics such as furosemide may increase the risk of ototoxicity.

Fluoroquinolones have wide clinical applications because of their broad spectrum of activity and relative safety.

◀ **Core Concept 27.11**

The fluoroquinolones were once reserved only for UTIs because of their toxicity. However, the newer fluoroquinolones are safer, have a broader spectrum of activity, and are used for a variety of infections. The fluoroquinolones are listed in Table 27.8.

The first drug in this class, nalidixic acid (NegGram), was approved in 1962, but its use is restricted to UTIs. Four generations of fluoroquinolones have since become available. All

Table 27.8 Fluoroquinolones

Drug	Route and Adult Dose	Remarks
besifloxacin (Besivance)	Ophthalmic: One drop in each affected eye q8h	For bacterial conjunctivitis
Pr ciprofloxacin (Cipro)	PO: 250–750 mg bid	For lung, skin, bone, and joint infections, and for anthrax; broad spectrum; IV form available
finafloxacin (Xtoro)	Eardrops: 4 drops in affected ear bid for 1 week	For otitis media
gatifloxacin (Zymar, Zymaxid)	Ophthalmic: 1 drop in affected eye q2–6h	For bacterial conjunctivitis
gemifloxacin (Factive)	PO: 320 mg daily	For respiratory infections
levofloxacin (Levaquin)	PO: 250–500 mg daily	For respiratory tract and skin infections; IV form available
moxifloxacin (Avelox, Moxeza, Vigamox)	PO/IV (Avelox): 400 mg daily Ophthalmic: One drop in affected eye tid (Vigamox) or bid (Moxeza)	PO: For sinus, skin, intraabdominal, and respiratory infections Ophthalmic: For bacterial conjunctivitis
nalidixic acid (NegGram)	PO: 500–1000 mg qid	For UTI
norfloxacin (Noroxin)	PO: 400 mg bid	For UTI; ophthalmic form available
ofloxacin (Floxin)	PO: 200–400 mg bid	For UTI, respiratory tract infections, and gonorrhea; otic drops available

Prototype Drug: Ciprofloxacin (Cipro)

Therapeutic Class: Antibacterial **Pharmacologic Class:** Fluoroquinolone, bacterial DNA synthesis inhibitor

Actions and Uses: Ciprofloxacin (Cipro), a second-generation fluoroquinolone, is the most widely used drug in this class. Ciprofloxacin inhibits bacterial replication and DNA repair and is more effective against gram-negative than gram-positive organisms. It is prescribed for respiratory infections, bone and joint infections, GI infections, ophthalmic infections, sinusitis, and prostatitis. It is rapidly absorbed after oral administration, and an IV form is available for severe infections. An extended-release form of the drug, Proquin XR, is administered for only 3 days and is approved for bladder infections.

Adverse Effects and Interactions: Ciprofloxacin is well tolerated by most patients, and serious adverse effects are uncommon. Nausea, vomiting, and diarrhea may occur in as many as 20% of patients. Ciprofloxacin may be administered with food to lessen adverse GI effects; however, it should not be taken with antacids or mineral supplements because drug absorption will be diminished. Some patients report headache and dizziness.

Using this drug with warfarin may increase warfarin's anticoagulant effects and result in bleeding. Antacids, ferrous sulfate, and sucralfate decrease the absorption of ciprofloxacin. Caffeine should be restricted to avoid excessive nervousness, anxiety, or tachycardia.

BLACK BOX WARNING:
Tendinitis and tendon rupture may occur, especially in patients over age 60; in kidney, heart, and lung transplant recipients; and in those receiving concurrent corticosteroid therapy. Fluoroquinolones may cause extreme muscle weakness in patients with myasthenia gravis.

fluoroquinolones have activity against gram-negative pathogens; the newer ones are significantly more effective against gram-positive microbes.

The fluoroquinolones are bactericidal and act by inhibiting bacterial DNA synthesis. These antibiotics are extensively used as alternatives to other antibiotics. Clinical applications include infections of the respiratory, GI, and gynecologic tracts, and some skin and soft-tissue infections.

The most widely used drug in this class, ciprofloxacin (Cipro), is a preferred drug for exposure to anthrax (*Bacillus anthracis*), a potential bioterrorist threat. If exposure to anthrax is *suspected*, 500 mg of ciprofloxacin is administered PO every 12 hours for 60 days. If exposure is *confirmed*, ciprofloxacin is immediately administered IV, 400 mg every 12 hours. Other antibiotics are also effective against anthrax, including penicillin, vancomycin, ampicillin, erythromycin, tetracycline, and doxycycline.

A major advantage of the fluoroquinolones is that most are well absorbed orally and may be administered either once or twice daily. They should not be taken together with multivitamins or mineral supplements because these interact to reduce the absorption of some fluoroquinolones by as much as 90%.

Fluoroquinolones are safe for most patients, with nausea, vomiting, and diarrhea being the most frequent adverse effects. The most serious adverse effects are dysrhythmias (for moxifloxacin) and potential hepatotoxicity. Fluoroquinolones have been shown to exhibit cartilage toxicity, resulting in an increased risk of tendonitis and tendon rupture, particularly of the Achilles tendon. The risk of tendon rupture is especially increased in patients over age 60 and those receiving concurrent corticosteroids. Because they may affect cartilage development, these drugs are not approved for children under age 18. In 2013, the U.S. Food and Drug Administration (FDA) issued a safety warning regarding an increased risk for peripheral neuropathy for fluoroquinolones taken by mouth or by injection. Patients should report symptoms such as numbness, weakness, or changes in sensation to pain, temperature, or touch to their healthcare provider immediately. Fluoroquinolones are pregnancy category C and their use should be avoided during pregnancy or in lactating patients.

Core Concept 27.12 ▶

Sulfonamides and urinary antiseptics are traditional drugs for urinary tract infections.

The discovery of the sulfonamides in the 1930s heralded a new era in the treatment of infectious disease. With their wide spectrum of activity, the sulfonamides significantly reduced deaths due to infections and earned their discoverer a Nobel Prize in medicine. The sulfonamides are listed in Table 27.9. Sulfonamides suppress bacterial growth by inhibiting folic acid, an essential substance in cellular metabolism.

Although initially very effective, several factors led to a significant decline in the use of sulfonamides. Their widespread availability over 70 years produced a substantial number

Table 27.9 Sulfonamides and Urinary Antiseptics

Drug	Route and Adult Dose	Remarks
SULFONAMIDES		
silver sulfadiazine	Topical: Apply cream 1–2 times per day	For prevention of sepsis in patients with serious burns
sulfadiazine	PO: 2–4 g daily in 4–6 divided doses	Also for malaria, toxoplasmosis, and prophylaxis of rheumatic fever
sulfadoxine–pyrimethamine (Fansidar)	PO: 1 tablet weekly (500 mg sulfadoxine, 25 mg pyrimethamine)	Also for prevention and treatment of malaria
sulfasalazine (Azulfidine)	PO: 1–2 g/day in four divided doses (max: 8 g/day)	Also for ulcerative colitis and rheumatoid arthritis
sulfisoxazole (Gantrisin)	PO: 2–4 g initially, followed by 1–2 g qid	For UTI; short acting; vaginal form available
Pr trimethoprim-sulfamethoxazole (Bactrim, Septra)	PO: 1 double-strength (DS) tablet (160 mg TMP/800 mg SMZ) bid	Combination drug; for UTI, Pneumocystis, and ear infections; IV form available
URINARY ANTISEPTICS		
fosfomycin (Monurol)	PO: 3 g sachet dissolved in 3–4 oz of water as a single dose	Bactericidal; for UTI
methenamine hippurate (Hiprex) methenamine mandelate	PO: Hippurate 1 g bid; mandelate 1 g qid	For chronic UTI; broad spectrum
nitrofurantoin (Furadantin, Macrobid, Macrodantin)	PO: 50–100 mg qid	For UTI; extended-release form available; interferes with bacterial enzymes

of resistant bacterial strains. The development of the penicillins, cephalosporins, and macrolides gave healthcare providers greater choices of safer drugs. Approval of the combination antibiotic trimethoprim–sulfamethoxazole (Bactrim, Septra, TMP-SMZ) marked a resurgence in the use of sulfonamides in treating UTIs. In communities with high resistance rates, trimethoprim–sulfamethoxazole is no longer a first-line drug, unless C&S testing determines it to be the most effective drug for the specific pathogen.

Prototype Drug: Pr *Trimethoprim–Sulfamethoxazole (Bactrim, Septra)*

Therapeutic Class: Antibacterial **Pharmacologic Class:** Sulfonamide, folic acid inhibitor

Actions and Uses: The combination of sulfamethoxazole (SMZ), a sulfonamide, with the anti-infective trimethoprim (TMP) is most often used in the pharmacotherapy of UTIs. It is also approved for the treatment of *Pneumocystis jiroveci* pneumonia, *Shigella* infections of the small bowel, traveler's diarrhea, acute otitis media, and acute exacerbations of chronic bronchitis.

Both SMZ and TMP are inhibitors of the bacterial metabolism of folic acid. Combining the two drugs produces a greater bacterial kill than would be achieved with either drug used separately. Another advantage of the combination is that development of resistance is lower than is observed when either of the drugs is used alone.

Adverse Effects and Interactions: Nausea and vomiting are the most frequent adverse effects of TMP–SMZ therapy. Hypersensitivity to the sulfonamide component is relatively common and usually manifests as skin rash, itching, and fever. This medication should be used cautiously in patients with pre-existing kidney disease, because sulfonamides can adversely affect renal function. Periodic laboratory evaluations are usually performed to identify early signs of adverse blood effects. Patients with AIDS experience a high incidence of adverse effects to this drug combination.

TMP and SMZ may increase the effects of oral anticoagulants. These drugs may also increase methotrexate toxicity. Potassium supplements should not be taken during therapy, unless directed by the healthcare provider.

Sulfonamides are classified by their route of administration: systemic or topical. Systemic medications, such as sulfisoxazole (Gantrisin) and trimethoprim–sulfamethoxazole, are readily absorbed when given PO and excreted rapidly by the kidney. Other sulfonamides such as silver sulfadiazine (Silvadene) are used only for topical infections. The topical sulfonamides are rarely used because many patients are allergic to substances containing sulfur. One drug in this class, sulfadoxine–pyrimethamine (Fansidar), has an exceptionally long half-life and is occasionally prescribed for malarial prophylaxis. Sulfasalazine (Azulfidine) is a sulfonamide with anti-inflammatory properties that is used to treat rheumatoid arthritis and ulcerative colitis.

In general, the sulfonamides are safe medications; however, some adverse effects may be serious. Adverse effects include the formation of crystals in the urine, allergic reactions, nausea, and vomiting. Although not common, potentially fatal blood abnormalities, such as aplastic anemia, acute hemolytic anemia, and agranulocytosis, can occur.

Urinary antiseptics are drugs given by the PO route for their antibacterial action in the urinary tract. The kidney concentrates the drugs; thus, their actions are specific to the urinary system. Urinary antiseptics reach therapeutic levels in the kidney tubules, and their anti-infective action continues as they travel to the urinary bladder. Although not considered first-line drugs for UTI, they serve important roles as secondary medications, especially in patients who present with infections resistant to TMP–SMZ or the fluoroquinolones.

Core Concept 27.13 ▶ A number of additional anti-infectives have distinct mechanisms of action and specific indications.

Some anti-infectives cannot be grouped into classes, or the class is too small to warrant separate discussion. That is not to diminish their importance in medicine; some of these anti-infectives are critical drugs for specific infections.

For example, clindamycin (Cleocin) is sometimes a preferred drug for abdominal infections caused by *Bacteroides* species. It is considered to be appropriate treatment when less toxic alternatives are not effective. Vancomycin (Vancocin) is an antibiotic usually reserved for severe infections from gram-positive organisms such as *S. aureus* and *Streptococcus pneumoniae.* It is often used after bacteria have become resistant to other, safer antibiotics. Vancomycin is the most effective drug for treating MRSA infections.

Of the miscellaneous antibiotics, several belong to a newer class of antibiotics called *carbapenems*. These drugs are bactericidal, given by the IV route, and have some of the broadest antimicrobial spectrums of any class of antibiotics. Imipenem (Primaxin), the most widely prescribed drug in this small class, is administered in a fixed-dose combination with cilastatin, which increases the serum levels of the antibiotic. Meropenem (Merrem IV) is approved only for peritonitis and bacterial meningitis. Ertapenem (Invanz) and doripenem are approved for the treatment of serious abdominopelvic infections and complicated UTI. Diarrhea, nausea, rashes, and thrombophlebitis at injection sites are the most frequent adverse effects of the carbapenems.

Several miscellaneous drugs represent newer classes of antibiotics. Linezolid (Zyvox) and Tedizolid (Sivextro) belong to a class called the oxazolidinones. Both of these drugs may be given by either the PO or IV route and are usually reserved for serious infections of the skin and skin structure, including MRSA infections.

Quinupristin–dalfopristin (Synercid) is a combination drug that is the first in an antibiotic class called streptogramins. This drug is primarily indicated for treatment of vancomycin-resistant *Enterococcus (VRE)* infections. Daptomycin (Cubicin) is the first in a newer class of antibiotics called the cyclic lipopeptides. It is approved for the treatment of serious skin and skin-structure infections such as major abscesses, postsurgical skin-wound infections, and infected ulcers. Table 27.10 lists some of these miscellaneous antibiotics and their dosages.

Prototype Drug: Pr *Vancomycin (Vancocin)*

Therapeutic Class: Antibiotic **Pharmacologic Class:** Bacterial cell wall synthesis inhibitor

Actions and Uses: Vancomycin is usually reserved for severe infections from gram-positive organisms such as *S. aureus* and *Streptococcus pneumoniae.* It is often used after bacteria have become resistant to other safer antibiotics. It is bactericidal, inhibiting bacterial cell wall synthesis. Because vancomycin was not used frequently during the first 30 years following its discovery, the incidence of vancomycin-resistant organisms is smaller than with other antibiotics. Vancomycin is the most effective drug for treating MRSA infections. Vancomycin-resistant strains of *S. aureus*, however, have begun to appear in recent years. Vancomycin is normally given IV because it is not absorbed from the GI tract.

Adverse Effects and Interactions: Frequent, minor side effects include flushing, hypotension, and itching and rash on the upper body, sometimes called **red man syndrome.** This syndrome can often be prevented by treating the patient with an antihistamine and infusing the drug over at least 60 minutes. More serious adverse effects are possible with higher doses, including nephrotoxicity and ototoxicity. Some patients experience an acute allergic reaction and even anaphylaxis.

Vancomycin adds to toxicity of aminoglycosides, amphotericin B, cisplatin, cyclosporine, polymyxin B, and other ototoxic and nephrotoxic medications. Cholestyramine and colestipol can decrease the absorption of vancomycin.

Table 27.10 Miscellaneous Anti-infectives

Drug	Route and Adult Dose	Remarks
CARBAPENEMS		
doripenem (Doribax)	IV: 500 mg every 8 hours (max: 500 mg every 8 hours)	Very broad spectrum; for serious abdominopelvic and skin infections, pneumonia, complicated UTI, and bacterial meningitis (meropenem)
ertapenem (Invanz)	IV/IM: 1 g/day	
imipenem-cilastatin (Primaxin)	IV: 250–500 mg tid–qid (max: 4 g/day)	
meropenem (Merrem IV)	IV: 0.5–1 g tid	
OTHER MISCELLANEOUS ANTIBIOTICS		
aztreonam (Azactam)	IM/IV: 0.5–2 g bid–qid (max: 8 g/day)	Monobactam class; for gram-negative aerobic bacteria
chloramphenicol	PO: 50 mg/kg qid	Broad spectrum; for typhoid fever and meningitis; IV form available
clindamycin (Cleocin)	PO: 150–450 mg qid	Bacteriostatic; effective against anaerobic organisms; topical, IM, and IV forms available
dalbavancin (Dalvance)	IV: 1000 mg followed 1 week later by 500 mg	Newer drug; bactericidal for serious skin infections
daptomycin (Cubicin)	IV: 4 mg/kg once every 24 hours for 7–14 days	Bactericidal; for serious skin infections
lincomycin (Lincocin)	PO: 500 mg tid–qid (max: 8 g/day)	Bacteriostatic; effective against anaerobic organisms; IM form available
linezolid (Zyvox)	PO: 600 mg bid (max: 1,200 mg/day)	For vancomycin-resistant *Enterococcus*; IV form available
metronidazole (Flagyl) (see the Prototype Drug box in Core Concept 28.7)	PO: 7.5 mg/kg qid	For serious infections with anaerobic bacteria; also for protozoan infections; IV form available
oritavancin (Orbactiv)	IV: One 1200 mg dose infused over 3 hours	Newer drug; bactericidal for serious skin infections
quinupristin-dalfopristin (Synercid)	IV: 7.5 mg/kg infused over 50 minutes every 8 hours	Streptogamins class; for serious infections resistant to vancomycin
spectinomycin (Trobicin)	IM: 2 g as single dose	Bacteriostatic; for gonorrhea
tedizolid (Sivextro)	PO/IV: 200 mg once daily for 6 days	Newer drug for serious skin infections
telavancin (Vibativ)	IV: 10 mg/kg over 60 minutes for 24 hours	For hospital-acquired pneumonia
telithromycin (Ketek)	PO: 800 mg daily	Ketolide class; for community-acquired respiratory tract infections
Pr vancomycin (Vancocin)	IV: 500 mg qid–1 g bid	For *S.aureus*-resistant infections; PO form available

Nursing Process Focus Patients Receiving Antibacterial Therapy

ASSESSMENT

Prior to administration:

- Obtain a complete health history, including neurological, GI, renal and liver conditions, past infections, allergies, drug history, and possible drug interactions.
- Acquire the results of a complete physical examination, including vital signs, height, weight, and any signs or symptoms of infection.
- Evaluate laboratory blood findings: complete blood count (CBC), electrolytes, lipid panel, and renal and liver function studies.
- Obtain specimens for C&S testing before initiating therapy.

POTENTIAL NURSING DIAGNOSES*

- *Acute Pain* related to tissue damage secondary to infection
- *Deficient Knowledge* related to a lack of information about disease process, transmission and drug therapy
- *Risk for Injury* related to tissue destruction and adverse effects of drug therapy

PLANNING: PATIENT GOALS AND EXPECTED OUTCOMES

The patient will:

- Experience therapeutic effects (reduction in symptoms related to the diagnosed infection).
- Be free from or experience minimal adverse effects from drug therapy.
- Verbalize an understanding of the drug's use, adverse effects, and required precautions.

(*Continued*)

Nursing Process Focus (*continued*)

IMPLEMENTATION

Interventions and (Rationales)	Patient Education/Discharge Planning
• Monitor signs and symptoms of infection, including vital signs. (Monitoring of patient signs and symptoms is used to determine antibacterial effectiveness or worsening of infection. Another drug or different dosage may be required.)	• Instruct the patient to notify the healthcare provider if there are changes in level of consciousness (LOC), if the fever does not return to normal parameters (under 38.2°C [100.8°F]), or if other symptoms persist or worsen.
• Administer medication correctly and evaluate the patient's knowledge of proper administration, especially monitoring for compliance with antibiotic therapy. (Partial doses, skipped doses, and shortened length of treatment encourage the recurrence of infection or development of resistant organisms.)	Instruct the patient to: • Take the medication on schedule. • Complete the entire prescription even if feeling better to prevent development of resistant bacteria. • Follow up with the healthcare provider after antibiotic therapy is completed.
• If drug is being given IV, monitor the site for signs and symptoms of tissue irritation, severe pain, and extravasation.	• Instruct the patient to immediately report pain or other symptoms of discomfort to the healthcare provider during IV infusion.
• Monitor for hypersensitivity reaction. (Immediate hypersensitivity reaction may occur within 2–30 minutes; accelerated reaction occurs in 1–72 hours; and delayed reaction after 72 hours.)	• Instruct the patient to discontinue the medication and inform the healthcare provider if symptoms of hypersensitivity reaction develop such as wheezing; shortness of breath; swelling of face, tongue, or hands; or itching or rash.
• Monitor for severe diarrhea. (The condition may occur due to superinfection or the possible adverse effect of specific antibiotics.)	Instruct the patient to: • Report any diarrhea that increases in frequency or amount, or that contains mucus or blood, to the healthcare provider. • Consult the healthcare provider before taking antidiarrheal drugs, which could cause retention of harmful bacteria. • Consume cultured dairy products with live active cultures, such as kefir, yogurt, or buttermilk, to help maintain normal intestinal flora.
• Monitor for superinfection, especially in elderly, debilitated, or immunosuppressed patients. (Increased risk for superinfections is due to elimination of normal flora.)	Instruct the patient to: • Report signs and symptoms of superinfection, such as fever; white patches in the mouth; itchy rash; loose, foul-smelling stools; or whitish thick vaginal discharge to the healthcare provider. • Use infection control measures such as frequent hand hygiene.
• Monitor intake of over-the-counter (OTC) products such as antacids, calcium supplements, iron products, and laxatives containing magnesium. (These products interfere with absorption of many antibiotics.)	• Advise the patient to consult with the healthcare provider before using OTC medications or herbal products.
• Monitor for photosensitivity and sensitivity of the skin to the sun. (Tetracyclines, fluoroquinolones, and sulfonamides can increase the patient's sensitivity to ultraviolet light and increase risk of sunburn.)	Encourage the patient to: • Avoid exposure to direct sunlight during and after therapy. • Wear protective clothing, sunglasses, and sunscreen when outdoors.
• Determine the interactions of the prescribed antibiotics with various foods and beverages. (Many antibiotics are associated with significant GI effects. Food or milk may impair absorption of some antibiotics such as macrolides.)	Instruct the patient regarding foods and beverages that should be avoided with specific antibiotic therapies: • No acidic fruit juices with penicillins • No alcohol intake with cephalosporins • No dairy or calcium products with tetracyclines
• Monitor for other adverse effects specific to various antibiotic therapies. (See each Core Concept for each antibiotic classification in this chapter.)	• Instruct the patient to report adverse effects specific to the antibiotic therapy prescribed.
• Continue to monitor periodic laboratory work: CBC, liver and renal function studies, C&S, peak and trough drug levels as applicable, and possibly a urinalysis. (Many antibiotics are renal or hepatic toxic. Periodic C&S are done to confirm effectiveness of therapy. Drug levels will be monitored with some drugs.)	Inform the patient: • About the importance and purpose of required laboratory tests. • To schedule follow-ups with the healthcare provider. • To help with renal function, increase fluid intake to 2000–3000 mL/day.

Interventions and (Rationales)	Patient Education/Discharge Planning
• Monitor for symptoms of ototoxicity. (Some antibiotics, such as the aminoglycosides and vancomycin, may cause vestibular or auditory nerve damage.)	Instruct the patient to notify the healthcare provider of: • Changes in hearing, ringing in the ears, or full feeling in the ears. • Nausea and vomiting with motion, ataxia, nystagmus, or dizziness.
• Monitor for symptoms of neurotoxicity. (Penicillins, cephalosporins, sulfonamides, aminoglycosides, and fluoroquinolones have an increased risk of neurotoxicity.)	• Instruct the patient to notify the healthcare provider if dizziness, drowsiness, severe headache, changes in LOC, or seizures occur.
EVALUATION OF OUTCOME CRITERIA	
Evaluate the effectiveness of drug therapy by confirming that patient goals and expected outcomes have been met (see "Planning"). *See Tables 27.3 through 27.10 for lists of drugs to which these nursing actions apply.*	

TUBERCULOSIS

TB is a highly contagious infection caused by the organism *Mycobacterium tuberculosis*. Although *M. tuberculosis* typically invades the lungs, it may travel to other body systems, particularly bone. The slow-growing mycobacteria activate cells of the immune response, which attempt to isolate the pathogens by creating a wall around them. The mycobacteria usually become dormant, lying inside cavities called **tubercles**. They may remain dormant during an entire lifetime, or they may become reactivated if the immune system becomes suppressed. When active, TB can be quite infectious, being spread by contaminated sputum. With the immune suppression characteristic of AIDS, the incidence of TB has greatly increased: As many as 20% of all patients with AIDS develop active TB.

Two other types of mycobacteria infect humans. *Mycobacterium leprae* is responsible for leprosy, a disease rarely seen in the United States. *M. leprae* is treated with multiple drugs, usually beginning with rifampin. *Mycobacterium avium* complex (MAC) causes an infection of the lungs, most commonly observed in patients with AIDS. The most effective drugs against MAC are the macrolides azithromycin (Zithromax) and clarithromycin (Biaxin).

The pharmacotherapy of tuberculosis requires special dosing regimens and schedules.

◀ Core Concept 27.14

Drug therapy of TB differs from that of most other infections. Mycobacteria have a cell wall that is resistant to penetration by anti-infective drugs. For medications to reach the microorganisms isolated in the tubercles, therapy must continue for 6–12 months. Although the patient may not be infectious this entire time and have no symptoms, it is critical that therapy continue the entire period. Some patients develop multidrug-resistant infections and require therapy for as long as 24 months.

A second feature of the pharmacotherapy of TB is that at least two—and sometimes four or more—antibiotics must be administered concurrently. During the 6- to 12-month treatment period, different combinations of drugs may be used. Multidrug therapy is necessary because the mycobacteria grow slowly, and resistance is common. Using multiple drugs and switching the combinations during the long treatment period lowers the potential for resistance and increases therapeutic success. Although many different drug combinations are used, a typical regimen for patients with no complicating factors includes the following:

- *Initial phase* 2 months of daily therapy with isoniazid (INH), rifampin (Rifadin, Rimactane), pyrazinamide (PZA), and ethambutol (Myambutol). If laboratory test results show that the strain is sensitive to the first three drugs, ethambutol is dropped from the regimen.
- *Continuation phase* 4 months of therapy with isoniazid and rifampin, two to three times per week.

Table 27.11 First-Line Antitubercular Drugs

Drug	Route and Adult Dose	Remarks
ethambutol (Myambutol)	PO: 15–25 mg/kg daily	Used in combination with other antituberculars
Pr isoniazid (INH, Nydrazid)	PO: 300 mg/day or 900 mg twice weekly for 6–9 months for latent TB or 15 mg/kg/day for active TB	Used in combination with other antituberculars; IM form available
pyrazinamide (PZA)	PO: 15–30 mg/kg once daily (max: 3 g/day)	Rifater is a fixed-dose combination of pyrazinamide with isoniazid and rifampin
rifabutin (Mycobutin)	PO: 300 mg once daily (for prophylaxis) or 5 mg/kg/day (for active TB) (max: 300 mg/day)	Very similar to rifampin and rifapentine
rifampin (Rifadin, Rimactane)	PO: 600 mg daily as a single dose or 900 mg twice weekly for 4 months	Used in combination with other antituberculars; IV form available; also for leprosy, *H. influenzae*, and meningococcus infections
rifapentine (Priftin)	PO: 600 mg twice a week for 2 months, then once a week for 4 months	Used in combination with other antituberculars

There are two broad categories of antitubercular drugs. One category consists of first-line drugs, which are generally the most effective and give the fewest adverse effects. Second-line medications, more toxic and less effective than the first-line drugs, are used when resistance develops. Table 27.11 lists the first-line drugs for therapy of TB.

Prototype Drug: Pr *Isoniazid (INH, Nydrazid)*

Therapeutic Class: Antituberculosis drug **Pharmacologic Class: Mycolic acid inhibitor**

Actions and Uses: Isoniazid is a drug of choice for the treatment of *M. tuberculosis* because decades of experience have shown it to have a superior safety profile and to be the most effective single drug for the disease. Isoniazid acts by inhibiting the synthesis of mycolic acid, an essential cell wall component of mycobacteria. It is bactericidal for actively growing organisms but bacteriostatic for dormant mycobacteria. It is selective for *M. tuberculosis.* Isoniazid may be used alone for chemoprophylaxis, or in combination with other antituberculosis drugs for treating active disease.

Adverse Effects and Interactions: The most common adverse effects of isoniazid are numbness of the hands and feet, rash, and fever. Peripheral neuropathy occurs in a significant percentage of patients and may be prevented by giving pyridoxine (vitamin B6) during therapy.

Aluminum-containing antacids should not be administered concurrently because they can decrease the absorption of isoniazid. When disulfiram is taken with INH, lack of coordination or psychotic reactions may result. INH reduces the effectiveness of azole antifungals; thus they should not be administered concurrently.

BLACK BOX WARNING:
Although rare, hepatotoxicity is a serious and sometimes fatal adverse effect; thus, the patient should be monitored carefully for jaundice, fatigue, elevated hepatic enzymes, or loss of appetite. Liver enzyme tests are usually performed monthly during therapy. Hepatotoxicity usually appears in the first 1–3 months of therapy but may occur at any time during treatment. Older adults and those with daily alcohol consumption are at greater risk of developing hepatotoxicity.

Nursing Process Focus Patients Receiving Antitubercular Drugs

ASSESSMENT

Prior to administration:

- Obtain a complete health history, including respiratory, neurological, renal and liver conditions, allergies, drug history, past infections, and possible drug interactions.
- Evaluate laboratory blood findings: CBC, electrolytes, and renal and liver function studies.
- Acquire the results of a complete physical examination, including vital signs and any signs or symptoms of infection.
- Collect information on the presence or history of the following: positive tuberculin skin test, sputum culture, or smear; close contact with person recently infected with TB; HIV infection, or AIDS; immunosuppressant drug therapy; alcohol abuse; cognitive ability to comply with long-term therapy.

POTENTIAL NURSING DIAGNOSES*

- *Infection* related to inadequate primary defenses, environmental exposure
- *Fatigue* related to presence of infection; adverse effects of drug therapy
- *Deficient Knowledge* related to a lack of information about drug therapy
- *Noncompliance* related to adverse drug effects, deficient knowledge, length of treatment, or cost of medication
- *Risk for Injury* related to tissue destruction and adverse effects of drug therapy

PLANNING: PATIENT GOALS AND EXPECTED OUTCOMES	
The patient will: • Experience therapeutic effects (an absence or reduction in TB symptoms). • Be free from or experience minimal adverse effects from drug therapy. • Verbalize an understanding of the drug's use, adverse effects, and required precautions.	
IMPLEMENTATION	
Interventions and (Rationales)	**Patient Education/Discharge Planning**
• Administer the medication correctly and evaluate the patient's knowledge of proper administration; monitor the patient's ability and motivation to comply with the therapeutic regimen. (Treatment must continue for the full-length of therapy to eliminate all *M. tuberculosis* organisms.)	Explain the importance of complying with the entire therapeutic regimen, including: • Taking all medications as directed by the healthcare provider. • Not discontinuing medication until so instructed. • Wearing a medical alert bracelet. • Keeping all appointments for follow-up care.
• Monitor for hepatic adverse effects. (Antituberculosis drugs, such as isoniazid and rifampin, cause hepatic impairment.)	• Instruct the patient to report yellow eyes and skin, loss of appetite, dark urine, and unusual tiredness.
• Monitor for neurologic adverse effects such as numbness and tingling of the extremities. (Antituberculosis drugs, such as isoniazid, cause peripheral neuropathy and depletion of vitamin B_6.)	Instruct the patient to: • Report numbness and tingling of extremities. • Take supplemental vitamin B_6 as ordered to reduce risk of adverse effects.
• Monitor for dietary compliance when patient is taking isoniazid. (Foods high in tyramine can interact with the drug and cause palpitations, flushing, and hypertension.)	• Advise patients taking isonlazid to avoid foods containing tyramine, such as aged cheese, smoked and pickled fish, beer and red wine, bananas, and chocolate.
• Monitor for other adverse effects specific to various antituberculosis drugs.	Instruct the patient to report to the healthcare provider any adverse effects specific to the antituberculosis therapy prescribed, such as: • Blurred vision or changes in color or vision field (ethambutol). • Difficulty in voiding (pyrazinamide). • Fever, yellowing of skin, weakness, dark urine (isoniazid, rifampin). • GI system disturbances (rifampin). • Changes in hearing (streptomycin). • Numbness and tingling of extremities (isoniazid). • Red discoloration of body fluids (rifampin). • Dark concentrated urine, weight gain, edema (streptomycin).
• Establish therapeutic environment to ensure adequate rest, nutrition, hydration, and relaxation. (Symptoms of TB are manifested when the immune system is suppressed.)	Instruct the patient: • About infection control measures, such as frequent hand hygiene, covering the mouth when coughing or sneezing, and proper disposal of soiled tissues. • To incorporate health-enhancing activities, such as adequate rest and sleep, intake of essential vitamins and nutrients, and drinking six to eight glasses of water a day.
• Collect sputum specimens as directed by the healthcare provider. (This will determine the effectiveness of the antituberculosis drug.)	• Instruct the patient in the technique needed to collect a quality sputum specimen.
EVALUATION OF OUTCOME CRITERIA	
Evaluate the effectiveness of drug therapy by confirming that patient goals and expected outcomes have been met (see "Planning"). *See Table 27.11 for a list of drugs to which these nursing actions apply.*	

*Herdman, T.H. & Kamitsuru, S. (Eds.), *Nursing Diagnoses: Definitions & Classification* 2015–2017. Copyright © 2014, 1994–2014 NANDA International. Used by arrangement by John Wiley & Sons, Inc. Companion website: www.wiley.com/go/nursingdiagnoses.

A third feature of anti-TB therapy is that drugs are used extensively for *preventing* the disease in addition to treating it. Chemoprophylaxis is common for close contacts or family members of patients recently infected with TB. Therapy usually begins immediately after a patient receives a positive tuberculin test. Patients with immunosuppression, such as those with AIDS or those receiving immunosuppressant drugs, may receive preventive treatment with anti-TB drugs. A short-term therapy of 2 months, consisting of a combination treatment with isoniazid and pyrazinamide, is approved for TB prophylaxis in patients positive for HIV.

Treatment guidelines strongly recommend that **directly observed therapy (DOT)** be used in the treatment of TB (CDC, 2012). DOT means that a healthcare worker or other trained individual administer the medications and watch the patient swallow the dose. This ensures that the medication is taken exactly as prescribed and decreases the risk for relapse, limits the spread of the infection in the community, and reduces the development of drug resistance that could result from erratic or partial treatment.

CONCEPT REVIEW 27.3

- How does drug therapy of TB differ from that of conventional anti-infective chemotherapy? What are the rationales for these differences?

Patients Need to Know

Patients treated for bacterial infections need to know the following:

In General

1. Take the entire prescription of anti-infective medication exactly as directed because partial doses, skipped doses, and shortened length of treatment encourage the development of resistant organisms.
2. Some antibiotics may cause GI upset. If this occurs, take the drug with food or milk as directed. Check the prescription label for specific directions.
3. Eating active-culture yogurt or buttermilk may decrease the risks for diarrhea and vaginitis associated with antibiotic destruction of normal flora.
4. Antibiotics are most effective if taken around the clock, rather than just during normal waking hours.

Regarding Penicillins

5. It may be necessary to stay in the office for at least 30 minutes after receiving an injection of penicillin so the healthcare providers can monitor for possible allergic reactions.
6. Avoid intake of caffeinated beverages, citrus fruits, and fruit juices for at least 1 hour before and 2 hours after taking oral penicillin to maximize the drug's absorption.

Regarding Sulfonamides and Tetracyclines

7. Take oral cephalosporins and oral lincomycin with food, and oral sulfonamides with food or milk, to decrease GI upset. Drink a glass of water with each dose of sulfonamide, tetracycline, lincomycin, or fluoroquinolone, and drink a total of 2–3 L of fluid a day.
8. Avoid sun or tanning exposure while taking sulfonamides and tetracyclines because these drugs cause photosensitivity and sun sensitivity.
9. Antacids, dairy products, iron, baking soda, and kaolin-pectin bind and inactivate tetracycline. Separate intake by 2 to 3 hours for full antibiotic effectiveness.
10. Sulfonamides, tetracycline, and other antibiotics may interfere with the effectiveness of oral contraceptives. Ask a healthcare provider about the advisability of using an additional form of contraception.

Safety Alert: Allergic Reactions and Antibiotics

After receiving her first dose of levofloxacin (Levaquin), Mrs. Jones reported itching and a slight swelling of the tongue and lips (angioedema). However, later that day she had no discomfort or presence of the previous symptoms. Prior to the initial administration of the drug, the nurse checked Mrs. Jones's chart for the presence of allergies. Now it is time for a second dose, and it is imperative that the nurse monitor her for an allergic reaction. Hypersensitivity reactions can worsen with each exposure to an antigen (the antibiotic). The next dose could cause a life-threatening anaphylactic response.

Chapter Review

Core Concepts Summary

27.1 Pathogens are organisms that cause disease by invading tissues or secreting toxins.

Pathogens can overwhelm natural immune defenses by growing extremely rapidly and invading normal tissues or by producing potent toxins. Bacteria are classified on the basis of their staining ability and structural and functional characteristics.

27.2 Anti-infective drugs are classified by their chemical structures or by their mechanisms of action.

Because of the large number of anti-infectives available, it is advantageous for the student to understand how to classify these drugs because medications in the same class exhibit similar pharmacologic activity. Anti-infective drugs are classified based on similarities in their chemical structures or by their mechanisms of action.

27.3 Anti-infective drugs act by selectively targeting a pathogen's metabolism or life cycle.

Bacteria multiply rapidly, and drugs have been designed to take advantage of this characteristic. Anti-infectives may be bactericidal or bacteriostatic, or both, depending on the organism and dose.

27.4 Acquired resistance is a major clinical problem that is worsened by improper use of anti-infectives.

Errors during replication result in random mutations of the bacterial DNA. Although rare, an occasional mutation may confer antibiotic resistance to a bacterium. Therapy with antibiotics kills the affected bacteria, leaving the resistant ones to multiply and spread within the patient. To limit this problem, antibiotics should be prescribed only when medically necessary.

27.5 Careful selection of the correct antibiotic is essential for effective pharmacotherapy and to limit adverse effects.

Culture and sensitivity tests are used to identify the type of bacteria present and determine which antibiotics are most effective. Until test results are obtained, the patient may be started on a broad-spectrum antibiotic. Because broad-spectrum drugs are more likely to affect the patient's normal flora, a narrow-spectrum drug may be prescribed after the organism is identified.

27.6 The penicillins are one of the oldest and safest groups of anti-infectives.

Penicillins have been widely used because of their high margin of safety and effectiveness. Some patients are allergic to this class of drugs, and many bacterial species have become resistant to penicillins, thus limiting their use.

27.7 The cephalosporins are similar in structure and function to the penicillins and are one of the most widely prescribed anti-infective classes.

The cephalosporins consist of a large class of antibiotics, classified by generation, that are considered alternatives to penicillin. In general, they are used for serious gram-negative infections and for patients who are resistant to or cannot tolerate the penicillins.

27.8 The tetracyclines have broad spectrums but are preferred drugs for few diseases.

The tetracyclines have a broader spectrum of action and produce more adverse effects than the penicillins. Their use is limited to a small number of diseases, such as Rocky Mountain spotted fever, typhus, cholera, Lyme disease, and chlamydial infections.

27.9 The macrolides are safe alternatives to penicillin for many infections.

The macrolides are generally prescribed when a patient is allergic to penicillin or has a penicillin-resistant infection. They produce few adverse effects.

27.10 The aminoglycosides are narrow-spectrum drugs that have the potential to cause serious toxicity.

The aminoglycosides are usually reserved for severe gram-negative infections of the urinary tract because they have the potential to cause serious adverse effects. Most of them are poorly absorbed from the GI tract and must be given parenterally.

27.11 Fluoroquinolones have wide clinical applications because of their broad spectrum of activity and relative safety.

Although fluoroquinolones are an older class of antibacterials, newer drugs in this class have been developed to greatly expand their use. They are effective oral alternatives to other antibiotics for both gram-negative and gram-positive organisms. Ciprofloxacin (Cipro) is one of the few drugs approved for the treatment of anthrax.

27.12 Sulfonamides and urinary antiseptics are traditional drugs for urinary tract infections.

In the 1930s, the sulfonamides revolutionized the treatment of infectious disease. Present-day use of these medications is limited by bacterial resistance. The fixed combination of trimethoprim–sulfamethoxazole (Bactrim, Septra) is an important drug in the pharmacotherapy of UTIs.

27.13 A number of additional anti-infectives have distinct mechanisms of action and specific indications.

A number of important antibiotics do not belong to any of the previous classes. The streptogramins and oxazolidinones are small groups of drugs having specific applications. Vancomycin is known as the "last chance" antibiotic for use when resistance has developed to most other anti-infectives.

27.14 The pharmacotherapy of tuberculosis requires special dosing regimens and schedules.

Drug therapy of TB involves taking multiple drugs for prolonged periods. Patients exhibiting a new, positive TB test are often given these drugs prophylactically, even if no signs of the disease are apparent.

REVIEW Questions

Answer the following questions to assess your knowledge of the chapter material, and go back and review any material that is not clear to you.

1. The patient is taking amoxicillin (Amoxil). Which of the following statements by the patient demonstrates that additional instruction is needed?
 1. "I will take this medication until it is gone."
 2. "I will call my doctor if I develop a fever or a rash."
 3. "Before I take my medication, I will avoid orange juice."
 4. "I will take the medication until I feel better."

2. Before administering cefazolin (Ancef), the nurse checks for a previous allergic reaction to:
 1. Yeasts.
 2. Penicillins.
 3. Sulfonamides.
 4. Macrolides.

3. When assisting with the development of a patient care plan, the nurse needs to include what information about tetracyclines?
 1. To take it with food or milk
 2. They are safe for use during pregnancy
 3. To take it 1 to 2 hours before or after meals
 4. That it has no adverse effects

4. The patient on aminoglycosides is monitored for:
 1. Nephrotoxicity.
 2. Hepatic failure.
 3. Superinfection.
 4. Hypertension and rash.

5. A nurse instructs the patient that if ciprofloxacin (Cipro) is taken with antacids, absorption is:
 1. Increased.
 2. Decreased.
 3. Not affected.
 4. Delayed.

6. A patient has been diagnosed with MRSA and is prescribed vancomycin. What information should be provided to the patient about possible adverse effects?
 1. Vancomycin may cause flushing.
 2. Adverse effects are infrequent.
 3. Vacomycin does not cause rashes.
 4. During therapy, hypertension may occur.

7. The patient with tuberculosis is taking isoniazid (INH). Which laboratory test should the nurse monitor?
 1. PT and PTT
 2. CBC
 3. BUN
 4. Liver enzymes

8. The most common adverse effects of penicillin G include(s): (Select all that apply.)
 1. Diarrhea.
 2. Nausea and vomiting.
 3. Pain at the injection site.
 4. Rash.
 5. Constipation

9. A patient at a rehabilitation center is prescribed erythromycin. The nurse is reviewing the patient's medication list, checking to see if there are medications that should not be taken with this antibiotic. One medication is found. What medication should not be taken with erythromycin?
 1. Lisinopril
 2. Ibuprofen
 3. Lasix
 4. Lovastatin

10. A patient is to receive Cipro 500 mg PO four times a day, for a week. The pharmacy sends Cipro 250 mg tablets. How many tablet(s) will the patient receive in 24 hours?
 1. Two tablets
 2. Four tablets
 3. Six tablets
 4. Eight tablets

CASE STUDY Questions

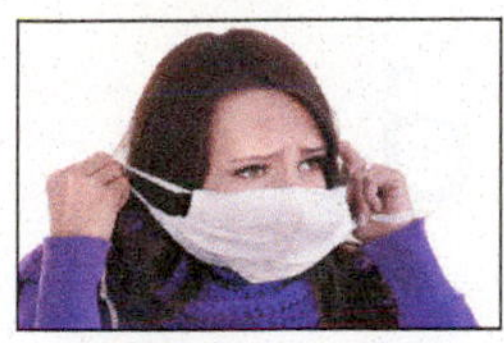

Remember Ms. Jackson, the patient introduced at the beginning of the chapter? Now read the remainder of the case study. Based on the information you have learned in this chapter, answer the questions that follow.

Ms. Shelly Jackson is a new patient at your clinic. Six months ago, she had a kidney transplant and is taking immunosuppressant drugs. Recently, she has been experiencing repeated bacterial infections due to resistant strains and has been switched to different antibiotics throughout the past 6 months. The healthcare provider suspects a kidney infection.

1. Ms. Jackson is admitted to the hospital and is administered gentamicin 300 mg daily by IV infusion. The nurse monitors which of the following tests?
   1. Input and output ratio
   2. Liver enzymes
   3. Visual acuity tests
   4. Fasting blood glucose levels

2. Gentamicin can cause:
   1. Anemia.
   2. Persistent headaches.
   3. Nausea and vomiting.
   4. Liver failure.

3. Ms. Jackson is showing signs of hearing loss due to gentamicin therapy and the healthcare provider is going to switch her antibiotic. The nurse anticipates which of the following medications being ordered?
   1. Sulfacetamide (Klaron)
   2. Silver sulfadiazine
   3. Trimethoprim–sulfamethoxazole (Septra)
   4. Vancomycin (Vancocin)

4. The adverse effects of sulfonamides include: (Select all that apply.)
   1. Increased sensitivity of skin to sunlight.
   2. Liver failure.
   3. Nausea and vomiting.
   4. Hypotension.

Answers and complete rationales for the Review and Case Study Questions appear in Appendix A.

REFERENCES

Centers for Disease Control and Prevention. (2012). *Self-study modules on tuberculosis: Module 9: Patient adherence to tuberculosis treatment.* Retrieved from http://www.cdc.gov/tb/education/ssmodules/module9/ss9reading2.htm

Herdman, T. H., & Kamitsuru, S. (Eds.). (2014). *NANDA International nursing diagnoses: Definitions and classification, 2015–2017.* Oxford, United Kingdom: Wiley-Blackwell.

SELECTED BIBLIOGRAPHY

Centers for Disease Control and Prevention. (2013). *CDC fact sheet: Incidence, prevalence and cost of sexually transmitted infections in the United States.* Retrieved from http://www.cdc.gov/std/stats/sti-estimates-fact-sheet-feb-2013.pdf

Centers for Disease Control and Prevention. (2014). *Antibiotic resistance threats in the United States, 2013.* Retrieved from http://www.cdc.gov/drugresistance/threat-report-2013

Centers for Disease Control and Prevention. (2014). *General information about MRSA in healthcare settings.* Retrieved from http://www.cdc.gov/mrsa/healthcare/index.html

Centers for Disease Control and Prevention. (2014). *New, simpler way to treat latent TB infection.* Retrieved from http://www.cdc.gov/features/tuberculosistreatment/index.html

Centers for Disease Control and Prevention. (2015). *Foodborne germs and illness.* Retrieved from http://www.cdc.gov/foodsafety/foodborne-germs.html

Centers for Disease Control and Prevention. (2015). *Get smart: Know when antibiotics work.* Retrieved from http://www.cdc.gov/getsmart/community/index.html

Centers for Disease Control and Prevention. (2015). *2015 sexually transmitted diseases treatment guidelines.* Retrieved from http://www.cdc.gov/std/tg2015

Custodio, H. T. (2014). *Hospital-acquired infections.* Retrieved from http://emedicine.medscape.com/article/967022-overview

D'Ambrosio, L., Centis, R., Sotgiu, G., Pontali, E., Spanevello, A., & Migliori, G. B. (2015). New anti-tuberculosis drugs and regimens: 2015 update. *ERJ Open Research, 1*(1), 00010-2015. doi:10.1183/23120541.00010-2015

Herchline, T. E. (2015). *Tuberculosis.* Retrieved from http://emedicine.medscape.com/article/230802-overview

Madigan, M. T., Martinko, J. M., Bender, K. S., Buckly, D. H., & Stahl, A. A. (2015). *Brock biology of microorganisms* (14th ed.). San Francisco, CA: Benjamin Cummings.

Laxminarayan, R., Duse, A., Wattal, C., Zaidi, A. K., Wertheim, H. F., Sumpradit, N., . . . Cars, O. (2013). Antibiotic resistance—the need for global solutions. *The Lancet Infectious Diseases, 13,* 1057-1098. doi.org/10.1016/S1473-3099(13)70318-9

Olans, R. N., Olans, R. D., & DeMaria, A. (2015). The critical role of the staff nurse in antimicrobial stewardship—unrecognized, but already there. *Clinical Infectious Diseases, 62,* 84–89. doi:10.1093/cid/civ697

Oliphant, C. M., & Eroschenko, K. (2015). Antibiotic Resistance, Part 2: Gram-negative pathogens. *The Journal for Nurse Practitioners, 11,* 79–86. doi.org/10.1016/j.nurpra.2014.10.008

Chapter 28

Drugs for Fungal, Viral, and Parasitic Diseases

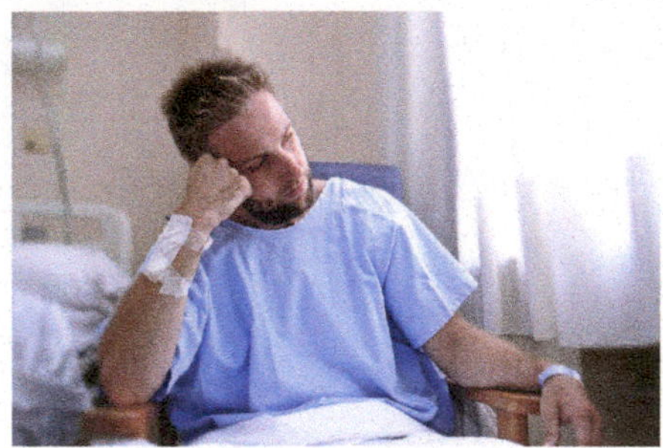

"Over the last several weeks, I've become really tired and achy all over. I feel like I have a fever all the time, my throat hurts, and my head hurts. I don't know why I'm not getting better."

Mark Engelstad

Core Concepts

28.1 Fungal infections are classified as superficial or systemic.

28.2 Systemic antifungal drugs are used for serious infections of internal organs.

28.3 Superficial infections of the skin, nails, and mucous membranes are effectively treated with topical and oral antifungal drugs.

28.4 Viruses are infectious agents that require a host to replicate.

28.5 Antiretroviral drugs do not cure HIV-AIDS, but they do help many patients live longer.

28.6 Antiviral drugs are available to treat herpes simplex, influenza, and viral hepatitis infections.

28.7 Infections caused by helminths and protozoans cause significant disease worldwide.

Drug Snapshot

The following drugs are discussed in this chapter:

Drug Classes	Prototype Drugs
Antifungal drugs for systemic infections	Pr amphotericin B (AmBisome, Fungizone, others)
Antifungal drugs for superficial infections	Pr nystatin (Mycostatin, Nystop, others)
Antiretroviral drugs for HIV-AIDS	Pr zidovudine (AZT, Retrovir)
Antiviral drugs for herpes simplex and influenza	Pr acyclovir (Zovirax)
Antiprotozoan and antihelminthic drugs	Pr metronidazole (Flagyl)

Learning Outcomes

After reading this chapter, the student should be able to:

1. Describe how fungal infections are classified.
2. Identify drugs used in the pharmacotherapy of systemic fungal infections.
3. Identify drugs used in the pharmacotherapy of superficial fungal infections.
4. Describe the characteristics of viruses.
5. Explain the outcomes expected for the pharmacotherapy of HIV-AIDS.
6. Identify antiviral drugs used in the pharmacotherapy of herpes simplex, influenza, and viral hepatitis.
7. Identify drugs used to treat protozoan and helminthic infections.

Key Terms

antiretrovirals (an-tie-RET-roh-veye-ral)
capsid (CAP-sid)
dysentery (DISS-en-tare-ee)
fungi (FUN-jeye)
helminths (HELL-minthz)
highly active antiretroviral therapy (HAART)
host
influenza (in-flew-EN-zah)
intracellular parasites
malaria (mah-LARE-ee-ah)
mycoses (my-KOH-sees)
protozoans (PRO-toh-ZOH-enz)
reverse transcriptase (ree-VERS trans-CRIP-tace)
superficial mycoses
systemic mycoses
viruses
yeasts (YEESTz)

Fungi, protozoans, and multicellular parasites are exceedingly more complex than bacteria. Most antibacterial drugs are ineffective against these organisms because their structure and biochemistry are so different from that of bacteria. Although there are fewer medications to treat these diseases, the available medications are usually effective.

Viruses, on the other hand, are nonliving particles that infect by entering a host cell and using the host's internal machinery to replicate themselves. Antiviral drugs are the least effective of all the anti-infective classes. Although the number of antiviral medications has increased dramatically in recent years, they are relatively ineffective at preventing or treating viral infections.

ANTIFUNGAL DRUGS

Fungal infections are classified as superficial or systemic.

◀ **Core Concept 28.1**

Fungi are single-celled or multicellular organisms that are much more complex than bacteria. Several species of fungi grow on skin and mucosal surfaces and are part of the normal host flora. The human body is remarkably resistant to infection by these organisms; people with healthy immune systems rarely experience serious fungal diseases. Patients with a weakened immune system, however, such as those infected with HIV, may acquire frequent fungal infections, some of which may require intensive drug therapy.

Fungal infections are called **mycoses**. Most exposure to pathogenic fungi occurs through inhalation of fungal spores or by handling contaminated soil. Thus, many fungal infections involve the respiratory tract, skin, hair, and nails. An additional common source of fungal infections, especially of the mouth or vagina, is overgrowth of normal host flora. **Yeasts**, which include the common pathogen *Candida albicans*, are single-celled fungi. Table 28.1 lists the most common fungal pathogens.

A simple and useful method of classifying fungal infections is to consider them as either superficial or systemic. **Superficial mycoses** typically affect the scalp, skin, nails, and mucous membranes such as the oral cavity and vagina. Mycoses of this type are often treated with topical drugs because the incidence of adverse effects is much lower with this route of administration.

myc = *fungus*
oses = *conditions*

Fast Facts Fungal, Viral, and Parasitic Diseases

- Although there are about 1.5 million species of fungi on the planet, only a few hundred are human pathogens.
- The most common source of fungal infections in immunocompromised patients is *Candida albicans*.
- About one of every six Americans age 14–49 are infected with genital herpes.
- More than 1.2 million Americans are currently living with HIV infections; about 50,000 new infections occur each year.
- In the United States, approximately 54% of new HIV infections occur in men who have sex with other men.
- Of the new HIV infections in women, 84% are acquired through heterosexual contact and 16% from injecting drug use.
- Since the beginning of the AIDS epidemic, more than 658,000 Americans have died of AIDS.
- About 198 million cases of malaria occur worldwide each year; about 1500 U.S. travelers acquire malaria abroad.

Table 28.1 Fungal Pathogens

Name of Fungus	Disease and Primary Organ System
SYSTEMIC	
Aspergillus fumigatus and others	Aspergillosis: opportunistic; most commonly affects the lungs but can spread to other organs
Blastomyces dermatitidis	Blastomycosis: begins in the lungs and spreads to other organs
Candida albicans and others	Candidiasis: most common opportunistic fungal infection; may occur in mucous membranes and nearly any organ
Coccidioides immitis	Coccidioidomycosis: begins in the lungs and spreads to the skin and other organs
Cryptococcus neoformans	Cryptococcosis: opportunistic; begins in the lungs but is the most common cause of meningitis in patients with AIDS
Histoplasma capsulatum	Histoplasmosis: begins in the lungs and spreads to other organs
Pneumocystis jiroveci	*Pneumocystis* pneumonia: opportunistic; primarily causes pneumonia but can spread to other organs
SUPERFICIAL	
Candida albicans and others	Candidiasis: affects the skin, nails, oral cavity (thrush), vagina
Epidermophyton floccosum	Athlete's foot (tinea pedis), jock itch (tinea cruris), and other skin disorders
Microsporum species	Ringworm of the scalp (tinea capitus)
Sporothrix schenckii	Sporotrichosis: affects primarily the skin and superficial lymph nodes
Trichophyton species	Affects the scalp, skin, and nails

Systemic mycoses are those affecting internal organs, typically the lungs, brain, and digestive organs. Although less common than superficial mycoses, systemic fungal infections often affect multiple body systems and are sometimes fatal to patients with suppressed immune systems. Mycoses of this type require aggressive oral or parenteral medications that produce more adverse effects than the topical drugs.

CORE CONCEPT 28.2 ▶ Systemic antifungal drugs are used for serious infections of internal organs.

Systemic or invasive fungal infections require intensive pharmacotherapy for extended periods. Amphotericin B and fluconazole are the most frequently prescribed drugs for these types of infections. Table 28.2 lists the primary antifungal drugs.

Serious opportunistic fungal disease can occur in patients whose immune systems are compromised, such as those with HIV-AIDS. Others who may experience systemic infections include patients receiving prolonged therapy with corticosteroids (see Chapter 25 and Chapter 33), those with extensive burns, those receiving antineoplastic drugs (see Chapter 29), and those who have recently received organ transplants (see Chapter 26). Pharmacotherapy of systemic mycoses may continue for several months to ensure complete removal of the pathogen.

Amphotericin B (AmBisome, Fungizone, others) has been the gold standard for treating systemic fungal infections since the 1960s. However, the newer *azole* drugs, such as fluconazole (Diflucan) and itraconazole (Sporanox), are safer and have become preferred drugs for the treatment of some systemic infections. Ketoconazole has also become a first-line drug for less severe systemic mycoses or for the prophylaxis of fungal infections. The *azole* drugs have a spectrum of activity similar to that of amphotericin B, are considerably less toxic, and have the major advantage that they can be administered orally. Several are available for both superficial and systemic mycoses.

Several other antifungals are available as treatment options for systemic mycoses. These include caspofungin (Cancidas) for aspergillosis and isovuconazonium (Cresemba), anidulafungin (Eraxis), and micafungin (Mycamine) for invasive candidiasis. These drugs are usually prescribed when amphotericin B and the systemic azoles have failed to produce an adequate response.

Table 28.2 Selected Antifungal Drugs

Drug	Route and Adult Dose	Remarks
Pr amphotericin B (AmBisome, Fungizone, others)	IV: 0.3–1.5 mg/kg/day, infused over 2–4 hours (max: 1.5 mg/kg/day)	Cream, lotion, and PO suspension forms available for topical mycoses; must infuse a test dose first
butenafine (Lotrimin, Mentax)	Topical: Apply daily for 4 weeks	For tinea infections
anidulafungin (Eraxis)	IV: Loading dose 100 mg on day 1 followed by 50 mg/day	For advanced candidiasis
caspofungin (Cancidas)	IV: 70 mg on day 1, followed by 50 mg qid for 30 days	Newer drug for invasive *Candida* and *Aspergillus* infections
ciclopirox cream, gel, shampoo (Loprox) or nail lacquer (Penlac)	Topical: Apply bid for 4 weeks	For skin and nail mycoses
flucytosine (Ancobon)	PO: 50–150 mg/kg in divided doses	For severe systemic infections such as candidiasis or cryptococcosis; IV form available
griseofulvin (Fulvicin)	PO: 500 mg microsize or 330–375 mg ultramicrosize daily	For ringworm and other skin and nail infections
micafungin (Mycamine)	IV: 50–150 mg/kg/day	For advanced candidiasis
naftifine (Naftin)	Topical: Apply cream daily or gel bid for 4 weeks	For tinea infections
Pr nystatin (Mycostatin, Nystop, others)	PO: 500,000–1,000,000 units tid	For candidiasis; vaginal tablet form available
tavaborole (Kerydin)	Topical: Apply once daily for 48 weeks	For toenail mycoses
terbinafine (Lamisil)	Topical: Apply daily or bid for 7 weeks; PO: 250 mg daily for 6–13 weeks	For skin and nail mycoses
tolnaftate (Aftate, Tinactin)	Topical: Apply bid for 4–6 weeks	For tinea infections
undecylenic acid (Fungi-Nail, Gordochom)	Topical: Apply once or twice daily	For tineas and other superficial mycoses
AZOLE ANTIFUNGALS		
butoconazole (Femstat, Gynazole)	Intravaginal: 1 applicator/day for 3 days	For vaginal mycoses
clotrimazole (Gyne-Lotrimin, Mycelex)	Topical: For skin mycoses apply bid for 4 weeks; for vaginal mycoses, insert 1 applicator/day intravaginally for 7 days	For vaginal and skin mycoses, tineas, and candidiasis; oral troche also available for oral candidiasis
econazole (Spectazole)	Topical: Apply bid for 4 weeks	For tineas and cutaneous candidiasis
fluconazole (Diflucan)	PO: 150 mg as a single dose for vaginal candidiasis PO: 100–400 mg daily for 2–4 weeks for other mycoses	For both systemic and superficial mycoses; IV form available for severe mycoses
isavuconazonium (Cresemba)	PO/IV: 372 mg/day	Newer azole for invasive aspergillosis and mucormycosis infections
itraconazole (Sporanox)	PO: 200 mg daily (max: 400 mg/day)	For severe systemic lung mycoses and superficial nail mycoses
ketoconazole (Nizoral)	PO: 200–400 mg daily	For severe systemic mycoses; topical form available for superficial mycoses
luliconazole (Luzu)	Topical: Apply daily for 2 weeks	For tinea infections
miconazole (Micatin, Monistat-3)	Topical: Apply bid for 2–4 weeks	For vaginal and skin mycoses; also available as vaginal suppositories and tampons
oxiconazole (Oxistat)	Topical: Apply daily for 2 months	For tinea infections
posaconazole (Noxafil)	PO: 100–200 mg tid	For prevention of invasive *Aspergillus* and *Candida* infections
sertaconazole (Ertaczo)	Topical: Apply bid for 4 weeks	For tinea pedis
sulconazole (Exelderm)	Topical: Apply once or twice daily for 2–6 weeks	For tinea infections
terconazole (Terazol)	Intravaginal: 1 applicator/day for 3–7 days	For vulvovaginal candidiasis
tioconazole (Vagistat)	Intravaginal: 1 applicator as single dose	For vulvovaginal candidiasis
voriconazole (Vfend)	IV: 3-6 mg/kg bid	For systemic aspergillosis and esophageal candidiasis; oral form available

CONCEPT REVIEW 28.1

- Why has the number of antifungal and antiviral drugs increased significantly over the past 20 years?

Prototype Drug: Amphotericin B (AmBisome, Fungizone, Others)

Therapeutic Class: Antifungal (systemic type) **Pharmacologic Class:** Polyene

Actions and Uses: Amphotericin B has a wide spectrum of activity and is effective against most of the fungi pathogenic to humans; thus, it is a preferred drug for many severe systemic mycoses. It acts by binding to fungal cell membranes and causing them to become permeable or leaky. Because amphotericin B is not absorbed from the gastrointestinal (GI) tract, it is normally given by IV infusion. Topical preparations are available for superficial mycoses. Several months of pharmacotherapy may be required for a complete cure. Unlike antibiotics, resistance to amphotericin B is not common.

To reduce the toxicity of amphotericin B, the original drug molecule has been formulated with several lipid molecules. These include liposomal amphotericin B (AmBisome), amphotericin B lipid complex (Abelcet), and amphotericin B cholesteryl sulfate complex (Amphotec). Because these newer forms are expensive, they are usually reserved for serious fungal infections.

Adverse Effects and Interactions: Amphotericin B can cause frequent and potentially serious adverse effects. Many patients develop fever and chills at the beginning of therapy, which subside as treatment continues. Phlebitis, or inflammation of the veins, is common during IV therapy. Some degree of nephrotoxicity is observed in most patients, and laboratory tests of kidney function are normally performed throughout the treatment period.

Amphotericin B interacts with many drugs. For example, therapy with aminoglycosides, vancomycin, carboplatin, and furosemide, which reduce renal function, is not recommended. Use with corticosteroids, skeletal muscle relaxants, and thiazole may cause hypokalemia. Use with digoxin increases the risk of digoxin toxicity in patients with preexisting hypokalemia.

CORE CONCEPT 28.3 ▶ Superficial infections of the skin, nails, and mucous membranes are effectively treated with topical and oral antifungal drugs.

Superficial fungal infections of the hair, scalp, nails, and the mucous membranes of the mouth and vagina are rarely medical emergencies. Infections of the nails and skin, for example, may be ongoing for months or even years before a patient seeks treatment. Unlike systemic fungal infections, superficial infections may occur in any patient, not just those who have suppressed immune systems.

Antifungal medications applied topically are much safer than their systemic counterparts because only small amounts are absorbed into the circulation. Many are available as over-the-counter (OTC) creams, gels, and solutions. Although a fungal infection may be diagnosed as superficial, oral antifungal drugs are occasionally prescribed along with topical medications to be certain that the infection is completely eliminated from the deeper skin layers. The length of pharmacotherapy varies widely among the different types of superficial mycoses. Vaginal infections are sometimes treated successfully with a single vaginal tablet of clotrimazole, whereas nail mycoses may require several months of therapy with itraconazole or terbinafine.

Adverse effects from topical antifungal therapy are generally minor and limited to the region being treated. If applied to the skin, irritation, redness, and itching may be experienced. Vaginal administration may cause burning, itching, or irritation. Antifungal drugs should not be applied to open sores or severely abraded skin because this may result in undesirable absorption of the drug and additional adverse effects. When applying topical antifungal medication, gloves should be worn to prevent transmission.

Prototype Drug: Nystatin (Mycostatin, Nystop, Others)

Therapeutic Class: Topical antifungal **Pharmacologic Class:** Polyene

Actions and Uses: Although it belongs to the same chemical class as amphotericin B, nystatin is available in a wider variety of formulations, including cream, ointment, powder, tablets, and lozenges. It is used as a topical drug against *Candida* infections of the vagina, skin, and mouth. It may also be used orally to treat candidiasis of the intestine because it travels through the GI tract without being absorbed. In topical forms, nystatin is often combined with triamcinolone, a corticosteroid that helps to reduce inflammation.

Adverse Effects and Interactions: When given topically, nystatin produces few adverse effects other than minor skin irritation. When given orally, it may cause diarrhea, nausea, and vomiting.

Nursing Process Focus Patients Receiving Superficial Antifungal Therapy

ASSESSMENT	POTENTIAL NURSING DIAGNOSES*
Prior to administration: • Obtain a complete health history, including skin, GI, renal and liver conditions, past infections, allergies, drug history, and possible drug interactions. • Acquire the results of a complete physical examination, including vital signs and any signs or symptoms of infection. • Evaluate laboratory blood findings: complete blood count (CBC), electrolytes, and renal and liver function studies.	• *Acute Pain* related to tissue damage secondary to infection • *Risk for Injury* related to adverse effect of drug therapy • *Deficient Knowledge* related to lack of information about drug therapy • *Impaired Skin Integrity* related to tissue damage and adverse effects of drug therapy

PLANNING: PATIENT GOALS AND EXPECTED OUTCOMES

The patient will:

- Experience therapeutic effects (healing of fungal infection).
- Be free from or experience minimal adverse effects from drug therapy.
- Verbalize an understanding of the drug's use, adverse effects, and required precautions.

IMPLEMENTATION

Interventions and (Rationales)	Patient Education/Discharge Planning
• Administer oral medication correctly and evaluate the patient's knowledge of proper administration. (Proper administration increases medication effectiveness.)	Instruct the patient to: • Complete all medication as prescribed. • Swish the oral suspension to coat all mucous membranes, and then swallow the medication. • Spit out the medication instead of swallowing if GI irritation occurs. • Allow troche to dissolve completely, rather than chewing or swallowing; it may take 30 minutes for it to dissolve completely. • Avoid food or drink for 30 minutes following administration. • Remove dentures prior to using the oral suspension. • Take ketoconazole with water, fruit juice, coffee, or tea to enhance dissolution and absorption.
• Administer topical medication correctlyand evaluate the patient's knowledge of proper administration. (Proper administration increases medication effectiveness.)	Instruct the patient to: • Use gloves when applying medication. • Avoid wearing tight-fitting undergarments if using ointment in the vaginal or groin area. • Avoid occlusive dressings. (Dressings increase moisture in the infected areas and encourage development of additional yeast infections.)
• Monitor for possible adverse effects or hypersensitivity.	Instruct the patient to report any of the following to the healthcare provider: • Burning, stinging, dryness, itching, erythema, urticaria, angioedema, and local irritation (for superficial drugs). • Symptoms of hepatic toxicity—jaundice, dark urine, light-colored stools, and pruritus. • Nausea, vomiting, and diarrhea. • Signs and symptoms of hypo- or hyperglycemia.
• Monitor for contact dermatitis with topical formulations. (This is related to the preservatives found in many of the formulations.)	• Instruct the patient to report any redness or skin rash.
• Encourage infection control practices. Ensure that the patient, family members, and other visitors also practice infection control techniques such as hand hygiene and avoiding the affected area (to prevent the spread of infection).	Instruct the patient to: • Clean the affected area daily. • Apply medication while wearing a glove. • Clean hands properly before and after application. • Change socks daily if rash is on the feet. • Avoid sharing personal care items with family members or guests.

EVALUATION OF OUTCOME CRITERIA

Evaluate the effectiveness of drug therapy by confirming that patient goals and expected outcomes have been met (see "Planning"). *See Table 28.2 for a list of drugs to which these nursing actions apply.*

*Herdman, T.H. & Kamitsuru, S. (Eds.), *Nursing Diagnoses: Definitions & Classification* 2015–2017. Copyright © 2014, 1994–2014 NANDA International. Used by arrangement by John Wiley & Sons, Inc. Companion website: www.wiley.com/go/nursingdiagnoses.

ANTIVIRAL DRUGS

CORE CONCEPT 28.4 ▶ Viruses are infectious agents that require a host to replicate.

Viruses are nonliving agents that infect bacteria, plants, and animals. Viruses contain none of the vital organelles that are present in the cells of living organisms. In fact, the structure of viruses is primitive compared to even the simplest cell. Surrounded by a protective protein coat or **capsid**, a virus contains only a few dozen genes—either in the form of ribonucleic acid (RNA) or deoxyribonucleic acid (DNA)—that contain the information needed for viral replication. Figure 28.1 shows the basic structure of one important virus: HIV.

intra = *within*
cellular = *cell*

Although nonliving and structurally simple, viruses are capable of remarkable feats. They infect an organism (the **host**), by entering a target cell and using the enzymes inside that cell to replicate. Thus, viruses are called **intracellular parasites**, meaning that they must be inside a host cell to cause infection. The host organism and cell are often very specific: It may be a single species of plant, bacteria, or animal, or even a single type of cell within that species. Most often, viruses that infect one species do not affect others, although cases have been documented in which viruses can mutate and cross species, as is likely the case for HIV.

Many viral infections, such as the rhinoviruses that cause the common cold, are self-limiting and require no medical treatment. Although symptoms may be annoying, the virus disappears in 7–10 days and causes no permanent damage if the patient is otherwise healthy. Other viruses, such as HIV, are in a class called *retroviruses* that can cause serious and ultimately fatal disease and require aggressive drug therapy. Antiviral therapy is extremely challenging because of the rapid mutation rate of viruses, which can quickly render drugs ineffective. Also complicating therapy is the intracellular nature of the virus, which makes it difficult for medications to find their targets without giving excessively high doses that injure normal cells. The three basic strategies used for antiviral pharmacotherapy are as follows:

- Prevent viral infections through the administration of vaccines (see Chapter 26).
- Treat active infections with drugs that interrupt an aspect of the virus's replication cycle, such as acyclovir (Zovirax).
- For long-term infections, use drugs that boost the patient's immune response (immunostimulants) so that the virus remains in latency and the patient symptom free.

CORE CONCEPT 28. 5 ▶ Antiretroviral drugs do not cure HIV-AIDS, but they do help many patients live longer.

Drugs for viral infections may be classified into those used to treat HIV-AIDS and those used for other viral disorders such as herpes and influenza. Antiviral medications used for HIV-AIDS are called **antiretrovirals** because they block the replication cycle of HIV, which is classified as a retrovirus. Antiretroviral medications for HIV-AIDS have been developed that slow the growth of HIV by different mechanisms. Doses of these medications are shown in Table 28.3.

The widespread appearance of HIV infection in 1981 created enormous challenges for public health and for the development of effective antiretroviral drugs. HIV-AIDS is unlike any other infectious disease because it is uniformly fatal and demands a continuous supply of new medications for the patients' survival. The challenges of HIV-AIDS have been met by the development of more than 20 antiretroviral drugs. Unfortunately, the initial hope of curing HIV-AIDS through antiretroviral therapy or vaccines has not been realized; none of these medications produces a cure for this disease. Once begun, antiretroviral therapy continues for the life of the patient because stopping the therapy results in a rapid rebound in HIV replication. HIV mutates extremely rapidly, and resistant strains develop so quickly that the creation of novel approaches to antiretroviral drug therapy must remain an ongoing process.

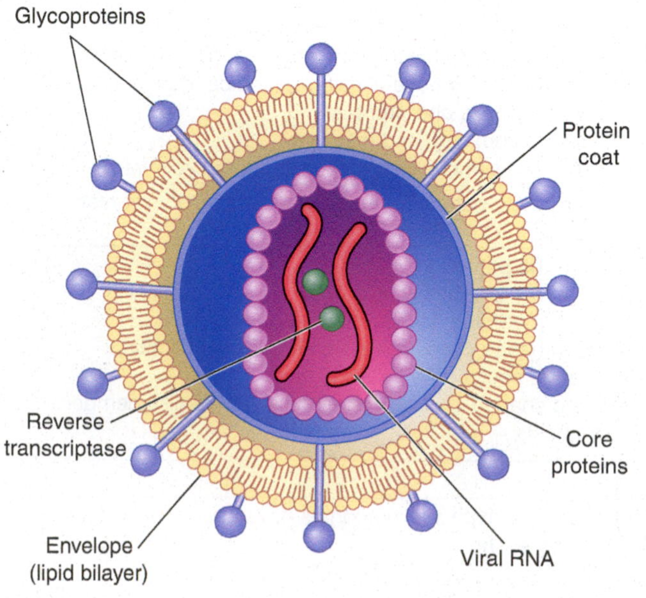

FIGURE 28.1 Structure of the human immunodeficiency virus (HIV).

Table 28.3 Antiretroviral Drugs for HIV-AIDS

Drug	Route and Adult Dose	Remarks
NONNUCLEOSIDE REVERSE TRANSCRIPTASE INHIBITORS (NNRTIs)		
delavirdine (Rescriptor)	PO: 400 mg tid	Second-line drug due to low effectiveness
efavirenz (Sustiva)	PO: 600 mg/day	First-line drug
etravirine (Intelence)	PO: 200 mg bid	Second-line drug due to effects on drug metabolism
nevirapine (Viramune)	PO: 200 mg/day once or twice daily	Second-line drug due to hepatotoxicity
rilpivirine (Edurant)	PO: 25 mg once daily	Newer, first-line drug
NUCLEOSIDE AND NUCLEOTIDE REVERSE TRANSCRIPTASE INHIBITORS (NRTIs)		
abacavir (Ziagen)	PO: 300 mg bid	First-line drug; hypersensitivity reactions can be serious
didanosine (Videx EC)	PO: 125–300 mg bid	Second-line drug for patients intolerant to AZT
emtricitabine (Emtriva)	PO: 200 mg daily	First-line drug
lamivudine (Epivir)	PO: 150 mg bid	First-line drug; also for chronic hepatitis B (Epivir-HBV).
stavudine (Zerit)	PO: 40 mg bid	Second-line drug; can cause serious mitochondrial toxicity
tenofovir (Viread)	PO: 300 mg/day	First-line drug
Pr zidovudine (AZT, Retrovir)	PO: 100-200 mg qid	Older, prototype drug; also for postexposure chemoprophylaxis; IV form available
PROTEASE INHIBITORS: THESE DRUGS ARE USUALLY COMBINED (BOOSTED) WITH RITONAVIR OR COLBICSTAT		
atazanavir (Reyataz)	PO: 100–400 mg/day	First-line drug
darunavir (Prezista)	PO: 800 mg/day	First-line drug
fosamprenavir (Lexiva)	PO: 700–1400/day with 100-200 mg ritonavir/day	First-line drug
idinavir (Crixivan)	PO: 800 mg tid	Second-line drug
lopinavir/ritonavir (Kaletra)	PO: 800/200 mg/day (four capsules)	First-line drug
nelfinavir (Viracept)	PO: 750 mg tid	Second-line drug due to severe diarrhea
ritonavir (Norvir)	PO: 600 mg bid	Used in small doses to boost the effectiveness of other PIs
saquinavir (Invirase)	PO: 1000 mg bid	Second-line drug due to resistance
tipranavir (Aptivus)	PO: 500 mg/day	Second-line drug due to possibility of intracranial hemorrhage
MISCELLANEOUS DRUGS FOR HIV		
dolutegravir (DTG, Tivicay)	PO: 50 mg/day	Newer integrase inhibitor
elvitegravir (Vitekta)	PO: 85–150 mg/day	Newer integrase inhibitor; first-line drug
enfuvirtide (Fuzeon)	Subcutaneous: 90 mg bid	Fusion inhibitor; usually for advanced HIV-AIDS
maraviroc (Selzentry)	PO: 150–600 mg bid	CCR5 receptor inhibitor; usually for advanced HIV-AIDS
raltegravir (Isentress)	PO: 400 mg bid	Integrase inhibitor; first-line drug

After initial exposure, HIV may remain dormant for several months to many years. During this *latent phase,* patients are asymptomatic and may not realize they are infected. Once a diagnosis is established, current guidelines recommend that antiretroviral therapy be initiated immediately. The advantage of starting therapy immediately, during the latent stage, is that it may delay the onset of acute symptoms and the progression to AIDS.

The decision to begin treatment immediately after diagnosis, however, has certain negative consequences. Medications for HIV-AIDS are expensive; treatment with some of the newer drugs may cost more than $60,000 per year. These drugs produce uncomfortable and potentially serious adverse effects that can reduce the quality of life. Therapy over many years promotes viral resistance; when the acute stage eventually develops, the medications may no longer be effective.

The therapeutic goals for the pharmacotherapy of HIV-AIDS include the following:

- Reduce HIV-related morbidity and prolong survival.
- Improve the quality of life.
- Restore and preserve natural functions of the immune system.
- Suppress plasma HIV viral load to the maximum extent possible.
- Prevent HIV transmission.

Although drug therapy for HIV-AIDS has not produced a cure, it has resulted in a number of therapeutic successes. For example, many patients with HIV are able to live symptom free with their disease for a much longer time because of antiretroviral therapy. Furthermore, the transmission of the virus from a mother infected with HIV to her offspring has been reduced dramatically because of drug therapy of the mother prior to delivery and of the baby immediately following birth. Overall deaths due to the infection have stabilized at approximately 50,000 annually. Unfortunately, this stabilization has not been observed in African countries. About 70% of people infected with HIV worldwide live in sub-Saharan Africa.

The standard treatment for HIV-AIDS includes aggressive treatment with three to four drugs at a time, a regimen called **highly active antiretroviral therapy (HAART)**. The goal of HAART is to reduce the amount of HIV in the plasma to its lowest possible level. It must be understood, however, that HIV is harbored in locations other than the blood, such as in lymph nodes; therefore, elimination of the virus from the blood is not a cure.

The replication of HIV is illustrated in Figure 28.2. Antiretroviral drugs are classified into groups based on how they inhibit HIV replication.

- *Nucleoside and nucleotide reverse transcriptase inhibitors (NRTIs and NtRTIs)* The oldest antiretroviral drug, zidovudine, belongs to the NRTI class. Drugs in this group are structurally similar to nucleosides, the building blocks of DNA. NRTIs inhibit the action of **reverse transcriptase**, the viral enzyme that converts viral RNA into viral DNA.
- *Nonnucleoside reverse transcriptase inhibitors (NNRTIs)* This class also inhibits the viral enzyme reverse transcriptase, but these drugs are not structurally similar to the building blocks of DNA. Instead, these drugs bind directly to the reverse transcriptase molecule and inhibit its ability to build viral DNA.
- *Protease inhibitors* These drugs block the final assembly of the HIV particle. They are effective at reducing plasma HIV to very low levels, although resistance develops quickly.
- *Miscellaneous drugs for HIV infection* Newer drugs are being developed as scientists discover more about the HIV replication cycle. Enfuvirtide (Fuzeon) blocks the fusion of HIV to the CD4 receptor on the lymphocyte. Integrase inhibitors such as raltegravir (Isentress) and dolutegravir (DTG, Tivicay) prevent HIV from inserting its genes into the human chromosome.

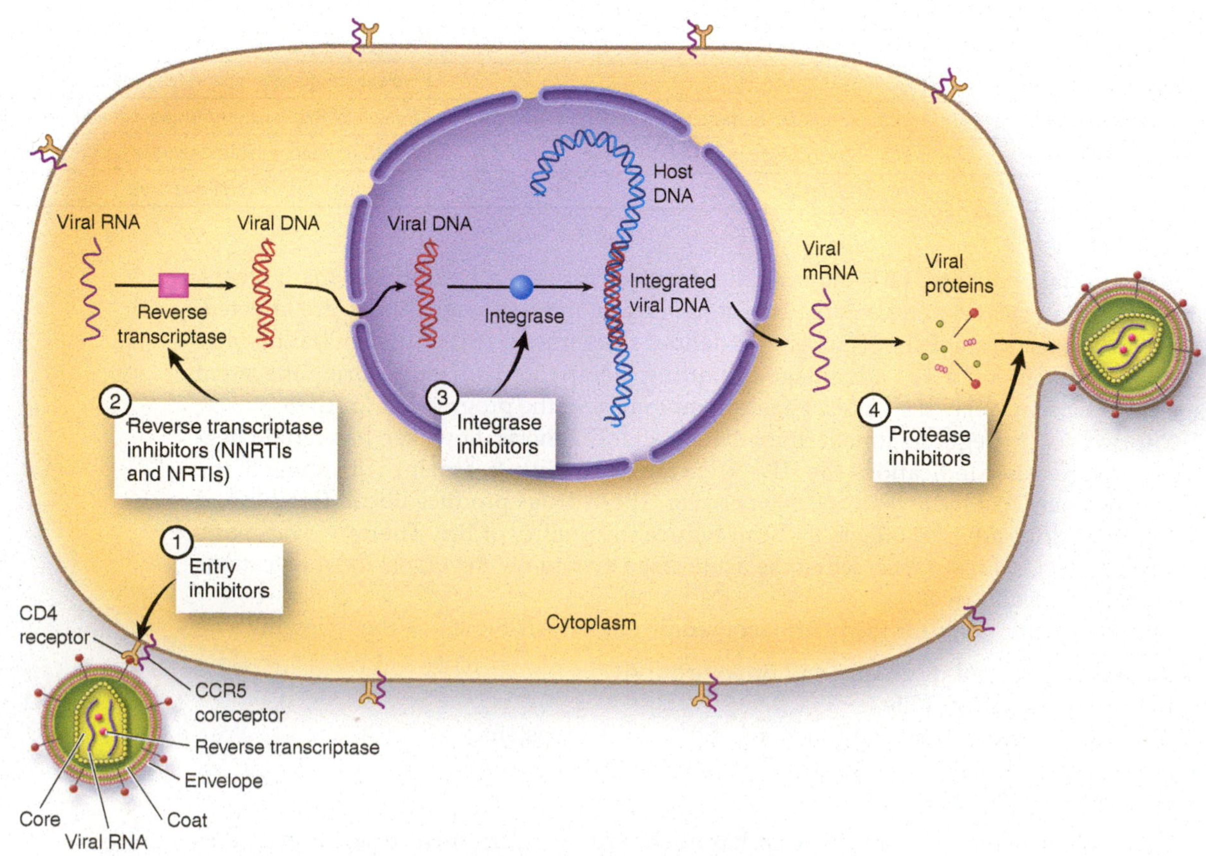

FIGURE 28.2 Replication of HIV.

Throughout the AIDS epidemic, regimens for treating the infection have continuously evolved. Healthcare providers should always review the latest medical literature before treating patients with HIV-AIDS. In current clinical practice, the following regimens have been shown to be the most successful choices for the initial therapy of HIV infection (Panel on Antiretroviral Guidelines for Adults and Adolescents, 2016):

- ***PI-based regimen:***
  - darunavir (ritonavir-boosted) + tenofovir + emtricitabine
- *Integrase inhibitor–based regimens:*
  - dolutegravir + abacavir + lamivudine (Triumeq)
  - dolutegravir (or raltegravir) + tenofovir + emtricitabine
  - elvitegravir (with cobicistat) + tenofovir + emtricitabine.

Prototype Drug: Pr *Zidovudine (AZT, Retrovir)*

Therapeutic Class: Antiretroviral **Pharmacologic Class:** Nucleoside reverse transcriptase inhibitor (NRTI)

Actions and Uses: Zidovudine was first discovered in the 1960s, and its antiviral activity was demonstrated prior to the AIDS epidemic. As the HIV reverse transcriptase enzyme begins to synthesize viral DNA, it mistakenly uses zidovudine as one of the building blocks, thus creating a defective DNA strand. Once incorporated, zidovudine slows synthesis of HIV, thereby reducing symptoms associated with this infection.

Because of its widespread use over the past 25 years, strains of HIV resistant to zidovudine are common. It is usually used in combination with other antiretrovirals because this slows the development of resistance and allows HIV to be attacked by several mechanisms. Combination products containing zidovudine include Combivir (zidovudine and lamivudine) and Trizivir (zidovudine, lamivudine, and abacavir).

Zidovudine is one of the few HIV-AIDS drugs that can prevent HIV infection. By administering zidovudine to a mother infected with HIV starting at 14 weeks of gestation and to the newborn for 6 weeks following delivery, the risk of transmission of the virus to the child can be significantly reduced. Zidovudine is also administered as prophylaxis to healthcare providers following an accidental needlestick or other exposure to HIV.

Adverse Effects and Interactions: Zidovudine can result in severe toxicity to blood cells at high doses. Many patients report GI symptoms such as anorexia, nausea, and diarrhea. Patients may experience fatigue and report generalized weakness. Headache will occur in the majority of patients taking zidovudine, and more serious CNS effects have been reported.

Zidovudine interacts with many drugs. Acetaminophen and ganciclovir may worsen bone marrow suppression. The following drugs may increase the risk of AZT toxicity: atovaquone, amphotericin B, aspirin, doxorubicin, fluconazole, methadone, and valproic acid.

Use with caution with herbal supplements such as St. John's wort, which may cause a decrease in antiretroviral activity.

BLACK BOX WARNING:
Rare cases of fatal lactic acidosis with hepatomegaly and steatosis have been reported with zidovudine use. Bone marrow suppression may result in neutropenia or severe anemia. Myopathy may occur with long-term use.

Although no drug or drug combination has yet been found to cure HIV-AIDS, some progress has been made on its prevention. In addition, manufacturers have compounded multiple drugs into single tablets for ease of use. Examples include Atripla (efavirenz, emtricitabine, and tenofovir), Combivir (lamivudine and zidovudine), Complera (emtricitabine, rilpivirene, and tenofovir), Epzicom (abacavir and lamivudine), Stribild (emtricitabine, tenofovir, elvitegravir, and cobicistat), Evotaz (atazanavir and colbicistat), and Prezcobix (darunavir and colbicistat).

Some progress has been made on preventing HIV infection through the use of medications. Truvada (emtricitabine and tenofovir) has been found to reduce the risk of acquiring HIV infection and may be recommended for people at very high risk for the disease. It is important for patients to be taught, however, that no drug combination is 100% effective and that established methods for HIV prevention such as abstinence, condoms, or other safe sex measures should always be implemented.

CONCEPT REVIEW 28.2

- Why are viral infections difficult to treat with current drugs?

Nursing Process Focus Patients Receiving Pharmacotherapy for HIV-AIDS

ASSESSMENT	POTENTIAL NURSING DIAGNOSES*
Prior to administration: • Obtain a complete health history, including cardiovascular, GI, neurological, skin, renal and liver conditions, past infections, allergies, sexual and drug history, and possible drug interactions. • Acquire the results of a complete physical examination, including vital signs, height, weight, lung sounds, level of consciousness (LOC), electrocardiogram (ECG), echocardiogram, and any signs of a current infection. • Evaluate laboratory blood findings: CBC, electrolytes, renal and liver function studies, amylase, glucose, and HIV viral load/CD4 count. • Obtain specimens for culture and sensitivity (C&S) testing before initiating therapy for possible bacterial infections.	• *Infection* related to compromised immune system • *Decisional Conflict* related to therapeutic regimen • *Fear* related to HIV diagnosis and a lack of knowledge about therapeutic regimen • *Deficient Knowledge* related to a lack of information about disease process, transmission, and drug therapy • *Ineffective Health Maintenance* related to the complexity of therapies (medications, counseling, diet) • *Risk for Injury* related to adverse effects of drug therapy

PLANNING: PATIENT GOALS AND EXPECTED OUTCOMES

The patient will:

- Experience therapeutic effects (a decrease in viral load and an increase in CD4 counts).
- Be free from or experience minimal adverse effects from drug therapy.
- Verbalize an understanding of the drug's use, adverse effects, and required precautions.
- Adhere to recommended treatment regimen.

IMPLEMENTATION

Interventions and (Rationales)	Patient Education/Discharge Planning
• Administer medication correctly, and evaluate the patient's knowledge of proper administration, especially monitoring the patient's ability and motivation to comply with treatment regimen. (Antiretroviral therapy continues for the life of the patient. Stopping the therapy results in a rapid rebound in HIV replication.)	Inform the patient: • That treatment for HIV-AIDS is a life-long, ongoing process. Stopping therapy will result in a rebound in the HIV viral replication. • Not to stop taking the drug regimen when feeling better. • To take according to the drug schedule. • Not to share doses with others. • To return to the healthcare provider if adverse effects make compliance to therapy difficult to continue.
• Monitor for symptoms of hypersensitivity reactions. (Abacavir may cause anaphylactic reaction.)	• Instruct the patient to discontinue the medication and inform the healthcare provider if symptoms of hypersensitivity reaction develop, such as wheezing; shortness of breath; swelling of face, tongue, or hands; or itching or rash.
• Monitor vital signs, especially temperature, and for symptoms of infection. Monitor white blood cell count. (Antiretroviral drugs such as delavirdine may cause neutropenia.)	Instruct the patient: • To report symptoms of infections such as fever, chills, sore throat, and cough to the healthcare provider. • On methods to minimize exposure to infection, such as frequent hand hygiene; avoiding crowds and people with colds, flu, and other infections; limiting exposure to children and animals; increasing fluid intake; emptying the bladder frequently; and coughing and deep breathing several times per day.
• Monitor the patient for signs of stomatitis. (Immunosuppression may result in the proliferation of oral bacteria.)	• Inform the patient to be alert for mouth ulcers and to report their appearance to the healthcare provider.
• Monitor blood pressure. (Antiviral drugs such as abacavir may cause significant decrease in blood pressure.)	Instruct the patient to: • Rise slowly from a lying or sitting position to minimize the effects of orthostatic hypotension. • Report changes in blood pressure.
• Monitor HIV RNA assay, CD4 counts, liver function, kidney function, CBC, blood glucose, and serum amylase and triglyceride levels. (Monitoring labs will aid in determining the effectiveness or drug toxicity.)	Instruct the patient: • On the purpose of required laboratory tests and scheduled follow-ups with the healthcare provider. • To monitor weight and the presence of swelling. • To keep all appointments for laboratory tests.

Interventions and (Rationales)	Patient Education/Discharge Planning
• Determine potential drug–drug and drug–food interactions. (Antiretroviral medications have multiple drug–drug interactions and must be taken as prescribed. Some antiretrovirals should not be taken with acidic fruit juice.)	Instruct the patient: • When to take the specific medication in relationship to food intake. • About foods or beverages to avoid when taking medication. • To take the medication exactly as directed; do not skip any doses. • To consult with the healthcare provider before taking any OTC medications or herbal supplements.
• Monitor the skin for rash; withhold medication, and notify the healthcare provider at the first sign of rash. (Several antiretroviral drugs may cause Stevens–Johnson syndrome, which may be fatal.)	• Advise the patient to check the skin frequently and to notify the healthcare provider at the first sign of any rash.
• Establish therapeutic environment to ensure adequate rest, nutrition, hydration, and relaxation. (Support of the immune system is essential in patients with HIV to minimize opportunistic infections.)	Advise the patient to incorporate the following health-enhancing activities: • Adequate rest and sleep • Proper nutrition that provides essential vitamins and nutrients • Intake of six to eight glasses of water per day.
• Monitor blood lipid levels. (Antiretroviral drugs such as raltegravir and dolutegravir may increase cholesterol and triglyceride levels.)	• Instruct the patient to report for all laboratory tests.
• Monitor for neurologic adverse effects such as numbness and tingling of the extremities. (Many NRTI drugs cause peripheral neuropathy.)	Instruct the patient to: • Report numbness and tingling of extremities. • Use caution when in contact with heat and cold due to possible peripheral neuropathy.
• Determine the effect of the prescribed antiretroviral drugs on oral contraceptives. (Many drugs reduce the effectiveness of oral contraceptives.)	• Instruct the patient to use an alternate form of birth control while taking antiretroviral medications.
• Provide resources for medical and emotional support. (Medications for the treatment of HIV-AIDS can be expensive.)	• Advise the patient on community resources and support groups.
• Determine the patient's understanding of the effect of the medication and impact on lifestyle activities. (Antiretroviral medications used for HIV-AIDS do not cure the disease; therefore, patients need to understand that lifestyle changes still need to occur.)	Advise the patient: • That the medication may decrease the level of HIV infection in the blood but will not prevent transmission of the virus. • To use barrier protection during sexual activity. • To avoid sharing needles. • To not donate blood.

EVALUATION OF OUTCOME CRITERIA

Evaluate the effectiveness of drug therapy by confirming that patient goals and expected outcomes have been met (see "Planning"). *See Table 28.3 for lists of drugs to which these nursing actions apply.*

*Herdman, T.H. & Kamitsuru, S. (Eds.), *Nursing Diagnoses: Definitions & Classification* 2015–2017. Copyright © 2014, 1994–2014 NANDA International. Used by arrangement by John Wiley & Sons, Inc. Companion website: www.wiley.com/go/nursingdiagnoses.

Antiviral drugs are available to treat herpes simplex, influenza, and viral hepatitis infections.

◀ **CORE CONCEPT 28.6**

Other than the drugs used to treat HIV, only a few antivirals are available to treat serious viral infections. These include drugs to treat infections with the herpesviruses, the influenza virus, and the hepatitis virus. Doses for these medications are shown in Table 28.4.

Treatment of Herpesvirus Infection

Herpes simplex viruses (HSVs) are a family of viruses that cause repeated, blisterlike lesions on the skin, genitals, and other mucosal surfaces. Herpesviruses are acquired through sexual intercourse or other direct physical contact with an infected person. The herpesvirus family includes the following:

- HSV-type 1—primarily causes infections of the eye, mouth, and lips, although genital infections are possible.
- HSV-type 2—primarily causes genital infections.

Table 28.4 Antiviral Drugs for Herpes and Influenza Infections

Drug	Route and Adult Dose	Remarks
HERPESVIRUS DRUGS		
Pr acyclovir (Zovirax)	PO: 400 mg tid	For HSV-1, HSV-2, and varicella-zoster; topical and IV forms available
cidofovir (Vistide)	IV: 5 mg/kg once weekly for 2 weeks	For cytomegalovirus retinitis in patients with AIDS; must give probenecid before and after infusion
docosanol (Abreva)	Topical: 10% cream applied to lesion up to five times/day	For herpes simplex lesions on the face and lips
famciclovir (Famvir)	PO: 500 mg tid for 7 days	For HSV-2 and varicella-zoster
foscarnet (Foscavir) ganciclovir (Cytovene)	IV: 40–60 mg/kg tid PO: 1 g tid IV: 5 mg/kg bid	For cytomegalovirus retinitis and treatment of acyclovir-resistant herpesvirus Preferred drug for cytomegalovirus; oral form available
penciclovir (Denavir)	Topical: 0.5 inch of ointment to each eye every 3 hours	For herpes simplex lesions on the face and lips
trifluridine (Viroptic)	Topical: One drop in each eye every 2 hours during waking hours (max: nine drops/day)	For herpes eye infections
valacyclovir (Valtrex)	PO: 1 g tid for 7 days (herpes zoster) or 1 g bid for 10 days (genital herpes)	For HSV-1, HSV-2, and varicella-zoster
INFLUENZA DRUGS		
amantadine (Symmetrel)	PO: 100 mg bid	For treatment and prevention of influenza A; also for Parkinson disease
oseltamivir (Tamiflu)	PO: 75 mg bid for 5 days	For treatment of influenza
peramivir (Rapivab)	IV: 600 mg once	Newer drug for influenza
rimantadine (Flumadine)	PO: 100 mg bid	For treatment and prevention of influenza
zanamivir (Relenza)	Inhalation: Two inhalations per day for 5 days	For influenza

- Cytomegalovirus (CMV)—affects multiple body systems, usually in patients with immunosuppression.
- Varicella-zoster virus—causes shingles (zoster) and chickenpox (varicella).
- Epstein-Barr virus—causes infectious mononucleosis and Burkitt's lymphoma (a form of cancer).

Following its initial entrance into the human host, HSV may remain in a latent, nonreplicating state in nerve cells for many years. Immunosuppression, physical challenge, or emotional stress can activate the virus and cause the characteristic lesions to reappear. *Initial* HSV-1 and HSV-2 infections are usually treated with oral antiviral therapy for 5 to 10 days. Topical drugs are available for application on active lesions, but they are not as effective as oral medications. Although *recurrent* herpes lesions are often mild and require no drug therapy, patients who experience frequent or severe recurrences may benefit from low doses of prophylactic antiviral therapy. It should be noted that the antiviral drugs used to treat herpesviruses do not cure the patient; the virus remains in the patient for life. Drugs for treating herpesviruses are listed in Table 28.4.

Prototype Drug: Pr *Acyclovir (Zovirax)*

Therapeutic Class: Antiviral for herpesviruses **Pharmacologic Class: Nucleoside analog**

Actions and Uses: The antiviral activity of acyclovir is limited to the herpesviruses, for which it is the preferred drug. It is most effective against HSV-1 and HSV-2 and effective only at high doses against CMV and varicella-zoster. By inhibiting viral DNA synthesis, acyclovir decreases the duration and severity of herpes episodes. Resistance has developed to the drug, particularly in patients with HIV-AIDS. When given for prophylaxis, it may decrease the frequency of active herpes episodes, but it does not cure the patient. It is available in topical form for placing directly on active lesions, in oral form for prophylaxis, and as an IV for particularly severe disease.

Adverse Effects and Interactions: There are few adverse effects to acyclovir when administered topically or orally. When given IV, the drug may cause painful inflammation of vessels at the site of infusion. Because nephrotoxicity is possible, especially when the drug is given by the IV route, kidney function should be carefully monitored.

Acyclovir interacts with several drugs. For example, probenecid decreases acyclovir elimination, and zidovudine may cause increased drowsiness and lethargy.

Treatment of Influenza Virus Infection

Influenza is a viral infection characterized by acute symptoms that include sore throat, sneezing, coughing, fever, and chills. The virus is easily spread via airborne droplets. In patients with compromised immune systems, an influenza infection may be fatal. Influenza viruses are designated with the letters A, B, or C.

The best approach to influenza infection is prevention through annual vaccination. Those who benefit greatly from vaccinations include residents of long-term care facilities, those with chronic cardiopulmonary disease, women who will be in their second or third trimester during the peak flu season, and healthy adults older than age 50. Adequate immunity is achieved about 2 weeks after vaccination and lasts for several months to a year. The Centers for Disease Control (CDC, 2016) recommends that people get vaccinated as soon as the vaccine becomes available in their community. Additional details on vaccines are presented in Chapter 26.

Antivirals may be used to prevent influenza or decrease the severity of influenza symptoms. The drug amantadine (Symmetrel) has been available for many years to prevent and treat influenza. Amantadine or rimantadine are approved against influenza type A, but not type B. Due to a high level of viral resistance to these drugs, the CDC (2016) no longer recommends that they be used for prophylaxis or treatment of influenza type A. Antivirals for influenza are shown in Table 28.4.

The *neuroamidase inhibitors* are used to treat active infections, and are effective against both influenza A and B. If given within 48 hours of the onset of symptoms, oseltamivir (Tamiflu) and zanamivir (Relenza) are reported to shorten the normal 7-day duration of influenza symptoms to 5 days. A newer drug in this class, peramivir (Rapivab), is available as a single dose by the IV route. Because these influenza antivirals produce only modest benefits for patients with an active infection, prevention through vaccination remains the best alternative.

Treatment of Viral Hepatitis Infection

Viral hepatitis is a common infection caused by several different viruses, the most common types being hepatitis A, hepatitis B, and hepatitis C. Although each has its own unique features, all hepatitis viruses cause inflammation and death of liver cells and produce similar symptoms. Acute symptoms include fever, chills, fatigue, anorexia, nausea, and vomiting. Chronic hepatitis may result in prolonged fatigue, jaundice, liver cirrhosis, and, ultimately, hepatic failure.

HEPATITIS A

Hepatitis A virus (HAV) infection in the United States is usually caused by eating food contaminated with the virus. The best treatment for HAV is prevention by the administration of HAV vaccine (Havrix, VAQTA). Because acute HAV infection is self-limiting, there is no specific therapy for the condition. Unlike the other hepatitis viruses, HAV infection is only an acute disease, and does not have a chronic form.

HEPATITIS B

Hepatitis B virus (HBV) is transmitted primarily through exposure to contaminated blood and body fluids. Major risk factors for HBV include injected drug abuse, sex with a partner infected with HBV, and sex between men. Healthcare workers are at risk because of accidental exposure to HBV-contaminated needles or body fluids.

Treatment of *acute* HBV infection is symptomatic because 90% of these infections resolve with complete recovery and do not progress to chronic disease. Symptoms of *chronic* HBV, however, may develop as long as 10 years following exposure. The final stage of the infection is hepatic cirrhosis. In addition, chronic HBV infections are associated with an increased risk of hepatocellular carcinoma.

The best treatment for HBV infection is prevention through vaccination with HBV vaccine (Recombivax HB, Engerix-B). Once the symptoms of chronic HBV appear, drug therapy is prolonged, often for as long as 48 weeks. Although a number of therapies exist for treating chronic HBV, the following are considered first-line therapies due to their effectiveness and acceptable safety profiles.

- Interferon alfa or peginterferon alfa: natural proteins that suppress viral replication and enhance body defenses.

- Tenofovir: resembles a building block for DNA; inhibits viral DNA synthesis.
- Entecavir (Baraclude): blocks viral DNA synthesis.

HEPATITIS C

Transmitted primarily through exposure to infected blood or body fluids, hepatitis C virus (HCV) is more common than HBV. HCV is the most common cause of the need for liver transplants. Unlike with HAV and HBV, no vaccine is available to prevent HCV.

Current pharmacotherapy for chronic HCV infection is rapidly evolving due to the development of several new drugs. The traditional treatment includes combinations of interferon (or peginterferon) and the antiviral ribavirin. In 2011, two new protease inhibitors, bocepprevir (Victrelis) and telaprevir (Incivek), were added to the traditional regimen. Since 2013 multiple drugs and drug combinations have been approved by the U.S. Food and Drug Administration (FDA). They represent a new generation of medications that inhibit viral proteins necessary for HCV to replicate. They include Simeprevir (Olysia), sofosbuvir (Sovaldi), ledipasvir, ombitasvir, paritaprevir, dasabuvir, daclarasvir (Daklinza), and Zapatier (grazoprevir and elbasvir). Newer combinations include Harvoni (sosofovir and ledipasvir), Viekira Pak (ombitasvir, dasabuvir, paritaprevir, and ritonavir), Epclusa (sosobuvir and velpatasvir), and Technivie (obitasvir, paritaprevir, and andritonavir).

ANTIPARASITIC DRUGS

CORE CONCEPT 28.7 ▶

Infections caused by helminths and protozoans cause significant disease worldwide.

proto = *first*
zoans = *animals*

Other pathogens that may infect humans include single-celled organisms, or **protozoans**, and multicellular animals such as mites, ticks, and worms. Some of these parasites thrive in conditions in which sanitation and personal hygiene are poor and population density is high. Although many of these diseases are rare in the United States and Canada, travelers to Africa, Asia, and South America may acquire infections overseas and return home with them. Table 28.5 lists selected antiparasitics. Scabicides and pediculicides are covered in Chapter 37.

With a few exceptions, antibiotic, antifungal, and antiviral drugs are ineffective against these complex organisms. Drugs prescribed for parasitic diseases may be classified as antimalarials, antiprotozoans (other than antimalarial drugs), antihelminthics, and scabicides/pediculicides.

Malaria is a disease caused by four species of the protozoan *Plasmodium*. Although rare in the United States and Canada, malaria is the second most common fatal infectious disease in the world, with 300 to 500 million cases occurring annually. The CDC recommends that travelers to infected areas receive prophylactic antimalarial drugs prior to and during their visit and for 1 week after leaving. Chloroquine (Aralen) is the preferred drug; however, most regions of the world have developed chloroquine-resistant strains of *Plasmodium*. Many of the newer drugs used in high malaria regions have not been approved by the FDA. Healthcare providers planning travel to these regions should consult the CDC website for the most current information on pharmacotherapy.

Other species of protozoans that cause significant disease worldwide include *Entamoeba*, *Giardia*, *Leishmania*, *Pneumocystis*, *Toxoplasma*, and *Trypanosoma*. Amebiasis is a disease caused by *Entamoeba histolytica*, commonly found in Africa, Latin America, and Asia, where it frequently causes serious disease. Although primarily an intestinal disease, *E. histolytica* can invade the liver, where it causes abscesses. The primary sign of amebiasis is a severe form of diarrhea known as amebic **dysentery**. Drugs used to treat amebiasis include those that act directly on amebas in the intestine and those that are administered for their systemic effects on the liver and other organs.

dys = *difficult or painful*
enter = *intestine*

Helminths consist of various species of parasitic worms, including hookworms, pinworms, roundworms, tapeworms, and flukes. Many of these worms attach to the mucosa of the human intestinal tract. Helminth diseases are quite common in areas of the world lacking high standards of sanitation. Helminth infections in the United States and Canada are generally neither common nor fatal, although drug therapy may be indicated. The most common helminth disease worldwide is caused by the roundworm *Ascaris*; however, infection by the

Table 28.5 Selected Drugs for Helminth and Protozoan Infections

Drug	Route and Adult Dose	Remarks
ANTIHELMINTHICS		
albendazole (Albenza)	PO: 400 mg bid (max: 800 mg/day)	Only antihelminthic drug active against all stages of the helminth life cycle
ivermectin (Stromectol)	PO: 150–200 mcg/kg for one dose	Preferred drug for many helminth infections
mebendazole (Vermox)	PO: 100 mg once or twice daily for 3 days	For whipworm, roundworm, hookworm, and pinworm
praziquantel (Biltricide)	PO: 5 mg/kg for one dose or 25 mg/kg tid	For schistosomiasis
pyrantel (Antiminth, Ascarel, Pin-X, Pinworm Caplets)	PO: 11 mg/kg for one dose (max: 1 g)	For hookworm and roundworm
ANTIMALARIALS		
artemether and lumefantrine (Coartem)	PO: 3–6 doses for 3 days (20 mg of artemether and 120 mg of lumefantrine per dose)	For chloroquine-resistant malaria
atovaquone and proguanil (Malarone)	PO (for prophylaxis): One tablet/day starting 1–2 days before travel, and continuing until 7 days after return	Atovaquone is also indicated for *Pneumocystis* pneumonia
chloroquine (Aralen)	PO: 600 mg initial dose, then 300 mg weekly	Preferred drug for malaria; also for amebiasis and rheumatoid arthritis; IM and IV forms available
hydroxychloroquine (Plaquenil) (see the Prototype Drug box in Core Concept 36.7)	PO: 620 mg initial dose, then 310 mg weekly	Also for rheumatoid arthritis and systemic lupus erythematosus
pyrimethamine (Daraprim)	PO: 25 mg once per week for 10 weeks	For malaria and toxoplasmosis
ANTIPROTOZOANS (NONMALARIAL)		
doxycycline (Vibramycin)	PO: 100 mg/day	For traveler's diarrhea; also for malaria prophylaxis; a tetracycline antibiotic
Pr metronidazole (Flagyl)	PO: 250–750 mg tid	For many parasitic infections; IV form available
paromomycin (Humatin)	PO: 25–35 mg/kg in divided doses for 5–10 days	For acute and chronic amebiasis; an aminoglycoside antibiotic
pentamidine (NebuPent, Pentam)	IV: 4 mg/kg daily for 14–21 days	For *Pneumocystis* pneumonia, trypanosomiasis, and leishmaniasis; IM and inhalation forms available
tinidazole (Tindamax)	PO: 2 grams per day for 3 days	For amebiasis, giardiasis, or trichomoniasis

pinworm *Enterobius* is more common in the United States. For ascariasis, oral mebendazole (Vermox) for 3 days is the standard treatment. Pharmacotherapy for enterobiasis includes a single dose of mebendazole, albendazole (Albenza), or pyrantel (Antiminth). To prevent the spread of these parasites, good hand hygiene techniques must be practiced.

CONCEPT REVIEW 28.3

- How do most patients in the United States and Canada acquire protozoan infections?

Prototype Drug: Pr *Metronidazole (Flagyl)*

Therapeutic Class: Anti-infective, antiprotozoan **Pharmacologic Class:** Drug that disrupts nucleic acid synthesis

Actions and Uses: Metronidazole is a preferred drug for amebiasis because it is effective against amebas in the intestine and in other organs. Metronidazole is also a drug of choice for two other protozoan infections: giardiasis from *Giardia lamblia* and trichonomiasis due to *Trichomonas vaginalis*.

Metronidazole is somewhat unique in that it also has antibiotic activity against anaerobic bacteria and thus is used to treat a number of respiratory, bone, skin, and CNS infections. Topical forms are used to treat rosacea, a disease characterized by reddening of the sebaceous glands in the skin around the nose and face. It is used in combination with bismuth and tetracycline to eradicate *H. pylori* infection, which is associated with peptic ulcer disease.

Adverse Effects and Interactions: Although adverse effects are relatively common, most are not serious enough to cause discontinuation of therapy. The most common adverse effects of metronidazole are anorexia, nausea, diarrhea, dizziness, and headache. Dryness of the mouth and an unpleasant metallic taste may be experienced.

Metronidazole interacts with several drugs. For example, oral anticoagulants increase hypoprothombinemia. In combination with alcohol and medications that contain alcohol, metronidazole may cause a disulfiram reaction. It may also elevate lithium levels.

BLACK BOX WARNING:
Metronidazole causes cancer in laboratory animals and should be used only for approved indications.

Patients Need to Know

Patients treated for fungal, viral, or parasitic infections need to know the following:

Regarding Antifungals

1. Avoid alcohol and other drugs toxic to the liver while taking azole-type antifungals.
2. Griseofulvin, used to treat superficial mycoses, can decrease the effectiveness of oral contraceptives. An alternative method of contraception is advised.
3. Older children and adult patients should swish oral antifungal drugs around in their mouths and swallow them. Caregivers should swab the mouths of infants and toddlers. Wait at least 10 minutes after antifungal treatment to put anything else in the mouth.
4. Rinse the mouth after use of corticosteroid inhalers to avoid a decrease in local immune defenses against oral candidiasis.
5. While taking antifungal drugs for a vaginal infection, refrain from sexual intercourse until the infection is resolved.
6. Wear gloves when applying topical medications.

Regarding Antivirals

7. When taking antivirals, it is important to report symptoms of hypersensitivity reactions.
8. When taking drugs for HIV-AIDS, avoid crowds and those with infections because many of these medications will suppress your immune system.

Regarding Antihelminthics and Antiprotozoans

9. Course of treatment depends on the nature of the infection or infestation, and the treatment plan is to be followed completely as prescribed.
10. Take showers instead of baths. Change underwear, linens, and towels daily.
11. Good hand hygiene practices are a must in the prevention of pinworms and roundworms.

Chapter Review

Core Concepts Summary

28.1 Fungal infections are classified as superficial or systemic.

Fungi are multicellular organisms. Because most are unaffected by antibiotics, they require different classes of medications. Fungal infections are usually a serious problem only in patients with compromised immune systems. Mycoses are classified as superficial or systemic.

28.2 Systemic antifungal drugs are used for serious infections of internal organs.

Systemic mycoses affect the internal organs and may require prolonged and aggressive drug therapy. Systemic antifungal drugs may cause serious adverse effects.

28.3 Superficial infections of the skin, nails, and mucous membranes are effectively treated with topical and oral antifungal drugs.

Superficial mycoses of the hair, skin, nails, and mucous membranes are very common, though rarely serious. Antifungals given topically as powders, troches, and ointments produce few adverse effects.

28.4 Viruses are infectious agents that require a host to replicate.

Viruses take over the cellular machinery of host cells and use it to replicate themselves. Although most viral infections require no pharmacotherapy, patients with infections by HIV, herpesviruses, and the influenza virus may benefit from drug treatment.

28.5 Antiretroviral drugs do not cure HIV-AIDS, but they do help many patients live longer.

Drugs used to treat HIV infections include the nucleoside and nonnucleoside reverse transcriptase inhibitors, protease inhibitors, and fusion inhibitors. These drugs may produce significant toxicity. Although they are not able to cure the disease, they may extend the symptom-free period.

28.6 Antiviral drugs are available to treat herpes simplex, influenza, and viral hepatitis infections.

Drug therapy is used to extend the latent period of genital herpes and to speed the recovery from active lesions. A few antivirals are available to prevent influenza, and these are most useful when combined with vaccines. New drugs have been developed to shorten the discomfort period for influenza symptoms, although these drugs have limited effectiveness.

28.7 Infections caused by helminths and protozoans cause significant disease worldwide.

Malaria is one of the most common infections in the world, and a significant number of drugs are available to disrupt the *Plasmodium* life cycle. Similarly, amebiasis is a common protozoan disease requiring intensive drug treatment. Diseases caused by helminths are common in areas of the world lacking adequate sanitation.

REVIEW Questions

Answer the following questions to assess your knowledge of the chapter material, and go back and review any material that is not clear to you.

1. The patient on amphotericin B must be monitored for:
   1. Ototoxicity.
   2. Hepatic toxicity.
   3. Nephrotoxicity.
   4. Anoxia.

2. The patient has oral candidiasis. Which of the following medications does the nurse expect to be ordered?
   1. Terbinafine (Lamisil)
   2. Clotrimazole (Mycelex)
   3. Ketoconazole (Nizoral)
   4. Nystatin (Mycostatin)

3. The patient with a fungal infection of the toenails asks how long treatment must occur. The best response would be:
   1. "Treatment is very quick, requiring only one tablet of clotrimazole."
   2. "Treatment will occur daily for 3 days."
   3. "Treatment will last for several months."
   4. "You will need to speak to your healthcare provider."

4. One of the residents at a local retirement center asks, "If I get the flu vaccine today, when will it start working?" The nurse responds that immunity is achieved:
   1. In about a day or two.
   2. Within a week after the vaccination.
   3. About 2 weeks after the vaccination.
   4. About 3 to 4 weeks after the vaccination.

5. A patient has just been diagnosed with genital herpes and has been prescribed acyclovir (Zovirax). The patient asks how this drug will help the condition. The nurse replies: (Select all that apply.)
   1. "It can be given to reduce the frequency of herpes episodes."
   2. "If taken correctly, this medication will cure the disease."
   3. "It decreases the duration and severity of herpes episodes."
   4. "In addition to treating herpes, it also can be used to treat viral influenza."
   5. "It is part of the medication regimen for the treatment of HIV."

6. The patient complains of flu-like symptoms that started 24 hours ago. Which of the following classes of medications would the nurse anticipate being ordered?
   1. Protease inhibitors
   2. Nonnucleoside reverse transcriptase inhibitors
   3. Nucleoside reverse transcriptase inhibitors
   4. Neuroamidase inhibitors

7. A patient has started taking metronidazole (Flagyl) for the treatment of a gastric ulcer caused by *H. pylori*. The nurse knows to monitor for which of the following adverse effects? (Select all that apply.)
   1. Constipation
   2. Anorexia
   3. A metallic taste
   4. Dryness of the mouth
   5. Headache

8. When applying topical antifungals, which of the following statements should be included in a patient teaching plan?
   1. No other antifungals should be administered.
   2. Gloves should be worn to prevent transmission.
   3. Antifungals should not be applied to open skin areas.
   4. Vital signs should be checked prior to administration.

9. A patient using clotrimazole as a vaginal antifungal may experience which of the following adverse effects? (Select all that apply.)
   1. Burning
   2. An increase in discharge
   3. Itching
   4. Irritation
   5. Ulceration

10. The nurse is providing education to a mother of a young patient about pinworms and roundworms. Which of the following should be included in this educational session?
    1. Good hand hygiene practices are important in preventing the spread of pinworms and roundworms.
    2. Play habits do not contribute to the transmission of pinworms and roundworms.
    3. It is not important that children wear shoes when playing outside.
    4. Once the child has had worms, reinfection cannot occur.

CASE STUDY Questions

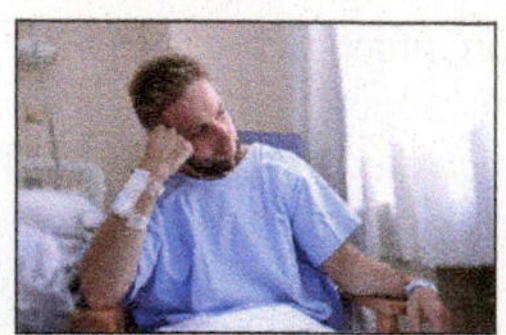

Remember Mr. Engelstad, the patient introduced at the beginning of the chapter? Now read the remainder of the case study. Based on the information you have learned in this chapter, answer the questions that follow.

Mark Engelstad, a 35-year-old computer technician, was seen at a local clinic because he had not been feeling well, stating, "Over the past several weeks, I've become really tired and achy all over. I feel like I have a fever all the time, my throat hurts, and my head hurts. I don't know why I'm not getting better." Additionally, he had not felt like eating and had lost a noticeable amount of weight. Because of his symptoms, he was admitted to the hospital for treatment and further testing. As a result, a diagnosis of HIV was confirmed. A medical specialist in HIV/AIDS prescribed the following antiretroviral drug regimen:

darunavir (ritonavir-boosted), protease inhibitors
tenofovir, nucleoside reverse transcriptase inhibitors (NRTIs)
emtricitabine, NRTIs

1. Mr. Engelstad has been started on his medication regimen. Which of the following is true regarding current HIV medication regimens?
   1. Complete cures are possible using highly active antiretroviral therapy.
   2. Drugs have been developed that are effective against multiple resistant HIV strains
   3. Antiretroviral drugs, used for HIV, can also treat many other viruses, such as the flu.
   4. They help patients to live symptom free, for a longer period of time.

2. Mr. Engelstad is given information on his medication regimen, which includes a list of the antiretroviral medications he will be taking. He asks the nurse, "What is an antiretroviral medication?" The best response is:
   1. "These medications strengthen the immune system of the body."
   2. "They interfere with the ability of the virus to enter a target cell."
   3. "These are antiviral drugs that block the viruses from replicating."
   4. "The medication binds to the proteins on the virus and destroys it."

3. Other important information to include when teaching Mr. Englestad about his medications includes: (Select all that apply.)
   1. Antiretroviral therapy will continue for the rest of his life.
   2. If the medications start causing problems, it is okay for him to stop taking them.
   3. He should notify the healthcare provider if any adverse effects make taking the medications difficult.
   4. He should keep all laboratory appointments so that effectiveness of drug therapy can be monitored.

4. Because Mr. Engelstad is taking four different antiretroviral medications, he must be monitored for anemia because he:
   1. Is most likely being abused.
   2. Is experiencing minor adverse reactions.
   3. Is not taking the medications as ordered.
   4. May be experiencing severe toxicity due to high doses of the drug.

Answers and complete rationales for the Review and Case Study Questions appear in Appendix A.

REFERENCES

Centers for Disease Control and Prevention. (2016). *Influenza antiviral medications: Summary for clinicians*. Retrieved from http://www.cdc.gov/flu/professionals/antivirals/summary-clinicians.htm

Herdman, T. H., & Kamitsuru, S. (Eds.). (2014). *NANDA International nursing diagnoses: Definitions and classification, 2015–2017*. Oxford, United Kingdom: Wiley-Blackwell.

Panel on Antiretroviral Guidelines for Adults and Adolescents, Department of Health and Human Services. (2016). *Guidelines for the use of antiretroviral agents in HIV-1-infected adults and adolescents*. Retrieved from http://aidsinfo.nih.gov/contentfiles/lvguidelines/AdultandAdolescentGL.pdf

SELECTED BIBLIOGRAPHY

Buggs, A.M. (2014). *Viral hepatitis*. Retrieved from http://emedicine.medscape.com/article/775507-overview

Centers for Disease Control and Prevention. (2015). *Hepatitis B FAQs for health professionals*. Retrieved from http://www.cdc.gov/hepatitis/HBV/HBVfaq.htm

Centers for Disease Control and Prevention. (2015). *HIV in the United States: At a glance*. Retrieved from http://www.cdc.gov/hiv/statistics/basics/ataglance.html

Centers for Disease Control and Prevention. (2015). *Malaria*. Retrieved from http://www.cdc.gov/malaria

Centers for Disease Control and Prevention. (2016). *Fungal diseases*. Retrieved from http://www.cdc.gov/fungal

Centers for Disease Control and Prevention. (2016). *Genital herpes—CDC fact sheet*. Retrieved from http://www.cdc.gov/std/herpes/stdfact-herpes.htm

Centers for Disease Control and Prevention. (2016) *Influenza (Flu)*. Retrieved from http://www.cdc.gov/flu

Derlet, R. W. (2015). *Influenza*. Retrieved from http://emedicine.medscape.com/article/219557-overview

Grohskopf, L. A., Sokolow, L. Z., Olsen, S. J., Bresee, J. S., Broder, K. R., & Karron, R. A. (2015). Prevention and control of influenza with Vaccines: Recommendations of the Advisory Committee on Immunization Practices, United States, 2015-16 influenza season. *Morbidity and Mortality Weekly Report*, *64*, 818–825.

Hidalgo, J. A. (2015). *Candidiasis*. Retrieved from http://emedicine.medscape.com/article/213853-overview

Macías, J., Neukam, K., Merchante, N., & Pineda, J. A. (2014). Latest pharmacotherapy options for treating hepatitis C in HIV-infected patients. *Expert Opinion on Pharmacotherapy, 15*, 1837–1848. doi:10.1517/14656566.2014.934810

Panel on Treatment of HIV-Infected Pregnant Women and Prevention of Perinatal Transmission. (2016). *Recommendations for use of antiretroviral drugs in pregnant HIV-1-infected women for maternal health and interventions to reduce perinatal HIV transmission in the United States*. Retrieved from https://aidsinfo.nih.gov/contentfiles/lvguidelines/perinatalgl.pdf

Perfect, J. R. & Andes, D. (2013). Antifungal therapy: Current concepts and evidence-based management. *Current Medical Research and Opinion*, *29*, 289–290. doi:10.1185/03007995.2012.761136

Pyrsopoulos, N. T. (2015). *Hepatitis B*. Retrieved from http://emedicine.medscape.com/article/177632-overview

Salvaggio, M. R. (2015). *Herpes simplex*. Retrieved from http://emedicine.medscape.com/article/218580-overview

Tosti, A. (2016). *Onychomycosis*. Retrieved from http://emedicine.medscape.com/article/1105828-overview

Chapter 29

Drugs for Neoplasia

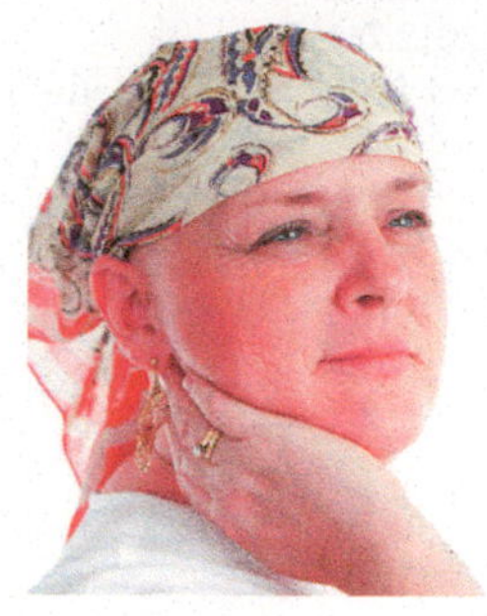

"I know they are helping with my cancer, but four different drugs? I guess it could be worse."

Ms. Patricia Novak

Core Concepts

29.1 Cancer is characterized by rapid, uncontrolled growth of cells.

29.2 The causes of cancer may be chemical, physical, or biological.

29.3 The three primary goals of chemotherapy are cure, control, and palliation.

29.4 To achieve a total cure, every malignant cell must be removed or killed.

29.5 Use of multiple drugs and special dosing schedules improves the success of chemotherapy.

29.6 Serious toxicity limits therapy with most of the antineoplastic drugs.

29.7 Alkylating drugs act by changing the structure of DNA in cancer cells.

29.8 Antimetabolites disrupt critical cellular pathways in cancer cells.

29.9 A few cytotoxic antibiotics are used to treat cancer rather than infections.

29.10 Some natural products kill cancer cells by preventing cell division.

29.11 Some hormones and hormone antagonists are effective against prostate and breast cancer.

29.12 Targeted therapies and some miscellaneous antineoplastic drugs are effective against specific tumors.

29.13 Adjunct medications are sometimes necessary to treat cancer symptoms and to reduce the intensity of adverse effects from antineoplastic drugs.

Drug Snapshot

The following drugs are discussed in this chapter:

Drug Classes	Prototype Drugs
Alkylating drugs	Pr cyclophosphamide (Cytoxan)
Antimetabolites	Pr methotrexate (Rheumatrex, Trexall)
Antitumor antibiotics	Pr doxorubicin (Adriamycin)
Natural products	Pr vincristine (Oncovin)
Hormones and hormone antagonists	Pr tamoxifen

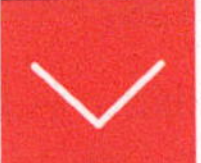

Learning Outcomes

After reading this chapter, the student should be able to:

1. Explain differences between normal cells and cancer cells.
2. Identify factors associated with an increased incidence of cancer.
3. Identify the primary goals of chemotherapy.
4. Explain why cancer is difficult to cure.
5. Explain how combination therapy and special dosing schedules increase the effectiveness of chemotherapy.
6. Describe the general adverse effects of antineoplastic drugs.
7. Explain the role of alkylating agents in the treatment of cancer.
8. Explain the role of antimetabolites in the treatment of cancer.
9. Explain the role of cytotoxic antibiotics in the treatment of cancer.
10. Explain the role of natural products in the treatment of cancer.
11. Explain the role of hormone and hormone antagonists in the treatment of cancer.
12. Explain the role of targeted therapies in the treatment of cancer.
13. Explain the role of adjunct medications in treating the adverse effects of cancer chemotherapy.

Key Terms

adenomas (AH-den-OH-mahz)
adjuvant chemotherapy (AD-ju-vent)
alkylation (AL-kill-AYE-shun)
alopecia (AL-oh-PEESH-ee-uh)
benign (bee-NINE)
cancer (KAN-sir)
carcinogens (kar-SIN-oh-jenz)
chemotherapy
folic acid (FOH-lik)
gliomas (glee-OH-muhz)
leukemia (lew-KEE-mee-ah)
lipomas (lip-OH-mahz)
liposomes (LIP-oh-sohms)
lymphomas (lim-FOH-mahz)
malignant (mah-LIG-nent)
metastasis (mah-TAS-tah-sis)
neoplasm (NEE-oh-PLAZ-um)
nitrogen mustards
palliation (PAL-ee-AYE-shun)
purines (PYUR-eenz)
pyrimidines (peer-IM-uh-deenz)
targeted therapies
taxanes (TAKS-anez)
topoisomerase (TOH-poh-eye-SOM-er-ase)
tumor (TOO-more)
tumor suppressor genes
vinca alkaloids (VIN-ka AL-kah-loids)

Cancer is one of the most feared diseases for a number of valid reasons. It may be silent, producing no symptoms until it is too advanced for a complete cure. It sometimes requires painful and disfiguring treatments. It may strike at an early age—even during childhood—depriving people of a normal lifespan. Perhaps worst of all, the medical treatment of cancer often cannot offer a cure, and progression to death is sometimes psychologically difficult for patients and their loved ones.

Despite its feared status, many advances have been made in the diagnosis, understanding, and treatment of cancer. Modern treatment methods result in a cure for nearly two of every three cancer patients and the 5-year survival rate has steadily increased for many types of cancer. This chapter examines the role of drugs in the treatment of cancer. Medications used to treat this disease are called anticancer drugs, antineoplastics, or cancer chemotherapeutic agents.

Core Concept 29.1 ▶ Cancer is characterized by rapid, uncontrolled growth of cells.

Cancer is a disease characterized by abnormal, uncontrolled cell division. Cell division is a normal process occurring extensively in most body tissues from conception to late childhood. At some point in time, however, most cells stop dividing at such a rapid rate. Indeed, some adult cells such as muscle cells and brain cells have a total lack of ability to divide. In other cells, the genes controlling growth can be turned back on whenever it is necessary to replace worn-out cells, as is the case for blood cells and cells lining the digestive tract.

Fast Facts Cancer

- It is estimated that more than 1,685,000 new cancer cases occur each year in the United States, with about 596,000 deaths (almost 1630 people every day).
- Although cancer occurs most frequently in older adults, over 10,000 new cases of childhood cancer occur annually.
- Leukemia is the most common childhood cancer and is responsible for about 30% of all cancers occurring before age 20.
- Lung cancer has the highest mortality rate in both women and men, being responsible for about 27% of all cancer deaths.
- Pancreatic cancer has the lowest 5-year survival rate at 8%. The highest 5-year survival rates are for cancers of the prostate, testes, and thyroid. The lowest survival rates are for pancreatic, lung, and liver cancers.
- Among ethnic groups, African Americans have the highest incidence and death rates for many types of cancers.

Source: Data from Cancer facts & figures 2016 by American Cancer Society.

Cancer is thought to result from the damage to genes controlling cell growth. Once damaged, the cell may become unresponsive to normal chemical signals checking its growth. The cancer cells lose their normal functions, divide rapidly, and invade surrounding cells. The abnormal cells often travel to distant sites, where they populate new tumors, a process called **metastasis**. Figure 29.1 illustrates the metastasis of cancer cells.

neo = *new*
plasm = *thing formed*

The word **tumor** means swelling, abnormal enlargement, or mass. **Neoplasm** is often used interchangeably with tumor. Tumors may be either benign or malignant.

adeno = *gland*
oma = *tumor*
lip = *fat*

Benign tumors grow slowly, do not metastasize, and rarely require drug treatment. Although they do not cause death, their growth may cause pressure on nerves, blood vessels, or other tissues. When this occurs, they may be surgically removed; they do not normally grow back. Examples include **adenomas**, which are benign tumors of glandular tissue, and **lipomas**, which are tumors of adipose tissue.

leuk = *white*
emia = *blood condition*

Malignant tumors are called cancer. The word **malignant** refers to a disease that grows rapidly worse, becomes resistant to treatment, and normally results in death. The two major divisions of malignant neoplasms are carcinomas and sarcomas. Other types include cancer of the blood-forming cells in bone marrow (**leukemia**), cancers of lymphatic tissue (**lymphomas**), and cancers of the central nervous system (CNS) (**gliomas**).

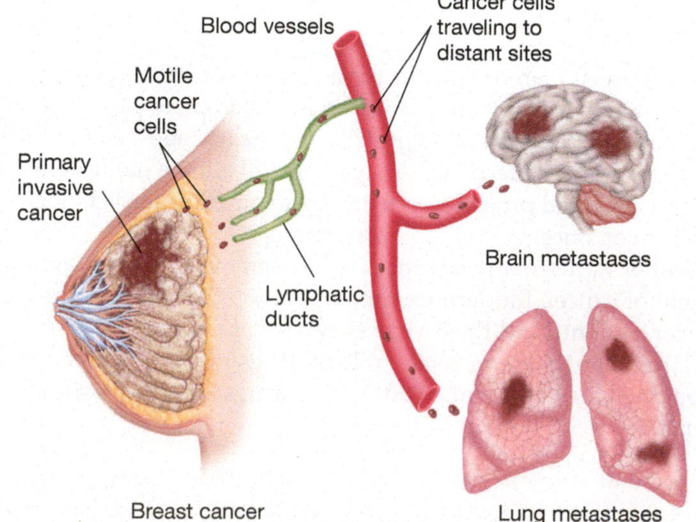

FIGURE 29.1 Invasion and metastasis by cancer cells.

The causes of cancer may be chemical, physical, or biological.

◀ Core Concept 29.2

A large number of factors have been found to cause cancer or to be associated with a higher risk for acquiring the disease. These factors are known as **carcinogens**.

Many chemical carcinogens have been identified. For example, chemicals in tobacco smoke are responsible for about one-third of all cancers in the United States. Some chemicals, such as asbestos and benzene, have been associated with a higher incidence of cancer in the workplace. The actual site of the cancer may be distant from the site of exposure, as is the case of bladder cancer caused by the inhalation of certain industrial chemicals.

A number of physical factors are also associated with cancer. For example, exposure to large amounts of x-rays is associated with a higher risk of leukemia. Ultraviolet (UV) light from the sun is a known cause of skin cancer, including melanoma.

Viruses are associated with about 15% of all human cancers. Examples include herpes simplex viruses types I and II, Epstein-Barr virus, human papillomavirus (HPV), cytomegalovirus, and human T-lymphotrophic viruses. Factors that suppress the immune system, such as HIV or drugs given after transplant surgery, may encourage the growth of cancer cells.

Some cancers have a strong genetic component. The fact that close relatives may acquire the same type of cancer suggests that the patient may have certain genes that predispose him or her to the condition. These abnormal genes interact with chemical, physical, and biological agents to promote cancer formation in the patient. Other genes, called **tumor suppressor genes**, may *inhibit* the formation of tumors. The *BRCA* gene is an example of a tumor suppressor gene that, once damaged, results in a significantly higher incidence of breast cancer. About 50% of women who have the BRCA mutation will develop breast cancer before age 70.

Fortunately, adopting healthy lifestyle habits may reduce the risk of acquiring cancer. The following list indicates some actions that healthcare providers can recommend to their patients to reduce their risk of cancer:

- Eliminate tobacco use and exposure to secondhand tobacco smoke.
- Maintain a healthy diet low in saturated fat and high in fresh vegetables and fruit.
- Choose most of the foods from plant sources, and increase fiber in the diet.
- Exercise regularly and keep body weight within optimal guidelines.
- Self-examine your body monthly for abnormal lumps and skin lesions.
- Avoid prolonged exposure to direct sunlight or wear protective clothing or sunscreen.
- For women, have periodic mammograms, according to the schedule recommended by their healthcare provider.
- For men, receive prostate screening, as recommended by their healthcare provider.
- Receive a screening colonoscopy, as recommended by the healthcare provider.
- Women who are sexually active or have reached age 21 should have a Pap test every 3–5 years, or as recommended by their healthcare provider.
- For preteen boys and girls, receive the HPV vaccine (Cervarix, Gardasil) according to the schedule recommended by the Centers for Disease Control and Prevention.

CONCEPT REVIEW 29.1

- What is the fundamental feature that makes a cancer cell different from a normal cell?

The three primary goals of chemotherapy are cure, control, and palliation.

◀ Core Concept 29.3

Pharmacotherapy of cancer is sometimes simply referred to as **chemotherapy**. Because oral and parenteral drugs are transported through the blood, chemotherapy has the potential to reach cancer cells in virtually any location. Chemotherapy has three general goals: cure, control, or palliation.

When diagnosed with cancer, the primary goal desired by most patients is to achieve a complete cure: permanent removal of all cancer cells from the body. The possibility for cure is much greater if a cancer is identified and treated in its early stages, when the tumor is small and localized to a well-defined region. Examples in which chemotherapy has been used successfully as curative treatments include Hodgkin lymphoma, certain leukemias, and choriocarcinoma.

When cancer has progressed and cure is not possible, a second goal of chemotherapy is to control or manage the disease. Although the cancer is not eliminated, preventing the growth and spread of the tumor may extend the patient's life. Essentially, the cancer is managed as a chronic disease, as is hypertension or diabetes.

In its advanced stages, cure or control of the cancer may not be achievable. For these patients, chemotherapy is used as **palliation**. Chemotherapy drugs are administered to reduce the size of the tumor, easing the severity of pain and other tumor symptoms, thus improving the quality of life.

Chemotherapy may be used alone or in combination with surgery or radiation therapy. Surgery is especially useful for removing solid tumors that are localized. Surgery lowers the number of cancer cells in the body so that radiation therapy and pharmacotherapy can be more successful. Surgery is not an option for cancer of the blood cells or when it would not be expected to extend a patient's lifespan or to improve the quality of life.

Approximately 50% of patients with cancer receive radiation therapy as part of their treatment. Radiation therapy is most successful for cancers that are localized. Radiation treatments are frequently prescribed postoperatively to kill cancer cells that may remain following an operation. Radiation is sometimes given as palliation for inoperable cancers to shrink the size of a tumor that may be pressing on vital organs and to relieve pain, difficulty breathing, or difficulty swallowing.

Adjuvant chemotherapy is the administration of antineoplastic drugs *after* surgery or radiation therapy. The purpose of adjuvant chemotherapy is to rid the body of any cancerous cells that were not removed during the surgery or to treat any microscopic metastases that may be developing. In a few cases, drugs are given as *chemoprophylaxis* with the goal of preventing cancer from occurring. For example, some patients who have had a primary breast cancer removed may receive tamoxifen, even if there is no evidence of metastases, because there is a high likelihood that the disease will recur. Chemoprophylaxis is uncommon, because most of these drugs have potentially serious adverse effects.

Core Concept 29.4 ▶

To achieve a total cure, every malignant cell must be removed or killed.

To cure a patient, it is believed that every single cancer cell must be eliminated from the body. Leaving even a single malignant cell could result in regrowth of the tumor. Eliminating every cancer cell, however, is a very difficult task.

Consider that a 1-cm breast tumor may contain 1 billion cancer cells before it is detected. A drug that kills 99% of these cells would be considered a very effective drug. Yet even with this fantastic achievement, 10 million cancer cells would still remain, any one of which could cause the tumor to return and kill the patient. The relationship between cell kill and chemotherapy is shown in Figure 29.2.

It is likely that no antineoplastic drug (or combination of drugs) will kill 100% of the tumor cells. The large burden of cancer cells, however, may be lowered sufficiently to permit the patient's immune system to control or eliminate the remaining cancer cells. Because the immune system is able to eliminate only a relatively small number of cancer cells, it is important that as many cancerous cells as possible be eliminated during treatment. This example reinforces the need to diagnose and treat tumors at an *early* stage, when the number of cancer cells is smaller.

Core Concept 29.5 ▶

Use of multiple drugs and special dosing schedules improve the success of chemotherapy.

Because of their rapid cell division, tumor cells express a high mutation rate. This causes the tumor to change its genetic make-up as it grows, resulting in hundreds of different clones with different growth rates and physiologic properties. An antineoplastic drug may kill only a small portion of the tumor, leaving some clones unaffected. Complicating the chances

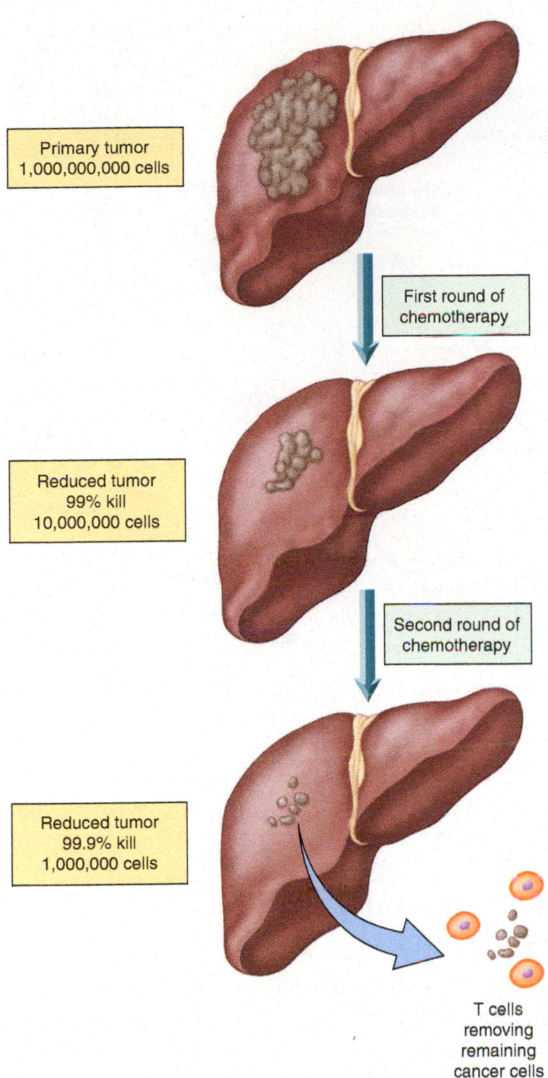

FIGURE 29.2 Cell kill and chemotherapy.

for a cure is that cancer cells often develop resistance to antineoplastic drugs. Thus a therapy that was very successful in reducing the tumor mass at the start of chemotherapy may become less effective over time.

A number of treatment strategies have been found to increase the effectiveness of anticancer drugs. In most cases, multiple medications from different antineoplastic classes are given concurrently during a course of chemotherapy. Multiple classes will affect different stages of the cancer cell's life cycle, as illustrated in Figure 29.3. This allows the tumor to be attacked through several mechanisms of action, thus increasing the cell kill percentage. Using multiple drugs also allows the dosages of each individual medication to be lowered, thereby reducing toxicity and slowing the development of resistance. Examples of common therapies include cyclophosphamide-methotrexate-fluorouracil (CMF) for breast cancer, cyclophosphamide-doxorubicin-vincristine (CAV) for lung cancer, and cyclophosphamide-doxorubicin-vincristine-prednisone (CHOP) for non-Hodgkin lymphoma. Each type of cancer requires its own individual protocol, which is continually being revised based on recent research.

Specific dosing schedules or cycles have been found to increase the effectiveness of antineoplastic drugs. For example, some anticancer drugs are given as single doses or perhaps a couple of doses over a few days. Several weeks may pass before the next series of doses. This gives normal cells time to recover from the adverse effects of the drugs, especially bone marrow suppression. It also allows tumor cells that may not have been replicating at the time of the first dose to begin dividing and become more sensitive to the next round of chemotherapy. The specific dosing schedule depends on the type of tumor, the stage of the disease, and the patient's overall condition.

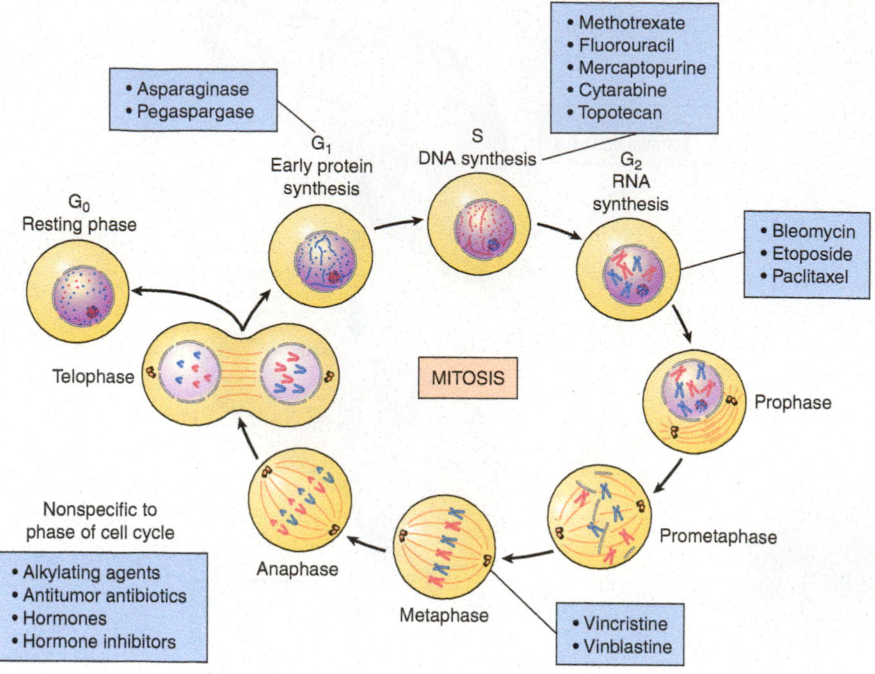

FIGURE 29.3 Antineoplastic drugs and the cell cycle.

CONCEPT REVIEW 29.2

- Why is it important to kill or remove 100% of the cancer cells to achieve a cure?

Core Concept 29.6 ▶

Serious toxicity limits therapy with most of the antineoplastic drugs.

Almost all anticancer drugs have the potential to cause serious toxicity. These drugs are often pushed to their maximum possible dosages so that the greatest tumor cell kill can be obtained. Such high dosages always result in adverse effects in the patient. A list of typical adverse effects of anticancer drugs is given in Table 29.1.

Normal tissues that are rapidly dividing in the adult are most susceptible to adverse effects. Hair follicles are damaged, resulting in hair loss or **alopecia**. The lining of the digestive tract is affected, sometimes resulting in bleeding, difficulty eating, or severe diarrhea. The vomiting center in the medulla of the brain is triggered by many antineoplastics, resulting in severe nausea and vomiting. Vomiting is often so severe that patients may be treated with antiemetic drugs such as ondansetron (Zofran) just prior to receiving the antineoplastic medication. Blood cells in the bone marrow may be destroyed, causing a reduction in the number of red blood cells (RBCs), white blood cells (WBCs), and platelets. Severe effects on blood cells may cause discontinuation of chemotherapy and lower the chances for a positive therapeutic outcome. Efforts to minimize this toxicity may include therapy with growth factors such as filgrastim (Neupogen) or sargramostim (Leukine). These drugs stimulate the production of WBCs within the bone marrow.

Antineoplastic drugs act by many mechanisms, most of which involve cell killing, or cytotoxicity. Classification is quite variable because some drugs kill cancer cells by several

Table 29.1 Adverse Effects of Anticancer Drugs

Blood Toxicity	GI Toxicity	Other Effects
Anemia (low RBC count)	Anorexia (loss of appetite)	Alopecia (loss of hair)
Leukopenia (low WBC count)	Bleeding	Fatigue
Thrombocytopenia (low platelet count)	Diarrhea	Fetal birth defects
	Nausea and vomiting	Opportunistic infections
	Stomatitis, ulceration and bleeding of the lips and gums	Sterility or loss of fertility

mechanisms and have characteristics from more than one class. Furthermore, the mechanisms by which some of these medications act are not completely understood. A simple method of classifying this complex class of drugs includes the following groups:

- Alkylating drugs
- Antimetabolites
- Antitumor antibiotics
- Natural products
- Hormones and hormone blockers
- Targeted therapies and miscellaneous drugs.

Alkylating drugs act by changing the structure of DNA in cancer cells.

◀ **Core Concept 29.7**

Alkylating drugs act by chemically binding to DNA and inhibiting cell division. They are some of the most widely used classes of antineoplastic drugs. Table 29.2 lists the alkylating drugs and their dosages.

The first alkylating drugs, the **nitrogen mustards**, were developed in secrecy as chemical warfare agents during World War II. Although the drugs in this class have very different chemical structures, all have the common characteristic of being able to form bonds or linkages with DNA. These agents physically attach to DNA, a process called **alkylation**. Alkylation changes the shape of DNA and prevents it from functioning normally. Although each alkylating drug attaches to DNA in a different manner, collectively they have the effect of inducing cell death, or at least slowing the replication of tumor cells. The alkylation may occur in any cancer cell; however, the killing action does not occur until the affected cell attempts to divide. Figure 29.4 illustrates the process of alkylation.

Table 29.2 Alkylating Drugs

Drg	Route and Adult Dose	Remarks
NITROGEN MUSTARDS		
bendamustine (Treanda)	IV: 90–120 mg/m^2 (variable schedule)	For chronic lymphocytic leukemia and non-Hodgkin lymphoma
chlorambucil (Leukeran)	PO: Initial dose 0.1–0.2 mg/kg daily; maintenance dose 4–10 mg daily	For chronic lymphocytic leukemia, non-Hodgkin lymphoma, and cancer of the breast and ovary
Pr cyclophosphamide (Cytoxan)	PO: Initial dose 1–5 mg/kg daily; maintenance dose 1–5 mg/kg every 7–10 days	For Hodgkin disease, non-Hodgkin lymphoma, leukemias, multiple myeloma, and cancer of the breast, ovary, and lung; IV form available
estramustine (Emcyt)	PO: 14 mg/kg/day in 3–4 divided doses	For palliative treatment of advanced prostate cancer
ifosfamide (Ifex)	IV: 1.2 g/m^2 daily for 5 consecutive days	For testicular cancer
mechlorethamine (Mustargen)	IV: 6 mg/m^2 on days 1 and 8 of a 28-day cycle	For Hodgkin disease, non-Hodgkin lymphoma, and lung cancer
melphalan (Alkeran)	PO: 6 mg daily for 2–3 weeks	For multiple myeloma
NITROSOUREAS		
carmustine (BiCNU, Gliadel)	IV: 200 mg/m^2 every 6 weeks	For Hodgkin disease, malignant melanoma, multiple myeloma, and brain cancer
lomustine (CeeNU)	PO: 130 mg/m^2 as a single dose	For Hodgkin disease and brain cancer
streptozocin (Zanosar)	IV: 500 mg/m^2 for 5 days	For pancreatic cancer
OTHER ALKYLATING DRUGS		
busulfan (Busulflex, Myleran)	PO: 4–8 mg daily	For chronic myelogenous leukemia; also available IV, prior to stem cell transplant
carboplatin (Paraplatin)	IV: 360 mg/m^2 every 4 weeks	For cancer of the ovary
cisplatin (Platinol)	IV: 20 mg/m^2 daily for 5 days	For testicular, bladder, ovarian, uterine, head, and neck carcinomas
dacarbazine (DTIC-Dome)	IV: 2–4.5 mg/kg daily for 10 days	For Hodgkin disease and malignant melanoma
oxaliplatin (Eloxatin)	IV: 85 mg/m^2 once every 2 weeks	For metastatic colorectal cancer
temozolomide (Temodar)	PO: 150 mg/m^2 daily for 5 consecutive days	For brain cancer
thiotepa (Thioplex)	IV: 0.3–0.4 mg/kg every 1–4 weeks	For Hodgkin disease and cancer of the bladder, breast, and ovary

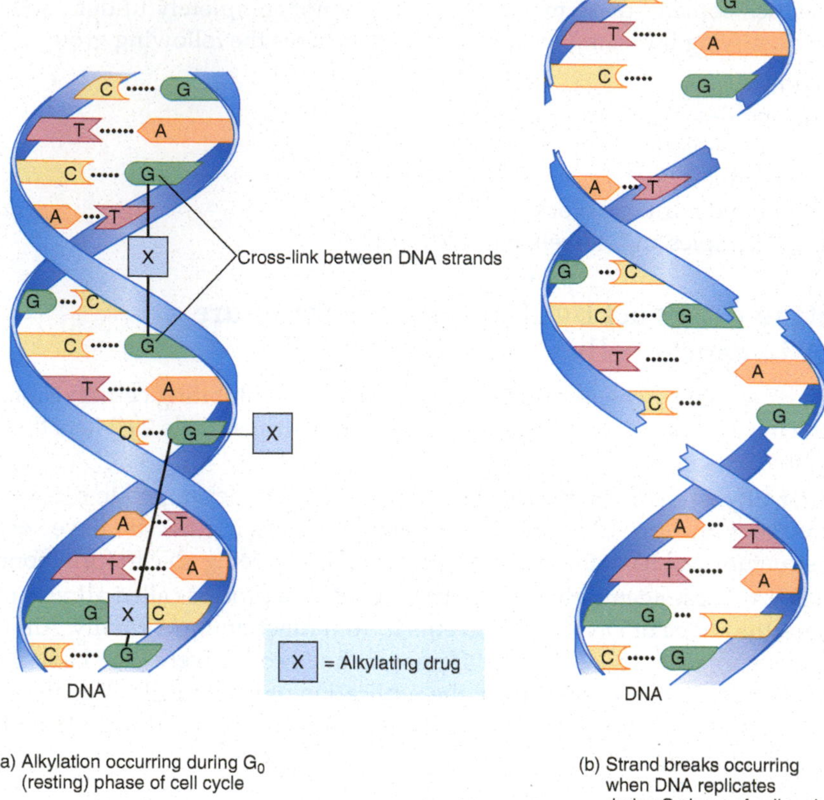

FIGURE 29.4 Mechanism of action of alkylating drugs.

Because blood cells are particularly sensitive to alkylating drugs, bone marrow suppression is the primary dose-limiting toxicity of these drugs. Within days of administration, the numbers of RBCs, WBCs, and platelets begin to decline. In addition to effects on the blood, cells lining the gastrointestinal (GI) tract are also damaged, resulting in nausea, vomiting, and diarrhea. Alopecia is expected from most of the alkylating drugs. As a delayed adverse effect, some patients treated with alkylating agents will develop acute leukemia 4 years or more after chemotherapy has been completed.

Prototype Drug: Pr *Cyclophosphamide (Cytoxan)*

Therapeutic Class: Antineoplastic Pharmacologic Class: Alkylating drug

Actions and Uses: Cyclophosphamide is a frequently prescribed alkylating agent. It is used alone or in combination with other drugs against a wide variety of cancers, including Hodgkin disease, leukemia, lymphoma, multiple myeloma, breast cancer, and ovarian cancer. Cyclophosphamide acts by attaching to DNA and disrupting cell replication, particularly in rapidly dividing cells. It is one of only a few anticancer drugs that are well absorbed when given orally.

Cyclophosphamide is a powerful immunosuppressant. Although this is considered an adverse effect during cancer chemotherapy, the drug is sometimes used to *intentionally* cause immunosuppression for the prophylaxis of organ transplant rejection and to treat severe rheumatoid arthritis and systemic lupus erythematosus (SLE).

Adverse Effects and Interactions: Bone marrow suppression is a potentially life-threatening adverse reaction that occurs during days 9–14 of therapy; the patient is at dangerous risk for severe infection and sepsis during this period. Thrombocytopenia is common; thus bleeding and bruising may be observed. Nausea, vomiting, and diarrhea are frequently experienced. Fifty percent of patients will develop baldness, although this effect is usually reversible. Patients should drink plenty of fluids and empty their bladder frequently to prevent hemorrhagic cystitis. Unlike other alkylating agents, cyclophosphamide causes little neurotoxicity.

Cyclophosphamide interacts with many drugs. For example, immunosuppressant agents may increase the risk of infections and promote the development of neoplasms. There is an increased chance of bone marrow toxicity if cyclophosphamide is used together with allopurinol. There is an increased risk of bleeding if given with anticoagulants.

If used with digoxin, decreased serum levels of digoxin occur. Phenobarbital, phenytoin, or glucocorticoids may lead to an increased rate of cyclophosphamide metabolism by the liver. Thiazide diuretic use with cyclophosphamide may lead to leukopenia. St. John's wort may increase the toxic effects of cyclophosphamide.

Antimetabolites disrupt critical cellular pathways in cancer cells.

◀ **Core Concept 29.8**

Rapidly growing cancer cells require large amounts of nutrients to build proteins and nucleic acids. Antimetabolites are drugs that chemically resemble essential building blocks of the cell. When cancer cells attempt to construct proteins or DNA, they use the antimetabolite drugs instead of the normal building blocks. By disrupting metabolic pathways in this manner, antimetabolites can kill cancer cells or slow their growth. For example, methotrexate interferes with the synthesis of folate. Folate is required for the synthesis of DNA, RNA, and protein in rapidly dividing cancer cells. The antimetabolites are listed in Table 29.3.

Table 29.3 Antimetabolites

Drug	Route and Adult Dose	Remarks
FOLIC ACID ANTAGONISTS		
Pr methotrexate (Rheumatrex, Trexall)	PO: 10–30 mg/day for 5 days	For acute lymphoblastic leukemia, choriocarcinoma, lymphoma, and cancer of the head, neck, testes, and bone; IV and IM forms available
pemetrexed (Alimta)	IV: 500 mg/m^2 on day 1 of each 21-day cycle	For malignant mesothelioma and non–small cell lung cancer
pralatrexate (Folotyn)	IV: 30 mg/m^2 administered over 3–5 minutes	For refractory T-cell lymphoma
PYRIMIDINE AND PURINE ANALOGS		
capecitabine (Xeloda)	PO: 2500 mg/m^2 daily for 2 weeks	For metastatic breast cancer and colon cancer
cladribine (Leustatin)	IV: 0.09 mg/m^2 for 7 days	For hairy cell leukemia
clofarabine (Clolar)	IV: 52 mg/m^2 for 5 days	For childhood acute lymphoblastic leukemia
cytarabine (Cytosar, Depot-Cyt)	IV: 200 mg/m^2 as a continuous infusion over 24 hours	For leukemias and lymphomas; subcutaneous and intrathecal forms available
fludarabine (Fludara)	IV: 25 mg/m^2 daily	For chronic lymphocytic leukemia
floxuridine (FUDR)	Intra-arterial: 0.1–0.6 mg/kg daily as a continuous infusion	For metastasis from the GI tract to the liver
fluorouracil (5-FU, Adrucil, Efudex)	IV: 12 mg/kg daily for 4 days	For cancer of the breast, colon, rectum, stomach, and pancreas; topical form available for basal cell carcinoma
gemcitabine (Gemzar)	IV: 1000 mg/m^2 every week	For advanced cancers of the pancreas, breast, ovaries, and lung
mercaptopurine (Purinethol)	PO: 2.5 mg/kg daily	For childhood acute leukemia
nelarabine (Arranon)	IV: 1500 mg/m^2 on days 1, 3, and 5; repeat every 21 days	For leukemias and lymphomas
pentostatin (Nipent)	IV: 4 mg/m^2 every other week	For hairy cell leukemia
thioguanine (Tabloid)	PO: 2 mg/kg daily	For remission induction in adult acute leukemia

Prototype Drug: Pr *Methotrexate (Rheumatrex, Trexall)*

Therapeutic Class: Antineoplastic **Pharmacologic Class:** Antimetabolite, folic acid analog

Actions and Uses: Methotrexate blocks folic acid metabolism in rapidly growing tumor cells. **Folic acid** is a water-soluble vitamin found in eggs, veal, liver, whole grains, and dark green vegetables. Folic acid is part of a coenzyme essential to the synthesis of nucleic acids.

Methotrexate is prescribed alone or in combination with other drugs for lymphoblastic leukemia, choriocarcinoma, lymphoma, and cancer of the head, neck, testes and bone. It is occasionally used to treat non-neoplastic disorders such as severe psoriasis, rheumatoid arthritis, and SLE that are unresponsive to safer medications.

Adverse Effects and Interactions: Methotrexate has many adverse effects, some of which can be life threatening and are described in the black box warning. In addition, hemorrhage and bruising due to low platelet counts are often observed. Nausea, vomiting, and anorexia are common. When methotrexate is given in high doses, leucovorin may be given within 24 hours to "rescue" normal cells from the toxic effects of the antimetabolite. Methotrexate is pregnancy category X.

Methotrexate interacts with several drugs. Bone marrow suppressants such as other antineoplastic drugs may cause increased effects; the patient will require a lower dose of methotrexate. When used with nonsteroidal anti-inflammatory drugs (NSAIDs), severe methotrexate toxicity may occur. Aspirin may interfere with excretion of methotrexate, leading to increased serum levels and toxicity. Administration with live oral vaccine may result in decreased antibody response and increased adverse reactions to the vaccine. Use with caution with herbal supplements, such as echinacea, which may interfere with the drug's immunosuppressant effects.

BLACK BOX WARNINGS:

Methotrexate combined with NSAIDs may cause severe and sometimes fatal bone marrow suppression, which is the primary dose-limiting toxicity of this drug. The drug is hepatotoxic and may cause liver cirrhosis. Ulcerative stomatitis and diarrhea require suspension of therapy because they may lead to intestinal bleeding or perforation. Potentially fatal opportunistic infections may occur during therapy. Pulmonary toxicity may result in acute or chronic interstitial pneumonitis at any dose level. Severe, sometimes fatal, dermatologic reactions such as toxic epidermal necrolysis and Stevens–Johnson syndrome (SJS) have been reported.

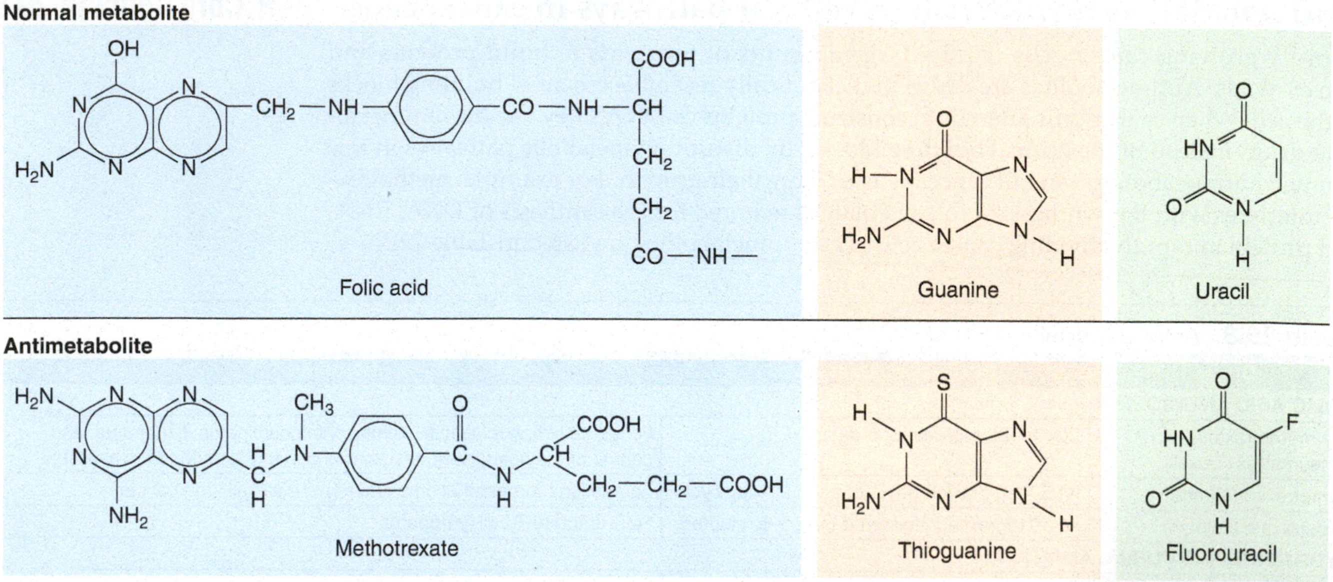

Normal metabolite

Folic acid | Guanine | Uracil

Antimetabolite

Methotrexate | Thioguanine | Fluorouracil

FIGURE 29.5 Structural similarities between antimetabolites and their natural counterparts.

Several of these antimetabolites resemble **purines** and **pyrimidines**, chemicals that are the building blocks of DNA and RNA. These antimetabolites are called purine or pyrimidine analogs. For example, floxuridine (FUDR) and fluorouracil (Adrucil) are able to block the formation of thymidylate, an essential chemical needed to make DNA. After becoming activated and incorporated into DNA, cytarabine (Cytosar) blocks DNA synthesis. Figure 29.5 illustrates the similarities of some of these analogs to their natural counterparts.

Core Concept 29.9 ▶

A few cytotoxic antibiotics are used to treat cancer rather than infections.

Antitumor antibiotics are drugs obtained from bacteria that have the ability to kill cancer cells. Although they are not widely prescribed, they are very effective against certain tumors. Table 29.4 lists the primary antitumor antibiotics.

Several substances isolated from bacteria have been found to possess antitumor properties. These chemicals are more toxic than the traditional antibiotics; thus, their use is restricted to treating specific cancers. All the antitumor antibiotics interact with DNA in a manner similar to the alkylating drugs. Because of this, their general actions and adverse

Table 29.4 Antitumor Antibiotics

Drug	Route and Adult Dose	Remarks
bleomycin (Blenoxane)	IV: 0.25–0.5 units/kg every 4–7 days	For squamous cell carcinoma, Hodgkin disease, lymphomas, and testicular cancer
dactinomycin (Cosmegen)	IV: 500 mcg/day for 5 days	For Wilms tumor and rhabdomyosarcoma
daunorubicin (Cerubidine)	IV: 30–60 mg/m^2 daily for 3–5 days	For leukemias and lymphomas
daunorubicin liposomal (DaunoXome)	IV: 40 mg/m^2 every 2 weeks	For Kaposi sarcoma
Pr doxorubicin (Adriamycin)	IV: 60–75 mg/m^2 as a single dose	For lymphomas, sarcomas, acute leukemia, and cancer of the breast, lung, testes, thyroid, and ovary
doxorubicin liposomal (Doxil, Evacet)	IV: 20 mg/m^2 every 3 weeks	For Kaposi sarcoma, refractory ovarian cancer, and refractory multiple myeloma
epirubicin (Ellence)	IV: 100–120 mg/m^2 as a single dose	For breast cancer
idarubicin (Idamycin)	IV: 8–12 mg/m^2 daily for 3 days	For acute myelogenous leukemia
mitomycin (Mutamycin)	IV: 2 mg/m^2 as a single dose	For cancer of the colon, stomach, lung, head and neck, rectum, bladder, pancreas, and breast; also for malignant melanoma
mitoxantrone (Novantrone)	IV: 12 mg/m^2 daily for 3 days	For acute nonlymphocytic leukemia

effects are similar to those of the alkylating drugs. Unlike the alkylating drugs, however, all the antitumor antibiotics must be administered IV or through direct instillation into a body cavity using a catheter. A major dose-limiting adverse effect of drugs in this class is bone marrow suppression.

Prototype Drug: Pr *Doxorubicin (Adriamycin)*

Therapeutic Class: Antineoplastic Pharmacologic Class: Antitumor antibiotic

Actions and Uses: Doxorubicin attaches to DNA, causing the double strands to be distorted, thus preventing cancer cell division. It is prescribed for solid tumors of the lung, breast, ovary, and bladder, and for certain types of leukemias and lymphomas. It is structurally similar to daunorubicin (Cerubidine). Doxorubicin is one of the most effective single drugs against solid tumors.

A novel delivery method for both doxorubicin and daunorubicin places the drug in small sacs, or lipid bilayer vesicles, called **liposomes**. The liposomal vesicle opens when it fuses with the plasma membrane of the cancer cell and releases the antitumor antibiotic. The goal is to deliver a higher concentration of drug directly to the cancer cells, thus sparing normal cells. Doxorubicin liposomal is approved for use in patients with Kaposi sarcoma, refractory ovarian tumors, and relapsed multiple myeloma.

Adverse Effects and Interactions: Doxorubicin has many adverse effects, some of which can be life threatening and are described in the black box warning. In addition, nausea, vomiting, diarrhea, and hair loss are common.

Doxorubicin interacts with many drugs. If digoxin is taken at the same time, the patient will have decreased serum digoxin levels. Phenobarbital leads to increased plasma clearance of doxorubicin and decreased effectiveness. Using doxorubicin with phenytoin may lead to decreased phenytoin levels and possible seizure activity. Liver toxicity may occur if mercaptopurine is taken at the same time. Using with verapamil may increase serum doxorubicin levels, leading to doxorubicin toxicity.

BLACK BOX WARNING:

Severe bone marrow suppression may occur, which is the major dose-limiting toxicity with doxorubicin. It may manifest as seriously low blood cell counts. Doxorubicin exhibits significant cardiotoxicity, which may be either acute or chronic. Cardiac adverse effects can be life threatening and may include sinus tachycardia, bradycardia, delayed heart failure, acute left ventricular failure, and myocarditis. Heart failure may occur months or years after the termination of therapy. Acute, IV infusion–related reactions may occur, including anaphylaxis. Severe local necrosis may result if extravasation occurs. Secondary malignancies, especially acute myelogenous leukemia, may occur 1 to 3 years following therapy.

Some natural products kill cancer cells by preventing cell division.

◀ **Core Concept 29.10**

Natural products are substances with anticancer properties that have been extracted from plants. The natural products used as antineoplastics are listed in Table 29.5.

Chemicals with antineoplastic activity have been isolated from a number of plants, including the common periwinkle (*Vinca rosea*), the Pacific yew, the mandrake plant (May apple), and the shrub *Campothecus acuminata.* Although structurally very different, drugs in this class have the common ability to arrest cell division; thus they are sometimes called *mitotic inhibitors.*

The **vinca alkaloids**, vincristine (Oncovin) and vinblastine (Velban), are older medications derived from the periwinkle plant. Their biological properties were described in folklore for many years in various parts of the world prior to their use as anticancer drugs.

Native Americans described uses of the May apple long before teniposide (Vumon) and etoposide (VePesid) were isolated from this plant and used for chemotherapy. These drugs are called **topoisomerase** inhibitors because they block the enzyme topoisomerase, an enzyme that helps repair DNA damage. This allows DNA damage to accumulate, eventually killing the tumor cell. Bone marrow suppression is a serious adverse effect of most natural product drugs. More recently isolated topoisomerase inhibitors include topotecan (Hycamtin), which is used to treat metastatic ovarian cancer and lung cancer, and irinotecan (Camptosar), which is indicated for metastatic cancer of the colon.

The **taxanes**, which include cabazitaxel (Jevtana), paclitaxel (Abraxane, Taxol), and docetaxel (Taxotere), were isolated from the Pacific yew, an evergreen found throughout the western United States. Paclitaxel is approved for metastatic ovarian and breast cancer and for Kaposi sarcoma; however, off-label uses include many other cancers. Bone marrow toxicity is usually the dose-limiting factor for the taxanes.

Table 29.5 Natural Products

Drug	Route and Adult Dose	Remarks
VINCA ALKALOIDS		
vinblastine (Velban)	IV: 3.7–18.5 mg/m^2 every week	For cancer of the breast and testes, and Hodgkin disease
Pr vincristine (Oncovin, Vincasar)	IV: 1.4 mg/m^2 every week (max: 2 mg/m^2)	For acute leukemias, Hodgkin disease, lymphosarcoma, neuroblastoma, Wilms tumor, lung and breast cancer, reticular cell carcinoma, and osteogenic sarcomas
vincristine liposome (Marquibo)	IV: 2.25 mg/m^2 once every week	For acute lymphoblastic leukemia
vinorelbine (Navelbine)	IV: 30 mg/m^2 every week	For lung cancer
TAXANES		
cabazitaxel (Jevtana)	IV: 25 mg/m^2 every 3 weeks	For prostate cancer
docetaxel (Taxotere)	IV: 60–100 mg/m^2 every 3 weeks	For ovarian cancer, metastatic breast and prostate cancer, advanced stomach cancer, and lung cancer
paclitaxel (Abraxane, Taxol)	IV: 135–175 mg/m^2 every 3 weeks	For Kaposi sarcoma, ovarian cancer, metastatic breast cancer, lung cancer, and certain other solid tumors
TOPOISOMERASE INHIBITORS AND OTHER NATURAL PRODUCTS		
eribulin (Halaven)	IV: 1.4 mg/m^2 on days 1 and 8 of a 21-day cycle	For metastatic breast cancer and liposarcoma; inhibits microtubule formation
etoposide (VePesid)	IV: 50–100 mg/m^2 daily for 5 days	For testicular and lung cancer, and choriocarcinomas; PO form available
irinotecan (Camptosar)	IV: 125 mg/m^2 every week for 4 weeks	For colorectal cancer
omacetaxine (Synribo)	Subcutaneous: 1.25 mg/m^2 for 14 days	For chronic myeloid leukemia; inhibits protein synthesis
teniposide (Vumon)	IV: 165 mg/m^2 every 3–4 days for 4 weeks	For acute lymphocytic leukemia
topotecan (Hycamtin)	IV: 1.5 mg/m^2 daily for 5 days	For ovarian cancer

Prototype Drug: Pr *Vincristine (Oncovin)*

Therapeutic Class: Antineoplastic Pharmacologic Class: Vinca alkaloid, plant extract

Actions and Uses: Vincristine affects rapidly growing cells by inhibiting their ability to complete mitosis. Although it must be given IV, a major advantage of vincristine is that it causes minimal immunosuppression. It is prescribed in combination with other antineoplastics for many different cancers (see Table 29.5). A newer form of vincristine (Marquibo), encased in a liposomal carrier, is approved for acute lymphoblastic leukemia.

Adverse Effects and Interactions: Vincristine has many adverse effects, some of which can be life threatening and are described in the black box warning. In addition, the major dose-limiting adverse effect of vincristine is neurotoxicity. Symptoms include numbness and tingling in the limbs, muscular weakness, loss of neural reflexes, and pain. CNS effects may include seizures, depression, hallucinations, and coma. Severe constipation is common. Reversible alopecia occurs in most patients.

Vincristine interacts with many drugs. Asparaginase used together with or before vincristine may cause increased neurotoxicity secondary to decreased liver clearance of vincristine. When used with digoxin, the patient may need an increased digoxin dose. Vincristine may decrease serum phenytoin levels, leading to increased seizure activity. Statin medications will increase the serum levels of vincristine. Use with St. John's wort can lower the serum levels of vincristine.

BLACK BOX WARNINGS:
Myelosuppression may be severe and predispose to opportunistic infections. Extravasation can cause intense pain, inflammation, and tissue necrosis. If extravasation occurs, treatment with warm compresses and hyaluronidase is recommended; cold compresses will significantly increase the toxicity of vinca alkaloids.

Core Concept 29.11 ▶ Some hormones and hormone antagonists are effective against prostate and breast cancer.

Use of hormones or hormone antagonists is a strategy that slows the growth of hormone-dependent tumors. Most hormone therapies are limited to treating hormone-sensitive tumors of the breast or prostate. The major hormones and hormone antagonists prescribed for cancer are given in Table 29.6.

The growth of certain tumors of reproductive tissues is greatly stimulated by natural hormones. Administering high doses of specific hormones or hormone antagonists can block these receptors and slow tumor growth. For example, administering the male hormone testosterone or the antiestrogen drug tamoxifen can slow specific types of breast cancer that depend on estrogen for growth. Tamoxifen is one of the most widely used drugs for this type of cancer. Administration of the female sex hormone estrogen slows the growth of prostate cancer. The

Table 29.6 Hormones and Hormone Antagonists

Drug	Route and Adult Dose	Remarks
HORMONES		
dexamethasone (Decadron, others)	PO: 0.25 mg bid–qid	For palliative treatment of leukemias and lymphomas
diethylstilbestrol (DES, Stilbestrol)	PO: 1–15 mg daily	For cancer of the prostate and breast
ethinyl estradiol (Estinyl, others)	PO: 1 mg tid for 2–3 months (breast cancer) or 0.15–3 mg/day (prostate cancer)	For cancer of the prostate and breast, and contraception
fluoxymesterone (Halotestin)	PO: 10 mg tid	For breast cancer
medroxyprogesterone (Depo-Provera, Provera) (see the Prototype Drug box in Core Concept 35.4)	IM: 400–1000 mg every week	For uterine and renal cancer, dysfunctional uterine bleeding, and contraception
megestrol (Megace)	PO: 40–160 mg bid–qid	For advanced cancer of the prostate and breast
prednisone (see the Prototype Drug box in Core Concept 25.5)	PO: 20–100 mg day	For acute leukemia, Hodgkin disease, lymphomas, and many inflammatory conditions
testosterone (Andro 100, Histerone, Testred, Delatest)	IM: 200–400 mg every 2–4 weeks	For breast cancer in women and hypogonadism in men
HORMONE ANTAGONISTS		
abiraterone (Zytiga)	PO: 1 g once daily in combination with prednisone	For prostate cancer
anastrozole (Arimidex)	PO: 1 mg daily	For advanced breast cancer
bicalutamide (Casodex)	PO: 50 mg daily	For metastatic prostate cancer
degarelix (Firmagon)	Subcutaneous: 240 mg loading dose followed by 80 mg every 28 days	For advanced prostate cancer
enzalutamide (Xtandi)	PO: 160 mg once daily	For metastatic prostate cancer
exemestane (Aromasin)	PO: 25 mg daily after a meal	For advanced breast cancer
flutamide (Eulexin)	PO: 250 mg tid	For prostate cancer
fulvestrant (Faslodex)	IM: 500 mg on days 1, 15, 29, then once a month thereafter	For metastatic breast cancer
goserelin (Zoladex)	Subcutaneous: 3.6 mg every 28 days	For prostate and breast cancer, dysfunctional uterine bleeding, and endometriosis
histrelin (Vantas)	Implant: One subcutaneous implant every 12 months (50 mg)	For palliation of advanced prostate cancer
letrozole (Femara)	PO: 2.5 mg daily	For advanced breast cancer
leuprolide (Eligard, Lupron, Viadur)	Subcutaneous: 1 mg daily	For palliation of advanced prostate cancer, endometriosis, and precocious puberty; IM depot form available
nilutamide (Nilandron)	PO: 150-300 mg/daily	For metastatic prostate cancer
raloxifene (Evista) (see the Prototype Drug box in Core Concept 36.4)	PO : 60 mg once daily	For prophylaxis of breast cancer; treatment of osteoporosis in postmenopausal women
Pr tamoxifen	PO (breast cancer): 20-40 mg/day PO (breast cancer prophylaxis): 20 mg daily	For breast cancer treatment and prophylaxis
toremifene (Fareston)	PO: 60 mg daily	For metastatic breast cancer
triptorelin (Trelstar)	IM: 3.75 mg once monthly, 11.25 mg q12wk or 22.5 mg q24wk	For palliation of advanced prostate cancer

other major class of hormones used for chemotherapy is the corticosteroids. When used for chemotherapy, the doses of these hormones are much higher than the levels normally found in the body. Additional indications for hormone pharmacotherapy are discussed in Chapter 32.

As a group, hormones and hormone antagonists are the least toxic of the antineoplastic classes. They can, however, cause serious adverse effects when given at high doses for prolonged periods. Because they rarely produce cancer cures when used singly, these drugs are normally given for palliation.

CONCEPT REVIEW 29.3

- Would a patient with breast cancer be given estrogen, or an estrogen antagonist? Explain your answer.

Prototype Drug: Pr *Tamoxifen*

Therapeutic Class: Antineoplastic **Pharmacologic Class:** Hormone, estrogen receptor blocker

Actions and Uses: Because it blocks estrogen receptors in cancer cells, tamoxifen is sometimes classified as an antiestrogen. Tamoxifen is effective against breast tumors that require estrogen for their growth. These susceptible cancer cells are known as estrogen receptor (ER)-positive cells. Tamoxifen is given orally and is a preferred drug for treating metastatic breast cancer in both men and women.

A unique feature of tamoxifen is that it is one of the few antineoplastics approved for prophylaxis of breast cancer—for high-risk patients who are at risk of developing the disease. In addition, it is approved as adjunctive therapy in women following mastectomy to decrease the potential for cancer in the other breast.

Adverse Effects and Interactions: Other than nausea and vomiting, tamoxifen produces little of the serious toxicity observed with other antineoplastics. Hot flashes, fluid retention, venous blood clots, and abnormal vaginal bleeding are relatively common. When used in men, the drug may cause a loss of libido and impotence.

Tamoxifen interacts with several drugs. For example, anticoagulants may increase the risk of bleeding. Using this drug with cytotoxic drugs may increase the risk of blood clots.

BLACK BOX WARNINGS:

The most serious problem associated with tamoxifen use is the increased risk of endometrial cancer. The benefits of tamoxifen outweigh the risks in women who are taking tamoxifen to *treat* breast cancer. The benefit versus risk is not as clear in women who are taking tamoxifen to *prevent* breast cancer. There is also a slightly increased risk of thromboembolic disease, including stroke, pulmonary embolism, and deep vein thrombosis (DVT), with the use of tamoxifen. The risk of a thromboembolic event is believed to be about the same as for oral contraceptives.

Core Concept 29.12 ▶ Targeted therapies and some miscellaneous antineoplastic drugs are effective against specific tumors.

Although they originate from normal cells, cancer cells are clearly different. Scientists have been quite productive in finding ways that cancer cells differ, and in developing drugs that take advantage of these differences. Dozens of new antineoplastic drugs are now available that target specific aspects of cancer cell physiology. These drugs, appropriately called **targeted therapies**, were developed with the hope that they would be more selective in their cell killing than existing drugs and thus cause fewer adverse effects in normal cells. Unfortunately, this has not always been the case.

Monoclonal antibodies (MABs) are types of targeted therapies that are engineered to attack only one specific type of tumor cell. Once the MAB binds to its target cell, the cancer cell dies or is marked for destruction by other cells of the immune response. For example, rituximab (Rituxan) is a MAB that binds to CD20, a surface protein present on cancerous B lymphocytes. Once bound, rituximab shatters the tumor cells. As is typical of MABs, the action of rituximab is very specific: It was designed to only affect tumor cells with the CD20 protein. The key point about MABs is that the tumor cells must possess the specific protein receptor; otherwise, the MAB will be ineffective.

The largest group of targeted therapies attack tyrosine kinase, a key enzyme for cell growth. The development of new targeted therapies for cancer is progressing at a rapid rate. These drugs, along with some miscellaneous antineoplastics, are shown in Table 29.7.

All targeted therapies, including the MABs, are very specific: They are designed to affect only cells with certain antibodies or proteins. The key point about targeted therapies is that the tumor cells must possess the specific antibody or protein; otherwise, the drug will be ineffective.

Core Concept 29.13 ▶ Adjunct medications are sometimes necessary to treat cancer symptoms and to reduce the intensity of adverse effects from antineoplastic drugs.

Antineoplastic drugs are only part of the arsenal of medications used to treat cancer patients. Adjunctive medications are those used to supplement the primary therapies. The three primary groups of drugs used as adjunctive therapy are opioid analgesics, antiemetics, and hematopoietic drugs.

Many types of cancer produce extreme pain, which affects the patient's quality of life. Indeed, pain management is one of the primary concerns of both patients and healthcare providers. Pain management proceeds up a ladder, starting with NSAIDs to the weak

Table 29.7 Selected Targeted Therapies and Miscellaneous Anticancer Drugs*

Drug	Route and Adult Dose	Remarks
altretamine (Hexalen)	PO: 65 mg/m^2/day	For ovarian cancer
arsenic trioxide (Trisenox)	IV: 0.15 mg/kg/day	For acute promyelocytic leukemia
axitinib (Inlyta)	PO: 5 mg bid	For advanced renal cancer
bevacizumab (Avastin)	IV: 5 mg/kg every 14 days	For metastatic colorectal cancer
bosutinib (Bosulif)	PO: 500 mg once daily	For chronic myelogenous leukemia
cetuximab (Erbitux)	IV: 400 mg/m^2 over 2 hours, then 250 mg/m^2 over 1 hour weekly	For metastatic colorectal cancer
dinutuximab (Unituxin)	IV: 17.5 mg/m^2/day for 4 days	For pediatric neuroblastoma
erlotinib (Tarceva)	PO: 150 mg once daily	For metastatic non–small cell lung cancer
gefitinib (Iressa)	PO: 250–500 mg/day	For advanced lung cancer
ibrutinib (Imbruvica)	PO: 420 mg (three 140-mg capsules) daily	For chronic lymphocytic leukemia
imatinib (Gleevec)	PO: 400–600 mg daily	For chronic myeloid leukemia after failure with interferon alfa therapy
interferon alfa-2 (Intron A) (see the Prototype Drug box in Core Concept 26.4)	Subcutaneous or IM: 2–3 million units daily for leukemia; 36 million units daily for Kaposi sarcoma	For hairy cell leukemia, Kaposi sarcoma, non-Hodgkin lymphoma, and malignant melanoma; also for chronic hepatitis B and C viral infections
ixazomib (Ninlaro)	PO: 4 mg on days 1, 8, and 15 of a 28-day cycle	For multiple myeloma
levamisole (Ergamisol)	PO: 50 mg tid for 3 days	For colon cancer
mitotane (Lysodren)	PO: 3–4 mg tid–qid	For adrenal cortex cancer
ofatumumab (Arzerra)	IV: 300 mg initial dose followed by 2000 mg weekly for 7 doses	Newer antineoplastic drug; for chronic lymphocytic leukemia
pazopanib (Votrient)	PO: 800 mg once daily	Newer antineoplastic drug; for advanced renal carcinoma
pegaspargase (Oncaspar, PEG-L-asparaginase)	IV: 2500 international units/m^2 every 14 days	For acute lymphocytic leukemia; IM form available
pertuzumab (Perjeta)	IV: 840 mg followed every 3 weeks thereafter by 420 mg	For metastatic breast cancer
pomalidomide (Pomalyst)	PO: 4 mg/day for 21 days	For multiple myeloma
procarbazine (Matulane)	PO: 2–4 mg/kg daily	For Hodgkin disease
regorafenib (Stivarga)	PO: 160 mg/day for the first 21 days of each 28-day cycle	For metastatic colorectal cancer and GI tumors
rituximab (Rituxan)	IV: 375 mg/m^2 daily as a continuous infusion	For non-Hodgkin lymphomas
sunitinib (Sutent)	PO: 50 mg once daily for 4 weeks followed by 2 weeks off	For gastrointestinal, advanced renal and pancreatic tumors
trastuzumab (Herceptin) and ado-trastuzumab (Kadcycla)	IV (Herceptin): 4 mg/kg as a single dose, then 2 mg/kg every week IV (Kadcycla): 3.6 mg/kg every 3 weeks	For metastatic breast cancer
vismodegib (Erivedge)	PO: 150 mg once daily	For advanced or metastatic basal cell carcinoma
ziv-aflibercept (Zaltrap)	IV: 4 mg/kg every 2 weeks	For metastatic colorectal cancer
zoledronic acid (Zometa)	IV: 4 mg over at least 15 minutes	For multiple myeloma, severe hypercalcemia caused by malignancy, and Paget disease

*This table includes a selected sample of drugs in this class. For a complete listing, see Adams & Urban, *Pharmacology: Connections to Nursing Practice*, 3rd ed., 2016. Hoboken, NJ: Pearson.

opioid analgesics (codeine) and eventually to the strongest opioids (morphine, fentanyl, hydromorphone). Drug combinations may be used to achieve optimal pain control. At high levels, opioids produce significant adverse effects (see Chapter 15).

Chemotherapy-induced nausea and vomiting (CINV) can be debilitating for patients. CINV can occur in the first few hours after the initiation of chemotherapy, or be delayed more than 24 hours. Antineoplastics are classified as their emetogenic potential and those with the highest potential require adjunctive therapy with antiemetics. The most effective drugs used for this purpose are in a class called serotonin receptor antagonists. Examples include palonosetron (Alxi) and ondansetron (Zofran, Zuplenz), which can be given as an orally disintegrating tablet. The antiemetic drugs are presented in Chapter 31.

Many antineoplastic drugs are toxic to bone marrow and can produce serious blood abnormalities. Some drugs are given during chemotherapy to limit or counteract this toxicity. Oprelvekin (Neumega) stimulates platelet production and helps to prevent severe thrombocytopenia. Epoetin alfa (Epogen, Procrit) stimulates RBC production and is used to limit **anemia** caused by certain antineoplastics. Administration of filgrastim (Neupogen) increases neutrophil production in patients with cancer whose bone marrow has been suppressed by antineoplastic drugs. Low WBC counts (neutropenia) often result in severe bacterial and fungal infections in patients during chemotherapy or following organ transplants. A prototype feature for epoetin alfa is presented in Chapter 24.

Nursing Process Focus Patients Receiving Antineoplastic Therapy

ASSESSMENT	POTENTIAL NURSING DIAGNOSES*
Prior to administration: • Obtain a complete health history, including GI, renal and liver conditions, allergies, drug history, past infections, and possible drug interactions. • Evaluate laboratory blood findings: complete blood count (CBC), platelets, electrolytes, uric acid, glucose, and renal and liver function studies. • Acquire the results of a complete physical examination, including vital signs, height, weight, and any diagnostic test dependent on type of antineoplastic therapy (audiology, cardiac, electromyography). • Determine neurologic status, including level of consciousness (LOC), mood, or sensory impairment. • Collect information about previous immunization and a history or presence of herpes zoster or chickenpox.	• *Infection* related to compromised immune system secondary to adverse effects of antineoplastic drugs and disease process • *Imbalanced Nutrition: Less than Body Requirements* related to nausea, vomiting, diarrhea, and anorexia secondary to adverse effects of drug therapy • *Impaired Skin Integrity* related to extravasation of antineoplastic drug therapy • *Fatigue* related to adverse effects of drug therapy • *Fear* related to lack of knowledge of disease process and effects of treatment regimen • *Deficient Knowledge* related to lack of information about drug therapy • *Risk for Disturbed Body Image* related to physical changes from the adverse effects of drug therapy or other treatment regimens

PLANNING: PATIENT GOALS AND EXPECTED OUTCOMES

The patient will:
- Experience therapeutic effects (a reduction in tumor mass or progression of abnormal cell growth).
- Experience minimal adverse effects from drug therapy.
- Verbalize an understanding of the drug's use, adverse effects, and required precautions.

IMPLEMENTATION

Interventions and (Rationales)	Patient Education/Discharge Planning
• Monitor immune status. Observe signs and symptoms for potential and actual infections, and monitor laboratory tests such as CBC, specifically WBC and neutrophil counts. (Most antineoplastic drugs cause immunosuppression neutropenia.)	Instruct the patient to: • Wash their hands frequently, using proper technique. • Immediately report profound fatigue, fever, sore throat, epigastric pain, coffee-grounds vomit, bruising, tarry stools, or frank bleeding to the healthcare provider. • Avoid crowded indoor places and persons with active infections. • Monitor vital signs daily, ensuring proper use of home equipment. • Take temperature every 4 hours, if symptoms indicate a need, and notify the healthcare provider if it goes above approved parameters. • Not use antipyretics unless approved by the oncology provider. • Not eat raw foods. Cook foods thoroughly or allow family members to prepare raw foods. • Anticipate fatigue and balance daily activities to prevent exhaustion.

Interventions and (Rationales)	Patient Education/Discharge Planning
• Monitor cardiac and respiratory status, including vital signs, heart and breath sounds, presence of edema, electrocardiogram (ECG), and laboratory testing. (Many antineoplastic agents, such as alkylating drugs, antimetabolites, and antitumor antibodies, have adverse effects that cause problems with the cardiac and respiratory systems.)	Instruct the patient: • To report immediately any problems with dyspnea; pain in the chest, arm, neck, or back; tachycardia; cough; frothy sputum; swelling; or activity intolerance to the healthcare provider. • To adhere to the laboratory testing regimen for serum blood level tests (CBC, clotting factors, chemistry panel), as directed. Alert laboratory personnel of chemotherapy use. • That heart changes may be a sign of drug toxicity; heart failure may not appear for up to 6 months after completion of doxorubicin therapy.
• Monitor nutritional status. Administer antiemetics 30–45 minutes prior to antineoplastic administration or at the first sign of nausea. (Profound nausea, dry heaves, and vomiting are common with antineoplastic therapy. Dry mouth can also occur. Dietary consultation may be needed.)	Instruct the patient to: • Report loss of taste sensation, appetite, nausea, or vomiting. • Consume frequent small, high calorie, and nutrient dense meals. Nutritional supplements may help. • Avoid foods with strong odors, spicy foods, high-roughage, and very hot or cold foods. • Avoid carbonated and acidic beverages, alcohol, and caffeine.
• Monitor for mucositis. (Antineoplastic drugs may cause significant mucositis because of their effects on rapidly dividing cells.)	Instruct the patient to: • Examine mouth daily for changes and report the presence of mouth redness, soreness, or ulcers. Also report any changes in quality of voice or swallowing ability. • Maintain regular dental exams. • Encourage frequent oral hygiene (after each meal and at bedtime), use of lip balm, and avoidance of alcohol-based mouthwash, which can be drying to the mucosa. • Use a soft toothbrush; avoid toothpicks.
• Monitor for diarrhea and constipation. (An adverse effect of many antineoplastic drugs is diarrhea although severe constipation may occur with vincristine use, especially among older adults.)	Instruct the patient to: • Report changes in bowel habits to the healthcare provider. • Report excessive diarrhea, especially if it contains blood or mucus. • Increase fluid intake 2–3 L a day to prevent constipation.
• Monitor liver function tests. (Antineoplastics are metabolized by the liver, increasing the risk of hepatotoxicity.)	Instruct the patient to: • Report nausea, vomiting, jaundice, abdominal pain, tenderness or bloating, or light or clay-colored stool to the healthcare provider. • Comply with laboratory testing regimen for serum blood level tests of liver enzymes, as directed.
• Monitor deep tendon reflexes (DTR), neurologic and sensory status, and LOC. (Alkylating drugs such as cyclophosphamide and natural product antineoplastics such as vincristine have neurologic adverse effects. Such neurologic changes may be irreversible.)	Instruct the patient to: • Report any changes in skin color, vision, hearing; numbness or tingling; staggering gait; changes in consciousness; or depressed mood to the healthcare provider.
• Monitor genitourinary status: intake and output, daily weights, and renal function tests. (Antineoplastic drugs may cause significant renal toxicity. Hormones, especially tamoxifen, increase the risk of endometrial cancer and may alter menstrual cycles in women and may produce impotence in men.)	Instruct the patient: • To report the following immediately to the healthcare provider: diminished urinary output; changes in thirst; changes in color, quantity, and character of urine (e.g., "cloudy," with odor or sediment); joint, suprapubic, abdominal, flank, or lower back pain; difficult urination; and weight gain • That doxorubicin will turn urine red-brown for 1 to 2 days after administration; blood in the urine may occur several months after cyclophosphamide has been discontinued. • To increase fluid intake to 2–3 L a day. • To report changes in menstruation, sexual functioning, or vaginal discharge. • To recognize the risk of endometrial cancer before taking tamoxifen.

(*Continued*)

Nursing Process Focus *(continued)*

Interventions and (Rationales)	Patient Education/Discharge Planning
• Monitor for hypersensitivity or other adverse reactions. (Antineoplastic drugs may cause significant hypersensitivity and allergic responses.)	• Instruct the patient to immediately report chest or throat tightness, difficulty swallowing, swelling (especially facial), abdominal pain, headache, or dizziness to the healthcare provider.
• Monitor hair and skin status. (Alopecia is associated with most antineoplastic drugs. Alkylating and antimetabolites may cause significant skin reactions, including SJS.)	Instruct the patient to: • Immediately report shedding or peeling of skin on hands and feet, rash, pruritus, acne, or boils to the healthcare provider. • Wear a cold gel cap during chemotherapy to minimize hair loss.
• Monitor for conjunctivitis. (Doxorubicin may cause conjunctivitis.)	• Instruct the patient or caregiver to immediately report eye redness, stickiness, weeping, or pain.
• Administer with caution to patients with diabetes mellitus. (Hypoglycemia may occur secondary to the combination of cyclophosphamide and insulin.)	Instruct the patient to: • Report any signs and symptoms of hypoglycemia (e.g., sudden weakness, tremors) to the healthcare provider. • Monitor blood glucose daily; consult the healthcare provider regarding reportable results (e.g., less than 70 mg/dL).
• Be aware of specific policies and procedures related to antineoplastic administration. (Intense education programs are usually required prior to administering chemotherapy drugs.)	• Provide the patient, family, and caregiver education and support when giving antineoplastic (chemotherapy) drugs.

EVALUATION OF OUTCOME CRITERIA

Evaluate the effectiveness of drug therapy by confirming that patient goals and expected outcomes have been met (see "Planning"). *See Tables 29.2–29.7 for lists of drugs to which these nursing actions apply.*

Patients Need to Know

Patients treated for cancer need to know the following:

1. If hair loss is expected, cut long hair and be fitted for a wig or hairpiece before starting treatment. Select hats, scarves, or turbans. Use mild shampoo and conditioner.
2. Limit sun exposure; wear sunscreen, sunglasses, and long sleeves when outdoors. When hair is lost, protect the scalp from sunburn with sunscreen or a hat.
3. Eat foods that appeal in small amounts at frequent intervals if appetite is decreased. A healthcare provider may provide an appetite stimulant such as megestrol (Megace).
4. Discuss drugs to control nausea with a healthcare provider if nausea is a problem. Drink liquids between meals rather than with food.
5. Because the mouth may become irritated or ulcerated, avoid alcohol-based mouthwash, and use plain water or a mild salt solution instead. Use a soft toothbrush. Avoid spicy foods and very hot or very cold food and drink. Ask about a mouth rinse prepared with Benadryl, Maalox, and Xylocaine to coat, soothe, and numb.
6. Because chemotherapy may decrease sperm production or increase the risk of genetic damage to sperm, consider sperm banking prior to receiving chemotherapy. Women may choose to harvest and store eggs if infertility is a risk factor with therapy.
7. Increase fluid intake to decrease the risk of kidney damage and uric acid crystal formation.
8. Avoid exposure to crowds and individuals with infections or recent vaccinations because the immune system may be less able to protect you. Report temperatures of 101°F (38°C) or higher.
9. Follow a neutropenic diet if WBC count is significantly reduced. Avoid raw fruits and vegetables, peppercorns, and raw fish and meat.
10. Report easy bruising, blood in the stool or urine, vomiting, severe fatigue, epigastric pain, and difficulty clotting. Many chemotherapeutic drugs reduce production platelets needed for clot formation.

Chapter Review

Core Concepts Summary

29.1 Cancer is characterized by rapid, uncontrolled growth of cells.

Cancer cells grow rapidly, seemingly unaffected by their host surroundings. Cancer cells continue dividing until they invade normal tissues and eventually metastasize. Benign neoplasms grow slowly and rarely result in death. Malignant neoplasms, also known as cancer, are fast growing and often fatal.

29.2 The causes of cancer may be chemical, physical, or biological.

Many environmental factors have been found to cause or promote cancer. The genetic make-up of the patient plays an important role in whether or not cancer will develop after exposure to carcinogens. Eliminating tobacco use and limiting the intake of saturated fats and alcohol are important factors in reducing the risk of developing cancer.

29.3 The three primary goals of chemotherapy are cure, control, and palliation.

Surgery, radiation, and chemotherapy are the therapies used for treating cancer. Antineoplastic drugs may also be administered as adjuvant or neoadjuvant chemotherapy, prophylaxis, or myeloablation.

29.4 To achieve a total cure, every malignant cell must be removed or killed.

A single cancer cell may be able to divide rapidly enough to kill its host. Therefore, to achieve a complete cure, every single cancer cell must be eliminated by surgery, radiation, drugs, or the patient's immune system.

29.5 Use of multiple drugs and special dosing schedules improve the success of chemotherapy.

Combinations of antineoplastic drugs are often used to attack cancer cells through several mechanisms and to allow lower doses than if a single drug were used. The schedule of drug administration is critical to the success of the chemotherapy.

29.6 Serious toxicity limits therapy with most of the antineoplastic drugs.

Antineoplastic drugs are among the most toxic medications available. Adverse effects are expected and may be severe. Whereas each drug has somewhat different toxicities, common adverse effects include thrombocytopenia, anemia, leukopenia, alopecia, severe nausea, vomiting, and diarrhea.

29.7 Alkylating drugs act by changing the structure of DNA in cancer cells.

Alkylating drugs are some of the oldest and most reliable of the antineoplastic drugs. By attaching to DNA, they prevent cancer cells from replicating.

29.8 Antimetabolites disrupt critical cellular pathways in cancer cells.

Antimetabolites block a specific step in cancer cell metabolism. By blocking the synthesis of critical cellular molecules, the drugs can slow the growth of cancer cells.

29.9 A few cytotoxic antibiotics are used to treat cancer rather than infections.

Antitumor antibiotics attach to the DNA of cancer cells, thereby inhibiting their growth. Their properties and adverse effects resemble those of the alkylating drugs.

29.10 Some natural products kill cancer cells by preventing cell division.

Natural products of the periwinkle plant and the Pacific yew have provided several important antineoplastic drugs. Drugs in this class also include the topoisomerase inhibitors.

29.11 Some hormones and hormone antagonists are effective against prostate and breast cancer.

A number of estrogens, androgens, corticosteroids, and hormone inhibitors have antitumor activity and are most often given for palliation. They are usually reserved for tumors of the breast or prostate.

29.12 Targeted therapies and some miscellaneous antineoplastic drugs are effective against specific tumors.

Targeted therapies include monoclonal antibodies that have been designed to affect some specific aspect of cancer cell physiology. While a large number of new targeted therapies have been marketed, they are only effective against specific cancers and most have significant adverse effects.

29.13 Adjunct medications are sometimes necessary to treat cancer symptoms and to reduce the intensity of adverse effects from antineoplastic drugs.

Adjunct medications are needed to reduce the intense pain, nausea, and drug adverse effects that can occur during cancer treatment. Adjuncts include opioid analgesics, antiemetics, and drugs to reduce bone marrow toxicity.

REVIEW Questions

Answer the following questions to assess your knowledge of the chapter material, and go back and review any material that is not clear to you.

1. The nurse administers antiemetic drugs to a patient receiving chemotherapy:
   1. Only when vomiting occurs.
   2. Once the treatment regimen is completed.
   3. Just prior to treatment.
   4. Only if the patient requests to be medicated.
2. The patient with testicular cancer is receiving cisplatin (Platinol) IV. The nurse plans to monitor for:
   1. Irreversible heart failure.
   2. Bone marrow suppression.
   3. Cardiac toxicity.
   4. Peripheral neuropathy.
3. Before a patient begins drug therapy with methotrexate, the nurse collects information regarding the use of other medications. What medication(s) would be of concern if the patient were to take it along with the methotrexate? (Select all that apply.)
   1. Aspirin
   2. Iron supplement
   3. Acetaminophen
   4. Nonsteroidal anti-inflammatory drug (NSAID)
   5. Live oral vaccines
4. The patient with breast cancer has been receiving IV doxorubicin (Adriamycin). The patient is now complaining of severe pain at the IV site. Which of the following most likely occurred?
   1. An allergic reaction
   2. Leaking at the IV site
   3. Loss of neural reflexes
   4. Development of a blood clot
5. A patient has started on tamoxifen as a treatment for cancer. The healthcare provider orders 20 mg, PO, daily, but it is only available in 10 mg tablets. How many tablets will the patient receive in a day? How many tablets in a week?
   1. 1 tablet a day, 7 tablets a week
   2. 2 tablets a day, 14 tablets a week
   3. 2 tablets a day, 10 tablets a week
   4. 4 tablets a day, 14 tablets a week
6. The patient on cyclophosphamide (Cytoxan) is taught:
   1. That alopecia is not irreversible.
   2. About signs and symptoms of neurotoxicity.
   3. About signs and symptoms of renal toxicity.
   4. That nausea, vomiting, and diarrhea frequently occur.
7. The nurse monitors a patient taking methotrexate for which of the following adverse effect(s)? (Select all that apply.)
   1. Cardiac dysthymias
   2. Bruising
   3. Decreased urinary output
   4. Diarrhea
   5. Nausea
8. A patient is about to start chemotherapy treatments. He will be taking rituximab (Rituxan), a type of monoclonal antibody. He asks the nurse how it works. The nurse tells him that this type of monoclonal antibody:
   1. Changes the structure of cancer cell's DNA, preventing them from replicating.
   2. Binds to surface proteins present on cancer cells and shatters them.
   3. Blocks a specific step in cancer cell metabolism.
   4. Attaches to the DNA of cancer cells, inhibiting their growth.
9. The nurse informs a patient with a decreased white blood cell count that he should:
   1. Use alcohol-based mouthwash for mouth sores.
   2. Increase liquid intake with meals.
   3. Avoid raw foods.
   4. Ask his healthcare provider about ordering megestrol (Megace).
10. The patient on tamoxifen must be checked for:
    1. Flu-like symptoms.
    2. Uterine cancer.
    3. Alopecia.
    4. Thrombocytopenia.

CASE STUDY Questions

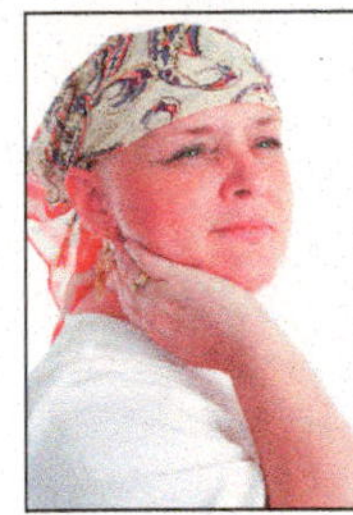

Remember Ms. Novak, the patient introduced at the beginning of the chapter? Now read the remainder of the case study. Based on the information you have learned in this chapter, answer the questions that follow.

Ms. Patricia Novak has arrived at the cancer center in her community. She is being treated for an invasive type of cancer. She is getting very tired of all the drugs she has to take, stating, "I know they are helping, but four different drugs? I guess it could be worse." Ms. Novak is receiving the following drugs:

1. *Vincristine (Oncovin)*
2. *Filgrastim (Neupogen)*
3. *Tamoxifen (Soltamox)*
4. *Epoetin alfa (Epogen)*

1. Ms. Novak knows that one of the medications boosts her immune system but can't remember which one. The medication is:
   1. Vincristine (Oncovin).
   2. Epoetin alfa (Epogen).
   3. Filgrastim (Neupogen).
   4. Tamoxifen.

2. Asked why Ms. Novak is taking epoetin alfa (Epogen), the nurse responds that it is being administered to:
   1. Boost Ms. Novak's immune system.
   2. Boost the number of her red blood cells.
   3. Reduce possible neurotoxicity.
   4. Kill her cancer cells.

3. During vincristine (Oncovin) therapy, the nurse must regularly monitor for:
   1. Blood glucose levels.
   2. Signs of peripheral neuropathy.
   3. Ototoxicity.
   4. Signs of confusion.

4. Because of the type of cancer she has and the type of antineoplastic drug she is taking, Ms. Novak complains of pain. The healthcare provider orders a pain medication. Understanding the pain management protocols, the nurse may expect to use what type of medication to achieve optimal pain control for Ms. Novak?
   1. A combination drug such as a nonsteroidal anti-inflammatory drug and codeine
   2. A strong opioid such as fentanyl
   3. A weak opioid such as codeine
   4. A nonsteroidal anti-inflammatory drug

Answers and complete rationales for the Review and Case Study Questions appear in Appendix A.

REFERENCE

Herdman, T. H., & Kamitsuru, S. (Eds.). (2014). *NANDA International nursing diagnoses: Definitions and classification, 2015–2017*. Oxford, United Kingdom: Wiley-Blackwell.

SELECTED BIBLIOGRAPHY

American Cancer Society. (2016). *What are the key statistics about breast cancer?* Retrieved from http://www.cancer.org/cancer/breastcancer/detailedguide/breast-cancer-key-statistics

American Cancer Society. (2016). *Cancer facts & figures 2016*. Retrieved from http://www.cancer.org/acs/groups/content/@research/documents/document/acspc-047079.pdf

Beard, C., & Beard, V. (2015, Sep 11). Re-examining current breast cancer screening: An analysis of the 2009 U.S. Preventive Services Task Force guidelines for breast cancer screening. *Women & Health*, 1–15. doi:10.1080/03630242.2015.1088115

Bourdeanu, L., & Liu, E. A. (2015). Systemic treatment for breast cancer: Chemotherapy and biotherapy agents. *Seminars in Oncology Nursing 31*, 156–162. doi:10.1016/j.soncn.2015.02.003

Gross, S., Rahal, R., Stransky, N., Lengauer, C., & Hoeflich, K. P. (2015). Targeting cancer with kinase inhibitors. *The Journal of Clinical Investigation, 125*, 1780–1789. doi:10.1172/JCI76094

Jordan, K., Jahn, F., & Aapro, M. (2015). Recent developments in the prevention of chemotherapy-induced nausea and vomiting (CINV): A comprehensive review. *Annals of Oncology, 26*, 1081–1090. doi:10.1093/annonc/mdv138

Rimawi, M. F., Schiff, R., & Osborne, C. K. (2015). Targeting HER2 for the treatment of breast cancer. *Annual Review of Medicine, 66*, 111–128. doi:10.1146/annurev-med-042513-015127

Sanchez Cuervo, M., Rojo Sanchis, A., Pueyo Lopez, C., Gomez de Salazar Lopez de Silanes, E., Gramage Caro, T., & Bermejo Vicedo, T. (2015). The impact of a computerized physician order entry system on medical errors with antineoplastic drugs 5 years after its implementation. *Journal of Clinical Pharmacy and Therapeutics, 40*, 550–554. doi:10.1111/jcpt.12305

Wagland, R., Richardson, A., Armes, J., Hankins, M., Lennan, E., & Griffiths, P. (2015). Treatment-related problems experienced by cancer patients undergoing chemotherapy: A scoping review. *European Journal of Cancer Care, 24*, 605–617. doi:10.1111/ecc.12246

Yarbro, C. H., Wujcik, D., & Gobel, B. H. (2017). *Cancer nursing: Principles and practice* (8th ed.). Sudbury, MA: Jones-Bartlett.

Unit 5

The Respiratory and Digestive Systems

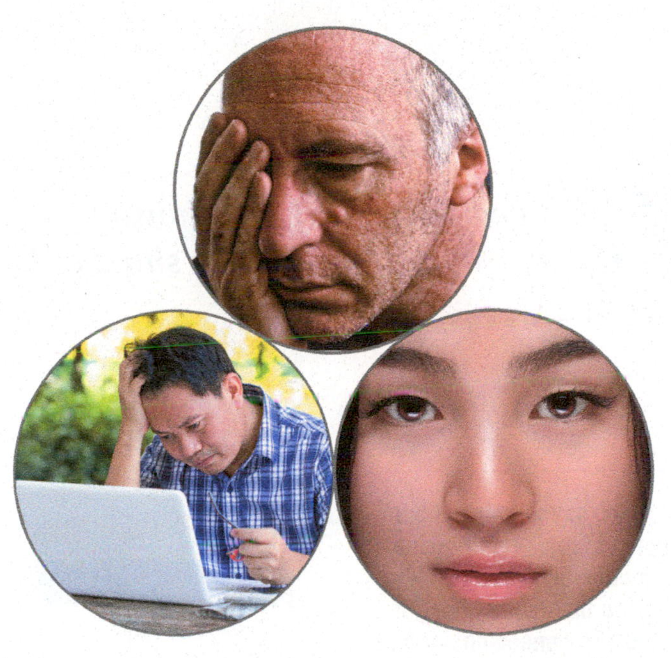

Unit Contents

Chapter 30

Drugs for Respiratory Disorders

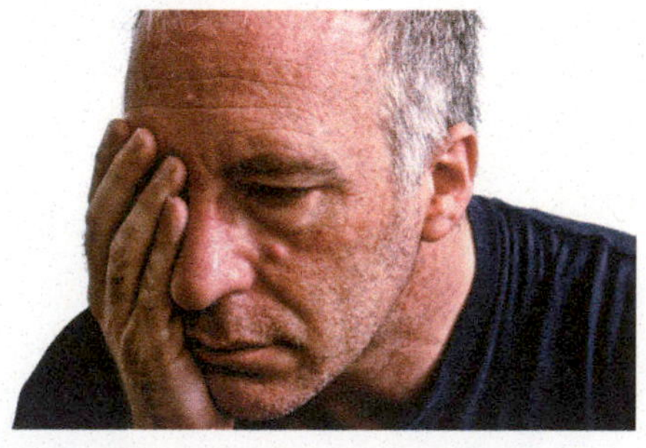

"I can't sleep at night with this cough, and I can hardly work without getting short of breath."
Mr. Michael Thomas

Core Concepts

30.1 **The respiratory system supplies oxygen for the body and provides protection against inhaled pathogens.**
30.2 **The inhalation route of drug administration quickly delivers medications directly to their sites of action.**
30.3 **Allergic rhinitis is characterized by sneezing, watery eyes, and nasal congestion.**
30.4 **Antihistamines are widely used to treat allergic rhinitis and other minor allergies.**
30.5 **Intranasal corticosteroids are first-line drugs for treating allergic rhinitis.**
30.6 **Decongestants are used to reduce nasal congestion caused by allergic rhinitis and the common cold.**
30.7 **Antitussives and expectorants are used to treat symptoms of the common cold.**
30.8 **Asthma is a chronic inflammatory disease characterized by bronchospasm.**
30.9 **Beta-adrenergic agonists are the most effective drugs for relieving acute bronchospasm.**
30.10 **Corticosteroids are the most effective drugs for the long-term prophylaxis of asthma.**
30.11 **Mast cell stabilizers, leukotriene modifiers, and monoclonal antibodies are alternative anti-inflammatory drugs for the prophylaxis of asthma.**
30.12 **Chronic obstructive pulmonary disease is a progressive disorder treated with multiple drugs.**

Drug Snapshot

The following drugs are discussed in this chapter:

Drug Classes	Prototype Drugs
Antihistamines (H_1-receptor blockers)	Pr diphenhydramine (Benadryl, others)
Intranasal corticosteroids	Pr fluticasone (Flonase, Veramyst)
Decongestants (sympathomimetics)	Pr oxymetazoline (Afrin, others)
Antitussives, expectorants, and mucolytics	
Beta-adrenergic drugs	Pr albuterol (Proventil HFA, Ventolin, VoSpire ER)
Anticholinergics	
Inhaled corticosteroids	
Xanthines	
Mast cell stabilizers	
Leukotriene modifiers	

Learning Outcomes

After reading this chapter, the student should be able to:

1. Identify major structures and functions associated with the respiratory system.
2. Explain why inhalation is an effective route of drug administration for respiratory medicines.
3. Describe common causes and symptoms of allergic rhinitis.
4. Explain the role of antihistamines in the treatment of allergic rhinitis and other allergies.
5. Explain the role of intranasal corticosteroids in the treatment of allergic rhinitis.
6. Explain the role of decongestants in the treatment of nasal congestion.
7. Explain the role of antitussives and expectorants in treating symptoms of the common cold.
8. Describe the inflammatory and bronchospasm components of asthma.
9. Explain the role of beta-adrenergic agonists in the treatment of asthma.
10. Explain the role of corticosteroids in the treatment of asthma.
11. Explain the role of mast cell stabilizers, leukotriene modifiers, and monoclonal antibodies in the treatment of asthma.
12. Identify the drugs that are used to bring symptomatic relief for patients with chronic obstructive pulmonary disease.

Key Terms

aerosol (AIR-oh-sol)
allergic rhinitis (rye-NYE-tis)
alveoli (al-VEE-oh-lie)
antitussives (anti-TUSS-ives)
asthma (AZ-muh)
bronchi (BRON-ky)
bronchioles (BRON-key-oles)
bronchoconstriction (BRON-koh-kun-STRIK-shun)
bronchodilation (BRON-koh-dye-LAY-shun)
bronchospasm (bron-koh-SPAZ-um)
chronic bronchitis (KRON-ik bron-KEYE-tis)
dry powder inhaler (DPI)
dyspnea
emphysema (em-fuss-EE-muh)
expectorants (eks-PEK-tor-entz)
H_1-receptor blocker
metered-dose inhalers (MDIs)
mucolytics
nebulizers (NEB-you-lyes-urz)
perfusion (purr-FEW-shun)
rebound congestion
respiration (res-purr-AY-shun)
status asthmaticus (STAT-us az-MAT-ik-us)
ventilation (ven-tah-LAY-shun)

The respiratory system is one of the most important organ systems; a mere 5 to 6 minutes without breathing may result in death. When functioning properly, the respiratory system filters incoming air and provides the body with the oxygen critical for all cells to function. The respiratory system also provides a means by which the body can rid itself of excess acids and bases, a topic that is covered in Chapter 18. The first portion of this chapter examines drugs used to treat conditions associated with the upper respiratory tract: allergic rhinitis, nasal congestion, and cough. The second portion presents the pharmacotherapy of asthma and conditions that affect the lower respiratory tract.

Core Concept 30.1 ▶ The respiratory system supplies oxygen for the body and provides protection against inhaled pathogens.

The primary function of the respiratory system is to bring oxygen into the body and to remove carbon dioxide. The process by which gases are exchanged is called **respiration**. The basic structures of the respiratory system are shown in Figure 30.1. This system is sometimes divided into two anatomic divisions: the upper and lower respiratory tracts.

Upper Respiratory Tract

The upper respiratory tract (URT) consists of the nose, nasal cavity, pharynx, and paranasal sinuses. These passageways warm, humidify, and clean the air before it enters the lungs. The URT traps and removes particulate matter and many pathogens before they reach the lower portions of the lungs, where they would be able to access the capillaries of the systemic circulation.

The nasal mucosa is a dynamic structure, richly supplied with vascular tissue, under the control of the autonomic nervous system. For example, certain drugs can reduce the thickness of the mucosal layer, thus widening the airway to allow more air to enter. The nasal mucosa is also a first line of immune defense. Up to a quart of nasal mucus is produced daily, and this fluid is rich with substances that are able to neutralize airborne pathogens. Unfortunately, these cells can overreact to some substances and cause symptoms typical of seasonal allergies, such as nasal congestion, watery eyes, and sneezing.

Lower Respiratory Tract

The lower respiratory tract (LRT) consists of the lungs and associated structures. Air leaving the URT travels into the trachea and **bronchi**, which divide into smaller and smaller passages called **bronchioles**. The bronchioles contain a considerable amount of smooth muscle that can make breathing easier by dilating, or more difficult by constricting. The bronchial tree ends in dilated sacs called **alveoli**. Although they have no smooth muscle, the alveoli are abundantly rich in capillaries. An extremely thin membrane in the alveoli allows gases to readily move between the internal environment of the blood and the inspired air. As oxygen crosses this membrane, it is exchanged for carbon dioxide, a cellular waste product that travels from the blood to the air. The lung is richly supplied with blood. Blood flow through the lung is called **perfusion**. The process of gas exchange is depicted in Figure 30.1.

Ventilation is the process of moving air into and out of the lungs. As the muscular diaphragm contracts and lowers in position, it creates a negative pressure that draws air into

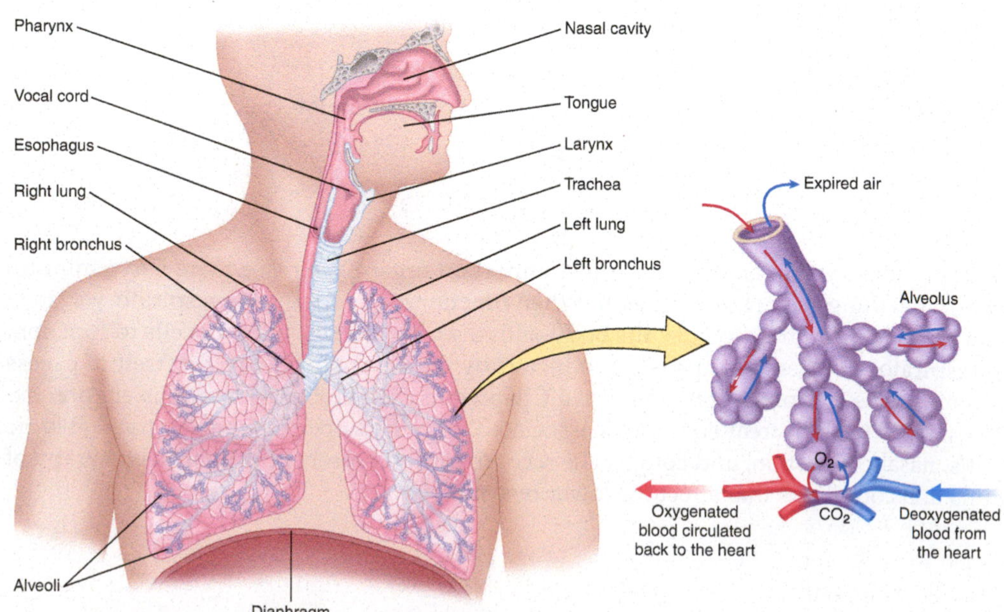

FIGURE 30.1 The respiratory system and the process of gas exchange.

the lungs. This process, known as inspiration, requires energy to produce the contraction. During expiration, the diaphragm relaxes and air leaves the lung passively, with no energy expenditure required. Ventilation is a purely mechanical process that occurs approximately 12–18 times per minute in adults, a rate determined by neurons in the brainstem. This rate may be modified by a number of factors, including emotions, fever, stress, and the pH of the blood.

CONCEPT REVIEW 30.1

- What is the difference between ventilation and perfusion?

The inhalation route of drug administration quickly delivers medications directly to their sites of action.

◀ **Core Concept 30.2**

The respiratory system offers a rapid and efficient mechanism for delivering drugs. The enormous surface area of the bronchioles and alveoli, and the rich blood supply to these areas, results in an almost instantaneous onset of action for inhaled substances.

Medications are delivered to the respiratory system by aerosol therapy. An **aerosol** is a suspension of very small liquid droplets or fine solid particles suspended within a gas. Aerosol therapy can give immediate relief for bronchospasm, an acute condition in which the airways become constricted (narrowed), leaving the patient gasping for breath. Drugs may also be given to loosen thick mucus in the bronchial tree. The major advantage of aerosol therapy is that it delivers the medications to their immediate site of action, thus reducing systemic adverse effects. To produce the same therapeutic action, an oral medication would need to be given at higher doses and would be distributed to all body tissues.

Drugs delivered by inhalation can produce *systemic* effects because there is always some degree of drug absorption across the respiratory membranes into the bloodstream. For example, anesthetics such as nitrous oxide and isoflurane (Forane) are delivered via the inhalation route and are rapidly distributed to cause central nervous system (CNS) depression, as presented in Chapter 16. Solvents such as paint thinners and glues are sometimes intentionally inhaled and can cause serious adverse effects on the nervous system and even death. In general, however, drugs administered by the inhalation route for respiratory conditions produce minimal systemic toxicity.

Several devices are used to deliver medications via the inhalation route. **Nebulizers** are small machines that vaporize a liquid drug into a fine mist that can be inhaled, often using a facemask. If the drug is a solid, it may be administered using a **dry powder inhaler (DPI)**. A DPI is a small device that is activated by the process of inhalation to deliver a fine powder directly to the bronchial tree. Turbuhalers and rotahalers are types of DPIs. **Metered-dose inhalers (MDIs)** are a third type of device commonly used to deliver respiratory medicines. MDIs use a propellant to deliver a measured dose of drugs to the lungs during each breath. The patient times the inhalation to the puffs of drug emitted from the MDI. Patients must be carefully instructed on the correct use of these devices because drug dose depends on their correct use. Patients should be advised to rinse their mouth thoroughly following drug use to reduce the potential for absorption of the drug across the oral mucosa because swallowing medication that has been deposited in the oral cavity may cause the drug to be absorbed in the gastrointestinal (GI) tract, causing potential adverse effects. When using MDIs, spacers are placed on the end of the inhaler to help reduce the amount of medicine deposited in the mouth and throat. Devices used to deliver respiratory drugs are shown in Figure 30.2.

The primary goal of drug therapy for many respiratory disorders is to keep the airways open. Drugs include bronchodilators, which directly open the airways, and anti-inflammatory drugs, which prevent their closure. Drugs may be used to act on excessive mucus blocking the airways, either by causing it to become thinner or by breaking up thick mucus plugs. These and other types of drugs used to treat respiratory disorders are illustrated in Figure 30.3.

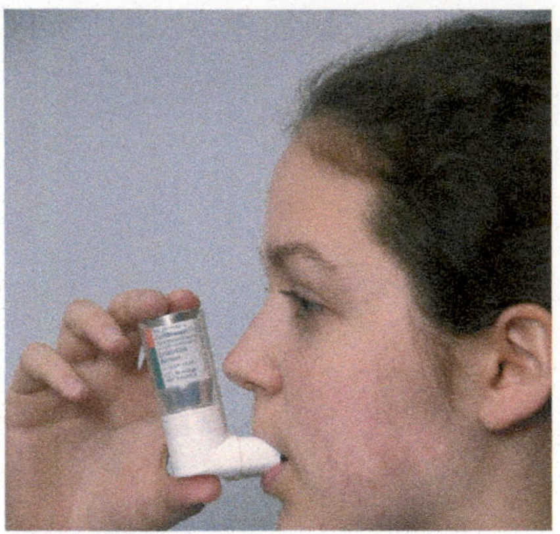
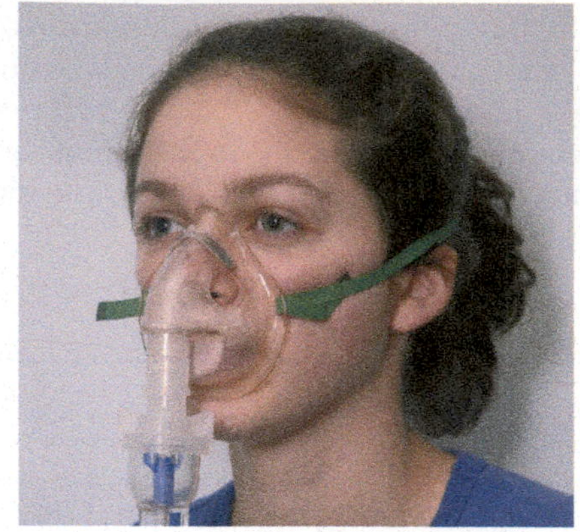
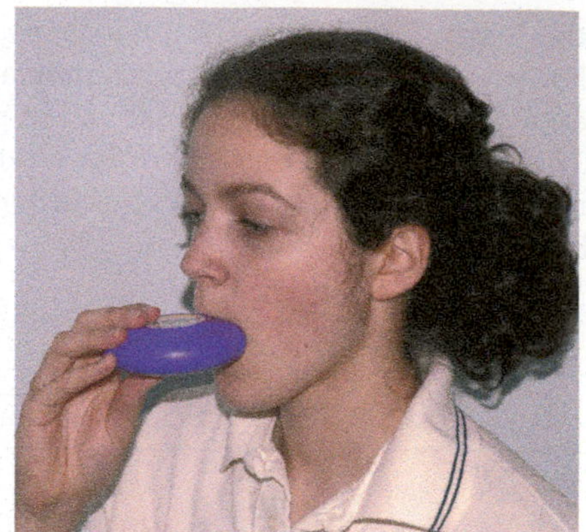

FIGURE 30.2 Devices used to deliver respiratory drugs.

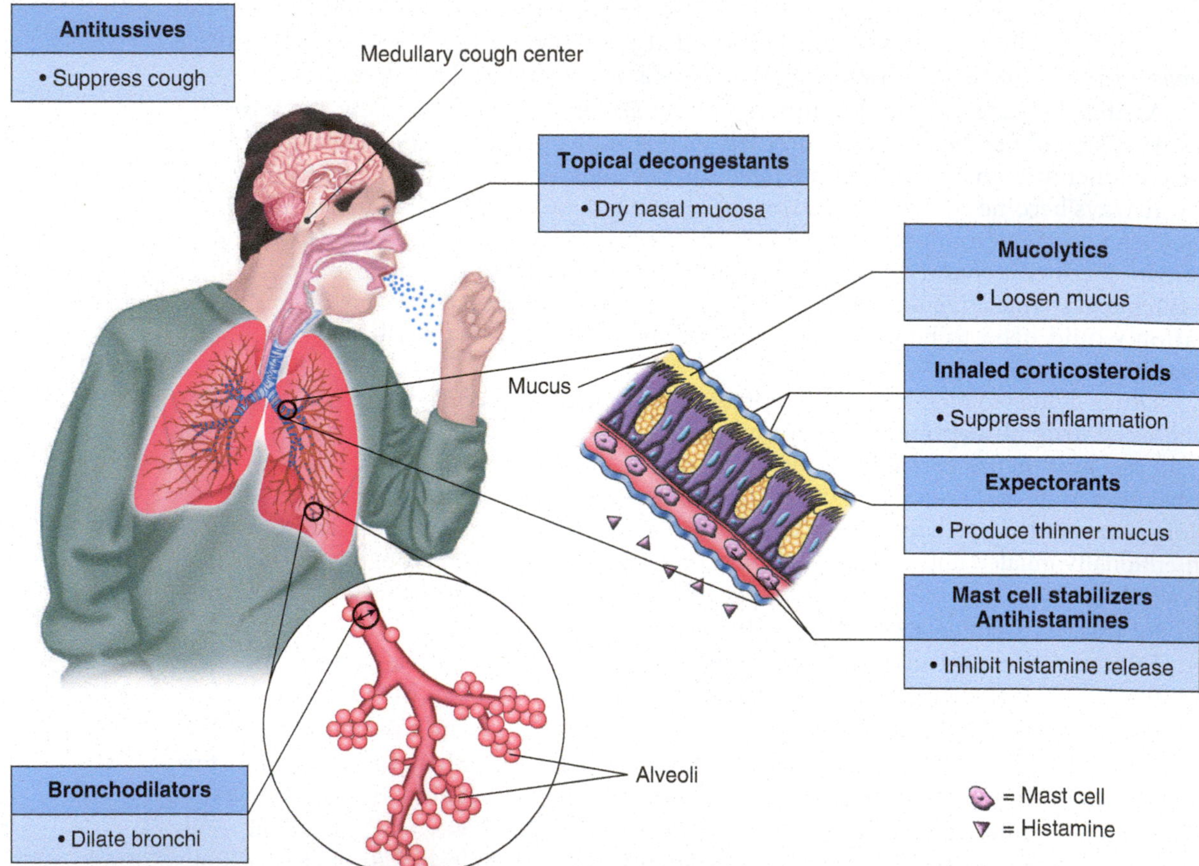

FIGURE 30.3 Drugs used to treat respiratory disorders.

CONCEPT REVIEW 30.2

- Name the three types of devices used to deliver drugs by the inhalation route. What are the differences among them?

ALLERGIC RHINITIS

Allergic rhinitis, or hay fever, is inflammation of the nasal mucosa due to exposure to allergens. Although not life threatening, allergic rhinitis is a condition affecting millions of patients, and pharmacotherapy is frequently necessary to control symptoms and to prevent secondary complications.

Allergic rhinitis is characterized by sneezing, watery eyes, and nasal congestion.

◀ **Core Concept 30.3**

The acute symptoms of allergic rhinitis resemble those of the common cold: tearing eyes, sneezing, nasal congestion, postnasal drip, and itching of the throat. Complications of allergic rhinitis may include loss of taste or smell, sinusitis, chronic cough, hoarseness, and middle ear infections in children.

As with other allergies, the cause of allergic rhinitis is exposure to an antigen. An antigen, or **allergen**, may be defined as anything that is recognized as foreign by the body's defense system. The specific allergen is often difficult to pinpoint; however, common agents include pollen from weeds, grasses, and trees; molds; dust mites; certain foods; and animal dander. Nonallergenic factors such as chemical fumes, tobacco smoke, or air pollutants such as ozone may contribute to the symptoms. Although some patients experience symptoms at specific times of the year, when pollen and mold are at high levels in the environment, others are bothered throughout the year.

The fundamental problem of allergic rhinitis is inflammation of the mucous membranes in the nose, throat, and airways. Chemical mediators of inflammation such as histamine are released and initiate the distressing symptoms. The pathophysiology of allergic rhinitis is illustrated in Figure 30.4.

Drugs used to treat allergic rhinitis are grouped into two basic categories: preventers and relievers. Preventers are used for prophylaxis and include antihistamines, intranasal corticosteroids, and mast cell stabilizers. Relievers are used to provide immediate, though temporary, relief for allergy symptoms once they have occurred. Relievers include the oral and intranasal sympathomimetics.

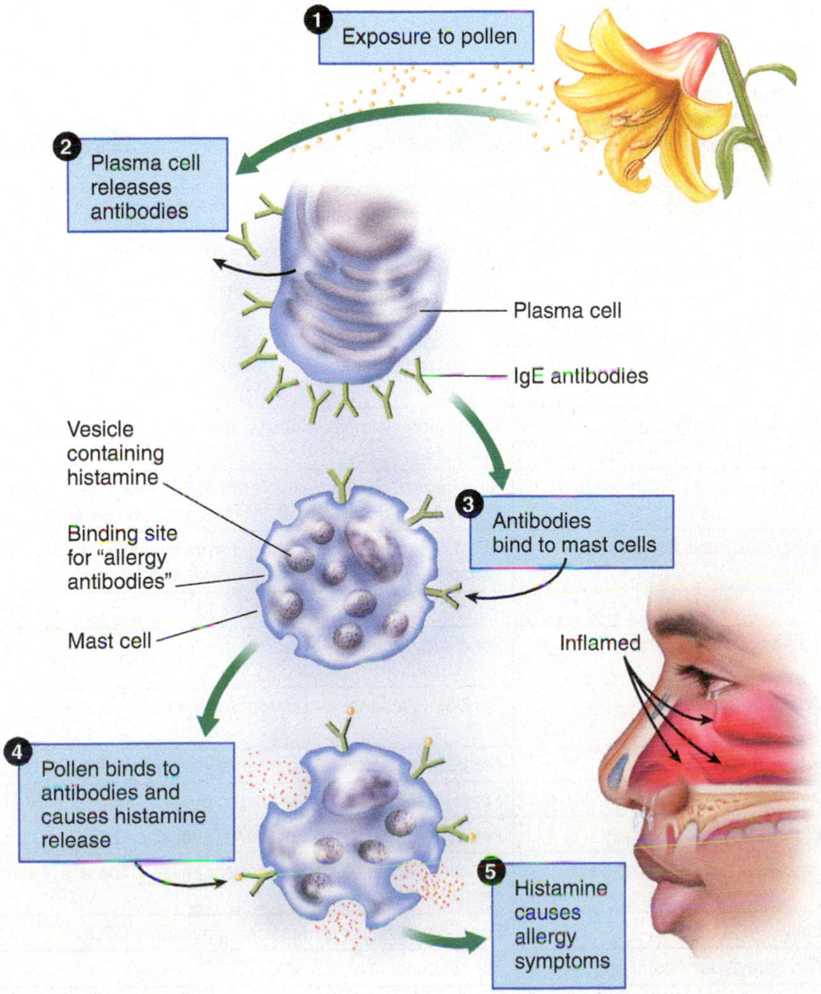

FIGURE 30.4
Pathophysiology of allergic rhinitis.

Fast Facts Allergies

- Allergies are believed to affect as many as 30% of adults and 40% of children.
- It is estimated that over 17 million adults experience allergic rhinitis (hay fever).
- Food allergies account for about 200,000 emergency department visits each year.
- The three most common allergies are peanut, milk and shellfish.

Source: From Asthma and Allergy Foundation of America (2016), Allergy Facts and Figure. Published by Asthma and Allergy Foundation of America.

Core Concept 30.4 ▶ Antihistamines are widely used to treat allergic rhinitis and other minor allergies.

Antihistamines are drugs that selectively block the actions of histamine at the H_1-receptor, thus alleviating allergic symptoms. Also called **H_1-receptor blockers**, several are available over the counter (OTC) and frequently used for relief of allergy symptoms, motion sickness, and insomnia. Common H_1-receptor blockers used to treat allergies and other disorders are listed in Table 30.1.

Because the term *antihistamine* does not specify which of the two histamine receptors is affected, *H_1-receptor blocker* is the more accurate term. Although a large number of H_1-receptor blockers are available for use, their effectiveness, therapeutic uses, and adverse effects are similar. A simple classification of these drugs is based on their ability to cause sedation. Older, first-generation H_1-receptor blockers have the potential to cause significant drowsiness, whereas the newer, second-generation drugs do not affect most patients. Care must be taken to avoid alcohol and other CNS depressants when taking antihistamines because their sedating effects may be additive.

The most common therapeutic use of H_1-receptor blockers is for the treatment of allergies. These drugs provide relief from the characteristic sneezing; runny nose; and

Table 30.1 H_1-Receptor Blockers (Antihistamines)

Drug	Route and Adult Dose	Remarks
FIRST-GENERATION DRUGS		
brompheniramine (Dimetapp, others)	PO (regular release): 4 mg tid–qid (max: 24 mg/day)	Less sedative effect than diphenhydramine; combined with other drugs for OTC use
chlorpheniramine (Chlor-Trimeton, others)	PO (regular release): 4 mg tid–qid (max: 24 mg/day)	Usually combined with a decongestant to treat cold, flu, and allergy symptoms; available OTC
clemastine (Tavist)	PO: 1.34–2.68 mg bid (max: 8.04 mg/day)	For allergic rhinitis, urticaria, and angioedema
dexchlorpheniramine (Dexchlor, Poladex, others)	PO: 2 mg every 4–6 hours (max: 12 mg/day)	For seasonal rhinitis and other allergy disorders
dimenhydrinate (Dramamine)	PO: 50–100 mg every 4–6 hours	For motion sickness, nausea, and vomiting; IV and IM forms available
Pr diphenhydramine (Benadryl, others)	PO: 25–50 mg tid–qid (max: 300 mg/day)	Also for motion sickness, Parkinson disease, vertigo, and as an OTC sleep aid; topical, IV, IM, and subcutaneous forms available
promethazine (Phenergan)	PO: 12.5–25 mg/day (max: 100 mg/day)	IV, IM, and rectal suppository forms available; also for preoperative sedation, motion sickness, nausea, and vertigo
SECOND-GENERATION DRUGS		
acrivastine with pseudoephedrine (Semprex-D)	PO: One capsule daily (8 mg acrivastine/ 60 mg pseudoephedrine)	For allergic rhinitis
azelastine (Astelin, Astepro)	Intranasal; One or two sprays daily per nostril	For both seasonal and perennial rhinitis
cetirizine (Zyrtec)	PO: 5–10 mg/day (max: 10 mg/day)	For both seasonal and perennial rhinitis; available OTC
desloratadine (Clarinex)	PO: 5 mg/day (max: 5 mg/day)	For allergic rhinitis and urticaria; the active metabolite of loratadine
fexofenadine (Allegra)	PO: 60 mg bid or 180 mg once daily	For allergic rhinitis and urticaria; available OTC
levocetirizine (Xyzal)	PO: 5 mg (1 tablet or 2 teaspoons) once daily	For allergic rhinitis and urticaria; similar to the active form of cetirizine
loratadine (Claritin)	PO: 10 mg daily	For allergic rhinitis and urticaria; available OTC
olopatadine (Patanase)	Intranasal: Two sprays per nostril bid	For seasonal allergic rhinitis

Table 30.2 Selected OTC Antihistamine Combinations

Brand Name	Antihistamine	Decongestant	Analgesic
Actifed Cold and Allergy tablets	chlorpheniramine	phenylephrine	—
Benadryl Allergy/Cold caplets	diphenhydramine	phenylephrine	acetaminophen
Chlor-Trimeton Allergy/Decongestant tablets	chlorpheniramine	pseudoephedrine	—
Dimetapp Children's Cold and Allergy	brompheniramine	phenylephrine	—
Sudafed PE Severe Cold tablets	diphenhydramine	phenylephrine	acetaminophen
Sudafed PE Sinus and Allergy tablets	chlorpheniramine	phenylephrine	—
Tavist Allergy tablets	clemastine	—	—
Triaminic Cold/Allergy	chlorpheniramine	phenylephrine	—
Tylenol Allergy Multisystem gels	chlorpheniramine	phenylephrine	acetaminophen
Tylenol PM gelcaps	diphenhydramine	—	acetaminophen

itching of the eyes, nose, and throat of allergic rhinitis. Many H_1-receptor blockers are used in OTC cold and sinus medicines, often in combination with decongestants and antitussives. Some common OTC antihistamine combinations used to treat allergies are listed in Table 30.2.

Antihistamines are most effective when taken to *prevent* allergic symptoms; their ability to treat allergy symptoms after they are present is limited. Their effectiveness may diminish with long-term use. It should be noted that during severe allergic reactions such as anaphylaxis, histamine is just one of several chemical mediators released; thus, H_1-receptor blockers are not very effective in treating this disorder.

Although most antihistamines are given orally, azelastine (Astelin, Astepro) and olopatadine (Patanase) are available by the intranasal route. Dymista is a newer combination that includes azelastine with fluticasone, an intranasal corticosteroid.

H_1-receptor blockers have been used to treat a number of non-allergy disorders. Motion sickness responds well to these medications. It is also one of the few classes of drugs available to treat vertigo, a form of dizziness that causes significant nausea. Some of the older antihistamines are marketed as OTC sleep aids, taking advantage of their ability to cause drowsiness. Diphenhydramine is used to treat tremors associated with Parkinson disease.

Prototype Drug: Pr *Diphenhydramine (Benadryl, Others)*

Therapeutic Class: Drug to treat allergies Pharmacologic Class: H_1-receptor blocker, antihistamine

Actions and Uses: Diphenhydramine is a first-generation H_1-receptor blocker whose primary use is to treat symptoms of allergy and the common cold, such as sneezing, runny nose, and tearing of the eyes. Diphenhydramine is often combined with an analgesic, a decongestant, or an expectorant in OTC cold and flu products. Diphenhydramine is also used as a topical drug to treat rashes, and IM and IV forms are available for severe allergic reactions. Other indications for diphenhydramine include Parkinson disease, motion sickness, and insomnia.

Adverse Effects and Interactions: First-generation H_1-receptor blockers such as diphenhydramine cause significant drowsiness, although this usually diminishes with long-term use. Occasionally, a patient will exhibit CNS stimulation and excitability rather than drowsiness. Excitation is more frequent in children than in adults. Anticholinergic effects such as dry mouth, tachycardia, and mild hypotension are seen in some patients.

Use of diphenhydramine with alcohol, CNS depressants, or monoamine oxidase inhibitors (MAOIs) may cause additive CNS depression. Use with other OTC cold preparations may increase anticholinergic adverse effects.

CONCEPT REVIEW 30.3

- Why are the antihistamines most effective if given *prior to allergen* exposure?

Nursing Process Focus Patients Receiving Antihistamine Therapy

ASSESSMENT	POTENTIAL NURSING DIAGNOSES*
Prior to administration: • Obtain a complete health history including respiratory, cardiovascular, renal, liver, thyroid, and skin conditions; experiences with anaphylaxis, asthma, or other allergies; drug history; and possible drug interactions. • Evaluate laboratory blood levels: complete blood count (CBC), renal, and liver function studies. • Acquire the results of a complete physical examination including vital signs, electrocardiogram (ECG), pulmonary function tests, breathing patterns, and neurologic status (level of consciousness [LOC]).	• *Ineffective Airway Clearance* related to difficulty swallowing and coughing • *Ineffective Breathing Pattern* related to retained secretions and discomfort • *Disturbed Sleep Pattern* related to somnolence or agitation • *Deficient Knowledge* related to a lack of information about drug therapy

PLANNING: PATIENT GOALS AND EXPECTED OUTCOMES

The patient will:

- Experience therapeutic effects (relief from allergic symptoms such as congestion, itching, or postnasal drip).
- Be free from or experience minimal adverse effects from drug therapy.
- Verbalize an understanding of the drug's use, adverse effects, and required precautions.

IMPLEMENTATION

Interventions and (Rationales)	Patient Education/Discharge Planning
• Auscultate breath sounds before administering drug therapy. Use with extreme caution in patients with asthma or chronic obstructive pulmonary disease (COPD). Keep resuscitative equipment accessible. (Anticholinergic effects of antihistamines may trigger bronchospasm.)	• Instruct the patient to immediately report wheezing or difficulty breathing. • Advise patients with asthma to consult the nurse regarding the use of injectable epinephrine in emergency situations.
• Administer the medication correctly and evaluate the patient's knowledge of proper administration. (Proper administration helps increase effectiveness of drugs. Mixing antihistamines with other medication may increase adverse effects such as drowsiness.)	Instruct the patient to: • Begin taking antihistamines before allergy season begins or at the earliest possible appearance of symptoms for best effects. • Follow directions on specific medication label. • Avoid mixing OTC antihistamines; always consult the healthcare provider before taking any OTC drugs or herbal supplements.
• Monitor vital signs (including ECG) before administering drug therapy. Use with extreme caution in patients with a history of cardiovascular disease. (Anticholinergic effects can increase heart rate and lower blood pressure. Fatal dysrhythmias and cardiovascular collapse have been reported in some patients receiving antihistamines.)	Instruct the patient to: • Immediately report dizziness, palpitations, headache, or chest, arm, or back pain accompanied by nausea, vomiting, or sweating to the healthcare provider. • Monitor vital signs daily, ensuring proper use of home equipment.
• Monitor thyroid function. Use with caution in patients with a history of hyperthyroidism. (Antihistamines exacerbate CNS-stimulating effects of hyperthyroidism and may trigger thyroid storm.)	• Instruct the patient to report immediately any nervousness or restlessness, insomnia, fever, profuse sweating, thirst, and mood changes to the healthcare provider.
• Monitor for vision changes. Use with caution in patients with narrow-angle glaucoma. (Antihistamines can increase intraocular pressure and cause photosensitivity.)	Instruct the patient to: • Report head or eye pain and visual changes immediately to the healthcare provider. • Wear dark glasses, use sunscreen, and avoid excessive sun exposure.
• Monitor neurologic status, especially LOC. Use with caution in patients with a history of seizure disorder. (Drugs may cause sedation, especially in older adults. Antihistamines can also lower the seizure threshold.)	Instruct the patient to: • Avoid driving or performing hazardous activities until the effects of the drug are known. • Immediately report to the healthcare provider any seizure activity, including any changes in character and pattern of seizures.
• Observe for signs of renal toxicity. Measure intake and output. Use with caution in patients with a history of kidney or urinary tract disease. (Antihistamines promote urinary retention.)	• Instruct the patient to immediately report flank pain, difficulty urinating, reduced urine output, and changes in the appearance of urine (cloudy, with sediment, odor) to the healthcare provider.

Interventions and (Rationales)	Patient Education/Discharge Planning
• Use with caution in patients with diabetes mellitus. Monitor serum glucose levels with increased dosing frequency. (Antihistamines decrease serum glucose levels.)	Instruct the patient to: • Immediately report symptoms of hypoglycemia. • Consult the healthcare provider regarding timing of glucose monitoring and reportable results (e.g., "less than 70 mg/dL").
• Monitor for GI adverse effects. Use with caution in patients with a history of GI disorders, especially peptic ulcers or liver disease. (Antihistamines block H_1-receptors, altering the mucosal lining of the stomach. These drugs are metabolized in the liver, increasing the risk of hepatotoxicity.)	Instruct the patient to: • Immediately report nausea, vomiting, anorexia, bleeding, chest or abdominal pain, heartburn, jaundice, or a change in the color or character of stools to the healthcare provider. • Avoid substances that irritate the stomach, such as spicy foods, alcoholic beverages, and nicotine; take the drug with food to avoid stomach upset.
• Monitor for anticholinergic-related effects such as dry mouth, thickened mucus, and nasal drying. (Mild anticholinergic effects are common and are usually treated symptomatically.)	Instruct the patient to: • Immediately report fever or flushing accompanied by difficulty swallowing or dry mouth to the healthcare provider. • Suck on hard candy to relieve dry mouth and maintain adequate fluid intake.

EVALUATION OF OUTCOME CRITERIA

Evaluate the effectiveness of drug therapy by confirming that patient goals and expected outcomes have been met (see "Planning"). *See Table 30.1 for a list of drugs to which these nursing actions apply.*

Intranasal corticosteroids are first-line drugs for treating allergic rhinitis.

◀ **Core Concept 30.5**

Corticosteroids, also known as glucocorticoids, are applied directly to the nasal mucosa to prevent symptoms of allergic rhinitis. When applied consistently, they decrease the secretion of inflammatory mediators, reduce tissue edema, and cause mild vasoconstriction. They have largely replaced antihistamines as preferred drugs in the treatment of chronic allergic rhinitis. The intranasal corticosteroids are listed in Table 30.3. When delivered by oral inhalation (not intranasal), some of these medications are also used to treat asthma.

Intranasal corticosteroids are administered with a metered-spray device that delivers a consistent dose of drug per spray. All have equal effectiveness and require 2 to 3 weeks of therapy before optimal benefits are attained. Because of this delayed effect, intranasal corticosteroids are most effective when taken *in advance* of expected allergen exposure. Three drugs in this class, fluticasone (Flonase Allergy Relief), budesonide (Rhinocort Allergy Spray), and triamcinolone (Nasacort Allergy 12h) are available OTC.

Intranasal corticosteroids produce none of the potentially serious adverse effects that are observed when these hormones are given orally. The most frequently reported adverse effects are a burning sensation in the nose immediately after spraying and drying of the nasal mucosa.

Prototype Drug: Pr *Fluticasone (Flonase, Veramyst)*

Therapeutic Class: Drug for allergic rhinitis **Pharmacologic Class:** Intranasal corticosteroid

Actions and Uses: Fluticasone is typical of the intranasal corticosteroids used to treat allergic rhinitis. Therapy usually begins with two sprays in each nostril twice daily and decreases to one dose per day. Fluticasone acts to decrease local inflammation in the nasal passages, thus reducing nasal stuffiness.

Adverse Effects and Interactions: Adverse effects of fluticasone are rare. Small amounts of the intranasal corticosteroids are sometimes swallowed, which increases their potential for causing systemic adverse effects. Nasal irritation and bleeding occur in a few patients.

Table 30.3 Intranasal Corticosteroids

Drug	Route and Adult Dose	Remarks
beclomethasone (Beconase AQ, Qnasl, QVAR)	Intranasal: 1–2 sprays in each nostril bid–qid	Oral inhaler available (Beclovent) for asthma
budesonide (Rhinocort)	Intranasal: Two sprays in each nostril bid	Oral inhaler available (Pulmicort) for asthma
ciclesonide (Omnaris, Zetonna)	Intranasal: Two sprays in each nostril bid (Omnaris) or once daily (Zetonna)	Oral inhaler available (Alvesco) for asthma
flunisolide	Intranasal: Two sprays in each nostril bid	Oral inhaler available (Aerospan) for asthma
Pr fluticasone (Flonase, Veramyst)	Intranasal: One spray in each nostril once (Veramyst) or twice (Flonase) daily	Oral inhaler available (Flovent) for asthma; topical form available (Cutivate) for dermatitis
mometasone (Nasonex)	Intranasal: Two sprays in each nostril daily	Oral inhaler available (Asmanex) for asthma; Topical form available (Elocon) for dermatologic use
triamcinolone (Nasacort AQ)	Intranasal: 2–4 sprays in each nostril qid	Oral inhaler available (Nasacort) for asthma; also available in IM, subcutaneous, intradermal, and intra-articular forms

Core Concept 30.6 ▶ Decongestants are used to reduce nasal congestion caused by allergic rhinitis and the common cold.

Decongestants are drugs that relieve nasal congestion. They are administered by either the oral or intranasal routes and are often combined with antihistamines in the pharmacotherapy of allergies or the common cold. Most decongestants are sympathomimetics—drugs that activate the sympathetic nervous system. Because sympathomimetics relieve only nasal congestion, they are often combined with antihistamines to control the sneezing and eye tearing of allergic rhinitis. Doses for the decongestants are given in Table 30.4.

Sympathomimetics are effective at relieving the nasal congestion associated with allergic rhinitis and the common cold. Both oral and intranasal preparations are available. The intranasal drugs such as oxymetazoline (Afrin, others) are available OTC as sprays or drops and produce an effective response within minutes. Because of their local action, intranasal sympathomimetics produce few systemic effects. The most serious, limiting adverse effect of the intranasal preparations is **rebound congestion**, a condition characterized by hypersecretion of mucus and worsened nasal congestion once the drug effects wear off. This rebound effect sometimes leads to a cycle of increased drug use as the condition worsens. Because of rebound congestion, intranasal sympathomimetics should be used for no longer than 3 to 5 days. Patients with allergic rhinitis who develop tolerance to the effects of decongestants should be gradually switched to intranasal corticosteroids because they do not cause rebound congestion.

Table 30.4 Decongestants

Drug	Route and Adult Dose	Remarks
naphazoline (Privine)	Intranasal: Two drops in each nostril every 3–6 hours	Also available as spray
Pr oxymetazoline (Afrin 12 hour, Neo-Synephrine 12 hour, others)	Intranasal: 2–3 sprays in each nostril bid for up to 3–5 days	Also available as drops
phenylephrine (Afrin 4–6 hours, Neo-Synephrine 4–6 hours, others) (see the Prototype Drug box in Core Concept 9.8)	Intranasal: One or two sprays in each nostril every 3–4 hours	Also available as drops, chewable tablets, and hemorrhoid cream; also available by the subcutaneous, IM, and IV routes for severe hypotension and shock
pseudoephedrine (Sudafed, others)	PO: 60 mg every 4–6 hours (regular release) or 120 mg bid (sustained release)	Produces little congestive rebound or irritation
tetrahydrozoline (Tyzine)	Intranasal: 2–4 drops in each nostril every 3 hours	Ophthalmic solution is available for allergic reactions of the eye
xylometazoline (Otrivin)	Intranasal: One or two sprays in each nostril bid (max: 3 doses/day)	Also available as drops

When administered *orally*, sympathomimetics do not produce rebound congestion. Their onset of action by this route, however, is much slower than the intranasal preparations, and they are less effective at relieving severe congestion. The possibility of systemic adverse effects is also greater with the oral drugs. Potential adverse effects include hypertension and CNS stimulation that may lead to insomnia or anxiety.

Pseudoephedrine was once the most common decongestant found in oral OTC cold and allergy medicines. Pseudoephedrine, however, is the starting chemical for the synthesis of illegal methamphetamine by drug traffickers. Although pseudoephedrine is still available without a prescription, pharmacists are required to monitor its distribution by keeping a log of patients' names and addresses and checking the photo identification of the buyer. Most manufacturers have reformulated their OTC cold medicines to contain phenylephrine rather than pseudoephedrine. A drug prototype feature for phenylephrine is included in Chapter 9.

CONCEPT REVIEW 30.4

- The sympathomimetics are the most effective drugs for relieving nasal congestion, but healthcare providers often prefer to prescribe antihistamines or intranasal corticosteroids. Why?

Prototype Drug: Pr *Oxymetazoline (Afrin, Others)*

Therapeutic Class: Decongestant **Pharmacologic Class:** Sympathomimetic

Actions and Uses: Oxymetazoline activates alpha-adrenergic receptors of the sympathetic nervous system. This stimulation causes arterioles in the nasal passages to constrict, producing a drying of the mucous membranes. Relief from the symptoms of nasal congestion occurs within minutes and lasts for 10–12 hours. The drug is administered with a metered-spray device or by nose drops.

Oxymetazoline (Visine LR) is also available as eyedrops. It causes vasoconstriction of vessels in the eye and is used to relieve redness and provide relief from dryness and minor eye irritations.

Adverse Effects and Interactions: Rebound congestion is common when oxymetazoline is used for longer than 3 to 5 days. Minor stinging and dryness in the nasal mucosa may be experienced. Systemic adverse effects are unlikely, unless a considerable amount of the medicine is swallowed. Patients with thyroid disorders, hypertension, diabetes, or heart disease should use sympathomimetics only on the direction of their healthcare provider. No clinically significant interactions have been found.

Antitussives and expectorants are used to treat symptoms of the common cold.

◀ **Core Concept 30.7**

In addition to congestion, cough is a symptom that causes patients to take OTC remedies or to seek medical attention. Cough is a reflex mechanism controlled by neurons in the cough center, located in the medulla oblongata of the brain. In diseases such as emphysema and bronchitis, or when liquids have been aspirated into the bronchi, it is not desirable to suppress the normal cough reflex. Because cough is merely a symptom, the therapeutic goal is to identify and treat the underlying disorder whenever possible.

There are many possible causes of cough, ranging from the acute cough of an upper respiratory infection to the chronic cough of tobacco smoking. Some drugs, such as the angiotensin-converting enzyme (ACE) inhibitors and beta-adrenergic blockers, can trigger persistent cough. In many cases, keeping the throat moist with sugar-free candy, cough drops, or frequent sips of water is sufficient to suppress cough. However, a dry, hacking, nonproductive cough can be irritating to the membranes of the throat and can deprive a patient of much-needed rest. It is these types of conditions in which therapy with drugs that control cough, or **antitussives**, may be warranted.

anti = *against*
tussive = *pertaining to a cough*

Opioids, the most effective class of antitussives, act by raising the cough threshold in the cough center, thereby decreasing both the frequency and the intensity of cough. Hydrocodone and codeine are effective opioid antitussives. Doses needed to suppress the cough reflex are low; thus there is minimal potential for dependence. Most codeine cough mixtures are classified as Schedule III, IV, or V drugs and are reserved for more serious cough conditions. The amount of codeine in cough mixtures is low and rarely causes serious adverse effects. However, care must be taken not to give these mixtures to patients allergic to codeine or other opioids. In addition, the drug must be kept secure from children because accidental overdose of opioids in infants can cause severe respiratory depression and even death. Opioids may be combined with other drugs such as antihistamines, decongestants, and nonopioid antitussives in the therapy of severe cold or flu symptoms.

The most frequently used OTC antitussive is dextromethorphan, which is included in most severe cold and flu preparations. Dextromethorphan is chemically similar to the opioids and also acts on the CNS to raise the cough threshold. Although it does not have the high abuse potential of opioids, dextromethorphan can cause slurred speech, dizziness, drowsiness, euphoria, and lack of motor coordination when taken in high amounts.

Benzonatate (Tessalon) is a nonopioid antitussive that does not act on the cough center. Instead, benzonatate has a local anesthetic-like effect on stretch receptors in the lung, which essentially interrupts the cough message. The patient must be instructed not to chew the soft capsules because they will cause numbness of the throat and tongue.

Expectorants are drugs that reduce the thickness or viscosity of bronchial secretions. They stimulate mucus flow, which thins bronchial secretions, allowing them to be removed with less forceful coughing. The most effective OTC expectorant is guaifenesin. Like dextromethorphan, guaifenesin produces few adverse effects and is a common ingredient in many OTC cold and flu preparations. Higher doses of guaifenesin are available by prescription. Nonprescription cough and cold products (including those containing guaifenesin) should not be used in children under 6 years of age.

muco = *mucus*
lytic = *destruction or disintegration*

Acetylcysteine (Mucomyst) is one of the few drugs available to directly loosen thick, viscous bronchial secretions by breaking down the chemical structure of mucus molecules. Drugs of this type are called **mucolytics**. Acetylcysteine is delivered by the inhalation route and is not available OTC. It is used in patients who have cystic fibrosis or other diseases that produce large amounts of thick bronchial secretions. Acetylcysteine (Acetadote) is also given as a 5% oral solution for acetaminophen overdose. When given within 24 hours of the overdose, acetylcysteine prevents acute liver damage by blocking the formation of toxic metabolites of acetaminophen.

ASTHMA

Asthma is a chronic pulmonary disease that has both inflammatory and bronchospasm components. Drugs are given to either decrease the frequency of asthmatic attacks or terminate attacks in progress. Asthma is one of the most common chronic conditions in the United States, affecting about 24 million people.

Core Concept 30.8 ▶

Asthma is a chronic inflammatory disease characterized by bronchospasm.

Asthma is characterized by chronic inflammation that occurs when potent mediators of the immune and inflammatory responses are released by mast cells lining the bronchi. The result of this inflammation is increased mucus secretion, which narrows the airways and makes breathing more difficult.

The second component of asthma is acute **bronchoconstriction** or **bronchospasm** during which bronchiolar smooth muscle contracts and the airway diameter narrows. This condition is illustrated in Figure 30.5. The inflammatory conditions in the airway make the smooth muscle hyperresponsive to a variety of stimuli. Stimuli such as breathing smoke, pollutants, or cold air may trigger acute bronchospasm. Specific triggers are

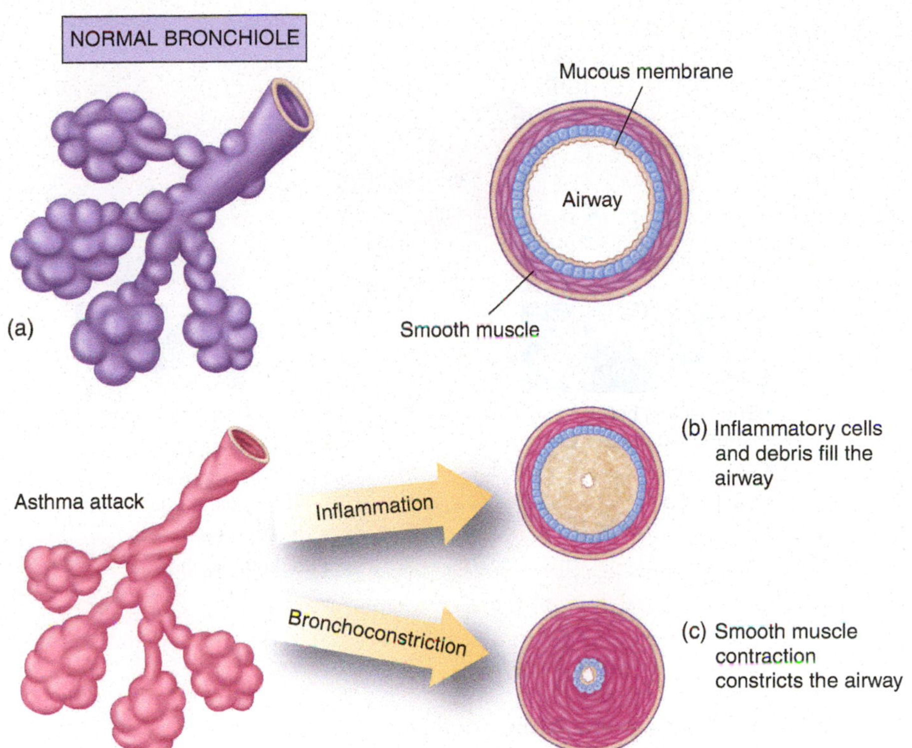

FIGURE 30.5 Changes in bronchioles during an asthma attack: (a) normal bronchiole, (b) inflammation obstructing the airway, and (c) constricted bronchiole in asthma attack.

listed in Table 30.5. Some patients experience bronchospasm on exertion, a condition called exercise-induced asthma.

The patient with asthma will exhibit symptoms such as evening cough, **dyspnea** (shortness of breath), chest tightness, and wheezing. Intervals between symptoms may vary from days to weeks to months. **Status asthmaticus** is a severe, prolonged form of asthma that is unresponsive to drug treatment and may lead to respiratory failure.

dys = *painful or difficult*
pnea = *breathing*

Table 30.5 Common Triggers of Asthma

Air pollutants	Tobacco smoke Ozone Nitrous and sulfur oxides Fumes from cleaning fluids or solvents Burning leaves
Allergens	Pollen from trees, grasses, and weeds Animal dander Household dust Mold
Chemicals and food	Drugs such as aspirin, ibuprofen, and beta blockers Sulfite preservatives Food such as nuts, monosodium glutamate (MSG), shellfish, and dairy products
Respiratory infections	Bacterial, fungal, and viral
Stress	Emotional stress or anxiety Exercise in dry, cold climates

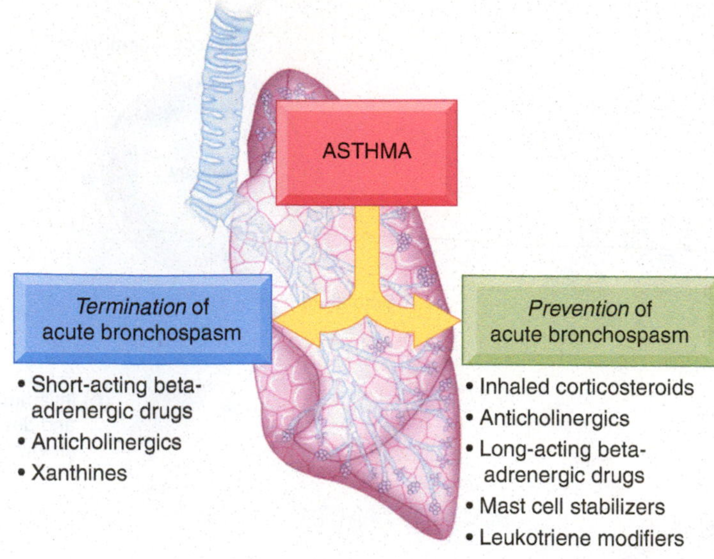

FIGURE 30.6 Drug classes used in the pharmacotherapy of asthma.

Because asthma has both a bronchoconstriction component and an inflammatory component, drug therapy of the disease focuses on one or both of these mechanisms. The goals of drug therapy are twofold: to terminate an acute bronchospasm in progress and to reduce the frequency of acute asthma attacks. Different drug classes are usually needed to achieve each of these goals. The various classes of drugs used for asthma are shown in Figure 30.6.

Core Concept 30.9 ▶ Beta-adrenergic agonists are the most effective drugs for relieving acute bronchospasm.

Recall from Chapter 9 that the smooth muscle lining the bronchioles is under the control of the autonomic nervous system. Changes in the airway diameter are made possible by the contraction or relaxation of the bronchiolar smooth muscle. During the fight-or-flight response, beta$_2$-adrenergic receptors of the sympathetic nervous system are activated, the bronchiolar smooth muscle relaxes, and **bronchodilation** results. This allows more air to reach the alveoli, thus increasing the oxygen supply to the body during periods of stress or exercise. In practical terms, drugs that enhance bronchodilation will cause the patient to breathe more easily; these are some of the most common medications for treating pulmonary disorders.

Bronchodilators are medications from several drug classes that are used to rapidly relieve the acute bronchospasm characteristic of an asthmatic attack. Although the beta-adrenergic drugs are the most commonly prescribed types of bronchodilators, theophylline and ipratropium may also be used. Bronchodilators used for asthma are listed in Table 30.6.

Beta-adrenergic drugs, or sympathomimetics, are the most effective drugs for the treatment of acute bronchospasm. In most cases, the drugs used for pulmonary disease are selective for beta$_2$-receptors in the lung; thus, they produce fewer cardiac adverse effects than the nonselective beta drugs. There are two basic classes of beta-adrenergic drugs, and each has different indications.

- *Short-acting beta agonists* Short-acting beta agonists (SABAs) are the most frequently prescribed drugs for aborting or terminating an acute asthma attack because they begin to act within minutes. Their effects, however, last only 2 to 6 hours.
- *Long-acting beta agonists* Because long-acting beta agonists (LABAs) take 20 to 60 minutes to act, they are not used to terminate bronchospasm. They are used in combination with inhaled corticosteroids for the prophylaxis of persistent asthma.

Table 30.6 Bronchodilators

Drug	Route and Adult Dose	Remarks
BETA-ADRENERGIC DRUGS		
Pr albuterol (Proventil HFA, Ventolin, VoSpire ER)	MDI: Two inhalations every 4–6 hours as needed (max: 12 inhalations/day) PO (extended release): 8 mg bid (max: 32 mg/day divided)	For asthma; relaxes bronchiolar smooth muscle; nebulizer form available
arformoterol (Brovana)	Nebulizer: 15 mcg bid (max: 30 mcg/day)	For COPD; long acting; similar to formoterol
formoterol (Foradil, Perforomist)	DPI: 12 mcg inhalation capsule bid (max: 24 mcg/day) Nebulizer: 20 mcg bid (max: 40 mcg/day)	For asthma prophylaxis and COPD; long acting
indacaterol (Arcapta neohaler)	Inhalation: One 75 mcg capsule daily using the Neohaler	For COPD
levalbuterol (Xopenex)	MDI: Two inhalations every 4–6 hours	For asthma; short acting; nebulizer and inhalations forms available
olodaterol (Stiverdi Respimat)	Inhalation: 2 inhalations daily	Newer drug for COPD
salmeterol (Serevent)	DPI: Two aerosol inhalations bid or one powder diskus bid	For asthma prophylaxis; long acting
terbutaline (Brethine)	PO: 2.5–5 mg tid (max: 15 mg/day) Subcutaneous: 250 mcg (may be repeated in 15 min)	Also used to delay preterm labor (off label)
ANTICHOLINERGICS		
aclidinium (Tudorza Pressair)	MDI: 400 mcg bid	For COPD
ipratropium (Atrovent)	MDI: Two inhalations qid (max: 12 inhalations/day) Nebulizer; 500 mcg every 6–8 hours	For COPD; intranasal form available for allergic rhinitis
tiotropium (Spiriva)	DPI: One capsule (18 mcg) /day using HandiHaler device	For COPD; inhalation form (Spiriva Respimat) available for asthma
umeclidinium (Incruse Ellipta)	DPI: 1 inhalation (62.5 mcg)/day	For COPD
XANTHINES		
aminophylline	PO/IV: 0.5-0.8 mg/kg/hr in 4 divided doses	Very similar to theophylline; dose individualized based on drug blood measurements
theophylline	PO: 300–600 mg/day in divided doses (max: 900 mg/day)	IV and extended-release form available

Fast Facts Asthma

According to the Asthma and Allergy Foundation of America (n.d.), every year in America:

- Children age 5 to 17 miss 10.5 million school days due to asthma.
- Adults miss more than 14 million days of work due to asthma.
- Two million people visit the emergency department due to asthma.
- About 439,000 people are admitted to a hospital due to asthma.
- About 3600 people die from asthma.

Prototype Drug: Pr *albuterol (Proventil HFA, Ventolin, VoSpire ER)*

Therapeutic Class: Beta$_2$-adrenergic agonist

Actions and Uses: Albuterol is a SABA that is used to relieve the bronchospasm of asthma. Its rapid onset and excellent safety profile have made inhaled albuterol a preferred drug for the termination of acute bronchospasm. In addition to relieving bronchospasm, the drug facilitates mucus drainage and can inhibit the release of inflammatory chemicals from mast cells. When inhaled 15 to 30 minutes prior to physical activity, it can prevent exercise-induced bronchospasm.

Albuterol is also available as extended-release tablets (VoSpire ER). The tablets have a longer onset of action and are not suitable for terminating acute asthma attacks.

Adverse Effects and Interactions: Serious adverse effects from inhaled albuterol are uncommon. Some patients experience palpitations, headaches, throat irritation, tremor, nervousness, restlessness, and tachycardia. Concurrent use with beta blockers will inhibit the bronchodilation effect of albuterol.

Inhaled beta-adrenergic drugs exhibit limited systemic toxicity because relatively small amounts of the drugs are absorbed. When given orally, a longer duration of action is achieved, but adverse effects such as tachycardia and tremor are more frequently experienced. Tolerance may develop to the therapeutic effects of the beta-adrenergic drugs; therefore, the patient must be instructed to seek medical attention if the drugs prove to be less effective with continued use.

As discussed in Chapter 9, blocking the parasympathetic nervous system produces similar effects to stimulation of the sympathetic nervous system. It is predictable then, that anticholinergic drugs would cause bronchodilation and have potential use in the pharmacotherapy of asthma and other pulmonary diseases. The most widely used drug in this class, ipratropium (Atrovent), is taken via inhalation to rapidly relieve bronchospasm. Because it is not readily absorbed from the lungs, it produces few adverse effects, although it is considered less effective than beta-adrenergic drugs. A nasal spray formulation of ipratropium (Atrovent) is indicated for the symptomatic relief of runny nose due to the common cold or allergic rhinitis.

Inhaled anticholinergics are more effective when used with other bronchodilators; Combivent is a combination of ipratropium and albuterol in a single MDI canister. Tiotropium (Spiriva) is a newer anticholinergic with a long duration of action that allows for once-daily dosing.

The third class of bronchodilators is the xanthines (sometimes called methylxanthines). Chemically related to caffeine, theophylline and aminophylline were preferred drugs for bronchoconstriction 20 years ago. Theophylline, however, has a narrow margin of safety and interacts with a large number of other drugs. Adverse effects such as nausea, vomiting, and CNS stimulation are relatively common, and dysrhythmias may occur at high doses. Having been largely replaced by safer and more effective drugs, the xanthines are now primarily used for the long-term oral prophylaxis of persistent asthma.

Nursing Process Focus Patients Receiving Bronchodilators

ASSESSMENT

Prior to administration:

- Obtain a complete health history, including respiratory, cardiovascular, renal and liver conditions, drug history, and possible drug interactions.
- Obtain information about experiences with anaphylaxis, asthma, allergies, and exposure to environmental irritants; effects of respiratory difficulties on sleep, eating, and performance of activities of daily living (ADLs).
- Evaluate laboratory blood findings: CBC, arterial blood gases (ABGs), and renal and liver function studies. Evaluate results of pulmonary function tests (peak expiratory flowmeter).
- Acquire the results of a complete physical examination, including vital signs, pulse oximetry, and symptoms related to respiratory deficiency, such as dyspnea, orthopnea, cyanosis, nasal flaring, adventitious lung sounds (wheezing), and weakness.

POTENTIAL NURSING DIAGNOSES*

- *Impaired Gas Exchange* related to bronchial constriction
- *Anxiety* related to difficulty in breathing
- *Deficient Knowledge* related to a lack of information about drug therapy
- *Ineffective Health Management* related to noncompliance with medication regimen, presence of adverse effects, and need for long-term medication use

PLANNING: PATIENT GOALS AND EXPECTED OUTCOMES

The patient will:

- Experience therapeutic effects (adequate oxygenation, improved lung sounds, and improved pulmonary function values).
- Be free from or experience minimal adverse effects from drug therapy.
- Verbalize an understanding of the drug's use, adverse effects, and required precautions.

IMPLEMENTATION

Interventions and (Rationales)	Patient Education/Discharge Planning
• Continue to monitor vital signs (including pulse and blood pressure, respiratory pattern, pulse oximetry, and lung sounds). Monitor periodic pulmonary function tests: peak expiratory flowmeter and ABGs. (Monitoring is necessary to determine drug effectiveness.)	Instruct the patient to: • Use medication as directed even if asymptomatic to prevent the onset of respiratory difficulties. • Report symptoms of deteriorating respiratory status such as increased dyspnea, breathlessness with speech, or orthopnea to the healthcare provider.

Interventions and (Rationales)	Patient Education/Discharge Planning
• Administer medication correctly and evaluate the patient's knowledge of proper use of the inhaler. (Proper administration techniques and use of equipment ensures correct dosage.)	Instruct the patient to: • Recognize the difference between long- and short-acting inhalers. • Use a spacer between MDI and mouth. • Shake or load the inhaler with tablet or powder. • If using a bronchodilator inhaler with a corticosteroid inhaler: Use the bronchodilator first to open the airway, wait 5 to 10 minutes, then take the corticosteroid. • Use the medication strictly as prescribed; do not "double up" on doses. • Rinse the mouth thoroughly following use. • Rinse inhaler and spacer with water daily.
• Observe for adverse effects specific to the medication used. (An increase in pulse rate, changes in blood pressure, or sensations of palpitations may occur with beta-adrenergic drugs.)	• Instruct the patient regarding adverse effects and to report specific drug adverse effects such as palpitations or fast heart rate and respirations.
• Maintain the environment free of respiratory contaminants such as dust, dry air, flowers, and smoke. (These substances may exacerbate bronchial constriction.)	Instruct the patient to: • Avoid respiratory irritants. • Maintain a "clean air environment." • Stop smoking and avoid secondhand smoke, if applicable.
• Maintain dietary intake adequate in essential nutrients and vitamins. (Dyspnea interferes with proper nutrition due to the added energy and effort required to breathe.)	Instruct the patient to: • Maintain nutrition with foods high in essential nutrients. • Consume small frequent meals to prevent fatigue.
• Ensure that the patient maintains adequate hydration of 3 to 4 L/day (to liquefy pulmonary secretions).	Instruct the patient to: • Consume 3 to 4 L of fluid per day if not contraindicated. • Avoid caffeine (increases CNS irritability).
• Provide emotional and psychosocial support during periods of dyspnea. (Providing support and remaining calm helps to reduce the anxiety brought on by respiratory difficulties.)	• Instruct the patient in relaxation and controlled breathing techniques.
• Monitor patient compliance. (Maintaining therapeutic drug levels is essential for effective therapy.)	• Inform the patient of the importance of ongoing medication compliance and follow-up.

EVALUATION OF OUTCOME CRITERIA

Evaluate the effectiveness of drug therapy by confirming that patient goals and expected outcomes have been met (see "Planning"). *See Table 30.6 for a list of drugs to which these nursing actions apply.*

*Herdman, T.H. & Kamitsuru, S. (Eds.), *Nursing Diagnoses: Definitions & Classification* 2015–2017. Copyright © 2014, 1994–2014 NANDA International. Used by arrangement by John Wiley & Sons, Inc. Companion website: www.wiley.com/go/nursingdiagnoses.

Corticosteroids are the most effective drugs for the long-term prophylaxis of asthma.

◀ **Core Concept 30.10**

The role of intranasal corticosteroids as first-line drugs in the treatment of allergic rhinitis is discussed in Core Concept 30.5. When given by the inhalation route, corticosteroids are also prime drugs for the prevention of asthma attacks.

Because asthma has a major inflammatory component, several classes of anti-inflammatory drugs are used for asthma prophylaxis. The inhaled corticosteroids are most frequently prescribed for this purpose, although mast cell stabilizers and leukotriene inhibitors are also effective. Doses of the anti-inflammatory drugs used for asthma are given in Table 30.7.

Corticosteroids are the most effective drugs available for the *prevention* of acute asthmatic episodes. When inhaled on a daily schedule, corticosteroids suppress inflammation without producing major adverse effects. Mucus production and edema are diminished, thus reducing airway obstruction. Patients should be informed that inhaled corticosteroids must be taken daily to produce their therapeutic effect and that these medications are not effective at terminating episodes in progress. Although symptoms will improve in the first 1 to 2 weeks of therapy, 4 to 8 weeks may be required for maximum benefit. For some patients, a SABA may be prescribed along with an inhaled corticosteroid because this permits the dose of the corticosteroid to be reduced by as much as 50%.

Table 30.7 Anti-Inflammatory Drugs for Asthma

Drug	Route and Adult Dose	Remarks
INHALED CORTICOSTEROIDS		
beclomethasone (Qvar)	MDI: One or two inhalations tid or qid (max: 320 mcg bid)	Intranasal form available for allergic rhinitis
budesonide (Pulmicort Flexhaler)	DPI: One or two inhalations daily (max: 720 mcg/day)	Intranasal form available for allergic rhinitis; oral form available for inflammatory bowel disease
ciclesonide (Alvesco)	MDI: One or two inhalations/day (max: 320–640 mcg/day)	For asthma prophylaxis; intranasal form available for allergic rhinitis
fluticasone (Arnuity Ellipta, Flovent Diskus)	MDI (Flovent Diskus): Two inhalations bid (max: 1000 mcg bid) MDI (Arnuity Ellipta): One inhalation/day (max: 200 mcg/day)	Intranasal form available for allergic rhinitis
mometasone (Asmanex)	DPI: One inhalation daily (max: two inhalations daily)	Intranasal form available for allergic rhinitis and topical form for skin inflammation
MAST CELL STABILIZER		
cromolyn	MDI: One inhalation qid	For exercise- or allergen-induced asthma prophylaxis; Intranasal form available OTC for allergic rhinitis; also for ophthalmic use
LEUKOTRIENE MODIFIERS		
montelukast (Singulair)	PO: 10 mg once daily	For allergic rhinitis and exercise- or allergen-induced asthma prophylaxis
roflumilast (Daliresp)	PO: 500 mcg once daily	For COPD
zafirlukast (Accolate)	PO: 20 mg bid	For asthma prophylaxis
zileuton (Zyflo)	PO (extended release): 1200 mg bid (max: 2400 mg/day)	For asthma prophylaxis

For severe, persistent asthma that is unresponsive to other treatments, oral corticosteroids may be prescribed. Treatment time is limited to the shortest length possible, usually 5 to 7 days. If taken for longer than 10 days, oral corticosteroids may produce significant adverse effects such as adrenal gland suppression, peptic ulcers, and hyperglycemia. Other uses and adverse effects of corticosteroids are presented in Chapters 25 and 32.

Core Concept 30.11 ▶

Mast cell stabilizers, leukotriene modifiers, and monoclonal antibodies are alternative anti-inflammatory drugs for the prophylaxis of asthma.

The mast cell stabilizers and leukotriene modifiers are second-line drugs for the treatment of asthma. These drugs are prescribed when bronchodilators and corticosteroids are unable to control asthma symptoms.

Cromolyn is an anti-inflammatory drug that inhibits the release of histamine from mast cells. Although not a preferred drug for asthma control, cromolyn is a safe alternative to the corticosteroids for preventing asthma attacks. For optimal effectiveness, cromolyn must be taken on a daily basis and not be used to terminate acute attacks. An intranasal form of cromolyn (Nasalcrom) is used in the treatment of seasonal allergies.

The leukotriene modifiers reduce inflammation and ease bronchoconstriction by modifying the action of leukotrienes, which are mediators of the inflammatory response in patients with asthma. Leukotriene modifiers are second-line drugs used for the management of persistent asthma that cannot be controlled with inhaled corticosteroids or SABAs.

The leukotriene modifiers are approved for the prophylaxis of chronic asthma; they are ineffective in relieving acute bronchospasm. They are all given orally. Zileuton and roflumilast have rapid onsets, whereas the other two leukotriene modifiers take as long as a week to provide therapeutic benefit. Adverse effects associated with the leukotriene modifiers include headache, cough, nasal congestion, GI upset, and psychiatric effects such as depression and suicidal thinking.

The final approach to managing asthma is through the use of immunomodulators. The two approved medications in this class, omalizumab (Xolair) and reslizumab (Cinqair), are monoclonal antibodies indicated for severe, persistent asthma that cannot be controlled through safer medications. Omalizumab attaches to a receptor on immunoglobulin E (IgE) to prevent inflammation and the body's response to allergen triggers. Reslizumab attaches to inerleukin-5, reducing the number of eosinophils that exacerbate asthma symptoms. Both drugs are given subcutaneously and care must be taken to observe the patient for anaphylaxis.

CONCEPT REVIEW 30.5

- Distinguish the classes of drugs that *prevent* asthma attacks from those that can *terminate* an attack in progress. Name at least one drug in each class.

CHRONIC OBSTRUCTIVE PULMONARY DISEASE

COPD includes progressive lung disorders primarily caused by tobacco smoking. COPD is a major cause of death and disability. Drugs may bring symptomatic relief but do not cure the disorders.

Chronic obstructive pulmonary disease is a progressive disorder treated with multiple drugs.

◀ **Core Concept 30.12**

The two primary disorders classified as COPD are chronic bronchitis and emphysema. Both are strongly associated with smoking tobacco products and, secondarily, air pollutants. In **chronic bronchitis**, excess mucus is produced in the respiratory tract due to inflammation and irritation from smoke or pollutants. The airway becomes partially obstructed with mucus, resulting in the classic signs of dyspnea and coughing; thus, wheezing and decreased exercise tolerance are additional clinical signs. Because microbes enjoy the mucus-rich environment, pulmonary infections are common. Gas exchange may be impaired.

bronch = *bronchus*
itis = *inflammation*

COPD is a progressive disease, with the terminal stage being **emphysema**. After years of chronic inflammation, the bronchioles lose their elasticity, and the alveoli dilate to maximum size to get more air into the lungs. The patient suffers from extreme dyspnea from even the slightest physical activity.

The goals of pharmacotherapy of COPD are to relieve symptoms and avoid complications of the condition. Most patients receive the same classes of bronchodilators and anti-inflammatory drugs that are used for asthma. Mucolytics and expectorants are sometimes used to reduce thick bronchial mucus and to aid in its removal. Long-term oxygen therapy assists breathing and has been shown to decrease mortality in patients with advanced COPD. Antibiotics may be prescribed for patients who experience multiple bouts of pulmonary infections.

Several newer agents and drug combinations have been recently approved specifically for the maintenance treatment of COPD. These include roflumilast (Daliresp), umeclidinium (Incruse ellipta), Anoro ellipta (umeclidinium with vilanterol, a LABA), Breo ellipta (vilanterol with a corticosteroid), Stiolto Respimat (tiotropium with olodaterol, a LABA), Bevespi Aerosphere (glycopyrrolate with formoterol, a LABA) and Utibron Neohaler (indacaterol with glycopyrrolate).

Patients should be taught to avoid taking any drugs that have beta-blocking activity or that otherwise cause bronchoconstriction. Respiratory depressants should be avoided. It is important to note that none of the pharmacotherapies offer a cure for COPD; they only treat the symptoms of a progressively worsening disease. The most important teaching point is to strongly encourage smoking cessation in these patients. Smoking cessation has been shown to slow the progression of COPD and to result in fewer respiratory symptoms.

Patients Need to Know

Patients treated for pulmonary disorders need to know the following:

In General

1. Because tolerance to some medications may occur, if medication is no longer effective, report to a healthcare provider. Do not take extra medication without notifying a healthcare provider.

Regarding Inhaled Medications

2. When using MDIs or DPIs, allow an interval of at least 1 minute to pass between puffs.
3. When taking more than one respiratory medicine, take the bronchodilator first. This opens the airways and increases the effectiveness of the second medication.
4. Rinse the mouth thoroughly following inhaler use to reduce the oral absorption of inhaled medicines.
5. Take inhaled corticosteroids on a regular basis. These medications are not effective at stopping an acute asthma attack once it has begun.
6. Do not use decongestant nasal sprays for more than 2 or 3 days unless instructed to do so by a healthcare provider.

Regarding Bronchodilators

7. Avoid caffeine-containing foods and beverages.
8. Immediately report any abnormalities in pulse rate, changes in blood pressure, or sensations of palpitations when taking beta-adrenergic stimulators.

Regarding Antihistamines and Decongestants

9. If taking antihistamines for the first time, avoid operating machinery or performing other tasks requiring alertness because drowsiness may occur.
10. Use hard candies, chewing gum, or ice chips to treat the dry mouth caused by some decongestants and antihistamines.
11. Stop taking antihistamines and notify a healthcare provider if excessive sedation, wheezing, chest tightness, bleeding, or bruising occurs.
12. Do not take OTC cold or allergy medicines containing antihistamines at the same time as prescription antihistamines.

Chapter Review

Core Concepts Summary

30.1 The respiratory system supplies oxygen for the body and provides protection against inhaled pathogens.

The URT warms the incoming air and reacts to particles or pathogens that attempt to enter the body. The LRT brings needed oxygen into the body and removes carbon dioxide through expiration. The process of moving air into and out of the lungs, or ventilation, is distinct from the process of gas exchange across the alveoli, a process known as respiration.

30.2 The inhalation route of drug administration quickly delivers medications directly to their sites of action.

Inhalation is frequently used as a route of drug administration for those medications targeted for the respiratory system. Nebulizers, DPIs, and MDIs are used to deliver drugs via the inhalation route.

30.3 Allergic rhinitis is characterized by sneezing, watery eyes, and nasal congestion.

Allergic rhinitis, also known as hay fever, is a chronic allergy triggered by a wide variety of antigens. The release of chemicals mediating the immune response can result in seasonal symptoms for some patients, and chronic, continuous symptoms for others.

30.4 Antihistamines are widely used to treat allergic rhinitis and other minor allergies.

The H_1-receptor blockers, or antihistamines, are used to treat allergies, motion sickness, and insomnia. Newer drugs in this class are nonsedating and offer the advantage of once-a-day dosing.

30.5 Intranasal corticosteroids are first-line drugs for treating allergic rhinitis.

Intranasal corticosteroids are the treatment of choice for allergic rhinitis because of their high effectiveness and wide margin of safety. When used by this route, they do not produce the serious adverse effects observed when they are given orally or parenterally.

30.6 Decongestants are used to reduce nasal congestion caused by allergic rhinitis and the common cold.

Oral and intranasal sympathomimetics are effective at relieving nasal congestion. The intranasal drugs act more rapidly and are more effective. Use of the intranasal preparations, however, is usually limited to 3 to 5 days because of the potential for rebound congestion.

30.7 Antitussives and expectorants are used to treat symptoms of the common cold.

Antitussives are effective at inhibiting the cough reflex. Although opioids are the most effective, there is some risk of physical dependence. Guaifenesin is an OTC drug used to increase bronchial secretions so that cough may be more productive. Mucolytics loosen mucus so that it may be more easily removed from the bronchial tree.

30.8 Asthma is a chronic inflammatory disease characterized by bronchospasm.

Asthma is a common disease characterized by bronchospasm and chronic airway inflammation. Exposure to a number of factors, including allergens, can cause an acute episode.

30.9 Beta-adrenergic agonists are the most effective drugs for relieving acute bronchospasm.

Inhaled beta$_2$-adrenergic drugs are preferred medications for relieving bronchospasm. Anticholinergics are sometimes used for bronchodilation, but fewer are available because of their incidence of adverse effects. Xanthines, once widely used in pulmonary medicine, are now second-choice drugs for relieving bronchospasm because of their higher potential for adverse effects.

30.10 Corticosteroids are the most effective drugs for the long-term prophylaxis of asthma.

Inhaled corticosteroids are the drugs of choice for asthma prophylaxis. The inhaled corticosteroids, even when used on a long-term basis, produce few adverse effects compared to oral corticosteroids.

30.11 Mast cell stabilizers, leukotriene modifiers, and monoclonal antibodies are alternative anti-inflammatory drugs for the prophylaxis of asthma.

Mast cell stabilizers such as cromolyn and the leukotriene modifiers are sometimes used for asthma prophylaxis, although they are not as effective as the corticosteroids. Monoclonal antibody therapy offers a novel approach to managing chronic asthma.

30.12 Chronic obstructive pulmonary disease is a progressive disorder treated with multiple drugs.

Chronic bronchitis and emphysema are two disorders of COPD that often require multiple drug therapy. Bronchodilators, expectorants, mucolytics, antibiotics, and oxygen may offer symptomatic relief.

REVIEW Questions

Answer the following questions to assess your knowledge of the chapter material, and go back and review any material that is not clear to you.

1. The patient is having an acute asthma attack. The nurse knows that which of the following drugs to be most appropriate?
   1. Albuterol (Proventil HFA)
   2. Budesonide (Pulmicort)
   3. Fluticasone (Flovent)
   4. Zafirlukast (Accolate)

2. Salmeterol (Serevent) has been added to your patient's treatment regimen for asthma. Which of the following is of highest priority for patients to know?
   1. Nausea and vomiting may be adverse effects.
   2. It is important to take this medication every day in order to prevent an asthma attack.
   3. The drug causes tremors.
   4. Avoid caffeine-containing foods and beverages.

3. A 24-year-old patient has just started taking Benadryl because of an allergic reaction. The nurse knows to monitor the patient for: (Select all that apply.)
   1. Drowsiness.
   2. Dry mouth.
   3. Tachycardia.
   4. Nausea.
   5. Mild hypotension.

4. The healthcare provider has ordered montelukast (Singulair). As the nurse begins to administer the medication, the patient asks how soon it will begin working. The nurse responds by answering:
   1. "The medication has a rapid onset—within 2 hours."
   2. "It will take about a week to become effective."
   3. "This medication is used to treat acute bronchospasms only."
   4. "Therapeutic benefits may take several weeks."

5. The patient asks what the difference is between antitussives and mucolytics. The nurse replies:
   1. "Antitussives loosen bronchial secretions, and mucolytics stimulate removal of bronchial secretions."
   2. "Antitussives suppress cough, whereas mucolytics loosen bronchial secretions."
   3. "The terms are interchangeable."
   4. "Both types of drugs work to loosen and remove secretions."

6. A patient with asthma states that it has become worse over the past few months. He continues to say that when an acute asthma attack occurs, budesonide (Pulmicort Turbuhaler) does not stop the episode. The nurse should advise the patient:
   1. To use four inhalations of budesonide instead of two.
   2. That budesonide must be taken on a regular schedule to work.
   3. To request a tablet form of corticosteroid, rather than an inhaler.
   4. To always clear his nose gently just prior to using budesonide.
7. The patient complains of numbness of the throat and tongue after taking benzonatate (Tessalon). The nurse instructs the patient:
   1. To swallow, not chew, the medication.
   2. To decrease the dosage of medication.
   3. To stop taking the medication immediately.
   4. That this is a common adverse effect that will subside over time.
8. The healthcare provider ordered albuterol 4 mg, three times a day. The available concentration is 2 mg in 5 mL. How many milliliters would be given per dose?
   1. 2 mL
   2. 5 mL
   3. 10 mL
   4. 20 mL
9. The nurse informs patients taking intranasal corticosteroids that they may experience which of the following adverse effects?
   1. Rebound congestion
   2. Intense burning sensation
   3. Drowsiness
   4. Anxiety
10. Wile planning an educational session for patients using Afrin, the nurse would include:
    1. Not to use it for longer than 3 to 5 days to prevent rebound congestion from occurring.
    2. The importance of monitoring for hypertension.
    3. To notify the healthcare provider if nervousness occurs.
    4. Not to take it with any other medications.

CASE STUDY Questions

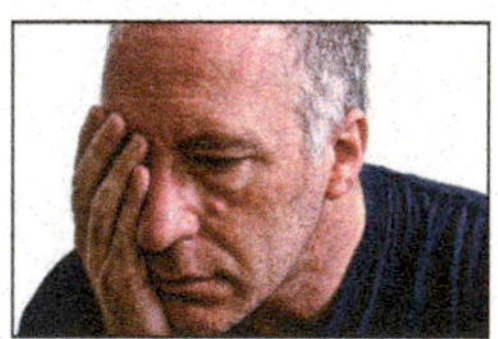

Remember Mr. Thomas, who was introduced at the beginning of the chapter? Now read the remainder of the case study. Based on the information you have learned in this chapter, answer the questions that follow.

Mr. Michael Thomas arrives at the office with what appears to be an acute upper respiratory tract infection. He tells the nurse, "I can't sleep at night with this cough, and I can hardly work without getting short of breath." On examination, he has a low-grade fever and dyspnea when walking. He is 60 years old, smokes a pack of cigarettes daily, and has a history of emphysema, although he doesn't usually take any medications. For his upper respiratory infection, the healthcare provider prescribes hydrocodone, guaifenesin, acetaminophen, and an ipratropium (Atrovent) inhaler.

1. Before leaving the doctor's office, Mr. Thomas asks which of his prescribed drugs will directly help him with his dyspnea. The nurse tells him that it is:
   1. Hydrocodone.
   2. Acetaminophen.
   3. Guaifenesin.
   4. Ipratropium.
2. He wants to know which of his prescriptions will help him "get the mucus up that's stuck in the back of my throat." The nurse tells him that ________ will help thin bronchial secretions, allowing them to be removed more easily.
   1. Hydrocodone
   2. Acetaminophen
   3. Guaifenesin
   4. Ipratropium
3. Mr. Thomas calls the office the next day, complaining that he is unable to drive his car because of excessive drowsiness. The nurse suspects that ________ is most likely causing this drowsiness.
   1. Hydrocodone
   2. Acetaminophen
   3. Guaifenesin
   4. Ipratropium
4. Mr. Thomas also has emphysema. The healthcare provider plans to continue him on guaifenesin and ipratropium. He also wants him to take an inhaled corticosteroid. The nurse expects that Mr. Thomas will be given a prescription for:
   1. Salmeterol.
   2. Tiotropium.
   3. Budesonide.
   4. Olopatadine.

Answers and complete rationales for the Review and Case Study Questions appear in Appendix A.

REFERENCES

Asthma and Allergy Foundation of America. (n.d.). *Asthma facts and figures*. Retrieved from http://www.aafa.org/page/asthma-facts.aspx

Herdman, T. H., & Kamitsuru, S. (Eds.). (2014). *NANDA International nursing diagnoses: Definitions and classification, 2015–2017*. Oxford, United Kingdom: Wiley-Blackwell

SELECTED BIBLIOGRAPHY

American Academy of Allergy, Asthma & Immunology (n.d.). *AAAAI allergy and asthma drug guide*. Retrieved from https://www.aaaai.org/conditions-and-treatments/drug-guide

Asthma and Allergy Foundation of America (n.d). *Allergy facts and figures*. Retrieved from http://www.aafa.org/page/allergy-facts.aspx

Barjaktarevic, I. Z., Arredondo, A. F., & Cooper, C. B. (2015). Positioning new pharmacotherapies for COPD. *International Journal of Chronic Obstructive Pulmonary Disease, 10*, 1427–1442. doi:10.2147/COPD.S83758

Calverley, P., & Vlies, B. (2015). New pharmacotherapeutic approaches for chronic obstructive pulmonary disease. *Seminars in Respiratory and Critical Care Medicine 36*, 523–542. doi:10.1055/s-0035-1556057

Centers for Disease Control and Prevention. (2016). *Asthma*. Retrieved from http://www.cdc.gov/nchs/fastats/asthma.htm

Jackson, K. D., Howie, L. D., & Akinbami, L. J. (2013). Trends in allergic conditions among children: United States, 1997–2011. *NCHS Data Brief, 121*. Retrieved from http://www.cdc.gov/nchs/data/databriefs/db121.pdf

Klimek, L., Mullol, J., Hellings, P., Gevaert, P., Mösges, R., & Fokkens, W. (2016). Recent pharmacological developments in the treatment of perennial and persistent allergic rhinitis. *Expert Opinion on Pharmacotherapy, 17*, 657–669. doi:10.1517/14656566.2016.1145661

Licari, A., Castagnoli, R., Bottino, C., Marseglia, A., Marseglia, G., & Ciprandi, G. (2016). Emerging drugs for the treatment of perennial allergic rhinitis. *Expert Opinion on Emerging Drugs, 21*, 57–67. doi:10.1517/14728214.2016.1139082

National Institute of Allergy and Infectious Diseases. (n.d.). *Food allergies: Quick facts*. Retrieved from https://www.niaid.nih.gov/topics/foodallergy/Pages/default.aspx

Restrepo, R. D. (2015). Year in review 2014: COPD. *Respiratory Care, 60*, 1057–1060. doi:10.4187/respcare.04227

Smith, S. M., Schroeder, K., & Fahey, T. (2014). Over-the-counter (OTC) medications for acute cough in children and adults in community settings. *Cochrane Database of Systematic Reviews 2014, 11*, Art. No.: CD001831. doi:10.1002/14651858.CD001831.pub5

Rosenberg, S. R., Kalhan, R., & Mannino, D. M. (2015). Epidemiology of chronic obstructive pulmonary disease: Prevalence, morbidity, mortality, and risk factors. *Seminars in Respiratory and Critical Care Medicine 36*, 457–469. doi:10.1055/s-0035-1555607

Tharpe, C. A., & Kemp, S. F. (2015). Pediatric allergic rhinitis. *Immunology and Allergy Clinics, 35*, 185–198. doi: http://dx.doi.org/10.1016/j.iac.2014.09.003

Chapter 31

Drugs for Gastrointestinal Disorders

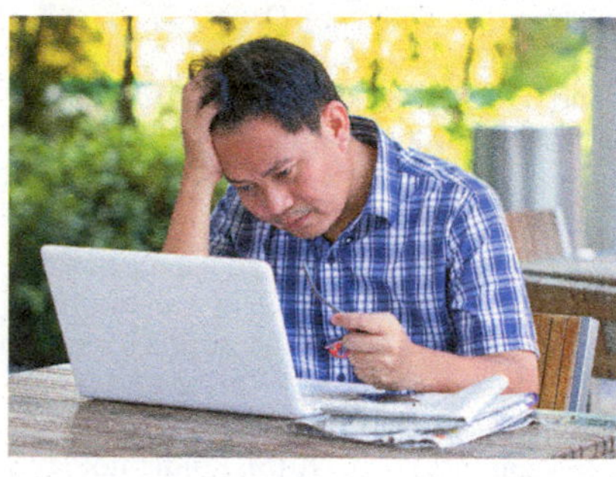

"An ulcer ... this is the last thing I need right now. My job is stressful enough."

Mr. Jeffery Han, stockbroker

Core Concepts

31.1 **The digestive system breaks down food, absorbs nutrients, and eliminates wastes.**

31.2 **Peptic ulcer disease is caused by erosion of the mucosal layer of the stomach or duodenum.**

31.3 **Peptic ulcer disease is treated by a combination of lifestyle changes and pharmacotherapy.**

31.4 **Proton-pump inhibitors are effective at reducing gastric acid secretion.**

31.5 **H_2-receptor blockers reduce the secretion of gastric acid.**

31.6 **Antacids rapidly neutralize stomach acid and reduce the symptoms of PUD and GERD.**

31.7 **Antibiotics are administered to eliminate *Helicobacter pylori*, the cause of many peptic ulcers.**

31.8 **Several miscellaneous drugs are also beneficial in treating peptic ulcer disease.**

31.9 **Laxatives are used to promote defecation.**

31.10 **Opioids are the most effective drugs for controlling severe diarrhea.**

31.11 **Antiemetics are prescribed to treat nausea, vomiting, and motion sickness.**

31.12 **Pancreatic enzymes are administered as replacement therapy for patients with pancreatitis or malabsorption syndromes.**

Drug Snapshot

The following drugs are discussed in this chapter:

Drug Classes	Prototype Drugs
Proton-pump inhibitors	Pr omeprazole (Prilosec)
H_2-receptor blockers	Pr ranitidine (Zantac)
Antacids	
Antibiotics for *H. pylori*	
Laxatives	Pr psyllium mucilloid (Metamucil, others)
Antidiarrheals	Pr diphenoxylate with atropine (Lomotil)
Antiemetics	Pr ondansetron (Zofran, Zuplenz)
Pancreatic enzyme replacements	

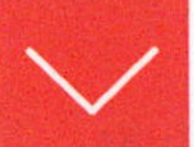

Learning Outcomes

After reading this chapter, the student should be able to:

1. Describe the major functions of the digestive system.
2. Identify common causes, signs, and symptoms of peptic ulcer disease and gastroesophageal reflux disease (GERD).
3. Describe general approaches to treating peptic ulcer disease and GERD.
4. Explain the role of proton pump inhibitors in the treatment of peptic ulcer disease and GERD.
5. Explain the role of H_2-receptor blockers in the treatment of peptic ulcer disease and GERD.
6. Explain the role of antacids in the treatment of peptic ulcer disease and GERD.
7. Explain the role of miscellaneous drugs in the treatment of peptic ulcer disease and GERD
8. Explain why two or more antibiotics are used concurrently in the treatment of *H. pylori*.
9. Compare and contrast the major classes of laxatives.
10. Identify the major drug classes used to treat diarrhea.
11. Identify the major drug classes used to treat nausea and vomiting.
12. Describe the pharmacotherapy of pancreatic insufficiency.

Key Terms

alimentary canal (AL-uh-MEN-tare-ee)
anorexia (AN-oh-REX-ee-uh)
antacid (an-TASS-id)
antiemetic (AN-tie-ee-MET-ik)
antiflatulents (an-tie-FLAT-u-lentz)
cathartic (kah-THAR-tik)
constipation (kon-stah-PAY-shun)
Crohn disease (KROHN)
defecation (def-ah-KAY-shun)
diarrhea
dietary fiber
digestion (dye-JES-chun)
emesis (EM-eh-sis)
emetics (ee-MET-ikz)
gastroesophageal reflux disease (GERD) (GAS-troh-ee-SOF-ah-JEEL REE-flux)
H^+, K^+-ATPase
H_2-receptor blocker
Helicobacter pylori (hee-lick-oh-BAK-tur py-LOR-eye)
inflammatory bowel disease (IBD)
pancreatic insufficiency
peptic ulcer
peristalsis (pair-ih-STAL-sis)
proton-pump inhibitors (PPIs)
triple therapy
ulcerative colitis (UL-sir-ah-tiv koh-LIE-tuss)
Zollinger–Ellison syndrome (ZOLL-in-jer ELL-ih-sun)

Very little of the food we eat is directly available for use as energy by our body. Food must be broken down, absorbed, and chemically modified before it is in a form useful to cells. The digestive system performs these functions and more. Some disorders of the digestive system are mechanical in nature, slowing or speeding up the transit of substances through the gastrointestinal tract. Other disorders are metabolic, affecting the secretion of digestive enzymes and fluids or the absorption of essential nutrients. Many signs and symptoms are nonspecific and may be caused by any number of different disorders. This chapter examines the drug therapy of common conditions affecting the digestive system.

Fast Facts Gastrointestinal Tract Disorders

- Sixty to 70 million Americans have a digestive disease.
- Patients with severe pancreatitis have about a 1 in 3 risk of dying from the disorder.
- About 4.5 million Americans are affected by peptic ulcer disease; there is a 1 in 10 lifetime risk of experiencing a duodenal ulcer.
- About 10% of Americans experience symptoms of gastroesophageal reflux disease on a daily basis.
- Inflammatory bowel disease most frequently occurs between ages 15 and 40, with the highest rates occurring in those of Jewish descent.
- Irritable bowel syndrome affects 10–15% of adults, with women about two times more likely to have the disorder.

Source: Data from National Institute of Diabetes and Digestive and Kidney Disorders (2014), Gardner, Anand, Patti, Rowe, and National Institute of Diabetes and Digestive and Kidney Disorders 2015.

Core Concept 31.1 ▶ The digestive system breaks down food, absorbs nutrients, and eliminates wastes.

The digestive system consists of two basic anatomic divisions: the alimentary canal and the accessory organs. The **alimentary canal**, or gastrointestinal (GI) tract, is a long, continuous, hollow tube that extends from the mouth to the anus. The accessory organs of digestion include the liver, gallbladder, and pancreas. The structure of the digestive system is shown in Figure 31.1.

Digestion is the process by which the body breaks down ingested food into small molecules that can be absorbed. The primary functions of the GI tract are to physically transport ingested food and to provide the necessary enzymes and surface area for chemical digestion and absorption. The inner surface is lined with a mucosa layer that secretes acids, bases, mucus, and enzymes important to digestion. The mucosa of the small intestine is lined with tiny projections called villi and microvilli that provide a huge surface area for the absorption of food and medications.

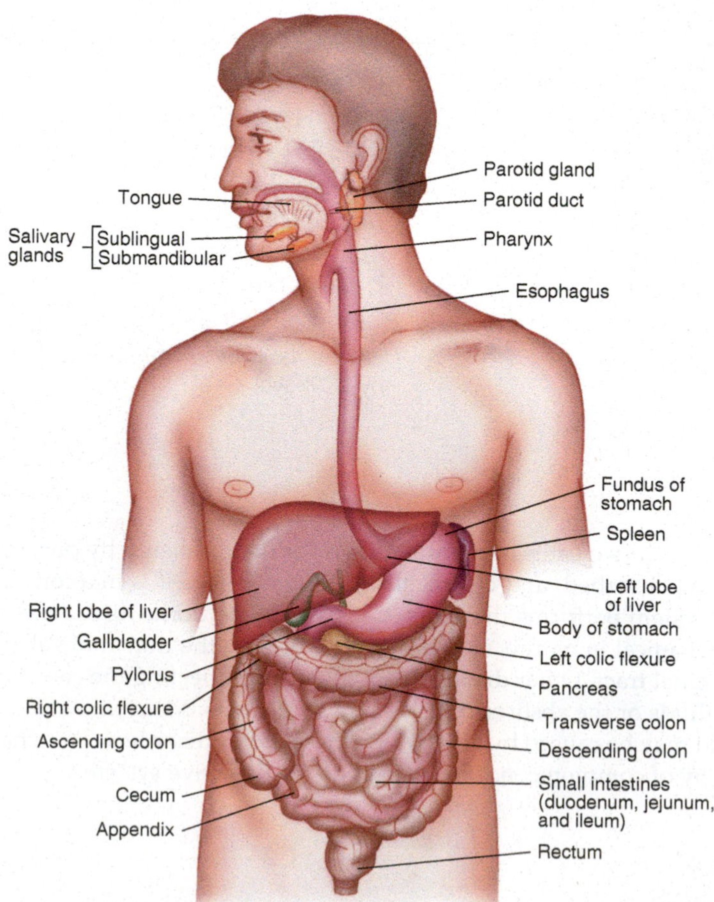

FIGURE 31.1 The digestive system.

Substances are propelled along the GI tract by the contractions of several layers of smooth muscle, a process known as **peristalsis**. The speed of transit is critical to the absorption of nutrients and water and for the removal of wastes. If peristalsis is too fast, substances will not have sufficient contact with the mucosa to be absorbed. In addition, the large intestine will not have enough time to absorb water, and diarrhea may result. Abnormally slow transit times may result in constipation or even obstructions in the small or large intestine.

peri = *around*
stalsis = *contraction*

To chemically break down ingested food, a large number of enzymes and other substances are required. Digestive enzymes are secreted by the salivary glands, stomach, small intestine, and pancreas. The liver makes bile, which is stored in the gallbladder until needed for lipid digestion. Because these digestive substances are not common targets for drug therapy, their discussion in this chapter is limited, and the student should refer to anatomy and physiology texts for additional information.

PEPTIC ULCER DISEASE

An ulcer is a sore or erosion of the mucosa of the GI tract. Although ulcers may occur in any portion of the GI tract, the duodenum is the most common site.

Peptic ulcer disease is caused by erosion of the mucosal layer of the stomach or duodenum.

◀ **Core Concept 31.2**

The term **peptic ulcer** refers to a lesion located in either the stomach (gastric) or small intestine (duodenal). The disorder is very common, affecting about 10% of the population at some point during their lifespan. Peptic ulcer disease (PUD) is associated with lifestyle factors such as cigarette smoking, stress, alcohol consumption, caffeine, and the use of drugs such as corticosteroids and nonsteroidal anti-inflammatory drugs (NSAIDs).

pept = *to digest*
ic = *pertaining to*

One to three liters of hydrochloric acid are secreted each day by cells in the stomach mucosa. Although this strong acid aids in the chemical breakdown of food and helps to protect the body from ingested microbes, it may be quite damaging to stomach cells. A number of natural defenses protect the stomach lining against this extremely acidic fluid. Certain cells lining the surface of the stomach secrete a thick mucus layer and bicarbonate, a basic ion that neutralizes acid and provides a protective function. On reaching the duodenum, the stomach contents are further neutralized by bicarbonate from pancreatic and biliary secretions. These natural defenses are depicted in Figure 31.2.

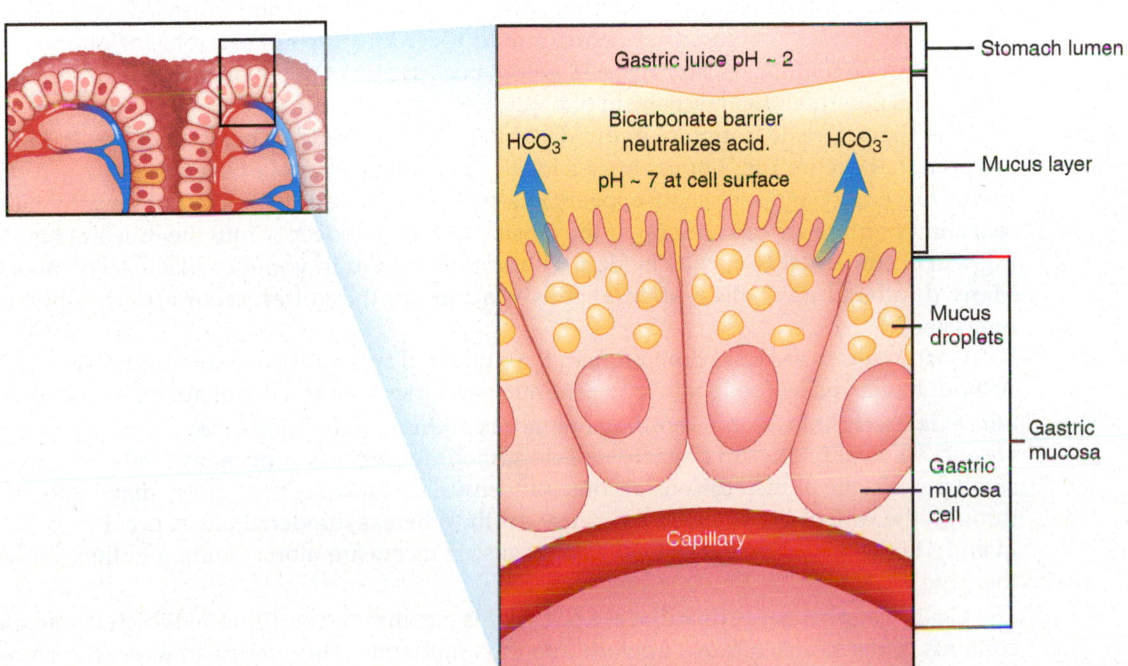

FIGURE 31.2 Natural defenses against stomach acid.

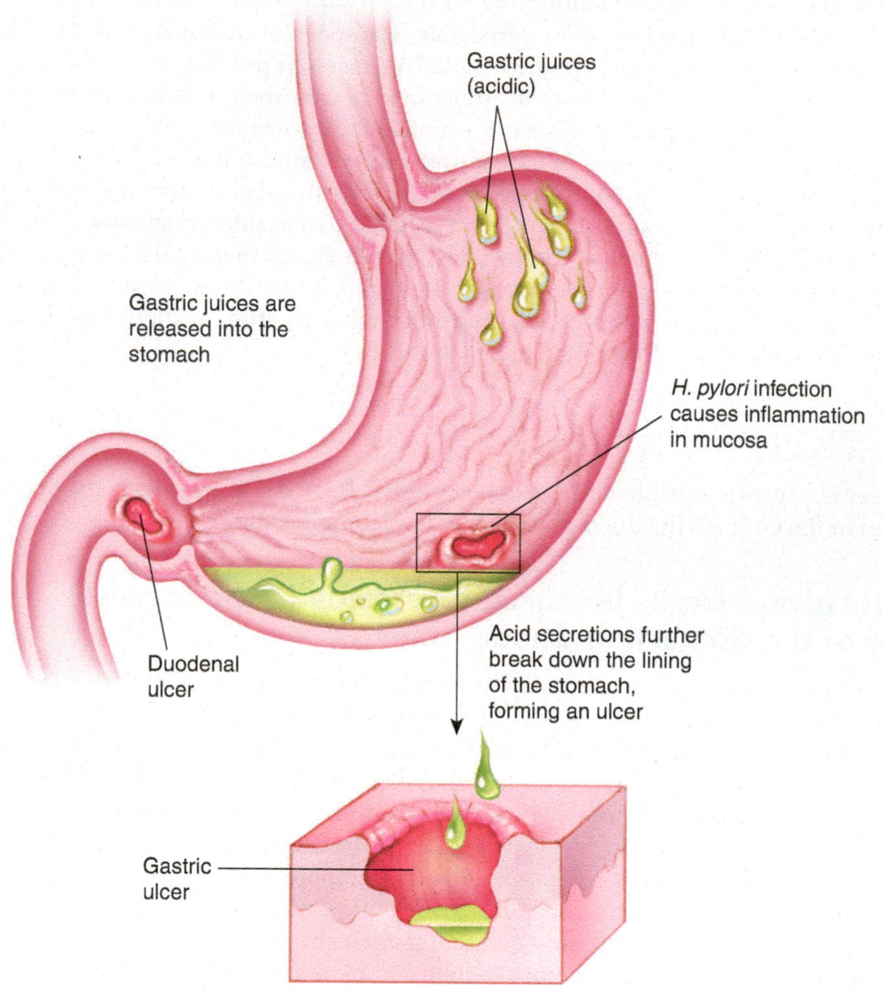

FIGURE 31.3 Mechanism of peptic ulcer formation.

It is well established that the primary cause of peptic ulcers is infection by the bacterium ***Helicobacter pylori***. In noninfected patients, the most common cause is therapy with NSAIDs. Secondary factors that contribute to ulcer and the subsequent inflammation include secretion of excess stomach acid and hyposecretion of adequate mucous protection. Figure 31.3 illustrates the mechanism of peptic ulcer formation.

The characteristic symptom of duodenal ulcer is a gnawing or burning upper abdominal pain that occurs 1 to 3 hours after a meal. The pain is worse between meals when the stomach is empty and it often disappears following ingestion of food. Nighttime pain, nausea, and vomiting are uncommon. If the erosion progresses deeper into the mucosa, bleeding will occur, and this may be evident as bright red blood in vomit or black, tarry stools. Many duodenal ulcers heal spontaneously, although they often recur after months of remission.

an = *without*
orexia = *appetite*

Gastric ulcers are less common than the duodenal type and have different symptoms. Although relieved by food, pain may continue even after a meal. Loss of appetite (known as **anorexia**), weight loss, and vomiting are more common. Remissions may be infrequent or absent. Medical follow-up of gastric ulcers sometimes proceeds for many years because a small percentage of the erosions become cancerous. The most severe ulcers may penetrate through the wall of the stomach and cause death. Whereas duodenal ulcers occur most frequently in the 30- to 50-year-old age group, gastric ulcers are more common in those older than age 60.

Gastroesophageal reflux disease (GERD) is a common condition in which the acidic contents of the stomach move upward into the esophagus. This causes an intense burning known as *heartburn* and may lead to ulcers in the esophagus. The cause of GERD is usually a loosening of the sphincter located between the esophagus and the stomach. GERD is strongly associated with obesity, and losing weight may eliminate the symptoms. Many of the drugs prescribed for peptic ulcers are also used to treat GERD.

Ulceration in the lower small intestine is known as **Crohn disease**, and erosions in the large intestine are called **ulcerative colitis**. These diseases are called **inflammatory bowel disease (IBD)**. Patients with these disorders experience abdominal cramping, diarrhea, and weight loss. Pharmacotherapy of IBD is usually with anti-inflammatory medications such as sulfasalazine (Azulfidine) or mesalamine (Asacol, Lialda, others). Severe cases may require immunosuppressant drugs such as corticosteroids, or immunomodulators such as infliximab (Remicade) or vedolizumab (Entyvio). A newer approach is to administer budesonide (Entocort EC, Uceris), a corticosteroid that is taken orally but is not absorbed. Budesonide produces anti-inflammatory actions directly on the intestine, with few or no systemic side effects.

CONCEPT REVIEW 31.1

- What are the similarities and differences between duodenal ulcers and gastric ulcers?

Peptic ulcer disease is treated by a combination of lifestyle changes and pharmacotherapy.

◀ **Core Concept 31.3**

Before starting drug therapy, patients are usually advised to change lifestyle factors that contribute to PUD. For example, eliminating tobacco, alcohol, and caffeine consumption, and reducing stress often allow the ulcer to heal, causing it to go into remission.

For patients requiring drug therapy, a wide variety of both prescription and over-the-counter (OTC) medications are available. These drugs fall into four primary classes, plus one miscellaneous group:

- Proton-pump inhibitors
- H_2-receptor blockers
- Antacids
- Antibiotics
- Miscellaneous drugs.

The treatment goals for pharmacotherapy are to provide immediate relief from symptoms, promote healing of the ulcer, and prevent recurrence of the disease. The choice of medication depends on the source of the disease (infectious versus inflammatory), the severity of symptoms, and the convenience of OTC versus prescription drugs. The most common therapy for the management of PUD is a combination of a proton-pump inhibitor plus two antibiotics. This approach, referred to as **triple therapy**, eliminates the cause of most peptic ulcers (*H. pylori*) while also reducing acid secretion. The mechanisms of action of the four major classes of drugs used to treat PUD are depicted in Figure 31.4.

Proton-pump inhibitors are effective at reducing gastric acid secretion.

◀ **Core Concept 31.4**

Proton-pump inhibitors act by blocking the enzyme responsible for secreting hydrochloric acid in the stomach. The proton-pump inhibitors are listed in Table 31.1.

Proton-pump inhibitors (PPIs) are the most effective medications available for reducing acid secretion and thus are preferred drugs for the treatment of PUD and GERD. These drugs reduce acid secretion by binding irreversibly to the enzyme **H^+, K^+-ATPase**. In the mucosal cells of the stomach, this enzyme acts as a pump to release acid (also called H^+, or protons) onto the surface of the GI mucosa. PPIs reduce acid secretion to a greater extent than do the H_2-receptor blockers and have a longer duration of action.

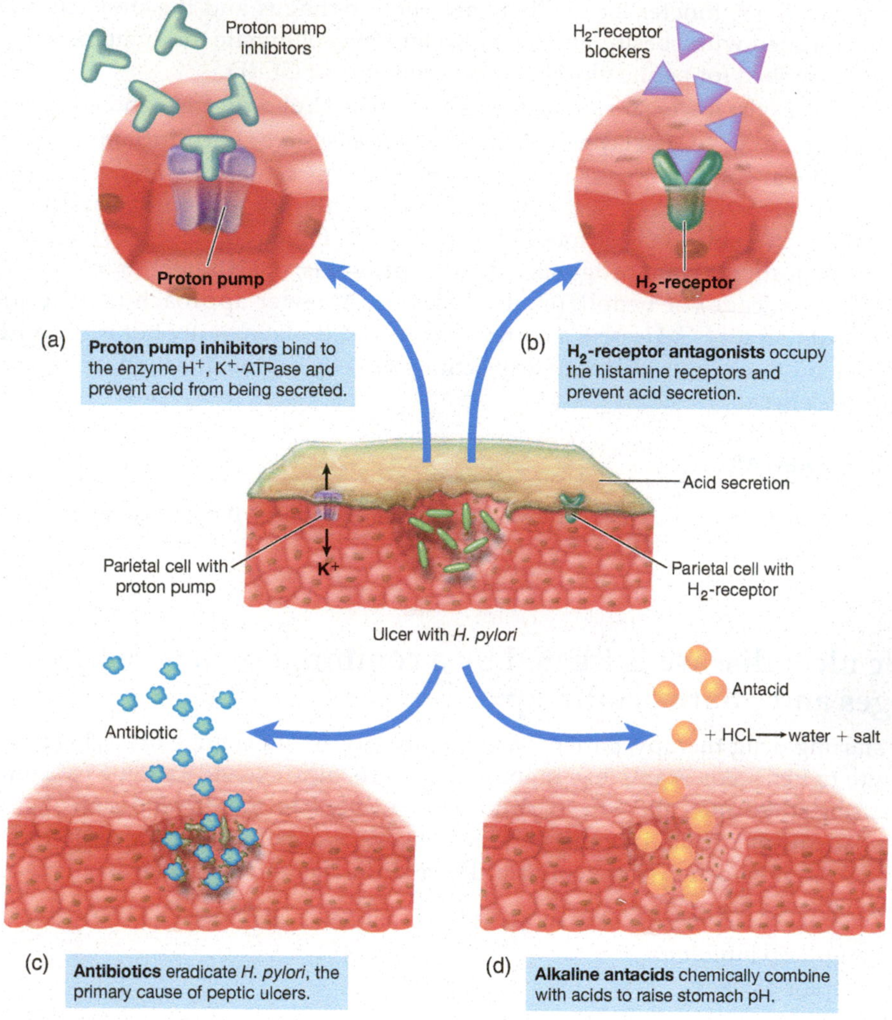

FIGURE 31.4 Mechanisms of action of antiulcer drugs: (a) Proton-pump inhibitors act by blocking acid secretion by the HCl pump; (b) H_2-receptor blockers act by decreasing acid secretion; (c) antibiotics act by removing *H. pylori*; (d) antacids act by neutralizing acids.

In addition to PUD, the PPIs are also indicated for GERD and for acid hypersecretory conditions such as Zollinger–Ellison syndrome. They may also be prescribed to *prevent* PUD in patients taking high doses of NSAIDs. As a component of triple therapy, PPIs are usually continued for 1 to 2 weeks. In refractory cases, therapy may continue for 4 to 8 weeks. The beneficial effects of PPIs last 3 to 5 days after therapy is stopped.

Adverse effects from short-term therapy with PPIs are uncommon. Headache, abdominal pain, diarrhea, nausea, and vomiting are the most frequently reported adverse effects. If taken for prolonged periods, PPIs may interfere with calcium absorption and cause osteoporosis and fractures.

Prototype Drug: Pr *Omeprazole (Prilosec)*

Therapeutic Class: Antiulcer drug Pharmacologic Class: Proton-pump inhibitor

Actions and Uses: Omeprazole was the first PPI approved for PUD; both prescription and OTC forms are available. Although this drug may take 2 hours to reach therapeutic levels, its effects last up to 72 hours. It is used for the short-term therapy of peptic ulcers and GERD. Most patients are symptom-free after 2 weeks of therapy. It is used for longer periods in patients who have chronic hypersecretion of gastric acid, a condition known as **Zollinger–Ellison syndrome**. Omeprazole is available in oral form only. Zegerid is a combination drug containing omeprazole and the antacid sodium bicarbonate.

Adverse Effects and Interactions: Adverse effects are generally minor and include headache, nausea, diarrhea, and abdominal pain. Long-term therapy can interfere with calcium absorption and result in fractures due to weakened bones.

Omeprazole interacts with several drugs. For example, using it together with diazepam, phenytoin, and central nervous system (CNS) depressants will cause increased blood levels of these drugs. Concurrent use with warfarin may increase the risk of bleeding.

Table 31.1 Drugs for Peptic Ulcer Disease

Drug	Route and Adult Dose	Remarks
PROTON-PUMP INHIBITORS		
esomeprazole (Nexium)	PO: 20–40 mg/day	Also for GERD and hypersecretory disorders; IV form available; available OTC for heartburn
lansoprazole (Prevacid)	PO: 15–60 mg/day	Also for GERD and hypersecretory disorders; Prevpac combines lansoprazole, amoxicillin, and clarithromycin; available OTC for heartburn
Pr omeprazole (Prilosec)	PO: 20–60 mg once or twice daily	Also for GERD and hypersecretory disorders; often used in combination with antibiotics for *Helicobacter* infections
pantoprazole (Protonix)	PO: 40 mg/day	Primarily for GERD and hypersecretory disorders; IV form available
rabeprazole (AcipHex)	PO: 20 mg/day	Also for GERD and hypersecretory disorders
H_2-RECEPTOR BLOCKERS		
cimetidine (Tagamet)	PO: 300 mg every 6 hours or 800 mg at bedtime or 400 mg bid with food	Also for GERD and hypersecretory disorders; IM and IV forms available; available OTC for heartburn
famotidine (Pepcid)	PO: 20 mg bid or 40 mg at bedtime	Also for GERD and hypersecretory disorders; IV form available; available OTC for heartburn
nizatidine (Axid)	PO: 150–300 mg at bedtime	Also for GERD
Pr ranitidine (Zantac)	PO: 100–150 mg bid or 300 mg at bedtime	Also for GERD and hypersecretory disorders; IM and IV forms available
ANTACIDS		
aluminum hydroxide (AlternaGEL, others)	PO: 600 mg tid–qid	Not absorbed; may cause constipation
calcium carbonate (Titralac, Tums)	PO: 1–2 g bid–tid	Also for calcium replacement therapy; may cause constipation
calcium carbonate with magnesium hydroxide (Mylanta Gel-caps, Rolaids)	PO: Two to four capsules or tablets prn (max: 12 tablets/day)	Common OTC therapy
magaldrate (Riopan)	PO: 540–1080 mg (5–10 mL suspension or one or two tablets) daily (max: 20 tablets or 100 mL/day)	Lower incidence of bowel adverse effects than magnesium or aluminum antacids
magnesium hydroxide (Milk of Magnesia)	PO: 5–15 mL or two to four tablets as needed up to four times daily	Also used as a laxative; may cause diarrhea
magnesium hydroxide and aluminum hydroxide with simethicone (Mylanta, Maalox Plus)	PO: 10–20 mL prn (max: 120 mL/day) or two to four tablets prn (max: 24 tablets/day)	Common OTC therapy
sodium bicarbonate ($NaHCO_3$) (see the Prototype Drug box in Core Concept 18.10)	PO: 325 mg–2 g one to four times per day	IV form available to treat metabolic acidosis and cardiac arrest

H_2-receptor blockers reduce the secretion of gastric acid.

◀ **Core Concept 31.5**

The discovery of the H_2-receptor blockers in the 1970s marked a major breakthrough in the treatment of PUD. Since then they have become available OTC and are widely used in the treatment of PUD and GERD. Doses of the H_2-receptor blockers are given in Table 31.1.

Histamine has two types of receptors: H_1 and H_2. Activation of H_1-receptors produces the classic symptoms of allergy, whereas the H_2-receptors are responsible for increasing acid secretion in the stomach. Cimetidine (Tagamet), the first **H_2-receptor blocker**, and other drugs in this class are quite effective at suppressing the volume and acidity of stomach acid. These drugs are also used to treat the symptoms of GERD.

Adverse effects of the H_2-receptor blockers are minor and rarely cause discontinuation of therapy. Patients taking high doses, or those with renal or hepatic disease, may experience confusion, restlessness, hallucinations, or depression. Patients should be advised not to take antacids at the same time as H_2-receptor blockers because the absorption of these drugs will be lessened.

Prototype Drug: Ranitidine (Zantac)

Therapeutic Class: Antiulcer drug **Pharmacologic Class:** H_2-receptor blocker

Actions and Uses: Ranitidine has become one of the most frequently used drugs in the treatment of PUD and GERD. It has a higher potency than cimetidine, which allows it to be administered once daily, usually at bedtime. Adequate healing of the ulcer takes 4 to 8 weeks. Patients with persistent disease may continue on drug maintenance for long periods to prevent recurrence. Gastric ulcers heal more slowly than duodenal ulcers and require longer drug therapy. IV and IM forms are available for the treatment of acute stress-induced bleeding ulcers. Ranitidine is available in a dissolving tablet form (EFFERdose) for treating GERD in children and infants older than 1 month of age.

Adverse Effects and Interactions: Adverse effects are uncommon and mild. Ranitidine does not cross the blood–brain barrier to any appreciable extent, so the confusion and CNS depression observed with cimetidine does not occur with ranitidine. Ranitidine has fewer drug–drug interactions than cimetidine. Although rare, severe reductions in the number of red and white blood cells and platelets are possible.

Ranitidine exhibits fewer drug–drug interactions than cimetidine. Ranitidine may reduce the absorption of cefpodoxime, ketoconazole, and itraconazole. Antacids should not be given within 1 hour of H_2-receptor antagonists because effectiveness may be decreased due to reduced absorption.

CONCEPT REVIEW 31.2

- Explain the following statement: All H_2-receptor blockers are antihistamines, but not all antihistamines are H_2-receptor blockers.

Nursing Process Focus Patients Receiving Drug Therapy for Peptic Ulcer Disease

ASSESSMENT

Prior to administration:

- Obtain a complete health history, including GI and liver conditions, nutrition, allergies, drug history, and possible drug interactions.
- Evaluate laboratory blood findings: complete blood count (CBC), electrolytes, renal, and liver function studies.
- Acquire the results of a complete physical examination, including vital signs, height and weight, pain, signs of bleeding, and level of consciousness (LOC).

POTENTIAL NURSING DIAGNOSES*

- *Deficient Knowledge* related to a lack of information about drug therapy
- *Acute Pain* related to tissue damage of the gastric mucosa or gastric inflammation and/or to ineffective drug therapy
- *Imbalanced Nutrition: Less than Body Requirements* related to adverse effects of drug

PLANNING: PATIENT GOALS AND EXPECTED OUTCOMES

The patient will:

- Experience therapeutic effects (diminished or absent gastric pain and bloating).
- Be free from or experience minimal adverse effects from drug therapy.
- Verbalize an understanding of the drug's use, adverse effects, and required precautions.

IMPLEMENTATION

Interventions and (Rationales)	Patient Education/Discharge Planning
• Administer medications correctly, and evaluate the patient's knowledge of proper administration. (Following guidelines with regard to meals and other medications will result in improved outcomes.)	Inform the patient to: • Take PPIs before meals, preferably before breakfast. • Shake liquid antacids well before pouring. • Take H_2-receptor antagonists and other medications at least 1 hour before antacids. Patients taking antacids should avoid taking other medications for at least 2 hours.
• Monitor the level of abdominal pain or discomfort (to assess effectiveness of drug therapy; it may take days to weeks before pain is controlled).	Advise the patient: • That pain relief may not occur for several days after beginning therapy. • To immediately report episodes of severe or increasing pain to the healthcare provider.
• Monitor patient use of alcohol. (Alcohol can increase gastric irritation.)	• Instruct the patient to avoid alcohol use.

Interventions and (Rationales)	Patient Education/Discharge Planning
• Discuss and monitor for possible drug interactions, including OTC drugs like antacids. (Antacids can decrease the effectiveness of other drugs taken concurrently.)	Instruct the patient to: • Consult with the healthcare provider before taking other medications or herbal products. • Avoid drugs that may cause stomach irritation, such as aspirin or NSAIDs.
• Institute effective safety measures regarding falls. (Drowsiness may occur when starting H_2-receptor blockers.)	• Instruct the patient to avoid driving or performing hazardous activities until drug effects are known.
• Explain the need for lifestyle changes. Provide consultation for dietitian and information on smoking cessation programs. (Smoking and certain foods increase gastric acid secretion.)	Encourage the patient to: • Adopt a healthy lifestyle: Eliminate alcohol and smoking, increase exercise, and choose low-fat foods. • Keep a food diary in order to identify foods that trigger discomfort. Avoid foods that cause stomach discomfort.
• Observe the patient for signs of GI bleeding. (Drugs used to treat PUD decrease gastric acidity, making the gastric environment less favorable for ulcer development, but they do not heal existing ulcers. Blood in the stool or emesis and abdominal pain may indicate a worsening condition.)	• Instruct the patient to immediately report to the healthcare provider any episodes of blood in the stool or vomitus, increase in abdominal discomfort, or diarrhea.
• Monitor CBC, electrolytes, liver function, and serum gastrin during long-term use of medications for PUD. (Abnormal liver function tests may indicate adverse effect of drug therapy. Long-term therapy with PPIs can lead to decreased calcium absorption. H_2 receptors can affect CBC values. Antacids may affect electrolytes such as sodium and phosphorus.)	• Inform the patient of the importance of keeping all scheduled doctor and laboratory visits.
• Monitor for pregnancy or breastfeeding. (Women who are breastfeeding should not take these medications.)	• Instruct the patient to report possible pregnancy and plans for breastfeeding to the healthcare provider.

EVALUATION OF OUTCOME CRITERIA

Evaluate the effectiveness of drug therapy by confirming that patient goals and expected outcomes have been met (see "Planning"). *See Table 31.1 for a list of drugs to which these nursing actions apply.*

Antacids rapidly neutralize stomach acid and reduce the symptoms of PUD and GERD.

◀ **Core Concept 31.6**

Antacids are alkaline substances that have been used for hundreds of years to neutralize stomach acid. Doses of the antacids are listed in Table 31.1.

Prior to the development of H_2-receptor blockers and PPIs, antacids were the mainstay of peptic ulcer and GERD pharmacotherapy. Indeed, many patients still use these inexpensive and readily available OTC medications. Antacids, however, are no longer recommended as the sole medication for PUD because they do not promote healing of the ulcer.

Antacids are alkaline, inorganic compounds of aluminum, magnesium, or calcium. Combinations of aluminum hydroxide and magnesium hydroxide are the most common type. Both aluminum hydroxide and magnesium hydroxide are bases that are capable of rapidly neutralizing stomach acid. A few products combine antacids and H_2-receptor blockers into a single tablet; for example, Pepcid Complete contains calcium carbonate, magnesium hydroxide, and famotidine.

Simethicone is sometimes added to antacid preparations because it reduces gas bubbles that cause bloating and discomfort. For example, Mylanta contains simethicone, aluminum hydroxide, and magnesium hydroxide. Simethicone is classified as an **antiflatulent** because it reduces gas. It also is available by itself in OTC products such as Gas-X and Mylanta.

anti = *against*
flatus = *gas in the GI tract*

Self-medication with antacids is safe when taken in doses directed on the labels. Although they act within 10 to 15 minutes, their duration of action is only 2 hours. Therefore, they must be taken often during the day. Products containing sodium, calcium, or magnesium can result in absorption of these minerals to the general circulation. When given in high doses, aluminum compounds may interfere with phosphate metabolism and cause constipation. Magnesium compounds may cause diarrhea. Patients should follow the label instructions very carefully and not take more than the recommended dosages.

Core Concept 31.7 ▶

Antibiotics are administered to eliminate *Helicobacter pylori*, the cause of many peptic ulcers.

The bacterium *H. pylori* is associated with 80% of all duodenal ulcers and 70% of all gastric ulcers. This organism has adapted well as a human pathogen by devising ways to neutralize the high acidity surrounding it and by making substances that allow it to stick tightly to the GI mucosa. *H. pylori* causes inflammation of the stomach mucosa by both increasing acid secretion and reducing bicarbonate secretion.

Because *H. pylori* infections can remain active for life if not treated, treatment for this infection is a primary goal of PUD management. Elimination of this organism causes ulcers to heal more rapidly and to remain in remission longer. The following antibiotics are commonly used for this purpose:

- amoxicillin (Amoxil)
- clarithromycin (Biaxin)
- metronidazole (Flagyl)
- tetracycline (Sumycin).

Two or more antibiotics are given concurrently (usually with a PPI) to increase the effectiveness of therapy and to lower the potential for bacterial resistance. Clarithromycin and amoxicillin are the preferred drugs. Antibiotic therapy generally continues for 7 to 14 days. Bismuth compounds (Pepto-Bismol, Tritec) are sometimes added to the antibiotic regimen. Although not antibiotics, bismuth compounds do inhibit bacterial growth and prevent *H. pylori* from adhering to the surface of the gastric mucosa. Dosages and additional information for these anti-infectives can be found in Chapter 27.

Core Concept 31.8 ▶

Several miscellaneous drugs are also beneficial in treating peptic ulcer disease.

Three additional drugs are beneficial in treating PUD. Sucralfate (Carafate) consists of sucrose (a sugar) plus aluminum hydroxide (an antacid). The drug produces a thick, gel-like substance that coats the ulcer, protecting it against further erosion and promoting healing. Very little of the drug is absorbed from the GI tract. Other than constipation, adverse effects are minimal. A major disadvantage of sucralfate is that it must be taken four times a day.

Misoprostol (Cytotec) is a prostaglandin-like substance that inhibits gastric acid secretion and stimulates the production of protective mucus. Its primary use is for the prevention of peptic ulcers in patients taking high doses of NSAIDs. Diarrhea and abdominal cramping are relatively common. Classified as a pregnancy category X drug, misoprostol is contraindicated during pregnancy. In fact, misoprostol is sometimes used to terminate pregnancies.

Metoclopramide (Reglan) is occasionally used for the short-term therapy of PUD in patients who fail to respond to first-line drugs. It is also approved to treat nausea and vomiting associated with surgery or cancer chemotherapy. Metoclopramide is available for the oral, IM, or IV routes. CNS adverse effects such as drowsiness, fatigue, confusion, and insomnia may occur in a significant number of patients.

CONCEPT REVIEW 31.3

- Is PUD considered an infection, an inflammation, or both?

CONSTIPATION

▶ Lifespan and Diversity

Constipation occurs more frequently in older adults because fecal transit time through the colon slows with aging; this population also exercises less and has more chronic disorders that cause constipation.

A major function of the large intestine is to reabsorb water from stools. If the waste material remains in the colon for an extended period, however, too much water will be reabsorbed, leading to small, hard stools. The normal frequency of bowel movements varies widely among individuals, from two to three per day to as few as one per week. A decrease in the frequency of bowel movements, known as **constipation**, is a common problem with a large number of different causes that include lack of exercise, insufficient food or fluid intake, and lack of sufficient insoluble **dietary fiber**. Certain medications such as opioids, antihistamines, certain antacids, and iron supplements promote constipation. Dietary adjustments and increased physical activity should be considered before drugs are used to treat constipation.

Laxatives are used to promote defecation.

◀ Core Concept 31.9

Occasional constipation does not require drug therapy. However, if the condition progresses to chronically infrequent and painful bowel movements accompanied by severe straining, pharmacotherapy may be beneficial. Also, pharmacotherapy may be indicated following surgical procedures to prevent the patient from straining or bearing down when attempting a bowel movement. Drugs are given to cleanse the bowel prior to surgery or for diagnostic procedures of the colon, such as a colonoscopy or barium enema.

Laxatives are drugs that promote emptying of the bowel, or **defecation**. **Cathartic** is a related term that implies a stronger and more complete bowel emptying. When taken in prescribed amounts, laxatives have few adverse effects. Selected medications used to treat constipation are listed in Table 31.2. These drugs are often classified into four primary groups and a miscellaneous category.

laxat = *to loosen*
ive = *nature of, quality of*

- *Bulk-forming laxatives* absorb water, thus adding size to the fecal mass. These are preferred drugs for the prevention and treatment of chronic constipation. They have a slow onset of action and are not used when a rapid and complete bowel evacuation is necessary.
- *Stimulant laxatives* promote peristalsis by irritating the bowel mucosa. Although drugs in this class are effective and act rapidly, they are more likely to cause diarrhea and cramping than the other types of laxatives. They should only be used occasionally because they may cause laxative dependence and depletion of fluid and electrolytes.
- *Saline and osmotic laxatives* cause water to be retained in the fecal mass, causing a more liquid stool. These drugs produce a bowel movement in 1 to 6 hours. The U.S. Food and Drug Administration (FDA) has issued a warning that saline laxatives may cause severe dehydration and electrolyte depletion.
- *Stool softeners and surfactant laxatives* cause more water and fat to be absorbed into the stools. They are most often used to *prevent* constipation, especially in patients who have undergone recent surgery.
- *Miscellaneous laxatives* act by mechanisms other than those just described. These include mineral oil and newer drugs for specific indications, such as naloxegol (Movantik) for opioid-induced constipation and linaclotide (Linzess) for irritable bowel syndrome (IBS) with constipation.

▶ Lifespan and Diversity

Because of their reduced food intake and diminished physical activity, older patients are most prone to laxative misuse. Healthcare providers should advise these patients to increase their fluid intake, fiber consumption, and level of exercise.

Table 31.2 Laxatives

Drug	Route and Adult Dose	Remarks
bisacodyl (Correctol, Dulcolax, others)	PO: 5–15 mg daily	Stimulant type; also available as a rectal suppository
calcium polycarbophil (Equalactin, FiberCon, others)	PO: 1 g/day	Bulk-forming type
castor oil (Emulsoil, Neoloid)	PO: 15–60 mL daily	Stimulant type; the only laxative to act on the small intestine
docusate (Colace, Surfak)	PO: 50–500 mg daily	Stool softener and surfactant type
linaclotide (Linzess)	PO: 145–290 mg/day	For IBS with constipation and chronic idiopathic constipation
lubiprostone (Amitiza)	PO: 8–24 mg bid	Stool softener type; for IBS with constipation and chronic idiopathic constipation
magnesium hydroxide (Milk of Magnesia)	PO: 20–60 mL daily	Saline type
methylcellulose (Citrucel)	PO: 5–20 mL tid in 8–10 oz water	Bulk-forming type
methylnaltrexone (Relistor)	Subcutaneous: 8 or 12 mg every other day	For opioid-induced constipation
mineral oil	PO: 45 mL bid	Miscellaneous type; lubricates the stools
naloxegol (Movantik)	PO: 25 mg once daily in the morning	For opioid-induced constipation
Pr psyllium mucilloid (Metamucil, others)	PO: 1–2 tsp in 8 oz water daily	Bulk-forming type; also used for diarrhea and as an aid in lowering blood cholesterol
senna (Ex Lax, Senokot, others)	PO: 8.6–17.2 mg/day	Stimulant type; considered an herbal product

Although laxatives are safe drugs when used as directed, there are several conditions and potential adverse effects that must be monitored carefully. Laxatives are contraindicated in any patient with a suspected bowel obstruction because their use could cause the bowel to perforate. If acute abdominal cramping or diarrhea occurs, laxatives should be discontinued. Patients should be advised not to overuse laxatives because the smooth muscle in the colon can lose its tone and cause chronic constipation.

Laxative abuse is the use of laxatives to lose weight or purge the body of toxins, conditions sometimes connected with eating disorders such as anorexia nervosa or bulimia. Abusers believe they can avoid the absorption of calories by speeding the transit of food through the body, usually with stimulant laxatives. However, the laxatives have no effect on calorie intake because they act on the large intestine, not the small intestine. Chronic use may cause dehydration and electrolyte imbalances. Larger and larger amounts of the drugs are needed to produce bowel movements, resulting in dependency. Healthcare providers should consult with behavior management specialists when abuse is suspected.

CONCEPT REVIEW 31.4

- Bismuth compounds are used to treat several digestive disorders. Describe these drugs and their uses.

Prototype Drug: Pr *Psyllium Mucilloid (Metamucil, Others)*

Therapeutic Class: Drug for constipation **Pharmacologic Class:** Bulk-type laxative

Actions and Uses: Like other bulk-forming laxatives, psyllium is an insoluble fiber that is indigestible and not absorbed from the GI tract. When taken with plenty of water, psyllium swells and increases the size of the fecal mass by drawing water into the intestine. The larger the size of the fecal mass, the more the defecation reflex will be stimulated to promote bowel movements. Several doses of psyllium may be needed to produce a therapeutic effect. More frequent doses of psyllium (7 g/day) may cause a small reduction in blood cholesterol level.

Adverse Effects and Interactions: Psyllium is a safe laxative and rarely produces adverse effects. It causes less cramping than the stimulant-type laxatives and produces a more natural bowel movement. If taken with insufficient water, it may cause obstructions in the esophagus or intestine. Psyllium may decrease absorption and the clinical effects of antibiotics, warfarin, digoxin, nitrofurantoin, and salicylates.

Nursing Process Focus Patients Receiving Laxative Therapy

ASSESSMENT

Prior to administration:
- Obtain a complete health history, including GI and liver conditions, nutrition, allergies, drug history, and possible drug interactions.
- Evaluate laboratory blood findings: CBC, electrolytes, and liver function studies.
- Acquire the results of a complete physical examination, including vital signs, height, weight, bowel elimination patterns, and bowel sounds.

POTENTIAL NURSING DIAGNOSES*

- *Diarrhea* related to adverse effect of drug therapy
- *Deficient Knowledge* related to a lack of information about drug therapy
- *Acute Pain* related to intestinal irritation or adverse effect of drug therapy

PLANNING: PATIENT GOALS AND EXPECTED OUTCOMES

The patient will:
- Experience therapeutic effects (relief from constipation).
- Be free from or experience minimal adverse effects from drug therapy.
- Verbalize an understanding of the drug's use, adverse effects, and required precautions.

IMPLEMENTATION

Interventions and (Rationales)	Patient Education/Discharge Planning
• Administer medications correctly and evaluate the patient's knowledge of proper administration. (Following guidelines will result in improved outcomes.)	Instruct the patient to: • Take medication as prescribed. • Expect results from medication within 2 to 3 days of the initial dose. • Increase fluids and dietary fiber, such as whole grains, fibrous fruits, and vegetables.

Interventions and (Rationales)	Patient Education/Discharge Planning
• Determine the patient's ability to swallow. (Bulk laxatives can swell and cause obstruction in the esophagus.)	• Instruct the patient to discontinue the medication and notify the healthcare provider if having difficulty swallowing.
• Monitor the patient's fluid intake. (Adequate fluid intake helps to prevent constipation or intestinal obstruction.)	Instruct the patient to: • Drink six 8-oz glasses of fluid per day. • Mix medication in a full 8 oz of liquid. • Drink at least 8 oz of additional fluid.
• Monitor frequency, volume, and consistency of bowel movements. (Changes in bowel habits can indicate a serious condition.)	Advise the patient to: • Discontinue laxative use if diarrhea occurs. • Notify the healthcare provider if constipation continues.

EVALUATION OF OUTCOME CRITERIA

Evaluate the effectiveness of drug therapy by confirming that patient goals and expected outcomes have been met (see "Planning"). *See Table 31.2 for a list of drugs to which these nursing actions apply.*

*Herdman, T.H. & Kamitsuru, S. (Eds.), *Nursing Diagnoses: Definitions & Classification* 2015–2017. Copyright © 2014, 1994–2014 NANDA International. Used by arrangement by John Wiley & Sons, Inc. Companion website: www.wiley.com/go/nursingdiagnoses.

DIARRHEA

Occasionally, the colon does not reabsorb enough water from the fecal mass, and stools become watery. **Diarrhea** is an increase in the frequency and fluidity of bowel movements. Like constipation, occasional diarrhea is a common, self-limiting disorder that does not require drug therapy. When prolonged or severe, especially in children, diarrhea can result in significant loss of body fluids, and medications may be indicated. Prolonged diarrhea may lead to acid–base or electrolyte disorders, as discussed in Chapter 18.

dia = *through/between*
rrhea = *flow/discharge*

Diarrhea is not a disease; it is a symptom of an underlying disorder. Diarrhea may be caused by certain medications, infections of the bowel, IBD, and substances such as lactose. Superinfections occurring during anti-infective therapy are common causes of diarrhea because they disrupt the normal microbial flora in the colon.

Opioids are the most effective drugs for controlling severe diarrhea.

◀ **Core Concept 31.10**

Drug therapy of diarrhea depends on the severity of the condition and whether a specific cause can be identified. If the cause is an infectious disease, then an antibiotic or antiparasitic drug such as metronidazole (Flagyl) is indicated. If the cause is inflammatory, anti-inflammatory drugs are needed. If the cause appears to be drug induced, the medication should be discontinued and another substituted.

Many antidiarrheals act by relaxing the colon's smooth muscle, thus relieving cramping. Slower transit through the large intestine allows for better-formed stools. The selection of a particular drug depends on the severity of the diarrhea. Some antidiarrheals are listed in Table 31.3.

Acute or long-lasting diarrhea can lead to serious and even life-threatening conditions. The opioids are first-line drugs for this type of diarrhea because of their rapid onset and effectiveness. At doses used for diarrhea, opioids do not produce dependence or serious

Prototype Drug: Pr *Diphenoxylate with Atropine (Lomotil)*

Therapeutic Class: Antidiarrheal **Pharmacologic Class:** Opioid

Actions and Uses: The primary antidiarrheal ingredient in Lomotil is diphenoxylate. Like other opioids, diphenoxylate slows peristalsis, resulting in additional water being reabsorbed from the colon and formation of more solid stools. It is effective for moderate to severe diarrhea. The atropine in Lomotil is not added for its anticholinergic effect; it is added to discourage patients from taking too much of the drug. Diphenoxylate is discontinued as soon as the diarrhea symptoms resolve.

Adverse Effects and Interactions: Unlike most opioids, diphenoxylate has no analgesic properties and has an extremely low potential for abuse. The drug is well tolerated at normal doses. Some patients experience dizziness or drowsiness, and care should be taken not to operate machinery until the effects of the drug are known. At higher doses, the anticholinergic effects of atropine may be observed, which include drowsiness, dry mouth, and tachycardia.

Other CNS depressants, including alcohol, will cause additive CNS depressant or sedative effects. Monoamine oxidase inhibitors (MAOIs) may cause hypertensive crisis. Alcohol and other CNS depressants may enhance CNS effects.

Table 31.3 Antidiarrheals

Drug	Route and Adult Dose	Remarks
bismuth salts (Pepto-Bismol)	PO: Two tablets or 30 mL prn	OTC adsorbent
camphorated opium tincture (Paregoric)	PO: 5–10 mL one to four times daily	Contains morphine: Schedule III drug; also used to prevent severe opioid withdrawal symptoms in neonates
difenoxin with atropine (Motofen)	PO: One to two mg after each diarrhea episode (max: 8 mg/day)	Opioid; Schedule IV drug
Pr diphenoxylate with atropine (Lomotil)	PO: One or two tablets or 5–10 mL tid–qid	Opioid; Schedule V drug
eluxadoline (Viberzi)	PO: 100 mg bid	For IBS with diarrhea
loperamide (Imodium)	PO: 4 mg as a single dose, then 2 mg after each diarrhea episode (max: 16 mg/day)	Opioid with no physical dependence; abuse is so low, it is not classified as a controlled substance
octreotide (Sandostatin)	Subcutaneous or IV: 100–600 mcg/day in two to four divided doses	For severe diarrhea associated with cancer
rifaximin (Xifaxan)	PO: 200–550 mg tid	For traveler's diarrhea and IBS with diarrhea

adverse effects. The most common opioid antidiarrheal is diphenoxylate (Lomotil), which is a Schedule V controlled substance. Loperamide (Imodium) is an opioid that carries no risk for dependence and is available OTC.

Nonopioid antidiarrheals include bismuth subsalicylate (Pepto-Bismol), which acts by binding and absorbing toxins. The psyllium and pectin preparations slow diarrhea by absorbing large amounts of fluid to form bulkier stools. Intestinal flora modifiers are supplements that help to correct the altered GI flora; a good source of healthy bacteria is yogurt with active cultures.

NAUSEA AND VOMITING

Nausea is an uncomfortable, subjective sensation that is sometimes accompanied by dizziness and an urge to vomit. Vomiting, or **emesis**, is a reflex primarily controlled by the vomiting center, which is located in the medulla oblongata of the brain. Nausea and vomiting are commonly associated with a wide variety of conditions such as food poisoning, early pregnancy, extreme pain, migraines, trauma to the head or abdominal organs, inner ear disorders, and emotional disturbances. Some drugs cause nausea or vomiting as an adverse effect. The most extreme example of this is the antineoplastic drugs, almost all of which cause some degree of nausea or vomiting. In treating nausea or vomiting, an important therapeutic goal is to remove the cause whenever feasible.

Core Concept 31.11 ▶ Antiemetics are prescribed to treat nausea, vomiting, and motion sickness.

Drugs from several pharmacologic classes are prescribed to prevent or treat nausea and vomiting. As shown in Table 31.4, antiemetic drugs belong to a number of different classes, including the following:

- Antipsychotics
- Antihistamines
- Serotonin-receptor blockers (also called 5HT-3 receptor antagonists)
- Corticosteroids (glucocorticoids)
- Benzodiazepines.

anti = *against*
emetic = *vomit*

Therapy with antineoplastic drugs is one of the most common reasons why **antiemetic** medications are prescribed. When cancer chemotherapy is initiated, it is common for a patient to receive three or more antiemetics.

To avoid losing antiemetic medication due to vomiting, many of these drugs are available through the IM, IV, transdermal, and suppository routes, as well as orally disintegrating tablets and soluble films. The most effective antiemetics for serious nausea and vomiting are serotonin-receptor blockers such as ondansetron (Zofran, Zuplenz).

Motion sickness is a disorder that affects a portion of the inner ear known as the vestibular apparatus that is associated with significant nausea. The most common drug used for

Table 31.4 Selected Antiemetics

Drug	Route and Adult Dose	Remarks
dexamethasone (Decadron)	IV: 10–20 mg before chemotherapy	Corticosteroid; also for inflammatory disorders, severe allergies, acute asthma, and neoplasia; IM, inhalation, and IV forms available
dimenhydrinate (Dramamine, others)	PO: 50–100 mg every 4 hours–qid (max: 400 mg/day)	Antihistamine; also used for allergies and cold or flu symptoms; IM and IV forms available
diphenhydramine (Benadryl, others) (see the Prototype Drug box in Core Concept 30.4)	PO: 25–50 mg tid–qid (max: 300 mg/day)	Antihistamine; also for allergies, Parkinson disease, and anaphylaxis; IM, IV, and topical forms available
dolasetron (Anzemet)	PO: 100 mg 1 hour before chemotherapy	Serotonin-receptor blocker; IV form available
doxylamine (Diclegis)	PO: 2 tablets daily at bedtime	Antihistamine combined with pyridoxine (vitamin B_6) for the nausea and vomiting of pregnancy
dronabinol oral solution (Syndros)	PO: 1.2–2.4 mg bid (max: 8.4 mg bid)	Cannabinoid (THC); for nausea and vomiting of chemotherapy; also for anorexia associated with weight loss in patients with AIDS
granisetron (Kytril, Sustol)	IV: 10 mcg/kg 30 minutes before chemotherapy	Serotonin-receptor blocker; oral form available
hydroxyzine (Atarax, Vistaril)	PO: 25–100 mg tid or qid	Antihistamine; also for anxiety and as a preoperative medication; IM form available
meclizine (Antivert, Bonine)	PO: 25–50 mg/day, 1 hour before travel	Antihistamine; for motion sickness and nausea associated with vertigo
methylprednisolone (Medrol, Solu-Medrol)	IV: Two doses of 125–500 mg 6 hours apart before chemotherapy	Corticosteroid; also for inflammatory disorders, severe allergies, acute asthma, and neoplasia; IM form available
metoclopramide (Reglan)	PO: 2 mg/kg 1 hour before chemotherapy	Phenothiazine-like; also for GERD and facilitation of small-bowel intubation; IV and IM forms available
netupitant and palonosetron (Akynzeo)	PO: 1 capsule (300 mg/0.5 mg)	Give 1 hour prior to chemotherapy with dexamethasone
Pr ondansetron (Zofran)	IV: 4 mg tid prn	Serotonin-receptor blocker; IM and PO forms available
prochlorperazine (Compazine)	PO: 5–10 mg tid or qid	Phenothiazine; also for treatment of psychoses; IM, IV, and suppository forms available
promethazine (Phenergan)	PO: 12.5–25 mg every 4 hours–qid	Both a phenothiazine and an antihistamine; also for allergic conditions and to provide sedation before or after surgery; IM, IV, and suppository forms available
rolapitant (Varubi)	PO: 180 mg	Give 1–2 hours prior to chemotherapy with dexamethasone and serotonin receptor antagonist
scopolamine (Isopto hyoscine, Transderm Scop)	Transdermal patch: 0.5 mg every 72 hours	Anticholinergic; oral, IV, IM, and subcutaneous forms available

motion sickness is scopolamine, which is administered as a transdermal patch placed behind the ear. Antihistamines such as dimenhydrinate (Dramamine) and meclizine are also effective but may cause significant drowsiness in some patients. Drugs used to treat motion sickness are most effective when taken 20 to 60 minutes before travel is expected.

On some occasions, it is desirable to *stimulate* the vomiting reflex with drugs called **emetics**. Indications for emetics include ingestion of poisons and overdoses of oral drugs. Ipecac syrup, given orally, or apomorphine, given subcutaneously, will induce vomiting in about 15 minutes. Drugs used to stimulate emesis should be used only in emergency situations under the direction of a healthcare provider.

Prototype Drug: Pr *Ondansetron (Zofran, Zuplenz)*

Therapeutic Class: Antiemetic **Pharmacologic Class:** Serotonin (5-HT3) receptor blocker

Actions and Uses: Ondansetron and other drugs in the serotonin-receptor blocker class have replaced other, older drugs for the treatment of serious nausea and vomiting. To prevent chemotherapy-induced nausea and vomiting, the medication is started at least 30 minutes prior to chemotherapy and continued for several days after.

Ondansetron acts by blocking serotonin receptors in the chemoreceptor trigger zone, an area of the brain responsible for nausea and vomiting. It is available by the PO, IV, IM, oral disintegrating tablet, and oral soluble film routes.

Adverse Effects and Interactions: The most common adverse effects are headache, dizziness, drowsiness, and diarrhea. Caution must be used when treating patients with cardiac abnormalities because ondansetron can prolong the QT interval and cause dysrhythmias. Ondansetron exhibits few drug interactions.

CAM Therapy | Ginger for Nausea

Ginger is obtained from the roots of the herb Zingiber officinale, which grows in a wide variety of places across the world. Active ingredients include aromatic oils that give the herb its characteristic scent and antiemetic activity. Because of its widespread use as a spice in Asian cooking, ginger is widely available in a number of forms, including tincture, tea, dried and fresh root, and capsules. Commercial products that use ginger as a flavoring include ginger cookies, gingerbread, and ginger ale. Consumers should check the product ingredients to be certain that the item truly contains ginger extract, rather than artificial ginger flavoring.

Ginger has been used in Chinese medicine for thousands of years. Indications relating to the digestive system include nausea, vomiting, morning sickness, and motion sickness. Studies have shown its effectiveness to be comparable to OTC medications.

Ginger is purported to have other significant benefits. The herb is said to have anti-inflammatory properties that are of benefit to patients with arthritis. It is sometimes given to patients with flu symptoms to help coughs and lower fever. Because of a possible effect on blood clotting, patients taking anticoagulants should avoid ginger unless otherwise directed by their healthcare provider.

PANCREATIC ENZYMES

In addition to secreting insulin, the pancreas is also responsible for producing essential digestive enzymes. Lack of secretion, or **pancreatic insufficiency**, will result in malabsorption disorders. Replacement therapy with pancreatic enzymes is sometimes necessary.

Core Concept 31.12 ▶ Pancreatic enzymes are administered as replacement therapy for patients with pancreatitis or malabsorption syndromes.

The pancreas secretes more than 1 L of pancreatic juice daily, which contains enzymes that split proteins, fats, and carbohydrates. Because these nutrients must be broken down into simpler molecules before they can be absorbed, lack of sufficient pancreatic juice can cause malabsorption syndromes. Lipase, the enzyme that digests fats, is most affected. The most common cause of pancreatic insufficiency is chronic pancreatitis, which is most often associated with alcoholism.

steato = *fat*
rrhea = *flow or discharge*

Symptoms of chronic pancreatitis include upper abdominal pain, loss of appetite, nausea, vomiting, and weight loss. *Steatorrhea*, the passing of bulky, foul-smelling fatty stools, occurs because dietary fats are passing through the GI tract without being broken down.

Pancrelipase (Cotazym, Pancrease, others) is a pancreatic enzyme supplement obtained from pigs that contains the necessary enzymes to digest fats, carbohydrates, and proteins. To avoid destruction by stomach acid, capsules are made with an enteric coating. Dosing is individualized to the degree of pancreatic insufficiency in each patient. Administration of the drug is timed to coincide with meals so that the enzymes are available when food reaches the duodenum. Overtreatment can cause nausea, vomiting, and diarrhea.

Patients Need to Know

Patients treated for digestive disorders need to know the following:

Regarding Antiulcer Medications

1. Do not smoke tobacco when taking H_2-receptor blockers because it interferes with the drug action.
2. Because drowsiness may occur when starting therapy with H_2-receptor blockers or PPIs, do not operate machinery, and do not use alcohol or other CNS drugs.

3. When taking medications for PUD, avoid drugs that may cause stomach irritation, such as aspirin or NSAIDs.
4. Shake liquid antacids well before pouring. Chewable tablets should be thoroughly chewed before swallowing.

Regarding Laxatives

5. Because bulk-forming laxatives and stool softeners may take several days for results, be patient and do not take more than prescribed.
6. Take bulk-forming laxatives with at least two full glasses of water because this aids in forming larger stools.
7. If constipation is a frequent problem, try drinking more fluids and adding fiber to the diet rather than taking laxatives on a continual basis. Foods rich in fiber include all fruits and vegetables, bran cereals, and whole grain breads.

Regarding Antiemetics

8. Before taking antiemetic medications, try other methods of relieving nausea, such as drinking flat carbonated beverages or weak tea or eating small amounts of crackers or dry toast.
9. When taking phenothiazines or antihistamines as antiemetics, use sugarless candy, gum, or ice chips to minimize dry mouth.
10. Recall that medications taken to suppress hunger produce only modest weight loss and are not effective without a reduced-calorie diet. True, sustained weight loss can only be achieved by modification of exercise and dietary habits.

Chapter Review

Core Concepts Summary

31.1 The digestive system breaks down food, absorbs nutrients, and eliminates wastes.

The alimentary canal provides a large surface area for the absorption of nutrients and drugs. Substances are propelled through the GI tract by peristalsis. Abnormally fast or slow peristalsis can affect nutrient, drug, and water absorption.

31.2 Peptic ulcer disease is caused by erosion of the mucosal layer of the stomach or duodenum.

Infection with *H. pylori* and pharmacotherapy with NSAIDs are the most common causes of peptic ulcers. A gnawing pain in the upper abdomen that is relieved by eating is the most common symptom of duodenal ulcer. Though less common, gastric ulcers may be more serious and require longer treatment and follow-up. GERD has symptoms similar to those of peptic ulcers and is treated with some of the same medications.

31.3 Peptic ulcer disease is treated by a combination of lifestyle changes and pharmacotherapy.

Before beginning drug therapy, the patient should eliminate tobacco and alcohol use and reduce stress levels because these changes will favor remission of PUD. Goals of drug therapy include relief of symptoms, promotion of ulcer healing, and prevention of recurrences.

31.4 Proton-pump inhibitors are effective at reducing gastric acid secretion.

Proton-pump inhibitors diminish gastric acid secretion by interfering with the enzyme H^+, K^+-ATPase, which is present in the mucosal cells in the stomach. Although very effective, use is usually limited to 2 months because of the possibility of long-term adverse effects.

31.5 H_2-receptor blockers reduce the secretion of gastric acid.

H_2-receptor blockers reduce the volume and acidity of stomach acid. Healing of duodenal ulcers occurs in 4 to 8 weeks, and adverse effects are uncommon.

31.6 Antacids rapidly neutralize stomach acid and reduce the symptoms of PUD and GERD.

Once preferred drugs for treating PUD, antacids are now primarily used to give immediate relief for the heartburn associated with GERD or peptic ulcers.

31.7 Antibiotics are administered to eliminate *Helicobacter pylori*, the cause of many peptic ulcers.

Elimination of *H. pylori* using combination therapy with different antibiotics has been found to promote more rapid ulcer healing and longer remissions.

31.8 Several miscellaneous drugs are also beneficial in treating peptic ulcer disease.

Sucralfate produces a gel-like substance that provides a protective coating for ulcers. Misoprostol inhibits gastric acid secretion and promotes the secretion of protective mucus.

31.9 Laxatives are used to promote defecation.

Laxatives are given to promote emptying of the colon. Laxatives act by stimulating peristalsis or by adding more bulk or water to the fecal mass.

31.10 Opioids are the most effective drugs for controlling severe diarrhea.

Diarrhea is treated by addressing its cause, which may include anti-inflammatory drugs or anti-infectives. Opioids are the most effective drugs for relieving severe diarrhea, but they have some abuse potential. OTC bismuth compounds can help with simple diarrhea.

31.11 Antiemetics are prescribed to treat nausea, vomiting, and motion sickness.

Symptomatic treatment of nausea and vomiting involves drugs from many different classes, including phenothiazines, antihistamines, corticosteroids, benzodiazepines, and serotonin-receptor blockers. Motion sickness can be controlled through medications such as transdermal scopolamine or dimenhydrinate (Dramamine).

31.12 Pancreatic enzymes are administered as replacement therapy for patients with pancreatitis or malabsorption syndromes.

Pancreatic insufficiency leads to the lack of breakdown and absorption of sufficient quantities of fats, carbohydrates, and proteins. This can lead to malabsorption syndromes. Pancrelipase and pancreatin are used to restore the deficient enzymes.

REVIEW Questions

Answer the following questions to assess your knowledge of the chapter material, and go back and review any material that is not clear to you.

1. A nurse is providing information about peptic ulcers to a group at a senior residential facility. She tells them that the primary cause of peptic ulcers is:
   1. Stress.
   2. Smoking.
   3. *H. pylori* bacteria.
   4. Family history.

2. The patient with a gastric ulcer has been started on ranitidine (Zantac). The nurse should include what information: (Select all that apply.)
   1. Drug therapy will extend over several weeks or months.
   2. The signs and symptoms of central nervous system depression.
   3. Drug therapy will extend over a few days.
   4. Antacids should not be given within 1 hour of taking H_2-receptor antagonists.
   5. A complete blood count (CBC) should be done periodically.

3. A patient has been experiencing acute diarrhea. In order to control this condition, the healthcare provider initially orders Lomotil 10 mL (2 teaspoons), four times a day. Every 5 mL (1 teaspoon) contains 2.5 mg of medication. How many milligrams of medication will the patient receive a day?
   1. 20 mg
   2. 15 mg
   3. 10 mg
   4. 2.5 mg

4. The nurse understands that it is important that the teaching plan for a patient on omeprazole (Prilosec) should include which of the following?
   1. This drug is safe for long-term use.
   2. This drug should not be taken for a prolonged period of time.
   3. Therapeutic effects may take weeks.
   4. This drug must be used with antacids to be effective.

5. After administering magnesium hydroxide (Mylanta) to a patient, the nurse monitors for:
   1. Diarrhea.
   2. Peripheral disease.
   3. Neuropathy.
   4. Respiratory disorders.

6. The nurse instructs patients using laxatives to:
   1. Use daily for best results.
   2. Not overuse them because they can cause chronic constipation.
   3. Decrease fluid intake.
   4. Decrease food intake.

7. A patient about ready to receive chemotherapy has an order for ondansetron (Zofran). When should the nurse administer the ondansetron?
   1. Every time the patient complains of nausea
   2. Thirty to 60 minutes before starting chemotherapy
   3. Only if the patient complains of nausea
   4. When the patient begins to experience vomiting during the chemotherapy

8. A patient, newly diagnosed with a peptic ulcer, needs more education when he states:
   1. "It's okay for me take aspirin if I get a headache."
   2. "Good thing I can eat raw foods. I love to go to the salad bar."
   3. "I should avoid the use of alcohol."
   4. "Right now I'm not feeling sick, but if I do feel nauseous, I can take an antiemetic."
9. The patient taking sucralfate (Carafate) should be monitored for:
   1. Constipation.
   2. Dizziness.
   3. Muscle pain.
   4. Diarrhea.
10. The patient demonstrates understanding about the medication pancrelipase (Cotazym) when she states:
    1. "I will take this medication with meals."
    2. "I will take this medication on an empty stomach."
    3. "I will only take this medication when I am eating carbohydrates."
    4. "If I develop nausea, vomiting, or diarrhea, I will increase my dosage."

CASE STUDY Questions

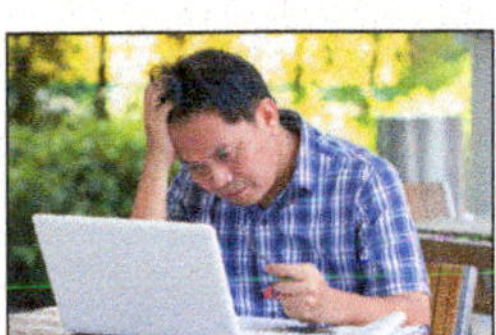

Remember Mr. Han, who was introduced at the beginning of the chapter? Now read the remainder of the case study. Based on the information you have learned in this chapter, answer the questions that follow.

Mr. Jeffery Han is a 32-year-old stockbroker with a very stressful job. He has just been diagnosed with a peptic ulcer. Although he is relieved to find out what has been causing "all this pain," he is not happy to learn he has an ulcer and states, "This is the last thing I need right now. My job is stressful enough." The healthcare provider prescribed omeprazole (Prilosec), clarithromycin, and amoxicillin, with OTC antacids as needed.

1. Mr. Han is confused about the function of each one of his new drugs. He asks the nurse about how each drug is going to help him "overcome" the ulcer. The nurse begins by explaining that part of the pain he is experiencing is due to inflammation caused by both the hydrochloric acid produced in his stomach and the presence of *H. pylori*, a bacteria. She also tells him that the medication responsible for blocking acid secretion is:
   1. Omeprazole.
   2. Antacid.
   3. Clarithromycin.
   4. Amoxicillin.
2. The nurse explains to Mr. Han that ________ was prescribed to eradicate the bacteria *H. pylori*. (Select all that apply.)
   1. Omeprazole
   2. Clarithromycin
   3. Amoxicillin
   4. Antacid
3. In the treatment of *H. pylori*, the nurse explains that the use of two or more antibiotics is essential to: (Select all that apply.)
   1. Lower the potential for bacterial resistance.
   2. Increase the effectiveness of therapy.
   3. Guarantee that the bacteria will be totally destroyed.
   4. Decrease the cost of future drug therapy.
4. Mr. Han had already been taking aluminum-based antacids for his pain but explains that he has started to experience constipation. In order to promote bowel movements, which of the following OTC medications would be beneficial for Mr. Han?
   1. Methylcellulose (Citrucel)
   2. Famotidine (Pepcid)
   3. Omeprazole (Prilosec)
   4. Bismuth salts (Pepto-Bismol)

Answers and complete rationales for the Review and Case Study Questions appear in Appendix A.

REFERENCE

Herdman, T. H., & Kamitsuru, S. (Eds.). (2014). *NANDA International nursing diagnoses: Definitions and classification, 2015–2017*. Oxford, United Kingdom: Wiley-Blackwell

SELECTED BIBLIOGRAPHY

Anand, B. S. (2015). *Peptic ulcer disease treatment & management*. Retrieved from http://emedicine.medscape.com/article/181753-treatment

Basch, E., Prestrud, A. A., Hesketh, P. J., Kris, M. G., Feyer, P. C., Somerfield, M. R., . . . Lyman, G. H. (2011). Antiemetics: American Society of Clinical Oncology clinical practice guideline update. *Journal of Clinical Oncology, 29*, 4189–4198. doi:10.1200/JCO.2010.34.4614

Gardner, T. B. (2015). *Acute pancreatitis*. Retrieved from http://emedicine.medscape.com/article/181364-overview

National Institute of Diabetes and Digestive and Kidney Disorders. (2014). *Digestive diseases statistics for the United States*. Retrieved from http://www.niddk.nih.gov/health-information/health-statistics/Pages/digestive-diseases-statistics-for-the-united-states.aspx

National Institute of Diabetes and Digestive and Kidney Disorders. (2015). *Definition and facts for irritable bowel syndrome.* Retrieved from http://www.niddk.nih.gov/health-information/health-topics/digestive-diseases/irritable-bowel-syndrome/Pages/definition-facts.aspx

Patti, M. G. (2016). *Gastroesophageal reflux disease*. Retrieved from http://emedicine.medscape.com/article/176595-overview

Petersen, B. (2014). Diagnosis and management of functional constipation: A common pediatric problem. *The Nurse Practitioner, 39*(8), 1–6. doi:10.1097/01.NPR.0000451909.40427.b0

Phillips R. S., Friend, A. J., Gibson, F., Houghton, E., Gopaul, S., Craig, J. V., & Pizer, B. (2016). Antiemetic medication for prevention and treatment of chemotherapy-induced nausea and vomiting in childhood. *Cochrane Database of Systematic Reviews, 2*, Art. No.: CD007786. doi:10.1002/14651858.CD007786.pub3

Rowe, W. B. (2016). *Inflammatory bowel disease*. Retrieved from http://emedicine.medscape.com/article/179037-overview

Siemens, W., Gaertner, J., & Becker, G. (2015). Advances in pharmacotherapy for opioid-induced constipation—A systematic review. *Expert Opinion on Pharmacotherapy, 16*, 515–532. doi:10.1517/14656566.2015.995625

Tageja, N., & Groninger, H. (2016). Chemotherapy-induced nausea and vomiting: An overview and comparison of three consensus guidelines. *Postgraduate Medical Journal, 92*, 34–40. doi:10.1136/postgradmedj-2014-132969

Tonore, T. B., Spree, D. C., & Abell, T. (2014). Cyclic vomiting syndrome: A common, underrecognized disorder. *Journal of the American Association of Nurse Practitioners, 26*, 340–347. doi:10.1002/2327-6924.12068

Chapter 32

Drugs for Nutritional Disorders and Obesity

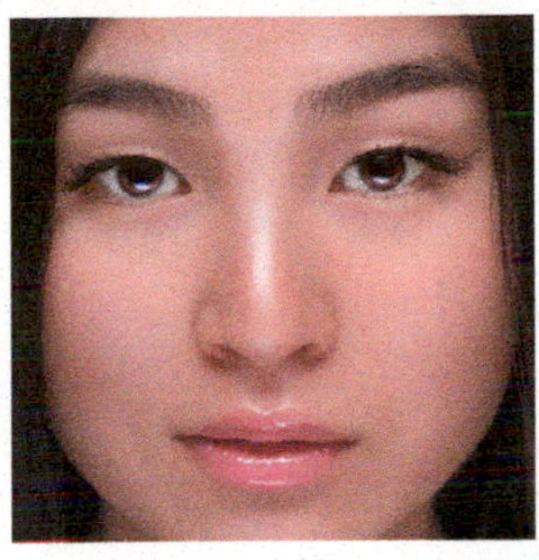

"I'm so busy, I don't eat very much so I take lots of vitamins and minerals. I figure it's better to take more than not enough."
Ms. Mei Chin

Core Concepts

32.1 Vitamins promote growth and maintain health and wellness.
32.2 Vitamins are classified as fat soluble or water soluble.
32.3 Recommended dietary allowances for vitamins have been established for the average healthy adult.
32.4 Vitamin therapy is indicated for specific conditions.
32.5 Mineral therapy is indicated for certain deficiency conditions.
32.6 Enteral and total parenteral nutrition are therapies that deliver essential nutrients to patients with deficiencies.
32.7 Anorexiants and lipase inhibitors are used for the short-term management of obesity.

Drug Snapshot

The following drugs are discussed in this chapter:

Drug Classes	Prototype Drugs
Vitamins	Pr cyanocobalamin (Nascobal)
Minerals	Pr ferrous sulfate (Feosol, Feostat, others)
Enteral nutrition	
Total parenteral nutrition	
Drugs for obesity	

Learning Outcomes

After reading this chapter, the student should be able to:

1. Identify the importance of vitamins and minerals to proper wellness and nutrition.
2. Explain how vitamins are classified.
3. Explain the rationale behind recommended dietary allowances.
4. Identify conditions for which vitamin therapy may be indicated.
5. Identify conditions for which mineral therapy may be indicated.
6. Compare and contrast the enteral and parenteral methods of providing nutrition.
7. Describe drug classes used in the management of obesity.

Key Terms

anorexiants (AN-oh-REX-ee-ants) enteral nutrition
hypervitaminosis
intrinsic factor
macrominerals (major minerals)
megaloblastic anemia
microminerals (trace minerals)
pernicious anemia (pur-NISH-us ah-NEE-mee-ah)
provitamins
recommended dietary allowances (RDAs)
total parenteral nutrition (TPN)
undernutrition
vitamins

Most people are able to obtain all necessary nutrients their body requires through a balanced diet. There are some conditions, however, in which dietary supplementation is necessary and will benefit the patient's health. This chapter focuses on these conditions and explores the role of vitamins, minerals, and nutritional supplements in pharmacology. In addition, the pharmacologic management of obesity is presented.

Core Concept 32.1 ▶ Vitamins promote growth and maintain health and wellness.

Vitamins are organic compounds required by the body in small amounts for growth and for the maintenance of normal metabolic processes. Since the discovery of thiamine in 1911, over a dozen vitamins have been identified. Because scientists did not know the chemical structures of the vitamins when they were discovered, they were assigned letters and numbers such as A, B_{12}, and C. These names are still widely used today.

pro = *before*
vitamin = *essential substance*

An important characteristic of vitamins is that, with the exception of vitamin D, human cells cannot synthesize them. They or their precursors—known as **provitamins**—must be supplied in the diet. A second important characteristic is that if the vitamin is not present in adequate amounts, the body's metabolism will be disrupted and disease will result. Furthermore, the symptoms of the deficiency can be reversed by the administration of the missing vitamin.

Vitamins serve diverse and important roles in human physiology. For example, the B complex vitamins are coenzymes essential to many metabolic pathways. Vitamin A is a precursor of retinal, a pigment needed for normal vision. Calcium metabolism is regulated by a hormone that is derived from vitamin D. Without vitamin K, abnormal prothrombin is produced, and blood clotting is affected. Patients having a low or unbalanced dietary intake, those who are pregnant, and those experiencing a chronic disease may benefit from vitamin therapy.

Fast Facts Vitamins, Minerals, and Dietary Supplements

- About 33% of Americans take a multivitamin supplement daily.
- Chronic use of loop or thiazide diuretics can lead to magnesium deficiency.
- Because vitamin B_{12} is present only in animal products, vegetarians must obtain this vitamin in fortified cereals, nutritional supplements, or yeast.
- Administration of folic acid (folate) during pregnancy has been found to reduce birth defects in the nervous system of the baby.
- Patients who never receive sun exposure may need vitamin D supplements.
- Heavy menstrual periods may result in considerable iron loss.
- Technically, vitamins and minerals cannot increase a patient's energy levels. Energy can be provided only by adding calories from carbohydrates, proteins, and fats.

Core Concept 32.2 ▶ Vitamins are classified as fat soluble or water soluble

A simple way to classify vitamins is by their ability to mix with water. Those that dissolve easily in water are called water-soluble vitamins. Examples include vitamin C and the B vitamins. Those that dissolve in lipids are called fat soluble or lipid soluble and include vitamins A, D, E, and K.

The difference in solubility affects the way the vitamins are absorbed by the gastrointestinal (GI) tract and stored in the body. The water-soluble vitamins are absorbed along with water in the digestive tract and readily dissolve in blood and body fluids. When excess water-soluble vitamins are ingested, they cannot be stored for later use and are simply excreted in the urine. Because they are not stored to any significant degree, they must be ingested daily; otherwise deficiencies will quickly develop.

Fat-soluble vitamins, however, cannot be absorbed in sufficient quantity in the small intestine unless they are ingested with other fats. These vitamins can be stored in large quantities in the liver and fat. Should the patient not ingest sufficient quantities, fat-soluble vitamins are removed from storage depots in the body as needed. Unfortunately, this storage ability can lead to dangerously high levels of the fat-soluble vitamins if they are taken in excessive amounts.

Recommended dietary allowances for vitamins have been established for the average healthy adult.

◀ **Core Concept 32.3**

Based on scientific research on humans and animals, the Food and Nutrition Board of the National Academy of Sciences has established levels for the intake of vitamins and minerals, called **recommended dietary allowances (RDAs)**. The RDA values represent the *minimum* amount of a vitamin or mineral needed daily to prevent a deficiency in most healthy adults. The RDAs are revised periodically to reflect the latest scientific research. Current RDAs for vitamins are listed in Table 32.1. A newer standard, the Dietary Reference Index (DRI), is sometimes used to represent the *optimal* level of nutrient needed to ensure wellness.

Vitamin, mineral, or nutritional supplements should never substitute for a balanced diet. Sufficient intake of proteins, carbohydrates, and fats is needed for proper health. Furthermore, although the label on a vitamin supplement may indicate that it contains 100% of the RDA for a particular vitamin, the body may absorb as little as 10% to 15% of the amount ingested. With the exception of vitamins A and D, it is not harmful for most patients to consume two to three times the recommended levels of vitamins. In cases where there is an increase in dietary needs, such as during pregnancy and growth periods, the RDAs will need adjustment and supplements may be needed to achieve optimal wellness.

▶ Lifespan and Diversity

Infancy and childhood are times of potential vitamin deficiency due to the high growth demands placed on the body.

Table 32.1 Vitamins

Vitamin	Function(s)	RDA Men	RDA Women	Common Cause(s) of Deficiency
A	Visual pigments, epithelial cells	900 RE*	700 RE	Prolonged dietary deprivation, particularly when rice is the main food source; pancreatic disease; cirrhosis
B complex: Biotin (B_7)	Coenzyme in metabolic reactions	30 mcg	30 mcg	Deficiencies are rare
Pr Cyanocobalamin (B_{12})	Coenzyme in nucleic acid metabolism	2.4 mcg	2.4 mcg	Lack of intrinsic factor, inadequate intake of foods from animal origin
Folic acid/folate (B_9)	Coenzyme in amino acid and nucleic acid metabolism	400 mcg	400 mcg	Pregnancy, alcoholism, cancer, oral contraceptive use
Niacin (B_3)	Coenzyme in metabolic reactions	16 mg	14 mg	Prolonged dietary deprivation, particularly when Indian corn (maize) or millet is the main food source; chronic diarrhea; liver disease; alcoholism
Pantothenic acid (B_5)	Coenzyme in metabolic reactions	5 mg	5 mg	Deficiencies are rare
Pyridoxine (B_6)	Coenzyme in amino acid metabolism	1.3-1.7 mg	1.3–1.5 mg	Alcoholism, oral contraceptive use, malabsorption diseases
Riboflavin (B_2)	Coenzyme in metabolic reactions	1.3 mg	1.1 mg	Inadequate consumption of milk or animal products, chronic diarrhea, liver disease, alcoholism
Thiamine (B_1)	Coenzyme in metabolic reactions	1.2 mg	1.1 mg	Prolonged dietary deprivation, particularly when rice is the main food source; hyperthyroidism, pregnancy, liver disease, alcoholism
C	Coenzyme and antioxidant	90 mg	75 mg	Inadequate intake of fruits and vegetables, pregnancy, chronic inflammatory disease, alcoholism; smokers require 35 mg more/day
D	Calcium and phosphate metabolism	15 mcg	15 mcg	Low dietary intake, inadequate exposure to sunlight
E	Antioxidant	15 TE**	15 TE	Premature infants, malabsorption diseases
K	Cofactor in blood clotting	120 mcg	90 mcg	Newborns, liver disease, long-term parenteral nutrition, certain drugs such as cephalosporins and salicylates

**RE = retinoid equivalents*

***TE = alpha-tocopherol equivalents*

Core Concept 32.4 ▶ Vitamin therapy is indicated for specific conditions.

hyper = *above*
vitamin = *vitamin*
osis = *condition*

▶ Lifespan and Diversity

Older patients who have less exposure to direct sunlight may need vitamin D supplements.

Most people who eat a normal, balanced diet obtain all the necessary nutrients without vitamin supplementation. Indeed, ingesting large amounts of vitamins is not only expensive but may be harmful to health. **Hypervitaminosis**, or toxic levels of vitamins, has been reported for vitamins A, C, D, E, B_6, niacin, and folic acid. In the United States, it is actually more common to observe syndromes of vitamin *excess* than those of vitamin *deficiency*. Most patients are unaware that taking too much of a vitamin or mineral can cause serious adverse effects.

Vitamin deficiencies have a number of causes. Table 32.1 lists the functions of the vitamins and some common causes of deficiencies. In the United States, deficiencies are most often the result of poverty, fad diets, chronic alcoholism, or prolonged parenteral feeding. Infants, pregnant women, nursing mothers, older adults, and those eating a vegan or vegetarian diet often require larger amounts of vitamins and minerals to maintain optimal health. Men and women can have different vitamin and mineral needs, as do persons who participate in vigorous exercise. Vitamin deficiencies in patients with chronic liver and kidney disease are well documented. Patients with alcohol or serious drug dependency are often deficient in the quality and quantity of their nutritional intake. In cases in which dietary needs are increased, the RDAs will need adjustment, and supplements are indicated to achieve optimal wellness.

Certain drugs affect vitamin metabolism. Alcohol is well known for its ability to inhibit the absorption of thiamine and folic acid; alcohol abuse is the most common cause of thiamine deficiency in the United States. Folic acid levels may be reduced in patients taking methotrexate (Rheumatrex, Trexall), sulfasalazine (Azulfidine), and certain antiepileptic medications such as phenytoin (Dilantin). Vitamin D deficiency can be caused by therapy with phenytoin, orlistat (Alli, Xenical), and corticosteroids. Inhibition of vitamin B_{12} absorption has been reported with a number of drugs, including omeprazole (Prilosec), metformin (glucophage), alcohol, and oral contraceptives.

megalo = *large*
blastic = *embryonic state*
an = *lack of*
emia = *blood condition*

One of the most important vitamin syndromes is deficiency of vitamin B_{12}. The most obvious consequence of B_{12} deficiency is a condition called **megaloblastic anemia**. If the B_{12} deficiency results from a lack of intrinsic factor, the condition is called **pernicious anemia**. In both conditions, insufficient vitamin B_{12} creates a lack of activated folic acid, which is essential for DNA synthesis and cell division. Lack of vitamin B_{12} also affects the nervous system, causing tingling or numbness in the limbs, mood disturbances, and even hallucinations in severe deficiencies. If the disease has been prolonged, symptoms may take longer to resolve, and some neurologic damage may be permanent.

▶ Lifespan and Diversity

Infants fed only breast milk receive insufficient amounts of vitamin D, which can result in rickets.

Vitamins are indicated for several additional conditions. Vitamin K is administered to patients with certain clotting disorders, as an antidote to warfarin (Coumadin) overdose, and to newborns, who frequently experience a deficiency of this vitamin. B complex vitamins such as folic acid, thiamine, and riboflavin are commonly administered to patients with chronic alcoholism. The role of vitamin D therapy in the pharmacotherapy of bone disorders is discussed in Chapter 36.

Prototype Drug: Pr *Cyanocobalamin (Nascobal)*

Therapeutic Class: Drug for anemia **Pharmacologic Class:** Vitamin supplement

Actions and Uses: Cyanocobalamin is a purified form of vitamin B_{12} that is administered in deficiency states. Vitamin B_{12} is not synthesized by either plants or animals; only bacteria perform this function. The most common cause of vitamin B_{12} deficiency is lack of **intrinsic factor**, which is secreted by stomach cells. Intrinsic factor is required for vitamin B_{12} to be absorbed from the intestine. Figure 32.1 illustrates the metabolism of vitamin B_{12}. Inflammatory diseases of the stomach or surgical removal of the stomach may result in deficiency of intrinsic factor.

Treatment of vitamin B_{12} deficiency is most often accomplished by weekly, biweekly or monthly intramuscular (IM) or subcutaneous injections. Parenteral administration rapidly reverses most signs and symptoms of B_{12} deficiency. Although oral supplements are available, they are effective only in patients who have sufficient intrinsic factor and normal absorption in the small intestine. The intranasal spray and gel formulations (Nascobal) provide for once-weekly dosage after normal vitamin B_{12} levels have been restored by IM preparations. Treatment of vitamin B_{12} deficiency may need to continue for the remainder of the patient's life.

Adverse Effects and Interactions: Adverse effects from cyanocobalamin are uncommon. Hypokalemia is possible; thus, serum potassium levels are monitored periodically.

Alcohol, aminosalicylic acid, neomycin, and colchicine may decrease absorption of oral cyanocobalamin. Chloramphenicol may interfere with therapeutic response to cyanocobalamin.

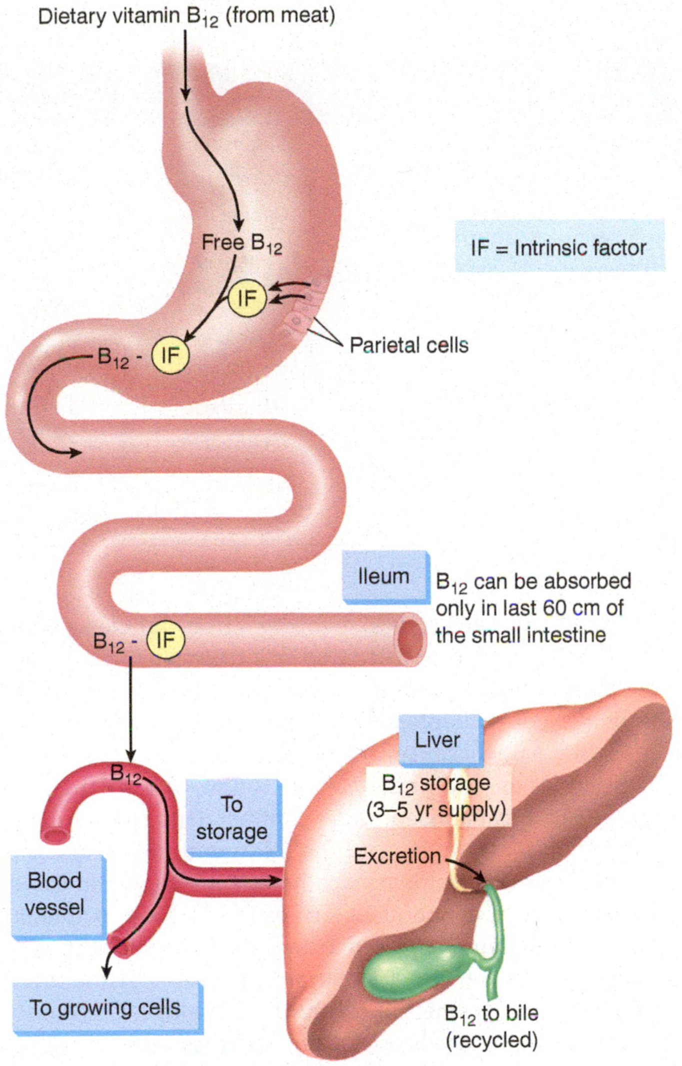

FIGURE 32.1 Metabolism of vitamin B_{12}.

CONCEPT REVIEW 32.1

- What are some conditions in which the RDA for a vitamin may not be sufficient?

Mineral therapy is indicated for certain deficiency conditions

◀ **Core Concept 32.5**

Minerals are inorganic substances that constitute about 4% of body weight. The most common minerals are the bone salts, calcium, and phosphorus, which make up about 75% of the total mineral content in the body. Minerals are classified as **macrominerals (major minerals)** or **microminerals (trace minerals)**, depending on how much is needed in the diet. The seven major minerals must be obtained daily from dietary sources in amounts of 100 mg or higher. Required daily amounts of the nine trace minerals are 20 mg or less. These minerals are listed in Table 32.2.

Minerals serve many important and diverse functions in the body. Some minerals, such as sodium and magnesium, appear primarily as ions in body fluids. Others, such as iron and cobalt, are usually bound to organic molecules. The functions of many of the minerals in human physiology, such as calcium, sodium, and potassium, are well known. The functions of some of the trace minerals, such as aluminum, silicon, arsenic, and nickel, are less understood.

Because minerals are needed in very small amounts for human metabolism, a balanced diet will supply the necessary quantities for most patients. Like vitamins, excess amounts of minerals can lead to toxicity, and patients should be advised not to exceed recommended doses. For example, arsenic, chromium, and nickel have been implicated as human carcinogens, and excess sodium intake can lead to water retention and hypertension.

▶ Lifespan and Diversity

For each decade after age 40, bone mass decreases approximately 3% to 5%. To avoid bone fractures, older adults must ensure a substantial dietary intake of calcium or take calcium supplements.

Table 32.2 Minerals

Macrominerals	Recommended Daily Intake (Adults)	Microminerals	Recommended Daily Intake (Adults)
Calcium	1000–1200 mg	Chromium	20–35 mcg
Chloride	1800–2300 mg	Cobalt	0.1 mcg
Magnesium	Men: 400–420 mg Women: 350–360 mg	Copper	900 mcg
Phosphorus	700 mg	Fluoride	3–4 mg
Potassium	4.7 g	Iodide	150 mcg
Sodium	1500 mg	Iron	Men: 8 mg Women: 8–18 mg
Sulfur	Not established	Manganese	1.8–5 mg
		Molybdenum	45 mg
		Selenium	55 mcg
		Zinc	8–11 mg

osteo = *bone*
por = *passage*
osis = *condition*

Mineral therapy is indicated for certain disorders. Iron-deficiency anemia is the most common nutritional deficiency in the world and is a primary indication for iron supplements. Women at high risk for osteoporosis are advised to consume extra calcium, either in their diet or as a supplement (see Chapter 36). Magnesium deficiencies are promptly treated with oral or IV magnesium salts because lack of sufficient amounts of this electrolyte can lead to weakness, dysrhythmias, and hypertension. Iodine-based drugs serve a number of functions, including use as topical antiseptics, as contrast drugs in radiologic procedures of the urinary and cardiovascular systems, and the treatment of thyroid abnormalities (see Chapter 33). Selected minerals used in pharmacotherapy are shown in Table 32.3.

Certain drugs affect mineral metabolism. For example, loop or thiazide diuretics can cause significant urinary potassium loss. Corticosteroids, oral contraceptives, and a number of other drugs can cause sodium retention. The uptake of iodine by the thyroid gland can be impaired by certain oral hypoglycemics and lithium (Eskalith). Oral contraceptives have been reported to lower the plasma levels of zinc and increase those of copper.

hemo = *blood*
globin = *protein*

CONCEPT REVIEW 32.2

- What is the difference between a vitamin and a mineral?

Prototype Drug: Pr *Ferrous Sulfate (Feosol, Feostat, Others)*

Therapeutic Class: Drug for anemia Pharmacologic Class: Iron supplement

Actions and Uses: Ferrous sulfate is an iron supplement. Iron is a mineral essential to the function of several biological molecules, the most significant of which is hemoglobin. Each molecule of hemoglobin in a red blood cell contains four iron atoms, each of which can bind reversibly to an oxygen atom. Sixty to eighty percent of all iron in the body is associated with hemoglobin.

After red blood cells die, nearly all of the iron in their hemoglobin is recycled for later use. Because of this recycling, very little iron is excreted; thus, dietary iron requirements in most individuals are small.

Iron deficiency is a common cause of anemia. The usual cause of iron-deficiency anemia is blood loss, such as may occur during menstruation or from peptic ulcers. Certain patients have an increased demand for iron, including those who are pregnant and those undergoing intensive athletic training. Ferrous sulfate is available in a wide variety of dosage forms to prevent or rapidly reverse symptoms of iron-deficiency anemia.

Adverse Effects and Interactions: The most common adverse effect of iron sulfate is GI upset. Although taking iron with meals will lessen GI upset, food can decrease the absorption of iron by as much as 70%. It is recommended that iron preparations be administered 1 hour before or 2 hours after a meal. However, if major gastric irritation is experienced, the iron may be taken with juice or small meals. Patients should be advised that iron preparations may darken stools and that this is a harmless adverse effect. Excessive doses of iron are very toxic, and patients should be advised to take their medication exactly as directed.

Antacids and food decrease the absorption of iron. Vitamin C increases the absorption of iron, whereas calcium (including dairy products) and bran block its absorption. Vitamin C may increase the absorption of ferrous sulfate.

Table 32.3 Selected Minerals Used for Pharmacotherapy

Drug	Route and Adult Dose	Remarks
potassium chloride (KCl) (see the Prototype Drug box in Core Concept 18.9)	PO: 10–100 mEq/day in divided doses IV: 10–40 mEq/h diluted to at least 10–20 mEq/100 mL of solution (max: 200–400 mEq/day)	Drug should be discontinued immediately if hyperkalemia is suspected.
sodium bicarbonate ($NaHCO_3$) (see the Prototype Drug box in Core Concept 18.10)	PO: 0.3–2 g once or twice daily	For treatment of metabolic acidosis, to enhance renal excretion of certain drugs, and as an antacid
CALCIUM		
calcium acetate (PhosLo)	PO: 2–4 tablets with each meal (each tablet contains 169 mg elemental calcium)	To prevent high blood phosphate levels in patients who are on dialysis
calcium carbonate (Rolaids, Tums, Os-Cal, others)	PO: 1–2 g bid–tid	For calcium supplementation and as an antacid
calcium citrate (Citracal)	PO: 1–2 g bid–tid	For calcium supplementation
calcium gluconate (Kalcinate)	PO: 1–2 g bid–qid	For calcium supplementation and to reverse cardiac signs of hyperkalemia
calcium lactate (Cal-Lac)	PO: 325–650 mg bid–tid before meals	To correct mild hypocalcemia
IRON		
ferrous fumarate (Feostat, others)	PO: 120–200 mg elemental iron /day	For iron supplementation
ferrous gluconate (Fergon, others)	PO: 60 mg elemental iron bid–qid	For iron supplementation
Pr ferrous sulfate (Feosol, others)	PO: 750–1500 mg/day in divided doses	For iron supplementation
iron dextran (Dexferrum, others)	IM/IV: Dose is individualized and determined from a table in the package insert (max: 100 mg [2 mL] of iron dextran within 24 hours)	For iron supplementation when oral administration is not indicated
MAGNESIUM		
magnesium chloride (Chloromag, Slow-Mag)	PO: 270–400 mg/day	For magnesium supplementation
magnesium hydroxide (Milk of Magnesia)	PO: 2.4-4.8 g/day for constipation	For constipation, hyperacidity, or magnesium supplementation
magnesium oxide (Mag-Ox, Maox, others)	PO: 400–1200 mg/day in divided doses as a supplement	For constipation, hyperacidity, or magnesium supplementation
magnesium sulfate (Epsom salt)	IV/IM: 1-5 g/day as a supplement	For constipation, to control seizures, or for magnesium supplementation
PHOSPHORUS		
potassium/sodium phosphates (K-Phos original, K-Phos MF, K-Phos neutral, Neutra-Phos-K, Uro-KP neutral)	PO: 250–1000 mg /day	For correction of phosphate deficiency and to lower urinary calcium concentration
ZINC		
zinc gluconate	PO: 20–100 mg	For correction of zinc deficiency
zinc sulfate (Orazinc, Zincate, others)	PO: 15–220 mg/day	For correction of zinc deficiency

Nursing Process Focus Patients Receiving Iron Supplements

ASSESSMENT

Prior to administration:

- Obtain a complete health history, including GI, renal and liver conditions; problems with anemia; prophylaxis during infancy, childhood, and pregnancy; allergies, drug history, and possible drug interactions.
- Evaluate laboratory blood findings: complete blood count (CBC) (specifically hematocrit and hemoglobin levels), electrolytes, and liver function studies.
- Acquire the results of a complete physical examination including vital signs, height, and weight.

POTENTIAL NURSING DIAGNOSES*

- *Deficient Knowledge* related to lack of information about drug therapy
- *Risk for Imbalanced Nutrition* related to inadequate iron intake
- *Risk for Injury* (weakness, dizziness, syncope) related to anemia

PLANNING: PATIENT GOALS AND EXPECTED OUTCOMES

The patient will:

- Experience therapeutic effects (an increase in hematocrit level and improvement in anemia-related symptoms).
- Be free from or experience minimal adverse effects from drug therapy.
- Verbalize an understanding of the drug's use, adverse effects, and required precautions.

IMPLEMENTATION

Interventions and (Rationales)	Patient Education/Discharge Planning
• Monitor vital signs, especially pulse. (Increased pulse is an indicator of decreased oxygen content in the blood.)	• Instruct the patient to monitor pulse rate and report irregularities and changes in rhythm to the healthcare provider.
• Monitor CBC to evaluate effectiveness of treatment. (Increases in hematocrit and hemoglobin values indicate increased red blood cell production.)	Instruct the patient: • On the need for initial and continuing laboratory blood monitoring. • To keep all laboratory appointments.
• Monitor changes in stool. (Supplement may cause constipation, change stool color, and cause false positives when stool is tested for occult blood.)	Instruct the patient: • That stool color may change, and that this is no cause for alarm. • On measures to relieve constipation, such as including fruits and fruit juices in the diet and increasing fluid intake and exercise.
• Plan activities and allow for periods of rest to help the patient conserve energy. (Diminished iron levels result in decreased formation of hemoglobin, leading to weakness.)	Instruct the patient to: • Rest when he or she is feeling tired, and avoid overexertion. • Plan activities to avoid fatigue.
• Administer oral forms of ferrous sulfate (iron) 1 hour before or 2 hours after meals with a full glass of water or juice for better absorption.	Instruct the patient: • Not to crush or chew sustained-release preparations; take with a full glass of water or juice. • That medication may cause GI upset and may be taken with food if this becomes a problem.
• Administer liquid iron preparations through a straw or place on the back of the tongue (to avoid staining the teeth).	Instruct the patient to: • Dilute liquid medication before using and use a straw to take the medication. • Rinse the mouth after swallowing to decrease the chance of staining the teeth.
• Monitor dietary intake to ensure adequate intake of foods high in iron.	• Instruct the patient to increase intake of iron-rich foods such as liver, egg yolks, brewer's yeast, wheat germ, and muscle meats.
• Monitor for potential of child access to the medication. (Iron poisoning can be fatal to young children.)	• Advise the parent to store iron-containing vitamins out of reach of children and in childproof containers.

EVALUATION OF OUTCOME CRITERIA

Evaluate the effectiveness of drug therapy by confirming that patient goals and expected outcomes have been met (see "Planning").

Core Concept 32.6 ▶ Enteral and total parenteral nutrition are therapies that deliver essential nutrients to patients with deficiencies.

When a patient is eating or drinking fewer nutrients than required for normal body growth and maintenance, **undernutrition** occurs. Undernutrition can also occur in certain malabsorption disorders of the intestinal tract. The two primary goals in treating undernutrition are to identify the specific type of deficiency and supply the missing nutrients. Nutritional supplements may be needed for short-term therapy or for the remainder of a patient's life.

Causes of undernutrition range from simple to complex and include the following:

- Advanced age
- HIV-AIDS
- Alcoholism
- Severe burns

- Cancer
- Chronic inflammatory bowel disease
- Eating disorders.

The most obvious cause for undernutrition is low dietary intake. Reasons for the inadequate intake must be carefully assessed. Patients may have no resources to purchase food and may be suffering from starvation. Clinical depression leads many patients to shun food. In terminal disease, patients may be comatose or otherwise unable to take food orally. Although the causes differ, patients with insufficient intake exhibit a similar pattern of general weakness, muscle wasting, and loss of subcutaneous fat.

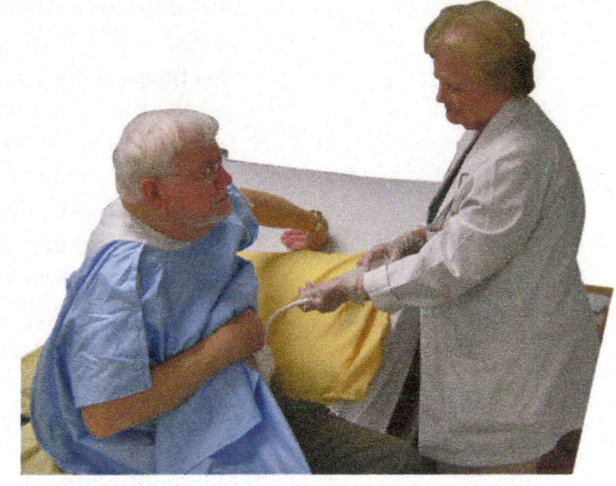

FIGURE 32.2 Nurse administering enteral nutrition through a feeding tube.

Many different types of nutritional supplements are available to assist patients suffering from undernutrition. Products administered via the GI tract, either orally or through a feeding tube, are called **enteral nutrition**. Oral feeding allows natural digestive processes to occur and requires less nursing care. Tube feeding is necessary when the patient has difficulty swallowing or is otherwise unable to take meals orally (Figure 32.2). An advantage of tube feeding is that the amount of enteral nutrition the patient is receiving can be precisely measured and recorded.

▶ Lifespan and Diversity

Older patients may have poor-fitting dentures or difficulty chewing or swallowing following a stroke.

The particular enteral product is chosen to address the specific nutritional needs of the patient. For example, some contain mixtures of amino acids and protein, whereas others contain primarily carbohydrates or fats. There are many different formulations of enteral products available, each designed to meet a specific nutrient need. Examples of enteral products include Vivonex T.E.N., Peptamen, Sustacal, Ensure-Plus, Casec, Polycose, Microlipid, and MCT Oil.

▶ Lifespan and Diversity

The absorption of food diminishes with age, and often the quantity of ingested food is reduced, leading to vitamin deficiencies in older patients.

Patients sometimes exhibit vomiting, nausea, or diarrhea when first receiving enteral nutrition. Therapy is often started slowly, with small quantities so that adverse effects can be assessed and prevented.

When the metabolic needs of the patient cannot be met through enteral nutrition, **total parenteral nutrition (TPN)**, which is also called parenteral nutrition, is indicated. For short-term therapy, peripheral vein PN may be used. Because of the risk of phlebitis, however, long-term therapy often requires central vein PN. Because the GI tract is not being used, patients with severe malabsorption disease may be successfully treated with TPN.

TPN is able to provide all the patient's nutritional needs with solutions containing amino acids, fats, carbohydrate (as dextrose), electrolytes, vitamins, and minerals. The particular formulation may be specific to the disease state, such as products for renal failure or hepatic failure. TPN is administered through an infusion pump so that nutrition can be precisely monitored. Patients in various settings such as acute care, long-term care, and home healthcare often benefit from TPN therapy.

Anorexiants and lipase inhibitors are used for the short-term management of obesity.

◀ Core Concept 32.7

Despite the public's desire for effective drugs to promote weight loss, there are few such drugs available. The approved drugs used for the treatment of obesity produce only modest weight loss.

Obesity may be defined as being more than 20% above ideal body weight or having a body mass index of 30 kg/m^2 or higher. Because of the prevalence of obesity in society and the difficulty that most patients experience when following weight-reduction plans for extended periods, drug manufacturers have long sought to develop safe drugs that cause weight loss.

Current pharmacologic strategies for weight management focus on two mechanisms: lipase inhibitors and anorexiants. Orlistat (Xenical) acts by inhibiting the enzyme lipase in the GI tract. This blocks the absorption of fats in the small intestine. Unfortunately, orlistat may also decrease absorption of other substances, including fat-soluble vitamins and warfarin (Coumadin). Orlistat produces only a small decrease in weight compared to placebos.

A second strategy to reduce weight is to block parts of the nervous system responsible for hunger with **anorexiants**, also called appetite suppressants. In the 1970s, amphetamine and dextroamphetamine (Dexedrine) were widely prescribed as anorexiants to reduce appetite. These drugs, however, are addictive, and amphetamines are rarely prescribed for this purpose today. In the 1990s, the combination of fenfluramine and phenteramine, known as fen-phen, was widely prescribed until fenfluramine was removed from the market for causing heart valve defects. Sibutramine (Meridia), once the most widely prescribed anorexiant for the short-term control of obesity, was removed from the market in 2010 due to an increased risk for heart attacks and strokes.

Phentermine, once part of the combination fen-phen, was approved in 2012 as a fixed dose combination with topiramate (Qysmia). Phenteramine decreases appetite but the precise mechanism of antiobesity action of topiramate (an antiepileptic) drug is unknown. Side effects of Qysmia include paresthesia, dizziness, dysgeusia, insomnia, constipation, and dry mouth. Because both drugs in Qysmia are pregnancy category X, effective contraception should be implemented in sexually-active women.

Also approved in 2012, lorcaserin (Belviq) is one of the newer anorexiants that is believed to act by activating serotonin receptors in the hypothalamus, causing a feeling of fullness or satiety. The drug is well tolerated, with headache and upper respiratory tract infection being the most common side effects. Like other antiobesity drugs, it should be combined with a regimen of diet and exercise for successful weight loss.

In 2014, two additional anorexiants were approved. Contrave is a combination of bupropion (an atypical antidepressant) and naltrexone (an opioid agonist). The combination reduces appetite by increasing dopamine activity and blocking opioid receptors in the brain. The drug carries a black box warning that it may cause suicidal behavior, and it is pregnancy category X.

Liraglutide (Saxenda) is indicated for weight management in obese patients with at least one comorbid condition, such as hypertension, dyslipidemia, or type 2 diabetes. The drug activates glucagon-like peptide (GLP-1) receptors, which regulates appetite in the brain, resulting in decreased calorie intake. The drug is administered daily by the subcutaneous route and carries a black box warning regarding the potential for thyroid carcinoma. It is interesting to note that liraglutide was previously approved by the trade name Tradjenta to treat type 2 diabetes. Despite being the same drug, Saxenda and Tradjenta are not considered interchangeable.

The newest of the approved weight loss products is actually an old one. Evekeo consists of amphetamine sulfate and is approved for the short-term management of obesity, as well as for narcolepsy and ADHD.

Patients Need to Know

Patients treated with vitamins, minerals, or herbs need to know the following:

In General

1. If receiving regular monthly injections of vitamin B_{12}, do not take additional oral supplements of vitamin B_{12} or folic acid without the advice of a healthcare provider.
2. Do not take more than the recommended doses of any vitamin or mineral without first checking with a healthcare provider. Although small amounts of these substances are beneficial, large amounts may be dangerous.
3. Ensure that diet is nutritionally adequate, adding foods that naturally supply the needed vitamins and minerals before taking supplements. See a dietitian for advice, particularly for special needs such as pregnancy or diabetes.
4. Avoid foods with high zinc or oxalate content if a calcium supplement is being taken because these may interfere with absorption. These foods include nuts, peas, beans, spinach, and soy products.
5. Know that niacin, or vitamin B_3, is also effective at lowering lipid levels. The dose for lowering cholesterol, however, is 2–3 g per day, whereas the vitamin dose is only 25 mg per day.
6. When providing a medical or drug history to the healthcare provider or dentist, always report vitamins, minerals, herbs, or dietary supplements being taken. If allergies to any dietary supplements are known, be sure to report these also.
7. Because liquid iron preparations can stain teeth, dilute these solutions with juice or water and rinse the mouth after taking the medication to reduce staining.
8. Take oral forms of ferrous sulfate (iron) 1 hour before or 2 hours after meals for better absorption. Take with a full glass of water or juice.

Safety Alert: Accidental Overdose of Vitamins and Other Medications

Accidental overdose of vitamins or other medications are of special concern in children. It has the ability to cause injury and death. Medications used for children, such as vitamins and cough medicine, may appeal to children because of their candy-like appearance. To avoid tragedy, nurses should teach caregivers not to refer to any medications as "candy" and to store all medications in a secure place out of the reach and sight of children, even if the containers have child-resistant caps.

Chapter Review

Core Concepts Summary

32.1 Vitamins promote growth and maintain health and wellness.

With the exception of vitamin D, vitamins cannot be synthesized by the body and must be provided in the diet. Although only small amounts of vitamins are needed, lack of sufficient quantity will result in disease.

32.2 Vitamins are classified as fat soluble or water soluble.

Water-soluble vitamins include vitamins C and B. Fat-soluble vitamins include vitamins A, D, E, and K. Water-soluble vitamins cannot be stored and must be ingested daily, whereas excess fat-soluble vitamins can be stored for later use.

32.3 Recommended dietary allowances for vitamins have been established for the average healthy adult.

RDA values represent the minimum amount of vitamin or mineral needed to prevent a deficiency in a healthy adult. These values must be adjusted for changes in health status, such as athletic training, pregnancy, or chronic disease.

32.4 Vitamin therapy is indicated for specific conditions.

Most people do not need vitamin supplementation, and excess intake may lead to hypervitaminosis. Indications for vitamin therapy include alcoholism, pregnancy or breast-feeding, chronic kidney or liver disease, therapy with certain drugs that affect vitamin metabolism, and reduced food intake in older patients.

32.5 Mineral therapy is indicated for certain deficiency conditions.

Like vitamins, most people receive all the minerals they need through a balanced diet. Certain conditions, such as osteoporosis or iron-deficiency anemia, warrant mineral pharmacotherapy.

32.6 Enteral and total parenteral nutrition are therapies that deliver essential nutrients to patients with deficiencies.

Enteral nutrition supplies patients all the essential nutrients via the oral route or through a feeding tube. For patients who cannot take oral supplements, nutrients are supplied parenterally by way of total parenteral nutrition.

32.7 Anorexiants and lipase inhibitors are used for the short-term management of obesity.

Only a few drugs are available for the management of obesity, and these drugs produce only modest weight loss. The lipase inhibitor orlistat and newer medications such as Contrave and liraglutide are approved to treat obesity when combined with increased physical activity and a weight management program.

REVIEW Questions

Answer the following questions to assess your knowledge of the chapter material, and go back and review any material that is not clear to you.

1. Vitamin B_{12} is indicated for which of the following conditions?
   1. Liver disease
   2. Chronic inflammatory bowel disease
   3. Pernicious anemia
   4. Inadequate exposure to sunlight

2. The nurse administers which vitamin for a patient experiencing warfarin (Coumadin) overdose?
   1. Vitamin A
   2. Vitamin D
   3. Vitamin E
   4. Vitamin K

3. For the patient taking ferrous sulfate, the nurse will provide what instructions?
   1. Do not take antacids with this medication.
   2. This medication can cause severe diarrhea.
   3. This medication should never be taken on an empty stomach.
   4. Blood pressure must be monitored closely.

4. The nurse monitors patients with a history of alcohol abuse for a ______ deficiency.
   1. Biotin
   2. Thiamine
   3. Niacin
   4. Riboflavin

5. The patient on a thiazide or loop diuretic, such as Lasix, is monitored for which electrolyte?
   1. Selenium
   2. Calcium
   3. Potassium
   4. Magnesium

6. The nurse instructs the patient taking liquid iron to:
   1. Swish the medication in his mouth for 1 minute.
   2. Take the medication with food.
   3. Avoid foods with high iron content.
   4. Rinse the mouth with water after swallowing.

7. The patient is exhibiting weakness, hypertension, and dysrhythmias. Which of the following will the nurse check?
   1. Calcium levels
   2. Magnesium levels
   3. Aluminum levels
   4. Chromium levels

8. The patient on Qysmia (phtereamine with topiramate) must be monitored for: (Select all that apply.)
   1. Constipation.
   2. Dizziness.
   3. Hypertension.
   4. Diarrhea.
   5. Dry mouth.

9. The patient's gastrointestinal tract is not functioning. Which type of feeding technique does the nurse expect to use to ensure the patient is receiving adequate nutrition?
   1. Oral
   2. Enteral
   3. Total parenteral nutrition
   4. Gastrointestinal

10. The patient has hypomagnesemia and is to receive an IV infusion of 350 mg of magnesium in 250 mL over 4 hours. How many milliliters per hour will the patient receive?
    1. 65.5 mL
    2. 50.5 mL
    3. 62.5 mL
    4. 55.5 mL

CASE STUDY Questions

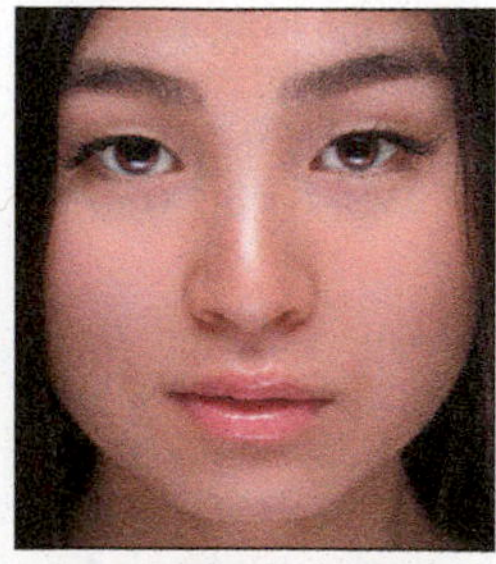

Remember Ms. Chin, who was introduced at the beginning of the chapter? Now read the remainder of the case study. Based on the information you have learned in this chapter, answer the questions that follow.

Ms. Mei Chin, a young woman, has come to the office for a routine check-up. While reviewing her medications, Ms. Chin tells the nurse that she has been taking multivitamins with minerals for the last year, and that lately, she has been taking four times the label dose because she does not eat very much and figures that "it's better to take more than not enough."

1. While teaching Ms. Chin about multivitamins, the nurse identifies which of the following as a water-soluble vitamin?
   1. A
   2. B complex
   3. D
   4. E

2. While continuing the discussion on the topic of multivitamins and minerals, Ms. Chin asks about the meaning of recommended daily allowance (RDA). The nurse responds:
   1. "It is the amount of nutrient required by all people."
   2. "It is the maximum amount of nutrient needed to prevent a deficiency in healthy adults."
   3. "It is the amount of nutrient needed by an average person."
   4. "It is the minimum amount of nutrient needed to prevent a deficiency in healthy adults."

3. Ms. Chin asks if she should be taking the multivitamins. The nurse collects what information before responding? (Select all that apply.)
   1. Weight
   2. Diet
   3. Presence of any chronic diseases
   4. Use of alcohol

4. Ms. Chin wants to continue taking the multivitamins, convinced that they are helping her. She says that sometimes she just does not feel like eating. The nurse tells Ms. Chin to:

1. Stop taking the multivitamins; her diet is good enough.
2. Continue taking four times the label dose until she starts to feel sick.
3. Not take more than the recommended dose until she speaks to the healthcare provider about the problems associated with her diet.
4. Discontinue taking four times the recommended dose; instead, take two times the recommended dose because she has not been eating well.

Answers and complete rationales for the Review and Case Study Questions appear in Appendix A.

REFERENCE

Herdman, T. H., & Kamitsuru, S. (Eds.). (2014). *NANDA International nursing diagnoses: Definitions and classification, 2015–2017*. Oxford, United Kingdom: Wiley-Blackwell

SELECTED BIBLIOGRAPHY

Apovian, C. M., Aronne, L. J., Bessesen, D. H., McDonnell, M. E., Murad, M. H., Pagotto, U., . . . Still, C. D. (2015). Pharmacological management of obesity: An endocrine society clinical practice guideline. *The Journal of Clinical Endocrinology & Metabolism, 100*(2), 342–362. doi:10.1210/jc.2014-3415

Bolzetta, F., Veronese, N., De Rui, M., Berton, L., Toffanello, E. D., Carraro, S., . . . Sergi, G. (2015). Are the recommended dietary allowances for vitamins appropriate for elderly people? *Journal of the Academy of Nutrition and Dietetics, 115*, 1789–1797. doi:10.1016/j.jand.2015.04.013

Chan, L. N. (2013). Drug-nutrient interactions. *Journal of Parenteral and Enteral Nutrition, 37*, 450–459. doi:10.1177/0148607113488799

Dawodu, S. T. (2015). *Nutritional management in the rehabilitation setting*. Retrieved from http://emedicine.medscape.com/article/318180-overview#a1

Kozeniecki, M., & Fritzshall, R. (2015). Enteral nutrition for adults in the hospital setting. *Nutrition in Clinical Practice, 30*, 634–651. doi:10.1177/0884533615594012

Kurien, M., Penny, H., & Sanders, D. S. (2015). Impact of direct drug delivery via gastric access devices. *Expert Opinion on Drug Delivery, 12*, 455-463. doi:10.1517/17425247.2015.966683

Kushner, R. F. (2014). Weight loss strategies for treatment of obesity. *Progress in Cardiovascular Diseases, 56*, 465–472. Doi:10.1016/j.pcad.2013.09.005

National Institutes of Health (n.d.). *Vitamin and mineral supplement fact sheets*. Retrieved from https://ods.od.nih.gov/factsheets/list-VitaminsMinerals

U.S. Department of Health and Human Services and U.S. Department of Agriculture. (2015). *Dietary guidelines for Americans 2015–2020*, eighth edition. Retrieved from http://health.gov/dietaryguidelines/2015/guidelines

Yanovski, S. Z., & Yanovski, J. A. (2014). Long-term drug treatment for obesity: A systematic and clinical review. *JAMA, 311*, 74–86. doi:10.1001/jama.2013.281361

Unit 6

The Endocrine and Reproductive Systems

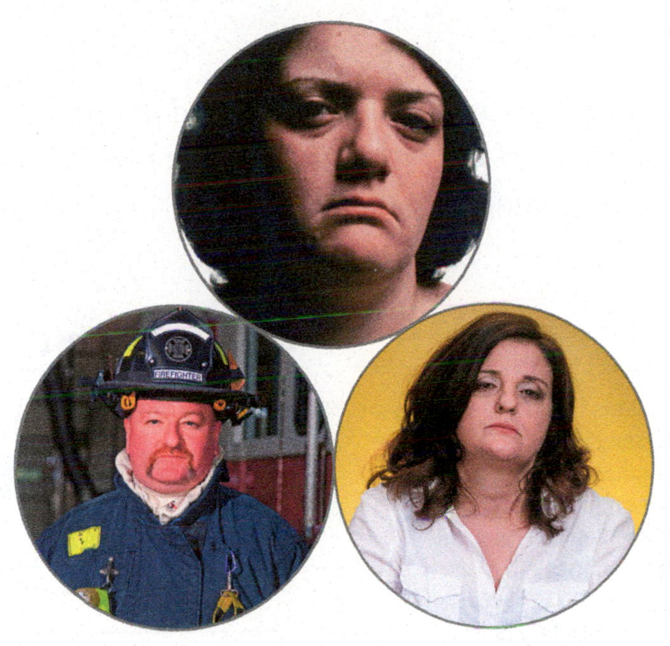

Unit Contents

Chapter 33

Drugs for Endocrine Disorders

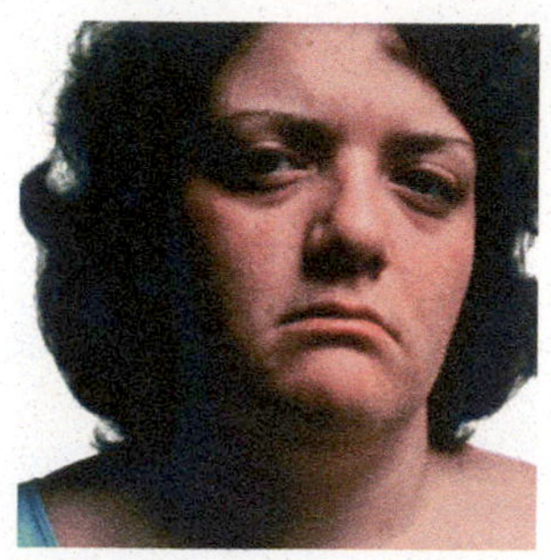

"I don't know why I'm so tired all the time. I've gained a lot of weight and am cold all the time too. Maybe it's just hormones."
Mrs. Helen Brookfield

Core Concepts

33.1 The endocrine system maintains homeostasis by using hormones as chemical messengers.
33.2 The hypothalamus and the pituitary gland secrete hormones that control other endocrine organs.
33.3 Hormones are used as replacement therapy, as antineoplastics, or as "antihormones" to block endogenous actions.
33.4 Of the many hypothalamic and pituitary hormones, several have clinical applications as drugs.
33.5 The thyroid gland controls the basal metabolic rate and affects virtually every cell in the body.
33.6 Thyroid disorders may be treated by administering thyroid hormone or by decreasing the activity of the thyroid gland.
33.7 Corticosteroids are released during periods of stress and influence carbohydrate, lipid, and protein metabolism in most cells.
33.8 Corticosteroids are prescribed for adrenocortical insufficiency and to dampen inflammatory and immune responses.

Drug Snapshot

The following drugs are discussed in this chapter:

Drug Classes	Prototype Drugs
Hypothalamic and Pituitary Drugs	Pr desmopressin (DDAVP, Stimate)
Thyroid Agents	Pr levothyroxine (Levothroid, Synthroid, others)
Antithyroid Agents	Pr propylthiouracil (PTU)
Corticosteroids	Pr hydrocortisone (Cortef, Hydrocortone, others)

Learning Outcomes

After reading this chapter, the student should be able to:

1. Describe the role of hormones in maintaining body homeostasis.
2. Explain how hypothalamic and pituitary hormones influence other endocrine glands and body tissues.
3. Categorize drugs used in the treatment of endocrine disorders based on their classifications and mechanisms of action.
4. Discuss the clinical applications of hypothalamic and pituitary drugs.

5. Discuss the primary functions of the thyroid gland, and identify the signs and symptoms of hypothyroidism and hyperthyroidism.
6. Explain the pharmacologic management of thyroid disorders with thyroid and antithyroid agents.
7. Explain important classes of hormones released from the adrenal cortex and their primary functions in the body.
8. Describe the signs and symptoms of Addison disease and Cushing syndrome, and explain the primary actions as well as the important adverse effects of corticosteroid drug therapy.

Key Terms

acromegaly (AKROW-megah-lee)
Addison disease (ADD-iss-un)
adrenal atrophy (AT-troh-fee)
adrenocorticotropic hormone (ACTH) (uh-dreen-oh-kor-tik-o-TRO-pik)
anterior pituitary
antidiuretic hormone (ADH) (ANT-eye-DYE-yure-EH-tick)
corticosteroids (KORT-ik-ko-STARE-oyd)
cretinism (KREE-ten-izm)
Cushing syndrome (KUSH-ing)
diabetes insipidus (die-uh-BEE-tees in-SIP-uh-dus)
dwarfism
follicular cells (fo-LIK-yu-lur)
glucocorticoids (glu-ko-KORT-ik-oyds)
gonadocorticoids (go-NAD-oh-KORT-ik-oyds)
Graves disease
hormones
hypothalamus (hi-po-THAL-ih-mus)
mineralocorticoids (min-ur-al-oh-KORT-ik-oyds)
myxedema (mix-uh-DEEM-uh)
negative feedback
parafollicular cells (par-uh-fo-LIK-u-lur)
pituitary gland (pit-TOO-it-air-ee)
posterior pituitary
releasing hormones
somatotropin (so-mat-oh-TROH-pin)
vasopressin (vaz-oh-PRESS-in)

Like the nervous system, the endocrine system is a major controller of homeostasis. Whereas a nerve may exert instantaneous control over a single muscle group or several glands, a hormone may affect thousands of body cells and take as long as several days to produce an optimal response. Hormonal balance must be maintained within a narrow range. Too little or too much of a hormone may produce profound changes in the body. This chapter examines common endocrine disorders and their pharmacotherapy. Drugs for diabetes mellitus are covered in Chapter 34. The reproductive hormones are covered in Chapter 35

endo = *within*
crine = *to secrete*

The endocrine system maintains homeostasis by using hormones as chemical messengers.

◀ Core Concept 33.1

Hormones are chemical messengers released in response to a change in the body's internal environment. For example, whenever the body's metabolic rate slows, the thyroid gland secretes thyroid hormone. When levels of calcium in the bloodstream fall, the parathyroid glands secrete parathyroid hormone (PTH). The various endocrine glands and their locations in the body are illustrated in Figure 33.1.

In the endocrine system, it is common for one hormone to control the secretion of another hormone. In addition, it is common for the last hormone or action in the pathway to provide feedback. Most endocrine glands work by feedback inhibition in which the last hormone or action in the pathway prevents the production and release of the first hormone. For example, as serum calcium level falls, PTH is released. PTH causes an increase in serum calcium level, which provides feedback to the parathyroid glands to shut off PTH secretion. This is a common feature of endocrine homeostasis known as **negative feedback**.

The hypothalamus and the pituitary gland secrete hormones that control other endocrine organs.

◀ Core Concept 33.2

Two endocrine structures in the brain deserve special recognition because they control many other endocrine glands. The **hypothalamus** secretes chemicals called **releasing hormones** that travel via blood vessels a short distance to an area immediately below, called the **pituitary gland**. These releasing factors tell the pituitary gland which hormone to release. After the pituitary releases the appropriate hormone, it travels to its target organ to

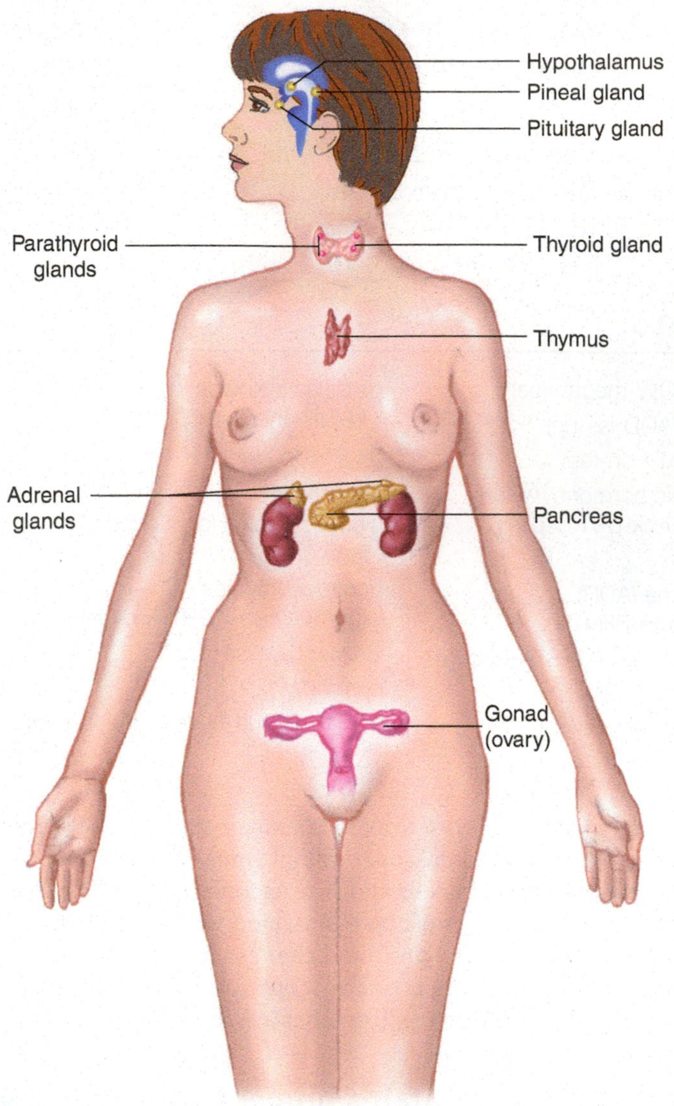

FIGURE 33.1 The endocrine system.

cause its effect. For example, the hypothalamus secretes thyrotropin-releasing hormone, which travels to the pituitary gland with the message to secrete thyroid-stimulating hormone (TSH). TSH then travels to its target organ—the thyroid gland—to stimulate the release of thyroid hormone.

adeno = *glandular tissue*
neuro = *neural tissue*
hypo = *under*
physis = *growth*

The pituitary gland comprises two distinct areas, the **anterior pituitary** or *adenohypophysis* and the **posterior pituitary** or *neurohypophysis*. The majority of hormones are released by *glandular tissue* of the adenohypophysis. Only a few hormones are released from *neural tissue* of the neurohypophysis. Selected hormones associated with the hypothalamus and pituitary gland are shown in Figure 33.2.

Core Concept 33.3 ▶

Hormones are used as replacement therapy, as antineoplastics, or as antihormones to block endogenous actions.

endo = *within*
genous = *generated from*

The goals of hormone pharmacotherapy vary widely. In many cases, the hormone is administered simply as replacement therapy for patients who are unable to secrete sufficient quantities of their own endogenous hormones. Examples of replacement therapy include the administration of thyroid hormone after the thyroid gland has been surgically removed or supplying insulin to a patient whose pancreas is not functioning. Replacement therapy usually supplies the same physiologically low-level amounts of the hormone that would normally be present in the body. A summary of selected endocrine disorders and their drug therapy is given in Table 33.1.

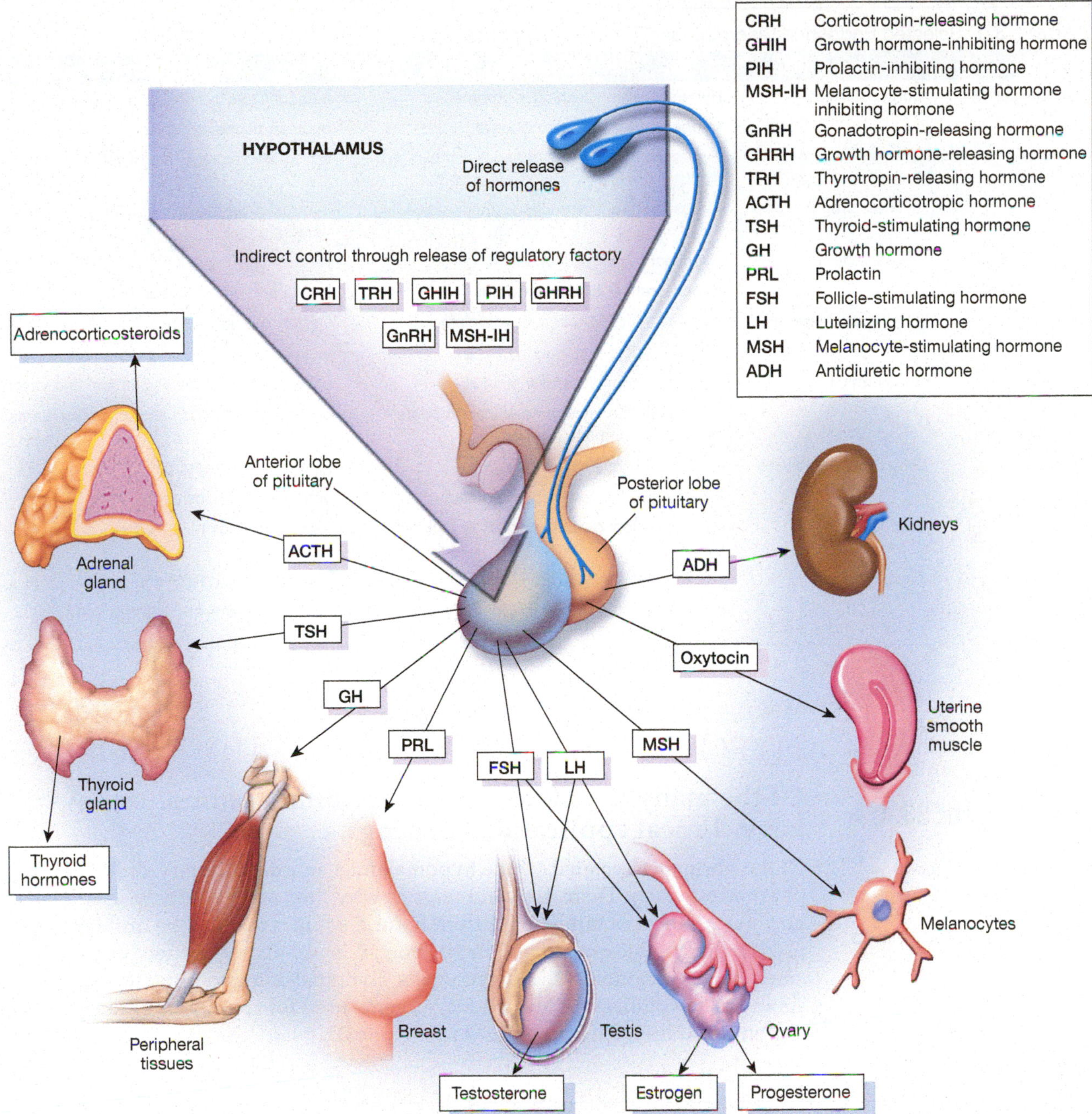

FIGURE 33.2 Hormones associated with the hypothalamus and pituitary gland.

Some hormones are used in cancer chemotherapy to shrink the size of hormone-sensitive tumors. Examples include testosterone for breast cancer and estrogen for testicular cancer. Exactly how these hormones produce their antineoplastic action is unknown. When used as antineoplastics, the doses of these hormones far exceed those levels normally present in the body (see Chapter 29).

Another goal of hormone therapy may be to produce an exaggerated response that is part of the normal action of the drug. Administering hydrocortisone to suppress inflammation takes advantage of the normal action of the corticosteroids but to a greater extent than would normally occur in the body. Supplying small amounts of estrogen or progesterone at specific times during the menstrual cycle can prevent ovulation and pregnancy.

Endocrine pharmacotherapy also involves the use of antihormones. These hormones block the actions of endogenous hormones. For example, propylthiouracil (PTU) is given to block the effects of an overactive thyroid gland. Tamoxifen (Nolvadex) is given to block the actions of estrogens in estrogen-dependent breast cancers (see Chapter 35).

Table 33.1 Selected Endocrine Disorders and Their Pharmacotherapy

Gland	Hormone(s)	Disorder	Drug Therapy Examples
Adrenal cortex	Corticosteroids	Hypersecretion: Cushing syndrome	ketoconazole (Nizoral) and mitotane (Lysodren)
		Hyposecretion: Addison disease	hydrocortisone, prednisone
Gonads	Ovaries: estrogen	Hyposecretion: menstrual and metabolic dysfunction	conjugated estrogens and estradiol
	Ovaries: progesterone	Hyposecretion: dysfunctional uterine bleeding	medroxyprogesterone (Provera, Others) and norethindrone
	Testes: testosterone	Hyposecretion: hypogonadism	testosterone
Pancreatic islets	Insulin	Hyposecretion: diabetes mellitus	insulin and oral antidiabetic agents
Parathyroid	Parathyroid hormone	Hypersecretion: hyperparathyroidism	surgery (no drug therapy)
		Hyposecretion: hypoparathyroidism	vitamin D and calcium supplements
Pituitary	Antidiuretic hormone	Hyposecretion: diabetes insipidus	desmopressin (DDAVP, Stimate) and vasopressin
		Hypersecretion: syndrome of inappropriate antidiuretic hormone (SIADH)	conivaptan (Vaprisol) and tolvaptan (Samsca)
	Growth hormone (GH)	Hyposecretion: small stature	somatropin (Genotropin, Others)
		Hypersecretion: acromegaly (adults)	octreotide (Sandostatin)
	Oxytocin	Hyposecretion: delayed delivery or lack of milk ejection	oxytocin (Pitocin)
Thyroid	Thyroid hormone (T_3 and T_4)	Hypersecretion: Graves disease	propylthiouracil (PTU) and I-131
		Hyposecretion: myxedema (adults), cretinism (children)	thyroid hormone and levothyroxine (T4)

HYPOTHALAMIC AND PITUITARY DISORDERS

Core Concept 33.4 ▶

Of the many hypothalamic and pituitary hormones, several have clinical applications as drugs.

diabetes = *siphon (urine passing through)*
mellitus = *sweetened*
insipidus = *tasteless (watered down)*

en = *in*
uresis = *to urinate*

Of the hormones secreted by the hypothalamus and the pituitary, only a few are used in pharmacotherapy. There are valid reasons why they are not widely used. Some of these hormones can be obtained only from natural sources and can be quite expensive when used in therapeutic quantities. Furthermore, it is usually more effective to give drugs that *directly* affect secretion at the target organs. Hypothalamic and pituitary agents are listed in Table 33.2. Hypothalamic and pituitary agents used for conditions of the male and female reproductive systems are presented in Chapter 35.

Table 33.2 Selected Hypothalamic and Pituitary Drugs

Drug	Route and Adult Dose	Remarks
HYPOTHALAMIC DRUG		
bromocriptine (Cycloset, Parlodel)	PO (Cycloset): 0.8–1.6 mg daily until max dose of 4.8mg/day PO: 1.25–2.5 mg/day for 3 days, then increase gradually to 30–60 mg/day	Blocks the release of prolactin; for treatment of acromegaly (overproduction of GH) and pituitary tumors; for signs and symptoms of Parkinson disease and type 2 diabetes mellitus
PITUITARY DRUGS		
Posterior Pituitary—ADH Drugs		
Pr desmopressin (DDAVP, Stimate)	IV/Subcutaneous: 2–4 mcg in divided doses PO: 0.2–0.4 mg/day	To control symptoms of diabetes insipidus; in children under 6 years old, for bed-wetting (enuresis); also used to treat von Willebrand disease
vasopressin	IM/Subcutaneous: 5–10 units two to four times per day IV: 0.2–0.4 units/min up to 1 unit/min	Human ADH; reduces urine output by targeting renal collecting tubules
Anterior Pituitary—GH and TSH Drugs		
lanreotide (Somatuline Depot)	Subcutaneous: 60–100 mg every 4 weeks	For long-term treatment of patients with acromegaly who cannot be treated with surgery or radiation

Drug	Route and Adult Dose	Remarks
mecasermin (Increlex)	Subcutaneous: 0.04–0.08 mg/kg bid. Must be administered within 20 minutes of a meal (max: 0.12 mg/kg bid)	Synthetic version of insulin-like growth factor (IGF-1); suppresses liver glucose production and stimulates glucose uptake; for long-term treatment of growth failure in children with antibodies that neutralize GH
octreotide (Sandostatin)	Subcutaneous/IV: 100–600 mcg/day in divided doses; after 2 weeks may switch to IM depot, 20 mg every 4 weeks	For acromegaly; also for severe diarrhea that occurs with intestinal tumors or metastatic carcinoid tumors (tumors already spread in the body)
pegvisomant (Somavert)	Subcutaneous: 40 mg loading dose, then 10 mg/day (max: 30 mg/day)	GH receptor antagonist (blocker) used in the treatment of patients with acromegaly who cannot be treated with surgery or radiation
somatropin (Genotropin, Humatrope, Norditropin, Nutropin, Saizen, Serostim, Zorbtive)	Humatrope: Subcutaneous: 0.006 mg/kg daily (max: 0.0125 mg/kg/day) Serostim: Subcutaneous: 4–6 mg/day Genotropin: Subcutaneous; 0.16–0.24 mg/kg/ week Norditropin: 0.024–0.034 mg/kg six to seven times per week	Form of recombinant human GH; also for HIV-associated wasting (Serostim)

Antidiuretic hormone (ADH) is one of the most important ways the body maintains fluid homeostasis. As its name implies, ADH conserves water in the body. ADH is secreted from the posterior pituitary gland when the hypothalamus senses that plasma volume has decreased or that the osmolality of the blood has become too high. ADH is also called **vasopressin**, because it has the ability to constrict blood vessels and raise blood pressure. A deficiency in ADH results in central **diabetes insipidus (DI)**, a rare condition characterized by the production of large volumes of very dilute urine, usually accompanied by increased blood sodium levels and increased thirst. Two ADH preparations are available for the treatment of DI: desmopressin (DDAVP) and vasopressin. Desmopressin is the most common drug for treating DI. Details regarding this drug are found in the Prototype Drug feature.

anti = *against*
diuretic = *urination agent*

osmolality = *concentration*

vaso = *blood vessel*
pressin = *tension*

Prototype Drug: Pr *Desmopressin (DDAVP, Stimate)*

Therapeutic Class: Antidiuretic hormone replacement; retains fluid in the body Pharmacologic Class: Antidiuretic hormone; vasopressin

Actions and Uses: Desmopressin is a synthetic form of human ADH that acts on the renal tubular cells to increase the reabsorption of water. It is used to control the acute symptoms of DI in patients who have insufficient ADH secretion. The oral route is preferred, although intranasal and parenteral forms are available. It has a duration of action of up to 20 hours, whereas vasopressin has a duration of only 2–8 hours. The drug is sometimes used to manage enuresis (bed-wetting that occurs during the night). Desmopressin is also available as a nasal spray (Stimate) to treat von Willebrand disease, a disorder of blood clotting.

Adverse Effects and Interactions: Desmopressin causes contraction of smooth muscle in the vascular system, uterus, and gastrointestinal (GI) tract. It also is used to manage bleeding in patients with hemophilia A. When taken an hour prior to bedtime, desmopressin lowers the production of urine during the night and thus is useful in the management of nocturnal enuresis (bed-wetting).

Desmopressin can cause symptoms of water intoxication: edema, weight gain, hypertension (HTN), drowsiness, headache, and listlessness, progressing to convulsions and coma. Patients are advised to weigh themselves daily. Other adverse effects include transient headache, nausea, mild abdominal pain and cramping, facial flushing, and pain or swelling at the injection site. Intranasal forms can cause nasal congestion, rhinitis, and epistaxis.

Desmopressin is contraindicated in patients with DI that is caused by kidney disease because the drug can worsen fluid retention and overload. It is used with caution in patients with coronary artery disease and HTN and in patients at risk for hyponatremia or thrombi.

Increased antidiuretic action can occur with carbamazepine, chlorpropamide, clofibrate, and nonsteroidal anti-inflammatory drugs (NSAIDs). Decreased antidiuretic action can occur with lithium, alcohol, heparin, and epinephrine.

Growth hormone (GH), also called **somatotropin**, stimulates the growth and metabolism of nearly every cell in the body. Deficiency of this hormone in children can cause *short stature*, a condition characterized by significantly decreased physical height compared with the norm of a specific age group. Severe deficiency results in **dwarfism**. Short stature is caused by many conditions other than GH deficiency, and often a specific cause cannot be

somato = *cells of the body*
tropin = *attraction toward*

dwarfism = *small stature*

identified. Treatment of this condition usually involves the administration of the GH. It is given subcutaneously, several times a week during periods of active growth. Therapy continues until the desired height is achieved or until the epiphyses close. The earlier the condition is treated, the better the chance that a child will grow to be a near-normal adult height. When hormone therapy is first initiated, the gain in growth is very rapid but then slows over time.

acro = *extremeties*
megaly = *enlarged*

Excess secretion of GH in adults is known as **acromegaly**. Acromegaly is a rare disorder caused by a GH-secreting tumor of the pituitary gland. Because the epiphyseal plates are closed in adults, bones become deformed rather than elongated with this disorder. The onset is gradual, with enlargement of the small bones of the hands and feet, face, and skull; broad nose, protruding lower jaw; and slanting forehead.

Treatment of acromegaly consists of a combination of surgery, radiation therapy, and pharmacotherapy to suppress GH secretion or block GH receptors. Pharmacotherapy is generally attempted only in patients who are unable to undergo surgical removal of the tumor. Octreotide (Sandostatin) is a synthetic GH *antagonist* (blocker) structurally related to GH–inhibiting hormone (somatostatin). Other choices to treat acromegaly include pegvisomant (Somavert), bromocriptine (Cycloset, Parlodel), and lanreotide (Somatuline Depot).

THYROID DISORDERS

Core Concept 33.5 ▶

The thyroid gland controls the basal metabolic rate and affects virtually every cell in the body.

The thyroid gland secretes hormones that affect nearly every cell in the body. Thyroid hormone increases basal metabolic rate, which is the baseline speed at which cells perform their functions. By increasing cellular metabolism, this hormone increases body temperature. Adequate secretion of thyroid hormone is also necessary for the normal growth and development in infants and children. **Cretinism** is the abnormal stunting of growth due to the lack of thyroid hormone, usually seen in infants born with a congenital condition where the thyroid gland is not working or did not develop appropriately. The thyroid strongly affects cardiovascular, respiratory, GI, and neuromuscular function.

The thyroid gland lies in the neck, just below the larynx and in front of the trachea. **Follicular cells** in the gland secrete thyroid hormone, which is actually a combination of two different hormones: thyroxine (tetraiodothyronine or T_4) and triiodothyronine (T_3). Iodine is essential for the synthesis of these hormones and is provided through the dietary intake of common iodized salt. T_3 is named for the three iodine atoms that make up its chemical structure; T_4 has four iodine atoms. **Parafollicular cells** in the thyroid gland secrete calcitonin, a hormone that is involved with calcium homeostasis (see Chapter 36).

Thyroid function is regulated in various ways. Thyroid-releasing hormone (TRH) from the hypothalamus stimulates the pituitary gland to secrete TSH. TSH then stimulates the thyroid gland to release thyroid hormone. As blood levels of thyroid hormone increase, negative feedback suppresses the secretion of TRH and TSH. High levels of iodine can also cause a temporary decrease in thyroid activity that can last for several weeks. One of the strongest stimuli for increased thyroid hormone production is reduced body metabolism. The negative feedback mechanism for the thyroid gland is shown in Figure 33.3.

Core Concept 33.6 ▶

Thyroid disorders may be treated by administering thyroid hormone or by decreasing the activity of the thyroid gland.

Disorders of the thyroid result from *hypofunction* or *hyperfunction* of the thyroid gland. Abnormal thyroid hormone levels may occur due to disease within the thyroid gland itself or be caused by abnormalities of the pituitary gland or hypothalamus. Thyroid disorders are quite common, and drug therapy is often indicated.

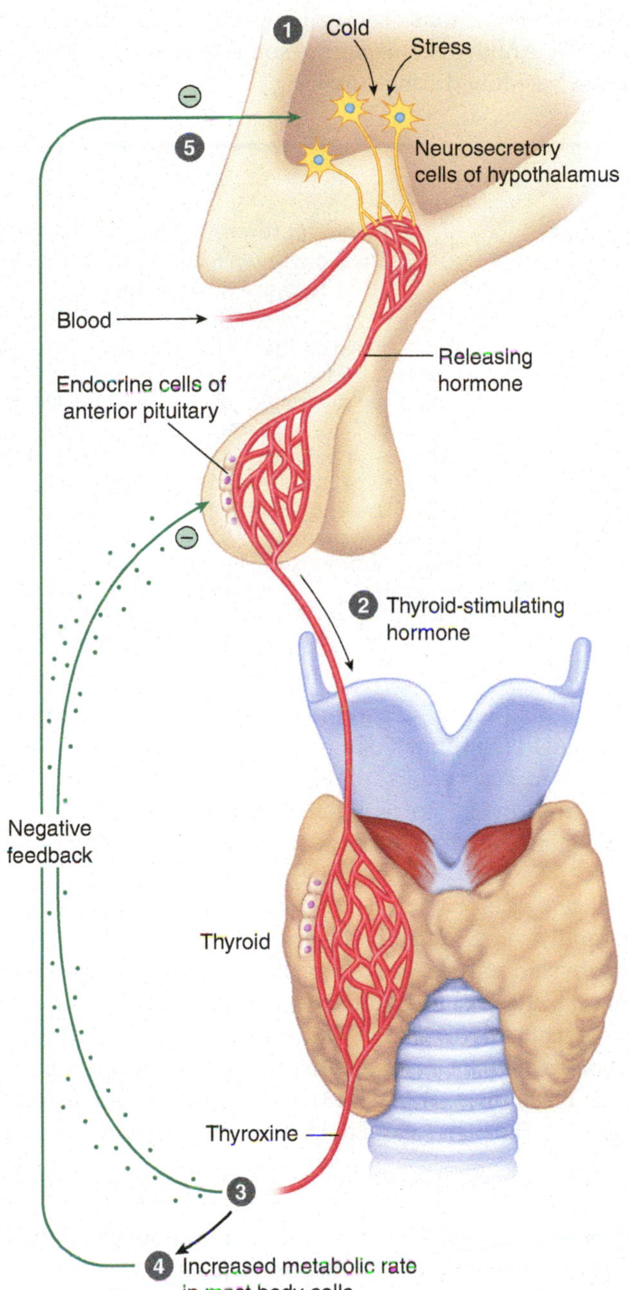

FIGURE 33.3 Feedback mechanisms of the thyroid gland: (1) stimulus; (2) release of TSH; (3) increased metabolic rate; (4) negative feedback.

Hypothyroidism is a common disease caused by insufficient secretion of either TSH or thyroid hormone. The most common type of hypothyroidism is Hashimoto's disease, an autoimmune disorder. Symptoms of severe hypothyroidism, also known in adults as **myxedema**, include slowed body metabolism, fatigue, slurred speech, bradycardia, weight gain, low body temperature, and intolerance to cold environments. If left untreated, severe hypothyroidism can result in coma or death. Low or absent thyroid function may be a consequence of autoimmune disease, surgical removal of the gland, or aggressive treatment with antithyroid drugs. Hypothyroidism is treated with natural or synthetic thyroid hormone.

Hypersecretion of thyroid hormone causes symptoms that are the opposite of hypothyroidism and results in increased body metabolism. The symptoms include nervousness, tremors, irritability, insomnia, tachycardia, palpitations, weight loss, hyperthermia, and heat intolerance. A particularly severe form of hyperthyroidism is called **Graves disease**. If the cause of the hypersecretion is found to be a tumor, the disease is corrected through surgical removal of the thyroid gland, or thyroidectomy. In less severe conditions, the patient may receive antithyroid medications or ionizing radiation to kill or inactivate some of the hyperactive thyroid cells. Antithyroid drugs are sometimes given 10 to 14 days prior to thyroidectomy to decrease bleeding during surgery.

Fast Facts Thyroid Disorders

- The two most common thyroid disorders, Graves disease and Hashimoto thyroiditis, are autoimmune diseases and may run in families.
- Women are 15–20 times more likely than men to develop Hashimoto thyroiditis.
- Hypothyroidism is 10 times more common in women than men; hyperthyroidism is 5–10 times more common in women.
- One of every 4000 babies is born without a working thyroid gland.
- About 15,000 new cases of thyroid cancer are diagnosed each year.
- Postpartum thyroiditis occurs in 5–9% of women after giving birth and may recur in future pregnancies.
- Both hyperthyroidism and hypothyroidism can affect a woman's ability to become pregnant; both also can cause miscarriages.

Source: Based on Toft, D. (2014). Graves' disease overview. What is Graves's disease; Akamizu, T., Amino, N., DeGroot, L. J. (2013). Hashimoto's thyroiditis; Baby's First Test. (2015). About newborn screening. Screening facts and Skugor, M. (2014). Hypothyroidism and hyperthyroidism; University of Maryland Medical Center. (2012). Hypothyroidism; Womens Health Advice.com (n.d.). Thyroid cancers; American Thyroid Association. (2014). Postpartum thyroiditis; American Association of Clinical Endocrinology. (n.d.) Thyroid awareness. The thyroid and pregnancy.

Because the thyroid gland is the organ most susceptible to nuclear and radiation exposure, thyroid dysfunction in the context of emergency preparedness is an important topic to consider. Symptoms of radiation exposure remain some of the most difficult to treat pharmacologically. Apart from the symptomatic treatment of *acute radiation syndrome*, taking potassium iodide (KI) tablets after an incident or a nuclear or biologic attack is the only recognized therapy.

Following a nuclear explosion, one of the resultant radioisotopes is iodine-131 (I-131). Because iodine is naturally concentrated in the thyroid gland, I-131 will immediately enter the thyroid and damage thyroid cells. If taken prior to, or immediately following a nuclear incident, KI can prevent up to 100% of the radioactive iodine from entering thyroid tissue. Unfortunately, KI only protects the thyroid gland from I-131. It has no protective effects on other body tissues, and it offers no protection against the dozens of other harmful radioisotopes generated by a nuclear blast. Interestingly, I-131 is also a medication used to shrink the size of overactive thyroid glands. The thyroid and antithyroid medications are listed in Table 33.3.

CONCEPT REVIEW 33.1

- If thyroid hormone is secreted by the thyroid gland, how can a deficiency in this hormone be caused by disease in the hypothalamus or pituitary gland?

Table 33.3 Thyroid and Antithyroid Agents

Drug	Route and Adult Dose	Remarks
THYROID AGENTS		
Pr levothyroxine (Levothroid, Synthroid, others)	PO: 100–400 mcg/day	Synthetic T_4; IV form available
liothyronine (Cytomel, Triostat)	PO: 25–75 mcg/day	Synthetic T_3
liotrix (Thyrolar)	PO: 12.5–30 mcg/day	Mixture of synthetic T_3 and synthetic T_4 in a 1:4 ratio
thyroid dessicated (Armour Thyroid, Thyrar, Thyroid USP)	PO: 60–100 mg/day	Obtained from animal thyroid glands
ANTITHYROID AGENTS		
methimazole (Tapazole)	PO: 5–15 mg tid	Ten times more potent than propylthiouracil
potassium iodide and iodine (Lugol's solution, Thyro-block)	PO: 0.1–1.0 mL tid	IV form available; Lugol's is a mixture of 5% elemental iodine and 10% potassium iodide
Pr propylthiouracil (PTU)	PO: 100–150 mg tid	May take 6–12 months for full therapeutic effect
radioactive iodide (I-131)	PO: 0.8–150 mCi (based on radiation quantity)	May take 2–3 months for full therapeutic effect

Prototype Drug: Pr *Levothyroxine (Levothroid, Synthroid, Others)*

Therapeutic Class: Thyroid hormone replacement; metabolic enhancer Pharmacologic Class: Thyroid hormone

Actions and Uses: Levothyroxine is a synthetic form of thyroxine (T_4) used for replacement therapy in patients with low thyroid function. Actions are those of thyroid hormone and include loss of weight, improved tolerance to environmental temperature, increased activity, and increased pulse rate. Blood levels of thyroid hormone are monitored carefully until the patient's symptoms stabilize. In order to closely approximate the body's own hormone level, levothyroxine should be taken in the morning, ideally at the same time each day. To achieve the proper level of thyroid function, doses may require periodic adjustments for several months or longer.

Adverse Effects and Interactions: The difference between a therapeutic dose of levothyroxine and one that produces adverse effects is quite narrow. Adverse effects of levothyroxine resemble symptoms of hyperthyroidism and include tachycardia, anxiety, tremors, insomnia, weight loss, and heat intolerance. Menstrual irregularities may occur in women. Long-term use of levothyroxine has been associated with osteoporosis in women.

Levothyroxine interacts with many other drugs. For example, cholestyramine and colestipol decrease the absorption and effectiveness of levothyroxine if taken too close together. Using it with epinephrine and norepinephrine increases the risk of cardiac insufficiency. Oral anticoagulants may increase hypoprothrombinemia.

High fiber foods may affect absorption. Herbal supplements such as lemon balm should be used cautiously. Lemon balm may interfere with thyroid hormone function.

Prototype Drug: Pr *Propylthiouracil (PTU)*

Therapeutic Class: Drug for hyperthyroidism Pharmacologic Class: Antithyroid agent

Actions and Uses: Propylthiouracil is administered to patients with hyperthyroidism, sometimes prior to surgery. It acts by interfering with the synthesis of T_3 and T_4. Because it does not affect thyroid hormone that has already been secreted, its action may be delayed from several days to as long as 6 to 12 weeks. Effects include a return to normal thyroid function: weight gain, reduction in anxiety, less insomnia, and slower pulse rate.

Adverse Effects and Interactions: Overtreatment with PTU produces symptoms of hypothyroidism. In addition, a small percentage of patients display blood changes such as decreased platelet counts, which may increase the risk of bruising and bleeding, and decreased white blood cell counts, which may increase the risk of infection and fever. Periodic laboratory blood counts and thyroid hormone values are necessary to establish the proper dosage.

Antithyroid medications interact with many other drugs. For example, PTU can reverse the effectiveness of drugs such as aminophylline, anticoagulants, and cardiac glycosides.

Nursing Process Focus Patients Receiving Thyroid Hormone Replacement

ASSESSMENT

Prior to administration:

- Obtain a complete health history, including cardiovascular, neurologic, renal and liver conditions; pregnancy, allergies, drug history, and possible drug interactions.
- Evaluate laboratory blood findings: complete blood count (CBC), electrolytes, lipid panel, renal and liver function studies, T_4, T_3, and TSH levels.
- Acquire the results of a complete physical examination, including vital signs, height, weight, and electrocardiogram (ECG).

POTENTIAL NURSING DIAGNOSES*

- *Activity Intolerance* related to decrease in levels of thyroid hormones
- *Fatigue* related to impaired metabolic status
- *Deficient Knowledge* related to a lack of information about drug therapy
- *Infective Health Maintenance* related to adverse effects of drug therapy
- *Risk for Infection* related to adverse effects of drug therapy

PLANNING: PATIENT GOALS AND EXPECTED OUTCOMES

The patient will:

- Experience therapeutic effects of drug regimen (normal thyroid levels).
- Be free from or experience minimal adverse effects from drug therapy.
- Verbalize an understanding of the drug's use, adverse effects, and required precautions.

IMPLEMENTATION

Interventions and (Rationales)	Patient Education/Discharge Planning
• Administer medication correctly, and evaluate the patient's knowledge of proper administration. In addition, monitor the patient for signs of decreased compliance with therapeutic regimen. (Proper administration and compliance helps to ensure adequate thyroid hormone levels and a decrease in adverse effects.)	• Instruct the patient about the disease, the importance of taking the medication regularly each day, and the importance of follow-up care.

(Continued)

Nursing Process Focus (*continued*)

Interventions and (Rationales)	Patient Education/Discharge Planning
• Monitor vital signs. (Changes in metabolic rate will be manifested as changes in blood pressure, pulse, and body temperature.)	Instruct the patient to: • Take and record pulse rate two to three times a week. • Report to the healthcare provider any dizziness, palpitations, and an intolerance to temperature changes.
• Monitor for symptoms related to hypothyroidism, such as fatigue, constipation, cold intolerance, lethargy, depression, and menstrual irregularities. (Decreasing symptoms will help determine effectiveness of hormone replacement hormone.)	• Instruct the patient about the signs of hypothyroidism and to report symptoms to the healthcare provider.
• Monitor for symptoms related to hyperthyroidism, such as nervousness, irritability, insomnia, tremors, tachycardia, palpitations, weight loss, hyperthermia, and heat intolerance. (Symptoms of hyperthyroidism may indicate overuse or adverse effects of hormone replacement medication.)	• Instruct the patient about the signs of hyperthyroidism and to report symptoms to the healthcare provider.
• Monitor T_3, T_4, and TSH levels. (This helps to determine need or effectiveness of drug therapy.)	Instruct the patient: • About the importance of ongoing monitoring of thyroid hormone levels. • To keep all laboratory appointments.
• Monitor blood glucose levels, especially in individuals with diabetes mellitus. (Thyroid hormones increase metabolic rate and may alter glucose utilization.)	• Instruct the patient with diabetes to monitor blood glucose levels and adjust insulin doses as directed by the healthcare provider.
• Provide supportive nursing care to cope with symptoms of hypothyroidism such as constipation, cold intolerance, and fatigue, until the drug has achieved therapeutic effect. (Providing care will ensure patient comfort and enable the nurse to monitor signs and symptoms.)	Instruct the patient to: • Increase fluid and fiber intake, as well as activity, to reduce constipation. • Wear additional clothing, and maintain a comfortable room environment for cold intolerance. • Plan activities and include rest periods to avoid fatigue.
• Monitor weight at least weekly. (Weight loss or gain may indicate disease process and helps to determine the effectiveness of drug therapy.)	Instruct the patient to: • Take and record weight weekly. • Report significant changes in weight to the healthcare provider.
• Unless approved by the healthcare provider, avoid iodine-containing foods such as soy sauce, tofu, milk, eggs, yogurt, and some fish. (Increasing or decreasing normal intake of these foods may result in adverse drug effects.)	• Provide dietary instruction on foods to avoid.

EVALUATION OF OUTCOME CRITERIA

Evaluate the effectiveness of drug therapy by confirming that patient goals and expected outcomes have been met (see "Planning"). *See* Table 33.3 *for a list of drugs to which these nursing actions apply.*

*Herdman, T.H. & Kamitsuru, S. (Eds.), *Nursing Diagnoses: Definitions & Classification* 2015–2017. Copyright © 2014, 1994–2014 NANDA International. Used by arrangement by John Wiley & Sons, Inc. Companion website: www.wiley.com/go/nursingdiagnoses.

ADRENAL DISORDERS

Core Concept 33.7 ▶

Corticosteroids are released during periods of stress and influence carbohydrate, lipid, and protein metabolism in most cells.

mineralo = *minerals (i.e., sodium, potassium)*

cortic/cortico = *cortex*
tropin/tropic = *attraction toward*
adreno = *adrenal glands*

Though small, the adrenal glands, located on top of each kidney, secrete hormones that affect almost every body tissue. These hormones help prepare the body to rapidly respond to stressful situations. Adrenal disorders include those resulting from either *excess* hormone production or *deficient* hormone production. The specific pharmacotherapy depends on which portion of the adrenal gland is being affected. There are two major portions of the adrenal glands: the outer cortex and the inner medulla. The outer cortex releases three important classes of hormones: the *mineralocorticoids*, *glucocorticoids*, and *androgens*. Collectively, these hormones are referred to as **corticosteroids** or *adrenocortical hormones*.

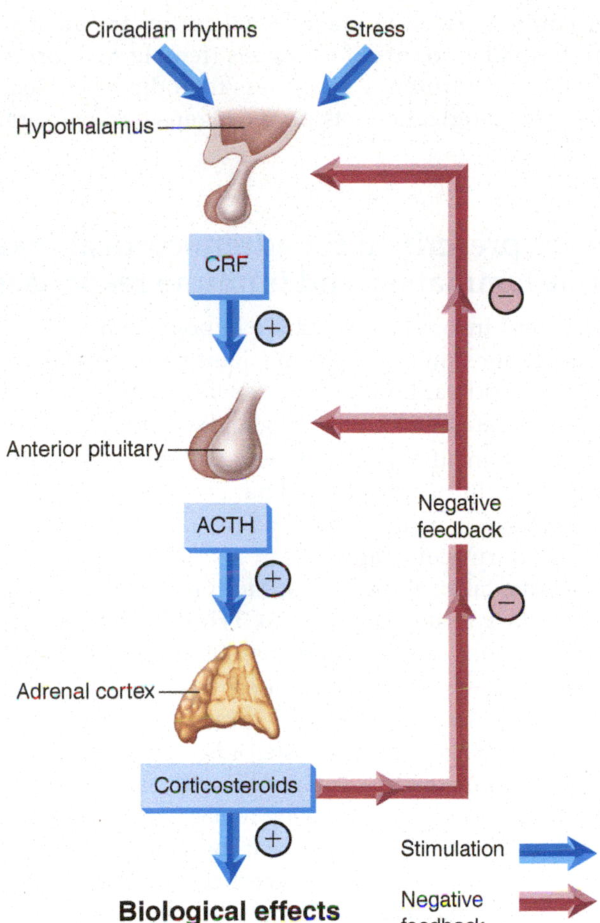

FIGURE 33.4 Feedback control of the adrenal cortex.

Control of corticosteroids begins with corticotropin-releasing factor (CRF), secreted by the hypothalamus. CRF travels to the pituitary, where it causes the release of **adrenocorticotropic hormone (ACTH)**. ACTH then travels through the bloodstream and reaches the adrenal cortex, causing the adrenal gland to release cortisol and other important corticosteroids. When the level of corticosteroids in the bloodstream rises, it provides negative feedback to the hypothalamus and pituitary to shut off further release of corticosteroids. This negative feedback mechanism is shown in Figure 33.4.

Aldosterone accounts for most of the **mineralocorticoids** secreted by the adrenal glands. Mineralocorticoids regulate the extracellular concentrations of mineral salts, particularly sodium and potassium, in the body. Aldosterone is the principle mineralocorticoid. The primary function of aldosterone is to regulate plasma volume by promoting sodium reabsorption and potassium secretion by the renal tubules. When plasma volume falls, the kidney secretes renin, which results in the production of angiotensin II. Angiotensin II then causes aldosterone secretion, which promotes sodium retention (*hypernatremia*) and water retention. Angiotensin II is also a potent vasoconstrictor responsible for hypertension (HTN). Attempts to modify this pathway led to the development of the angiotensin-converting enzyme (ACE) inhibitor class of medications, which are often preferred drugs for treating HTN and heart failure. ACE inhibitors interfere with the conversion of angiotensin I to angiotensin II within pulmonary circulation (see Chapters 19 and 20).

hyper = *elevated*
natri = *sodium*
emia = *blood levels*
tension = *blood pressure*

Cortisol is one of numerous **glucocorticoids** secreted from the outer portion, or cortex, of the adrenal gland. Glucocorticoids affect the metabolism of nearly every cell in the body. During long-term stress, these hormones increase the level of blood glucose (*hyperglycemia*) and promote the breakdown of proteins and lipids for energy (*gluconeogenesis*). They have a potent anti-inflammatory effect, and they suppress the immune response (Chapters 25 and 26).

gluco/glyc = *sugar*
al/oid = *resembling*

neo = *new*

gonado = *gonads (e.g., sex organs)*
andro = *male hormones*
estro = *female hormones*
gens/genesis = *synthesized*

The **gonadocorticoids** secreted by the adrenal cortex are mostly androgens (male sex hormones), though small amounts of estrogens (female sex hormones) are also produced. The amounts of these hormones are far less than the levels secreted by either the testes or ovaries.The physiological effects of androgens and estrogens are detailed in Chapter 35.

Core Concept 33.8 ▶

Corticosteroids are prescribed for adrenocortical insufficiency and to dampen inflammatory and immune responses.

Symptoms of adrenocortical insufficiency include hypoglycemia, unusual fatigue, orthostatic hypotension, darkening skin pigmentation, joint pain, and GI disturbances such as anorexia, vomiting, and diarrhea. Low plasma levels of cortisol, accompanied by high plasma levels of ACTH, indicate that the adrenal gland is not responding to ACTH stimulation. *Primary* adrenocortical insufficiency, known as **Addison disease**, is quite rare and includes a deficiency of both glucocorticoids and mineralocorticoids. *Secondary* adrenocortical insufficiency is more common than primary and can occur when corticosteroids are suddenly withdrawn during pharmacotherapy.

a = *without*
trophy = *nourishment*

When corticosteroids are taken as medications for prolonged periods, they provide negative feedback to the pituitary to stop secreting ACTH. Without stimulation by ACTH, the adrenal cortex shrinks and stops secreting endogenous corticosteroids, a condition known as **adrenal atrophy**. The goal of replacement therapy is to achieve the same physiologic level of corticosteroids in the blood that would be present if the adrenal glands were functioning properly. Abrupt withdrawal of corticosteroids may cause adrenal crisis, a medical emergency, requiring immediate treatment. Gradual withdrawal of corticosteroids is considered in some cases; however, patients requiring replacement therapy generally must take corticosteroids their entire lifetime, and concurrent therapy with a mineralocorticoid such as fludrocortisone (Florinef) is essential. Selected corticosteroids are listed in Table 33.4.

In addition to treating adrenal insufficiency, corticosteroids are prescribed for a large number of nonendocrine disorders. Their ability to suppress inflammatory and immune responses quickly and effectively gives them tremendous therapeutic utility to treat a diverse set of conditions, including shock, swelling, post-transplant surgery, some cancers, allergies, asthma, inflammatory bowel disease, and some rheumatic and skin disorders.

Cushing syndrome occurs when high levels of corticosteroids are present in the body over a prolonged period. Although hypersecretion of these hormones can be due to

Table 33.4 Selected Corticosteroids

Drug	Route and Adult Dose	Remarks
SHORT ACTING		
cortisone	PO: 20–300 mg/day	IM form available; has mineralocorticoid activity
Pr hydrocortisone (Cortef, Solu-Cortef)	PO: 10–320 mg/day in divided doses IV/IM; 15–800 mg/day in divided doses (max: 2 g/day)	Topical form available; has both glucocorticoid and mineralocorticoid activity
INTERMEDIATE ACTING		
methylprednisolone (Depo-Medrol, Medrol, Medrol Dosepak, others)	PO: 2–60 mg one to four times per day	IV and IM forms available; has little mineralocorticoid activity
prednisolone	PO: 5–60 mg one to four times per day	IV and IM forms available; has little mineralocorticoid activity
prednisone (see the Prototype Drug box in Core Concept 25.5)	PO: 5–60 mg one to four times per day	Has little mineralocorticoid activity
triamcinolone (Aristospan, Kenalog)	PO: 4–48 mg one to two times per day	IV, intra-articular, subcutaneous, topical, inhalation, and IM forms available; has little mineralocorticoid activity
LONG ACTING		
betamethasone (Celestone, Diprolene, others)	PO: 0.6–7.2 mg/day IM: 0.5–9 mg/day	IV, topical, and IM forms available; has little mineralocorticoid activity
dexamethasone	IM: 8–16 mg bid–qid PO: 0.25–4 mg bid–qid	IV, ophthalmic, topical, intranasal, inhalation, and IM forms available; has little mineralocorticoid activity
fludrocortisone (Florinef)	PO: 0.1–0.2 mg/day	Has strong mineralocorticoid activity

pituitary (due to excess ACTH) or adrenal tumors, the most common cause of Cushing syndrome is long-term therapy with high doses of systemic corticosteroids. Signs and symptoms include adrenal atrophy, behavioral changes, changes in vision, osteoporosis, HTN, increased risk of infections, delayed wound healing, acne, peptic ulcers, fluid retention, weight gain, and a redistribution of fat around the face (moon face), abdomen, shoulders, and neck (buffalo hump).

CONCEPT REVIEW 33.2

- Why does administration of corticosteroids for extended periods result in adrenal atrophy?

Prototype Drug: Pr *Hydrocortisone (Cortef, Hydrocortone, Others)*

Therapeutic Class: Adrenal hormone replacement; drug for moderate to severe asthma and allergies, and antineoplastic therapy **Pharmacologic Class:** Systemic corticosteroid

Actions and Uses: Structurally identical to the natural hormone cortisol, hydrocortisone is a synthetic corticosteroid that is the drug of choice for treating adrenocortical insufficiency. When used for replacement therapy, it is given at physiologic doses. Once proper dosing is achieved, its therapeutic effects should mimic those of natural corticosteroids. Hydrocortisone is also available for the treatment of inflammation, allergic disorders, and many other conditions. Intra-articular injections may be given to decrease severe inflammation in affected joints.

Adverse Effects and Interactions: When used at physiologic doses for replacement therapy, adverse effects of hydrocortisone should not be evident. The patient and the healthcare professional must be vigilant, however, in observing for signs of Cushing syndrome, which can develop with high doses. If taken for longer than 2 weeks, hydrocortisone should be discontinued gradually.

Hydrocortisone interacts with many drugs. For example, barbiturates, phenytoin, and rifampin may increase liver metabolism, thus decreasing hydrocortisone levels. Estrogens increase the effects of hydrocortisone. NSAIDs increase the risk of ulcers. Cholestyramine and colestipol decrease hydrocortisone absorption. Diuretics and amphotericin B increase hypokalemia. Anticholinesterase drugs may produce severe weakness. Hydrocortisone may cause a decrease in immune response to vaccines and toxoids. Patients with diabetes should be advised to check their blood glucose levels more frequently. Hydrocortisone may cause a rise in blood glucose levels, especially in patients with diabetes.

Herbal supplements, such as aloe and buckthorn (a laxative), may cause potassium deficiency.

Nursing Process Focus Patients Receiving Systemic Corticosteroid Therapy

ASSESSMENT

Prior to administration:

- Obtain a complete health history, including cardiovascular, respiratory, neurologic, renal, and liver conditions; pregnancy, allergies, drug history, and possible drug interactions.
- Evaluate laboratory blood findings: CBC, electrolytes, glucose, lipid panel, renal and liver function studies.
- Acquire the results of a complete physical examination, including vital signs, height, and weight.

POTENTIAL NURSING DIAGNOSES*

- *Deficient Knowledge* related to a lack of information about drug therapy
- *Risk for Infection* related to immunosuppression
- *Risk for Injury* related to adverse effects of drug therapy
- *Risk for Imbalanced Fluid Volume* related to fluid retention properties of corticosteroids
- *Risk for Electrolyte Imbalance* related to adverse drug effects of drug therapy
- *Risk for Unstable Blood Glucose Level* related to adverse effects of drug therapy

PLANNING: PATIENT GOALS AND EXPECTED OUTCOMES

The patient will:

- Experience therapeutic effects (decreased signs and symptoms of inflammation or allergic response).
- Be free from or experience minimal adverse effects from drug therapy.
- Verbalize an understanding of the drug's use, adverse effects, and required precautions.

(*Continued*)

Nursing Process Focus *(continued)*

IMPLEMENTATION

Interventions and (Rationales)	**Patient Education/Discharge Planning**
• Administer medication correctly, and evaluate the patient's knowledge of proper administration. Do not stop drug abruptly; taper off over a 1- to 2-week period. Monitor the patient's compliance with the drug regimen. (Improper use can cause an increase in adverse effects. Sudden discontinuation of these drugs can precipitate an adrenal insufficiency.)	Instruct the patient to: • Not stop taking corticosteroids abruptly and to notify the healthcare provider if unable to take the drug for more than 1 day. • Use the self-administering tapering dose pack properly. • Take oral medications with food.
• Monitor vital signs. (Corticosteroids may cause increase in blood pressure and tachycardia because of increased blood volume and potential vasoconstriction effect.)	Instruct the patient: • To report tachycardia, blood pressure over 140/90, dizziness, palpitations, or headaches to the healthcare provider. • How to use blood pressure monitoring equipment properly.
• Monitor for infection. Protect the patient from potential infections. (Corticosteroids increase susceptibility to infections by suppressing the immune response.)	Instruct the patient to: • Avoid people with infections. • Report signs of infection: fever, cough, sore throat, joint pain, increased weakness, rash, white patches in mouth, and malaise to the healthcare provider. • Consult with the healthcare provider before taking any immunizations.
• Monitor for symptoms of Cushing syndrome, such as moon face, "buffalo hump" contour of shoulders, weight gain, muscle wasting, and increased deposits of fat in the trunk. (Symptoms may indicate excessive use of corticosteroids.)	Instruct the patient: • To weigh self daily. • That initial weight gain is expected; provide the patient with weight-gain parameters that warrant reporting. • That there are multiple adverse effects to therapy and changes in health status should be reported to the healthcare provider.
• Monitor blood glucose levels. (Corticosteroids cause an increase in glucose formation [gluconeogenesis] and a decrease in glucose utilization, causing hyperglycemia.)	Instruct the patient to: • Report symptoms of hyperglycemia, such as excessive thirst, copious urination, and insatiable appetite to the healthcare provider. • Adjust insulin dose based on blood glucose level, as directed by the healthcare provider.
• Monitor skin and mucous membranes for lacerations, abrasions, or breaks in integrity. (Corticosteroids impair wound healing.)	Instruct the patient to: • Examine skin daily for cuts and scrapes and to cover any injuries with sterile bandage. • Watch for symptoms of skin infection such as redness, swelling, and drainage. • Notify the healthcare provider of any nonhealing wound or symptoms of infection.
• Monitor GI status for evidence of ulcers, GI bleeding. (Corticosteroids decrease gastric mucus production and predispose patients to peptic ulcers.)	Instruct the patient to: • Report GI adverse effects such as heartburn, dizziness, abdominal pain, blood in emesis, or tarry stools to the healthcare provider. • Take drug with food or milk to decrease GI irritation. • Avoid or eliminate alcohol.
• Continue to monitor periodic laboratory work: CBC, electrolytes glucose, lipid panel, liver and renal function studies. (Corticosteroids can cause hypernatremia and hypokalemia.)	Instruct the patient to: • Consume a diet high in protein, calcium, and potassium but low in fat and concentrated simple carbohydrates. • Keep all laboratory appointments.
• Monitor changes in the musculoskeletal system. (Corticosteroids decrease bone density and strength and cause muscle atrophy and weakness.)	Instruct the patient: • That the drug may cause weakness in bones and muscles; avoid strenuous activity that may cause injury. • To participate in weight-bearing exercise or physical activity to help maintain bone and muscle strength. • To maintain adequate calcium in diet.

Interventions and (Rationales)	Patient Education/Discharge Planning
• Monitor emotional status. (Corticosteroids may produce mood and behavior changes such as depression or feeling of invulnerability.)	• Instruct the patient that mood changes may be expected and to report excessive mood swings or unusual changes in mood to the healthcare provider.
• Monitor vision periodically. (Corticosteroids may cause increased intraocular pressure and an increased risk of glaucoma and cataracts.)	Inform the patient to: • Have regular eye exams twice a year. • Immediately report any eye pain, halos, inability to focus, or diminished or blurring vision to the healthcare provider.
• Weigh patient daily, and report increasing peripheral edema. (Daily weight is an accurate measure of fluid status.)	• Instruct the patient to weigh self daily at the same time every day and to report a gain of 2 lb (1 kg) per day or presence of or increase in edema.
EVALUATION OF OUTCOME CRITERIA	
• Evaluate the effectiveness of drug therapy by confirming that patient goals and expected outcomes have been met (see "Planning"). *See* Table 33.4 *for a list of drugs to which these nursing actions apply.*	

*Herdman, T.H. & Kamitsuru, S. (Eds.), *Nursing Diagnoses: Definitions & Classification* 2015–2017. Copyright © 2014, 1994–2014 NANDA International. Used by arrangement by John Wiley & Sons, Inc. Companion website: www.wiley.com/go/nursingdiagnoses.

Patients Need to Know

Patients treated for endocrine disorders need to know the following:

Regarding Hypothalamic and Pituitary Drugs

1. Patients taking GH should record height and weight weekly. Records should be brought to the healthcare provider each visit.
2. A diary of nighttime sleep habits and any bed-wetting should be kept and provided to the healthcare provider.

Regarding Thyroid Medications

3. Pulse rates should be taken regularly because they are a good indicator of the effectiveness of thyroid medications. If the pulse rate consistently exceeds 100 or any other significant change is noted, contact the healthcare provider.
4. Because finding the correct dosage of thyroid hormone often takes several months, do not change the prescribed dose without being advised to do so by a healthcare provider.

Regarding Corticosteroids

5. When taking oral corticosteroids for more than 2 weeks, do not miss doses or discontinue the drug without consulting a healthcare provider.
6. See a healthcare provider if any infections, cuts, or injuries appear to be healing too slowly while on corticosteroids.
7. If taking hydrocortisone for replacement therapy, take the medication between 6:00 a.m. and 9:00 a.m. because this is the time when natural corticosteroids are released.

Chapter Review

Core Concepts Summary

33.1 The endocrine system maintains homeostasis by using hormones as chemical messengers.

Hormones are secreted by endocrine glands in response to changes in the internal environment. The hormones act on their target cells to return the body to homeostasis. Negative feedback prevents the body from overresponding to internal changes.

33.2 The hypothalamus and the pituitary gland secrete hormones that control other endocrine organs.

The hypothalamus secretes releasing hormones that signal the anterior pituitary gland to release its hormones. Pituitary hormones travel throughout the body to affect many other organs.

33.3 Hormones are used as replacement therapy, as antineoplastics, or as "antihormones" to block endogenous actions.

Hormones are often given as replacement therapy to patients who are not able to secrete sufficient quantities of endogenous hormones. In high doses, several hormones may be used as antineoplastics. Hormones may also be used therapeutically to block natural physiologic effects.

33.4 Of the many hypothalamic and pituitary hormones, several have clinical applications as drugs.

ADH, or vasopressin, increases water reabsorption in the kidney and is used to treat diabetes insipidus. GH, or somatotropin, is used to increase the height of children with growth hormone deficiencies.

33.5 The thyroid gland controls the basal metabolic rate and affects virtually every cell in the body.

TSH released from the pituitary gland stimulates release of thyroid hormone. The thyroid gland secretes thyroid hormone, which is essential for normal growth and development. Adequate hormone levels are necessary for infants, children, and adults. Thyroid hormone is a combination of two different hormones, thyroxine and triiodothyronine, both of which require iodine for their synthesis.

33.6 Thyroid disorders may be treated by administering thyroid hormone or by decreasing the activity of the thyroid gland.

Hypothyroidism produces symptoms such as slowed body metabolism, slurred speech, bradycardia, weight gain, low body temperature, and intolerance to cold environments. Administration of thyroid hormone reverses these effects. Hyperthyroid patients exhibit the opposite symptoms. Hyperthyroidism may be treated with drugs that kill or inactivate thyroid cells.

33.7 Corticosteroids are released during periods of stress and influence carbohydrate, lipid, and protein metabolism in most cells.

The adrenal cortex secretes corticosteroids in response to stimulation by ACTH from the pituitary gland. Corticosteroids affect the metabolism of nearly every cell in the body and have potent anti-inflammatory effects.

33.8 Corticosteroids are prescribed for adrenocortical insufficiency and to dampen inflammatory and immune responses.

Corticosteroids are given to patients whose adrenal glands are unable to produce adequate amounts of these hormones and for a wide variety of other conditions. When used at high doses, oral therapy is limited because of the potential for producing Cushing syndrome and adrenal atrophy.

REVIEW Questions

Answer the following questions to assess your knowledge of the chapter material, and go back and review any material that is not clear to you.

1. The patient, who has been diagnosed with adrenal insufficiency, has been started on corticosteroids. The nurse explains that at high doses, and if taken for long periods of time, these drugs may cause symptoms like those seen in _______________.
   1. Cushing syndrome.
   2. Graves disease.
   3. Diabetes insipidus.
   4. Diabetes mellitus.

2. The nurse is assisting a patient with chronic adrenal insufficiency to make a medication plan for an upcoming camping trip. He is taking hydrocortisone (Cortef) and fludrocortisones (Florinef) as replacement therapy. Which detail does this patient need to remember?
   1. Take his blood pressure once or twice a day.
   2. Avoid crowded indoor areas to avoid infections.
   3. Have his vision check before he leaves.
   4. Make sure to carry extra medication in case there is a delay in getting home.

3. A patient is being treated with propylthiouracil (PTU) for hyperthyroidism while awaiting a thyroidectomy. What symptoms will the nurse tell the patient to report to the healthcare provider?
   1. Tinnitus, altered taste, thickened saliva
   2. Insomnia, nightmares, night sweats
   3. Sore throat, chills, low-grade fever
   4. Dry eyes, decreased blinking, reddened conjunctiva

4. The healthcare provider ordered vasopressin 5 units subcutaneously, bid, for a patient. The pharmacy has vasopressin 20 units/mL. How many milliliters will be administered per dose?
   1. 0.5 mL
   2. 0.25 mL
   3. 0.75 mL
   4. 1 mL

5. The patient has been on methylprednisolone (Medrol) for an exacerbation of asthma. Which of the following instructions to the patient is of the highest priority?
   1. "This medication may cause weight gain."
   2. "Do not stop taking this medication abruptly."
   3. "This medication can cause sleeplessness."
   4. "This medication may cause restlessness."

6. An older adult with chronic bronchitis has been taking a low dose of dexamethasone for several months. In order to reduce the risk of osteoporosis, an adverse effect, the nurse instructs the patient to: (Select all that apply.)
   1. Perform weight-bearing exercises at least three to four times a week.
   2. Increase dietary intake of calcium and vitamin D enriched foods.
   3. Remain sedentary except during periods of exercise.

4. Increase fluid intake, including carbonated sodas, but avoid alcohol.
5. Participate in highly strenuous activities.

7. A patient will be started on desmopressin (DDAVP) for treatment of diabetes insipidus. Which instruction should the nurse include in the patient teaching plan?
   1. Drink plenty of fluids, especially those high in calcium.
   2. Avoid close contact with children or pregnant women for 1 week after administration of the drug.
   3. Obtain and record your weight daily.
   4. Wear a mask if around children and pregnant women.

8. The patient has been started on desmopressin (DDAVP). The nurse understands the medication is effective when the patient's:
   1. Urinary output increases.
   2. Blood pressure falls below 90/60.
   3. Blood sugar level is between 80 and 120 mg/dL.
   4. Urinary output decreases.

9. The nurse should inform the parents of a child who has been prescribed somatropin (Humatrope) that:
   1. The drug must be given by injection.
   2. The drug must be given regularly to prevent mental deficiencies.
   3. If the drug is given during late adolescence, it could add 6 to 8 inches to the child's height.
   4. Daily laboratory monitoring will be required during the first weeks of therapy.

10. A nurse is helping to prepare a teaching plan for a patient who will be discharged on the corticosteroid methylprednisolone (Medrol Dosepak) after a significant response to poison ivy. The nurse includes information about which of the following adverse effects of this medication? (Select all that apply.)
    1. Tinnitus
    2. Edema
    3. Visual changes
    4. Lower abdominal pain
    5. Mood changes

CASE STUDY Questions

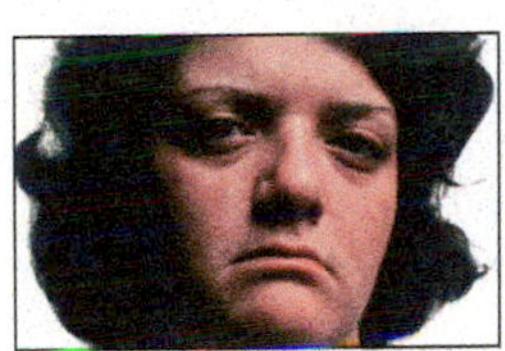

Remember Mrs. Brookfield, the patient introduced at the beginning of the chapter? Now read the remainder of the case study. Based on the information you have learned in this chapter, answer the questions that follow.

Mrs. Helen Brookfield is a 42-year-old mother of two children who works full time at a department store. She has been feeling very tired, gaining weight, and says she feels cold all the time. Because of this, she saw her healthcare provider several weeks ago. At that visit, the healthcare provider ordered some laboratory tests, including T3, T4, and TSH. She has returned to the office today to discuss her continuing symptoms and laboratory results. Her vital signs are 94/60, 58 (pulse), and a temperature of 97.4°F (36.3°C). Her weight has increased 30 pounds over the past 6 months, but she says that her appetite has decreased. The symptoms and laboratory results indicate that she has hypothyroidism. She is prescribed levothyroxine (Synthroid) 100 mcg/day.

1. The nurse explains to Mrs. Brookfield that the adverse effects of levothyroxine (Synthroid) are: (Select all that apply.)
   1. Constipation.
   2. Weight gain.
   3. Tachycardia.
   4. Insomnia.

2. The nurse also instructs Mrs. Brookfield:
   1. To take the pill in the afternoon with a high fiber snack to prevent stomach upset.
   2. To eat plenty of fruits and vegetables to replace nutrients.
   3. To take the dose in the morning before breakfast, as close to the same time each day as possible.
   4. That the drug may be taken every other day if diarrhea occurs.

3. Mrs. Brookfield has been on levothyroxine (Synthroid) 100 mcg/day. The nurse recognizes the medication is being effective when the:
   1. Patient sleeps more hours per day.
   2. Patient's weight increases.
   3. Patient's pulse rate increases.
   4. Patient states she feels tired.

4. A month later, Mrs. Brookfield reports feeling nervous and is having occasional palpitations and tremors. These symptoms may indicate that:
   1. Mrs. Brookfield is still experiencing symptoms of hypothyroidism, and the dose may need to be increased.
   2. Mrs. Brookfield's thyroid is now functioning normally, and levothyroxine is no longer needed.
   3. Mrs. Brookfield has developed diabetes and needs further evaluation.
   4. Mrs. Brookfield is experiencing symptoms of hyperthyroidism, and the drug dosage needs to be decreased.

Answers and complete rationales for the Review and Case Study Questions appear in Appendix A.

REFERENCE

Herdman, T. H., & Kamitsuru, S. (Eds.). (2014). *NANDA International nursing diagnoses: Definitions and classification, 2015–2017*. Oxford, United Kingdom: Wiley-Blackwell

SELECTED BIBLIOGRAPHY

Akamizu, T., Amino, N., DeGroot, L. J. (2013). *Hashimoto's thyroiditis*. Retrieved from http://www.ncbi.nlm.nih.gov/books/NBK285557

Almandoz, J. P., & Gharib, H. (2012). Hypothyroidism: Etiology, diagnosis, and management. *Medical Clinics of North America, 96*, 203–221. doi:10.1016/j.mcna.2012.01.005

American Association of Clinical Endocrinology. (n.d.) *Thyroid awareness. The thyroid and pregnancy*. Retrieved from http://www.thyroidawareness.com/the-thyroid-and-pregnancy

American Thyroid Association. (2014). *Postpartum thyroiditis*. Retrieved from http://www.thyroid.org/wp-content/uploads/patients/brochures/Postpartum_Thyroiditis_brochure.pdf

Baby's First Test. (2015). *About newborn screening. Screening facts*. Retrieved from http://www.babysfirsttest.org/newborn-screening/screening-facts

Crawford, A., & Harris, H. (2013). Tipping the scales: Understanding thyroid imbalances. *Nursing Critical Care, 8*(1), 23–28. doi:10.1097/01.CCN.0000418818.21604.22

Falorni, A., Minarelli, V., & Morelli, S. (2013). Therapy of adrenal insufficiency: An update. *Endocrine, 43*, 514–528. doi:10.1007/s12020-012-9835-4

Fatourechi, V. (2014). Hyperthyroidism and thyrotoxicosis. In F. Bandier, H. Gharib, A. Golbert, L. Griz, & M. Faria (Eds.), *Endocrinology and diabetes: A problem-oriented approach* (pp. 9–21). New York, NY: Springer. doi:10.1007/978-1-4614-8684-8_2

Feelders, R. A., & Hofland, L. J. (2013). Medical treatment of Cushing's disease. *The Journal of Clinical Endocrinology & Metabolism, 98*, 425–438. doi:10.1210/jc.2012-3126

Gorman, L. S. (2012). The adrenal gland: Common disease states and suspected new applications. *Clinical Laboratory Science: Journal of the American Society for Medical Technology, 26*(2), 118–125.

Griffing, G. T. (2015). *Addison disease clinical presentation*. Retrieved from http://emedicine.medscape.com/article/116467-clinical

Khardori, R. (2014). *Diabetes insipidus*. Retrieved from http://emedicine.medscape.com/article/117648-overview

Marieb, E. N., & Hoehn, K. (2017). *Human anatomy and physiology* (10th ed.). San Francisco, CA: Benjamin Cummings.

Nguyen, H. (2015). *Iatrogenic Cushing syndrome*. Retrieved from http://emedicine.medscape.com/article/117365-overview

Orlander, P. R. (2015). *Hypothyroidism*. Retrieved from http://emedicine.medscape.com/article/122393-overview

Skugor, M. (2014). *Hypothyroidism and hyperthyroidism*. Retrieved from http://www.clevelandclinicmeded.com/medicalpubs/diseasemanagement/endocrinology/hypothyroidism-and-hyperthyroidism

Silverthorn, D. U. (2016). *Human physiology: An integrated approach* (7th ed.). San Francisco, CA: Benjamin Cummings.

The New York Times. (n.d.). *Chronic thyroiditis (Hashimoto's disease) in-depth report*. Retrieved from http://www.nytimes.com/health/guides/disease/chronic-thyroiditis-hashimotos-disease/print.html

Toft, D. (2014). *Graves' disease overview. What is Graves' disease?* Retrieved from http://www.endocrineweb.com/conditions/graves-disease/graves-disease-overview

University of Maryland Medical Center. (2012). *Hypothyroidism*. Retrieved from http://umm.edu/health/medical/reports/articles/hypothyroidism

Vellanki, P. (n.d.). *Hypothyroidism: Potential symptoms and causes of an underactive thyroid gland*. Retrieved from http://www.endocrineweb.com/conditions/hypothyroidism/hypothyroidism-potential-symptoms-causes-underactive-thyroid-gland

Womens Health Advice.com (n.d.). *Thyroid cancers*. Retrieved from http://www.womens-health-advice.com/thyroid/cancer.html

Chapter 34

Drugs for Diabetes Mellitus

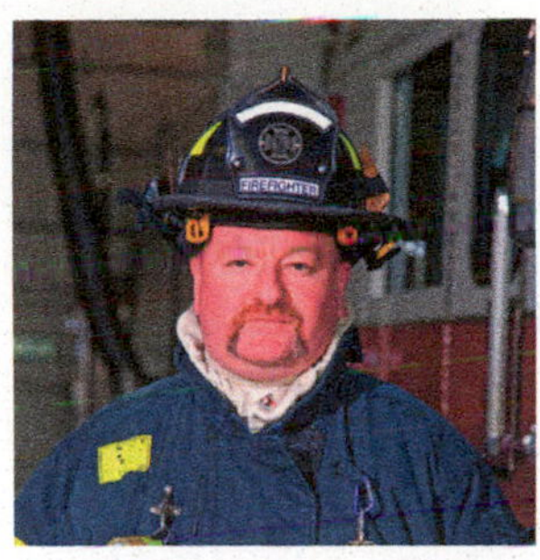

"I've always felt okay but recently I've been feeling sluggish. Now I learn that my sugar levels are high."
Mr. Brian Jones

Core Concepts

34.1 **The pancreas is responsible for the regulation of blood glucose levels.**
34.2 **Type 1 diabetes is caused by a deficiency of insulin.**
34.3 **Insulin replacement therapy is required for type 1 diabetes.**
34.4 **Type 2 diabetes is the most common form of the disorder.**
34.5 **Antidiabetic drugs are prescribed after diet and exercise have failed to reduce blood glucose to normal levels.**

Drug Snapshot

The following drugs are discussed in this chapter:

Drug Classes	Prototype Drugs
Insulin	Pr regular insulin (Humulin R, Novolin R)
Antidiabetic drugs for type 2 diabetes	Pr metformin (Fortamet, Glucophage, Glumetza, others)

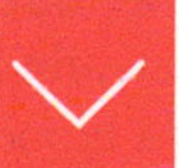

Learning Outcomes

After reading this chapter, the student should be able to:

1. Explain how blood glucose levels rise and fall and are stabilized with insulin and glucagon.
2. Explain the cause of type 1 diabetes mellitus.
3. Identify representative types of insulin, and explain their mechanisms of drug action, primary actions, and important adverse effects.
4. Explain the cause of type 2 diabetes mellitus.
5. Identify the representative drug classes used to treat type 2 diabetes mellitus, and explain their mechanisms of drug action, primary actions, and important adverse effects.

Key Terms

diabetic ketoacidosis (DKA) (KEY-toe-assi-doh-sis)
glucagon (GLUE-kah-gon)
hyperglycemic effect (hi-pur-gli-SEEM-ik)
hypoglycemic effect (hi-po-gli-SEEM-ik)
incretin enhancers (in KREE tin)
incretin mimetics
incretins
insulin (IN-sule-in)
insulin analogs (ANNAH-logs)
insulin resistance
islets of Langerhans (EYE-lits of LANG-gur-hans)
ketoacids (KEY-toe-ass-ids)
type 1 diabetes mellitus (die-uh-BEE-tees MEL-uh-tiss)
type 2 diabetes mellitus

Diabetes is one of the leading hormone disorders in the United States. Mortality due to diabetes has been steadily increasing, causing concern among public health officials and the general public. Diabetes can lead to serious complications, including heart disease, stroke, blindness, kidney failure, and amputations. Since healthcare providers frequently care for patients with diabetes, it is imperative that its treatment and possible complications are well understood.

Core Concept 34.1 ▶

The pancreas is responsible for the regulation of blood glucose levels.

exo = *out/away from*
crine = *to secrete*
endo = *within*

Located behind the stomach and between the duodenum and spleen, the pancreas is an organ that is essential to the function of both the digestive and the endocrine systems. It is responsible for the secretion of enzymes that assist in the chemical digestion of nutrients in the duodenum. This is the *exocrine* function of the pancreas. Clusters of cells in the pancreas, called **islets of Langerhans**, are responsible for the secretion of the hormones glucagon and insulin. This is the pancreas's *endocrine* function (Figure 34.1).

Glucose is one of the body's most essential molecules. The body prefers to use glucose as its primary energy source: The brain relies almost exclusively on glucose for its energy needs. Because of this need, blood levels of glucose must remain relatively constant throughout the day. Although many factors contribute to maintaining a stable blood glucose level, the two pancreatic hormones play major roles: **Insulin** acts to *decrease* blood glucose levels, and **glucagon** acts to *increase* blood glucose levels (Figure 34.2).

gluco = *glucose*

Following a meal, the pancreas recognizes the rising blood glucose level and releases insulin. Without insulin, glucose stays in the bloodstream and is not able to enter cells of the body. Cells may be virtually surrounded by glucose but they are unable to use it until insulin arrives. Insulin acts like a gateway for the entry of glucose into the cell. Thus, insulin is said to have a **hypoglycemic effect**, because its presence causes glucose to *leave* the bloodstream, and therefore blood glucose *falls*. Some of the glucose is stored as glycogen in the liver, where it can be converted back to glucose between meals.

hypo = *lowered*
glyc = *sugar*
emic = *blood*

The pancreas also secretes glucagon, which has the *opposite* effect of insulin. When levels of blood glucose fall, glucagon is secreted. Glucagon's primary function is to maintain adequate blood levels of glucose between meals. Glucagon increases blood glucose levels

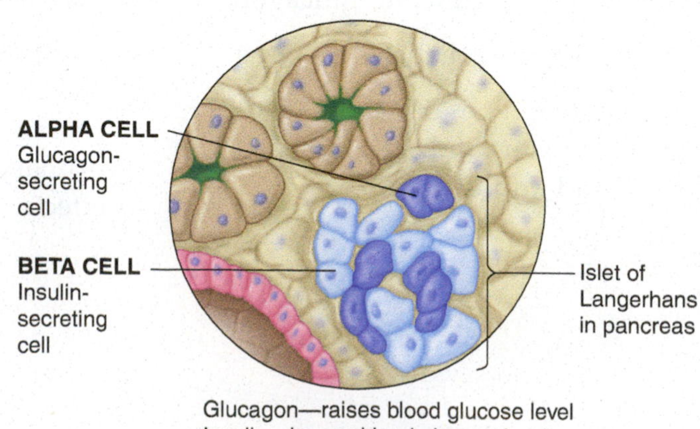

FIGURE 34.1 Microscopic view of glucagon- and insulin-secreting cells in the islets of Langerhans.

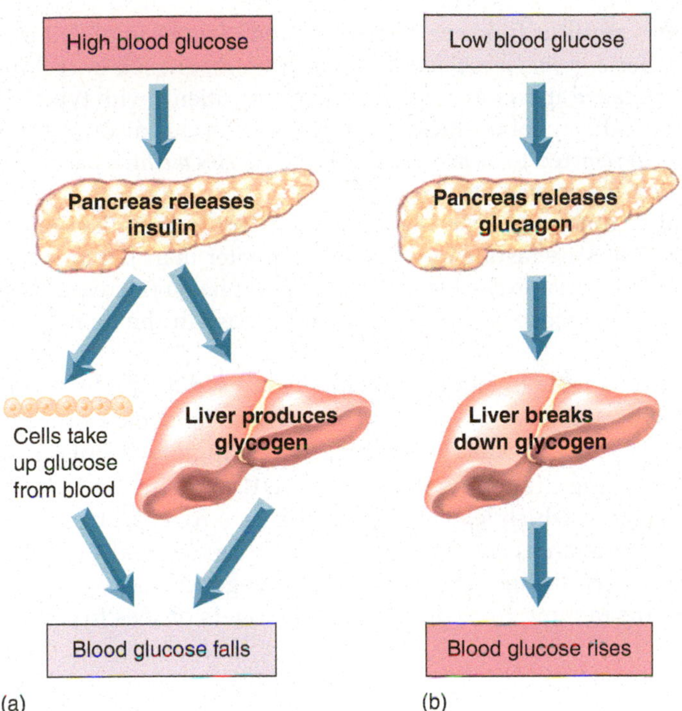

FIGURE 34.2 Insulin, glucagon, and blood glucose levels.

by increasing the breakdown of glycogen into glucose. Decreasing glycogen synthesis enhances the synthesis of glucose. Thus, glucagon has a **hyperglycemic effect**, because it causes glucose in the bloodstream to *rise*. The physiological actions of glucagon are essentially opposite of insulin.

hyper = *elevated*

TYPE 1 DIABETES MELLITUS

Type 1 diabetes is caused by a deficiency of insulin.

◀ **Core Concept 34.2**

Diabetes mellitus (DM) is a metabolic disorder in which there is deficient insulin secretion or decreased sensitivity of insulin receptors on target cells. Without insulin present, glucose is prevented from entering the cells and builds to high levels in the blood; thus, hyperglycemia is the hallmark characteristic of DM. The causes of DM include a combination of genetic and environmental factors. The recent increase in the frequency of the disease is probably the result of trends toward more inactive and stressful lifestyles and increasing consumption of foods with higher calories. Prediabetes is a condition in which blood glucose levels are higher than normal but not high enough to be classified as diabetes. According to the International Diabetes Federation, diabetes and obesity are among the biggest public health challenges of the 21st century.

Fast Facts **Diabetes Mellitus**

- Over 29 million Americans or 9.3% of the population have diabetes. Millions of people are unaware that they have the disease.
- It is estimated that 12 million women aged 20 years and older have diabetes, and approximately 27 million have prediabetes.
- Gestational diabetes affects about 2% to 10% of all pregnant women in the United States each year.
- Diabetes is the seventh leading cause of death; the risk of death among people with diabetes is twice that of people of similar age without diabetes.
- Diabetes is a major cause of retinopathy leading to blindness in adults.
- Diabetes is responsible for about 60% of nontraumatic lower-limb amputations; over 73,000 amputations are performed each year on patients with diabetes.

Source: Based on Centers for Disease Control and Prevention. (2014). 2014 Diabetes National Statistics Report; Centers for Disease Control and Prevention. (n.d.). Women at High Risk for Diabetes: Physical Activity, Healthy Eating, and Weight Loss; Centers for Disease Control and Prevention. (2014) National Diabetes Statistics Report: Estimates of Diabetes and Its Burden in the United States.

dia = *through (e.g., siphon)*
betes = *to go*
mellitus = *sweet*

Type 1 diabetes mellitus is one of the most common diseases of childhood. Type 1 DM was previously called *juvenile-onset diabetes*. It is often diagnosed in children between the ages of 11 and 13. Because approximately one-fourth of patients with type 1 DM develop the disease in adulthood, this is not the most accurate name for this disorder. This type of diabetes is also sometimes referred to as *insulin-dependent diabetes mellitus* because with this disorder the pancreas *does not produce insulin*.

poly = *excessive*
phagia = *hunger*
dipsia = *thirst*

glucos = *glucose*
uria = *urination*

keto = *ketone chemical compound (e.g., acetone)*
acids/acidosis = *state of lowered pH*

The signs and symptoms of type 1 DM are consistent from patient to patient. The typical signs and symptoms are fasting blood glucose greater than 126 mg/dL on at least two separate occasions, polyuria (excessive urination), polyphagia (increased hunger), polydipsia (increased thirst), glucosuria (high levels of glucose in the urine), weight loss, and fatigue.

When glucose is unable to enter cells, lipids are used as the primary energy source and **ketoacids** are produced as waste products. These ketoacids can give the patient's breath an acetone-like, fruity odor. More importantly, high levels of ketoacids lower the pH of the blood, causing **diabetic ketoacidosis (DKA)**. Untreated DM produces long-term damage to arteries, which leads to heart disease, stroke, kidney disease, and blindness. Lack of adequate circulation to the feet may cause death of tissues leading to gangrene of the toes, requiring amputation. Nerve degeneration, or neuropathy, is common, with symptoms ranging from tingling in the fingers or toes to complete loss of sensation of a limb.

Core Concept 34.3 ▶ Insulin replacement therapy is required for type 1 diabetes.

Patients with type 1 DM are severely deficient in insulin production; thus, insulin replacement therapy is required in normal physiological amounts. Insulin is also required for those with type 2 diabetes who are unable to manage their blood glucose levels with diet, exercise, and antidiabetic drugs.

Because normal insulin secretion varies greatly in response to daily activities such as eating and exercise, glucose monitoring and insulin administration must be carefully planned along with proper meal planning and lifestyle habits. The desired outcome of insulin therapy is to prevent the long-term consequences of the disorder by strictly maintaining blood glucose levels within the normal range. Poor compliance (not properly monitoring glucose levels or skipping insulin injections) can lead to continuing hyperglycemia and even death. Illness and stress can also cause an increase in blood glucose levels.

Many types of insulin are available, differing in their source, time of onset and peak effect, and duration of action. Almost all insulin today is human insulin obtained through recombinant DNA technology. Pharmacologists have modified human insulin to create forms that have a more rapid onset of action or a more prolonged duration of action. These modified forms are called **insulin analogs**. All the different types of insulin are administered by the subcutaneous route and are listed in Table 34.1.

Table 34.1 Types of Insulin: Actions and Administration

Drug	Action	Onset	Peak	Duration	Administration
insulin aspart (NovoLog)	Rapid	15 minutes	1–3 hours	3–5 hours	Subcutaneous; 5–10 minutes before a meal
insulin lispro (Humalog)	Rapid	5–15 minutes	0.5–1 hours	3–4 hours	Subcutaneous; 5–10 minutes before a meal
insulin glulisine (Apidra)	Rapid	15–30 minutes	1 hours	3–4 hours	Subcutaneous; 15 minutes before a meal or within 20 minutes after starting a meal
Pr insulin regular (Humulin R, Novolin R)	Short	30–60 minutes	2–4 hours	5–7 hours	Subcutaneous; 30–60 minutes before a meal; IV in emergencies
insulin isophane (NPH, Humulin N, Novolin N, ReliOn N)	Intermediate	1–2 hours	4–12 hours	18–24 hours	Subcutaneous; 30 minutes before first meal of the day and 30 minutes before evening meal, if necessary
insulin detemir (Levemir)	Long	Gradual: over 24 hours	6–8 hours	To 24 hours	Subcutaneous; with evening meal or at bedtime
insulin glargine (Lantus)	Long	Gradual: over 24 hours	N/A	To 24 hours	Subcutaneous; once daily, given at the same time each day

Doses of insulin are highly individualized for the precise control of blood glucose levels in each patient. Some patients require two or more injections daily for proper diabetes management. If mixing insulin, such as rapid- or short-acting with an intermediate-acting, the rapid or short-acting insulin is always drawn into the syringe first. For ease of administration, some of these combinations are marketed in cartridges containing premixed solutions. Important, however, is the fact that onset, peak, and duration times for each insulin are different within the same medication injection:

- Humulin 70/30 and Novolin 70/30: contain 70% NPH insulin and 30% regular insulin.
- Humulin 50/50: contains 50% NPH insulin and 50% regular insulin.
- NovoLog Mix 70/30: contains 70% insulin aspart protamine and 30% insulin aspart.
- Humalog Mix 75/25: contains 75% insulin lispro protamine and 25% insulin lispro.

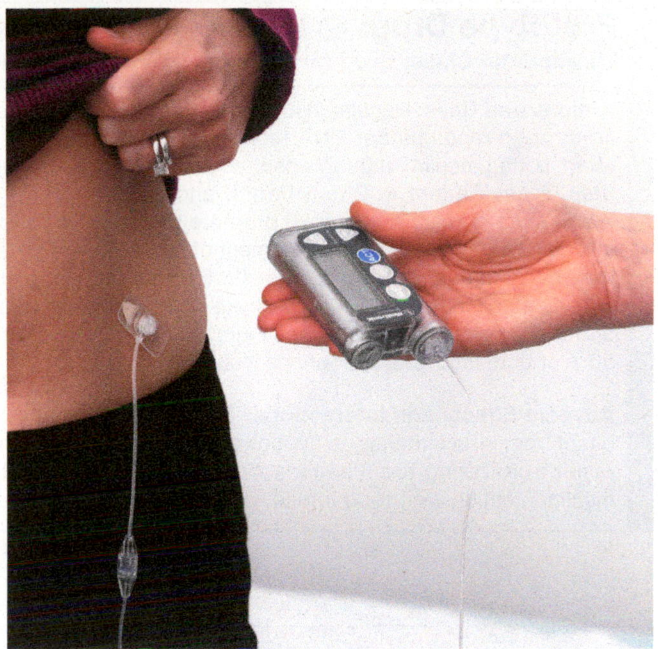

FIGURE 34.3 Insulin pump programmed to release insulin at predetermined intervals throughout the day.

Some patients may have an insulin pump (Figure 34.3). This pump is usually abdominally anchored and is programmed to release small subcutaneous doses of insulin into the abdomen at predetermined intervals, with larger amounts administered manually at mealtime if necessary. Most pumps contain an alarm that sounds to remind patients to take their insulin.

Adverse effects of insulin may include allergic reactions, redness at the site of injection, and changes in fat tissue (lipodystrophy) in the areas of body where injections are given more frequently. However, the most common adverse effect of insulin therapy is overtreatment—when insulin removes too much glucose from the blood, resulting in hypoglycemia. This occurs when a patient with type 1 diabetes has more insulin in the blood than is needed to balance the amount of glucose in the blood. Hypoglycemia may occur when insulin levels peak; during exercise, stress, or illness; when the patient receives too much insulin due to medication error; or if the patient skips a meal. Signs and symptoms of hypoglycemia include the sudden onset of pale, cool, and moist skin; confusion; mild tremors; and dizziness, usually with blood glucose of less than 50 mg/dL.

Giving food or drinks containing glucose (sugar) can reverse mild to moderate hypoglycemia symptoms. Patients are encouraged to routinely carry candy or other readily absorbable carbohydrates, such as crackers, to take at the first signs of a drop in blood glucose. For serious hypoglycemia, glucose can be administered via the IV route. In addition, the hormone glucagon is also used in emergency treatment. Glucagon can be administered IV, IM, or subcutaneously. Unstable diabetics can carry a glucagon pen for emergency use as well.

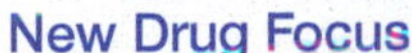

New Drug Focus

WILL GLUCAGON NASAL SPRAY REPLACE GLUCAGON INJECTIONS?

Families often fear what will happen if their diabetic loved one takes too much insulin. If not properly monitored, insulin can lower blood sugar to an unsafe level, and the patient risks becoming unresponsive or unconscious. Until recently, in an emergency situation, the only way to quickly raise blood glucose levels was to either have access to an emergency injection kit or take immediate action like drinking or ingesting something sweet. With intranasal glucagon, emergency treatment will be much easier to accomplish. Patients or caregivers will not have to mix or reconstitute vials of powder. Even if a patient is unable to self-administer, one-step glucagon nasal spray can raise blood sugar levels up to 200 mg/dL within 10 minutes. This product has already completed Phase III clinical trials, and U.S. Food and Drug Administration (FDA) approval is expected in 2016.

Prototype Drug: Pr *Regular Insulin (Humulin R, Novolin R)*

Therapeutic Class: Drug for diabetes mellitus **Pharmacologic Class:** Hypoglycemic drug

Actions and Uses: Regular insulin is prepared as human insulin through recombinant DNA technology. It is classified as short-acting insulin, with an onset of action of 30 to 60 minutes, a peak effect at 2 to 3 hours, and a duration of 5 to 7 hours. Its primary action is to promote the entry of glucose into cells. For the emergency treatment of acute ketoacidosis, it may be given subcutaneously or IV. Regular insulin is also available as Humulin 70/30 (a mixture of 30% regular insulin and 70% isophane insulin) or as Humulin 50/50 (a mixture of 50% of both regular and isophane insulin).

Adverse Effects and Interactions: The most serious adverse effect from insulin therapy is hypoglycemia. Hypoglycemia may result from taking too much insulin, not properly timing the insulin injection with food intake, or skipping a meal. Dietary carbohydrates must be in the blood when insulin is injected; otherwise the drug will remove too much glucose, and signs of hypoglycemia—tachycardia, confusion, sweating, and drowsiness—will result. If severe hypoglycemia is not quickly treated with glucose, convulsions, coma, and death may follow.

Regular insulin interacts with many drugs. For example, the following substances may increase hypoglycemic effects: alcohol, salicylates, monoamine oxidase inhibitors (MAOIs), and anabolic steroids. The following substances may decrease hypoglycemic effects: corticosteroids, thyroid hormones, and epinephrine. Serum glucose levels may be increased with furosemide or thiazide diuretics. Symptoms of hypoglycemic reaction may be hidden if beta blockers are used at the same time.

Use cautiously with herbal supplements such as garlic and ginseng, which may increase the hypoglycemic effects of insulin.

Nursing Process Focus Patients Receiving Insulin Therapy

ASSESSMENT

Prior to administration:

- Obtain a complete health history, including cardiovascular, vision, skin, neurologic, renal, and liver conditions; allergies; drug history; and possible drug interactions.
- Evaluate laboratory blood findings: complete blood count (CBC), electrolytes, lipid panel, liver and renal function studies, glucose, and glucated hemoglobin (HbA1C).
- Acquire the results of a complete physical examination, including vital signs, height, and weight; presence of paresthesia of hands or feet; ulceration of lower extremities; and condition of skin at insulin injection sites.
- Obtain a dietary history, including type of foods eaten, caloric intake, number of meals and snacks, and fluid types.
- Determine knowledge of diabetic medications, adverse effects, self-administration, and blood glucose monitoring.

POTENTIAL NURSING DIAGNOSES*

- *Deficient Knowledge* related to a lack of information about the disease process, medications, and need for lifestyle changes
- *Ineffective Health Management* related to noncompliance with medication regimen, presence of adverse effects, and lifelong need for medication
- *Noncompliance* related to the complexity of the medication regimen, lifestyle changes, and adverse effects of drug therapy
- *Risk for Unstable Blood Glucose Level* related to lack of diabetes management, unhealthy diet, inadequate glucose monitoring, or improper use of medication
- *Risk for Injury* related to blood glucose elevations, impaired circulation, or adverse effects of drug therapy
- *Risk for Imbalanced Nutrition* related to disease process and adverse effects of drug therapy
- *Risk for Infection* related to blood glucose elevations and impaired circulation

PLANNING: PATIENT GOALS AND EXPECTED OUTCOMES

The patient will:

- Experience therapeutic effects (stable blood glucose levels).
- Be free from or experience minimal adverse effects from drug therapy.
- Verbalize an understanding of the drug's use, adverse effects, and required precautions.
- Demonstrate an understanding of lifestyle modifications necessary for successful maintenance of drug therapy.

IMPLEMENTATION

Interventions and (Rationales)	Patient Education/Discharge Planning
• Monitor blood glucose several times a day, usually before meals. Hold or provide insulin per healthcare provider's protocols. (Daily glucose levels will assist in maintaining stable blood glucose.)	• Instruct the patient how to monitor blood glucose, including use of equipment, and when to notify the healthcare provider.
• Administer insulin as prescribed, at meal or insulin peak times. In addition, evaluate the patient's knowledge of proper administration. (Administering insulin at meal or peak times will assist in maintaining stable blood glucose levels.)	Inform patient or caregivers: • Of proper administration techniques for the type of insulin ordered. Have the patient communicate understanding of how the insulin medication should be administered to keep glucose levels stable. • That peak insulin levels and proper food sources are needed to prevent both hyper and hypoglycemia. • Of the need to rotate insulin injection sites on a weekly basis to prevent tissue damage.

IMPLEMENTATION	
• Ensure dietary needs are met based on weight and current glucose levels. Consult with a dietitian as needed (Adequate caloric amounts of carbohydrates, proteins, and fats influence the amount of insulin needed for glucose control).	• Advise the patient to monitor food choices and follow the recommended diet plan. • Provide written materials on dietary recommendations for future reference.
• Increase frequency of blood glucose monitoring if the patient is experiencing fever, nausea, vomiting, or diarrhea. (Illness usually requires adjustments in insulin doses.)	Instruct the patient to: • Increase blood glucose monitoring when experiencing fever, nausea, vomiting, or diarrhea. • Notify the healthcare provider if unable to eat normal meals for a possible change in insulin dose.
• Continue to monitor periodic laboratory work: CBC, electrolytes, glucose, HbA1C, lipid profile, liver and renal function studies. (Insulin can cause potassium to move into the cell and may cause hypokalemia. Periodic monitoring assists in determining glucose control, need for medication changes, and any indicators of complications.)	Inform the patient: • About the need to keep laboratory appointments. • To report to the healthcare provider the first sign of heart irregularity.
• Monitor weight on a routine basis. (Changes in weight will alter insulin needs.)	• Instruct the patient to weigh self on a routine basis at the same time each day and to report to the healthcare provider any significant changes (e.g., plus or minus 10 lb [5 kg]).
• Monitor vital signs. (Increased pulse and blood pressure are early signs of hypoglycemia. Patients with diabetes may have circulatory problems or impaired kidney function that can increase blood pressure.)	• Ensure that the patient knows how to take blood pressure and pulse and to report significant changes.
• Check for signs of hypoglycemia, especially around the time of insulin peak activity. If symptoms occur, provide quick-acting carbohydrate source (juice or simple sugar), and then recheck blood glucose. (Taking a simple sugar will raise blood sugar immediately.)	Advise the patient: • To always carry a quick-acting carbohydrate source in case symptoms of hypoglycemia occur. • If unsure whether symptoms are hypo or hyper, treat as hypoglycemia, wait 10–15 minutes, then check glucose level. • If symptoms are not relieved or glucose is below 70 mg/dL, notify the healthcare provider.
• Encourage the patient to increase physical activity gradually but continue to monitor blood glucose level before and after exercise. (Exercise assists muscle cells to use glucose more efficiently, lowering blood glucose. Effects may last up to 48 hours after activity, increasing the risk of hypoglycemia.)	Inform the patient: • About the benefit of exercise. • To check blood glucose before and after exercise and to keep a simple sugar on his or her person while exercising. • To eat some form of simple sugar or complex carbohydrate before strenuous exercise as prophylaxis against hypoglycemia.
• Ensure the proper storage of insulin to maintain potency. Opened vials may be stored at room temperature for up to 1 month, avoiding direct sunlight and heat. Store unopened vials in refrigerator. Discard any vial if any changes in solution are noted or if insulin has expired.	• Inform the patient about proper storage of insulin.

EVALUATION OF OUTCOME CRITERIA

Evaluate the effectiveness of drug therapy by confirming that patient goals and expected outcomes have been met (see "Planning"). *See* Table 34.1 *for a list of drugs to which these nursing actions apply.*

TYPE 2 DIABETES MELLITUS

Type 2 diabetes is the most common form of the disorder.

◀ **Core Concept 34.4**

Type 2 diabetes mellitus is the more common form of the disorder. Because type 2 DM first appeared in middle-aged adults, it has been referred to as *adult-onset diabetes* or *maturity-onset diabetes*. These are inaccurate descriptions, however, because increasing numbers of children are being diagnosed with type 2 DM. Type 2 is more common in patients who are overweight and those with low HDL-cholesterol and high triglyceride levels. Patients with type 2 DM are often asymptomatic and may have the condition for years before their diagnosis.

asymptomatic = *without having symptoms*

Unlike patients with type 1 diabetes, some patients with type 2 are capable of secreting insulin, although in amounts that are too small. However, the fundamental problem in type 2 is that insulin receptors in the target tissues have become unresponsive to the hormone, a phenomenon called **insulin resistance**. Essentially, the pancreas produces sufficient amounts of insulin, but target cells do not recognize it. In addition, the liver increases its production of glucose, compounding the problem of hyperglycemia. Whereas patients with type 1 diabetes must take insulin, those with type 2 diabetes are usually controlled with antidiabetic drugs. In severe, unresponsive cases, insulin may also be necessary for patients with type 2 diabetes.

With aging, cells become more resistant to insulin, blood glucose levels rise, and the pancreas responds by secreting even more insulin. Eventually, the hypersecretion of insulin causes beta cell exhaustion and ultimately leads to beta cell death. As type 2 DM progresses, it becomes a disorder characterized by insufficient insulin levels as well as insulin resistance. The long-term consequences of untreated type 1 and type 2 diabetes are the same.

The activity of insulin receptors can be increased by physical exercise and lowering the level of circulating insulin. In fact, adhering to a healthy diet and a regular exercise program has been shown to reverse insulin resistance and delay or prevent the development of type 2 DM. Many patients with type 2 diabetes are obese and need a medically supervised plan to help them reduce weight gradually and exercise safely. These are important lifestyle changes for such patients; they will need to maintain these changes for the remainder of their lives.

Core Concept 34.5 ▶ Antidiabetic drugs are prescribed after diet and exercise have failed to reduce blood glucose to normal levels.

Type 2 DM is usually controlled with noninsulin antidiabetic drugs. These drugs are sometimes referred to as *oral hypoglycemic drugs* but this is an inaccurate name because some are given by the subcutaneous route and some do not cause hypoglycemia.

incretin = *gut-derived*

The primary groups of antidiabetic drugs for type 2 DM are classified by their chemical structures and their mechanisms of action. These include alpha-glucosidase inhibitors, biguanides, incretin enhancers, meglitinides, sulfonylureas, and thiazolidinediones (or glitazones). Therapy with type 2 antidiabetic drugs is not effective for persons with type 1 DM. Antidiabetic drugs for type 2 DM are listed in Table 34.2.

Table 34.2 Antidiabetic Drugs for Type 2 Diabetes

Drug	Route and Adult Dose	Drug Class Remarks
ALPHA-GLUCOSIDASE INHIBITORS		
acarbose (Precose)	PO: 25–100 mg tid (max: 300 mg/day)	These drugs block an intestinal enzyme that breaks down complex carbohydrates into simple sugars. Avoid use in patients with chronic intestinal diseases; use cautiously in patients with renal impairment.
miglitol (Glyset)	PO: 25–100 mg tid (max: 300 mg/day)	
BIGUANIDE		
Pr metformin Immediate release (Glucophage, Riomet) Extended release (Fortamet, Glucophage XR, Glumetza)	PO: 500 mg bid or 850 mg once daily; increase to 1000–2550 mg in divided doses per day (max: 2.55 g/day) Fortamet: 1000 mg once daily (max: 2.5 g/day) Glumetza: 1000–2000 mg once daily (max: 2 g/day) Glucophage XR: 500 mg once daily (max: 2 g/day)	Immediate-release forms and extended-release forms are available. Lactic acidosis is a potential complication with this medication.
INCRETIN MIMETICS (GLP-1 AGONISTS)		
albiglutide (Tanzeum)	Subcutaneous: 30–50 mg once weekly	These drugs target a chemical called glucagon-like peptide (GLP). Insulin release is stimulated and glucagon release is inhibited. Nausea, diarrhea, headaches, and dizziness are common symptoms due to falling blood glucose levels. These drugs decrease appetite and promote weight loss. They should be taken or injected prior to meals.
exenatide (Byetta)	Subcutaneous: 5–10 mcg one to two times per day 60 minutes prior to a meal	
dulaglutide (Trulicity)	Subcutaneous: 0.75–1.5 mg once weekly	
liraglutide (Victoza)	Subcutaneous: 0.6–1.8 mg once daily	
INCRETIN ENHANCERS (DPP-4 INHIBITORS)		
alogliptin (Nesina)	PO: 25 mg once daily	These drugs prevent the breakdown of natural incretins, allowing the hormone levels to rise and produce a greater antidiabetic response.
linagliptin (Tradjenta)	PO: 5 mg once daily	
saxagliptin (Onglyza)	PO: 2.5–5 mg once daily	
sitagliptin (Januvia)	PO: 100 mg once daily	

Drug	Route and Adult Dose	Drug Class Remarks
MEGLITINIDES		
nateglinide (Starlix)	PO: 60–120 mg tid	These drugs stimulate the release of insulin from pancreatic islet cells similar to sulfonylurea drugs.
repaglinide (Prandin)	PO: 0.5–4 mg bid–qid (max: 16 mg/day)	
SODIUM-GLUCOSE CO-TRANSPORTER (SGLT) INHIBITOR		
canagliflozin (Invokana)	PO: 100 mg once daily (300 mg/day) taken before first meal	These drugs block the action of SGLT2, an enzyme in the kidney tubule causing glucose to be reabsorbed from kidney filtrate. Blocking of this co-transporter enzyme leads to more glucose being excreted in the urine. Drugs in this class have been under review by the FDA due to increased risk of bone fractures and decreased bone density in some patients.
dapagliflozin (Farxiga)	PO: 5–10 mg once daily in the morning with or without food	
empagliflozin (Jardiance)	PO: 10–25 mg once daily in the morning with or without food	
SULFONYLUREAS, FIRST GENERATION		
chlorpropamide (Diabinese)	PO: 100–250 mg/day (max: 750 mg/day)	These drugs stimulate the release of insulin from pancreatic islet cells. Symptoms are hypoglycemia, weight gain, GI distress, and liver toxicity.
tolazamide (Tolinase)	PO: 100–500 mg one to two times per day (max: 1 g/day)	
tolbutamide (Orinase)	PO: 250–1500 mg one to two times per day (max: 3 g/day)	
SULFONYLUREAS, SECOND GENERATION		
glimepiride (Amaryl)	PO: 1–4 mg/day (max: 8 mg/day)	Adverse effects are similar to first-generation sulfonylureas except that there are fewer drug–drug interactions. These drugs should be taken 30 minutes before breakfast.
glipizide (Glucotrol)	PO: 2.5–20 mg one to two times per day (max: 40 mg/day)	
glyburide (DiaBeta, Micronase)	PO: 1.25–10 mg one to two times per day (max: 20 mg/day)	
glyburide micronized (Glynase)	PO: 0.75–12 mg one to two times per day (max: 12 mg/day)	
THIAZOLIDINEDIONES		
pioglitazone (Actos)	PO: 15–30 mg/day (max: 45 mg/day)	These drugs have been under review by the FDA due to the increased risk of heart failure with drugs in this class.
rosiglitazone (Avandia)	PO: 2–4 mg one to two times per day (max: 8 mg/day)	
MISCELLANEOUS DRUGS		
bromocriptine (Cycloset)	PO: 0.8–4.8 mg/day upon awakening	Approved for Parkinson disease, pituitary adenoma, acromegaly, and women with amenorrhea and infertility caused by inappropriate augmentation of prolactin secretion.
colesevelam (Welchol)	PO: 1.875 g (3 tablets) every 12 h or 3.75 g (6 tablets) once daily	Used along with diet, exercise, and efforts to lose weight and reduce cholesterol in the bloodstream

The alpha-glucosidase inhibitors, which include acarbose (Precose) and miglitol (Glyset), act by blocking enzymes in the small intestine that are responsible for breaking down complex carbohydrates into monosaccharides. Because carbohydrates must be in the monosaccharide form to be absorbed, digestion of glucose is delayed.

Metformin (Glucophage) is the only drug in the biguanide drug class. Combinations of drugs with metformin have been developed to maximize the therapeutic effects and minimize adverse effects. Examples of selected drug combinations are: ACTOplus (pioglitazone+metformin); Avandamet (rosiglitazone+metformin); Glucovance (glyburide+metformin); Janumet (sitagliptin+metformin); Jentadueto (linagliptin+metformin); Metaglip (glipi ide+metformin); and PrandiMet (repaglinide+metformin)

Several antidiabetic drugs act by mimicking or enhancing the effect of incretins within the GI tract. **Incretins** are hormones secreted by the mucosa of the small intestine following a meal, when blood glucose is elevated. Incretins signal the pancreas to increase insulin secretion and the liver to stop producing glucagon. Both of these actions lower blood glucose levels. In addition, these drugs decrease food intake by increasing the feeling of satiety (fullness), and they also delay gastric emptying, which slows glucose absorption.

hypox = *lowered oxygen*
emia = *blood levels*

satiety = *state of fullness*

Albiglutide (Tanzeum), exenatide (Byetta, Bydureon), and liraglutide (Victoza) are injectable drugs that mimic the effects of incretins. Thus, these drugs are called **incretin mimetics**. They accomplish their actions by activating a receptor called GLP-1. Activation of the GLP-1 receptor causes the same types of effects as the natural incretin hormone.

Prototype Drug: Metformin (Fortamet, Glucophage, Glumetza, Others)

Therapeutic Class: Antidiabetic drug **Pharmacologic Class:** Hypoglycemic drug; biguanide

Actions and Uses: Metformin is a preferred antidiabetic drug for managing type 2 DM because of its effectiveness and safety. It is used alone or in combination with other oral hypoglycemics or insulin. It is approved for use in children age 10 or above in immediate release and extended-release forms.

Metformin reduces glucose levels by decreasing the hepatic production of glucose and reducing insulin resistance. It does not promote insulin release from the pancreas. A major advantage of the drug is that it does not cause hypoglycemia. The drug's actions do not depend on stimulating insulin release, so it is able to lower glucose levels in patients who no longer secrete insulin. In addition to lowering blood glucose levels, it lowers triglyceride and total and low-density lipoprotein (LDL) cholesterol levels, and it promotes weight loss.

Metformin is used off-label to treat women with polycystic ovary syndrome. Women with this syndrome have insulin resistance and high serum insulin levels.

Adverse Effects and Interactions: The most common adverse effects are GI related and include nausea, vomiting, abdominal discomfort, metallic taste, diarrhea, and anorexia. It may also cause headache, dizziness, agitation, and fatigue. Unlike the sulfonylureas, metformin rarely causes hypoglycemia or weight gain.

Metformin is contraindicated in patients with impaired renal function. It is also contraindicated in patients with heart failure, liver failure, history of lactic acidosis, or concurrent serious infection. It is contraindicated for 2 days prior to and 2 days after receiving IV radiographic contrast.

Alcohol increases the risk for lactic acidosis. Captopril, furosemide, and nifedipine may increase the risk for hypoglycemia. The following drugs may decrease renal excretion of metformin: amiloride, cimetidine, digoxin, dofetilide, midodrine, morphine, procainamide, quinidine, ranitidine, triamterene, trimethoprim, and vancomycin. Acarbose may decrease blood levels of metformin. Use with other antidiabetic drugs potentiates hypoglycemic effects. Metformin decreases the absorption of vitamin B_{12} and folic acid. Garlic and ginseng may increase hypoglycemic effects.

BLACK BOX WARNING:
Lactic acidosis is a rare, though potentially fatal, adverse effect of metformin therapy. The risk for lactic acidosis is increased in patients with renal insufficiency or any condition that puts them at risk for increased lactic acid production, such as liver disease, severe infection, excessive alcohol intake, shock, or hypoxemia.

The second group of drugs, **incretin enhancers**, are the dipeptidyl peptidase-4 (DPP-4) inhibitors. Alogliptin (Nesina), linagliptin (Tradjenta), saxagliptin (Onglyza), and sitagliptin (Januvia) prevent the breakdown of natural incretins, allowing the hormone levels to rise and produce a greater response. These drugs are given orally and are effective at lowering blood glucose with few adverse effects. They work well with other antidiabetic drugs and do not cause hypoglycemia.

The meglitinides, repaglinide (Prandin) and nateglinide (Starlix), act by stimulating the release of insulin from the pancreas in a manner similar to that of the sulfonylureas. Both drugs in this class have short durations of action of 2 to 4 hours, and they are well tolerated.

In 2013, the FDA approved canagliflozin (Invokana), the first in a new class of drugs called the sodium-glucose co-transporter (SGLT) inhibitors. Inhibiting the SGLT2 receptor in the kidney allows more glucose to leave the blood and be excreted via the urine. This drug has the advantage of promoting weight loss. Two additional drugs in this class, dapagliflozin (Farxiga) and empagliflozin, were approved in 2014 and have very similar actions and adverse effects. Recently approved fixed dose combinations include Invokamet (metformin with canagliflozin) and Xigduo XR (metformin with and dapagliflozin).

The first oral hypoglycemics available, sulfonylureas are divided into first- and second-generation categories. Although drugs from both generations are equally effective at lowering blood glucose, the second-generation drugs exhibit fewer drug–drug interactions. The sulfonylureas act by stimulating the release of insulin from pancreatic islet cells and by increasing the sensitivity of insulin receptors on target cells.

The thiazolidinediones, or glitazones, reduce blood glucose by decreasing insulin resistance and by inhibiting hepatic production of glucose. Optimal lowering of blood glucose may take 3 to 4 months of therapy. Liver function should be monitored, because thiazolidinediones may be hepatotoxic. Drugs in this class contain black box warnings. In 2013, an FDA panel of experts voted to modify or remove measures that limited patient access to rosiglitazone. Under the FDA's risk-evaluation management strategy (REMS), this drug remains under close scrutiny due to the risk of fluid retention and heart problems observed in some patients.

Two other miscellaneous drugs include bromocriptine and colesevelam. Bromocriptine was originally approved to treat Parkinson disease, pituitary adenoma, acromegaly, and amenorrhea and infertility in women caused by excessive prolactin secretion. The drug acts on the central nervous system to increase levels of the neurotransmitter dopamine.

Approved for type 2 diabetes as Cycloset, the exact mechanism by which it improves glycemic control remains unclear. More often used to treat hyperlipidemia, colesevelam (Welchol) is also indicated for type 2 diabetes. Being a nonabsorbed bile acid sequestrant, colesevelam can inhibit the absorption of other drugs, including fat-soluble vitamins.

CONCEPT REVIEW 34.1

- Why are noninsulin antidiabetic drugs ineffective for treating type 1 diabetes?

Nursing Process Focus Patients Receiving Pharmacotherapy for Type 2 Diabetes

ASSESSMENT	POTENTIAL NURSING DIAGNOSES*
Same as for patients receiving insulin (see Core Concept 34.3), so abbreviated here. Prior to administration: • Obtain a complete health history. • Evaluate laboratory blood findings. • Acquire the results of a complete physical examination. • Obtain a dietary history. • Determine knowledge of diabetic medications and blood glucose monitoring.	Same as for patients receiving insulin (see Core Concept 34.3), so abbreviated here. • *Deficient Knowledge* • *Ineffective Health Management* • *Noncompliance* • *Risk for Unstable Blood Glucose Level* • *Risk for Injury* • *Risk for Imbalanced Nutrition* • *Risk for Infection*

PLANNING: PATIENT GOALS AND EXPECTED OUTCOMES

The patient will:

- Experience therapeutic effects (stable blood glucose levels).
- Be free from or experience minimal adverse effects from drug therapy.
- Verbalize an understanding of the drug's use, adverse effects, and required precautions.
- Demonstrate an understanding of lifestyle modifications necessary for successful maintenance of drug therapy.

IMPLEMENTATION

Interventions and (Rationales)	Patient Education/Discharge Planning
• Monitor blood glucose at least daily. (Daily glucose levels will assist in maintaining stable blood glucose.)	• Instruct the patient how to monitor blood glucose, including use of equipment, and when to notify the healthcare provider.
• Administer medication correctly (at appropriate time according to type of medication ordered), and evaluate the patient's knowledge of proper administration. (Most oral antidiabetic medications are given at or around meal times. Maintaining levels of medication will assist in maintaining stable blood glucose levels.)	Inform patient or caregivers about: • Correct administration time for type of medication ordered. • Peak medication levels and proper food sources needed to prevent both hyperglycemia and hypoglycemia. Provide written materials for future reference.
• Monitor for signs of lactic acidosis if the patient is receiving a biguanide. (Mitochondrial oxidation of lactic acid is inhibited, and lactic acidosis may result.)	• Instruct the patient to report signs of lactic acidosis, such as hyperventilation, muscle pain, fatigue, and increased sleeping to the healthcare provider.
• Continue to monitor periodic laboratory work: CBC, electrolytes, glucose, HbA1C, lipid profile, liver and renal function studies. (Periodic monitoring assists in determining glucose control, need for medication changes, and any indicators of complications. These drugs are metabolized in the liver and may cause elevations in AST and LDH.)	Instruct the patient: • On sulfonylureas to immediately report any nausea, vomiting, yellow skin, pale or clay colored stools, abdominal pain, or dark urine to the healthcare provider. • Taking biguanides to immediately report any drowsiness, malaise, decreased respiratory rate, or general body aches to the healthcare provider. • About the need to keep laboratory appointments.
• Ensure dietary needs are met based on weight and current glucose levels. Avoid alcohol. (Patients taking sulfonylurea or biguanides should avoid alcohol entirely to prevent an antabuse-like reaction.)	Advise the patient to: • Monitor food choices and follow recommended diet plan. Provide written materials on dietary recommendations for future reference. • Abstain from alcohol and to avoid liquid over-the-counter (OTC) medications, which may contain alcohol.

(Continued)

Nursing Process Focus (*continued*)

Interventions and (Rationales)	Patient Education/Discharge Planning
• Monitor for edema, blood pressure, and lung sounds in patients taking thiazolidiones. (These drugs may cause edema and worsening heart failure.)	• Instruct the patient to immediately report to the healthcare provider any signs of edema of the hands or feet, dyspnea, or excessive fatigue.
• Increase the frequency of blood glucose monitoring if the patient is experiencing fever, nausea, vomiting, or diarrhea. (Illness may affect blood glucose levels and usually requires adjustments in medication.)	• Instruct the patient to report the first signs of fatigue, muscle weakness, and nausea. • Discuss the importance of adequate rest and healthy routines.
• Check for signs of hypoglycemia, especially around the time of insulin peak activity. If symptoms occur, provide a quick-acting carbohydrate source (juice or simple sugar), and then recheck blood glucose. (Using a simple sugar will raise blood sugar immediately.) Also monitor carefully patients who also take beta blockers, because early signs of hypoglycemia may not be apparent.	Inform the patient: • Of the signs and symptoms of hypoglycemia, such as hunger, irritability, and sweating. • At first sign of hypoglycemia, to check blood glucose and eat a simple sugar; if symptoms do not improve, call 911. • If necessary, to monitor blood glucose before breakfast and supper. • Not to skip meals and to follow a diet specified by the healthcare provider.
• Monitor weight, weighing at the same time of day each time. (Changes in weight will affect the amount of drug needed to control blood glucose.)	• Instruct the patient to weigh self each week, at the same time of day, and report any significant loss or gain.
• Encourage the patient to increase physical activity gradually but continue to monitor blood glucose level before and after exercise. (Exercise assists muscle cells to use glucose more efficiently, lowering blood glucose.)	Inform the patient: • About the benefit of exercise. • To check blood glucose before and after exercise and to keep a simple sugar on his or her person while exercising. • To eat some form of simple sugar or complex carbohydrate before strenuous exercise as prophylaxis against hypoglycemia.
• Monitor hypersensitivity and allergic reactions. (Anaphylactic reactions are possible.)	• Advise the patient of the importance of immediately reporting symptoms such as skin rashes, itching, swelling of the tongue or face, flushing, dizziness, syncope, wheezing, throat tightness, or shortness of breath to the healthcare provider.
• Determine pregnancy status. (Some oral antidiabetic medications are category C and must be stopped during pregnancy. Due to increasing the metabolic needs of pregnancy, insulin therapy may be needed.)	• Advise female patients of childbearing age to inform the healthcare provider if pregnancy is suspected.

EVALUATION OF OUTCOME CRITERIA

Evaluate the effectiveness of drug therapy by confirming that patient goals and expected outcomes have been met (see "Planning"). *See* Table 34.2 *for a list of drugs to which these nursing actions apply.*

Patients Need to Know

Patients treated for DM need to know the following:

1. When administering insulin, meals should not be skipped. If self-injecting insulin, carefully follow all instructions provided by the healthcare provider to avoid injury or infection. Opened vials may be stored at room temperature for up to 1 month, avoiding direct sunlight and heat. Store unopened vials in refrigerator. Discard any vial if any changes in the solution are noted or if insulin has expired.
2. Check with a healthcare provider before beginning a vigorous exercise program. Often, insulin doses should be reduced or extra food should be ingested just prior to intense exercise.
3. Know the time of peak action of any insulin, because that is when the risk for hypoglycemic adverse effects is greatest.
4. The right amount of insulin must be available to cells when glucose is available in the blood. Without insulin present, glucose from a meal can build up to high levels in the blood, causing hyperglycemia and possible coma.
5. When taking antidiabetic drugs, report to your healthcare provider immediately any signs of hypoglycemia, such as weakness, sweating, dizziness, tremor, anxiety, or tachycardia. Mild symptoms may be treated with small amounts of sugar in the form of candy or fruit juice.

6. Always take antidiabetic drugs the same time each day. When self-monitoring blood glucose, recall that normal values are 80–120 mg/dL before meals and 100–140 mg/dL before bedtime.
7. Read the directions for all medications very carefully because many drug–drug interactions are possible. Medications such as corticosteroids, thiazide diuretics, and sympathomimetics can raise blood glucose levels and inhibit the effects of insulin.

Safety Alert: Use of Multidose Medication Pens

The FDA (2015) warns that multidose insulin pens, and pens for other injectable medicines, never be shared among patients, even if the needle is changed. The practice of sharing pens can result in cross contamination causing the spread of disease. All medication pens should be clearly labeled with the patient's name or other identifying information.

Chapter Review

Core Concepts Summary

34.1 The pancreas is responsible for the regulation of blood glucose levels.

The pancreas is both an endocrine and an exocrine gland. The islets of Langerhans are responsible for secretion of insulin and glucagon. Insulin is released when blood glucose increases, and glucagon is released when blood glucose decreases.

34.2 Type 1 diabetes is caused by a deficiency of insulin.

Type 1 DM is caused by an absolute lack of insulin secretion due to autoimmune destruction of pancreatic islet cells. If untreated, it results in serious, chronic conditions affecting the cardiovascular and nervous systems.

34.3 Insulin replacement therapy is required for type 1 diabetes.

Type 1 DM is treated by dietary restrictions, exercise, and insulin therapy. The many types of insulin preparations vary as to their onset of action, time to peak effect, and duration. Doses of insulin are highly individualized in each patient.

34.4 Type 2 diabetes is the most common form of the disorder

Type 2 DM is caused by a lack of sensitivity of insulin receptors at the target cells and a deficiency in insulin secretion. If untreated, the same chronic conditions result as in type 1 DM. Most people with type 2 DM are older adults; more obese children and adolescents are being diagnosed.

34.5 Antidiabetic drugs are prescribed after diet and exercise have failed to reduce blood glucose to normal levels.

Type 2 DM is controlled through lifestyle changes and oral hypoglycemic drugs. Various classes of drugs are available for the pharmacotherapy of type 2 DM: alpha-glucosidase inhibitors, biguanides, incretin mimetics, incretin enhancers, meglitinides, sodium-glucose co-transporter (SGLT) inhibitors, sulfonylureas, thiazolidinediones, and miscellaneous drugs. Combinations of antidiabetic drugs maximize therapeutic effects and minimize adverse effects.

REVIEW Questions

Answer the following questions to assess your knowledge of the chapter material, and go back and review any material that is not clear to you.

1. While collecting information from a patient, the nurse notes which of the following symptoms of type 1 diabetes? (Select all that apply.)
   1. Poly
   2. phagia
   3. Polyuria
   4. Polydipsia
   5. Weight gain
   6. Weight loss
2. When administering insulin, what route is used?
   1. Oral
   2. Intradermal
   3. Subcutaneous
   4. Intramuscular

3. A patient who has just been prescribed an incretin enhancer (oral hypoglycemic medication) asks how it works. The nurse informs the patient that these types of medications:
   1. Decrease the uptake of glucose by body cells.
   2. Stimulate insulin release from the pancreas.
   3. Increase insulin production by the pancreas.
   4. Decrease the amount of insulin produced by the pancreas.
4. A patient receives NPH and regular insulin every morning. The nurse verifies that the patient understands that there are two different peak times to be aware of for this insulin combination. The reason why the nurse continues to evaluate the patient's understanding in this instance is because:
   1. The patient needs to plan the next insulin injection around the peak times.
   2. Additional insulin may be needed at peak times to avoid hyperglycemia.
   3. It is best to plan exercise or other activities around the peak insulin activity.
   4. The risk for hypoglycemia is greatest around the peak of insulin activity.
5. The nurse is evaluating the patient's knowledge about the use and effects of insulin. Which of the following statements indicates that the patient needs additional information?
   1. "If I experience hypoglycemia, I should drink half a cup of apple juice."
   2. "My insulin needs may increase when I have an infection."
   3. "I must draw the NPH insulin first if I am mixing it with regular insulin."
   4. "If my blood glucose levels are above 140 mg/dL, I should notify my healthcare provider."
6. The healthcare provider starts a patient on 500 mg, PO, twice a day. The pharmacy provides scored 1000 mg tablets. How many tablets will the patient take in 1 day?
   1. One tablet
   2. Two tablets
   3. One and one-half tablets
   4. One-half tablet
7. The patient with diabetes has decided to start an exercise program. He remembers that the nurse told him that exercise:
   1. Increases glucose in the blood thus increasing the need for insulin just after exercise.
   2. Decreases glucose in the blood thus decreasing the need for more insulin just after exercise.
   3. Does not affect glucose or the need for insulin.
   4. Decreases glucose in the blood thus increasing the need for insulin after exercise.
8. The nurse informs a group of patients, newly diagnosed with type 1 diabetes mellitus, that the following factors can influence the amount of insulin needed to control blood glucose levels: (Select all that apply.)
   1. Exercise.
   2. Diet.
   3. Illness.
   4. Sleep.
   5. Weight.
9. The nurse administers glipizide (Glucotrol):
   1. Subcutaneously only.
   2. After meals.
   3. At bedtime.
   4. Just before breakfast.
10. The nurse plans to administer glargine (Lantus) to a patient with type 1 diabetes:
    1. Before meals.
    2. With meals.
    3. Only at bedtime.
    4. At the same time each day.

CASE STUDY Questions

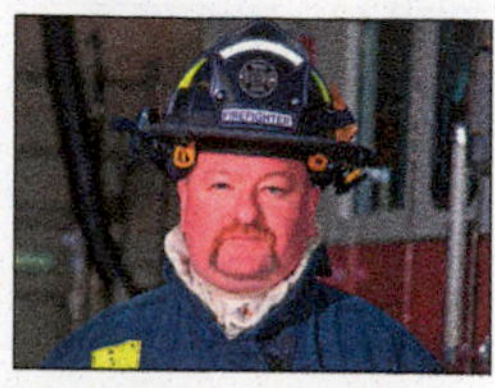

Remember Mr. Jones, the patient introduced at the beginning of the chapter? Now read the remainder of the case study. Based on the information you have learned in this chapter, answer the questions that follow.

Mr. Brian Jones is a 45-year-old firefighter who smokes and is somewhat overweight. Over the past 5 years, he has begun to develop slightly elevated blood pressure as determined by annual physical exams. He knows he should lose weight and is concerned about his energy level. He has always felt "okay" despite the fact that he smokes, but recently he has begun to feel sluggish and wonders what's going on. He thinks to himself, "Maybe I'm just getting older." At this current visit to the doctor, laboratory results reveal a fasting blood glucose level of 136 mg/dL. His blood pressure is 150/90 mmHg. Mr. Jones has not been taking medications for any reported disorders.

1. Mr. Jones is told that his blood glucose level is above the normal range, a condition known as hyperglycemia. In helping to determine factors that influenced his test results, the nurse asks him about: (Select all that apply.)
   1. His daily diet.
   2. His level of stress.
   3. How long he has smoked.
   4. How long he has had hypertension.
2. Mr. Jones is told that he has the symptoms of type 2 DM. He wants to know how it can be controlled. The nurse tells him that it can be controlled by: (Select all that apply.)
   1. Regular exercise.
   2. Oral antidiabetic medications.
   3. Maintaining current weight.
   4. Better coping skills to deal with stress.

3. Mr. Jones is started on metformin and asks the nurse about adverse effects. The nurse states that some of the adverse effects of metformin are: (Select all that apply.)
   1. Constipation.
   2. Diarrhea.
   3. Abdominal discomfort.
   4. Headaches.
4. Mr. Jones also has high blood pressure and is going to be prescribed medication. The nurse understands that several blood pressure drugs—captopril, furosemide, and nifedipine—may cause a(n):
   1. Increased risk for hypoglycemia.
   2. Decreased renal excretion.
   3. Increased renal excretion.
   4. Decreased risk for hypoglycemia.

Answers and complete rationales for the Review and Case Study Questions appear in Appendix A.

REFERENCES

Herdman, T. H., & Kamitsuru, S. (Eds.). (2014). *NANDA International nursing diagnoses: Definitions and classification, 2015–2017*. Oxford, United Kingdom: Wiley-Blackwell.

U. S. Food and Drug Administration. (2015). *FDA drug safety communication: FDA requires label warnings to prohibit sharing of multi-dose diabetes pen devices among patients*. Retrieved from http://www.fda.gov/Drugs/DrugSafety/ucm435271.htm

SELECTED BIBLIOGRAPHY

American Diabetes Association. (2016). *Statistics about diabetes*. Retrieved at http://www.diabetes.org/diabetes-basics/statistics/?referrer=https://www.google.com

American Diabetes Association. (2016). *Standards of medical care in diabetes—2016*. Retrieved from http://professional.diabetes.org/ResourcesForProfessionals.aspx?typ=17&cid=84160&pcid=84160

Anguita, M. (2013). Next generation of diabetes drugs arriving, but approach with caution. *Nurse Prescribing, 11*, 58–60. doi:10.12968/npre.2013.11.2.58

Bennett, W. L., Maruthur, N. M., Singh, S., Segal, J. B., Wilson, L. M., Chatterjee, R., . . . Bolen, S. (2011). Comparative effectiveness and safety of medications for type 2 diabetes: An update including new drugs and 2-drug combinations. *Annals of Internal Medicine, 154*, 602–613. doi:10.7326/0003-4819-154-9-201105030-00336

Centers for Disease Control and Prevention. (2014). *2014 Diabetes national statistics report*. Retrieved from http://www.cdc.gov/diabetes/data/statistics/2014statisticsreport.html

Centers for Disease Control and Prevention. (2014). *2014 national diabetes statistics report: Estimates of diabetes and its burden in the United States*. Retrieved at http://www.cdc.gov/diabetes/pdfs/data/2014-report-estimates-of-diabetes-and-its-burden-in-the-united-states.pdf

Centers for Disease Control and Prevention. (n.d.). *Women at high risk for diabetes: Physical activity, healthy eating, and weight loss*. Retrieved at http://www.cdc.gov/diabetes/pubs/pdf/womenHighRiskDiabetes.pdf

Maruthur, N. M., Tseng, E., Hutfless, S., Wilson, L. M., Suarez-Cuervo, C., Berger, Z., . . . Bolen, S. (2016). Diabetes medications as monotherapy or metformin-based combination therapy for type 2 diabetes: A systematic review and meta-analysis. *Annals of Internal Medicine, 164*, 740–751. doi:10.7326/M15-2650

Nathan, D. M. (2014). The diabetes control and complications trial/epidemiology of diabetes interventions and complications study at 30 years: Overview. *Diabetes Care, 37*, 9–16. doi:10.2337/dc13-2112

Powers, A. C., & D'Alessio, D. (2011). Endocrine pancreas and pharmacotherapy of diabetes mellitus and hypoglycemia. In L. L. Brunton, B. A. Chabner, & B. C. Knollman (Eds.), *Gordon and Gilman's the pharmacological basis of therapeutics* (12th ed., pp. 1237–1274). New York, NY: McGraw-Hill.

Rickels, M. R., Ruedy, K. J., Foster, N. C., Piché, C., Dulude, H., Sherr, J., . . . Beck, R. (2016). Intranasal glucagon for treatment of insulin induced hypoglycemia in adults with type 1 diabetes: A randomized, cross-over non-inferiority study. *Diabetes Care, 39*, 264–270. doi:10.2337/dc15-1498

Rotenstein, L. S., Kozak, B. M., Shivers, J. P., Yarchoan, M., Close, J., & Close, K. L. (2012). The ideal diabetes therapy: What will it look like? How close are we? *Clinical Diabetes, 30*, 44–53. doi:10.2337/diaclin.30.2.44

Tseng, C. H., Lee, K. Y., Tseng, F. H. (2015). An updated review on cancer risk associated with incretin mimetics and enhancers. *Journal of Environmental Science and Health Part C Environmental Carcinogenesis & Ecotoxicology Reviews, 33*, 67–124. doi:10.1080/10590501.2015.1003496

Wang, S. S. (2015). *Metabolic syndrome*. Retrieved from http://emedicine.medscape.com/article/165124-overview

Chapter 35

Drugs for Disorders and Conditions of the Reproductive System

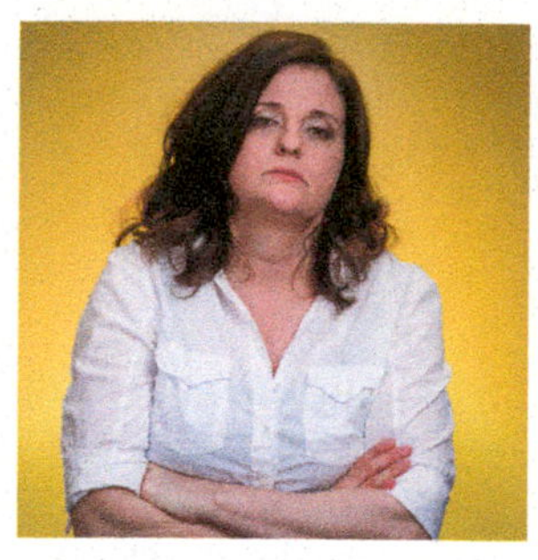

"I can't wait until all this stops. My periods hurt so bad and last so long. It just makes me tired."
Ms. Marge Philips

Core Concepts

35.1 The hypothalamus, pituitary, and gonads control reproductive function in both men and women.
35.2 Oral contraceptives and extended-release formulations are drugs used in low doses to prevent pregnancy.
35.3 Hormone replacement therapy provides estrogen to treat postmenopausal symptoms, but benefits may not outweigh risks.
35.4 Conjugated estrogens and progestins are prescribed for dysfunctional uterine bleeding, endometrial cancer, and postmenopausal symptoms.
35.5 Oxytocics and tocolytics are drugs that influence uterine contractions and labor.
35.6 Androgens are used to treat hypogonadism in males.
35.7 Erectile dysfunction is a common disorder successfully treated with drug therapy.
35.8 In its early stages, benign prostatic hyperplasia is successfully treated.

Drug Snapshot

The following drugs are discussed in this chapter:

Drug Classes	Prototype Drugs
Oral Contraceptives and extended-release formulations	Pr estradiol with norethindrone (Ortho-Novum, others)
Hormone replacement therapy (HRT)	Pr estrogen, conjugated (Cenestin, Enjuvia, Premarin)
Drugs for dysfunctional uterine bleeding	Pr medroxyprogesterone (Depo-Provera, Depo-SubQ-Provera, Provera)
Uterine stimulants and relaxants	Pr oxytocin (Pitocin)
Androgens	Pr testosterone
Drugs for erectile dysfunction	Pr sildenafil (Viagra)
Drugs for benign prostatic hyperplasia	Pr finasteride (Proscar)

Learning Outcomes

After reading this chapter, the student should be able to:

1. Describe the roles of the hypothalamus, pituitary, and sex organs in maintaining female and male reproductive function.
2. Explain the mechanisms by which estrogens and progestins prevent conception.

3. Describe the role of drug therapy in the treatment of menopausal and postmenopausal symptoms.
4. Discuss the uses of hormones in the therapy of dysfunctional uterine bleeding, endometrial cancer, and symptoms experienced after menopause in some women.
5. Compare and contrast the use of uterine stimulants and relaxants in the treatment of patients giving birth and after delivery of the baby.
6. Identify the reasons for pharmacotherapy with androgens.
7. Describe the pharmacotherapy of erectile dysfunction.
8. Describe the pharmacotherapy of benign prostatic hyperplasia.

Key Terms

amenorrhea (ah-men-oh-REE-ah)
androgens (AN-droh-jens)
benign prostatic hyperplasia (BPH) (bee-NINE pros-TAT-ik hy-PURR-plays-she-ah)
breakthrough bleeding
corpora cavernosa (KORP-us kav-ver-NOH-sah)
corpus luteum (KORP-us LUTE-ee-uhm)
dysfunctional uterine bleeding
endometrial carcinoma (en-doh-MEE-tree-ahl CAR-sin-OH-mah)
endometriosis (en-doh-MEE-tree-oh-sis)
estrogen (ES-troh-jen)
follicle-stimulating hormone (FSH)
gonadotropin-releasing hormone (GnRH) (go-NAD-oh-TROPE-en)
hormone replacement therapy (HRT)
hypogonadism (hy-poh-GO-nad-izm)
impotence (IM-poh-tense)
libido (lih-BEE-do)
luteinizing hormones (LH) (LEW-ten-iz-ing)
menopause (MEN-oh-paws)
menorrhagia (men-oh-RAGE-ee-uh)
oligomenorrhea (ol-ego-men-oh-REE-uh)
ovulation (ov-you-LAY-shun)
oxytocics (ox-ee-TOH-sicz)
oxytocin (ox-ee-TOH-sin)
postmenopausal bleeding (POST-men-oh-pause-ahl)
premenstrual syndrome (PMS) (PREE-men-stroo-ahl)
progesterone (pro-JESS-ter-own)
prolactin (pro-LAK-tin)
prostaglandins (pros-tah-GLAN-dins)
testosterone (test-AHST-erh-own)
tocolytics (toh-koh-LIT-ikz)
virilization (veer-you-lih-ZAY-shun)

Hormones from the pituitary gland and the gonads provide for the growth and continued maintenance of the male and female reproductive systems. Reproductive hormones impact virtually every body system function, including coagulation, blood vessels, bone, muscles, overall body growth, and behavior. Hormonal therapy of the female reproductive system is used to achieve a variety of therapeutic goals, ranging from replacement therapy after menopause, to prevention of pregnancy, to milk production. The pharmacologic treatment of reproductive disorders in men is less complex because hormonal secretion in men is relatively constant throughout the adult lifespan. This chapter examines hormones and drugs used to treat disorders and conditions associated with the reproductive system.

The hypothalamus, pituitary, and gonads control reproductive function in both men and women.

◄ **Core Concept 35.1**

Regulation of the reproductive system is achieved by hormones from the hypothalamus, pituitary gland, and sex organs. The hypothalamus secretes **gonadotropin-releasing hormone (GnRH)**, which travels a short distance to the pituitary to stimulate the secretion of **follicle-stimulating hormone (FSH)** and **luteinizing hormone (LH)**. Both of these pituitary hormones, when released, target the reproductive organs. The hormonal changes that occur during the ovarian and uterine cycles are illustrated in Figure 35.1.

gonads/gonado = *sex organs*
tropin = *attraction toward*

luteum/luteinizing = *yellowing (color of developing structures)*

During a woman's reproductive years and under the influence of FSH and LH, several ovarian follicles begin the maturation process each month. On approximately day 14 of the ovarian cycle, a surge of LH secretion causes one follicle to expel its oocyte, a process called **ovulation**. The ruptured follicle, minus its oocyte, remains in the ovary and is transformed into the hormone-secreting **corpus luteum**. The expelled oocyte begins its journey through the uterine tube and eventually reaches the uterus. If conception does not occur, the outer lining of the uterus degenerates and is shed to the outside during menstruation.

corpus = *body*
oocyte = *egg cell*

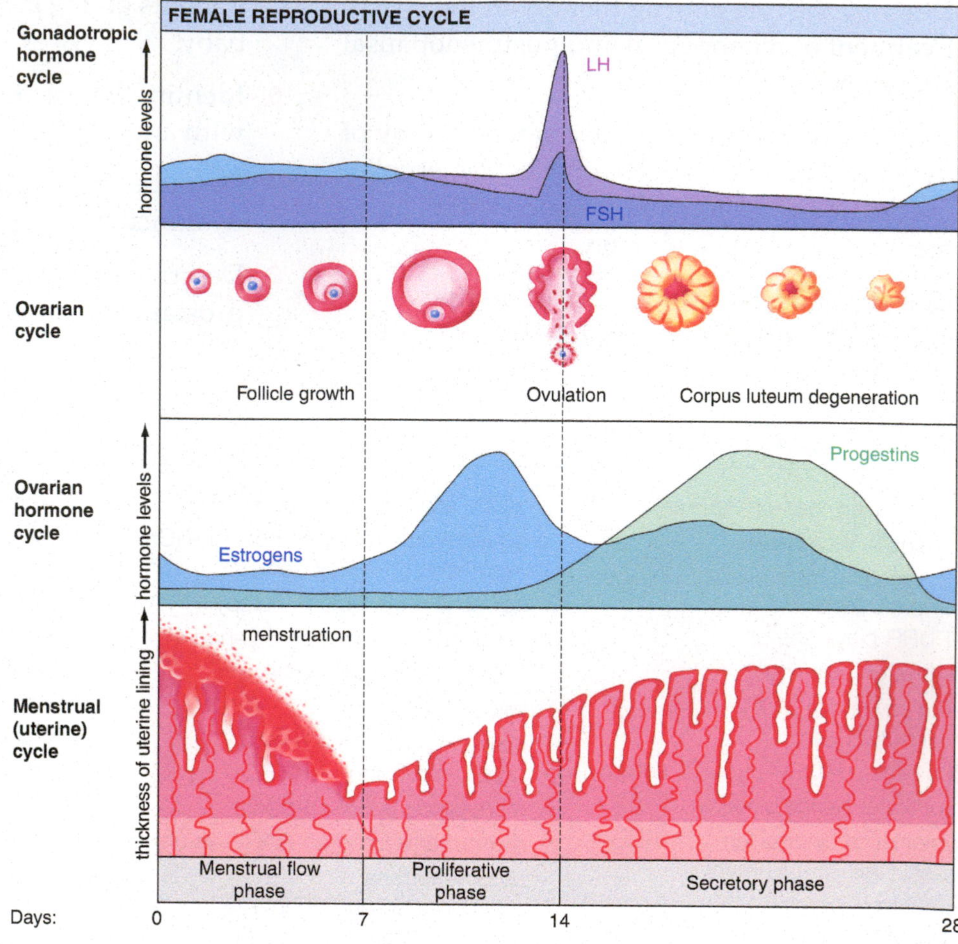

FIGURE 35.1 Hormonal changes during the ovarian and uterine cycles.

estro = *desire*
gen = *forming*

pro = *before*
gest = *gestation*

As ovarian follicles mature, they secrete the female sex hormones **estrogen** and **progesterone**. Estrogen is responsible for the maturation of the female reproductive organs and for the appearance of secondary sex characteristics. In addition, estrogen has numerous metabolic effects on nonreproductive tissues in the body. When women enter menopause at about age 50 to 55, the ovaries stop secreting estrogen.

In the last half of the monthly cycle, the corpus luteum secretes progesterone. In combination with estrogen, progesterone promotes breast development and regulates the monthly changes in the uterus. Under the influence of estrogen and progesterone, the uterine lining thickens in preparation for receiving a fertilized egg. High progesterone and estrogen levels in the final part of the uterine cycle provide negative feedback to shut off GnRH, FSH, and LH secretion. This negative feedback loop is illustrated in Figure 35.2.

The same pituitary hormones that control reproductive function in women also affect men. FSH regulates sperm production. LH regulates the production of testosterone. If the level of testosterone in the blood rises above normal, negative feedback to the pituitary shuts off the secretion of LH and FSH.

testo = *testis*
erone/sterone = *sterol chemical compound*

Testosterone is the primary male sex hormone responsible for male secondary sex characteristics. Unlike the 28-day cyclic secretion of estrogen and progesterone in women, testosterone secretion is relatively constant. Beginning in puberty, testosterone production increases rapidly and is maintained at a high level until late adulthood, after which it slowly declines.

CONTRACEPTIVES

Core Concept 35.2 ▶

Oral contraceptives and extended-release formulations are drugs used in low doses to prevent pregnancy.

The most widespread pharmacologic use of the female sex hormones is for the prevention of pregnancy. When used appropriately, they are nearly 100% effective. When contraceptives are taken orally, they are referred to as oral contraceptives (OCs). Many OCs contain a

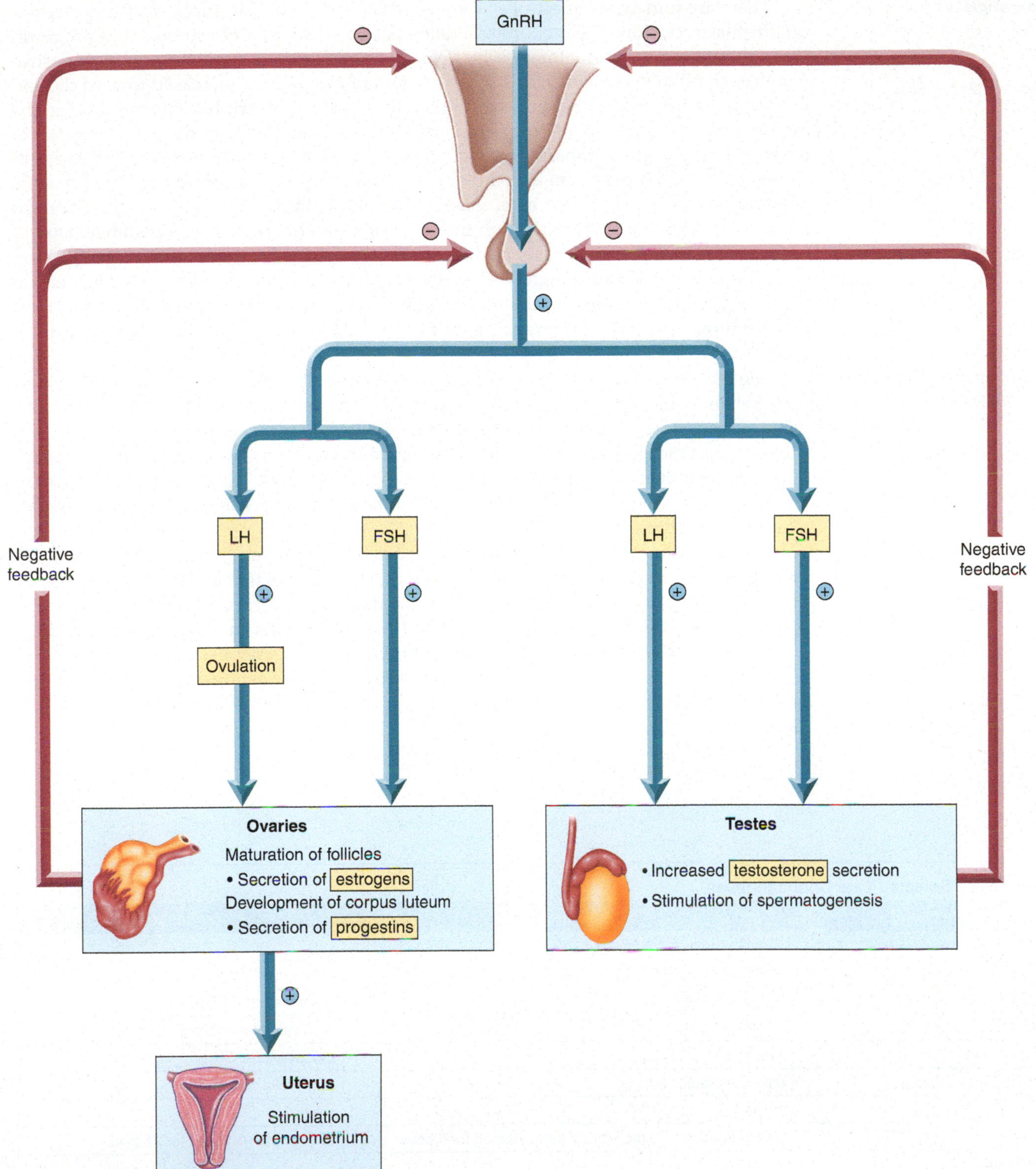

FIGURE 35.2 Hormonal control over male and female reproductive hormones.

combination of estrogen and progestin, although a few contain only progestin. The most common estrogen used in these preparations is ethinyl estradiol, and the most common progestin is norethindrone.

The estrogen–progestin OCs prevent ovulation, which is required for conception to occur. These hormones act by providing negative feedback to the pituitary gland that shuts down secretion of LH and FSH. Without these pituitary hormones, the egg cannot mature, and ovulation is prevented. The estrogen–progestin agents also make the lining of the uterus less favorable to receiving an embryo.

mono = *single*
bi = *two*
tri = *three*
quadra = *four*
phasic = *dosing level(s)*

There are four types of estrogen–progestin OCs: monophasic, biphasic, triphasic, and quadriphasic version. The monophasic delivers a constant dose of estrogen and progestin throughout the 21-day treatment cycle. With biphasic formulations, the amount of estrogen in each pill remains constant, but the amount of progestin is increased toward the end of the treatment cycle to better nourish the uterine lining. In triphasic formulations, the amounts of both estrogen and progestin vary in three distinct phases during the treatment cycle. Natazia, a quadraphasic contraceptive, contains a synthetic estrogen called estradiol valerate and a progestin called dienogest; it is the first drug containing this specific combination. Natazia has not been tested in women with obesity, and since OCs are less effective in obesity, this medication may well not be effectual in this instance. Due to increased risks of heart disease, healthcare providers are discouraged from prescribing oral OCs to patients with a high BMI. All four types of OC formulations are equally efficacious, although a common problem, and most likely the most common reason for treatment failure (pregnancy), is forgetting to take the medication daily. Selected OCs are listed in Table 35.1.

dys = *abnormal or unhealthy*
meno = *monthly*
rrhea = *flow*

thrombo = *stationary blood clot*
embolytic = *circulating blood clot*

The most common adverse effects of estrogen–progestin OCs are nausea, breast tenderness, weight gain, and breakthrough bleeding. Less common serious effects include edema, gallbladder disease, abdominal cramps, changes in urinary function, dysmenorrhea, fatigue, skin rash, headache, and vaginal candidiasis. Cardiovascular adverse effects, the most serious of all, include hypertension and thromboembolic disorders. The estrogen component of the pill can lead to venous and arterial thrombosis, which can result in pulmonary, myocardial, and thrombotic strokes.

The progestin-only OCs, sometimes called *minipills*, prevent pregnancy primarily by producing a thick, viscous mucus at the entrance to the uterus that prevents penetration by sperm. A thicker mucosal lining inhibits implantation of a fertilized egg. Progestin-only agents are less effective than estrogen–progestin combinations and produce a higher incidence of menstrual irregularities. Because of this, they are generally reserved for women who are at high risk for adverse effects from estrogen. Unlike estrogens, progestins are not associated with a higher risk of thromboembolic events, and they have no effect on breast cancer.

Table 35.1 Selected Oral Contraceptives

Trade Name	Estrogen	Progestin
MONOPHASIC		
Desogen	ethinyl estradiol: 30 mcg	desogestrel: 0.15 mg
Loestrin 1.5/30 Fe	ethinyl estradiol: 30 mcg	norethindrone: 1.5 mg
Ortho-Cyclen-28	ethinyl estradiol: 35 mcg	norgestimate: 0.25 mg
Yasmin	ethinyl estradiol: 30 mcg	drospirenone: 3 mg
Zovia 1/50E-21 and 28	ethinyl estradiol: 50 mcg	ethynodiol diacetate: 1 mg
BIPHASIC		
Mircette	ethinyl estradiol: 20 mcg for 21 days; 10 mcg for 5 days	desogestrel: 0.15 mg for 21 days
TRIPHASIC		
Pr Ortho-Novum 7/7/7-28	ethinyl estradiol: 35 mcg	norethindrone: 0.50, 0.75, 0.1 mg
Ortho Tri-Cyclen-28	ethinyl estradiol: 35 mcg	norgestimate: 0.18, 0.215, 0.25 mg
Trivora-28	ethinyl estradiol: 30, 40, 30 mcg	levonorgestrel: 0.05, 0.075, 0.125 mg
QUADRAPHASIC		
Natazia	ethinyl valerate: 3, 2, 2, 1 mg	dienogest: 0, 2, 2, 0 mg
PROGESTIN ONLY		
Micronor	None	norethindrone: 0.35 mg
Nor-Q.D.	None	norethindrone: 0.35 mg

Some contraceptives are available as topical, intradermal, or injectable formulations. Several long-term hormonal formulations are available. These extended-duration contraceptives are equally effective in preventing pregnancy and have the same basic safety profile as OCs. Examples of alternative formulations are:

- Depot injections: Depo-Provera (IM injection of medroxyprogesterone) and Depo-SubQ-Provera (subcutaneous injection of medroxyprogesterone) provide up to 3 months of contraception.
- Implants: Implanon is a single rod containing the progestin etonogestrel that is inserted under the skin of the upper arm and provides up to 3 years of contraception.
- Transdermal patches: Ortho Evra is a transdermal patch containing ethinyl estradiol and norelgestromin that provides 7 days of contraception.
- Vaginal route: NuvaRing is a 2-inch-diameter ring containing estrogen and progestin that is inserted into the vagina to provide 3 weeks of contraceptive protection.
- Intrauterine route: Mirena is a polyethylene cylinder placed in the uterus that releases levonorgestrel to provide 5 years of contraception. Skyla is smaller than Mirena and may last up to 3 years.
- Extended regimen OCs: Seasonale in tablet form containing levonorgestrel and ethinyl estradiol is taken for 84 consecutive days, followed by 7 inert tablets (without hormones).

Emergency contraception (EC) is the *prevention* of pregnancy following unprotected intercourse. The treatment goal for EC is to provide effective and immediate contraception. Two different medications are approved for EC: Levonorgestrel (Plan B) and ulipristal (Ella).

Plan B is approved for purchase over the counter (OTC). Dosing for Plan B involves taking 0.75 mg of levonorgestrel in two doses, 12 hours apart. Plan B One Step includes a single 1.5 mg dose. The drug acts in a manner similar to OCs; it prevents ovulation and also alters the lining of the uterus so that implantation does not occur. If implantation has already occurred, Plan B will not terminate the pregnancy. Plan B must be taken as soon as possible after unprotected intercourse; if taken more than 120 hours later, it becomes less effective. Adverse effects are mild and may include nausea, vomiting, abdominal pain, fatigue, headache, menstrual changes, diarrhea, dizziness, and breast tenderness. Ulipristal (Ella) is a single-dose product for EC that requires a prescription. One advantage of ulipristal is that it retains its effectiveness for 5 days following unprotected sex.

Prototype Drug: Pr *Estradiol with Norethindrone (Ortho-Novum, Others)*

Therapeutic Class: Oral Contraceptive **Pharmacologic Class:** Estrogen/Progestin

Actions and Uses: Ortho-Novum is typical of the monophasic OCs, containing fixed amounts of estrogen and progesterone for 21 days followed by placebo tablets for 7 days. It is nearly 100% effective at preventing conception. If a dose is missed, the patient should take the dose as soon as possible, or take two tablets the next day. If two consecutive doses are missed, conception is possible, and the patient should use other birth control methods until the regular dosing schedule is reestablished.

Adverse Effects and Interactions: Like most OCs, Ortho-Novum can increase the risks of thromboembolic disease: the potential for blood clots, hemorrhage, pulmonary embolism, or stroke. It should be used with caution in women with hypertension because it has the potential to raise blood pressure. Bleeding in the early or mid-menstrual cycle is relatively common.

Ethinyl estradiol interacts with many drugs. For example, rifampin, some antibiotics, barbiturates, anticonvulsants, and antifungals decrease efficacy of oral contraceptives, so the risks of breakthrough bleeding and pregnancy are higher

BLACK BOX WARNING:

Cigarette smoking increases the risk of serious cardiovascular adverse effects in women who are taking OCs containing estrogen. This risk increases dramatically in women over the age of 35. The absolute risks associated with OC use and smoking are greater because of the steeply rising incidence of arterial diseases. The combination of smoking and OC use among such women is associated with increased risk of stroke, acute myocardial infarction, and venous thromboembolism.

Nursing Process Focus Patients Receiving Contraceptive Therapy

ASSESSMENT

Prior to administration:

- Obtain a complete health history, including genitourinary, sexual, cardiovascular (especially hypertension or thromboembolic), thyroid, renal and liver conditions; pregnancy (or lactating); allergies; drug history; and possible drug interactions.
- Gather information about lifestyle, such as cigarette smoking and diet.
- Evaluate laboratory blood findings: complete blood count (CBC), electrolytes, lipid panel, renal, coagulation, and liver function studies.
- Acquire the results of a complete physical examination, including vital signs, height, weight, and menstrual pain

POTENTIAL NURSING DIAGNOSES*

- *Deficient Knowledge* related to a lack of information about drug therapy
- *Infective Health Maintenance* related to noncompliance with medication regimen or adverse drug effects
- *Excess Fluid Volume* related to adverse drug effects
- *Risk for Ineffective Peripheral Tissue Perfusion* related to adverse drug effects

PLANNING: PATIENT GOALS AND EXPECTED OUTCOMES

The patient will:

- Experience therapeutic effects (effective birth control).
- Be free from or experience minimal adverse effects from drug therapy.
- Verbalize an understanding of the drug's use, adverse effects, and required precautions.

IMPLEMENTATION

Interventions and (Rationales)	Patient Education/Discharge Planning
• Administer medication correctly and evaluate the patient's knowledge of proper administration. (Incorrect use may lead to pregnancy.)	Instruct the patient to: • Take the pill at the same time every day. • Not omit, increase, or decrease doses without consulting a healthcare provider. Omitting or decreasing doses increases the chance of pregnancy. • For estrogen–progestin combinations: Take a missed dose as soon as remembered. If two consecutive doses are missed, take the two missed pills on the day remembered and the next two pills on the following day. Then follow the remaining schedule of pills but use additional birth control until the regular schedule is reestablished. • Contact the healthcare provider if two consecutive periods are missed because pregnancy may have occurred.
• Monitor for the occurrence of breakthrough bleeding. (Spotting may occur, especially with low-dose hormone therapy, at mid-cycle. Any continuous, unusual, or heavy bleeding may indicate adverse effects, pregnancy loss, or disease and should be reported.)	• Inform the patient that spotting may occur with low-dose hormone therapy at mid-cycle but to report any unusual changes in the amount of bleeding or if bleeding continues.
• Monitor for thrombophlebitis or other thromboembolic disease. (Estrogen predisposes to thromboembolic disorders by increasing levels of clotting factors.)	• Instruct the patient to immediately report to the healthcare provider any pain in the calves, limited movement in the legs, dyspnea, sudden severe chest pain, headache, seizures, anxiety, or fear.
• Monitor for cardiac disorders: Take vital signs, especially pulse and blood pressure. (These drugs can increase blood levels of angiotensin and aldosterone, which increase blood pressure.)	Instruct the patient to: • Report immediately signs of possible cardiac problems such as chest pain, dyspnea, edema, tachycardia or bradycardia, and palpitations. • Monitor blood pressure regularly. • Report any symptoms of hypertension such as headache, flushing, fatigue, dizziness, palpitations, tachycardia, and nosebleeds.
• Encourage the patient not to smoke. (Smoking increases the risk of thromboembolic disease.)	Instruct the patient to be aware that: • The combination of OCs and smoking greatly increases the risk of cardiovascular disease, especially myocardial infarction (MI). • The risk increases with age (> 35) and with the number of cigarettes smoked (15 or more per day).

Interventions and (Rationales)	Patient Education/Discharge Planning
• Monitor liver function tests, lipid profile studies, and thyroid studies periodically. (These drugs are associated with an increased risk of gallbladder disease and a rare risk of liver toxicity.)	Instruct the patient to: • Return periodically for laboratory tests. • Report any symptoms of abdominal or right upper quadrant discomfort, yellowing of the skin or sclera, fatigue, anorexia, darkened urine, or clay-colored stools to the healthcare provider.
• Monitor for the development of breast or other estrogen-dependent tumors. (Estrogen may cause tumor growth or proliferation.)	• Instruct the patient to immediately report to the healthcare provider if a first-degree relative is diagnosed with any estrogen-dependent tumor.
• Encourage compliance with follow-up treatment. (Follow-up is necessary to avoid serious adverse effects.)	Instruct the patient to: • Schedule annual Pap smears. • Perform breast self-exams (BSEs) monthly, and obtain routine mammograms as recommended by the healthcare provider.

EVALUATION OF OUTCOME CRITERIA

Evaluate the effectiveness of drug therapy by confirming that patient goals and expected outcomes have been met (see "Planning"). *See Table 35.1 for a list of drugs to which these nursing actions apply.*

*Herdman, T.H. & Kamitsuru, S. (Eds.), *Nursing Diagnoses: Definitions & Classification* 2015–2017. Copyright © 2014, 1994–2014 NANDA International. Used by arrangement by John Wiley & Sons, Inc. Companion website: www.wiley.com/go/nursingdiagnoses.

CAM Therapy | Dong Quai for Premenstrual Syndrome

Since antiquity, dong quai has been recognized as an important herb for women's health in Chinese medicine. Obtained from *Angelica sinensis*, a small plant that grows in China, dong quai contains a number of active substances that are said to exert analgesic, antipyretic, anti-inflammatory, and antispasmodic activity. The dried root is available as capsules, tablets, teas, and tinctures.

The reproductive effects of dong quai may be due to active substances that have estrogenic activity. These estrogenic ingredients act as a "uterine tonic" to improve the overall hormonal balance of the female reproductive system. Dong quai is used to treat the symptoms of premenstrual syndrome, as well as irregular menstrual periods and painful menstruation.

Dong quai has also been used for its cardiovascular effects. It is claimed to increase circulation by dilating blood vessels. Because some of the active ingredients of dong quai may have anticoagulant activity, patients taking warfarin (Coumadin) or high doses of aspirin should not take the herb without notifying their healthcare provider.

MENOPAUSE

Hormone replacement therapy provides estrogen to treat postmenopausal symptoms, but benefits may not outweigh risks.

◀ **Core Concept 35.3**

post = *after*
meno = *monthly*
pause/pausal = *stopping*

Menopause is the permanent cessation of menstruation, resulting in a lack of estrogen secretion by the ovaries. Menopause is neither a disease nor a disorder, but a natural consequence of aging that is often accompanied by unpleasant symptoms that include hot flashes, night sweats, irregular menstrual cycles, vaginal dryness, and bone mass loss.

Over the past 50 years, healthcare providers have commonly prescribed **hormone replacement therapy (HRT)** for menopause. HRT supplies physiological doses of estrogen, sometimes combined with a progestin, to treat unpleasant symptoms of menopause and to prevent the long-term consequences of estrogen loss.

Studies have raised questions regarding the safety of HRT for menopause. Data suggest that patients may have an increased risk of coronary artery disease, stroke, and venous thromboembolism. Combination HRT increases breast cancer risk even when used for only a short time. Estrogen-only HRT increases the risk of ovarian cancer and also breast cancer, especially when used for a number of years. Women are encouraged to discuss alternatives with their healthcare provider. Undoubtedly, research will continue to provide valuable information on the long-term effects of HRT. Until then, the choice of HRT to treat menopausal symptoms will remain a highly individualized one between the patient and her healthcare provider.

UTERINE ABNORMALITIES

Core Concept 35.4 ▶

Conjugated estrogens and progestins are prescribed for dysfunctional uterine bleeding, endometrial cancer, and postmenopausal symptoms.

Conjugated estrogens are *combined* estrogens, and these, along with progestins, treat a variety of conditions. **Dysfunctional uterine bleeding** is a condition in which hemorrhage occurs on a noncyclic basis or in abnormal amounts. It is the most frequent health problem reported by women and is a common reason for hysterectomy. Other types of uterine abnormalities include the following:

hyster = *womb or uterus*
ectomy = *excision*

endo = *inside (e.g., uterus lining)*
metri/metrial = *measure*
osis = *abnormal*

oligo = *scanty*
meno = *month*
rrhagia = *excessive*
rrhea = *flow*

- **Amenorrhea**—absence of menstruation
- **Endometriosis**—abnormal location of endometrial tissues
- **Oligomenorrhea**—infrequent menstruation
- **Menorrhagia**—prolonged or excessive menstruation
- **Breakthrough bleeding**—hemorrhage between menstrual periods
- **Premenstrual syndrome (PMS)**—symptoms develop during the luteal phase
- **Postmenopausal bleeding**—hemorrhage following menopause
- **Endometrial carcinoma**—cancer of the endometrium

Dysfunctional uterine bleeding is often caused by a hormonal imbalance between estrogen and progesterone. Rather than rising and falling on a normal 28-day cycle, estrogen levels remain constant, resulting in chronic stimulation of the uterine lining. Without the presence of adequate amounts of progestins (progesterone-like hormones) to limit and stabilize growth of the uterine lining, irregular and prolonged bleeding occurs.

The primary indication for conjugated estrogens has been to treat moderate to severe symptoms of menopause, which include irregular menstrual cycles and extreme uterine bleeding. Progestins are the drugs most commonly used for treating uterine abnormalities. Administration of a progestin in a pattern starting 5 days after the onset of menses and continuing for the next 20 days can sometimes reestablish a normal, monthly cyclic pattern. OCs may also be prescribed for this disorder. Progestins are also occasionally prescribed for the treatment of metastatic endometrial carcinoma. In cases like this, progestins are used for total patient care, usually in combination with other antineoplastics. Conjugated estrogens and selected progestins with their dosages are listed in Table 35.2.

CONCEPT REVIEW 35.1

osteo = *bone*
porosis = *porous condition*

- Why is a progestin usually prescribed along with estrogen in oral contraceptives and when treating postmenopausal symptoms?

Prototype Drug: Pr *Estrogen, conjugated (Cenestin, Enjuvia, Premarin)*

Therapeutic Class: Hormone replacement therapy **Pharmacologic Class:** Estrogen

Actions and Uses: Conjugated estrogens (Premarin) contain a mixture of different natural estrogens. Conjugated estrogen A (Cenestin) and conjugated estrogen B (Enjuvia) contain a mixture of 9–10 different synthetic plant estrogens. Conjugated estrogens exert several positive metabolic effects, including an increase in bone density and a reduction in LDL cholesterol. It may also lower the risk of coronary artery disease and colon cancer in some patients.

Adverse Effects and Interactions: Adverse effects of conjugated estrogens include nausea, fluid retention, edema, breast tenderness, abdominal cramps, and bloating. Conjugated estrogens are contraindicated in pregnant patients and in women with breast cancer. Caution should be used when treating patients with a history of thromboembolic disease, hepatic impairment, or abnormal uterine bleeding.

Drug interactions include a decreased effect of tamoxifen and anticoagulants. The effects of estrogen may be decreased if taken with barbiturates, and there is a possible increased effect of tricyclic antidepressants.

BLACK BOX WARNING:
Estrogens, when used alone, have been associated with a higher risk of endometrial cancer in postmenopausal women. Although adding a progestin may exert a protective effect by lowering the risk of uterine cancer, studies suggest that progestin may increase the risk of breast cancer following long-term use.

Table 35.2 Drugs for Hormone Replacement Therapy and Uterine Abnormalities

Drug	Route and Adult Dose	Remarks
ESTROGENS		
estradiol (Alora, Climara, Divigel, Elestrin, Estraderm, Estrace, others)	PO (Estrace): 0.5–2 mg daily Transdermal patch: 1 patch once weekly (Climara) or twice weekly (Alora, Estraderm) Topical gel (Divigel, Elestrin): 0.25–1 g/day applied to the upper thigh or arm Intravaginal cream (Estrace): Insert 1–4 g/day	Systemic estrogens come in pill form, skin patches, gels, creams, and sprays. Low-dose vaginal preparations of estrogen are available in cream, tablet, and ring form. Estradiol valerate IM injection is a long-acting estrogen dissolved in sterile oil solution.
estradiol valerate (Delestrogen)	IM: 10–20 mg every 4 weeks	
Pr estrogen, conjugated (Cenestin, Enjuvia, Premarin)	PO: 0.3–1.25 mg/day for 21 days each month	
estropipate (Ogen)	PO: 0.75–6 mg/day for 21 days each month Intravaginal cream (Ogen): Insert 2–4 g/day	
PROGESTINS		
Pr medroxyprogesterone (Depo-Provera, Depo-SubQ-Provera, Provera)	PO: 5–10 mg daily on days 1–12 of the menstrual cycle IM (Depo-Provera): 150 mg daily for 3 months. Give the first dose during the first 5 days of the menstrual period Subcutaneous (Depo-SubQ-Provera): 104 mg daily for 3 months. Give the first dose during the first 5 days of the menstrual period	Synthetic versions of progestin are generally provided as high-dose pills or birth control pills. Injectable forms are also available. Treatments help restore hormonal balance.
norethindrone (Micronor, Norlutin, Nor-Q.D.)	PO (for amenorrhea): 5–20 mg/day on days 5–25 of the menstrual cycle	
progesterone (Crinone, Endometrin, Prochieve, Prometrium)	Amenorrhea or functional uterine bleeding: IM: 5–10 mg/day Assisted reproductive technology: Intravaginal: 90 mg gel once daily or 100 mg tablets bid–tid	
ESTROGEN–PROGESTIN COMBINATIONS		
Conjugated estrogens with medroxyprogesterone (Premphase, Prempro)	PO: Premphase: Estrogen 0.625 mg/daily on days 1–28; add 5 mg medroxyprogesterone daily on days 15–28 PO: Prempro: Estrogen 0.3 mg and medroxyprogesterone 1.5 mg daily Intravaginal cream: Insert 1/2 to 2 g daily for 3–6 months	Conjugated estrogens combined with progestins are prescribed to help women treat symptoms of menopause. Preparations are also used to treat certain menstrual disorders and to prevent osteoporosis (bone loss) in women.
estradiol with norgestimate (Prefest)	PO: 1 mg estradiol for 3 days, followed by 1 mg estradiol combined with 0.09 mg norgestimate for 3 days.	
ethinyl estradiol with norethindrone acetate (Activella)	PO: 1 tablet daily, which contains 0.5–0.1 mg of estradiol and 0.5–1 mg norethindrone Transdermal patch; 1 patch, twice weekly	

Prototype Drug: Pr *Medroxyprogesterone (Depo-Provera, Depo-SubQ-Provera, Provera)*

Therapeutic Class: Drug for endometriosis and dysfunctional uterine bleeding and endometriosis

Pharmacologic Class: Progestin

Actions and Uses: Medroxyprogesterone is a synthetic progestin with a prolonged duration of action. As with its natural counterpart, the primary target tissue for medroxyprogesterone is the endometrium of the uterus. It inhibits the effect of estrogen on the uterus, thus restoring normal hormonal balance. Indications include dysfunctional uterine bleeding, secondary amenorrhea, and contraception.

Medroxyprogesterone may also be given by sustained release IM (Depo-Provera) or subcutaneous (Depo-SubQ-Provera) depot injection. This is available in two doses: a lower dose for contraception and a higher dose for the alleviation of inoperable metastatic uterine or renal carcinoma.

Adverse Effects and Interactions: The most frequent adverse effects of medroxyprogesterone are breast tenderness, breakthrough bleeding, and other menstrual irregularities. Weight gain, depression, hypertension, nausea, vomiting, dysmenorrhea, and vaginal candidiasis may also occur. The most serious adverse effect is an increased risk for thromboembolic disease.

Medroxyprogesterone is contraindicated during pregnancy and in women with known or suspected carcinoma of the breast. Caution should be used when treating patients with a history of thromboembolic disease, hepatic impairment, or undiagnosed vaginal bleeding.

BLACK BOX WARNING:
Progestins combined with conjugated estrogens may increase the risk of stroke, deep venous thrombosis (DVT), MI, pulmonary emboli, and invasive breast cancer.

LABOR AND BREASTFEEDING

Core Concept 35.5 ▶ Oxytocics and tocolytics are drugs that influence uterine contractions and labor.

oxytocic = *oxytocin-related*
toco = *contraction*
lytic = *arrested*

Several drugs are used to manage uterine contractions and to stimulate lactation. **Oxytocics** are drugs that *stimulate* uterine contractions to promote the induction of labor. **Tocolytics** are used to *inhibit* uterine contractions during premature labor. These drugs are listed in Table 35.3.

The most widely used oxytocic is the natural hormone **oxytocin**, which is secreted by the posterior portion of the pituitary gland. The target organs for oxytocin are the uterus and the breast. As the growing fetus distends the uterus, oxytocin is secreted in increasingly larger amounts, thus promoting labor and the delivery of the baby. This process is referred to as *positive feedback*.

post = *after*
partum = *childbirth*

In postpartum women, oxytocin is released in response to suckling, which causes milk to be *ejected* (let down) from the mammary glands. Oxytocin does not increase the *volume* of milk production. This function is provided by the pituitary hormone **prolactin**, which increases the synthesis of milk.

Several prostaglandins, including dinoprostone (Cervidil, Prepidil) and carboprost (Hemabate), are also used as uterine stimulants. Unlike most hormones, which travel through the blood to affect distant tissues, **prostaglandins** are local hormones that act directly at the site where they are secreted. These drugs are used to initiate labor, dilate the cervix prior to delivery, and control hemorrhage following delivery.

preterm = *before term*

Tocolytics are given as uterine relaxants to suppress preterm labor. This option is carefully weighed against harm to the mother and the baby. Risks to the baby involve an elevated heart rate, circulatory collapse, and respiratory paralysis. Risk to the mother is elevated blood pressure. Of the tocolytics listed in Table 35.3, only hydroxyprogesterone (Makena) is approved for this indication; the others are used off-label.

Table 35.3 Uterine Stimulants and Relaxants

Drug	Route and Adult Dose	Remarks
OXYTOCIC		
Pr oxytocin (Pitocin)	IV: To control postpartum bleeding: 10–40 units per infusion pump in 1000 mL of IV fluid IV: To induce labor: 0.5–2 milliunits/min, gradually increasing the dose at 30–60 minute intervals until contraction pattern is established	Rapidly causes uterine contractions and induces labor; postpartum bleeding is controlled due to its stimulatory effect on uterine smooth muscle
ERGOT ALKALOID		
methylergonovine (Methergine)	PO: 0.2–0.4 mg bid–qid	Ergot alkaloids help to prevent and control bleeding after delivery of the baby
PROSTAGLANDINS		
carboprost (Hemabate)	IM: 250 mcg repeated at 1½- and 3½-hour intervals if indicated by uterine response	Prostaglandins make uterine muscles contract; during the uterine cycle, they naturally help the uterus shed its lining; clinically, these drugs are for refractory postpartum uterine bleeding
dinoprostone (Cervidil, Prepidil)	Intravaginal: 10 mg	
TOCOLYTICS		
magnesium sulfate	IV: 1–4 g in 5% dextrose by slow infusion (initial max dose = 10–14 g/day, then no more than 30–40 g/day at a max rate of 1–2 g/hour)	These drugs inhibit uterine contractions in pregnant women at risk for preterm labor. Drugs are from different classes: magnesium sulfate (mineral supplement), hydroxyprogesterone (progestin), nifedipine (calcium channel blocker), and terbutaline (beta-adrenergic drug)
hydroxyprogesterone (Makena)	IM: 250 mg once weekly, beginning at 16 week gestation and continuing until week 37	
nifedipine (Adalat, Procardia)	PO: Initial dosage of 20 mg, followed by 20 mg after 30 minutes (max:160 mg/day) After 72 hours, if still required, long-acting nifedipine 30–60 mg daily can be used	
terbutaline (Brethine)	IV: 2.5–10 mcg/min (max: 17.5–30 mcg/min) PO: Maintenance dose: 2.5–10 mg every 4–6 hours	

CONCEPT REVIEW 35.2

- What is the difference between the effects of prolactin and oxytocin on the breast?

Prototype Drug: Pr *Oxytocin (Pitocin)*

Therapeutic Class: Drug to induce labor; uterine stimulant Pharmacologic Class: Oxytocic

Actions and Uses: Oxytocin (Pitocin), identical to the natural hormone secreted by the posterior pituitary gland, is a preferred drug for inducing labor. It is timed to the final stage of pregnancy, after the cervix has dilated, membranes have ruptured, and presentation of the fetus has occurred. Oxytocin may also be administered to reduce postpartum hemorrhage after expulsion of the placenta.

Adverse Effects and Interactions: The most common adverse effects of oxytocin are elevated blood pressure; rapid, painful uterine contractions; and fetal tachycardia. Serious complications in the mother may include uterine rupture, seizures, or coma. Risk of uterine rupture increases in women who have delivered five or more children.

BLACK BOX WARNING:
Oxytocin is not indicated for the *elective* induction of labor (the initiation of labor in a pregnant patient who has no medical reason for induction).

HYPOGONADISM

Androgens are used to treat hypogonadism in males.

◀ Core Concept 35.6

andro = *male*
gen = *forming*

hypo = *reduced*
gonadism = *sex hormone function*

Androgens are male sex hormones. Testosterone is the primary androgen. Lack of sufficient testosterone secretion by the testes can result in male **hypogonadism**, the reduced function of gonads or sex organs in the body. Hypogonadism may be congenital or acquired later in life. When the condition is caused by a testicular disorder, it is called *primary* hypogonadism. Without sufficient FSH and LH secretion by the pituitary, the testes will lack their stimulus to produce testosterone. This condition is known as *secondary* hypogonadism. Lack of FSH and LH secretion may have a number of causes, including Cushing syndrome (negative feedback from corticosteroids), thyroid disorders, and estrogen-secreting tumors.

Symptoms of male hypogonadism include a diminished appearance of the secondary sex characteristics of men: sparse axillary (armpit) hair, less facial and pubic hair; increased subcutaneous fat; and small testicular size. In adult men, lack of testosterone can lead to erectile dysfunction, low sperm counts, and decreased **libido** or *interest in sex*. In young men, lack of sufficient testosterone secretion may lead to delayed puberty.

libido = *sexual desire*

Pharmacotherapy of hypogonadism includes replacement therapy with testosterone or other androgens. Within days or weeks of initiating therapy, androgens improve libido and correct erectile dysfunction resulting from low testosterone levels. Male sex characteristics reappear, a condition called *masculinization* or **virilization**. Therapy with androgens is targeted to return serum testosterone to normal levels. Above-normal levels serve no therapeutic purpose and increase the risk of adverse effects. High levels of androgens may cause abnormal growth of body hair, testicular shrinkage, altered sex drive, development of breasts, infertility, severe acne on the face and back, and possible mood swings involving rage or depression.

virilization = *appearance of male characteristics*

Testosterone is available in a variety of formulations to better meet individual patient preferences and lifestyles:

- Implantable pellets (subcutaneous): Testopel includes one to six pellets implanted on the anterior abdominal wall.
- Intramuscular (IM): Testosterone cypionate (Depo-Testosterone), testosterone undecanoate (Aveed), and testosterone enanthate (Delatestryl).
- Testosterone buccal system: Striant tablet is applied to the gum area just above the front teeth, producing a continuous supply of testosterone in the bloodstream.
- Transdermal testosterone gel: Androgel, Fortesta, Vogelexo, and Testim are applied once daily to the upper arms, shoulders, or abdomen. The drug is absorbed across the skin and into the bloodstream.
- Transdermal testosterone patch: Androgen patch is applied directly to the upper arm, thigh, back, or abdomen.
- Testosterone intranasal gel: Natesto is applied one spray in each nostril, three times daily.

Selected androgens with indications for men are listed in Table 35.4.

Table 35.4 Selected Androgens and Anabolic Steroids

Drug	Route and Adult Dose	Remarks
fluoxymesterone (Halotestin)	PO: 5 mg one to four times per day	Replacement therapy for deficiency of endogenous testosterone, primary and secondary hypogonadism, or delayed puberty
methyltestosterone (Android, Testred, Virilon)	PO: 10–50 mg/day Buccal: 5–25 mg/day	Primary hypogonadism, testicular failure, hypogonadotropic hypogonadism, and delayed puberty
nandrolone (Durabolin, Hybolin)	IM: 50–200 mg/week	Management of anemia due to renal insufficiency, to increase hemoglobin and red cell mass
oxandrolone (Oxandrin)	PO: 2.5–20 mg/day divided bid-qid for 2–4 weeks	To promote weight gain in debilitated patients and for the relief of the bone pain accompanying osteoporosis
oxymetholone (Anadrol-50)	PO: 1–5 mg/kg/day	Treatment of anemias caused by deficient red cell production, aplastic anemias, and myelofibrosis
Pr testosterone (buccal: Striant); (transdermal patch: Androderm); (topical gels: Androgel, Fortesta, Testim); (implantable pellets: Testopel)	Buccal: 30 mg/12 hours Transdermal: Apply 1–2 patches daily (max: 5 mg/day) Gel: Apply 5 g daily (max 10 g) IM: 50–400 mg every 2–4 weeks Pellets: 150–450 mg every 6 months (each pellet is 75 mg)	Primary therapy is for delayed puberty and hypogonadism; other indications are described in the Prototype Drug feature
testosterone cypionate (Depo-Testosterone)	IM: 50–400 mg every 2–4 weeks	Replacement therapy for deficiency of endogenous testosterone
testosterone enanthate (Delatestryl)	IM: 50–400 mg every 2–4 weeks	Replacement therapy for deficiency of endogenous testosterone, primary hypogonadism, secondary hypogonadism, and delayed puberty

Prototype Drug: Pr *Testosterone*

Therapeutic Class: Male hypogonadism drug Pharmacologic Class: Androgen

Actions and Uses: The primary therapeutic use of testosterone is for the treatment of hypogonadism in men. The administration of testosterone to young men who have an abnormally delayed puberty will stimulate normal secondary sex characteristics to appear, including enlargement of the sexual organs, facial hair, and a deepening of the voice. In adult men, testosterone administration will increase libido and restore masculine characteristics that may be deficient.

Adverse Effects and Interactions: An obvious adverse effect of testosterone therapy is virilization, or appearance of masculine characteristics. Salt and water are often retained, causing edema. Liver damage is a rare, although potentially serious, adverse effect. Acne and skin irritation are common during therapy.

Testosterone interacts with many drugs. For example, when taken with oral anticoagulants, testosterone may increase hypoprothrombinemia. Insulin requirements may decrease, and the risk of liver toxicity may increase when used with echinacea.

BLACK BOX WARNING:
Virilization in women and children may occur following secondary exposure. Signs of virilization may include any of the following: deepening of the voice, hirsutism, oily skin, and male-pattern baldness.

ERECTILE DYSFUNCTION

Core Concept 35.7 ▶

Erectile dysfunction is a common disorder successfully treated with drug therapy.

corpora = *bodies*
cavernosa = *cavernous*

Penile erection has both neuromuscular and vascular components. Autonomic nerves dilate arterioles leading to the major erectile tissues of the penis, called the **corpora cavernosa**. The corpora have vascular spaces that fill with blood to cause rigidity. In addition, constriction of veins draining blood from the corpora allows the penis to remain rigid long enough for successful penetration. After ejaculation, the veins dilate, blood leaves the corpora, and the penis quickly loses its rigidity. Organic causes of erectile dysfunction may include damage to the nerves or blood vessels involved in the erection reflex.

Erectile dysfunction, or **impotence**, is a common disorder in men. The defining characteristic of this condition is the consistent inability to either obtain an erection or to sustain an erection long enough to achieve successful intercourse.

The incidence of erectile dysfunction increases with age, although it may occur in an adult male of any age. Certain diseases, most notably atherosclerosis, diabetes, kidney disease, stroke, and hypertension, are associated with a higher incidence of the condition. Smoking increases the risk of erectile dysfunction. Psychogenic causes may include depression, fatigue, guilt, or fear of sexual failure. A number of common drugs cause impotence as an adverse effect, including thiazide diuretics, phenothiazines, selective serotonin reuptake inhibitors (SSRIs), tricyclic antidepressants (TCAs), beta- and alpha-adrenergic blockers, and angiotensin-converting enzyme (ACE) inhibitors. Low testosterone secretion can cause an inability to develop an erection due to loss of libido.

psycho = *the mind*
genic = *generated from*

The development of sildenafil (Viagra), an inhibitor of the enzyme phosphodiesterase-5 (PDE-5), revolutionized the medical therapy of erectile dysfunction. The PDE-5 inhibitors do not *cause* an erection; they merely *enhance* the erection resulting from physical contact or other sexual stimuli by increasing blood flow and maintaining relaxation of the smooth muscle in the penis.

Three additional PDE-5 inhibitors have been approved by the U.S. Food and Drug Administration (FDA). Vardenafil (Levitra) acts by the same mechanism as sildenafil but has a faster onset and slightly longer duration of action. Tadalafil (Cialis) acts within 30 minutes and has a prolonged duration lasting from 24 to 36 hours. Tadalafil is also used for the treatment of benign prostatic hyperplasia (BPH). The newest of the drugs in this class, avanafil (Stendra), has the same properties as the others but is claimed to have a faster onset of action. Drugs for erectile dysfunction are listed in Table 35.5.

CONCEPT REVIEW 35.3

- Why do you think that sildenafil is used to treat erectile dysfunction instead of testosterone?

Lifespan and Diversity

Erectile dysfunction affects about one in four men older than age 65.

Table 35.5 Drugs for Erectile Dysfunction

Drug	Route and Adult Dose	Remarks
avanafil (Stendra)	PO: 100 mg approximately 30 minutes before intercourse (max: 200 mg once per day)	The PDE-5 inhibitors do not cause an erection; they merely enhance the erection by increasing blood flow and maintaining relaxation of the smooth muscle in the penis. These drugs alter the body's response to sexual stimulation by enhancing the effect of nitric oxide, a chemical that is normally released during stimulation. Nitric oxide causes relaxation of the muscles in the penis, which allows for better blood flow to the penis.
Pr sildenafil (Viagra)	PO: 50 mg approximately 30–60 minutes before intercourse (max: 100 mg once per day)	
tadalafil (Cialis)	PO: 10 mg approximately 30 minutes before intercourse (max: 20 mg once per day) Once-daily dosing: 2.5–5 mg daily	
vardenafil (Levitra, Staxyn)	PO (film coated tablet or orally disintegrating tablet): 10 mg approximately 1 hour before intercourse (max: 20 mg/day)	

Prototype Drug: Pr *Sildenafil (Viagra)*

Therapeutic Class: Drug for erectile dysfunction Pharmacologic Class: Phosphodiesterase-5 inhibitor

Actions and Uses: Sildenafil acts by dilating blood vessels (vasodilation) and relaxing the erectile tissues in the penis, called the *corpora cavernosa*, which allows increased blood flow into the organ. The increased blood flow results in a firmer and longer-lasting erection in about 70% of men taking the drug.

Adverse Effects and Interactions: The most serious adverse effects with sildenafil occur in men who are concurrently taking organic nitrates, common drugs that also dilate blood vessels and are used in the therapy of angina. The combination of these drugs causes a marked increase in vasodilation, causing a drop in blood pressure and decreased blood flow to the heart, possibly causing a heart attack. Minor adverse effects include headache, flushing, and nasal congestion.

Cimetidine, erythromycin, and ketoconazole increase serum levels of sildenafil and require lower drug doses. Protease inhibitors (ritonavir, amprenavir, and others) will cause increased sildenafil levels, which may lead to toxicity. Rifampin may decrease sildenafil levels, leading to decreased effectiveness.

BENIGN PROSTATIC HYPERPLASIA

In its early stages, benign prostatic hyperplasia is successfully treated.

Core Concept 35.8

Benign prostatic hyperplasia (BPH) is the most common benign neoplasm in men. It is characterized by enlargement of the prostate gland. This decreases the outflow of urine by

benign = *mild*
hyper = *over*
plasia = *growth*

noct = *nighttime*
uria = *urine*

▶ Lifespan and Diversity

BPH affects 50% of men older than ag e 60 and 90% of men older than age 80.

obstructing the urethra, causing difficult urination. Symptoms include increased urinary frequency (usually with small amounts of urine), increased urgency to urinate, excessive nighttime urination (nocturia), decreased force of the urine stream, and a sensation that the bladder is not completely empty. BPH is illustrated in Figure 35.3.

Early in the course of the disease, drug therapy may relieve some symptoms. Only a few drugs are available for the treatment of BPH. These drugs are listed in Table 35.6.

Table 35.6 Drugs for Benign Prostatic Hyperplasia

Drug	Route and Adult Dose	Remarks
ALPHA$_1$-ADRENERGIC BLOCKERS		
alfuzosin (Uroxatral)	PO: 10 mg/day (max: 10 mg/day)	When activated, the alpha$_1$-adrenergic receptors compress the urethra and provide resistance to urine outflow from the bladder. Alpha$_1$blockers counter urethral compression.
doxazosin (Cardura)	PO (Regular-release): 1–8 mg/day (max: 8 mg/day)	
doxazosin (Cardura XL)	PO (Extended-release): 4–8 mg/day (max: 8 mg/day)	
silodosin (Rapaflo)	PO: 8 mg once daily	
tamsulosin (Flomax)	PO: 0.4 mg 30 minutes after a meal (max: 0.8 mg/day)	
terazosin (Hytrin)	PO: Start with 1–5 mg/day (max: 20 mg/day)	
5-ALPHA-REDUCTASE INHIBITORS		
dutasteride (Avodart)	PO: 0.5 mg once daily	5-Alpha-reductase inhibitors block the action of the enzyme that converts testosterone into dihydrotestosterone, a promoter of prostate growth. The size of the prostate is therefore reduced.
Pr finasteride (Proscar)	PO: 5 mg once daily	

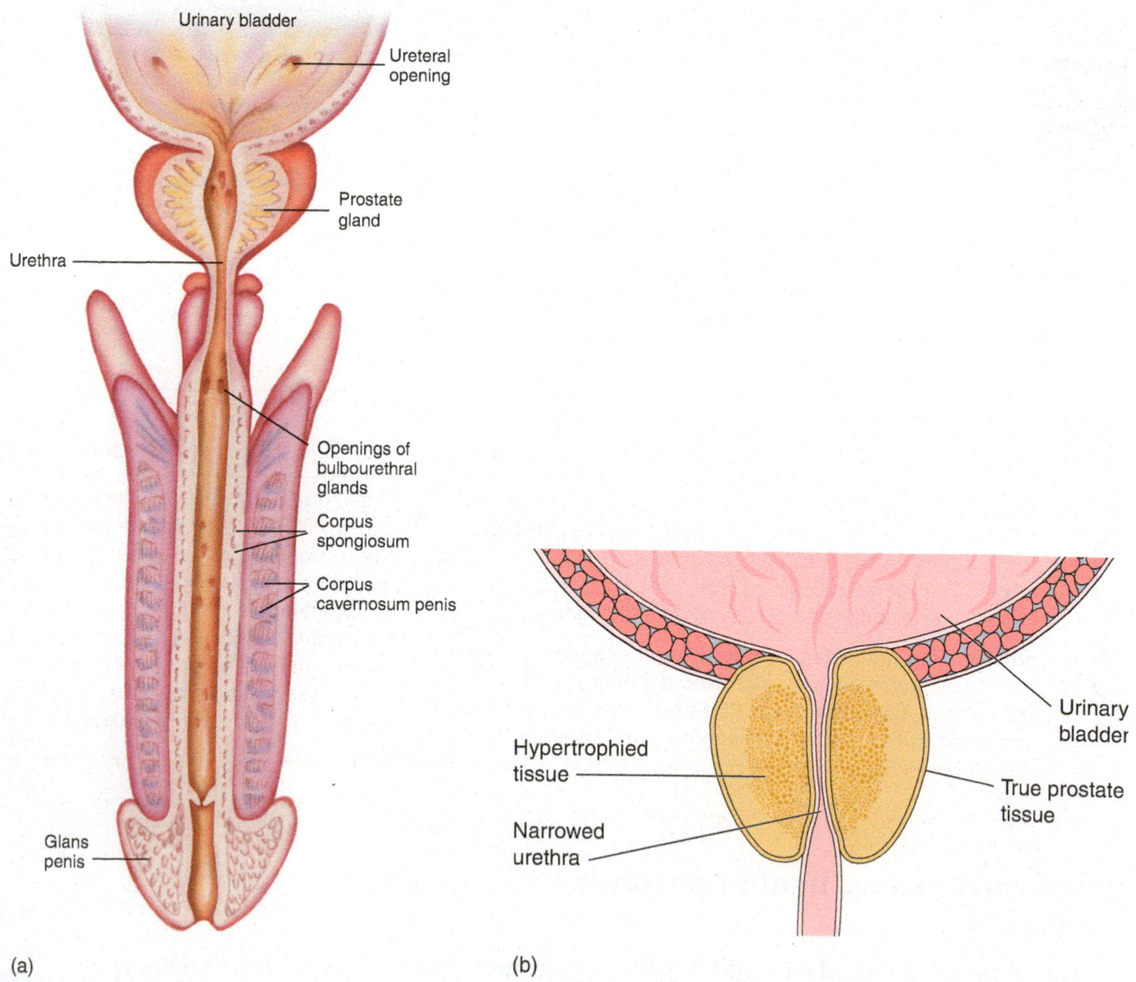

FIGURE 35.3 Benign prostatic hyperplasia (BPH): (a) normal prostate with penis; (b) benign prostatic hyperplasia.

Prototype Drug: Pr *Finasteride (Proscar)*

Therapeutic Class: Drug for benign prostatic hyperplasia Pharmacologic Class: 5-Alpha-reductase enzyme inhibitor

Actions and Uses: Finasteride acts by inhibiting 5-alpha reductase, the enzyme responsible for converting testosterone to one of its metabolites. This metabolite causes growth of prostate cells and promotes enlargement of the gland. Finasteride shrinks enlarged prostates and helps to restore urinary function. It is most effective in patients with larger prostates. This drug is also marketed as Propecia, which is prescribed to promote hair regrowth in patients with male-pattern baldness. Doses of finasteride are five times higher when prescribed for BPH than when prescribed for baldness.

Adverse Effects and Interactions: Finasteride causes various types of sexual dysfunction in some patients, including impotence, diminished libido, and ejaculatory dysfunction.

No clinically significant drug interactions have been established. Use with caution with herbal supplements. For example, saw palmetto may increase the effects of finasteride.

Patients Need to Know

Patients treated for purposes of regulating reproductive processes need to know the following:

Regarding Oral and Extended-release Contraceptives

1. If taking or applying contraceptives, schedule frequent medical checkups. Take blood pressure periodically and report any persistent changes to a healthcare provider.
2. Discontinue OCs, estrogen, or progestins immediately if pregnancy is suspected. Continued use may injure the fetus.
3. Inform the healthcare provider if contraceptives are taken or applied. Some drugs decrease their effectiveness and this could result in pregnancy. Drugs that reduce effectiveness of contraceptives include several common antibiotics and antiseizure medications.
4. A balanced diet is important when taking OCs, because these drugs may lower levels of folic acid and vitamin B_6.

Regarding Hormone Replacement Therapy

5. Before beginning HRT, a baseline mammogram should be performed. Monthly breast self-examinations should be conducted in addition to an annual exam by a healthcare provider.

Regarding Erectile Dysfunction Medications

6. If taking antihypertensive drugs, monitor blood pressure carefully when taking sildenafil. An increased risk of hypotension is possible.

Regarding Androgens

7. When taking androgens, expect virilization to occur. Prolonged erections, known as *priapisms*, should be reported to a healthcare provider immediately. This is a sign of overdose, and permanent damage to the penis may result.

Chapter Review

Core Concepts Summary

35.1 The hypothalamus, pituitary, and gonads control reproductive function in both men and women.

Estrogens are secreted by ovarian follicles and are responsible for maturation of the sex organs and the secondary sex characteristics of the female. Progestins are secreted by the corpus luteum and prepare the endometrium for implantation. Testosterone is secreted by the testes and is responsible for the growth and maintenance of the male reproductive system. The sex hormones are controlled by GnRH from the hypothalamus and FSH and LH from the pituitary gland.

35.2 Oral contraceptives and extended-release formulations are drugs used in low doses to prevent pregnancy.

Most hormonal contraceptives contain low doses of estrogens and progestins. Nearly 100% effective, these drugs prevent conception by blocking ovulation. Long-term formulations offer greater flexibility of administration. Oral and extended-duration contraceptives are safe for the majority of women, but they have some potentially serious adverse effects. Antibiotics, antifungals, barbiturates, and antiseizure medications can interfere with the effectiveness of hormonal agents.

35.3 Hormone replacement therapy provides estrogen to treat postmenopausal symptoms, but benefits may not outweigh risks.

Estrogen–progestin combinations are used for hormone replacement therapy during and after menopause. Their long-term use may have serious adverse effects, including increased risk of MI, stroke, breast cancer, and blood clots.

35.4 Conjugated estrogens and progestins are prescribed for dysfunctional uterine bleeding, endometrial cancer, and postmenopausal symptoms.

Dysfunctional uterine bleeding is often the result of an imbalance between progesterone and estrogen secretion. Administration of progestins may reestablish a normal cyclic menstrual pattern. Progestins are also used to treat endometrial cancer. Conjugated estrogens treat postmenopausal symptoms.

35.5 Oxytocics and tocolytics are drugs that influence uterine contractions and labor.

Oxytocics are drugs that stimulate uterine contractions and induce labor. Oxytocin, methylergonovine (ergot alkaloid), and prostaglandins are examples of uterine stimulants. Tocolytics slow uterine contractions to delay labor.

35.6 Androgens are used to treat hypogonadism in males.

Administration of testosterone promotes the appearance of masculine characteristics, a desirable action in men with hypogonadism. Anabolic steroids are testosterone-like drugs that may produce serious and permanent adverse effects.

35.7 Erectile dysfunction is a common disorder successfully treated with drug therapy.

Erectile dysfunction is a common disorder with many possible physiologic and psychogenic causes. Sildenafil is effective at promoting more rigid and longer-lasting erections. It is contraindicated in patients taking organic nitrates.

35.8 In its early stages, benign prostatic hyperplasia is successfully treated.

BPH results in urinary difficulties that may be treated by drug therapy or surgery. Alpha$_1$-blockers relax smooth muscle in the urethra to promote urine flow. 5-Alpha-reductase inhibitors reduce the size of the prostate to reduce pressure on the urethra. Goals are to minimize urinary obstruction, increase urine flow, and minimize complications.

REVIEW Questions

Answer the following questions to assess your knowledge of the chapter material, and go back and review any material that is not clear to you.

1. The healthcare provider tells the patient that the type of birth control where the estrogen level remains constant throughout the cycle but the progestin level increases toward the end of the menstrual cycle is called:
   1. Monophasic.
   2. Biphasic.
   3. Triphasic.
   4. Quadriphasic.

2. Before a patient begins taking sildenafil (Viagra), the nurse asks which of the following questions?
   1. "Are you currently taking any medications for angina?"
   2. "Do you have a history of diabetes?"
   3. "Have you ever had an allergic reaction to dairy products?"
   4. "Have you ever been treated for migraine headaches?"

3. When planning patient care, the nurse understands that medroxyprogesterone (Prempro) would be contraindicated for which of the following patients?
   1. A 37-year-old woman with dysfunctional uterine bleeding
   2. A 65-year-old woman diagnosed with metastatic uterine cancer
   3. A 40-year-old woman with a history of deep vein thrombosis
   4. A healthy 21-year-old who needs birth control

4. The patient states she had sexual intercourse yesterday and is concerned she may be pregnant. She is requesting emergency prevention. The healthcare provider knows that which of the following drugs may be ordered?
   1. Oxytocin
   2. Levonorgestrel
   3. Medroxyprogesterone
   4. Magnesium sulfate

5. The patient is being given oxytocin (Pitocin). The nurse evaluates her response to the drug, looking specifically for the possibility of: (Select all that apply.)
   1. Uterine rupture.
   2. Seizures.
   3. Fetal dysrhythmias.
   4. Hypotension.
   5. Hypertension.

6. A patient, seeking information about testosterone replacement therapy, asks about its application and possible complications. The nurse informs him that complications of testosterone therapy may include:
   1. Renal failure.
   2. Hepatic failure.
   3. Decreased cholesterol levels.
   4. Maturation of male sex organs.

7. Your patient states that she has forgotten to take her birth control pills for the last 2 days. You should instruct her to:
   1. Take her missed pills immediately.
   2. Get back on schedule as soon as possible.
   3. Use additional birth control measures until a regular schedule is established with the birth control pills.
   4. Get a home pregnancy kit.
8. The healthcare provider ordered testosterone cypionate (Depo-Testosterone), 50 mg, IM, every 2 weeks. The label on the vial states 100 mg/mL. How many milligrams will the nurse administer over an 8-week period of time?
   1. 100 mg
   2. 400 mg
   3. 300 mg
   4. 200 mg
9. A patient states that she is experiencing menopausal symptoms and asks for advice regarding hormone replacement therapy (HRT). The healthcare provider's best response is:
   1. "HRT is dangerous and should never be prescribed."
   2. "HRT is perfectly safe, with no risks."
   3. "You are not a candidate for HRT."
   4. "You need to discuss risks versus benefits of HRT with your healthcare provider."
10. Your patient with benign prostatic hyperplasia is complaining of feeling like he "cannot empty his bladder." You suspect that the healthcare provider will order which of the following?
    1. Finasteride (Propecia)
    2. Sildenafil (Viagra)
    3. Estrogen
    4. Finasteride (Proscar)

CASE STUDY Questions

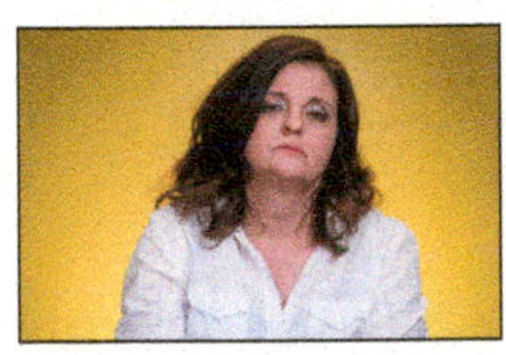

Remember Ms. Philips, the patient introduced at the beginning of the chapter? Now read the remainder of the case study. Based on the information you have learned in this chapter, answer the questions that follow.

Ms. Marge Philips, a 42-year-old female, enters the clinic with complaints of lower abdominal pain and irregular menstrual bleeding with prolonged menstruation. Blood pressure and pulse are slightly elevated. She states that she has had problems with frequently being tired. Other than her current complaint, she has no health problems or concerns. Ms. Philips last physical exam was 1 year ago. She is diagnosed with dysfunctional uterine bleeding and is prescribed Depo-Provera.

1. After the diagnosis is confirmed, the nurse knows that __________ is a common method of treating dysfunctional uterine bleeding.
   1. Use of condoms
   2. Visiting the doctor only when the pain gets really bad
   3. Possible use of oral contraceptives
   4. Screening of sexual partner
2. In order to determine if Ms. Philips is a good candidate for the medication, Depo-Provera, the nurse asks Ms. Philips if she:
   1. Has diabetes.
   2. Is planning on losing weight.
   3. Has a diet high in protein.
   4. Is planning on becoming pregnant.
3. Ms. Philips is to begin the oral contraceptive, Depo-Provera, as a means to control the uterine bleeding. The nurse informs her: (Select all that apply.)
   1. That smoking increases the risk of serious cardiovascular adverse effects.
   2. That it is okay to miss taking the medication for several days in a row.
   3. To notify her healthcare provider if two or more consecutive periods are missed.
   4. That caffeine will be beneficial.
4. The nurse also informs Ms. Philips that the adverse effects of Depo-Provera are: (Select all that apply.)
   1. Weight loss.
   2. Breast tenderness.
   3. Loss of appetite.
   4. Breakthrough bleeding.

Answers and complete rationales for the Review and Case Study Questions appear in Appendix A.

REFERENCE

Herdman, T. H., & Kamitsuru, S. (Eds.). (2014). *NANDA International nursing diagnoses: Definitions and classification, 2015–2017*. Oxford, United Kingdom: Wiley-Blackwell

SELECTED BIBLIOGRAPHY

Bedell, S., Nachtigall, M., & Naftolin, F. (2014). The pros and cons of plant estrogens for menopause. *The Journal of Steroid Biochemistry and Molecular Biology, 139*, 225–236. doi:10.1016/j.jsbmb.2012.12.004

Centers for Disease Control and Prevention (2015). *Contraceptive use.* Retrieved from http://www.cdc.gov/nchs/fastats/contraceptive.htm

Centers for Disease Control and Prevention. (2016). *Prostate cancer.* Retrieved from http://www.cdc.gov/cancer/prostate

Ensari, T. A., & Pal, L. (2015). Update on menopausal hormone therapy. *Current Opinion in Endocrinology Diabetes and Obesity. 22,* 475–482. doi:10.1097/MED.0000000000000207

Estephan, A. (2015*). Dysfunctional uterine bleeding in emergency medicine.* Retrieved from http://emedicine.medscape.com/article/795587-overview#a0104

Hawksworth, D. J., & Burnett, A. L. (2015). Pharmacotherapeutic management of erectile dysfunction. *Clinical Pharmacology and Therapeutics. 98,* 602–610. doi:10.1002/cpt.261

Levin, E. R., & Hammes, S. R. (2011). Estrogens and progestins. In L. L. Brunton, B. A. Chabner, & B. C. Knollman (Eds.), *Goodman and Gilman's the pharmacological basis of therapeutics* (12th ed., pp. 1163–1194). New York, NY: McGraw-Hill.

Nappi, R. E., & Cucinella, L. (2015). Advances in pharmacotherapy for treating female sexual dysfunction. *Expert Opinion on Pharmacotherapy, 16,* 875–887. doi:10.1517/14656566.2015.1020791

Ribaudo, G., Pagano, M. A., Bova, S., & Zagotto, G. (2016). New therapeutic applications of phosphodiesterase 5 inhibitors (PDE5-Is). *Current Medicinal Chemistry, 23,*1239–1249 doi:10.2174/0929867323666160428110059

Schimmer, B. P., & Parker, K. L. (2011). Contraception and the pharmacotherapy of obstetrical and gynecological disorders. In L. L. Brunton, B. A. Chabner, & B. C. Knollman (Eds.), *Goodman and Gilman's the pharmacological basis of therapeutics* (12th ed., pp. 1833–1852). New York, NY: McGraw-Hill.

Unit 7

The Skeletal System, Integumentary System, and Eyes and Ears

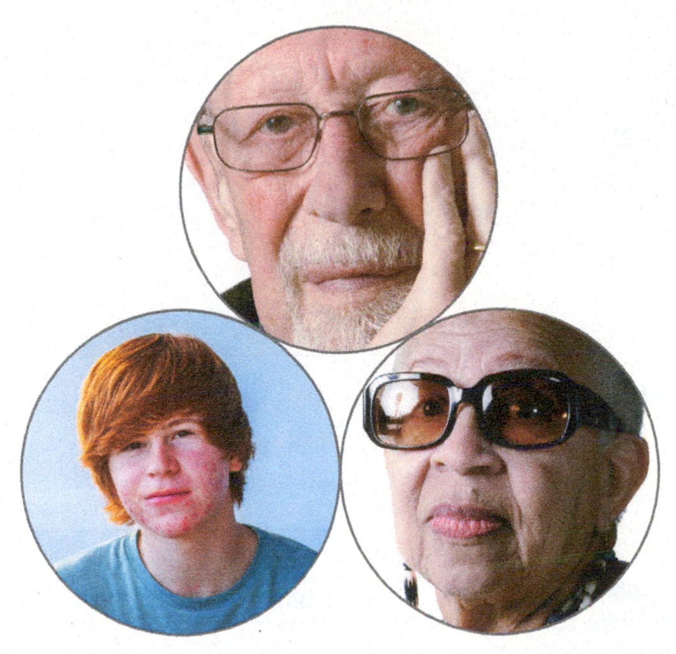

Unit Contents

Chapter 36

Drugs for Bone and Joint Disorders

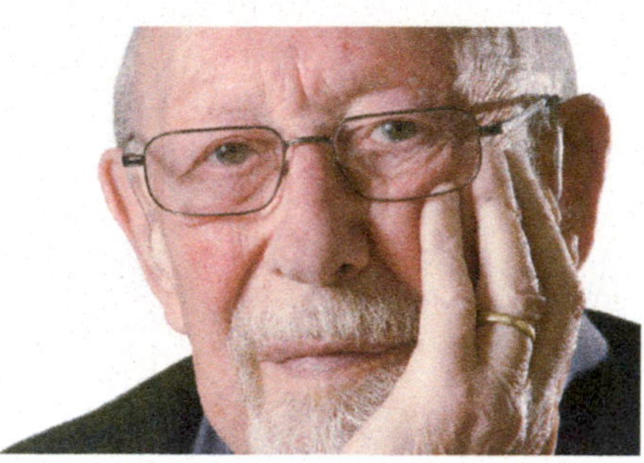

"I can't even work in the garden anymore. My joints ache so badly, and I don't understand what's going on with my big toe."

Mr. Steven Hurtt

Core Concepts

36.1 **Adequate levels of calcium, vitamin D, parathyroid hormone, and calcitonin are necessary for bone and body homeostasis.**

36.2 **Hypocalcemia is a serious condition that requires immediate therapy.**

36.3 **Osteomalacia and rickets are successfully treated with calcium salts and vitamin D supplements.**

36.4 **Treatment for osteoporosis includes calcitonin, selective estrogen-receptor modulators, and bisphosphonates.**

36.5 **Treatment for Paget disease includes biologic therapies and bisphosphonates.**

36.6 **Analgesics and anti-inflammatory drugs are important components of pharmacotherapy for osteoarthritis.**

36.7 **Immunosuppressants and disease-modifying drugs are additional therapies used to treat rheumatoid arthritis.**

36.8 **Pharmacotherapy for gout requires drugs that control uric acid levels.**

Drug Snapshot

The following drugs are discussed in this chapter:

Drug Classes	Prototype Drugs
DRUGS FOR HYPOCALCEMIA	
Calcium supplements	Pr calcium salts
DRUGS FOR METABOLIC BONE DISORDERS	
Vitamin D therapy	Pr calcitriol (Calcijex, Rocaltrol)
Selective estrogen-receptor modulators (SERMs)	Pr raloxifene (Evista)
Bisphosphonates	Pr alendronate (Fosamax)
DRUGS FOR JOINT DISORDERS	
Disease-modifying antirheumatic drugs (DMARDs)	Pr hydroxychloroquine (Plaquenil)
Drugs for gout	Pr allopurinol (Lopurin, Zyloprin)

Learning Outcomes

After reading this chapter, the student should be able to:

1. Describe the roles of calcium, vitamin D, parathyroid, and calcitonin in maintaining bone health.
2. Explain the importance of treating hypocalcemia.

3. Describe the pharmacologic management of disorders caused by calcium and vitamin D deficiency such as osteomalacia and rickets.
4. Explain drug treatments for weak and fragile bones such as osteoporosis and Paget disease.
5. Explain drug treatments directly related to weak bones and joints such as osteoarthritis, rheumatoid arthritis, and gout.

Key Terms

acute gouty arthritis (ah-CUTE GOW-ty are-THRYE-tis)
autoantibodies (AW-tow-ANN-tee-BAH-dees)
biologic response modifiers (BEYE-oh-LAH- jick)
bisphosphonates (bis-FOSS-foh-nayts)
bone deposition
bone resorption (ree-SORP-shun)
calcifediol (kal-SIF-eh-DYE-ol)
calcitonin (kal-sih-TOH-nin)
calcitriol (kal-si-TRY-ol)
cholecalciferol (KOH-lee-kal-SIF-er-ol)
disease-modifying antirheumatic (ANTY-roo-MAT-ik) drugs (DMARDs)
gout (GOWT)
metabolic bone disorders (meh-tuh-BAHL-ik)
osteoarthritis (OA) (OSS-tee-oh-are-THRYE-tis)
osteomalacia (OSS-tee-oh-muh-LAY-shee-uh)
osteoporosis (OSS-tee-oh-poh-ROH-sis)
Paget disease (PAH-jet)
rheumatoid arthritis (RA) (ROO-mah-toyd are-THRYE-tis)
selective estrogen-receptor modulators (SERMs)
uricosurics (YOUR-ik-cose-youriks)

The skeletal system and joints are at the core of movement and must be free from any defect that would destabilize the other body systems. For nerves, muscles, and bones to function well, the body needs adequate levels of calcium. Disorders associated with bones and joints affect a patient's ability to fulfill daily activities and lead to immobility.

This chapter focuses on the pharmacotherapy of skeletal disorders such as osteomalacia, osteoporosis, and Paget Disease, described as **metabolic bone disorders**, and the joint disorders, arthritis and gout. It stresses the importance of calcium balance and the action of vitamin D as they relate to the proper structure and function of bones and joints. Drugs are important because major mobility problems would occur without intervention.

Adequate levels of calcium, vitamin D, parathyroid hormone, and calcitonin are necessary for bone and body homeostasis.

◀ **Core Concept 36.1**

As shown in Figure 36.1, calcium levels in the bloodstream are controlled by two endocrine glands: the parathyroid glands and the thyroid gland. The parathyroid glands secrete parathyroid hormone (PTH), and the thyroid gland secretes calcitonin. PTH stimulates bone cells called *osteoclasts*. Osteoclasts break down bone tissue into its mineral components, a process called **bone resorption**. Once the bone is broken down, calcium is released for transport in the bloodstream and is used elsewhere in the body. The opposite of this process is **bone deposition**, or bone building. **Calcitonin** stimulates the building of bones by adding calcium to bone tissue.

Vitamin D is unique among vitamins in that the body is able to synthesize it from precursor molecules. The inactive form of vitamin D, called **cholecalciferol**, is synthesized in the skin from cholesterol. Exposure of the skin to sunlight or ultraviolet light increases the level of cholecalciferol in the bloodstream. Cholecalciferol can also be obtained from milk or other foods that are fortified with vitamin D. Figure 36.2 illustrates the metabolism of vitamin D.

Once cholecalciferol is absorbed or formed in the body, it is converted to an intermediate vitamin form called **calcifediol**. Enzymes in the kidneys metabolize calcifediol to **calcitriol**, the active form of vitamin D. Patients with extensive kidney disease are unable to synthesize adequate levels of calcitriol. The primary function of calcitriol is to increase calcium absorption from the gastrointestinal (GI) tract. Dietary calcium is absorbed better in the presence of PTH and active vitamin D.

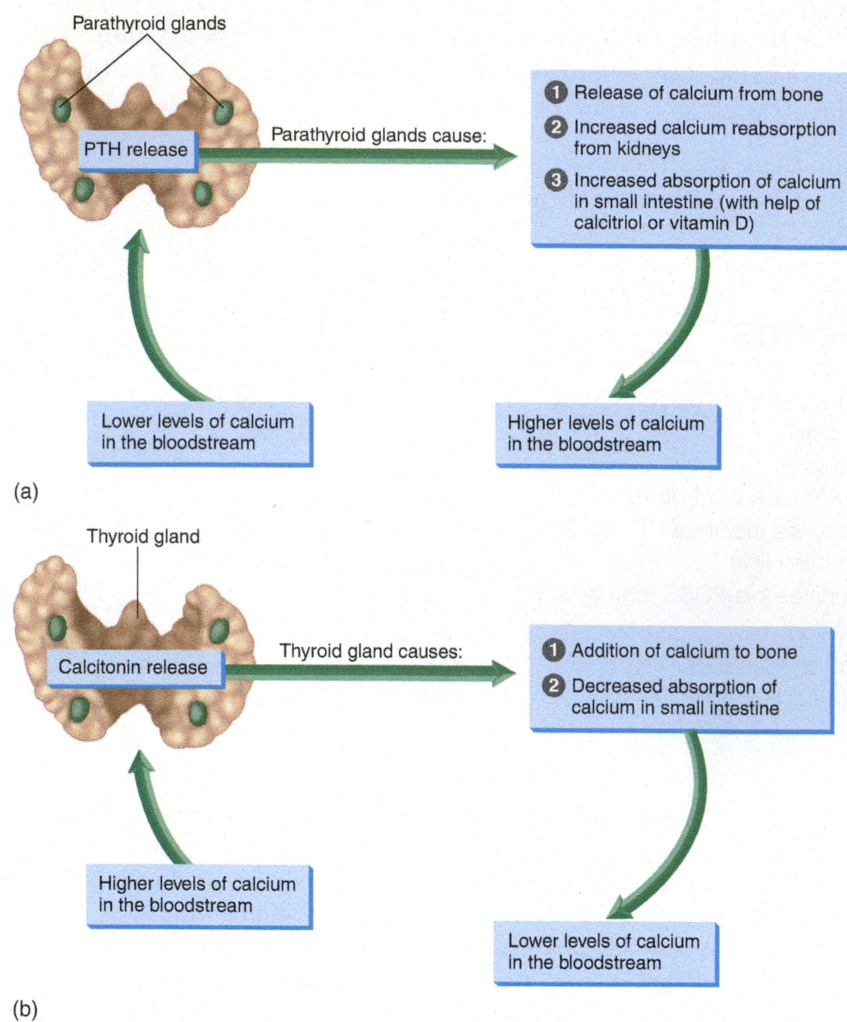

FIGURE 36.1 (a) Parathyroid hormone (PTH); (b) calcitonin action.

hyper = *elevated*
hypo = *lowered*
calc = *calcium*
emia = *blood level*

The importance of proper calcium balance in the body cannot be overstated. Calcium ions influence the excitability of all neurons. When calcium concentrations are too high (hypercalcemia), sodium permeability decreases across cell membranes. This is dangerous because nerve conduction depends on the proper influx of sodium into cells. When calcium levels in the bloodstream are too low (hypocalcemia), cell membranes become hyperexcitable. If hypocalcemia becomes severe, seizures or muscle spasms may result. Calcium is also important for the normal functioning of other body processes such as blood coagulation and neurotransmitter release, and stability of the entire skeletal system.

HYPOCALCEMIA

Core Concept 36.2 ▶

Hypocalcemia is a serious condition that requires immediate therapy.

Hypocalcemia, or lowered levels of calcium in the blood, is associated with a range of conditions, including poor nutrition, seizures, muscle spasms, and endocrine and bone disorders. Hypocalcemia is not a disease, but a sign of underlying pathology; therefore, diagnosis of the cause of hypocalcemia is essential. One common cause is hyposecretion of PTH, which occurs when the thyroid and parathyroid glands are surgically removed. Digestive-related malabsorption disorders and vitamin D deficiencies also result in hypocalcemia. In cases of hypocalcemia, healthcare providers should assess for the adequate intake of calcium-containing foods. With hypocalcemia, numbness and tingling of the extremities may occur, and convulsions are possible. Symptoms of hypocalcemia are nerve and muscle excitability. Muscle twitching, tremor, or cramping may be evident. A patient may be confused or behave abnormally.

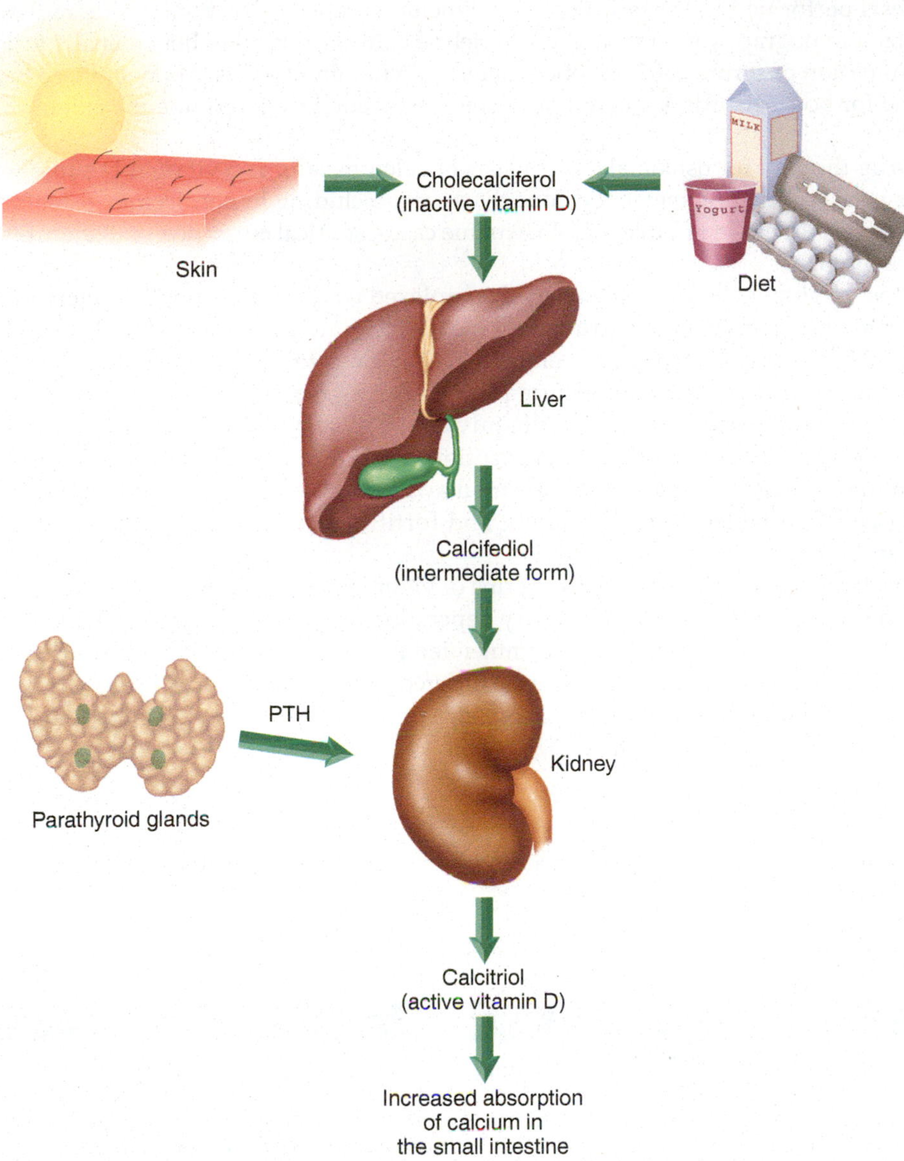

FIGURE 36.2 Pathway for vitamin D activation.

Therapies for calcium disorders involve calcium salts, vitamin D supplements, bisphosphonates, and miscellaneous drugs. Severe hypocalcemia requires IV administration of calcium salts, whereas less severe hypocalcemia can often be reversed with oral supplements.

OSTEOMALACIA AND RICKETS

Osteomalacia and rickets are successfully treated with calcium salts and vitamin D supplements

◀ Core Concept 36.3

Osteomalacia, referred to as *rickets* in children, is a metabolic bone disorder characterized by softening of bones without alteration of basic bone structure, although with noticeable deformities observed in the chest and leg areas. The cause of osteomalacia and rickets is a lack of vitamin D and calcium in the diet, usually as a result of kidney failure or malabsorption of calcium from the GI tract.

Signs and symptoms of osteomalacia include hypocalcemia, muscle weakness, muscle spasms, and diffuse bone pain, especially in the hip area. Patients may also experience pain in the arms, legs, and spinal column. Classic signs of rickets in children include bowlegs and a pigeon breast. Children may also develop a slight fever and become restless at night.

Tests performed to verify osteomalacia include bone biopsy; bone radiographs; computerized tomography (CT) scan of the vertebral column and other bone density tests; and determination of serum calcium, phosphate, and vitamin D levels. Many of these tests are routine for bone disorders and are performed as needed to determine the extent of bone health.

Drug therapy for osteomalacia consists of calcium salts and vitamin D supplements. Drugs used for treating metabolic bone disorders, including hypocalcemia, osteomalacia, and rickets, are shown in Table 36.1. In extreme cases, surgical correction of disfigured limbs may be required.

Most calcium salts are in the form of complexed calcium, meaning that elemental calcium is bound to an array of surrounding molecules. Calcium salts are often compared on the basis of their ability to release elemental calcium into the bloodstream. The supplement is more potent when the calcium product has a greater ability to release elemental calcium into the bloodstream. A milliequivalent (mEq) is the unit used to describe the amount of electrolyte available for absorption. Therefore, the higher the mEq, the more potent the calcium salt. Elemental calcium may be obtained from dietary sources such as dark green vegetables, canned salmon, and fortified products, including tofu, orange juice, and milk.

Inactive, intermediate, and active forms of vitamin D are also available. The amount of vitamin D a patient needs will often vary depending on how much he or she is exposed to sunlight. After age 70, the average recommended intake of vitamin D increases from 400 to 600 units per day. A laboratory test may be ordered to determine proper levels of vitamin D. Because vitamin D is needed to absorb calcium from the GI tract, many supplements combine vitamin D and calcium into a single tablet.

CONCEPT REVIEW 36.1

- Identify the major drug therapies used for hypocalcemia, osteomalacia, and rickets.

Table 36.1 Calcium Salts and Vitamin D Therapy

Drug	Route and Adult Dose	Remarks
CALCIUM SALTS (The higher the mEq, the more potent the calcium salt)		
calcium acetate (PhosLo)	PO: 1–2 g bid–tid	One gram calcium acetate equals 250 mg (12.6 mEq) elemental calcium; phosphate binder used to treat hypophosphatemia in kidney dialysis patients
calcium carbonate (Rolaids, Tums, others)	PO: 1–2 g bid–tid	One gram calcium carbonate equals 400 mg (20 mEq) elemental calcium
calcium chloride	IV: 0.5–1 g by slow infusion (1 mL/min)	One gram calcium chloride equals 272 mg (13.6 mEq) elemental calcium; may be irritating to body tissues
calcium citrate (Citracal)	PO: 1–2 g bid–tid	One gram calcium citrate equals 210 mg (12 mEq) elemental calcium
calcium gluconate (Kalcinate)	PO: 1–2 g bid–tid IV: 0.5–4 g by slow infusions (1 g/hour)	One gram calcium gluconate equals 90 mg (4.5 mEq) elemental calcium
calcium lactate (Cal-Lac)	PO: 100–200 mg tid with meals	One gram calcium lactate equals 130 mg (6.5 mEq) elemental calcium
calcium phosphate tribasic (Posture)	PO: 1–2 g bid–tid	One gram calcium phosphate equals 390 mg (19.3 mEq) elemental calcium
VITAMIN D SUPPLEMENTS		
Pr calcitriol (Calcijex, Rocaltrol)	PO: 0.25 mcg/day IV: 0.5 mcg three times per week at the end of dialysis	For hypocalcemia in chronic renal failure and with hypoparathyroidism
doxercalciferol (Hectorol)	PO: 10 mcg, three times per week (max: 60 mcg/week) IV: 4 mcg, three times per week at the end of dialysis (max: 18 mcg/week)	For hyperparathyroidism in patients with chronic kidney disease or in patients on dialysis
ergocalciferol (Calciferol, Drisdol)	PO: 25–125 mcg/day for 6–12 weeks	For osteomalacia; also used for vitamin D-dependent rickets and hypoparathyroidism
paricalcitol (Zemplar)	PO: 1 mcg/day or 4 mcg three times per week IV: 0.04–0.1 mcg/kg, every other day during dialysis (max: 24 mcg/kg)	For the prevention and treatment of hyperparathyroidism in patients with chronic kidney disease

Prototype Drug: *Calcium salts*

Therapeutic Class: Calcium supplement for hypoparathyroidism, osteoporosis, and rickets
Pharmacologic Class: Reverses hypocalcemia

Actions and Uses: Calcium salts are used to correct hypocalcemia and to treat osteoporosis and rickets. The objective of calcium therapy is to return serum levels of calcium to normal. People at high risk for developing these conditions include postmenopausal women, those with little physical activity over a prolonged period, and patients taking certain medications such as corticosteroids, immunosuppressive drugs, and some antiseizure medications.

Adverse Effects and Interactions: The most common adverse effect of calcium salts is hypercalcemia, which is brought on by taking too much of these supplements. Symptoms include drowsiness, lethargy, weakness, headache, anorexia, nausea and vomiting, increased urination, and thirst. IV administration of calcium may cause hypotension, bradycardia, dysrhythmia, and cardiac arrest.

When taking other medications, patients should wait for at least 1 hour before taking calcium supplements or medications such as Mylanta and Maalox. Magnesium antacids or supplements may compete with GI absorption. Calcium salts taken with cardiac glycosides increases the risk of dysrhythmias. Calcium decreases the absorption of tetracyclines.

Prototype Drug: *Calcitriol (Calcijex, Rocaltrol)*

Therapeutic Class: Drug for osteoporosis, osteomalacia, and rickets
Pharmacologic Class: Vitamin D, reverses hypocalcemia

Actions and Uses: Calcitriol is the active form of vitamin D and is available in both oral and IV formulations. It promotes the intestinal absorption of calcium and elevates serum levels of calcium. This medication is used when patients have impaired kidney function or have hypoparathyroidism. Calcitriol reduces bone resorption and is useful in treating rickets. The effectiveness of calcitriol depends on the patient receiving an adequate amount of calcium; therefore, it is usually prescribed in combination with calcium supplements.

Adverse Effects and Interactions: Common adverse effects include hypercalcemia, headache, weakness, dry mouth, thirst, increased urination, and muscle or bone pain. Thiazide diuretics may increase the effects of vitamin D, causing hypercalcemia. Too much vitamin D may cause dysrhythmias in patients who are receiving cardiac glycosides. Magnesium antacids or supplements should not be given together with calcitriol because of the increased risk of hypermagnesemia.

OSTEOPOROSIS

Treatment for osteoporosis includes calcitonin, selective estrogen-receptor modulators, and bisphosphonates.

◀ Core Concept 36.4

Osteoporosis is the most common metabolic bone disorder. This disorder is usually asymptomatic until the bones become brittle enough to fracture or a vertebra collapses. In some cases, a lack of dietary calcium and vitamin D contribute to bone deterioration. In other cases, osteoporosis is due to disrupted bone homeostasis.

Simply stated, the homeostatic imbalance with osteoporosis is that bone resorption outpaces bone deposition, and patients begin to develop weak bones. This is generally considered an aging disorder. Following are the risk factors for osteoporosis:

- Postmenopausal status
- High alcohol or caffeine consumption
- Anorexia nervosa
- Tobacco use
- Physical inactivity
- Testosterone deficiency, particularly in older men
- Lack of adequate vitamin D or calcium in the diet
- Drugs such as corticosteroids, some anticonvulsants, and immunosuppressants that lower calcium levels in the bloodstream.

The most common risk factor associated with the development of osteoporosis is the onset of menopause. When women reach menopause, estrogen secretion declines and bones become weak and fragile. One theory to explain this occurrence is that normal levels of estrogen may limit the lifespan of osteoclasts, the bone cells that resorb bone. When estrogen levels become low, osteoclast activity is no longer controlled, and bone demineralization accelerates, resulting in loss of bone density. In women with osteoporosis, fractures often occur in the hips, wrists, forearms, or spine. The metabolism of calcium in osteoporosis is illustrated in Figure 36.3.

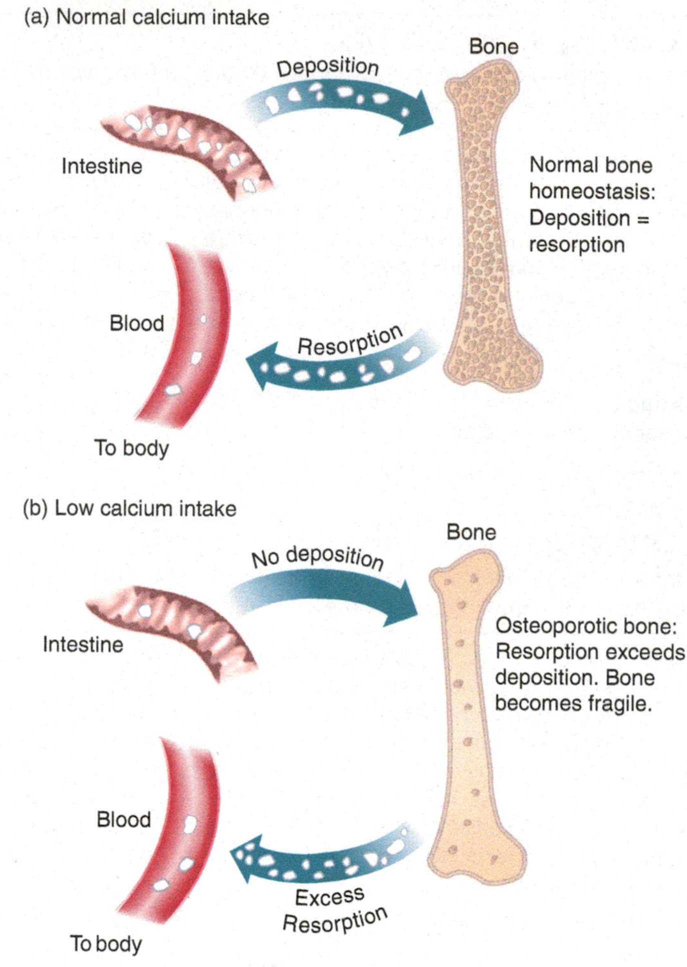

FIGURE 36.3 Calcium metabolism in osteoporosis: (a) bone deposition equals bone resorption; (b) bone resorption outpaces bone deposition.

Many drug therapies are available for osteoporosis. These include calcium and vitamin D therapy, hormone therapy with estrogen, estrogen-receptor modulators, calcitonin, statins, slow-release sodium fluoride, and bisphosphonates. Many of these drug classes are also used for other bone disorders or conditions unrelated to the skeletal system. Selected drugs for osteoporosis and related bone disorders are listed in Table 36.2.

Calcitonin

Calcitonin is a naturally occurring hormone secreted by the thyroid gland when blood calcium becomes elevated. It is involved in the process of bone building by opposing the effects of the PTH and inhibiting osteoclast activity in the bone. As a medication, calcitonin is obtained from salmon and is approved for the treatment of osteoporosis in women who are more than 5 years postmenopausal. It is available by nasal spray or subcutaneous injection. Calcitonin increases bone density and reduces the risk of vertebral fractures. Adverse effects are generally minor; the nasal formulation may irritate the nasal mucosa and allergies are possible. Parenteral forms may produce nausea and vomiting. In addition to treating osteoporosis, calcitonin is indicated for Paget disease and hypercalcemia.

Selective Estrogen-Receptor Modulators

Selective estrogen-receptor modulators (SERMs) bind to estrogen receptors and comprise a class of drugs used in the prevention and treatment of osteoporosis. SERMs may be estrogen agonists or antagonists, depending on the specific drug and the tissue involved. In the uterus and breasts, raloxifene (Evista) blocks estrogen receptors; thus, it has no estrogen-like proliferative effects on these tissues that might promote cancer. It is one of the few drugs available for the prevention of breast cancer in postmenopausal women at high risk for the disease. Evista decreases bone resorption, thus increasing bone density and making fractures less likely. Like estrogen, it has a cholesterol-lowering effect.

Table 36.2 Bone Resorption Inhibitors and Selected Drugs

Drug	Route and Adult Dose	Remarks
BIOLOGIC THERAPIES		
bazedoxifene with conjugated estrogens (Duavee)	PO: 20 mg/0.45 mg (1 tablet) daily	Newer drug to prevent osteoporosis that combines a selective estrogen-receptor modulator with estrogens
calcitonin–salmon (Fortical, Miacalcin)	Hypercalcemia: Subcutaneous/IM: calcitonin-salmon, 4 units/kg bid Osteoporosis: Intranasal: 1 spray/day (200 international units) in one nostril, alternating nostrils each day	Calcium regulating hormone; for hypercalcemia and postmenopausal osteoporosis
cinacalcet (Sensipar)	PO: Start with 30 mg once daily; may increase until target PTH of 150–300 mg/mL (max: 300/day)	For secondary hyperparathyroidism
denosumab (Prolia, Xgeva)	Subcutaneous (Prolia): 60 mg every 6 months	For postmenopausal osteoporosis in women at high risk for fracture (Prolia) or prevention of skeletal-related adverse events in patients with bone metastases (Xgeva)
Pr raloxifene (Evista)	PO: 60 mg daily	Selective estrogen-receptor modulator (SERM); for prevention and treatment of osteoporosis in postmenopausal women and breast cancer prophylaxis
teriparatide (Forteo)	Subcutaneous: 20 mcg/day	PTH (rDNA origin); for osteoporosis in postmenopausal women; for male patients with high risk of fractures
BISPHOSPHONATES		
Pr alendronate (Fosamax)	Osteoporosis treatment: PO: 10 mg daily; Osteoporosis prevention: PO: 5 mg daily; Paget disease: PO 40 mg daily for 6 months	For osteoporosis in men and women; for Paget disease
etidronate (Didronel)	PO: 5–10 mg/kg daily for 6 months or 11–20 mg/kg daily for 3 months	For Paget disease
ibandronate (Boniva)	PO: 2.5 mg daily or 150 mg once monthly	For treatment and prevention of postmenopausal osteoporosis
pamidronate (Aredia)	IV: 30–90 mg infused over 4–24 hours	For Paget disease and hypercalcemia of malignancy
risedronate (Actonel)	PO: 5 mg daily or 35 mg once weekly or 75 mg daily for 2 consecutive weeks	For prevention and treatment of osteoporosis and Paget disease
tiludronate (Skelid)	PO: 400 mg daily taken with 6–8 ounces of water 2 hours before or after food for 3 months	For Paget disease
zoledronate (Reclast, Zometa): also called zoledronic acid	IV: 4–5 mg, may be repeated in 7 days	For hypercalcemia; treatment of steroid-induced or postmenopausal osteoporosis, bone metastases, and Paget disease

Prototype Drug: Pr *Raloxifene (Evista)*

Therapeutic Class: Treatment of postmenopausal osteoporosis in women

Pharmacologic Class: Bone resorption inhibitor, selective estrogen-receptor modulator

Actions and Uses: Raloxifene is a SERM. It decreases bone resorption and increases bone mass and density by acting through the estrogen receptor. Raloxifene is primarily used for the prevention of osteoporosis in postmenopausal women. It is also one of the few drugs used for the prevention of breast cancer in women at high risk for invasive breast cancer. This drug also reduces serum total cholesterol and low-density lipoprotein (LDL) without lowering high-density lipoprotein (HDL) or triglycerides.

Adverse Effects and Interactions: Common adverse effects are hot flashes, migraine headache, flu-like symptoms, endometrial disorder, breast pain, and vaginal bleeding. Patients should not take cholesterol-lowering drugs or estrogen replacement therapy concurrently with this medication.

Absorption is reduced by cholestyramine. Patients taking raloxifene, along with warfarin, should have their prothrombin time (PT) and international normalized ratio (INR) tested when starting or stopping this medication

BLACK BOX WARNING:
Raloxifene increases the risk of venous thromboembolism and death from strokes. Women with a history of venous thromboembolism should not take this drug.

Bisphosphonates

The most common drug class used to treat osteoporosis is the **bisphosphonates**. These drugs are very similar to pyrophosphate, a natural inhibitor of bone resorption. Bisphosphonates inhibit bone resorption by suppressing osteoclast activity, thereby increasing bone density and reducing the incidence of fractures. Examples include alendronate (Fosamax), etidronate

(Didronel), ibandronate (Boniva), pamidronate (Aredia), risedronate (Actonel, Atelvia), tiludronate (Skelid), and zoledronate (Reclast, Zometa). Although primarily used to treat osteoporosis in postmenopausal women, drugs in this class are also used to treat Paget disease, osteoporosis in men, hypercalcemia and metastases due to bone cancer, multiple myeloma, and breast cancer. Adverse effects include GI problems such as nausea, vomiting, abdominal pain, and esophageal irritation; therefore, patients are advised to remain in an upright position for 30 minutes after taking these medications. All the bisphosphonates carry a warning that they may rarely cause osteonecrosis, a complete and irreversible destruction of the jawbone. Because these drugs are poorly absorbed, they should be taken on an empty stomach, as tolerated by the patient. Once-weekly dosing may give the same bone-density benefits as daily dosing because of these drugs' extended duration of action.

CONCEPT REVIEW 36.2

- What are the major drug therapies used for the treatment of osteoporosis and related bone disorders?

Prototype Drug: Pr *Alendronate (Fosamax)*

Therapeutic Class: Drug for osteoporosis **Pharmacologic Class:** Bone resorption inhibitor, bisphosphonate

Actions and Uses: Alendronate is approved for the following indications: prevention of osteoporosis in postmenopausal women, treatment of glucocorticoid-induced osteoporosis in both women and men, to increase bone mass in men with osteoporosis, and treatment of symptomatic Paget disease in both women and men. Alendronate is also used off-label for treating hypercalcemia due to malignancy. Therapeutic effects may take from 1 to 3 months to appear and may continue for several months after therapy is discontinued. All doses must be taken on an empty stomach, preferably in a fasting state 2 hours before breakfast.

Adverse Effects and Interactions: Common adverse effects of alendronate are diarrhea, nausea, vomiting, esophageal irritation, and a metallic or altered taste perception. Pathologic fractures may occur if the drug is taken longer than 3 months. Calcium supplements may decrease absorption of alendronate; therefore, use of these drugs together should be avoided. Food–drug interactions are common. Milk and other dairy products and medications, such as calcium, iron, antacids, and other mineral supplements, must be reviewed before beginning bisphosphonate therapy because they have the potential to decrease the effectiveness of bisphosphonates. Blood levels of the enzyme alkaline phosphatase are lowered with this drug.

Nursing Process Focus Patients Receiving Pharmacotherapy for Osteoporosis

ASSESSMENT	POTENTIAL NURSING DIAGNOSES*
Prior to administration: • Obtain a complete health history, including musculoskeletal, GI, cardiovascular, neurologic, thyroid, parathyroid, renal, and liver conditions; allergies; drug history; and possible drug interactions. • Evaluate laboratory blood findings: complete blood count (CBC), electrolytes, lipid panel, T_3, T_4 and TSH, and renal and liver function studies. Vitamin D levels may be obtained. • Acquire the results of a complete physical examination, including vital signs, height, and weight. • Collect a dietary history, noting adequacy of essential vitamins, minerals, and nutrients obtained through food sources. • Obtain a history of current symptoms and effect on activities of daily living (ADLs).	• *Deficient Knowledge* related to a lack of information about drug therapy • *Infective Health Maintenance* related to lifestyle changes or adverse drug effects • *Risk for Injury* related to disease process and adverse drug effects • *Risk of Falls* related to disease process and adverse drug effects

PLANNING: PATIENT GOALS AND EXPECTED OUTCOMES

The patient will:
- Experience therapeutic effects (a gain or maintenance of adequate bone density).
- Be free from or experience minimal adverse effects from drug therapy.
- Verbalize understanding of the drug's use, adverse effects, and required precautions.

IMPLEMENTATION	
Interventions and (Rationales)	**Patient Education/Discharge Planning**
• Administer medication correctly, and evaluate the patient's knowledge of proper administration. (Incorrect use may decrease absorption of medication.)	Instruct the patient: • About the proper administration method guidelines. • That bisphosphonates should be taken on an empty stomach, and to remain in a sitting position after taking medication.
• Review dietary history and discuss food source options, correcting any calcium and vitamin D deficiencies. (Adequate amounts of calcium, vitamin D, and magnesium are needed for bone health. If taking bisphosphonates, a review of foods and medications should be done because calcium-rich foods, medication, and supplements may decrease absorption of bisphosphonates.)	Inform the patient: • To consume adequate amounts of calcium, vitamin D, and magnesium from food. • That milk and other calcium-rich foods and medications (such as antacids and calcium supplements) must be reviewed before beginning bisphosphonate therapy.
• Monitor for adverse effects of medications. Bisphosphonates may cause GI irritation. SERMs increase the risk of venous thromboembolism and death from strokes. (Women with a history of thrombosis should not take this medication.)	Inform the patient that: • Bisphosphonates may cause esophageal and gastric irritation, abdominal pain, and nausea; to report immediately the onset of nausea or abdominal pain to the healthcare provider. • SERMs may cause hot flashes, migraines, flu-like symptoms, endometrial problems, breast pain, and increase the risk of forming blood clots. Discontinue 3 days prior to surgery. • Intranasal administration of calcitonin may cause nasal irritation and allergies.
• Review and monitor the use of other medications. (Concurrently using some medications with those used for osteoporosis may cause adverse effects or impact absorption.)	Instruct the patient: • Not to take cholesterol-lowering drugs or estrogen replacement therapy concurrently with SERMs. • If taking raloxifene along with warfarin, PT/INR should be tested when starting or stopping. • Calcium supplements should not be used with bisphosphonates.
• Continue to monitor periodic laboratory tests, especially calcium, magnesium, phosphorus, and creatinine. Assess for signs or symptoms of hypo- or hypercalcemia. (These electrolytes should remain or return to normal limits. Increased creatinine levels may require discontinuation of medication.)	Instruct the patient to: • Return periodically for laboratory tests. • Report any symptoms of hypocalcemia (muscle spasms, facial grimacing, tingling sensations of hands or feet) or hypercalcemia (increased bone pain, anorexia, nausea, vomiting, constipation, thirst, lethargy, or fatigue) to the healthcare provider.
• Increase fluid intake, avoiding caffeine, soda, and alcohol. (Some kidney stones are composed of calcium; increasing fluid intake decreases the risk of kidney stone formation. Caffeine diminishes the absorption of calcium.)	Instruct the patient to: • Increase fluid intake to 2 L/day. • Avoid excessive caffeine because it diminishes the absorption of calcium. • Limit or eliminate alcohol.
• Monitor for compliance with recommended lifestyle, for example, diet, exercise, and medication regimen. (Bone remodeling occurs over several months. The patient may discontinue the drug because of perceived lack of results.)	Inform the patient: • To engage in weight-bearing exercises, three to five times a week. • To acquire a minimum of 5–30 minutes of daily sun exposure for vitamin D synthesis. • That the therapeutic effects of the medication(s) may take 1 to 3 months and to continue taking the drug as prescribed to ensure full effect.

EVALUATION OF OUTCOME CRITERIA

Evaluate the effectiveness of drug therapy by confirming that patient goals and expected outcomes have been met (see "Planning"). *See Table 36.2 for a list of drugs to which these nursing actions apply.*

PAGET DISEASE

Core Concept 36.5 ▶

Treatment for Paget disease includes biologic therapies and bisphosphonates.

Paget disease, or *osteitis deformans*, is a chronic, progressive condition characterized by enlarged and abnormal bones. This condition is among the most common metabolic bone disorders. With this disorder, the processes of bone resorption and bone formation occur at a high rate. Excessive bone turnover causes the new bone to be weak and brittle, which may result in deformity and fractures. The patient may be asymptomatic or have only vague, nonspecific complaints for many years. Symptoms include pain of the hips and femurs, joint inflammation, headaches, facial pain, and hearing loss if bones around the ear cavity are affected. Nerves along the spinal column may be pinched in the compressed vertebrae.

Paget disease is sometimes confused with osteoporosis because some of the symptoms are similar. In fact, medical treatments for osteoporosis are similar to those for Paget disease. The cause of Paget disease, however, is quite different. Blood levels of the enzyme alkaline phosphatase are elevated because of the extensive bone turnover. Detection of this enzyme in the blood often provides early confirmation of the disease. Calcium blood levels are also increased. The symptoms of Paget disease can be treated successfully when diagnosis is made early. If the diagnosis is made late in the disease's progression, permanent skeletal abnormalities may develop, and other disorders may appear, including arthritis, kidney stones, and heart disease.

Bisphosphonates are the preferred pharmacotherapy for Paget disease. Therapy is usually cyclic: Bisphosphonates are administered until serum alkaline phosphatase levels return to normal; then a drug-free period of several months follows. When serum alkaline phosphatase levels become elevated, therapy is begun again. The pharmacologic goals are to slow the rate of bone reabsorption and encourage the deposition of strong bone. Calcitonin nasal spray is used as an option for patients who cannot tolerate bisphosphonates. Surgery may be indicated in cases of severe bone deformity, degenerative arthritis, or fracture. Patients with Paget disease should receive adequate daily dietary intake of calcium and vitamin D. Sufficient exposure to sunlight is also important.

CONCEPT REVIEW 36.3

- Identify two important disorders characterized by weak and fragile bones. What are the major drug therapies used in their treatments?

OSTEOARTHRITIS

Core Concept 36.6 ▶

Analgesics and anti-inflammatory drugs are important components of pharmacotherapy for osteoarthritis.

Arthritis is a general term meaning inflammation of a joint. There are several types of arthritis, each having somewhat different characteristics based on the etiology. Because joint pain is common to both metabolic bone and joint disorders, analgesics and anti-inflammatory drugs are important components of pharmacotherapy. A few additional drugs are specific to the particular pathologies.

osteo = *bone*
arthr = *joint*
itis = *associated disease, often linked with inflammation*

Osteoarthritis (OA) is a degenerative disease in which the cartilage at articular joint surfaces wears away. Like osteoporosis, this condition is considered to be an aging disorder. It is not accompanied by the degree of inflammation associated with other forms of arthritis. Signs are localized pain and stiffness, joint and bone enlargement, and limitations in movement. The cause of OA is thought to be excessive wear and tear of weight-bearing joints; the knee, spine, and hip are particularly affected.

The goals of pharmacotherapy for OA include reduction of pain and inflammation. The initial treatment of choice is acetaminophen. This drug should be used cautiously in geriatric patients and patients with chronic renal failure. For patients whose pain is unrelieved or untreatable by acetaminophen, nonsteroidal anti-inflammatory drugs (NSAIDs), including naproxen and ibuprofen, are usually given. Tramadol (Ultram) is a non-NSAID option for the treatment of moderate to severe pain. Although classified as an opioid, tramadol does

CAM Therapy | Glucosamine and Chondroitin for Osteoarthritis

Glucosamine sulfate is a natural substance that is an important building block of cartilage. With aging, glucosamine is lost with the natural thinning of cartilage. As cartilage wears down, joints lose their normal cushioning ability, resulting in the pain and inflammation of OA. Glucosamine sulfate is available as an OTC dietary supplement. Some studies have shown it to be more effective than a placebo in reducing mild arthritis and joint pain. It is claimed to promote cartilage repair in the joints. Although reliable long-term studies are not available, glucosamine is marketed as a safe and inexpensive alternative to prescription anti-inflammatory drugs.

Chondroitin sulfate is another dietary supplement claimed to promote cartilage repair. It is a natural substance that forms part of the matrix between cartilage cells. Chondroitin is usually combined with glucosamine in specific arthritis formulas.

not have abuse potential and is not a scheduled drug. Opioids such as codeine may be combined with acetaminophen for severe pain.

Many patients with OA use over-the-counter (OTC) topical creams, gels, sprays, patches, or ointments that include salicylates (Aspercreme and Sportscreme), capsaicin (Capzasin), and counterirritants (Ben-Gay and Icy Hot). These therapies are well tolerated and produce few adverse effects. Pennsaid is a prescription, topical form of the NSAID diclofenac that is rubbed on the knee for symptoms of OA.

One approach to treating patients with moderate OA who do not respond adequately to analgesics is sodium hyaluronate (Hyalgan), a chemical normally found in high amounts within synovial fluid. Administered by injection directly into the knee joint, this drug replaces or supplements the body's natural hyaluronic acid that deteriorated because of the inflammation of OA. By coating the articulating cartilage surface, Hyalgan helps provide a barrier that prevents friction and further inflammation of the joint.

RHEUMATOID ARTHRITIS

Immunosuppressants and disease-modifying drugs are additional therapies used to treat rheumatoid arthritis.

◀ **Core Concept 36.7**

rheuma = *watery discharge*
toid = *associated*

auto = *self-directed*
anti = *against*
bodies = *things*

Rheumatoid arthritis (RA) is a systemic autoimmune disorder that causes disfigurement and inflammation of multiple joints that usually occurs at an earlier age than OA. RA is the second most common form of arthritis and has an autoimmune etiology. In RA, **autoantibodies**, called rheumatoid factors, activate other inflammatory substances called complement proteins and draw leukocytes into an area where they attack normal cells. This results in ongoing injury and formation of inflammatory fluid within the joints. Joint capsules, tendons, ligaments, and skeletal muscles may also be affected. Unlike OA, which causes local pain in affected joints, patients with RA may develop systemic manifestations that include infections, pulmonary disease, pericarditis, abnormal numbers of blood cells, and symptoms of metabolic dysfunction such as fatigue, anorexia, and weakness.

The goals for the pharmacotherapy of RA include management of pain and inflammation and slowing the progress of the disease. The same classes of analgesics and anti-inflammatory drugs used to treat OA are used to manage RA. If inflammation is especially severe, short-term therapy with corticosteroids may be indicated (see Chapter 33).

Additional drugs are sometimes prescribed to manage the immune aspects of RA. Research has shown that the progression of tissue damage can be slowed by the use of **disease-modifying antirheumatic drugs (DMARDs)**. DMARDs may require several months of treatment before maximum therapeutic effects are achieved. Because many of these drugs can be toxic, patients should be closely monitored. Adverse effects vary depending on the type of drug. There are many DMARDs available, and these drugs are listed in Table 36.3.

Pharmacotherapy for RA occurs in a stepwise manner. Patients who have mild to moderate disease start on monotherapy with a nonbiologic DMARD, usually hydroxychloroquine (Plaquenil), methotrexate (Rheumatrex, Trexall), leflunomide (Arava), or sulfasalazine (Azulfidine). If symptoms have not improved or have worsened after 3 months of

Table 36.3 Disease-Modifying Antirheumatic Drugs (DMARDs)

Drug	Route and Adult Dose	Remarks
NONBIOLOGIC THERAPIES		
azathioprine (Azasan, Imuran)	PO: 1–2.5 mg/kg/day once or in divided doses bid	Immunosuppressant and anti-inflammatory; may cause bone marrow depression
Pr hydroxychloroquine (Plaquenil)	PO: 400–600 mg/day	Also used for acute malaria and malaria suppression
leflunomide (Arava)	PO: loading dose: 100 mg/day for 3 days then 10–20 mg daily	Immunomodulator with anti-inflammatory effects; may cause Stevens–Johnson syndrome
methotrexate (Rheumatrex, Trexall) (see the Prototype Drug box in Core Concept 29.8)	PO: 7.5 mg once/wk or 2.5–5 mg every 12 hours for three doses each week (max 20 mg/week)	Folic acid blocker; antineoplastic and immunosuppressant; may cause liver toxicity, sudden death, and pulmonary fibrosis
sulfasalazine (Azulfidine)	PO: 1–2 g daily in divided doses (max: 8 g/day)	Also for ulcerative colitis
BIOLOGIC THERAPIES (BIOLOGIC RESPONSE MODIFIERS)		
abatacept (Orencia)	IV: 500–1000 mg given on 0, 2, and 4 weeks, then every 4 weeks thereafter	Immune modulating drug; inhibits T lymphocyte activation
adalimumab (Humira)	Subcutaneous: 40 mg every other week	Tumor necrosis factor blocker
anakinra (Kineret)	Subcutaneous: 100 mg per day	Interleukin-1 receptor blocker
certolizumab pegol (Cimzia)	Subcutaneous: 400 mg initially and at weeks 2 and 4, followed by 200 mg every other week	Tumor necrosis factor blocker
etanercept (Enbrel)	Subcutaneous: 25 mg twice weekly; or 0.08 mg/kg or 50 mg once weekly	Tumor necrosis factor blocker
golimumab (Simponi)	Subcutaneous: 50 mg once monthly	Injectable man-made protein that binds to tumor necrosis factor and blocks its action
infliximab (Remicade)	IV: 3 mg/kg followed by 3 mg/kg 2 weeks and 6 weeks after initial dose and then every 8 weeks	Tumor necrosis factor-alpha blocker used in combination with methotrexate
rituximab (Rituxan)	IV: 1000 mg every 2 weeks for a total of two doses (give a corticosteroid 30 minutes prior to treatment)	Also indicated for the treatment of non-Hodgkin lymphoma
tocilizumab (Actemra)	IV: 4–8 mg/kg every other week	Interleukin-6 receptor blocker
tofacitinib (Xeljanz)	PO: 5 mg bid	Inhibits an enzyme called janus kinase (JAK), which drives the inflammatory process in RA

monotherapy, a second DMARD is added to the regimen. A third DMARD may be added for patients with persistent disease.

Patients with severe RA or who have not responded to nonbiologic therapies may receive biologic therapies also called **biologic response modifiers**. These biologic agents, most of which are monoclonal antibodies, block steps in the inflammatory cascade, reduce joint inflammation, and slow the progression of joint damage. Adalimumab (Humira), etanercept (Enbrel), certolizumab (Cimzia), golimumab (Simponi), and infliximab (Remicade) are tumor necrosis factor (TNF) blockers. TNF is a naturally occurring cytokine produced by macrophages and activated T cells that mediates inflammation and modulates cellular immune responses. Combinations of biologic and nonbiologic agents may be necessary for some patients.

cyto = *cell*
kine = *mediator*

Prototype Drug: Pr *Hydroxychloroquine (Plaquenil)*

Therapeutic Class: Disease-modifying antirheumatic drug (DMARD), rheumatoid drug
Pharmacologic Class: Protein synthesis inhibitor, inhibitor of DNA and RNA polymerase

Actions and Uses: Hydroxychloroquine is prescribed for RA and lupus erythematosus in patients who have not responded well to other anti-inflammatory drugs. This drug relieves the severe inflammation characteristic of these disorders. For full effectiveness, hydroxychloroquine is most often prescribed with salicylates and glucocorticoids. This drug has also been used for prophylaxis and treatment of malaria.

Adverse Effects and Interactions: Adverse symptoms include GI disturbances, loss of hair, headache, and mood and mental changes. Hydroxychloroquine has possible ocular effects that include blurred vision, photophobia, diminished ability to read, and blacked out areas in the visual field.

Antacids with aluminum and magnesium may prevent absorption. This drug interferes with the patient's response to the rabies vaccine. Hydroxychloroquine may increase the risk of liver toxicity when administered with drugs that are toxic to the liver. It also may lead to increased digoxin levels. Alcohol use should be eliminated during therapy because it may increase the risk of liver toxicity.

Fast Facts **Arthritis and Joint Disorders**

- Between 20 million and 40 million patients in the United States are affected by OA.
- After age 40, more than 90% of the population has symptoms of OA in major weight-bearing joints. After 70 years of age, almost all patients have symptoms of OA.
- Of the world's population, 1% has RA, which most often affects patients between 30 and 50 years of age. Women are three to five times more likely to develop RA than men.
- Between 1% and 3% of the U.S. population is affected by gout. Most of the patients are men between the ages of 30 and 60. Women are more likely to be affected after menopause.

CONCEPT REVIEW 36.4

- Identify the major types of arthritis. What are the general differences between these disorders?

GOUT

Pharmacotherapy for gout requires drugs that control uric acid levels.

◀ **Core Concept 36.8**

Gout, a form of acute arthritis, is a metabolic disorder caused by the accumulation of uric acid in the bloodstream or joint cavities. This disorder is extremely painful. Gout occurs when excretion of uric acid by the kidneys is reduced. One metabolic step important to the pharmacotherapy of this disease is the conversion of hypoxanthine (part of the chemical structure of the genes found with the body's cells) to uric acid by the enzyme xanthine oxidase. An elevated blood level of uric acid is called *hyperuricemia*.

hyper = *elevated*
uric = *uric acid*
emia = *blood level*

Gout may be classified as primary or secondary. *Primary gout*, caused by genetic errors in uric acid metabolism, is most commonly observed in Pacific Islanders. *Secondary gout* is caused by diseases or drugs that increase the metabolic turnover of nucleic acids or that interfere with uric acid excretion. Examples of drugs that may cause gout include thiazide diuretics, aspirin, cyclosporine, and alcohol (when ingested on a chronic basis). Conditions that can cause secondary gout include diabetic ketoacidosis, kidney failure, and diseases associated with a rapid cell turnover, such as leukemia, hemolytic anemia, and polycythemia.

Acute gouty arthritis occurs when needle-shaped uric acid crystals accumulate in joints, resulting in red, swollen, and inflamed tissue. Attacks have a sudden onset; often occur at night; and may be triggered by diet, injury, or other stresses. Gouty arthritis most often occurs in the big toes, heels, ankles, wrists, fingers, knees, and elbows. About 90% of patients with gout are men.

NSAIDs are the preferred drugs for treating the pain and inflammation associated with acute gout attacks. Indomethacin (Indocin) and naproxen (Naprosyn) are NSAIDs that have been widely used for acute gout. Corticosteroids may be used to treat exacerbations of acute gout, particularly when the symptoms are in a single joint, and the medication can be delivered intra-articularly.

Uric acid-inhibiting drugs treat the gouty condition (Table 36.4). The use of colchicine (Colcrys) has declined, although it may still be prescribed for patients whose symptoms cannot be controlled with NSAIDs. Low doses may be prescribed for gout prophylaxis.

Most patients with acute gouty arthritis will experience subsequent attacks within 1 to 2 years after the first attack. Thus, long-term prophylactic therapy with drugs that lower serum uric acid is often initiated. This can be accomplished through three strategies.

One strategy to prevent hyperuricemia is to use **uricosurics**, drugs that increase the excretion of uric acid by blocking its reabsorption in the kidney. The uricosuric drugs used for gout prophylaxis include probenecid (Probalan) and sulfinpyrazone (Anturane).

uricos = *uric acid excretion*
urics = *impact on urination*

A second strategy for preventing hyperuricemia is to reduce the formation of uric acid. The traditional drug for gout prophylaxis, allopurinol (Lopurin, Zyloprim), blocks the enzyme xanthine oxidase, thus reducing the formation of uric acid. A newer antigout drug, febuxostat (Uloric), acts by the same mechanism as allopurinol but is safer for patients with renal impairment because it is not excreted by the kidneys.

Table 36.4 Drugs for Gout and Gouty Arthritis

Drug	Route and Adult Dose	Remarks
Pr allopurinol (Lopurin, Zyloprim)	PO (primary): 100 mg daily (max: 800 mg/day) PO (secondary): 200–800 mg daily	For both primary and secondary hyperuricemia and prevention of gout flare-up
colchicine (Colcrys)	PO: 0.5–1.2 mg followed by 0.5–0.6 mg every 1–2 hours until pain relief (max: 1.2 mg/day)	For acute gouty attack; may cause gastric upset at higher doses; IV form available
febuxostat (Uloric)	PO: 40–80 mg once daily	For management of chronic hyperuricemia in patients with gout
pegloticase (Krystexxa)	IV: 8 mg every 2 weeks	For chronic gout; enzyme that metabolizes uric acid
probenecid (Benemid, Probalan)	PO: 250 mg bid for 1 week; then 500 mg bid (max: 3 g/day)	For gout; also used as an adjunctive drug for penicillin or cephalosporin therapy
rasburicase (Elitek)	IV: 0.2 mg/kg over 30 minutes for up to 5 days	For management of plasma uric acid levels in pediatric patients with leukemia; recombinant urate-oxidase produced by a genetically modified *Saccharomyces cerevisiae* (yeast) strain; may cause hypersensitivity reactions
sulfinpyrazone (Anturane)	PO: 100–400 mg bid	For gout; also used for inhibition of platelet aggregation

A third strategy for preventing hyperuricemia is to convert uric acid to a less toxic form. Two drugs are available that act by this mechanism. Rasburicase (Elitek) is an enzyme produced through recombinant DNA technology that is used to reduce uric acid levels in patients who are receiving cancer chemotherapy. Approved in 2010, pegloticase (Krystexxa) is a synthetic enzyme that metabolizes uric acid to an inert substance. It is used to lower uric acid levels in patients with chronic gout who have not responded to conventional therapies.

CONCEPT REVIEW 36.5

- Identify drug therapies used to treat the major arthritic and joint disorders.

Prototype Drug: Pr *Allopurinol (Lopurin, Zyloprim)*

Therapeutic Class: Antigout drug **Pharmacologic Class:** Inhibitor of uric acid formation, xanthine oxidase blocker

Actions and Uses: Allopurinol reduces the production of uric acid, controlling the buildup of uric acid that causes severe gout. Therefore, it reduces the risk of acute gout attacks. It is also approved to prevent recurrent kidney stones in patients with elevated uric acid levels. It may be used prophylactically to reduce the severity of the elevated uric acid blood levels associated with antineoplastic and radiation therapies, both of which increase blood uric acid levels by promoting nucleic acid degradation. This drug takes 1 to 3 weeks to bring blood uric acid levels to within the normal range.

Adverse Effects and Interactions: The most frequent and serious adverse effects are skin rash and rare cases of fatal toxic epidermal necrolysis and Stevens–Johnson syndrome. Other possible adverse effects include drowsiness, headache, vertigo, nausea, vomiting, abdominal discomfort, malaise, diarrhea, retinopathy, and thrombocytopenia.

Alcohol may inhibit the renal excretion of uric acid. Ampicillin and amoxicillin may increase the risk of skin rashes. An enhanced anticoagulant effect may be seen with the use of warfarin. The risk of ototoxicity is increased when allopurinol is used with thiazides and angiotensin-converting enzyme (ACE) inhibitors. Aluminum antacids taken concurrently with allopurinol may decrease its effects. An increased effect may be seen with phenytoin and anticancer drugs, necessitating the need for altered doses of these medications.

Patients Need to Know

Patients taking drugs for bone or joint disorders need to know the following:

In General

1. When receiving treatment for problems with mobility, it often takes several weeks for effectiveness to begin. Follow the advice of a healthcare provider in order to achieve full therapeutic effect.

Regarding Calcium and Bone-Regulating Medications

2. When taking calcium or vitamin D supplements, be aware of the signs and symptoms of hypercalcemia. Check with the healthcare provider or pharmacist before taking supplements of any kind. In some cases, only proper diet and sunshine are needed for successful therapy.
3. Calcium may react with some foods or interfere with the absorption of iron and bisphosphonates.

4. Be familiar with the risks and long-term effects of vitamin D therapy, corticosteroids, hormone therapy involving estrogen, and estrogen-receptor modulators. Major undesirable adverse effects could occur in some cases.
5. Know how to use a nasal spray if taking calcitonin by this method.
6. Be aware that some vitamins may interfere with the pharmacologic effects of calcitonin.
7. Some medications cause GI discomfort. Most drugs like these can be taken after meals or with milk to minimize discomfort.

Regarding Arthritic and Joint-Related Medications

8. Report any unfavorable symptoms such as bone pain, restricted mobility, inflammation, or fracture to a healthcare provider. Report any muscle pain because muscles that have not been moved for a while may feel stiff and tender.
9. When taking some antigout medications, drink plenty of fluids to avoid kidney stones. To ensure proper fluid balance, monitor intake and output of fluids.
10. When taking probenecid, avoid taking aspirin because it interferes with the drug's action. Take acetaminophen instead.

Safety Alert: Soundalike Drug Names

Nurses need to counsel patients about ways to avoid a self-medication error when taking medications that are "soundalike" drugs, such as Celebrex and Celexa. Confusing drugs with similar names accounts for about approximately 10% of all medication errors, according to the U.S. Food and Drug Administration (FDA). Patients could ask the pharmacist to package the "soundalikes" in distinctly different containers or to label the bottles with large letters describing the drug's use, like PAIN PILL and ANTIDEPRESSANT.

Chapter Review

Core Concepts Summary

36.1 Adequate levels of calcium, vitamin D, parathyroid hormone, and calcitonin are necessary for bone and body homeostasis.

One of the most important minerals in the body responsible for proper nerve conduction, muscle contractions, and bone formation is calcium. Calcium homeostasis is controlled by two important hormones, PTH and calcitonin. These hormones influence major body targets: the bones, kidneys, and GI tract. They direct the processes of bone resorption and bone deposition. Active vitamin D increases calcium absorption from the GI tract and helps to keep proper calcium balance in the body.

36.2 Hypocalcemia is a serious condition that requires immediate therapy.

Hypocalcemia, or lowered calcium levels in the bloodstream, is a sign of an underlying disorder; therefore, identifying its cause is essential. Signs of hypocalcemia are nerve and muscle excitability, muscle twitching, tremor, or cramping. These conditions are often reversed with calcium salts. Calcium salts consist of complexed and elemental calcium. Elemental calcium is also obtained from dietary sources.

36.3 Osteomalacia and rickets are successfully treated with calcium salts and vitamin D supplements.

Osteomalacia, called rickets in children, is a disorder characterized by softening of bones without alteration of basic bone structure. Drug therapy for children and adults consists of calcium and vitamin D supplements.

36.4 Treatment for osteoporosis includes calcitonin, selective estrogen-receptor modulators, and bisphosphonates.

Osteoporosis, or weak bones caused by disrupted bone homeostasis, is the most common metabolic bone disease. The onset of menopause is the most frequent risk factor. Many drug therapies are available for this disorder, including calcium and vitamin D supplements, calcitonin, SERMs, and bisphosphonates.

36.5 Treatment for Paget disease includes biologic therapies and bisphosphonates.

Paget disease is a chronic progressive condition characterized by enlarged and abnormal bones. Although the cause of Paget disease is different from that of osteoporosis, medical treatments are similar. Bisphosphonates are drugs primarily used in the pharmacotherapy of this disorder.

36.6 Analgesics and anti-inflammatory drugs are important components of pharmacotherapy for osteoarthritis.

The initial pharmacotherapy goals for OA are to reduce pain and inflammation. Acetaminophen and NSAIDs may be taken. Tramadol and opioids may be combined with acetaminophen for severe pain. OTC topical creams, gels, sprays, patches, or ointments may be used. For patients with moderate OA who do not respond to analgesics, sodium hyaluronate may be applied.

36.7 Immunosuppressants and disease-modifying drugs are additional therapies used to treat rheumatoid arthritis.

RA is the second most common form of arthritis and has an autoimmune etiology. Pharmacotherapy for RA includes the same classes of analgesics and anti-inflammatory drugs, plus DMARDs and immunosuppressants.

36.8 Pharmacotherapy for gout requires drugs that control uric acid levels.

Gout is caused by an accumulation of uric acid in the bloodstream. Gout may be classified as a primary or secondary condition. Acute gouty arthritis occurs when needle-shaped uric acid crystals accumulate in the joints. The goals of gout pharmacotherapy include termination of acute attacks and prevention of future attacks with several approaches to control uric acid levels.

REVIEW Questions

Answer the following questions to assess your knowledge of the chapter material, and go back and review any material that is not clear to you.

1. There are many trade names for certain medications. The trade name of a medication that lowers serum alkaline phosphatase is:
   1. Azulfidine.
   2. Fosamax.
   3. Colchicine.
   4. Benemid.

2. The patient on raloxifene (Evista) has had warfarin (Coumadin) ordered. The nurse incorporates what laboratory test into the plan of care?
   1. Platelets
   2. White blood count
   3. Sodium
   4. Prothrombin time and international normalized ratio (PT/INR)

3. The patient taking calcitriol should be monitored for:
   1. Dysrhythmias.
   2. Hypercalcemia.
   3. Fluid overload.
   4. Flu-like symptoms.

4. For the patient diagnosed with gout, the nurse would most likely administer which medication?
   1. Calcitriol (Calcijex, Rocaltrol)
   2. Azathioprine (Imuran)
   3. Allopurinol (Lopurin, Zyloprim)
   4. Raloxifene (Evista)

5. Because esophageal irritation can occur, the nurse instructs the patient to remain in an upright position for 30 minutes after taking which medication?
   1. Allopurinol (Lopurin)
   2. Calcitonin
   3. Alendronate (Fosamax)
   4. Raloxifene (Evista)

6. A patient is about to begin taking calcitonin and asks if this drug has any adverse effects. The healthcare provider tells the patient that it may cause:
   1. Nasal irritation.
   2. Headaches.
   3. Watery eyes.
   4. Sinus infection.

7. A patient has been taking hydroxychloroquine (Plaquenil) for rheumatoid arthritis. Which of the following symptoms may be an adverse effect?
   1. Cardiac dysrhythmias
   2. Joint stiffness
   3. Blurred vision
   4. Decreased muscle strength

8. The nurse is speaking at the local community center about vitamin and mineral supplements. She tells the audience that a milliequivalent (mEq) is the unit used to describe the amount of electrolyte available to the bloodstream; the higher the mEq, the more potent the calcium salt. To demonstrate their new knowledge, the nurse has the group choose the calcium salts with the greatest potency. Which do they choose?
   1. Calcium chloride
   2. Calcium citrate

3. Calcium phosphate
4. Calcium gluconate

9. The nurse would include calcitonin in the plan of care for patients with: (Select all that apply.)
   1. Paget disease.
   2. Hypercalcemia.
   3. Hypocalcemia.
   4. Osteoporosis.
   5. Osteoarthritis.

10. The healthcare provider has ordered tocilizumab (Actemra), 5 mg/kg, to be given IV. The patient weighs 121 pounds and is to receive 275 mg in a 250 mL bag of solution to be delivered over 4 hours. How many milliliters will the patient receive in 1 hour?
    1. 60 mL
    2. 62 mL
    3. 61.5 mL
    4. 62.5 mL

CASE STUDY Questions

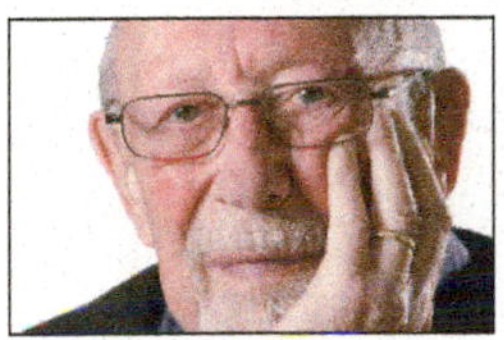

Remember Mr. Hurtt, the patient introduced at the beginning of the chapter? Now read the remainder of the case study. Based on the information you have learned in this chapter, answer the questions that follow.

Mr. Steven Hurtt is a 67-year-old white male. In an office visit, Mr. Hurtt complains of joint pain in the knees, ankles, toes, and shoulders. Over the last several years, he has taken aspirin for overall pain. Laboratory tests and physical examination yield the following information: small nodules found sporadically under the skin, acute swelling of the knees, redness of the big toe, and elevated uric acid and white blood cell (WBC) count in the blood. Mr. Hurtt is diagnosed with gouty arthritis and is prescribed allopurinol (Lopurin).

1. Mr. Hurtt asks how allopurinol works. The nurse explains that it works by:
   1. Decreasing the deposits of uric acid in the joint spaces.
   2. Reducing the pain associated with joint inflammation by uric acid crystals.
   3. Increasing renal excretion of uric acid.
   4. Reducing the production of uric acid.

2. Since Mr. Hurtt is starting on allopurinol, the nurse informs him that this medication has several possible adverse effects that he needs to know about. These effects include: (Select all that apply.)
   1. Headache.
   2. Vertigo.
   3. Toxic epidermal necrolysis.
   4. Skin rash.

3. Mr. Hurtt asks why he should avoid drinking alcohol while he is taking allopurinol. The nurse responds by telling him that alcohol:
   1. Significantly increases the drug levels of allopurinol.
   2. Interferes with the absorption of antigout medications.
   3. Raises uric acid levels.
   4. Causes the urine to become more alkaline.

4. Which of the following statements demonstrates that Mr. Hurtt needs additional instruction?
   1. "I will take my allopurinol as prescribed by my healthcare provider."
   2. "I will stop having alcoholic beverages."
   3. "I will avoid high purine foods."
   4. "I will continue taking my aspirin."

Answers and complete rationales for the Review and Case Study Questions appear in Appendix A.

REFERENCE

Herdman, T. H., & Kamitsuru, S. (Eds.). (2014). *NANDA International nursing diagnoses: Definitions and classification, 2015–2017.* Oxford, United Kingdom: Wiley-Blackwell.

SELECTED BIBLIOGRAPHY

Bethel, M. (2015). *Osteoporosis.* Retrieved from http://emedicine.medscape.com/article/330598-overview

Buch, M. H., & Emery, P. (2011). New therapies in the management of rheumatoid arthritis. *Current Opinion in Rheumatology, 23,* 245–251. doi:10.1097/BOR.0b013e3283454124

Centers for Disease Control and Prevention. (2015). *Gout.* Retrieved from http://www.cdc.gov/arthritis/basics/gout.html

Centers for Disease Control and Prevention. (2015). *Rheumatoid arthritis.* Retrieved from http://www.cdc.gov/arthritis/basics/rheumatoid.htm

Centers for Disease Control and Prevention. (2016). *Arthritis facts.* Retrieved from http://www.cdc.gov/arthritis/press/factsheet.htm

Centers for Disease Control and Prevention. (2016). *Arthritis-related statistics*. Retrieved from http://www.cdc.gov/arthritis/data_statistics/arthritis-related-stats.htm

Duque, G. (2013). Osteoporosis in older persons: Current pharmacotherapy and future directions. *Expert Opinion on Pharmacotherapy, 14*, 1949–1958. doi:10.1517/14656566.2013.822861

Gennari, L., Merlotti, D., Rendina, D., Gianfrancesco, F., Esposito, T., & Nuti, R. (2014). Paget's disease of bone: Epidemiology, pathogenesis and pharmacotherapy. *Expert Opinion on Orphan Drugs, 2*, 591–603. doi:10.1517/21678707.2014.904225

Islam, M. J., Yusuf, M. A., Hossain, M. S., & Ahmed, M. (2013). Updated management of osteoarthritis: A review. *Journal of Science Foundation, 11*, 49–55. doi:10.3329/jsf.v11i2.21597

Lawrence, R. C., Felson, D. T., Helmick, C. G., Arnold, L. M., Choi, H., Deyo, R. A., . . . National Arthritis Data Workgroup. (2012). Estimates of the prevalence of arthritis and other rheumatic conditions in the United States, Part II. *Arthritis and Rheumatism, 58*, 26–35. doi:10.1002/art.23176

Mayo Clinic. (n.d.). *Rheumatoid arthritis treatment*. Retrieved from http://www.mayoclinic.org/diseases-conditions/rheumatoid-arthritis/diagnosis-treatment/treatment/txc-20197400

National Institute of Arthritis and Musculoskeletal and Skin Diseases. (2016). *Handout on health: Rheumatoid arthritis*. Retrieved from http://www.niams.nih.gov/Health_Info/Rheumatic_Disease

National Osteoporosis Foundation. (n.d.). *Bone health basics: Get the facts*. Retrieved from https://www.nof.org/prevention/general-facts

Owens, G. M. (2015). Optimizing Rheumatoid Arthritis Therapy: Using Objective Measures of Disease Activity to Guide Treatment. *American Health and Drug Benefits, 8*, 354–360.

World Health Organization. (n.d.). *Chronic rheumatic conditions*. Retrieved from http://www.who.int/chp/topics/rheumatic/en

Chapter 37

Drugs for Skin Disorders

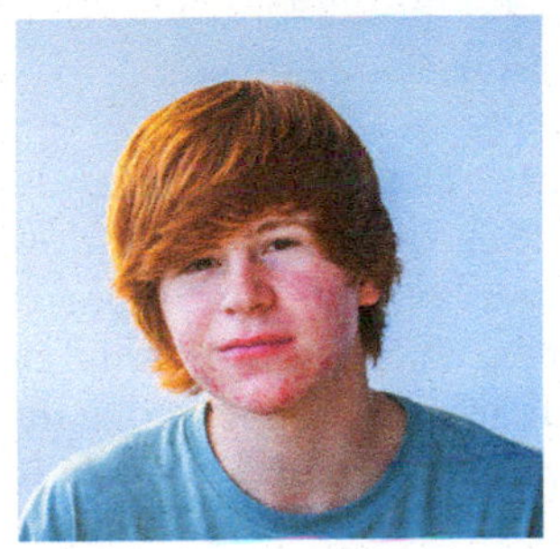

"I don't think I can go to the game this weekend. Can anything be done to get rid of these zits by Friday?"

Burt Nicholson

Core Concepts

37.1 **Layers of skin provide protection to the body.**

37.2 **The major causes of skin disorders are injury, aging, inherited factors, and other medical conditions.**

37.3 **Scabicides and pediculicides treat parasitic mite and lice infestations.**

37.4 **The goal of drug therapy for sunburn is to eliminate discomfort until healing occurs.**

37.5 **Acne and rosacea are treated by a combination of over-the-counter and prescription drugs.**

37.6 **Topical corticosteroids are used mainly to treat dermatitis and related symptoms.**

37.7 **Several topical and systemic medications are used to treat psoriatic symptoms.**

Drug Snapshot

The following drugs are discussed in this chapter:

Drug Classes	Prototype Drugs
DRUGS FOR SKIN PARASITES	
Scabicides and pediculicides	Pr permethrin (Acticin, Elimite, Nix)
DRUGS FOR SUNBURN AND MINOR SKIN IRRITATION	
Topical anesthetics	Pr benzocaine (Americaine, Anbesol, others)
DRUGS FOR ACNE AND ROSACEA	
Topical medications	Pr tretinoin (Avita, Retin-A, Tretin-X)
DRUGS FOR DERMATITIS AND ECZEMA	
DRUGS FOR PSORIASIS	

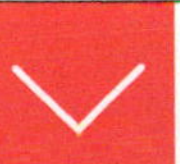

Learning Outcomes

After reading this chapter, the student should be able to:

1. Identify important skin layers, and explain how superficial skin cells must be replaced after they become damaged or lost.
2. Describe major symptoms associated with stress and injury to the skin versus those associated with a patient's changing age or health.
3. Describe popular treatments used in conjunction with available drug therapies to treat skin disorders, and identify the major actions, primary actions, and important adverse effects of the following types of drugs: scabicides, pediculicides, topical anesthetics, and topical medications, as well as antibiotics, retinoids, keratolytic agents, corticosteroids, emollients, and psoralens.

Key Terms

closed comedones (KOME-eh-dones)
dermatitis (dur-mah-TIE-tiss)
eczema (ECK-zih-mah)
emollients
erythema (ear-ih-THEE-mah)
keratinization (keh-RAT-en-eye zay-shun)
keratolytic agents (keh-RAT-oh-lih-tik)
open comedones
papules (PAP-yools)
pediculicides (puh-DIK-you-lih-sides)
pruritus (proo-RYE-tus)
psoralens (SOR-uh-lenz)
psoriasis
pustules (PUSS-chools)
retinoids (RETT-ih-noydz)
retinol (RETT-in-nall)
rosacea (roh-ZAY-shee-uh)
scabicides (SKAY-bih-sides)
scabies (SKAY-beez)
seborrhea (seb-oh-REE-ah)
urticaria (EHR-tik-air-ee-ah)

The integumentary system consists of the skin, hair, nails, sweat glands, and oil glands. The organ in the body with the largest surface area is the skin. It is considered a window to the body's health. The skin provides an effective barrier between extreme conditions of the outside environment and the body's internal tissues. At times, changes in external or internal conditions can damage the skin. When this happens, drug therapy can improve the skin's condition. The relationship between the integumentary system and other systems in the body is shown in Figure 37.1.

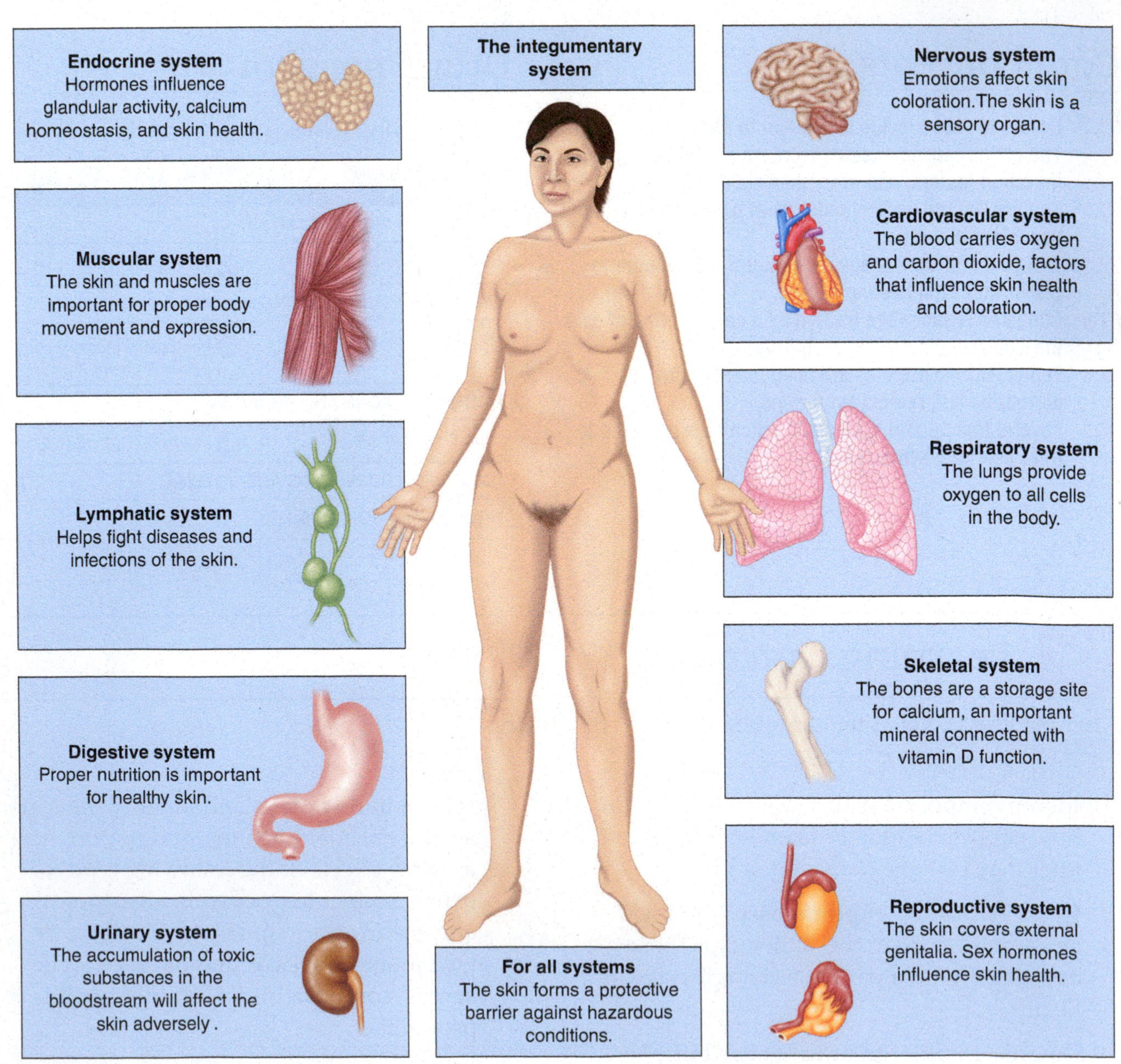

FIGURE 37.1 The integumentary system (skin) and how the other body systems affect it.

The purpose of this chapter is to examine the broad scope of skin disorders and the medications used for skin therapy. Particular attention is given to drugs that are of direct benefit to lice and mite infestations, sunburn, acne, inflammation, and dry, scaly skin.

Layers of skin provide protection to the body.

◀ **Core Concept 37.1**

epi = *on top of*
hypo = *below*
dermis = *the skin*
sub = *underneath*
cutaneous = *skin-related*

The integument has two major layers: the epidermis and the dermis. It also has a subcutaneous layer called the hypodermis. Each layer of the integument is distinct in form and function and determines how drugs are injected or applied to the surface of the skin (see Chapter 3).

The most superficial skin layer is the epidermis. Depending on its thickness, the epidermis has either four or five sublayers. The strongest and outermost sublayer is the stratum corneum, or horny layer. It is called this because of the abundance of the protein keratin, also found in the hair, hooves, and horns of many vertebrate mammals. Not every part of the skin has a large amount of keratin—only those areas that are subject to mechanical stress—for example, the soles of the feet and the palms of the hands.

The deepest sublayer of the epidermis is the stratum basale, also called the stratum germinativum. It supplies the epidermis with new cells after older superficial cells have been damaged or lost by normal wear. Cells must migrate over their lifetime to the outermost layers of the skin, where they eventually fall off. As these cells are pushed to the surface, they are flattened and covered with a water-insoluble material, forming a protective seal. The average time it takes for a cell to move from the basale layer to the outer body surface is about 3 weeks. Specialized cells called *melanocytes* within the deeper layers of the epidermis secrete the dark pigment melanin, which offers a degree of protection from the sun's ultraviolet rays.

The next major layer of skin, the dermis, is made up of dense, irregular connective tissue, which has an irregular arrangement of thick collagen fibers. The dermis provides a foundation for the epidermis and appendages such as hair and nails. Most receptor nerve endings, sweat glands, oil glands, and blood vessels are found within the dermis.

Below the dermis, the subcutaneous layer composed mainly of adipose tissue or fat cushions, insulates, and provides a source of energy for the body. The hypodermis is involved with maintaining homeostasis, regulating body temperature, and storing energy in the form of lipids.

The major causes of skin disorders are injury, aging, inherited factors, and other medical conditions.

◀ **Core Concept 37.2**

prur = *itching*
itus = *condition*

Skin that is dry, cracked, scaly, or inflamed represents a disturbance in the outermost skin layer. **Pruritus**, or itching, is a general symptom often associated with dry, scaly skin, or it may be a symptom of infestation with mites and lice. **Urticaria**, commonly referred to as *hives*, is recognized as raised, red, itchy bumps. Most commonly, urticaria is caused by an allergic reaction. Many drugs, especially antibiotics, can cause urticaria and pruritus as side effects. Although most drug allergies of the skin require only symptomatic treatment with over-the-counter (OTC) medications, some are severe. Toxic epidermal necrolysis (TEN) is a life-threatening drug reaction that results in massive death of skin cells and separation of the epidermis from the dermis.

Burns are a unique type of stress that may affect all layers of the skin. They are classified according to the degree of skin damage. First-degree burns affect only the outer layers of the epidermis, are characterized by redness, and are analogous to sunburn. Second-degree burns affect most of the epidermis and part of the dermis, resulting in inflammation and blisters. Third-degree burns are full-thickness burns; all layers of the skin are damaged. With full-thickness burns, the skin cannot regenerate, and skin grafting is required.

eryth = *red*
ema = *appears*

Inflammation, a characteristic of burns and other traumatic disorders, occurs when damage to the skin is extensive. Signs accompanying inflammation include **erythema** or redness, irritation, and pain. Symptoms including bleeding, bruises, and infections may accompany trauma to deeper tissues.

Not all skin disorders are associated with injury or infection. Many common skin disorders are related to inherited factors or the normal aging process. Sometimes the skin may appear unhealthy because of a disease process occurring in a different organ system, such as yellowing of the skin (jaundice) that occurs from liver damage. In many cases, the cause of the skin condition may be unknown. Common symptoms associated with a range of conditions are presented in Table 37.1. Although the causes and symptoms of skin conditions are very diverse, a simple method of classifying them is shown in Table 37.2.

Most skin conditions are not debilitating and require only intermittent drug therapy. A few irritating disorders are of particular importance to patients who require treatment on an outpatient basis. Examples include lice infestation, minor sunburn, and acne. Eczema, dermatitis, and psoriasis are more serious disorders requiring therapy for a longer time. Figure 37.2 shows examples of regions of the body where irritating symptoms most likely appear.

CONCEPT REVIEW 37.1

- Identify the skin layers protecting the body. Give examples of layers specifically affected by minor or major external stresses. What skin disorders are not related to the external environment? How would you categorize most skin disorders?

Table 37.1 Signs and Symptoms of Skin Conditions Associated with a Patient's Changing Health, Age, or Weakened Immune System

Symptom	Description
Delicate skin, wrinkles, and hair loss	Many degenerative changes occur in the skin; some are found in older patients; others are genetically related (fragile epidermis, wrinkles, reduced activity of oil and sweat glands, male pattern baldness, poor blood circulation); hair loss may also be linked to some medical procedures, such as radiation and chemotherapy.
Discoloration of the skin	Discoloration is often a sign of another medical disorder (for example, anemia, cyanosis, fever, jaundice, or Addison disease); some medications have photosensitive properties, making a patient's skin sensitive to the sun and causing erythema.
Scales, patches, and itchy areas	Some symptoms may be related to a combination of genetics, stress, and immunity; other symptoms may be related to a fast turnover of skin cells; some symptoms develop for unknown reasons.
Seborrhea, oily skin and bumps	Conditions are usually associated with a younger age group; examples include cradle cap in infants and an oily face, chest, arms, and back in teenagers and young adults; pustules, cysts, papules, and nodules represent lesions connected with oily skin.
Tumors	Tumors may be genetic or may occur because of exposure to harmful agents or conditions.
Warts, skin marks, and moles	Some skin marks are congenital; others are acquired or may be linked to environmental factors.

Table 37.2 Classification of Skin Disorders

Disorder	Example
Infectious disorders	Bacterial infections: boils, impetigo, and infected hair follicles Fungal infections: ringworm, athlete's foot, jock itch, and nail infections Parasitic infections: ticks, mites, and lice Viral infections: cold sores, fever blisters (herpes simplex), chickenpox, warts, shingles (herpes zoster), measles (rubeola), and German measles (rubella)
Inflammatory disorders	Injury and exposure to the sun Combination of overactive glands, increased hormone production, or infection such as acne and rosacea Disorders marked by itching, cracking, and discomfort, such as atopic dermatitis, contact dermatitis, seborrheic dermatitis, stasis dermatitis, and psoriasis.
Neoplastic	Malignant skin cancers: squamous cell carcinoma, basal cell carcinoma, and malignant melanoma (the most dangerous). Benign neoplasms: include keratosis and keratoacanthoma.

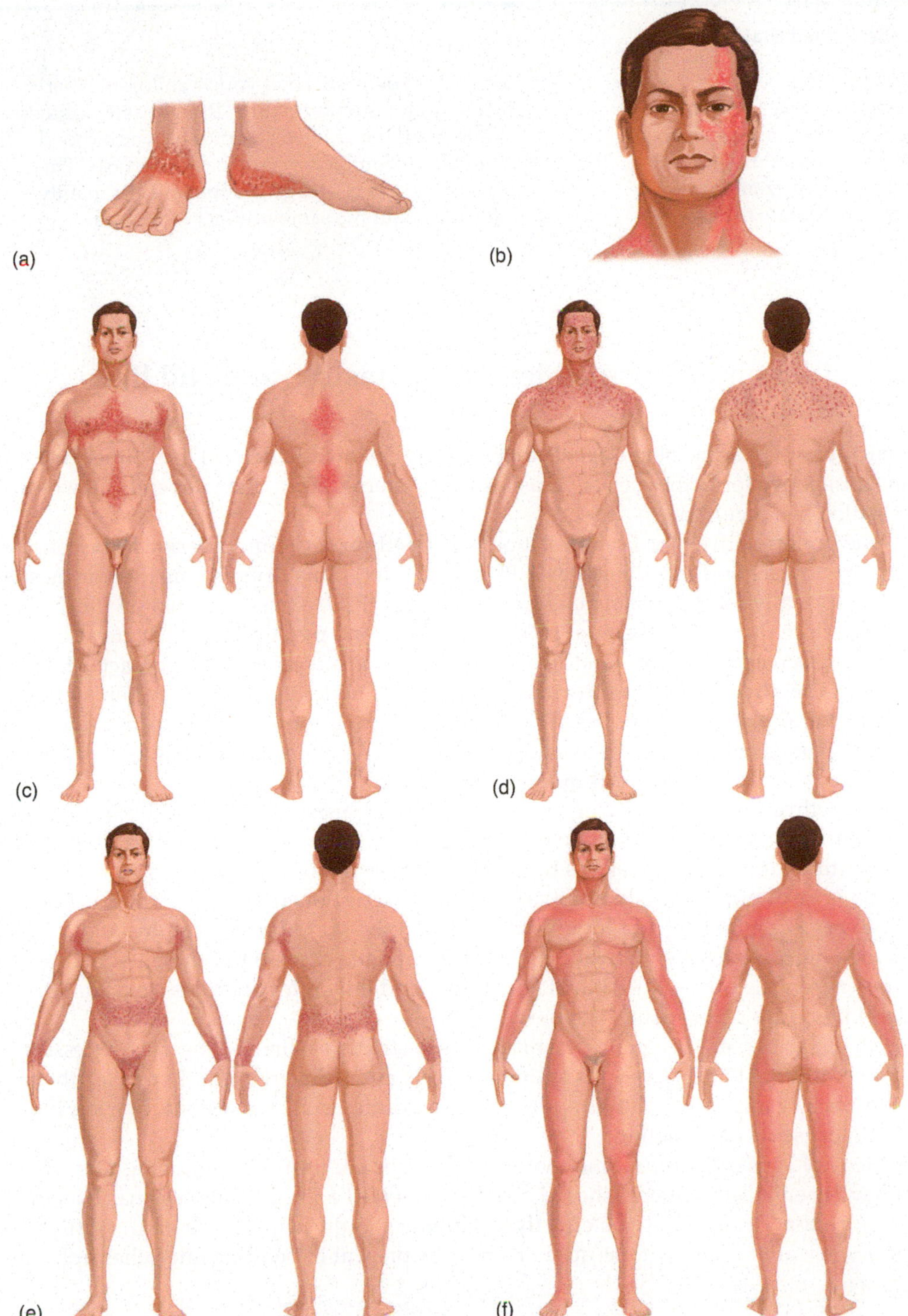

FIGURE 37.2 Anatomical distribution of common skin disorders: (a) contact dermatitis due to footwear, (b) cosmetics, (c) seborrheic dermatitis, (d) acne, (e) scabies, (f) sunburn.

SKIN PARASITES

Common skin parasites include mites and lice. Mites cause a skin disorder called **scabies**, based on their scientific name, *Sarcoptes scabiei*. Scabies is an eruption of the skin caused by the female mite burrowing into the skin and laying eggs. This causes intense itching, most commonly between the fingers, on the extremities, and around the trunk and pubic area. Scabies is readily spread among family members and sexual partners.

Lice, scientific name *Pediculus*, are another type of skin parasite readily passed on by infected clothing or close personal contact. Lice often infest the pubic area or the scalp and lay eggs that attach to body hairs.

Fast Facts **Skin Disorders in the United States**

- An estimated 6 to 11 million children between the ages of 3 and 11 are infected with lice each year.
- Nearly 40 to 50 million people have some form of acne, making it the most common skin disease.
- More than 31.6 million people have eczema, and at least 17.8 million people have moderate to severe eczema or atopic dermatitis.
- Ten percent of infants and young children experience symptoms of dermatitis. Roughly 60% of these infants continue to have symptoms in adulthood.
- More than 7.5 million people have psoriasis. This disorder occurs in all age groups—adults mainly—affecting about the same number of men as women.

Core Concept 37.3 ▶

Scabicides and pediculicides treat parasitic mite and lice infestations.

Scabicides are pharmacologic agents that kill mites; **pediculicides** kill lice. Either treatment may be effective for both types of parasites. The preferred drug often depends on where the infestation has occurred.

The preferred drug for lice infestation is permethrin, a chemical derived from chrysanthemum flowers and formulated as a 1% liquid (Nix). This drug is considered the safest agent, especially for infants and children. Pyrethrin (RID, others) is a related product also obtained from the chrysanthemum plant. Permethrin and pyrethrins, which are also widely used as insecticides on crops and livestock, kill lice and their eggs on contact. Malathion (Ovide) is an alternative drug treatment. Because of toxicity concerns, patients often ask about natural or home remedies. There are many common remedies for pediculicides, including vinegar, cranberry juice, and plant oils such as olive and coconut. Even Listerine mouthwash can help with lice or mite infestation.

Permethrin is a preferred drug for scabies. The 5% permethrin cream (Elimite) is applied to the entire skin surface and allowed to remain for 8 to 14 hours before bathing. Itching may continue for several weeks as the dead mites are removed from the skin. Crotamiton (Eurax) is an alternative scabicide available by prescription as a 10% cream. Approved in 2012, ivermectin (Sklice) is a lotion that is left on the scalp for 10 minutes and does not require a nit comb following treatment. Because lindane (Kwell) has the potential to cause serious nervous system toxicity, it is now prescribed only after other less toxic drugs have failed to produce a therapeutic response.

All scabicides and pediculicides must be used strictly as directed, because excessive use has the potential to cause serious systemic effects and skin irritation. Drugs for the treatment of lice or mites must not be applied to the mouth, open skin lesions, or eyes, because this will cause severe irritation.

Lice lay eggs called *nits*. Fine-toothed nit combs are useful in removing nits after the lice have been killed. Patients should comb the infested area after the hair has been dried. To ensure that drug therapy is effective, patients should inspect hair shafts daily for at least 1 week after treatment. Because nits may be present in bedding and other upholstery

Prototype Drug: Pr *Permethrin (Acticin, Elimite, Nix)*

Therapeutic Class: Antiparasitic drug **Pharmacologic Class:** Scabicide, pediculicide

Actions and Uses: Nix is marketed as a cream or shampoo to kill head and crab lice. It will also kill mites and eradicate their ova. A 1% lotion is approved for lice and 5% lotion for mites. The medication should be allowed to remain on the hair and scalp 10 minutes before removal. Patients should be aware that itching may last up to 2 or 3 weeks even after parasites have been killed. Successful elimination of parasitic infestations should include removing the nits with a comb, washing bedding, and cleaning or removing objects that have been in contact with the head or hair.

Adverse Effects and Interactions: Permethrin causes few systemic effects. Local reactions may occur and include pruritus, rash, transient tingling, burning, stinging, erythema, and edema of the infested area.

Contraindications include hypersensitivity to pyrethrins, chrysanthemums, sulfites, or other preservatives. Permethrin should be used cautiously on inflamed skin, in those with asthma, or in lactating women. No significant clinical drug interactions have been documented.

material, all material coming in close contact with the patient should be washed or treated with the medication.

CONCEPT REVIEW 37.2

- Name examples of medications used to treat mite and lice infestations. What precautions should be taken when using these medications?

Nursing Process Focus Patients Receiving Pharmacotherapy for Lice or Mite Infestation

ASSESSMENT	POTENTIAL NURSING DIAGNOSES*
Prior to drug administration: • Obtain a complete health history, including age, dermatological conditions, social history and close contacts, allergies, drug history, and possible drug interactions. • Examine skin areas to be treated for signs of infestation (e.g., lice or nits in hair, reddened track areas between web of fingers, around the belt or elastic lines), irritation, excoriation, or drainage.	• *Deficient Knowledge* related to a lack of information about condition and drug therapy regimen • *Impaired Health Maintenance* related to treatment regimen • *Risk for Impaired Skin Integrity* related to infestation or adverse effects of drug therapy • *Risk for Poisoning* related to adverse effects of drug therapy

PLANNING: PATIENT GOALS AND EXPECTED OUTCOMES

The patient will:
- Experience therapeutic effects (free of lice or mites).
- Be free from or experience minimal adverse effects from drug therapy.
- Verbalize an understanding of how lice and mites are spread; proper administration of medication; necessary household hygiene; and the need to notify household members, sexual partners, and other close contacts (such as classmates) about infestation.

IMPLEMENTATION

Interventions and (Rationales)	Patient Education/Discharge Planning
• Apply medication correctly and evaluate the patient's and caregiver's knowledge of proper administration. (Everyone in the household with mites or lice should be treated at the same time. Proper application is critical to eliminate the infestation.)	Instruct the patient and family members: • That all skin lotions, creams, and oil-based hair products should be removed completely before applying medication. • To apply the drug per package directions and allow it to remain in the hair or on the skin for the prescribed length of time (approximately 10 minutes). • To use a fine-toothed comb to remove any remaining dead lice or mites. • That eyelashes can be treated with the application of petroleum jelly once a day for 1 week. Use a fine-toothed comb to remove mites. • To recheck affected hair or skin daily for at least 1 to 2 weeks after treatment.
• Monitor the skin and head areas for infestation over the next 1 to 2 weeks. Reinfestations may appear within 1 week, and retreatment may be necessary. (Monitoring helps to determine proper medication administration technique and compliance with prevention protocols.)	Instruct the patient and family members to: • Monitor for nits on hair shafts; lice on skin or clothes, inner thigh areas, and seams of clothes that come in contact with axilla, neckline, or beltline. • Monitor for mites between the fingers, on the extremities, in the axillary and gluteal folds, around the trunk, and in the pubic area.
• Monitor household for signs of infestation. Inform the patient and others living in the home about proper care of clothing and equipment. (Contaminated articles can cause reinfestation.)	Instruct the patient and family members to: • Wash all bedding and clothing in hot water, and to dry-clean all nonwashable items that came in close contact with the patient. • Vacuum furniture or fabric that cannot be cleaned, and seal children's toys in plastic bags for 2 weeks. • Not share personal care items such as combs, brushes, and towels. • Clean combs and brushes, and rinse thoroughly after every use.

EVALUATION OF OUTCOME CRITERIA

Evaluate the effectiveness of drug therapy by confirming that patient goals and expected outcomes have been met (see "Planning").

*Herdman, T.H. & Kamitsuru, S. (Eds.), *Nursing Diagnoses: Definitions & Classification* 2015–2017. Copyright © 2014, 1994–2014 NANDA International. Used by arrangement by John Wiley & Sons, Inc. Companion website: www.wiley.com/go/nursingdiagnoses.

SUNBURN AND MINOR SKIN IRRITATION

Core Concept 37.4 ▶

The goal of drug therapy for sunburn is to eliminate discomfort until healing occurs.

Sunburn, a common problem among the general public, is associated with factors such as light skin complexion and lack of proper sun protection. Nonpharmacologic approaches to sun protection include the appropriate use of sunscreens, sunglasses, and sufficient clothing. Limiting the amount of time spent directly in the sun is essential to avoiding sunburn. Many dangers result from sun exposure, including eye injury and skin cancer. Some of these disorders may not appear until years after the exposure.

Pharmacologic treatments for sunburn may not be necessary. Remaining calm until the minor irritation passes is one common approach to mild sunburn. In cases in which pharmacologic intervention is necessary, drugs for sunburn and minor irritation include mild lotions and topical anesthetics such as benzocaine (Solarcaine, others), dibucaine (Nupercainal), and tetracaine (Pontocaine). These are used to provide temporary relief of painful symptoms. Some of these medications may also provide minor relief from insect bites and pruritus. In cases of more lengthy sun exposure, more potent pain medications may be administered (see Chapters 15 and 25), or tetanus toxoid might be administered to prevent infection (see Chapter 27).

Prototype Drug: Pr *Benzocaine (Americaine, Anbesol, Others)*

Therapeutic Class: Agent for sunburn pain and minor skin irritations **Pharmacologic Class:** Local anesthetic, sodium channel blocker

Actions and Uses: Benzocaine provides temporary relief for pain and discomfort in cases of sunburn, pruritus, minor wounds, and insect bites. Its pharmacologic action is caused by local anesthesia of skin receptor nerve endings. Preparations are also available to treat the skin and other areas such as the ear, mouth, throat, rectal, and genital areas.

Adverse Effects and Interactions: Benzocaine should not be used for treatment of patients with open lesions, traumatized mucosal areas, or a history of drug sensitivity. Benzocaine may interfere with the activity of some antibacterial sulfonamides. Patients should use preparations only in areas of the body for which the medication is intended.

CONCEPT REVIEW 37.3

- What is the major purpose of drugs used to treat sunburn, insect bites, and related injuries? What major class of drugs would be used for this purpose?

ACNE AND ROSACEA

sebor = *oil*
rhea = *flow*

Acne, sometimes called *acne vulgaris*, is a common condition found most often in adolescents and young adults. The disorder usually begins 1 or 2 years before puberty and is caused by overproductive oil glands or **seborrhea**. Acne is also caused by abnormal **keratinization** or development of the horny layer of the epithelial tissue of skin. This activity results in blocked oil glands. Administration of androgens or testosterone-like hormones may cause extensive acne by increasing keratinization and the production of sebum (oil). Following this, the bacterium *Propionibacterium acnes* grows within gland openings and modifies the sebum into an acidic and irritating substance. As a result, small inflamed bumps appear on the surface of the skin. Aggravating factors can trigger or make worse an existing case of acne. These include changing hormone levels, some medications (corticosteroids, androgens, or lithium), foods (chocolate, dairy, or carbohydrate-rich products), and stress.

Blackheads, or **open comedones**, are a type of acne in which sebum has plugged the oil gland, causing it to become black because of the presence of melanin granules. Whiteheads, or **closed comedones**, are a type of acne that develops just beneath the surface of the skin and appears white rather than black. In more severe cases of acne, deeper bumps called *nodules* may appear and become very painful because of the intense inflammation and pus found within pore pockets.

Another skin disorder characterized by inflammation but without pus is **rosacea**. Unlike pimples or **pustules**—the technical name given to pus-filled bumps—rosacea is characterized by small **papules** or inflammatory bumps that swell, thicken, and become very painful. Characteristic of rosacea is its swelling just beneath the surface of the skin. The face of a patient with rosacea may take on a flushed appearance, particularly around the nose and cheek area. Rosacea is exacerbated by many factors, including sunlight, stress, increased temperature, and agents that dilate facial blood vessels such as alcohol, spicy foods, and warm beverages.

Acne and rosacea are treated by a combination of over-the-counter and prescription drugs.

◀ **Core Concept 37.5**

Most acne drugs slow down the turnover of skin cells, especially those surrounding pore openings. Some inhibit bacterial growth because they are combined with antibiotics such as doxycycline and tetracycline (see Chapter 27). Some drugs must be used carefully because of their ability to dramatically reduce oil gland activity and skin cell turnover. Important medications for acne and rosacea are summarized in Table 37.3.

Benzoyl peroxide (Clearasil, Fostex, others) is one of the primary OTC medications used to treat acne. This medication may be dispensed as a lotion, cream, or gel and is available in various concentrations. Benzoyl peroxide decreases symptoms of acne by inhibiting bacterial growth and suppressing the turnover of skin cells at the pore's opening. Applied directly to affected skin, it is relatively safe, with redness, irritation, and drying being the most common adverse effects. Patients usually see some improvement in the first week, but it may take weeks, even a month or longer, to notice the full effect. Sometimes benzoyl peroxide is combined with antibiotics to directly fight bacterial infections. When acne is particularly severe, resorcinol, salicylic acid, or sulfur may be used as additional treatments to promote shedding of old skin. These are called **keratolytic agents**.

kerato = *horny layer*
lytic = *loosening*

Retinoids are vitamin A–like compounds used for acne. Vitamin A provides improved resistance to bacterial infection by reducing oil production and the occurrence of clogged

Table 37.3 Drugs for Acne and Rosacea

Drug	Remarks
OTC MEDICATION—TOPICAL PREPARATION	
benzoyl peroxide (Clearasil, Fostex, others)	Often combined with erythromycin or clindamycin to fight bacterial infection (see Chapter 27)
PRESCRIPTION MEDICATIONS—TOPICAL	
adapalene (Differin)	Retinoid-like compound used to treat acne formation
azelaic acid (Azelex, Finacea, others)	For mild to moderate inflammatory acne and rosacea
brimonidine (Mirvaso)	For persistent facial erythema of rosacea
clindamycin and tretinoin (Veltin, Ziana)	Combination product with an antibiotic and retinoid in a gel base, for mild to moderate acne
ivermectin (Soolantra)	For inflammatory lesions of rosacea
metronidazole (Metrogel, MetroCream)	For inflammatory papules and pustules of rosacea
sulfacetamide sodium (Cetamide, Klaron, others)	For sensitive skin; sometimes combined with sulfur to promote peeling, as in rosacea; also used for conjunctivitis
tazarotene (Avage, Tazorac)	A retinoid drug that may also be used for plaque psoriasis; has antiproliferative and anti-inflammatory effects
Pr tretinoin (Avita, Retin-A, others)	A retinoid used to prevent clogging of pore follicles associated with acne; the oral form (Vesanoid) is used to treat acute promyelocytic leukemia and wrinkles
PRESCRIPTION MEDICATIONS—ORAL	
doxycycline (Vibramycin, others)	Antibiotic (see Chapter 27)
ethinyl estradiol and norgestimate	Oral contraceptives are sometimes used for acne treatment; combination drugs may be helpful, for example, ethinyl estradiol plus norgestimate or Ortho Tri-Cyclen-28 (see Chapter 35)
isotretinoin	A retinoid used for severe acne with cysts or acne formed in small, rounded masses; pregnancy category X
minocycline (Minocin, others)	Antibiotic (see Chapter 27)
tetracycline (see the Prototype Drug box in Core Concept 27.8)	Antibiotic (see Chapter 27)

pores. Retinoids are not recommended during pregnancy because of possible harmful effects to the fetus. A common reaction to retinoids is sensitivity to sunlight.

Some drugs may be taken in combination with or in lieu of other acne medications, including doxycycline, tetracycline, and ethinyl estradiol. Doxycycline and tetracycline are antibiotics used to inhibit bacterial growth (see Chapter 27). Oral contraceptives containing ethinyl estradiol may be used to help clear the skin of acne by suppressing oil production (see Chapter 35).

The two most effective treatments for rosacea are topical metronidazole (Metrogel, MetroCream) and azelaic acid (Azelex, Finacea). Alternative medications include topical clindamycin (Cleocin-T, ClindaMax) and sulfacetamide. Tetracycline antibiotics are beneficial to patients with rosacea with multiple pustules or with ocular involvement. Severe, resistant cases may respond to isotretinoin.

CONCEPT REVIEW 37.4

- What is the major purpose of drugs used to treat acne and related skin conditions? Give examples of both topical and systemic medications. Which medications are OTC, and which are prescription medications?

Prototype Drug: Pr *Tretinoin (Avita, Retin-A, Others)*

Therapeutic Class: Antiacne drug **Pharmacologic Class:** Retinoid receptor drug, vitamin derivative

Actions and Uses: The topical forms of tretinoin are indicated for control of mild to moderate acne vulgaris. Symptoms take 4 to 8 weeks to improve, and maximum therapeutic benefit may take up to 5 or 6 months. This drug is most often reserved for cystic acne or severe keratinization disorders. Renova is a tretinoin cream approved to treat fine facial wrinkles.

The principal action of tretinoin is regulation of skin growth and cell turnover. As cells from the germinativum grow toward the skin's surface, skin cells are lost from the pore openings, and their replacement is slowed down. Tretinoin also decreases oil production by reducing the size and number of oil glands.

Adverse Effects and Interactions: Tretinoin is a natural derivative of **retinol** or vitamin A. Thus, vitamin A supplements, which increase toxicity, should be avoided.

Common adverse effects are skin irritation (such as a burning or stinging sensation, redness, and crusting), conjunctivitis (visual disturbance), dry mouth, inflammation of the lip, dry nose, increased serum concentrations of triglycerides, bone and joint pain, and photosensitivity. Additive phototoxicity can occur if tretinoin is used concurrently with other phototoxic drugs such as tetracyclines, fluoroquinolones, or sulfonamides.

Using tretinoin together with hypoglycemic agents may lead to loss of glycemic control as well as increased risk of cardiovascular disease due to elevated triglyceride levels.

BLACK BOX WARNING:
Patients with acute promyelocytic leukemia (APL) are at high risk for serious adverse effects: fever, weakness, fatigue, dyspnea, weight gain, peripheral edema, respiratory insufficiency, pneumonia, and rapidly evolving leukocytosis, which is associated with a high risk of life-threatening complications. There is a high risk that infants will be severely deformed if this drug is administered during pregnancy.

DERMATITIS AND ECZEMA

dermat = *skin*
itis = *inflammation*
atopic = *out of place*

Dermatitis is a general term that refers to superficial inflammatory disorders of the skin. **Eczema**, also called *atopic dermatitis*, is a skin disorder with symptoms resembling an allergic reaction, including inflammation, itching, and rash. Long-term itching and scaling may cause the skin to appear thickened and leathery. Exposure to environmental irritants may make these symptoms worse. Other conditions, including stress, too little or too much moisture, and extreme temperature fluctuations, may worsen symptoms. Blisters and other lesions may also develop. In infants and small children, lesions usually begin on the face and progress to other parts of the body. The skin may become raw and infected from scratching.

Contact dermatitis is a delayed type of allergic reaction resulting from exposure to specific allergens—for example, perfume, cosmetics, detergents, latex, or jewelry. Accompanying the allergic reaction may be various degrees of cracking, bleeding, or small blisters.

Seborrheic dermatitis is a disorder caused by overactive oil glands. This condition is sometimes seen in newborns and in teenagers after puberty. Oily and scaly patches of skin appear in areas of the face, scalp, chest, back, or pubic area. Bacterial infection or dandruff may accompany these symptoms.

Stasis dermatitis is seen more commonly in older women. It is found primarily in the lower extremities. Redness and scaling may be observed in areas where venous circulation is impaired or where deep venous blood clots have formed.

Topical corticosteroids are used mainly to treat dermatitis and related symptoms.

◀ Core Concept 37.6

Topical corticosteroids are used in cases of dermatitis and eczema to treat symptoms of inflammation, burning, and pruritus. In conjunction with other medical therapies, topical corticosteroids are also used for the treatment of psoriasis.

Topical corticosteroids are the most effective treatment for dermatitis. As seen in Table 37.4, there are many varieties of corticosteroids supplied at different levels of potency. Creams, lotions, solutions, gels, and pads are specially formulated to cross skin membranes.

CAM Therapy | Aloe Vera for Skin Conditions

Aloe vera is derived from the gel inside the leaf of the aloe plant, which is a member of the lily family. Used medicinally for thousands of years, aloe vera contains over 70 active substances, including amino acids, minerals, vitamins, and enzymes. Aloe vera is best known for its ability to soothe and heal minor skin irritations, cuts, and burns. For the most part, scientific studies have confirmed its benefit for these conditions. It can be found as an ingredient in many products, including soaps, lotions, creams, and sunblocks. Some evidence suggests it may be useful in treating genital herpes lesions and moderate plaque psoriasis. Although oral formulations can be found, these are not recommended because they can cause serious gastrointestinal (GI) side effects.

Table 37.4 Selected Topical Corticosteroids for Dermatitis and Related Symptoms

Generic Name	Trade Names
VERY HIGH POTENCY	
betamethasone dipropionate	Diprolene
clobetasol	Temovate
diflorasone	Maxiflor
halobetasol	Ultravate
HIGH POTENCY	
amcinonide	Cyclocort
fluocinonide	Lidex
halcinonide	Halog
MEDIUM POTENCY	
betamethasone benzoate	Uticort
betamethasone valerate	Valisone
clocortolone	Cloderm
desoximetasone, cream	Topicort
fluocinolone acetonide	Synalar
flurandrenolide, cream	Cordran
fluticasone propionate, cream	Cutivate
hydrocortisone valerate	Westcort
mometasone furoate	Elocon
prednicarbate	Dermatop
triamcinolone acetonide	Aristocort, Kenalog
LOWER POTENCY	
alclometasone dipropionate	Aclovate
desonide	Desonate, DesOwen, Verdeso
dexamethasone	-
hydrocortisone	Cortizone, Hycort

These medications are especially intended for the relief of local inflammation and itching. In cases of long-term use, however, adverse effects such as irritation, redness, and thinning of the skin membranes may occur. If absorption occurs, topical corticosteroids may produce undesirable systemic effects, including adrenal insufficiency, mood changes, serum imbalances, and bone defects, as discussed in Chapter 25.

PSORIASIS

Psoriasis is a chronic, noninfectious inflammatory skin disorder that affects 1% to 2% of the U.S. population each year. Psoriasis is characterized by red patches of skin covered with flaky, silver-colored scales called *plaques*. The reason for the appearance of plaques is an extremely fast skin turnover rate. The skin reacts as if it has been injured, but skin cells reach the surface much more quickly than usual, in about 4 days, or six to seven times faster than usual. The reason for this kind of reaction is not known, although scientists believe that it may be a genetic immune reaction. Plaques are ultimately shed from the skin's surface, while the underlying skin becomes inflamed and irritated.

Core Concept 37.7 ▶

Several topical and systemic medications are used to treat psoriatic symptoms.

emolli = *to soften*
ent = *causing*

Because psoriatic symptoms may be extreme, numerous drugs are employed to soothe the patient's symptoms, including **emollients**, topical corticosteroids, and immunosuppressants. Drugs used in the treatment of psoriasis are provided in Table 37.5.

Topical corticosteroids, such as betamethasone or hydrocortisone, are the primary, initial treatment for psoriasis because they are effective, safe, and inexpensive. Topical corticosteroids reduce the inflammation associated with fast skin turnover. Therapy usually begins with the high potency corticosteroids and switches to moderate- and low-potency agents after the initial symptoms have been controlled.

Other topical drugs are retinoid-like compounds such as calcipotriene (Dovonex) and tazarotene (Tazorac). These drugs provide the same benefits as topical corticosteroids, but they exhibit fewer side effects. Calcipotriene produces elevated levels of calcium in the bloodstream, so this medication is not used on an extended basis. Enstilar is a newer drug that consists of a combination of calcipotriene and beclomethasone.

Some patients have severe psoriasis that is resistant to topical drugs, so systemic therapy must be used. Systemic medications for psoriasis include acitretin (Soriatane), adalimumab (Humira), alefacept (Amevive), apremilast (Otezla), etanercept (Enbrel), infliximab (Remicade), secukinumab (Consentyx), and ustekinumab (Stelara). These drugs are taken orally to inhibit skin cell growth. Methotrexate (Rheumatrex, Trexall), an anticancer drug taken in tablet form, also inhibits cell growth (see Chapter 29). Other medications that have been used for different disorders but may provide relief of severe psoriatic symptoms are hydroxyurea and cyclosporine (Sandimmune, Neoral). Cyclosporine is an immunosuppressant, discussed in Chapter 26.

Other skin therapy techniques may be used with or without psoriasis medications. These include various forms of tar treatment (coal tar) and a material called anthralin. Both substances are applied to the skin's surface and are not considered first-line therapies. Tar and anthralin inhibit DNA synthesis and arrest abnormal cell growth.

Ultraviolet B (UVB) and ultraviolet A (UVA) phototherapy are techniques used in cases of severe psoriasis. UVB therapy is less hazardous than UVA therapy. UVB light has a wavelength similar to sunlight; it reduces widespread lesions that normally resist topical treatments. With close supervision, this type of phototherapy can be administered at home. Keratolytic pastes are often applied between treatments. The second type of phototherapy is often referred to as PUVA (psoralen plus ultraviolet light) therapy because **psoralens** are often administered in conjunction with phototherapy. Psoralens are oral or topical agents that, when exposed to UV light, produce a photosensitive reaction. This reaction seems to provide benefit to the patient by reducing the number of lesions, but unpleasant adverse effects such as headache, nausea, and skin sensitivity may occur, limiting the effectiveness of this therapy. Immunosuppressant drugs such as cyclosporine are not used in conjunction with PUVA therapy because they increase the risk of skin cancer.

Table 37.5 Drugs for Psoriasis and Related Disorders

Drug	Route and Adult Dose	Remarks
TOPICAL MEDICATIONS		
anthralin (Dritho-Scalp)	Topical: Apply to lesions of the scalp as directed	Second-line therapy after tolerance to corticosteroids has developed
calcipotriene (Dovonex)	Topical: Apply to lesions once or twice daily up to 8 weeks	Synthetic form of vitamin D_3; may raise the level of calcium in the body to unhealthy levels
coal tar (Balnetar, Cutar, others)	Topical: Apply to lesions daily or as directed	Second-line therapy after tolerance to corticosteroids has developed
salicylic acid (Salax, Neutrogena, others)	Topical: Apply to lesions (concentrations ranging from 2–10%) as directed	Wide range of delivery: creams, foams, gels, lotions, ointments, pads, plasters, shampoos, soaps, and skin solutions
tazarotene (Tazorac)	Acne: Topical: Apply thin film to clean, dry area daily Plaque psoriasis: Topical: Apply a thin film daily in the evening	Topical retinoid; less toxic than corticosteroids; also approved for facial wrinkles and acne
SYSTEMIC MEDICATIONS		
acitretin (Soriatane)	PO: 10–50 mg/day with the main meal	Retinoid; pregnancy category X drug
adalimumab (Humira)	Subcutaneous: 40–80 mg every other week	Tumor necrosis factor blocker; also for rheumatoid arthritis and Crohn disease
alefacept (Amevive)	IM: 15 mg once weekly for 12 weeks	Engineered immunosuppressant drug
apremilast (Otezla)	PO: Begin with 10 mg per day and increase over 6 weeks to 30 mg bid	Phosphodiesterase-4 (PDE-4) inhibitor for the treatment of moderate-to-severe plaque psoriasis
cyclosporine (Gengraf, Neoral, Sandimmune) (see the Prototype Drug box in Core Concept 26.5)	PO: 1.25 mg/kg bid (max: 4 mg/kg/day)	Immunosuppressant drug; also to prevent transplant rejection and for rheumatoid arthritis
etanercept (Enbrel)	Subcutaneous: 50 mg twice weekly (given 3–4 days apart); maintenance dose 50 mg/week	Also for rheumatoid arthritis
infliximab (Remicade)	IV: 5 mg/kg with additional doses 2 and 6 weeks after the initial infusion, then every 8 weeks thereafter	Tumor necrosis factor blocker; also for rheumatoid arthritis, Crohn disease, and ulcerative colitis
hydroxyurea	PO: 80 mg/kg every 3 days or 20–30 mg/kg daily	Alternative treatment for psoriasis; oral cancer medication
ixekizumab (Taltz)	Subcutaneous: 160 mg initially, then 80 mg at weeks 2, 4, 6, 8, and 12	Newer drug; interleukin-17A inhibitor
methotrexate (Otrexup Rheumatrex, Trexall) (see the Prototype Drug box in Core Concept 29.8)	PO: 2.5–5 mg bid × 3 doses each week (max: 25–30 mg/week) Subcutaneous (Otrexup): 7.5–20 mg once/week	Also for rheumatoid arthritis and neoplasia
secukinumab (Consentyx)	Subcutaneous: 150–300 mg at weeks 0, 1, 2, 3, 4 followed by 300 mg every 4 weeks	Interleukin-17A inhibitor approved for adults with ankylosing spondylitis and psoriatic arthritis
ustekinumab (Stelara)	Subcutaneous: 45–90 mg initially and 4 weeks later, followed by 45–90 mg every 12 weeks	Interleukin blocker

CONCEPT REVIEW 37.5

- In most cases, which drug category is used to treat symptoms of dermatitis and psoriasis? What other drug therapies and techniques are used to provide a measure of relief for these symptoms?

Patients Need to Know

Patients taking medications for skin disorders need to know the following:

1. Inform family members, sexual partners, school personnel, and any other persons with whom close contact has occurred about skin infestations. Treat clothes, bed linens, and personal items properly to avoid reinfestation.
2. Be informed and understand the proper way to apply medication or to remove nits if necessary. Scabicides and pediculicides should not be applied to the face, mouth, or eyes, or open skin lesions.
3. For acne and related disorders, apply medication only to areas where it is supposed to be applied. Follow instructions in package inserts and do not deviate from the precautions communicated by the healthcare provider.
4. Do not share skin medications with family or friends. Be familiar with medication adverse effects, especially those of retinoids, retinoid-like products, or medications used to treat severe skin disorders.

5. Use medications only during the time for which they are intended. With extended use, some medications (e.g., corticosteroids) may cause adverse effects. Take a medication suitable for the disorder; avoid those that are too potent or not potent enough.
6. Give medications a chance to work. Some systemic medications must be taken exactly as prescribed without skipping or stopping early.
7. Avoid contact with objects or drugs that are known to cause allergy or dermatitis. Try to avoid scratching, if possible. For severe skin disorders, see a dermatologist.

Chapter Review

Core Concepts Summary

37.1 Layers of skin provide protection to the body.

Two layers of skin and one underlying layer protect the body: the epidermis, dermis, and hypodermis. The most superficial layer is the epidermis, in which skin cells are replenished every 3 weeks. New cells arise from the bottom layer of the epidermis, called the germinativum, and are pushed to the outermost layer.

37.2 The major causes of skin disorders are injury, aging, inherited factors, and other medical conditions.

Many symptoms are associated with skin stress and injury. Others are associated with a patient's changing age or health. Skin disorders fit into three main categories: infectious, inflammatory, and cancerous disorders.

37.3 Scabicides and pediculicides treat parasitic mite and lice infestations.

Mites affect the skin and hair, whereas lice remain localized in hairy regions of the body. Both conditions are treatable with medications. Scabicides kill mites; pediculicides kill lice.

37.4 The goal of drug therapy for sunburn is to eliminate discomfort until healing occurs.

Local anesthetics are the primary medication used to treat mild sunburn and irritation. Often drugs are used for temporary relief of minor discomfort; in some cases, drugs may not be needed at all.

37.5 Acne and rosacea are treated by a combination of over-the-counter and prescription drugs.

Blackheads, whiteheads, and rosacea are disorders in which pores become blocked, inflamed, or infected because of accelerated skin processes. Topical drugs for acne are those that inhibit bacterial growth (antibiotics) or promote shedding of old skin (keratolytic agents). Vitamin A–like compounds (retinoids) provide an improved resistance to bacterial infections by reducing oil production and the occurrence of clogged pores.

37.6 Topical corticosteroids are used mainly to treat dermatitis and related symptoms.

Dermatitis is treated by agents that reduce symptoms of inflammation, itchiness, flaking, cracking, bleeding, and lesions. Topical corticosteroids are the primary drug treatment for dermatitis. Potency depends on the type of drug formulation and whether it is packaged as a cream, lotion, solution, gel, or pad.

37.7 Several topical and systemic medications are used to treat psoriatic symptoms.

Psoriasis is a chronic disorder characterized by extreme discomfort and flaky areas called plaques. The treatments for psoriasis include topical corticosteroids, retinoid-like compounds, drugs that arrest skin cell growth, and immunosuppressants. Skin therapy techniques are also used, including keratolytic agents, coal tar, anthralin, psoralens, and phototherapy.

REVIEW Questions

Answer the following questions to assess your knowledge of the chapter material, and go back and review any material that is not clear to you.

1. Which of the following is true regarding the use of benzocaine for a minor skin irritation?
   1. It cannot be used for sunburns.
   2. It should not be used on open lesions.
   3. It causes blisters.
   4. It can be used on open sores.

2. The nurse is helping to create a teaching plan for a patient prescribed desoximetasone (Topicort) for atopic dermatitis. Which adverse effect will be included in that plan?
   1. Localized pruritus and hives
   2. Hair loss in the application area
   3. Worsening of acne
   4. Skin irritation and redness in the application area

3. The nurse and a patient are discussing how to eliminate lice. The patient is given a shampoo-like medication that is applied and rinsed from the body within 10 minutes after application. This medication is:
   1. Lindane.
   2. Crotamiton.
   3. Cortizone.
   4. Permethrin.

4. The patient is complaining of discomfort related to minor sunburn. Which of the following medications would be included in a plan of care for someone who has minor sunburn?
   1. Benzocaine (Solarcaine)
   2. Cortizone
   3. Benzoyl peroxide
   4. Doxycycline

5. The nurse is providing information at a high school health fair. Many of the students ask for information on acne treatment. The nurse tells them that __________ is available but it is extremely important that women who are pregnant do not take this medication.
   1. Hydrocortisone
   2. Tretinoin
   3. Benzoyl peroxide
   4. Benzocaine

6. The patient using topical corticosteroids will need to be monitored for which of the following systemic effects? (Select all that apply.)
   1. Mood changes
   2. Bone defects
   3. Liver toxicity
   4. Adrenal insufficiency
   5. Skin irritation

7. A patient with rosacea has been treating her condition with over-the-counter medications, but they have worsened her condition. The healthcare provider understands the patient may need:
   1. Calcipotriene (Dovonex).
   2. Metronidazole (Metrogel).
   3. Acitretin (Soriatane).
   4. Cyclosporine (Sandimmune, Neoral).

8. Some patients with acne may need medications that promote the shedding of old skin. These medications are known as:
   1. Pediculicides.
   2. Keratolytic agents.
   3. Retinoids.
   4. Corticosteroids.

9. The skin on the elbow of a newly diagnosed patient with psoriasis is covered with red plaques and scales. The patient finds it very embarrassing and wants to know the most cost effective medication that can help her. The nurse understands that the initial and inexpensive medication is:
   1. Betamethasone.
   2. Doxycycline.
   3. Cyclosporine.
   4. Benzocaine.

10. A patient weighing 198 pounds is to receive the initial infused dose of infliximab (Remicade), 5 mg/kg. How many milligrams will the patient receive?
    1. 45 mg
    2. 90 mg
    3. 450 mg
    4. 990 mg

CASE STUDY Questions

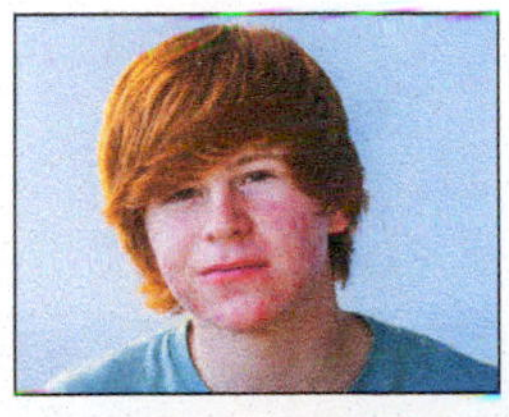

Remember Burt Nicholson, the patient introduced at the beginning of the chapter? Now read the remainder of the case study. Based on the information you have learned in this chapter, answer the questions that follow.

Burt Nicholson is a 16-year-old White male with a family history of various allergy disorders. He is complaining of general irritation and sores around the face, neck, and upper back. Upon examination, a severe case of acne and moderate erythema are observed on the chin, cheeks, and forehead. No excessive oil is noted. Although areas around the neck and upper back are inflamed, these do not appear to be infected. Burt states that he is so embarrassed about his skin, it is impacting his social life. He also says that he has tried many different OTC medications but nothing seems to work. Burt is diagnosed with acne vulgaris.

1. The nurse asks Burt which medications he tried. He says that he cannot remember all of them but is sure he tried benzoyl peroxide, which he stopped using after a week because his acne was still visible. The nurse responds by saying:
   1. "The cream should have worked within that first week."
   2. "Improvements begin in the first week but the full effects may take several weeks to a month or longer."
   3. "Acne is very difficult to treat. It may take several months before you see improvements."
   4. "If your acne is not gone by now, you may need an antibiotic."

2. The healthcare provider wants Burt to try the benzoyl peroxide again, but because Burt's skin is red and inflamed, the nurse suspects that a(n) __________ will also be prescribed.
   1. Metronidazole
   2. Benzocaine
   3. Corticosteroid
   4. Antibiotic

3. Other medication options are discussed. Burt is informed that he could also take tretinoin, a retinoid antiacne medication. When asked how the medication works, the nurse responds that tretinoin:

1. Sheds the outer layer of the skin.

2. Decreases oil production by reducing the size and number of oil glands.

3. Inhibits bacterial growth.

4. Reduces inflammation.

4. The nurse continues to tell Burt that tretinoin may cause the following adverse effects: (Select all that apply.)

1. Swelling around the lips

2. Dry mouth and nose

3. Photosensitivity (sensitivity to light)

4. Skin irritation such as burning and redness

Answers and complete rationales to the Review and Case Study Questions appear in Appendix A.

REFERENCE

Herdman, T. H., & Kamitsuru, S. (Eds.). (2014). *NANDA International nursing diagnoses: Definitions and classification, 2015–2017*. Oxford, United Kingdom: Wiley-Blackwell.

SELECTED BIBLIOGRAPHY

American Academy of Dermatology. (n.d.). *Acne*. Retrieved from https://www.aad.org/media/stats/conditions

American Academy of Dermatology. (n.d.). *Psoriasis*. Retrieved from https://www.aad.org/public/diseases/scaly-skin/psoriasis

Bradby, C. (2014). *Atopic dermatitis in emergency medicine*. Retrieved from http://emedicine.medscape.com/article/762045-overview#a0199

Centers for Disease Control and Prevention. (2013). *Epidemiology and risk factors*. Retrieved from http://www.cdc.gov/parasites/lice/head/epi.html

The Children's Hospital of Philadelphia. (n.d.). *Atopic dermatitis in childhood*. Retrieved from http://www.chop.edu/conditions-diseases/atopic-dermatitis-children#.V1xggPkrIhc

Guenther, L. C. (2016). *Pediculosis and pthiriasis (lice infestation)*. Retrieved from http://emedicine.medscape.com/article/225013-overview#a0156

Meffert, J. (2015). *Psoriasis*. Retrieved from http://emedicine.medscape.com/article/1943419-overview

National Eczema Association. (n.d.). *Eczema prevalence in the United States*. Retrieved from https://nationaleczema.org/research/eczema-prevalence

National Psoriasis Foundation. (n.d.). *Facts about psoriasis*. Retrieved from https://www.psoriasis.org/teens/about-psoriasis

Radtke, M. A., Reich, K., Spehr, C., & Augustin, M. (2015). Treatment goals in psoriasis routine care. *Archives of Dermatological Research, 307*, 445–449. doi:10.1007/s00403-014-1534-y

Rao, J. (2015). *Acne vulgaris*. Retrieved from http://emedicine.medscape.com/article/1069804-overview

Tüzün, Y., Wolf, R., Kutlubay, Z., Karakuş, Ö., & Engin, B. (2014). Rosacea and rhinophyma. *Clinics in Dermatology, 32*, 35–46. doi:10.1016/j.clindermatol.2013.05.024

Chapter 38

Drugs for Eye and Ear Disorders

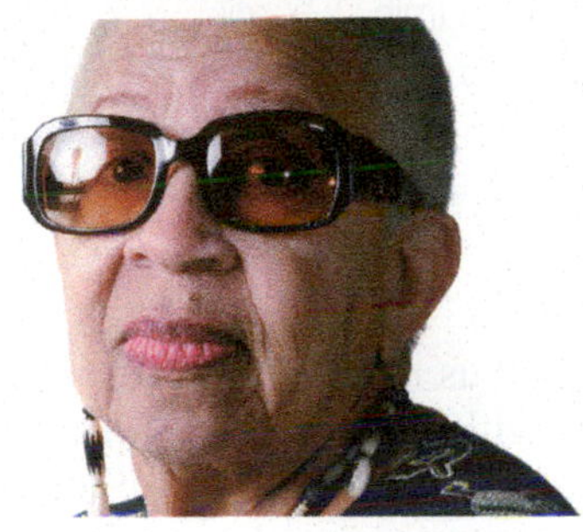

"Moving is so stressful, and it's worse because I haven't had any help. I'm not even sure where I packed my medication so I've been having problems seeing."

Ms. Mary Saunders

Core Concepts

38.1 Knowledge of basic eye anatomy is essential for an understanding of eye disorders and drug therapy.

38.2 Glaucoma is one of the leading causes of blindness.

38.3 Glaucoma therapy focuses on adjusting the circulation of aqueous humor.

38.4 Antiglaucoma medications may increase the outflow of aqueous humor.

38.5 Antiglaucoma medications may decrease the formation of aqueous humor.

38.6 Drugs provide relief for minor eye conditions and are used for eye exams.

38.7 Otic preparations treat infections, inflammation, and earwax buildup.

Drug Snapshot

The following drugs are discussed in this chapter:

Drug Classes	Prototype Drugs
DRUGS FOR GLAUCOMA	
Drugs that increase the outflow of aqueous humor	Pr latanoprost (Xalatan)
Drugs that decrease the formation of aqueous humor	Pr timolol (Betimol, Timoptic, others)
DRUGS FOR EYE EXAMINATIONS AND MINOR EYE CONDITIONS	
DRUGS FOR EAR CONDITIONS	

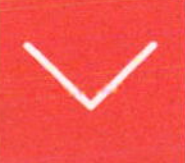

Learning Outcomes

After reading this chapter, the student should be able to:

1. Describe important anatomy relevant to disorders of the eyeball.
2. Identify the major risk factors associated with closed-angle glaucoma and open-angle glaucoma, and explain how increased intraocular pressure may cause blindness.
3. Explain the two major mechanisms by which drugs reduce intraocular pressure.
4. Identify important drugs that increase the outflow of aqueous humor and discuss primary actions and possible adverse effects.

5. Identify important drugs that decrease the formation of aqueous humor and discuss primary actions and possible adverse effects.
6. Identify examples of drugs that dilate or constrict pupils, relax ciliary muscles, constrict ocular blood vessels, or moisten eye membranes.
7. Identify examples of drugs that treat conditions of the ear.

Key Terms

closed-angle glaucoma (glaw-KOH-mah)
cycloplegia (sy-kloh-PLEE-jee-ah)
cycloplegic drugs (sy-kloh-PLEE-jik)
external otitis (oh-TYE-tiss)
glaucoma (glaw-CO-muh)
mastoiditis (mass-toy-DYE-tuss)
miosis (my-OH-sis)
mydriasis (mih-DRY-uh-siss)
mydriatic drugs (mih DRY-atik)
open-angle glaucoma (glaw-KOH-mah)
otitis media (oh-TYE-tuss MEE-dee-ah)
tonometry (toh-NAHM-uh-tree)

The senses of vision and hearing provide the primary means for us to communicate with the world around us. Disorders affecting the eye and ear can result in problems with self-care, mobility, safety, and communication. The eye is vulnerable to a variety of conditions, many of which can be prevented, controlled, or reversed with proper pharmacotherapy. The first part of this chapter covers drugs used for the treatment of glaucoma and those used routinely by ophthalmic healthcare providers. The remaining part of the chapter presents drugs used for treatment of common ear disorders, including infections, inflammation, and the buildup of earwax.

Core Concept 38.1 ▶

Knowledge of basic eye anatomy is essential for an understanding of eye disorders and drug therapy.

To understand eye disorders and drug action, a firm knowledge of basic ocular anatomy is required. As shown in Figure 38.1, the anterior segment is found at the front of the eyeball. It contains a watery fluid called *aqueous humor*. The anterior segment has two divisions: the anterior chamber and the posterior chamber. In the posterior chamber (Figure 38.2), aqueous humor originates from an important muscle structure called the *ciliary body*. From there,

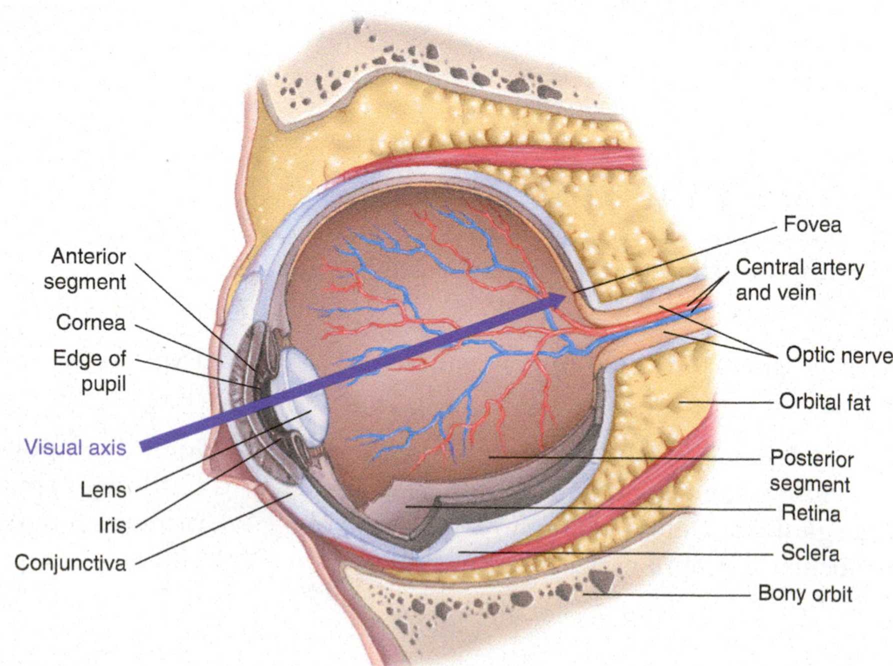

FIGURE 38.1 Internal structures of the eye.

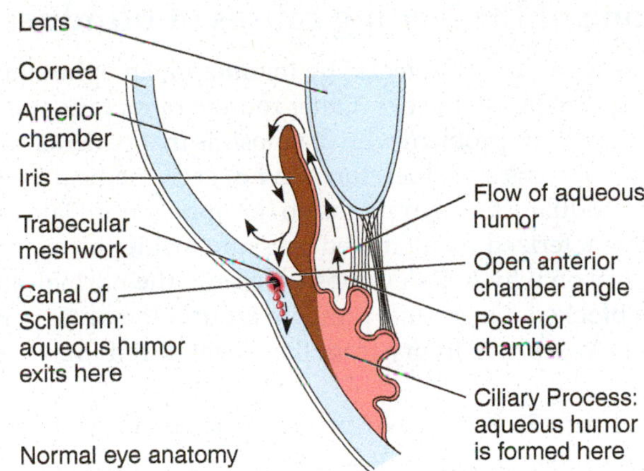

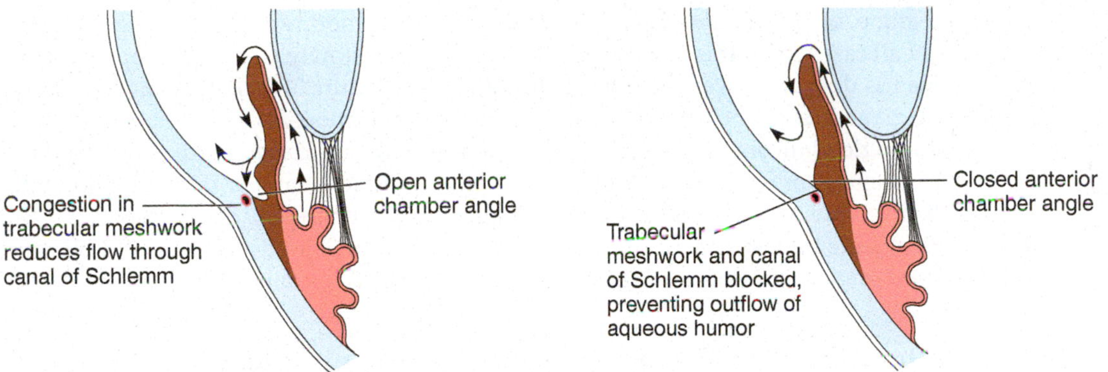

(a) Open-angle glaucoma: slowly rising intraocular pressure (b) Closed-angle glaucoma: rapidly rising intraocular pressure

FIGURE 38.2 Forms of primary adult glaucoma: (a) In chronic, open-angle glaucoma, the anterior chamber angle remains open, but drainage of aqueous humor through the canal of Schlemm is impaired; (b) in acute, narrow closed-angle glaucoma, the angle of the iris and anterior chamber is smaller, obstructing the outflow of aqueous humor.

it flows through the pupil and into the anterior chamber. Within the anterior chamber and around the periphery is a network of spongy connective tissue called *trabecular meshwork.* Connected to the trabecular meshwork is an opening called the canal of Schlemm, where aqueous humor drains from the anterior chamber.

trabecular = *strut-like*

GLAUCOMA

Glaucoma is an eye disorder that is characterized by gradual changes in peripheral vision, possibly advancing to blindness. In some cases, glaucoma is genetic; in other cases, glaucoma may be caused by eye trauma or disease. Some medications may contribute to the development of glaucoma, including long-term use of topical corticosteroids, some antihypertensives, antihistamines, and antidepressants. The major risk factors associated with the development of glaucoma include high blood pressure, migraine headaches, high levels of nearsightedness or farsightedness, and older age.

Fast Facts Glaucoma

- More than 3 million Americans have glaucoma. More than 120,000 have developed blindness due to this disorder.
- Individuals of African heritage are affected more by glaucoma than any other ethnic group.
- Glaucoma is most common in people older than 60 years of age.
- Acute glaucoma is often caused by head trauma, cataracts, tumors, or hemorrhage.
- Chronic simple glaucoma accounts for 90% of all glaucoma cases.

Core Concept 38.2 ▶

Glaucoma is one of the leading causes of blindness.

tono = *pressure*
metry = *measurement*

The presence of glaucoma may be detected by **tonometry**, an ophthalmic technique for measuring increased pressure inside the eye. Other routine refractory and visual field tests may uncover glaucoma signs. One problem with diagnosis is that patients with glaucoma typically do not experience symptoms and, therefore, do not seek medical attention. In some cases, glaucoma occurs so gradually that symptoms do not appear until late in the disease process.

intra = *inside*
ocular = *eye*

Glaucoma is characterized by increased pressure inside the eyeball, termed *intraocular pressure* (IOP). The reason why IOP develops is because the normal flow of aqueous humor in the eye becomes blocked. Over time, pressure around the optic nerve can build, leading to blindness. In some cases, eye injury from the elevated IOP may be sudden, but in most cases it is gradual.

As shown in Figure 38.2, the two principal types of glaucoma are **closed-angle glaucoma** and **open-angle glaucoma**. Both disorders result from the same problem: Pressure inside the eyeball leads to progressive damage of the optic nerve. The differences between these two disorders include how quickly the IOP develops.

Open-angle, or *chronic simple glaucoma,* is the most common type, accounting for more than 90% of all cases. With this disorder, IOP develops more slowly. It is called "open angle" because the iris does not cover the trabecular meshwork (Figure 38.2a). If discovered early, open-angle glaucoma can be treated successfully with medications.

Closed-angle glaucoma, sometimes referred to as *acute glaucoma,* is usually caused by stress, impact injury, or medications. Pressure inside the anterior chamber increases suddenly because the iris is pushed over the area where the aqueous fluid normally drains (Figure 38.2b). Symptoms include intense headaches, difficulty concentrating, bloodshot eyes, and blurred vision. Closed-angle glaucoma requires immediate intervention (usually surgical).

Core Concept 38.3 ▶

Glaucoma therapy focuses on adjusting the circulation of aqueous humor.

Treatment for glaucoma focuses on reducing the amount of aqueous humor formed or unblocking its drainage. Complete blockage of flow, as may occur with acute glaucoma, is a medical emergency that requires surgery to return the iris to its original position. For chronic glaucoma, drug therapy is employed to either *increase the outflow of aqueous humor* (canal of Schlemm location) or *decrease the formation of aqueous humor* (ciliary body location).

CONCEPT REVIEW 38.1

- Which components of the eye are specifically affected by glaucoma? Why is glaucoma such a dreaded eye disease? Drug therapy for glaucoma centers around which major approach?

Core Concept 38.4 ▶

Antiglaucoma medications may increase the outflow of aqueous humor.

miotic = *constricting pupil*

Drugs increasing the outflow of aqueous humor include miotics, sympathomimetics, and prostaglandins. All of these drugs are available as ophthalmic solutions. These drugs are summarized in Table 38.1.

Although antiglaucoma drugs are not designed to directly alter pupil diameter, they often produce this effect because of their physiologic properties. Cholinergic direct- and indirect-acting drugs cause *constriction* of pupils or **miosis**. Sympathomimetics are drugs that activate the sympathetic nervous system and cause *dilation* of pupils or **mydriasis** (see Chapter 9). Prostaglandins do not affect pupil diameter, but instead they directly dilate trabecular meshwork within the anterior chamber of the eye.

Prostaglandins

Prostaglandins are the preferred drugs for glaucoma therapy because they have long durations of action and produce fewer side effects than drugs from other classes. In resistant cases, they may be combined with drugs from other classes. Drugs in this class increase

Table 38.1 Antiglaucoma Drugs That Increase the Outflow of Aqueous Humor

Drug	Route and Adult Dose	Remarks
DIRECT- AND INDIRECT-ACTING CHOLINERGICS (MIOTIC DRUGS)		
carbachol (Miostat)	One or two drops 0.75–3% solution in the lower conjunctival sac every 4 hours tid	Cholinergic drug; less useful in glaucoma than other drugs; causes stinging of the eyes
echothiophate (Phospholine Iodide)	One drop of 0.03% solution bid	Irreversible acetylcholinesterase inhibitor; use cautiously due to an intense and persistent miosis and ciliary-muscle contraction that may occur
pilocarpine (Isopto Carpine, Pilopine)	Acute glaucoma: One drop 1–2% solution for 3–6 doses Chronic glaucoma: One drop 0.5–4% solution bid	Cholinergic drug
NONSELECTIVE SYMPATHOMIMETICS (MYDRIATIC DRUGS)		
dipivefrin HCl (Propine)	One drop 0.1% solution bid	Converted to epinephrine in the eye
PROSTAGLANDINS		
bimatoprost (Lumigan)	One drop 0.03% solution daily in the evening	Should not be used concurrently with latanaprost
Pr latanoprost (Xalatan)	One drop (1.5 mg) solution daily in the evening	May increase brown pigment in the iris
tafluprost (Zioptan)	One drop of 0.0015% solution in the evening	May increase brown pigment in the iris
travoprost (Travatan)	One drop 0.004% solution daily in the evening	Maximum effect after about 12 hours

aqueous humor outflow by reducing congestion in trabecular meshwork. Their main side effect is a change in pigmentation, usually a change to a brown iris color in patients with lighter colored eyes. These medications cause **cycloplegia** (blurred vision), local irritation, and stinging of the eyes. Because of these effects, prostaglandins are normally administered just before the patient goes to bed. Although prostaglandins can be irritating to the eyes, they usually do not prevent the patient from falling asleep.

cyclop = *round eye*
plegia = *paralysis*

Prototype Drug: Pr *Latanoprost (Xalatan)*

Therapeutic Class: Antiglaucoma drug Pharmacologic Class: Prostaglandin, reducer of IOP

Actions and Uses: Latanoprost is a prostaglandin analog believed to reduce IOP by increasing the outflow of aqueous humor. The recommended dose is one drop in the affected eye(s) in the evening. It is metabolized to its active form in the cornea, reaching its peak effect in about 12 hours. It is used to treat open-angle glaucoma and elevated IOP.

Adverse Effects and Interactions: Adverse effects include ocular symptoms such as conjunctival edema, tearing, dryness, burning, pain, irritation, itching, sensation of a foreign body in the eye, photophobia, and visual disturbances. The eyelashes on the treated eye may grow, thicken, and darken. Changes may occur in pigmentation of the iris of the treated eye and in the periocular skin. The most common systemic adverse effect is a flu-like upper respiratory infection. Rash, asthenia, or headache may occur.

Latanoprost interacts with thimerosal: If mixed with eyedrops containing thimerosal, precipitation may occur.

Direct- and Indirect-Acting Cholinergics (Miotic Drugs)

Carbachol (Miostat) and pilocarpine (Isopto Carpine, Pilopine HS) directly activate the cholinergic receptors, producing various responses in the eye, including dilation of trabecular meshwork, so that the canal of Schlemm can absorb more aqueous humor. When more aqueous humor is absorbed, IOP is reduced. Adverse effects include temporary cycloplegia. Cholinergic drugs are generally used in patients with open-angle glaucoma who have not responded to other medications. Echothiophate iodide (Phospholine iodide) is an indirect-acting cholinergic drug. It produces the same effects as direct-acting drugs, except that it blocks cholinesterase, the enzyme responsible for breaking down the natural neurotransmitter acetylcholine.

Nonselective Sympathomimetics (Mydriatic Drugs)

Dipivefrin (Propine) is a sympathomimetic drug. Dipivefrin is converted to epinephrine; epinephrine produces mydriasis, increased outflow of aqueous humor, and the subsequent fall of IOP. As discussed in Chapter 21, when epinephrine is released into the general circulation, it increases blood pressure and heart rate. Because of the potential for systemic adverse effects, this drug is rarely prescribed for the treatment of glaucoma.

Core Concept 38.5 ▶ Antiglaucoma medications may decrease the formation of aqueous humor.

Although prostaglandins are preferred drugs for glaucoma, other medications may be needed to bring IOP to normal levels. Beta-adrenergic blockers, alpha$_2$-adrenergic drugs, carbonic-anhydrase inhibitors, and osmotic diuretics are drug classes that decrease the formation of aqueous humor. These are summarized in Table 38.2.

Table 38.2 Antiglaucoma Drugs That Decrease the Formation of Aqueous Humor

Drug	Route and Adult Dose	Remarks
BETA-ADRENERGIC BLOCKERS		
betaxolol (Betoptic)	One drop 0.5% ophthalmic solution bid	Beta$_1$-blocker; reduces blood pressure, heart rate
carteolol (Ocupress)	One drop 1% ophthalmic solution bid	Nonspecific beta blocker; causes bronchoconstriction
levobunolol (Betagan)	One or two drops 0.25–0.5% ophthalmic solution once or twice daily	Nonspecific beta blocker
metipranolol (OptiPranolol)	One drop 0.3% ophthalmic solution bid	Nonspecific beta blocker
Pr timolol (Betimol, Timoptic, others)	One or two drops of 0.25–0.5% ophthalmic solution bid; gel (salve): apply daily	Nonspecific beta blocker
ALPHA$_2$-ADRENERGIC DRUGS		
apraclonidine (Iopidine)	One drop 0.5% ophthalmic solution bid	Should not be used within 14 days of monoamine oxidase inhibitor (MAOI) administration
brimonidine tartrate (Alphagan)	One drop 0.2% ophthalmic solution tid	Should not be used within 14 days of MAOI administration
CARBONIC ANHYDRASE INHIBITORS		
acetazolamide (Diamox)	PO: 250 mg one to four times per day	Oral diuretic; sulfonamide; also for seizures, high altitude sickness, and renal impairment
brinzolamide (Azopt)	One drop 1% ophthalmic solution tid	Sulfonamide
dorzolamide (Trusopt)	One drop 2% ophthalmic solution tid	Sulfonamide
methazolamide (Neptazane)	PO: 50–100 mg bid or tid	Oral sulfonamide; less diuretic activity than acetazolamide
OSMOTIC DIURETICS		
isosorbide (Ismotic)	PO: 1–3 g/kg bid–qid	Used before and after eye surgery
mannitol (Osmitrol)	IV: 1.5–2 mg/kg as a 15–25% solution over 30–60 minutes	Raises osmotic pressure, causing diuresis; IV medication

Beta-Adrenergic Blockers

Beta-blocking drugs include betaxolol (Betoptic), carteolol (Ocupress), levobunolol (Betagan), metipranolol (OptiPranolol), and timolol (Betimol, Timoptic, others). The exact mechanism by which these drugs produce their effects is not fully understood. However, they all reduce IOP effectively without the ocular adverse effects of other autonomic drugs. Beta blockers do not alter pupil diameter or produce cycloplegic effects. The doses of ophthalmic beta blockers are generally not high enough to enter the general circulation. Systemic adverse effects, if they occur, include bronchoconstriction, bradycardia, and hypotension.

hypo = *reduced*
tensive = *tension*

Prototype Drug: Pr *Timolol (Betimol, Timoptic, Others)*

Therapeutic Class: Antiglaucoma drug **Pharmacologic Class:** Beta-adrenergic blocker, reducer of IOP, ocular hypotensive drug

Actions and Uses: Timolol is a nonselective beta-adrenergic blocker available as a 0.25% or 0.5% ophthalmic solution. Timolol reduces elevated IOP in chronic open-angle glaucoma by reducing the formation of aqueous humor. The usual dose is one drop in the affected eye(s) twice a day. Timoptic XE allows for once-a-day dosing. Treatment may require 2 to 4 weeks for maximum therapeutic effect. It is also available in tablets, which are prescribed to treat mild hypertension.

Cosopt PF is a solution of timolol with dorzolamide, a carbonic-anhydrase inhibitor. Combigan combines timolol with brimonidine, an alpha adrenergic agonist.

Adverse Effects and Interactions: The most common adverse effects are local burning and stinging on instillation. In most patients there is no significant systemic absorption to cause adverse effects as long as timolol is applied correctly. If significant systemic absorption occurs, however, drug interactions could occur. Anticholinergics, nitrates, reserpine, methyldopa, or verapamil use could lead to hypotension and bradycardia. Indomethacin and thyroid hormone use could lead to decreased antihypertensive effects of timolol. Epinephrine use could lead to hypertension followed by severe bradycardia. Theophylline use could lead to decreased bronchodilation.

Alpha$_2$-Adrenergic Drugs

Alpha$_2$-adrenergic drugs are less frequently prescribed than the other antiglaucoma medications. These medications include apraclonidine (Iopidine) and brimonidine (Alphagan). The most significant adverse effects are headache, drowsiness, dry mucosal membranes, blurred vision, and irritated eyelids.

Carbonic Anhydrase Inhibitors

Carbonic anhydrase inhibitors may be administered topically or by mouth (PO) to reduce IOP. Usually these medications are used as a second choice if beta blockers are not effective. Examples include acetazolamide (Diamox), brinzolamide (Azopt), dorzolamide (Trusopt), and methazolamide (Neptazane). These medications are more effective in cases of open-angle glaucoma. Patients must be cautioned when taking these medications because they are sulfonamides—drugs that may cause an allergic reaction. All of these drugs are diuretics, which means they can reduce IOP rather quickly and dramatically, altering serum electrolytes with continuous treatment.

Osmotic Diuretics

Osmotic diuretics are used in cases of eye surgery or acute closed-angle glaucoma. Examples include isosorbide (Ismotic) and mannitol (Osmitrol). Because they have an ability to reduce plasma volume very quickly (see Chapter 19), they may produce unpleasant adverse effects, including headache, tremors, dizziness, dry mouth, fluid and electrolyte imbalance, and thrombophlebitis (venous clot formation) near the site of IV administration.

thrombo = *clot*
phleb = *vein*
itis = *inflammation*

CONCEPT REVIEW 38.2

- Describe two major approaches for controlling IOP in patients with glaucoma. What major drug classes are used in each case?

New Drug Focus

GLAUCOMA, RHO KINASE (ROCK) INHIBITORS, AND ADENOSINE AGONISTS

Two new drug classes are showing promise in the area of antiglaucoma drug research. Rho kinase (ROCK) inhibitors and adenosine agonists are drugs that target the anterior chamber of the eyeball. ROCK inhibitors relax trabecular meshwork cells and contract inner cells of the canal of Schlemm. They work by uncoupling actin from myosin, two proteins important for ciliary muscle contraction, and they shrink cells that block the outflow of aqueous humor. Adenosine agonists enhance extracellular matrix turnover in the trabecular meshwork, essentially achieving the same effect as ROCK inhibitors, increasing the outflow of aqueous humor. One unpleasant side effect for both drug classes is hyperemia (red eyes). Researchers are exploring different ways to address this unpleasant side effect.

Nursing Process Focus Patients Receiving Pharmacotherapy for Glaucoma

ASSESSMENT	POTENTIAL NURSING DIAGNOSES*
Prior to drug administration: • Obtain a complete health history, including cardiovascular, respiratory, thyroid, and renal conditions; eye trauma or infection; allergies; drug history; and possible drug interactions. • Acquire the results of physical examination focusing on vital signs, visual acuity, visual fields (peripheral and central), presence of halos, blurred vision, and ocular pain.	• *Self-Care Deficit* related to impaired vision • *Acute Pain* related to disease process or adverse drug effects • *Deficient Knowledge* related to a lack of information about drug therapy • *Risk for Injury* related to visual acuity deficits or adverse drug effects

(Continued)

Nursing Process Focus (*continued*)

PLANNING: PATIENT GOALS AND EXPECTED OUTCOMES

The patient will:

- Experience therapeutic effects (normal eye pressure and no progression of visual impairment).
- Be free from or experience minimal adverse effects from drug therapy.
- Verbalize understanding of the drug's use, adverse effects, and required precautions.

IMPLEMENTATION

Interventions and (Rationales)	Patient Education/Discharge Planning
• Administer ophthalmic solutions correctly and evaluate patient's knowledge of correct administration. (Using proper technique ensures that medication stays within the eye and helps to prevent complications.).	Instruct the patient in the proper administration of eyedrops to: • Remove contact lenses prior to administering eyedrops and wait 15 minutes before reinsertion. • Wash hands prior to eyedrop administration. • Avoid touching the tip of the container to the eye, which may contaminate the solution. • Administer the eyedrop in the conjunctival sac. • Apply pressure over the lacrimal sac for 1 minute to decrease systemic absorption. • Wait 5 minutes before administering other ophthalmic solutions. • Schedule glaucoma medications around daily routines such as waking, mealtimes, and bedtime to lessen the chance of missed doses.
• Monitor visual acuity, blurred vision, pupillary reactions, extraocular movements, and ocular pain. (Periodic monitoring helps to determine the effectiveness of drug therapy.)	• Instruct the patient to report to the healthcare provider any changes in vision, eye pain, light sensitivity, halos around lights, or headache.
• Monitor the patient for specific contraindications for the prescribed drug. (There are many physiologic conditions for which ophthalmic solutions may be contraindicated.)	• Instruct the patient to inform the healthcare provider of all health-related problems and prescribed and over-the-counter (OTC) medications.
• Provide for eye comfort such as an adequately lighted room. (Ophthalmic drugs such as beta blockers used in the treatment of glaucoma can cause miosis and difficulty seeing in low-level lighting.)	• Caution the patient about driving or other activities in low-lighting conditions or at night until the effects of the drug are known.
• Monitor for conjunctivitis and lid reactions. (These may indicate adverse reactions to the drug or infection due to improper administration.)	• Review with the patient the correct medication administration technique. • Instruct the patient to report itching, drainage, edema, ocular pain, sensation of a foreign body in the eye, photophobia, and visual disturbances to the healthcare provider.
• Monitor the color of the iris and periorbital tissue of the treated eye. (Prostaglandins can change the color of the iris over time.)	Inform the patient that: • More brown color may appear in the iris and in the periorbital tissue of the treated eye only. • Any pigmentation changes develop over months to years.
• Monitor vital signs periodically for systemic absorption of ophthalmic preparations. (Systemic ophthalmic drugs such as beta blockers and cholinergic drugs may cause serious cardiovascular complications such as hypertension or bradycardia.)	Instruct the patient to: • Take and record vital signs weekly. • Immediately report palpitations, chest pain, shortness of breath, and irregularities in pulse and blood pressure to the healthcare provider.
• Monitor and adjust environmental lighting to aid in patient's comfort. (People who have glaucoma are sensitive to excessive light, especially extreme sunlight.)	Instruct the patient to: • Adjust environmental lighting as needed to enhance vision or reduce ocular pain. • Wear darkened glasses as needed.
• Encourage compliance with the treatment regimen. (Noncompliance may result in total loss of vision.)	Instruct the patient: • To comply with the medication schedule for eyedrop administration. • About the importance of regular follow-up care with the ophthalmologist. • That IOP readings should be done prior to beginning treatment and periodically during treatment.

EVALUATION OF OUTCOME CRITERIA

Evaluate the effectiveness of drug therapy by confirming that patient goals and expected outcomes have been met (see "Planning"). *See Tables 38.1 and 38.2 for lists of drugs to which these nursing actions apply.*

*Herdman, T.H. & Kamitsuru, S. (Eds.), *Nursing Diagnoses: Definitions & Classification* 2015–2017. Copyright © 2014, 1994–2014 NANDA International. Used by arrangement by John Wiley & Sons, Inc. Companion website: www.wiley.com/go/nursingdiagnoses.

EYE EXAMINATIONS AND MINOR EYE CONDITIONS

Drugs provide relief for minor eye conditions and are used for eye exams.

◀ **Core Concept 38.6**

Drugs for minor eye irritation and injury come from a broad range of classes, including antimicrobials, local anesthetics, corticosteroids, and nonsteroidal anti-inflammatory drugs (NSAIDs). A range of drug preparations may be used, including drops, salves, optical inserts, and injectable formulations. Some drugs only provide moisture to the eye's surface. For example, bepotastine (Bepreve) is an antihistamine approved for twice daily dosing for itching associated with allergic conjunctivitis. Other drugs penetrate and affect a specific area of the eye.

Some drugs are specifically designed for ophthalmic examinations. These include **cycloplegic drugs** to relax ciliary muscles and **mydriatic drugs** to dilate the pupils. Caution must be used when administering anticholinergic mydriatics because these drugs can increase IOP and worsen glaucoma. In addition, anticholinergic drugs have the potential for producing adverse effects of the central nervous system such as confusion, unsteadiness, or drowsiness in adults. These effects are especially prevalent in older adults. Children generally become restless and spastic. Examples of cycloplegic, mydriatic, lubricant, and corneal edema drugs are listed in Table 38.3.

mydriatic = *dilating pupil*

CONCEPT REVIEW 38.3

- List examples of commonly used drugs for minor eye irritation and injury. What are the major actions of cycloplegic and mydriatic drugs?

Table 38.3 Drugs for Eye Examinations and for Moistening Eye Membranes

Drug	Route and Adult Dose	Remarks
MYDRIATICS: SYMPATHOMIMETICS		
phenylephrine (Neo-Synephrine) (see the Prototype Drug Box in Core Concept 9.8)	One drop 2.5% or 10% solution before eye exam	Decongestant and vasoconstriction properties; smaller doses provide temporary relief of eye redness; also for pupil dilation in closed-angle glaucoma
CYCLOPLEGICS: ANTICHOLINERGICS		
atropine (Atro-Pen) (see the Prototype Drug Box in Core Concept 9.7)	One drop 0.5% solution daily	Also provided as ointment; should not be administered to patients with glaucoma; effects may be prolonged
cyclopentolate (Cyclogyl, Pentalair)	One drop 0.5–2% solution 40–50 minutes before procedure	Not for patients with glaucoma; causes burning and irritation; possible central adverse effects with higher doses
homatropine (Isopto Homatropine, others)	One or two drops 2% or 5% solution before eye exam	Not for patients with glaucoma; effects may be prolonged after treatment
scopolamine hydrobromide (Isopto Hyoscine)	One or two drops 0.25% solution 1 hour before eye exam	Not for patients with glaucoma; effects may be prolonged after treatment; possible central adverse effects with higher doses
tropicamide (Mydriacyl, Tropicacyl)	One or two drops 0.5–1% solution before eye exam	Not for patients with glaucoma; central adverse effects with higher doses
LUBRICANTS CAUSING VASOCONSTRICTION		
naphazoline (Albalon, Allerest, ClearEyes, others)	One to three drops 0.1% solution every 3–4 hours prn	OTC and prescription medications available
oxymetazoline (OcuClear, Visine LR)	One or two drops 0.025% solution qid	OTC and prescription medications available
tetrahydrozoline (Murine Plus, Visine, others)	One or two drops 0.05% solution bid–tid	Primarily OTC medication
GENERAL PURPOSE LUBRICANTS		
lanolin alcohol (Lacri-lube)	Apply a thin film to the inside of the eyelid	Mixed with mineral oil and petroleum jelly as a salve
polyvinyl alcohol (Liquifilm, others)	One or two drops prn	Artificial tear solution
DRUGS FOR CORNEAL EDEMA AND ITCHING		
sodium chloride hypertonicity ointment (Muro 128 5% Ointment)	Apply a thin film to the inside of the eyelid; instill one drop into the affected eye(s) bid	Ophthalmic ointment for corneal edema; mixed with lanolin, mineral oil, purified water, and white petrolatum as a salve; for itching associated with allergic conjunctivitis

EAR CONDITIONS

The ear has two major sensory functions: hearing and maintenance of equilibrium and balance. Three important structural areas—the external ear, middle ear, and inner ear—carry out these functions (Figure 38.3).

externa = *outside*
ot = *ear*
itis = *inflammation*
media = *middle*

interna = *inside*

Otitis, inflammation of the ear, most often occurs in the external and middle ear compartments. **External otitis** or *otitis externa*, commonly referred to as swimmer's ear, is inflammation of the external ear; **otitis media** is inflammation of the middle ear. External ear infections most often occur with water exposure. Middle ear infections most often occur with upper respiratory infections, allergies, or auditory tube irritation. Of all ear infections, the most difficult ones to treat are infections of the inner ear (*otitis interna*). **Mastoiditis**, or inflammation of the mastoid sinus, can be a serious problem because if left untreated, it can result in hearing loss.

Core Concept 38.7 ▶

Otic preparations treat infections, inflammation, and earwax buildup.

Combination drugs effectively treat many different types of ear conditions, including infections, earaches, edema, and earwax.

The basic treatment for ear infection is essentially the same as in all places of the body: antibiotics. Topical antibiotics in the form of eardrops may be administered for external ear infections. Ciprofloxacin (Cipro HC otic, Cetraxal) is a very common topical antibiotic used for ear infections. Adverse reactions can occur with this medication. These include rashes; white patches in the mouth; vaginal itching or discharge; and itching, pain, or mild irritation within the ear.

Systemic antibiotics (see Chapter 27) may be needed in cases in which external ear infections are extensive or in cases of middle or inner ear infections. Medications for pain, edema, and itching may also be necessary. Corticosteroids are often combined with antibiotics or with other drugs when inflammation is present. Examples of these drugs are listed in Table 38.4.

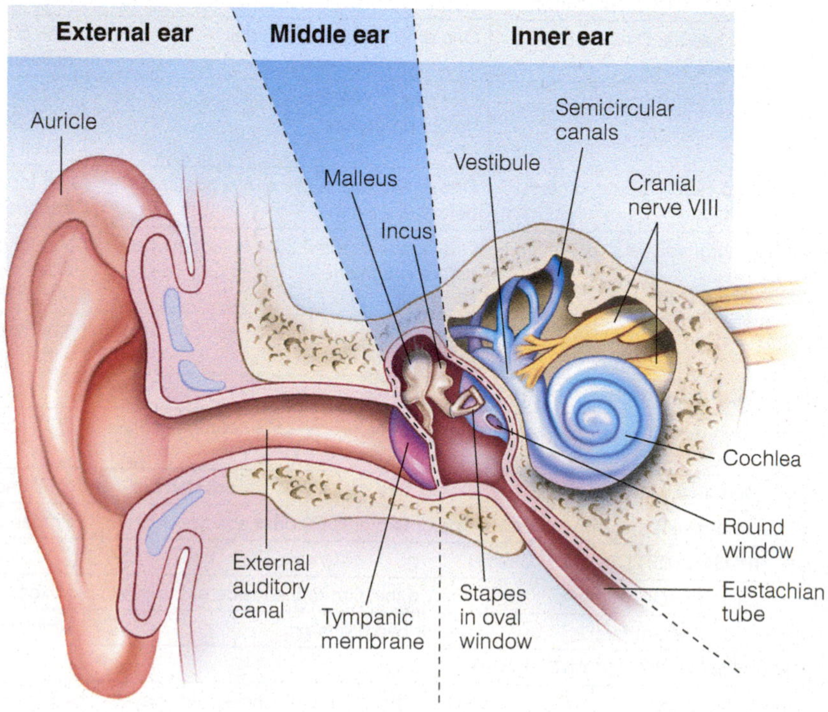

FIGURE 38.3 Structures of the external ear, middle ear, and inner ear.

Table 38.4 Otic Preparations

Drug	Route and Adult Dose	Remarks
acetic acid and hydrocortisone (Vosol HC)	Three to five drops in the affected ear every 4–6 hours for 24 hours, then five drops tid–qid	Combination of acetic acid and glucocorticoid; for general ear infections and inflammation
benzocaine and antipyrine (Auralgan)	Fill the ear canal with solution tid for 2–3 days	For acute otitis media and the removal of earwax; reduces earache associated with the infection
carbamide peroxide (Debrox)	One to five drops 6.5% solution bid for 4 days	To soften, loosen, and remove excessive earwax; OTC medication
ciprofloxacin and dexamethasone (CiproDex)	Four drops of the suspension instilled into the affected ear bid for 7 days	Combination of fluoroquinolone antibiotic and corticosteroid; for ear infections and inflammation
ciprofloxacin and hydrocortisone (Cipro HC)	Three drops of the suspension instilled into the affected ear bid for 7 days	Combination of fluoroquinolone antibiotic and corticosteroid; for ear infections and inflammation
polymyxin B, neomycin, and hydrocortisone (Cortisporin)	Four drops in the ear tid–qid	Combination of antibiotics and glucocorticoid; for general ear or mastoid infections and inflammation; some patients may develop dermatitis as a result of sensitivity to neomycin

Mineral oil, earwax softeners, and commercial products are also used for proper ear health. When earwax accumulates, it narrows the ear canal and may interfere with hearing. This is especially true for older patients who are not able to properly groom themselves. Healthcare providers working with younger and older patients are trained to take appropriate measures when removing impacted earwax.

CONCEPT REVIEW 38.4

- Identify the areas of the ear where microbial infections are most likely to occur. What kind of otic preparations treat infections, inflammation, and earwax buildup?

Patients Need to Know

Patients taking medications for eye and ear disorders need to know the following:

Regarding Eye Medications

1. Have regular eye exams after the age of 40.
2. Do not strain or lift heavy objects if risk for glaucoma is present. Any effort that might produce eyestrain should be avoided.
3. Make sure that all allergies or sensitivities, including those to sulfa drugs, are known to the healthcare providers.
4. Do not take OTC medications that are formulated to decrease redness of the eye for longer than 24 hours. Use eye lubricants instead. Persistent irritation should be reported immediately.
5. Keep eye solutions clear and sterile; do not actually touch the eye when instilling drops.

Regarding Ear Medications

6. Take precautions to keep the ear canal dry when in or around water for an extensive time. Use appropriate earplugs or a bathing cap.
7. Apply 2% acetic acid to the ear canal after swimming. Acetic acid acts as a drying agent and restores the ear canal to its normal acidic condition.
8. Antibiotics (with or without steroids) may be needed to treat swimmer's ear. Consult a healthcare provider.
9. Do not place objects such as cotton swabs in the ear canal; use a bulb syringe approved for removing debris and warm water. Use any cerumen dissolving agent responsibly.

Chapter Review

Core Concepts Summary

38.1 Knowledge of basic eye anatomy is essential for an understanding of eye disorders and drug therapy.

The anterior chamber of the eye is the place where aqueous humor is circulated. Aqueous humor originates from the ciliary body located in the posterior chamber and drains into the canal of Schlemm found in the anterior chamber.

38.2 Glaucoma is one of the leading causes of blindness.

Glaucoma develops because the flow of aqueous humor in the anterior eye chamber becomes disrupted, leading to increasing intraocular pressure (IOP). Two principal types of glaucoma are closed-angle glaucoma and open-angle glaucoma.

38.3 Glaucoma therapy focuses on adjusting the circulation of aqueous humor.

Glaucoma therapy generally works by increasing the outflow of aqueous humor or decreasing aqueous humor formation.

38.4 Antiglaucoma medications may increase the outflow of aqueous humor.

Drugs that increase the outflow of aqueous humor include miotics, sympathomimetics, prostaglandins, and prostamides. Prostaglandins are the preferred class of drugs for glaucoma treatment.

38.5 Antiglaucoma medications may decrease the formation of aqueous humor.

Medications that decrease the formation of aqueous humor include beta blockers, $alpha_2$-adrenergic drugs, carbonic-anhydrase inhibitors, and osmotic diuretics.

38.6 Drugs provide relief for minor eye conditions and are used for eye exams.

Mydriatic or pupil-dilating drugs and cyclopegic or ciliary-muscle relaxing drugs are routinely used for eye examinations. Some drugs constrict local blood vessels. Others lubricate the eyes.

38.7 Otic preparations treat infections, inflammation, and earwax buildup.

Combination drugs provide relief of conditions associated with the external, middle, and inner ear. Drugs include antibiotics, corticosteroids, and earwax dissolving drugs.

REVIEW Questions

Answer the following questions to assess your knowledge of the chapter material, and go back and review any material that is not clear to you.

1. A patient is at the optometric office for an eye examination. She is told that the healthcare provider will have to dilate her pupils with ___________ eyedrops so he can see the back of the eye.
   1. Miotic
   2. Mydriatic
   3. Constricting
   4. Corticosteroids

2. In a plan of care, a patient is to receive a drug that relieves pressure in the eye by increasing the outflow of aqueous humor. This drug would be:
   1. Timolol (Timoptic).
   2. Betaxolol (Betoptic).
   3. Pilocarpine (Ocusert).
   4. Ciprofloxacin (Cipro).

3. The patient is informed that the medication used to relieve the pressure in her eye by decreasing production of aqueous humor is:
   1. Timolol (Timoptic).
   2. Atropine sulfate.
   3. Pilocarpine (Ocusert).
   4. Ciprofloxacin (Cipro).

4. The patient has been given a prescription for acetazolamide (Diamox) 250 mg PO every 4 hours. What is the total amount of Diamox the patient will take in a 24-hour period?
   1. 250 mg
   2. 500 mg
   3. 750 mg
   4. 1000 mg

5. A patient has an ear infection and is taking Cipro. If he also had inflammation, which of the following class of drug would be added?
   1. Corticosteroids
   2. Aluminum sulfate and calcium acetate (Domeboro)
   3. Osmotic diuretics
   4. Carbonic-anhydrase inhibitors

6. Prior to administering eardrops, the nurse should inform the patient that:
   1. The solution should stay in the ear for 1 hour.
   2. The solution will be removed within 1 hour.
   3. There may be a decrease in hearing for a few minutes.
   4. The medication will take effect immediately.

7. A patient has just been prescribed ciprofloxacin for an ear infection. The nurse tells her that the drug can cause adverse reactions. The symptoms can include: (Select all that apply.)
   1. Rash.
   2. White patches in the mouth.
   3. Pain within the ear.
   4. Total loss of hearing.
   5. Vaginal itching.
8. In the plan of care for patients with glaucoma, the rationale for giving anti-glaucoma medications would be to reduce the pressure within the eye by:
   1. Decreasing aqueous humor production and increasing outflow of aqueous humor.
   2. Increasing aqueous humor production and decreasing outflow of aqueous humor.
   3. Decreasing aqueous humor production and decreasing outflow of aqueous humor.
   4. Increasing aqueous humor production and increasing outflow of aqueous humor.
9. The patient started on travoprost (Travatan) is instructed that:
   1. This medication is administered in the morning only.
   2. Due to pupil constriction, visual acuity may be affected.
   3. This medication may change the pigmentation of the iris.
   4. Due to dilation of the pupils, visual acuity may be affected.
10. If the patient is allergic to sulfonamides, the nurse understands that he should not take:
    1. Methazolamide (Neptazane).
    2. Betaxolol (Betoptic).
    3. Carteolol (Ocupress).
    4. Beta blockers.

CASE STUDY Questions

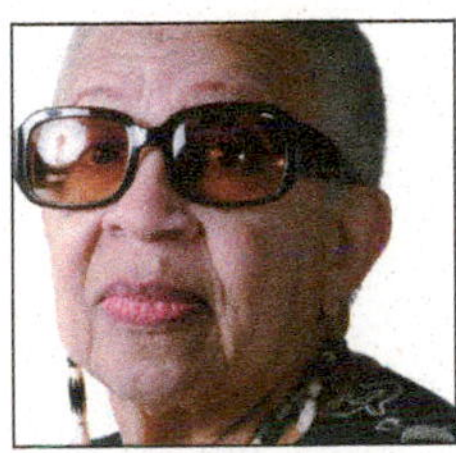

Remember Ms. Saunders, the patient introduced at the beginning of the chapter? Now read the remainder of the case study. Based on the information you have learned in this chapter, answer the questions that follow.

Ms. Mary Saunders is a 65-year-old African American woman presenting with severe pain in the right eye, headache, and blurred vision. She has a history of primary hypertension and glaucoma. Her blood pressure is 140/90 mmHg. No other obvious signs are noted. In the course of the examination, she mentions that she has recently relocated. It has been a particularly stressful time because she has not had much help from her family. She has not been using her antiglaucoma medication, the beta blocker timolol (Timoptic).

1. The nurse and Ms. Saunders begin to discuss the importance of using the glaucoma medication. The nurse explains that if left untreated pharmacologically, glaucoma could lead to:
   1. Mydriasis.
   2. Cycloplegia.
   3. Blindness.
   4. Vertigo.
2. Ms. Saunders states she knows that she should be applying her medication but has some concerns. She asks the nurse if timolol can cause any problems. The nurse responds that the most common adverse effect of timolol (Timoptic) is:
   1. Burning and stinging.
   2. Sinus irritation.
   3. Bronchoconstriction.
   4. Edema around the eyes.
3. In addition to the discussion about adverse effects, the nurse tells Ms. Saunders that it is not advisable to take the following drugs with timolol (Timoptic): (Select all that apply.)
   1. Epinephrine.
   2. Ciprofloxacin.
   3. Nitrates.
   4. Corticosteroids.
4. Ms. Saunders wants to know how long it would be before she could tell if the medication was working. The nurse tells her it would take about:
   1. 1 week.
   2. Up to 2 weeks.
   3. 2 to 4 weeks.
   4. 1 to 2 months.

Answers and complete rationales for the Review and Case Study Questions appear in Appendix A.

REFERENCE

Herdman, T. H., & Kamitsuru, S. (Eds.). (2014). *NANDA International nursing diagnoses: Definitions and classification, 2015–2017*. Oxford, United Kingdom: Wiley-Blackwell

SELECTED BIBLIOGRAPHY

American Association for Pediatric Ophthamology and Strabismus. (n.d.). *Dilating eye drops*. Retrieved from http://www.aapos.org/terms/conditions/43

Gemenetzi, M., Yang, Y., & Lotery, A. J. (2012). Current concepts on primary open-angle glaucoma genetics: A contribution to disease pathophysiology and future treatment. *Eye, 26*, 355–369. doi:10.1038/eye.2011.309

Glaucoma Research Foundation. (2015). *Glaucoma facts and stats*. Retrieved from http://www.glaucoma.org/glaucoma/glaucoma-facts-and-stats.php

Karmel, M. (n.d). *Glaucoma pipeline drugs: Targeting the trabecular meshwork*. Retrieved from http://www.aao.org/eyenet/article/glaucoma-pipeline-drugs-targeting-trabecular-meshw

Lieberthal, A. S., Carroll, A. E., Chonmaitree, T., Ganiats, T. G., Hoberman, A., Jackson, M. A., . . . Tunkel, D. E. (2013). The diagnosis and management of acute otitis media. *Pediatrics, 131*(3), e964–e999. doi:10.1542/peds.2012-3488

Newman-Casey, P. A., Weizer, J. S., Heisler, M., Lee, P. P., & Stein, J. D. (2013). Systematic review of educational interventions to improve glaucoma medication adherence. *Seminars in Ophthalmology 28*, 191–201. doi:10.3109/08820538.2013.771198

Saxby, C., Williams, R., & Hickey, S. (2013). Finding the most effective cerumenolytic. *The Journal of Laryngology & Otology, 127*, 1067–1070. doi.10.1017/S0022215113002375

Tehrani, S. (2015). Gender difference in the pathophysiology and treatment of glaucoma. *Current Eye Research, 40*, 191–200. doi:10.3109/02713683.2014.968935

Venekamp, R. P., Sanders, S., Glasziou, P. P., Del Mar, C. B., & Rovers, M. M. (2013). Antibiotics for acute otitis media in children. *Cochrane Database of Systematic Reviews, 1*, Art. No.: CD000219. doi:10.1002/14651858.CD000219.pub3

Appendix A

Complete Answers and Rationales to Review and Case Study Questions

Chapter 1

Review Answers

1. Answer: 4. Core Concept: 1.1. Rationale: Pathophysiology is the study (ology) of the nature (physio) of disease (patho). This includes how disease changes the function of the body. Pharmacology is defined by how drugs enter and travel through the body (option 1). Pharmacotherapy is defined by how drugs improve the health of the human body (option 2). Option 3 describes drug actions. Cognitive Level: Understanding. Client Need: N/A. Nursing Process: N/A.
2. Answer: 3. Core Concept: 1.3. Rationale: Biologics are naturally occurring agents produced in animal cells, in microorganisms, or by the body itself. Herbs, natural extracts, vitamins, and minerals are a part of natural therapies (option 1). Traditional drugs are chemically produced or synthesized in a laboratory (option 2). Biologics are widely used in drug therapy (option 4). Cognitive Level: Understanding. Client Need: N/A. Nursing Process: N/A.
3. Answer: 1. Core Concept: 1.2. Rationale: LPNs and LVNs cannot prescribe medication. The scope of practice for LPN and LVNs includes educating patients about their medications (option 2), ensuring drug laws are upheld (option 3), and assisting patients with medication management (option 4). Cognitive Level: Understanding. Client Need: Safe and Effective Care. Nursing Process: Implementation.
4. Answers: 1, 2, and 4. Core Concept: 1.4. Rationale: Patients should know that self-treatment with OTC drugs can be ineffective, that OTC drugs can react with foods, prescriptions, or other OTC drugs, and that they can cause serious adverse effects. In addition, patients should know that it is important to read and follow instructions. Option 3 is incorrect because the potential for further injury or disease is a consideration even when taking OTC medications. Option 5 is incorrect because a medication that works well for some people (friends) may not work for the patient. Cognitive Level: Understanding. Client Need: Physiological Integrity/Pharmacological Therapies. Nursing Process: Planning.
5. Answer: 2. Core Concept: 1.5. Rationale: Pharmaceutics is the science of preparing and dispensing of medications. Pharmacology is the study of medicine (option 1). Therapeutics is the branch of medicine concerned with disease prevention and treatment (option 3). Healthcare includes all the activity included in maintaining or restoring health (option 4). Cognitive Level: Remembering. Client Need: N/A. Nursing Process: N/A.
6. Answer: 2. Core Concept: 1.6. Rationale: The Food, Drug, and Cosmetic Act was the first law preventing the marketing of drugs that had not been thoroughly tested before they were marketed. Although the Pure Food and Drug Act of 1906 (option 1), the Prescription Drug User Fee Act of 1992 (option 3), and the FDA Modernization Act of 1997 (option 4) made significant contributions to the safety and availability of medications, the focus of these acts was different. Cognitive Level: Remembering. Client Need: N/A. Nursing Process: N/A.

7. Answer: 2. Core Concept: 1.8. Rationale: The clinical investigation stage of the drug approval process is the longest because it takes place in three different phases and involves the testing (research) of medications using humans with certain diseases. Drugs are evaluated for drug dosages, effectiveness, safety within certain populations, and adverse effects. The results of research must be presented to the FDA before the drug is allowed to proceed to the next stage. The preclinical stage involves basic scientific research (option 1). The NDA submission and review follows the clinical investigation stage and is not the longest (option 3). Postmarketing studies continue to monitor drug effects and are not typically the longest stage (option 4). Cognitive Level: Remembering. Client Need: N/A. Nursing Process: N/A.
8. Answer: 4. Core Concept: 1.9. Rationale: The Prescription Drug User Fee Act (1992) allowed the FDA to obtain extra income, which enabled it to hire more personnel in order to handle a greater number of drug applications more efficiently. This action resulted in cutting application review times by half. The Pure Food and Drug Act of 1906 (option 1), the Sherley Amendment (option 2), and the Public Health Service Act (option 3) did not affect application review time. Cognitive Level: Remembering. Client Need: N/A. Nursing Process: N/A.
9. Answer: 4. Core Concept: 1.7. Rationale: Part of the FDA Modernization Act (1997) included closer monitoring of drugs for death or serious injury. As a result of the monitoring, warnings were placed within a "black box" on drug packaging inserts. Black box warnings are not used to provide general information (option 1). The warnings do not list the ingredients in a medication (option 2) nor are they located on the drug container label (option 3). Black Box warnings are located on drug package inserts. Cognitive Level: Remembering. Client Need: N/A. Nursing Process: N/A.
10. Answers: 1–3. Core Concept: 1.10. Rationale: Each of the following options has been identified as a serious agent used in bioterrorist threats: anthrax, incapacitating chemicals, and radiation. The viruses that cause the common cold and sexually transmitted infections are not considered agents used in bioterrorist threats (options 4 and 5). Cognitive Level: Remembering. Client Need: N/A. Nursing Process: N/A.

Chapter 2

Review Answers

1. Answer: 1. Core Concept: 2.1. Rationale: Therapeutic drug classification focuses on what a drug does clinically. Pharmacologic drug classification (option 2) focuses on a drug's mechanism of action, and the term *chemical* focuses on the actual composition of a drug (option 3). Therefore, option 4 is incorrect because there is only 1 correct answer. Cognitive Level: Remembering. Client Need: N/A. Nursing Process: N/A.
2. Answer: 2. Core Concept: 2.1. Rationale: Mechanism of action refers to how specific medications affect the body. Therapeutic usefulness (option 1) describes the usefulness of a medication in treating a condition. Clinical focus (option 4) describes the use of drugs in a clinical setting. How a medication produces its effects on the body is its mechanism of action, not a model for other drugs (option 3). Cognitive Level: Remembering. Client Need: N/A. Nursing Process: N/A.
3. Answer: 4. Core Concept: 2.2. Rationale: Drugs are only given one name for both the chemical and generic drug categories; therefore, options 1 and 2 are incorrect because they list only one of these. Option 3 is incorrect because a drug may have many trade names, depending on the number of manufacturers. Cognitive Level: Remembering. Client Need: N/A. Nursing Process: N/A.
4. Answer: 4. Core Concept: 2.2. Rationale: The drug trade name is given by the drug developer, which has ownership (propriety) of the particular drug. Chemical drug names (option 1) are difficult to remember but are always considered in pharmacotherapy and

are used in part in some drug names. Option 2, matching an active ingredient with a trade name drug, is challenging because of the increasing number of combination drugs on the market. Option 3 is incorrect because trade names are usually capitalized and generic names are written in lower case. Cognitive Level: Remembering. Client Need: N/A. Nursing Process: N/A.

5. Answer: 4. Core Concept: 2.3. Rationale: The inert ingredients in a trade name drug and its generic form can differ. This difference can affect bioavailability, affecting the drug's reaction in the body. Drug formulations for trade name drugs are not always the same as their generic equivalents (option 1). In fact, ingredients may be more tightly compressed either in trade name drugs or in generic drugs, making option 2 incorrect. Option 3 is incorrect because generic drugs are not always best for treatment, despite their lower costs. Cognitive Level: Understanding. Client Need: N/A. Nursing Process: N/A.

6. Answer: 1, 3, 4, 5. Core Concept: 2.3. Rationale: It is important that the nurse understands that generic drugs cannot be substituted for drugs on the negative formulary list because of concern over the bioavailability of generic drugs and possible adverse effects on patient outcomes (option 1). The trade name drug must be dispensed as written on the prescription (option 3). The list was formed because of concern over the bioavailability of generic drugs and possible adverse effects on patient outcomes (Option 4). However, the efforts of consumer advocacy groups have led to changes in the lists (option 5). Option 2 is incorrect because the use of and drugs included on negative formulary lists are not consistent throughout the United States. Cognitive Level: Understanding. Client Need: Physiological Integrity/Pharmacological Therapies. Nursing Process: Data Collection.

7. Answer: 2. Core Concept: 2.4. Rationale: Physical dependence is the result of repeated use of a drug leading to physical changes and adaptations within the nervous system. When the drug is no longer available, the individual experiences physical signs of discomfort. Addiction (option 1) is the overwhelming feeling that drives someone to use a drug. Psychological dependence (option 3) is the intense emotional desire for continued drug use. Withdrawal (option 4) refers to the physical and psychological signs and symptoms a person experiences when the drug is no longer taken or available. Cognitive Level: Remembering. Client Need: N/A. Nursing Process: N/A.

8. Answer: 2. Core Concept: 2.4. Rationale: The Controlled Substance Act restricted the use of drugs that have significant potential for abuse. This law did not introduce drugs into the marketplace (option 1), restrict the use of all drugs that have abuse potential (option 3), or allow patients to obtain refills for Schedule II drugs without a visit to their healthcare provider (option 4). Cognitive Level: Remembering. Client Need: N/A. Nursing Process: N/A.

9. Answer: 3. Core Concept: 2.4. Rationale: Schedule IV drugs (option 3) have a relatively lower abuse and dependency potential than Schedules II and III drugs (options 1 and 2). Whereas Schedule IV drugs always require a prescription, some Schedule V drugs (option 4) do not require a prescription. Cognitive Level: N/A. Client Need: N/A. Nursing Process: N/A.

10. Answer: 3. Core Concept: 2.5. Rationale: A pregnant woman may take drugs classified within pregnancy category A or B. They have been shown to be relatively safe. Drugs within all other categories have been shown to have some adverse effect on the fetus, especially category X drugs (option 1), which have been shown to have a significant risk to both the woman and the fetus. Drugs in category D (option 4) may cause harm but can be provided if the benefit of the drug outweighs the risks. All medications, including herbs or dietary substances (option 2), must be reported to the healthcare provider because some of them can have adverse effects on the fetus. Cognitive Level: Remembering. Client Need: Physiological Integrity/Pharmacological Therapies. Nursing Process: Planning.

Chapter 3

Review Answers

1. Answer: 3. Core Concept: 3.7. Rationale: The stethoscope, large syringe, and water are all needed to administer medication by way of the nasogastric route. These pieces of equipment are not needed to administer medication through the transdermal (skin) route (option 1), the IV route (option 2), or the rectal route (option 4). Cognitive Level: Understanding. Client Need: Physiological Integrity/Pharmacological Therapies. Nursing Process: Implementation.
2. Answer: 2. Core Concept: 3.7. Rationale: Crushing XR medications alters the way they are delivered to and absorbed by the body. XR medications are not necessarily distasteful when crushed (option 1). When taken orally, crushing these medications should not cause obstructions (option 3). Some oral medications that are not XR can be crushed without affecting bioavailability (option 4). Cognitive Level: Understanding. Client Need: Physiological Integrity/Pharmacological Therapies. Nursing Process: Planning.
3. Answer: 1. Core Concept: 3.9. Rationale: Aspiration of the syringe is a safety technique done while giving an IM injection to ensure that the needle is in the muscle and not in a blood vessel (option 1). Aspiration (option 2) should not produce an air pocket and is not used to avoid hitting a nerve (option 3) or to remove air from the syringe (option 4). Cognitive Level: Understanding. Client Need: Physiological Integrity/Pharmacological Therapies. Nursing Process: Implementation.
4. Answer: 3. Core Concept: 3.9. Rationale: Administering medication via the IV route is the fastest way for it to reach the target tissue and begin working (onset) because the medication is injected directly into the circulatory system. Administering medications through the transdermal (option 1), IM (option 2), and ophthalmic (option 4) routes allows for the onset of the medication at different rates but not faster than being directly administered into the circulatory system. Cognitive Level: Remembering. Client Need: N/A. Nursing Process: N/A.
5. Answer: 1. Core Concept: 3.4. Rationale: The term *STAT* means immediately. Single (option 2), prn (option 3), and standing orders (option 4) do not indicate that an order needs to be done immediately. Cognitive Level: Application. Client Need: Physiological Integrity/Pharmacological Therapies. Nursing Process: Implementation.
6. Answer: 1. Core Concept: 3.2. Rationale: In this case, the nurse is checking for information found on the label—the right medication (option 1). The right documentation (option 2), patient (option 3), and time of delivery (option 4) are all parts of the six rights of drug administration but they are not involved in checking the medication label. Cognitive Level: Application. Client Need: Physiological Integrity/Pharmacological Therapies. Nursing Process: Implementation.
7. Answer: 5. Core Concept: 3.1. Rationale: Nurses should know and understand the medication they give (option 1), including its intended use (option 2), how the patient's age or disease state may affect the drug's pharmacotherapeutic response (option 3), and any side or adverse effects it may cause (option 4). Therefore, option 5 is the correct answer. Cognitive Level: Understanding. Client Need: Physiological Integrity/Pharmacological Therapies. Nursing Process: Data Collection.
8. Answer: 4. Core Concept: 3.4. Rationale: The information on the MAR does not include the actual classification of the medication(s) ordered. It does includes the date the medication is to be administered (option 1), the route of administration (option 2), and the dose to be administered (option 3). Cognitive Level: Knowledge. Client Need: N/A. Nursing Process: N/A.
9. Answer: 4. Core Concept: 3.5. Rationale: This is a conversion question between the metric system and the household system: 4–5 mL equals 1 teaspoon (option 4). Options 1, 2, and 3 are not equal to 5 mL. Cognitive Level: Application. Client Need: Physiological Integrity/Pharmacological Therapies. Nursing Process: Implementation.

10. Answer: 3. Concept: 3.8. Rationale: It is sometimes desirable for topical drugs (such as nitrates) to be absorbed into the systemic system. A local effect of a topical medication requires that it stay within the area of application (option 1). The type of medication applied to the skin comes in the form of creams, lotions, gels, powders, and sprays (option 4). Therefore, nurses should always wear gloves when preparing and administering the medication to prevent accidental absorption into their skin (option 2). Cognitive Level: Remembering. Client Need: Physiological Integrity/Pharmacological Therapies. Nursing Process: N/A.

Chapter 4

Review Answers

1. Answer: 3. Core Concept: 4.4. Rationale: The liver is the primary organ involved in metabolism. Patients with advanced liver disease usually need to receive lower doses than normal because their liver is unable to metabolize drugs to their inactive forms. The liver is not usually involved in the absorption (option 1), distribution (option 2), or excretion (option 4) of drugs. Cognitive Level: Understanding. Client Need: Physiological Integrity/Pharmacological Therapies. Nursing Process: Planning.
2. Answer: 2. Core Concept: 4.6. Rationale: The drug is to be given twice a day because of its half-life. This is done to maintain a therapeutic level of medication to the target cells. Option 1 is incorrect because taking the drug only once a day may not be enough to maintain therapeutic levels. The nurse should know about this mechanism of action to be able to answer the patient's question (option 3). Even though the initial dose of the drug may not be enough to maintain a therapeutic level over a period of time, it is still effective for a short time, and therefore is not blocked (option 4). Cognitive Level: Applying. Client Need: Physiological Integrity/Pharmacological Therapies. Nursing Process: Implementation.
3. Answers: 3 and 4. Core Concepts: 4.8 and 4.9. Rationale: Some medications act as *antagonists,* binding to receptors and producing responses that block agonists. Other medications act as *agonists,* binding to receptors and causing a cellular response that usually results in a therapeutic action. Drug effectiveness is determined by the desired outcome. It is possible that a drug could be more effective at a lower dose than another drug used for the same purpose (option 1). Efficacy refers to the ability of a drug to produce a more intense response as its concentration is increased. It is not solely reliant on drug dosing but on the drug's ability to meet the intended outcome (options 2 and 5). Cognitive Level: Analyzing. Client Need: Physiological Integrity/Pharmacological Therapies. Nursing Process: Planning.
4. Answer: 3. Core Concept: 4.8. Rationale: Agonists bind with a receptor to produce a therapeutic response. Antagonists (option 1) or blockers (option 4) bind to receptors, producing responses to block agonists. The term *facilitate* (option 2) is used to describe the action of agonists; such agonists are facilitators of cellular action. Level: Remembering. Client Need: Physiological Integrity/Pharmacological Therapies. Nursing Process: Planning.
5. Answer: 2. Core Concept: 4.2. Rationale: The presence of food in the digestive tract slows the absorption of any drugs taken orally. The presence of food does not cause drugs to be absorbed more rapidly (option 1), or to become either neutralized or activated by gastric enzymes (options 3 and 4). Cognitive Level: Understanding. Client Need: Physiological Integrity/Pharmacological Therapies. Nursing Process: Evaluation.
6. Answers: 1, 2, 3, and 5. Core Concept: 4.7. Rationale: Drug interactions can occur when two or more drugs are taken within a specific time frame of each other or when certain drugs are taken with specific foods (options 1 and 2). The route of administration greatly influences the rate of drug absorption—that is, IV drugs act more quickly because they

are placed directly into the bloodstream and bypass the necessity for absorption across the GI tract (option 3). Diseases of the liver or kidney impact drug effectiveness because of their role in the breakdown and excretion of medications (option 5). As long as the patient takes the medication as ordered by their healthcare provider, time of day has little impact on drug effectiveness (option 4). Cognitive Level: Analyzing. Client Need: Physiological Integrity/Pharmacological Therapies. Nursing Process: Planning.

7. Answer: 2. Core Concept: 4.3. Rationale: Only fat-soluble substances will pass the blood–brain barrier. Option 1 is incorrect because some antibiotics can easily cross the blood–brain barrier. Half-life of the drug is not determined by its ability to cross the blood–brain barrier (option 3). Antibiotics are usually absorbed easily from the GI tract (option 4). Cognitive Level: Understanding. Client Need: Physiological Integrity/Pharmacological Therapies. Nursing Process: Planning.

8. Answer: 3. Core Concept: 4.4. Rationale: The *first-pass effect* occurs when the liver metabolizes the drug to a less active form before it is distributed to the rest of the body and target organs. In some cases, this effect can inactivate more than 90% of an orally administered drug before it can reach the general circulation. Option 1 is incorrect because half-life is the length of time required for a drug's concentration in the plasma to decrease by one half. Potency refers to a drug's strength at a certain concentration or dose (option 2). The rate of elimination is defined as the amount of drug removed from the body by normal physiologic processes within a period of time (option 4). Cognitive Level: Remembering. Client Need: Physiological Integrity/Pharmacological Therapies. Nursing Process: Data Collection.

9. Answers: 1, 2, and 4. Core Concept: 4.5. Rationale: Drugs are removed from the body mainly by the kidneys, but also by bile or glandular activity, and the respiratory tract. Sweat glands are less effective at excreting drugs than other organs (option 3), and drugs are not usually excreted through the skin (option 5). Cognitive Level: Applying. Client Need: Physiological Integrity/Pharmacological Therapies. Nursing Process: Implementation.

10. Answer: 3. Core Concept: 4.5, Lifespan and Diversity. Rationale: Metabolic enzyme activity is reduced in older patients, making them more sensitive to medications than other patients. Drug doses for this age group are often reduced to compensate for the differences in metabolic rates. Drug dosages are not increased (option 1). Increasing (option 2) or decreasing (option 4) the number of times an older patient takes their medication does not directly affect metabolism. Cognitive Level: Analyzing. Client Need: Physiological Integrity/Pharmacological Therapies. Nursing Process: Planning.

Chapter 5

Review Answers

1. Answer: 1. Core Concept: 5.1. Rationale: During assessment/data collection; the nurse collects data about the patient prior to implementation of medication administration. Option 2 (planning), option 3 (implementing), and option 4 (evaluating) are incorrect because the nurse is collecting information. Cognitive Level: Applying. Client Need: Health Promotion and Maintenance. Nursing Process: Data Collection.

2. Answer: 3. Core Concept: 5.4. Rationale: During the implementation phase, it is the nurse's responsibility to both administer medication correctly and teach patients about medications they are taking. Option 1 is incorrect because it describes more general nursing actions not related to medication. Option 2 includes evaluating, which is another step of the nursing process. Option 4 describes the evaluation step. Cognitive Level: Understanding. Client Need: Physiological Integrity/Pharmacological Therapies. Nursing Process: Implementation.

3. Answer: 2. Core Concept: 5.5. Rationale: The main goal of administering a drug is to achieve a therapeutic effect, such as to relieve a symptom or cure a disease, with no or minimal adverse effects. Therefore, acquiring evidence of a drug's therapeutic effects is the most important role of the nurse in the evaluation phase of the nursing process. Patient satisfaction (option 1), minor adverse drug effects (option 3), and the possibility of noncompliance (option 4) are not as important as the therapeutic effect of the drug. Cognitive Level: Understanding. Client Need: Physiological Integrity/Pharmacological Therapies. Nursing Process: Evaluation.

4. Answer: 1, 3, 4, and 5. Core Concept: 5.1. Rationale: Before administering a medication, it is the nurse's responsibility to collect data about: drug allergies (option 1) to avoid giving the patient a drug that causes adverse effects; history of renal or hepatic disease (option 3) because these organs are involved in the excretion and metabolism of drugs; and the patient's physical examination information (option 4), in order to determine if they have any conditions that might contraindicate the administration of a specific drug. In addition, if administering an oral medication, the patient's ability to swallow properly must be determined (option 5). Option 2 is not applicable during the data collection phase because the drug had not yet been given. Cognitive Level: Understanding. Client Need: Health Promotion and Maintenance. Nursing Process: Data Collection.

5. Answer: 3. Core Concept: 5.4. Rationale: Implementation; the nurse is putting the plan of care into action by preparing and giving the patient ordered medication. Option 1 (data collection) would occur before planning and implementation. Option 2 (planning) would occur before implementation. Option 4 (evaluation) would occur after administering the drug. Cognitive Level: Applying. Client Need: Physiological Integrity/ Pharmacological Therapies. Nursing Process: Implementation.

6. Answer: 3. Core Concept: 5.2. Rationale: The second phase of the nursing process, nursing diagnosis, involves the analysis of data, identification of a patient's response to health problems, and the formulation of diagnostic statements such as *Activity Intolerance*. Option 1 (data collection) is done prior to diagnosing. Option 2 (implementation) is performing the nursing actions. Option 4 (planning) occurs after the nursing diagnoses have been identified. Cognitive Level: Understanding. Client Need: Health Promotion and Maintenance. Nursing Process: Nursing Diagnosis.

7. Answer: 4. Core Concept: Introduction. Rationale: The nursing process is a systematic approach to problem solving that is used to determine the benefits and risks of the use of medications. Option 1 is a limited assessment, not the nursing process. Option 2 describes documentation, not the nursing process. Option 3 is incorrect because the nursing process is not limited to textbook knowledge. Cognitive Level: Understanding. Client Need: Safe and Effective Care Environment/Coordinated Care. Nursing Process: All phases.

8. Answer: 3. Core Concept: Introduction. Rationale: The scope of practice for LPNs and LVNs is to contribute to each phase of the nursing process under the direction of the RN. Option 1 is incorrect because the LPN or LVN always works under the direction of the RN. Option 2 is incorrect because the LPN or LVN works with the RN, not the healthcare provider on the plan of care. Option 4 is incorrect because the LPN or LVN collaborates with the RN and is not completely dependent. Cognitive Level: Understanding. Client Need: Safe and Effective Care. Nursing Process: All phases.

9. Answer: 2. Core Concept: 5.3. Rationale: In the planning phase, the team lays out the necessary teaching and actions that will need to be performed. Option 1 is incorrect because the nurse is planning, not collecting data. Option 3 is incorrect because the nurse is not yet implementing the plan of care. Option 4 is incorrect because the nurse has not performed actions that need to be evaluated. Cognitive Level: Applying. Client Need: Safe and Effective Care Environment/Coordinated Care. Nursing Process: Planning.

10. Answer: 2. Core Concept: 5.2. Rationale: Etiology means the "cause" of an identified problem, in this case, anxiety. When formulating a problem statement, the nursing diagnosis (or problem) is followed by the etiology (cause) after the words "related to." Option 1 (insomnia) is the nursing diagnosis, not the etiology. Option 3 (difficulty falling asleep) is a manifestation of insomnia. Option 4 (difficulty staying asleep) is evidence of insomnia. Cognitive Level: Understanding. Client Need: Health Promotion and Maintenance. Nursing Process: Nursing Diagnosis.

Chapter 6

Review Answers

1. Answer: 4. Core Concept: 6.4. Rationale: Whenever an order is unclear, the nurse should contact the prescriber for clarification and have the order rewritten to prevent errors. Options 1, 2, and 3 are incorrect. Having another nurse clarify the order will not necessarily ensure that the dose is correct for the patient's condition. Although the pharmacist and a drug guide may provide the nurse with the usual dose for most patients, they do not take into consideration the patient's disease condition, weight, or other variables that may affect the drug's pharmacokinetics. Cognitive Level: Applying. Client Need: Physiological Integrity/Pharmacological Therapies. Nursing Process: Implementation.
2. Answers: 1, 3, 5. Core Concept: 6.3. Rationale: After giving an incorrect medication to a patient, the nurse should notify the healthcare provider or the prescribing provider, document the error in the critical incident or occurrence report used by the health care agency, and observe the patient for adverse reactions to the medication. Options 2 and 4 are incorrect. The error should be documented whether the patient experiences adverse effects or not. The hospital legal department is not notified by the nurse but may be apprised of the error through regular summaries by the agency's risk management department. Cognitive Level: Applying. Client Need: Physiological Integrity/Pharmacological Therapies. Nursing Process: Implementation.
3. Answer: 3. Core Concept: 6.2. Rationale: Pharmacies maintain records of all prescriptions, and by filling all prescriptions at one pharmacy, the pharmacist can review previously and currently prescribed medications for duplication or interactions. Options 1, 2, and 4 are incorrect. Information provided on the internet may vary in quality or may be from non–healthcare sources. Delaying to take new prescriptions may be harmful if necessary drugs such as antibiotics are ordered. A trade-name drug does not ensure the safety of the medication. Cognitive Level: Applying. Client Need: Physiological Integrity/Pharmacological Therapies. Nursing Process: Implementation.
4. Answer: 4. Core Concept: 6.4. Rationale: Returning when the patient is available ensures that the medications are taken and provides an opportunity to assess for medication effects or to teach the patient about the medications. Options 1, 2, and 3 are incorrect. Medications should not be left at the bedside unless ordered to do so and should never be given to anyone other than the patient. If a patient refuses a medication, the reason for doing so must be documented. In this case, the patient has not refused the medication and the nurse should return after the patient is available to give it. Cognitive Level: Applying. Client Need: Physiological Integrity/Pharmacological Therapies. Nursing Process: Implementation.
5. Answer: 1. Core Concept: 6.4. Rationale: The nurse should always validate a questionable order or drug when the patient or family member expresses concern. Options 2, 3, and 4 are incorrect. The nurse should verify the order and contact the provider if needed. The medication should not be given until verified. Although medications purchased by the healthcare agency may vary in appearance depending on the vendor the drug was purchased from, the nurse should withhold the medication until it is verified as being the correct drug and dose. Cognitive Level: Applying. Client Need: Physiological Integrity/Pharmacological Therapies. Nursing Process: Implementation.

6. Answer: 2. Core Concept: 6.4. Rationale: An RCA seeks to prevent recurrence of errors, including medication errors, by analyzing what happened, why it happened, and what can be done to prevent it from happening again. Options 1, 3, and 4 are incorrect. Although these may be important questions to ask to ensure that procedures are followed and the patient is receiving cost-effective care and had a good outcome from that care, they are not part of an RCA. Cognitive Level: Understanding. Client Need: Safe and Effective Care Environment. Nursing Process: Evaluation.
7. Answer: 3. Core Concept: 6.4. Rationale: Obtaining information about a patient's allergies and medication history prior to medication administration is the nurse's task during the assessment or data collection phase of the nursing process. Options 1 and 2, having the patient ask questions and provide information (outcomes) about medications, are usually done during teaching sessions (the implementation phase of the nursing process). Planning the times for medication administration is done during the planning phase of the nursing process (option 4). Cognitive Level: Applying. Need: Physiological Integrity/Pharmacological Therapies. Nursing Process: Data Collection.
8. Answers: 1, 2, 3, and 4. Core Concepts: 6.2 and 6.4. Rationale: The nurse must ensure that the correct drug is being given, the dose is correct through proper drug calculation, and the correct route of administration is used. Additionally, the nurse must verify the patient's name prior to actual administration. While it is important that the patient's home address be accurate in facility records, it is not necessary to check this information when administering medications (option 5). Cognitive Level: Understanding. Client Need: Physiological Integrity/Pharmacological Therapies. Nursing Process: Implementation.
9. Answer: 3. Core Concept: 6.3. Rationale: The *primary* purpose of completing an incident report after a medication error has occurred is to do an RCA, which will help prevent future errors. The primary purpose of an incident report is not to blame anyone specifically (option 1). Neither is it to gather information for risk management procedures (option 2) or to determine the competence of a nurse (option 4). Cognitive Level: Applying. Client Need: Safe and Effective Care Environment. Nursing Process: Implementation.
10. Answer: 4. Core Concept: 6.3. Rationale: When a medication error has been identified, the nurse should call the primary or prescribing healthcare provider. Because of the error, new patient orders may be given. Documentation of the error on the patients chart (option 1) or on an incident report (option 2) should be done according to institutional policy and only after the healthcare provider has been notified. Giving both the 6:00 a.m. and the 12:00 p.m. dose at the same time (option 3) would double the prescribed dose, and the medication error of "giving the wrong dose" will have occurred. Cognitive Level: Applying. Client Need: Physiological Integrity/Pharmacological Therapies. Nursing Process: Implementation.

Chapter 7

Review Answers

1. Answers: 1–3. Core Concept: 7.4. Rationale: Ginseng (option 1) and ginger (option 2) increase the effects of anticoagulants, thus increasing bleeding potential. St. John's wort (option 3) decreases the effectiveness of anticoagulants. Valerian (option 4) and Echinacea (option 5) have not been shown to have any effect on warfarin. Cognitive Level: Understanding. Client Need: Physiological Integrity/Pharmacological Therapies. Nursing Process: Data Collection.
2. Answer: 2. Core Concepts: 7.1 and 7.2. Rationale: Patients who use herbal therapies want to increase feelings of wellness and ensure that they are being treated holistically. Patients would not typically use herbal therapies for the following reasons: because the use of herbal therapies does not prevent the overuse of prescription medications (option 1),

because herbal therapies do not undergo the strict testing and regulation of prescription drugs (option 3), and because there is no proof that herbal therapies are "so much safer" than man-made drugs (option 4). Cognitive Level: Understanding. Client Need: Health Promotion and Maintenance. Nursing Process: Data Collection.

3. Answer: 2. Core Concept: 7.6. Rationale: It is the nurse's responsibility to ensure patients understand that herbal products should be used with caution, one reason being that the labeling of herbal therapies is not regulated like prescription drugs and therefore may not be reliable. The other options are incorrect because herbal products are not approved under FDA regulations (option 1) and even though herbal therapies can be purchased without a prescription, it does not mean that they have only a few side effects (option 3). In addition, manufacturers of herbal products do not have to demonstrate the safety or effectiveness of their product (option 4). Cognitive Level: Understanding. Client Need: Physiological Integrity/Pharmacological Therapies. Nursing Process: Planning.

4. Answer: 1. Core Concept: 7.5. Rationale: An example of a specialty supplement is *Lactobacillus acidophilus*. Ginseng (option 2), garlic (option 3), and *Ginkgo biloba* (option 4) are all herbal supplements. Cognitive Level: Remembering. Client Need: N/A. Nursing Process: N/A.

5. Answer: 3. Core Concept: 7.4. Rationale: Some CAM therapies, especially herbal therapies, can interact with prescription and OTC medications. Although manufacturers of herbal products are not required to prove safety, CAM therapies have not been shown to be dangerous when used as recommended (option 1). The use of CAM therapies does not ensure that additional treatment may not be needed (option 2). Furthermore, some CAM therapies have been reported to be helpful (option 4). Cognitive Level: Understanding. Client Need: Physiological Integrity/Pharmacological Therapies. Nursing Process: Data Collection.

6. Answer: 2. Core Concept: 7.5. Rationale: The actions of specialty supplements are more specific than herbal products and are generally used for treating specific, targeted conditions. Because of their actions, specialty supplements are not used to treat a diverse range of conditions (option 1). Furthermore, specialty supplements are not used based on the effectiveness of prescription medications (option 3) or used when the body does not make sufficient quantities (option 4). Cognitive Level: Remembering. Client Need: Health Promotion and Maintenance. Nursing Process: Planning.

7. Answer: 2. Core Concept: 7.6. Rationale: The DHSEA ensures that herbal products are labeled as "dietary supplements." The DHSEA is not responsible for strict product testing (option 1), sending the herbal product to the FDA for evaluation (option 3), or ensuring the safety of herbal products (option 4). Cognitive Level: Remembering. Client Need: N/A. Nursing Process: N/A.

8. Answer: 4. Core Concept: 7.4. Rationale: The nurse checks for the use of ginseng because it can increase digoxin toxicity. St John's wort (option 1) and Valerian (option 2) have not been shown to interact with digoxin. Fish oil (option 3) is a specialty supplement, not an herbal supplement. Cognitive Level: Applying. Client Need: Physiological Integrity/Pharmacological Therapies. Nursing Process: Data Collection.

9. Answer: 3. Core Concept: 6.5. Rationale: The nurse should provide information on chondroitin and glucosamine. These are the preferred specialty supplements for joint problems such as arthritis. Garlic and soy (option 1) are herbal supplements. Garlic reduces blood cholesterol, and soy helps to relieve menopausal symptoms and prevent cardiovascular disease. Fish oil (option 2) and DHEA (option 4) are specialty supplements. Fish oil is used to reduce blood cholesterol and enhance brain function. DHEA is used to boost immune function and memory. Cognitive Level: Applying. Client Need: Physiological Integrity/Pharmacological Therapies. Nursing Process: Implementation.

10. Answer: 4. Core Concept: 7.2. Rationale: Echinacea enhances the immune system, providing anti-inflammatory effects. Soy (option 1) helps relieve menopausal symptoms and prevent cardiovascular disease, saw palmetto (option 2) helps relieve urinary problems related to the prostate, and cranberry (option 3) helps prevent urinary tract infections. Cognitive Level: Remembering. Client Need: N/A. Nursing Process: N/A.

Chapter 8

Review Answers

1. Answer: 3. Core Concept: 8.1. Rationale: Alcohol and nicotine are the most commonly abused drugs. The other drug options (1, 2, and 4) are not used more than alcohol or nicotine. Cognitive Level: Remembering. Client Need: N/A. Nursing Process: N/A.
2. Answer: 2. Core Concept: 8.9. Rationale: An overdose of cocaine can cause dysrhythmias, convulsions, stroke, and even death. Irritability, restlessness, abdominal cramping (option 1); insomnia (option 3); and delirium, extreme fatigue, hunger, and headaches (option 4) are not usually attributed to an overdose of cocaine. Cognitive Level: Applying. Client Need: Physiological Integrity/Pharmacological Therapies. Nursing Process: Data Collection.
3. Answer: 4. Core Concept: 8.5. Rationale: Tolerance is a biological condition that occurs when the body adapts to a substance, requiring higher doses of a drug to achieve the same effects as prior lower doses. Toxicity (option 1) refers to a harmful accumulation of a substance within the blood. Resistance (option 2) is an increased ability to withstand an assault. Immunity (option 3) is the development or administration of protection against antigens. Cognitive Level: Applying. Client Need: Physiological Integrity/Pharmacological Therapies. Nursing Process: Data Collection.
4. Answer: 1. Core Concept: 8.6. Rationale: Methadone is the drug of choice to help those addicted to opioids such as heroin (option 2) or morphine. Diazepam (option 3) and alprazolam (option 4) are benzodiazepines, CNS depressants, commonly used for depression. Cognitive Level: Understanding. Client Need: Physiological Integrity/Pharmacological Therapies. Nursing Process: Planning.
5. Answer: 2. Core Concept: 8.7. Rationale: Marijuana has been shown to have few physically addictive qualities, whereas heroin (option 1), alcohol (option 3), and cocaine (option 4) can cause physical addiction. Cognitive Level: Remembering. Client Need: Physiological Integrity/Pharmacological Therapies. Nursing Process: Planning.
6. Answer: 2. Core Concept: 8.9. Rationale: Methyphenidate (Ritalin) is classified as a schedule II drug. Drugs in this class have a high potential for abuse and can lead to severe psychological or physical dependence. Drugs in Class III (option 3) and Class IV (option 4) have a lesser chance of abuse and addiction than Schedule II drugs. Schedule I (option 1) drugs have no currently accepted medical use in the United States and have a high potential for abuse. Cognitive Level: Remembering. Client Need: Physiological Integrity/Pharmacological Therapies. Nursing Process: Planning.
7. Answer: 3. Core Concept: 8.9. Rationale: Increased heart rate, dilated pupils, elevated body temperature, and sweating are all signs of cocaine use. Marijuana (option 1) slows motor activity, decreases coordination, and causes paranoia or euphoria. Heroin (option 2) produces brief, intense euphoria, constricted pupils, and increased ability to withstand pain. Amphetamine (option 4) use produces exhilaration, increased blood pressure and respirations, and reduced appetite. Cognitive Level: Applying. Client Need: Physiological Integrity/Pharmacological Therapies. Nursing Process: Data Collection.
8. Answer: 1. Core Concept: 8.6. Rationale: Patients who use barbiturates may exhibit drowsiness, lack of muscle coordination, and decreased respiration. Euphoria and irritability (option 2) are signs of cocaine use. Increased pain threshold and hallucinations

(option 3) are signs of using hallucinogens. Increased blood pressure and respirations (option 4) are signs of CNS stimulant use. Cognitive Level: Applying. Client Need: Physiological Integrity/Pharmacological Therapies. Nursing Process: Data Collection.

9. Answer: 3. Core Concepts: 8.3 and 8.4. Rationale: A person who is physically dependent on a drug and discontinues its use will go through signs of withdrawal. Intense craving (option 1) and an overwhelming need for the drug (option 2) can occur with either psychological or physical dependency. Some drugs produce the side effect of tolerance (option 4), the need to have higher doses to produce the initial effect of the drug. Cognitive Level: Understanding. Client Need: Physiological Integrity/Pharmacological Therapies. Nursing Process: Data Collection.

10. Answer: 2. Core Concept: 8.6. Rationale: Disulfiram is used to prevent the use of alcohol. Patients need to know that if they drink alcohol and use disulfiram, they may experience shortness of breath, nausea, vomiting, and headaches. Not even a small amount of alcohol should be ingested (option 1). Disulfiram is not safe during pregnancy (option 3), and it actually inhibits alcohol metabolism (option 4). Cognitive Level: Applying. Client Need: Physiological Integrity/Pharmacological Therapies. Nursing Process: Implementation.

Chapter 9

Review Answers

1. Answer: 4. Core Concept: 9.7. Rationale: Atropine may increase intraocular pressure and therefore is contraindicated for patients with glaucoma (a disorder of increased pressure in the eye). Pilocarpine (option 1), betaxolol (option 2), and timolol (option 3) can be used for the treatment of glaucoma. Cognitive Level: Understanding. Client Need: Physiological Integrity/Pharmacological Therapies. Nursing Process: Planning.

2. Answer: 2. Core Concept: 9.6. Rationale: Cholinergic drugs mimic the effects of the parasympathetic nervous system and reduce intraocular pressure in patients with glaucoma. Adrenergic drugs (option 1) are primarily used for their effects on the heart, bronchial tree, and nasal passages. Adrenergic blockers (option 3) are primarily used in the treatment of the cardiovascular system disorders such as HTN, and cholinergic blockers (option 4) are used to dry secretions and treat asthma. Cognitive Level: Understanding. Client Need: Physiological Integrity/Pharmacological Therapies. Nursing Process: Planning.

3. Answer: 4. Core Concept: 9.8. Rationale: An adrenergic drug, phenylephrine (Neo-Synephrine) stimulates alpha$_1$-receptors and is used to dry nasal secretions. Prolonged intranasal use can cause burning of the mucosa and rebound congestion. Albuterol (option 1) and salmeterol (option 3) are beta-adrenergic drugs used to treat bronchospasm. Neostigmine (option 2) is a cholinergic drug used to treat myasthenia gravis. Cognitive Level: Applying. Client Need: Physiological Integrity/Pharmacological Therapies. Nursing Process: Implementation.

4. Answer: 3. Core Concept: 9.7. Rationale: Oxybutynin (Ditropan), a cholinergic drug, is used to treat urinary urgency and incontinence. Dicyclomine (option 1) and scopolamine (option 4) are used to treat irritable bowel syndrome. Ipratropium (option 2) is used to treat asthma. Cognitive Level: Applying. Client Need: Physiological Integrity/Pharmacological Therapies. Nursing Process: Implementation.

5. Answers: 1, 2, and 5. Core Concept: 9.9. Rationale: Alpha-adrenergic blockers cause vasodilation and decreased blood pressure. Because of the drugs' hypotensive action, they may also cause dizziness (lightheadedness). This class of medications does not cause an increase in blood pressure (option 3) or vasoconstriction (option 4). Cognitive Level: Applying. Client Need: Physiological Integrity/Pharmacological Therapies. Nursing Process: Implementation.

6. Answer: 2. Core Concept: 9.9. Rationale: Lopressor is a cardioselective beta$_1$-blocker used to treat HTN, HF, and MI. Alpha blockers (option 1) relax the smooth muscle of the vessels, causing vasodilation and lowered blood pressure. Cholinergic drugs (option 3) mimic the effects of the parasympathetic system and are used for a variety of different disorders such as irritable bowel syndrome, incontinence, and Alzheimer disease. Cholinergic blockers (option 4) are used primarily to dry secretions and treat asthma. Cognitive Level: Remembering. Client Need: Physiological Integrity/Pharmacological Therapies. Nursing Process: Data Collection.

7. Answer: 3. Core Concept: 9.9. Rationale: Atenolol (Tenormin) is a cardioselective beta$_1$-blocker used to treat HTN and angina. The primary effect of this class of medication includes lowering heart rate, thus decreasing blood pressure. Because of this effect, the nurse should obtain the patient's pulse and blood pressure before administering the drug. Atenolol does not affect respirations (options 1 and 2) or temperature (option 4). Cognitive Level: Applying. Client Need: Physiological Integrity/Pharmacological Therapies. Nursing Process: Implementation.

8. Answer: 3. Core Concept: N/A. Rationale: 20 mg (the order) ÷ 10 mg × 5 mL (amt. supplied) = 10 mL × 3 times a day = 30 mL/day. Options 1, 2, and 4 are a result of miscalculations and therefore incorrect. Cognitive Level: Applying. Client Need: Physiological Integrity/Pharmacological Therapies. Nursing Process: Implementation.

9. Answer: 4. Core Concept: 9.8. Rationale: The nurse informs the patient that prolonged overuse of phenylephrine nasal spray can cause rebound congestion. When taken as a nasal spray, this selective alpha$_1$-adrenergic drug has few systemic effects, although it produces local (nasal) effects. If taken parenterally, phenylephrine stimulates the sympathetic nervous system and can cause an increase in heart rate and restlessness. Therefore, it does not decrease heart rate (option 1), decrease blood pressure (option 2), or cause drowsiness (option 3). Cognitive Level: Applying. Client Need: Physiological Integrity/Pharmacological Therapies. Nursing Process: Implementation.

10. Answer: 3. Core Concept: 9.7. Rationale: An effect of cholinergic blockers (anticholinergics) is the drying of secretions; therefore, the nurse should monitor the patient for having a dry mouth. These drugs do not cause diaphoresis (option 1), confusion (option 2), or an increase in urination (option 4). Cognitive Level: Understanding. Client Need: Physiological Integrity/Pharmacological Therapies. Nursing Process: Evaluation.

Case Study Answers

1. Answer: 3. Core Concept: 9.6. Rationale: Bethanechol, a cholinergic drug, is used to treat urinary retention. It stimulates smooth muscle contraction of the urinary tract, causing the bladder to return to normal functioning. This medication does not have any influence (an increase or decrease) on the amount of urine produced (options 1 and 4) and does not inhibit smooth muscle contraction (option 2). Cognitive Level: Applying. Client Need: Physiological Integrity/Pharmacological Therapies. Nursing Process: Implementation.

2. Answers: 2, 3, and 4. Core Concept: 9.6. Rationale: The nurse should inform Mrs. Wheaton that one of the possible adverse effects of bethanechol is hypotension and she should avoid abrupt position changes to prevent fainting. Increased salivation and sweating (option 3) are other adverse effects that Mrs. Wheaton should know about. In addition, because bethanechol will cause her to urinate, she should be near a bathroom after taking it (option 4). As previously mentioned, there are adverse effects; therefore, option 1 is incorrect. Cognitive Level: Applying. Client Need: Physiological Integrity/Pharmacological Therapies. Nursing Process: Implementation.

3. Answer: 4. Core Concept: 9.9. Rationale: Prazosin is an alpha-adrenergic blocker. It lowers blood pressure by relaxing the smooth muscle of the vessels and decreasing peripheral resistance. Prazosin is not classified as a cholinergic drug (option 1), a cholinergic blocker

(option 2), or an adrenergic drug (option 3). Cognitive Level: Understanding. Client Need: Physiological Integrity/Pharmacological Therapies. Nursing Process: Planning.

4. Answers: 1, 2, and 3. Core Concept: 9.9. Rationale: Mrs. Wheaton should be taught that Prazosin can cause dizziness when changing positions, an increase in heart rate, and nasal congestion. It is not known to cause nausea (option 4). Cognitive Level: Applying. Client Need: Physiological Integrity/Pharmacological Therapies. Nursing Process: Implementation.

Chapter 10

Review Answers

1. Answer: 4. Core Concept: 10.4. Rationale: Rebound insomnia occurs when a patient abruptly discontinues medications used for sleeping. Panic disorder (option 1) is characterized by intense feelings of immediate apprehension, fearfulness, terror, or impending doom, accompanied by increased autonomic nervous system activity. Long-term insomnia (option 2) is caused by intense emotional and mood-related illnesses such as depression, manic disorders, or chronic pain. Behavioral insomnia (option 3) is usually attributed to stress caused by a hectic lifestyle or the inability to resolve day-to-day conflicts within the home or workplace. Cognitive Level: Understanding. Client Need: Physiological Integrity/Pharmacological Therapies. Nursing Process: Evaluation.
2. Answer: 2. Core Concept: 10.9. Rationale: Buspirone (BusSpar), a CNS drug, may take several weeks to become fully effective. This drug will not give immediate relief (option 1) and, until the drug is allowed to become fully effective, drug dosages will not be increased (option 3). In addition, it is too early to determine if the patient may need any additional medication to help with their anxiety (option 4). Cognitive Level: Applying. Client Need: Physiological Integrity/Pharmacological Therapies. Nursing Process: Implementation.
3. Answer: 3. Core Concept: All. Rationale: The purpose of a sedative is to allow the patient to sleep. It would be disruptive to wake the patient to give this medication (option 1) or to notify the healthcare provider just because the patient is sleeping (option 2). The missed sedative should not be given with the next dose, essentially doubling the dose, because it may cause adverse effects (option 4). Instead, the nurse should hold the dose and document the reason. Cognitive Level: Applying. Client Need: Physiological Integrity/Pharmacological Therapies. Nursing Process: Implementation.
4. Answer: 3. Core Concept: 10.9. Rationale: The effects of zolpidem (Ambien) can be felt approximately 30 minutes after taking; therefore it should be taken just before going to bed. The patient does not need to take it several hours before bedtime, use it for at least a week, or use it on a long-term basis to benefit from the drug's effects (options 1, 2, and 4). Cognitive Level: Applying. Client Need: Physiological Integrity/Pharmacological Therapies. Nursing Process: Implementation.
5. Answer: 2. Core Concept: 10.8. Rationale: The use of barbiturates can lead to dependence. The nurse is concerned that a patient who takes barbiturates for sleeplessness and suddenly stops will experience severe withdrawal symptoms. Stopping barbiturate use should not lead to respiratory depression (option 1), hypotension (option 3), or shock (option 4). Cognitive Level: Understanding. Client Need: Physiological Integrity/Pharmacological Therapies. Nursing Process: Evaluation.
6. Answer: 4. Core Concept: 10.5. Rationale: Because sedatives relax patients in order to reduce anxiety and facilitate sleep, the nurse should ensure patient safety by making sure the patient's call light is within their reach. As a general rule, patients should be oriented to their surroundings, but after taking a sedative, a patient will be drowsy and may not remember what they are told (option 1). Sedatives, if given as prescribed, should not cause respiratory dysfunction (option 2). Shutting off the lights and closing

the door may increase the patient's confusion and anxiety and does not allow the nurse to properly monitor the patient (option 3). Cognitive Level: Applying. Client Need: Safe and Effective Care Environment. Nursing Process: Implementation.

7. Answers: 1, 2, 4, and 5. Core Concept: 10.5. Rationale: Benzodiazepines, antidepressants, barbiturates, and OTC antihistamine sleep aids can be used to treat anxiety and insomnia. Antipsychotics are used to treat psychoses such as hallucinations, delusions, and disorganized thoughts (option 3). Cognitive Level: Remembering. Client Need: Physiological Integrity/Pharmacological Therapies. Nursing Process: Planning.
8. Answer: 2. Core Concept: 10.6. Rationale: The nurse should inform patients to avoid using alcohol if taking CNS depressants, because alcohol (also a depressant) can enhance the effect of the medication. Nicotine, chocolate, and tea (options 1, 3, and 4) can act as stimulants. Cognitive Level: Understanding. Client Need: Physiological Integrity/Pharmacological Therapies. Nursing Process: Planning.
9. Answer: 1. Core Concept: 10.7. Rationale: While alprazolam (option 1), clonazepam (option 3) and lorazepam (option 4) are used for phobias and panic disorders, only alprazolam (Xanax) is also used for GAD. Estazolam (option 2) is used for insomnia. Cognitive Level: Remembering. Client Need: Physiological Integrity/Pharmacological Therapies. Nursing Process: Planning.
10. Answer: 1. Core Concept: 10.7. Rationale: Adverse effects of lorazepam (Ativan) may include drowsiness, sedation, amnesia, weakness, disorientation, sleep disturbance, blurred vision, and ataxia. Euphoria (option 2), astigmatism (option 3), and tachypnea (option 4) are not adverse effects of this medication. Cognitive Level: Applying. Client Need: Physiological Integrity/Pharmacological Therapies. Nursing Process: Evaluation.

Case Study Answers

1. Answer: 4. Core Concept: 10.6. Rationale: Although Celexa (option 1), Lexapro (option 2), Prozac (option 3), and Paxil (option 4) are all used for depression, only Paxil is also used for PTSD. Cognitive Level: Remembering. Client Need: Physiological Integrity/Pharmacological Therapies. Nursing Process: Planning.
2. Answer: 4. Core Concept: 10.6. Rationale: The nurse should monitor Ms. Reynolds for weight gain, possibly caused by changes in appetite and metabolism. Diarrhea (option 1), hypotension (option 2), and hallucinations (option 3) are not adverse effects of SSRIs. Cognitive Level: Applying. Client Need: Physiological Integrity/Pharmacological Therapies. Nursing Process: Evaluation.

Chapter 11

Review Answers

1. Answer: 4. Core Concept: 11.3. Rationale: Adverse effects of SSRIs include the possibility of sexual dysfunction. The patient taking an SSRI does not have to avoid tyramine-containing foods (option 1). Hypertension (option 2) and tremors (option 3) are not associated with SSRIs. Cognitive Level: Understanding. Client Need: Physiological Integrity/Pharmacological Therapies. Nursing Process: Planning.
2. Answer: 3. Core Concept: 11.3. Rationale: If a patient taking an MAOI eats foods containing tyramine, it enters the bloodstream and displaces norepinephrine, resulting in a sudden increase in norepinephrine that causes acute hypertension. Other symptoms can occur within minutes of ingesting the food and include occipital headache, stiff neck, flushing, palpitations, profuse sweating, and nausea. Calcium channel blockers may be given as an antidote to reduce blood pressure. Demerol, a narcotic (option 1); dextromethorphan, a cough suppressant (option 2); and carbamazepine, an anticonvulsant (option 4), are not used to treat hypertensive crisis. Cognitive Level: Understanding. Client Need: Physiological Integrity/Pharmacological Therapies. Nursing Process: Planning.

3. Answer: 4. Core Concept: 11.5. Rationale: Lithium is taken as a salt; therefore, it mixes in the bloodstream like sodium chloride, so conditions in which sodium is lost (e.g., dehydration) can cause the kidneys to reabsorb the lithium salts back into the blood, producing increasing serum levels of lithium (lithium toxicity) and the associated adverse effects of an overdose. Dehydration does not lower serum lithium levels (option 1) or increase the effectiveness of lithium (option 2). Increasing the dosage (option 3) would increase the risk for lithium toxicity or worsen an existing condition. Cognitive Level: Applying. Client Need: Physiological Integrity/Pharmacological Therapies. Nursing Process: Implementation.
4. Answer: 1. Core Concept: 11.6. Rationale: A common adverse effect of methylphenidate, a CNS stimulant, is weight loss. Methylphenidate does not cause hypotension (option 2), renal toxicity (option 3), or extreme euphoria (option 4). Cognitive Level: Understanding. Client Need: Physiological Integrity/Pharmacological Therapies. Nursing Process: Evaluating.
5. Answer: 1. Core Concept: 11.5. Rationale: Excessive sweating or an increase in urination may cause dehydration, a condition that can cause lithium to build up in the bloodstream (toxicity). Options 2–4 are incorrect because although vomiting can lead to dehydration, having a dry mouth and being hypotensive do not necessarily indicate dehydration. While constipation may be a sign of dehydration, having blurred vision, an increase in appetite, an increase in energy, a decrease in memory, or being hypertensive are not usually associated with dehydration. Cognitive Level: Understanding. Client Need: Physiological Integrity/Pharmacological Therapies. Nursing Process: Evaluating.
6. Answer: 2. Core Concept: 11.3. Rationale: While taking imipramine (Tofranil), the patient should avoid standing up too quickly as this medication may cause orthostatic hypotension due to vasoconstriction of the blood vessels. The use of alcohol should be discouraged while taking imipramine because it may cause increased sedation (option 1). As with most drugs used for depression, therapeutic effectiveness of this drug may take weeks after the initial administration (option 3). If a dose is missed, the patient should not double up on the next dose as this may increase the likelihood of adverse effects (option 4). Cognitive Level: Applying. Client Need: Physiological Integrity/Pharmacological Therapies. Nursing Process: Implementation.
7. Answer: 2. Core Concept: 11.3. Rationale: The patient taking phenelzine (Nardil), an MAOI, should avoid eating foods containing tyramine. These foods include smoked or pickled meats, aged cheeses, yogurt, soy sauce, yeast, avocados, chocolate, pineapple, and alcoholic beverages. Eggs (option 1), onions (option 3), and apples (option 4) do not contain tyramine. Cognitive Level: Applying. Client Need: Physiological Integrity/Pharmacological Therapies. Nursing Process: Implementation.
8. Answer: 3. Core Concept: N/A. Rationale: 25 mg (the order) ÷ 50 mg × 1 tablet (amt. supplied) = ½ tablet daily for the first week. Options 1, 2, and 4 are a result of miscalculations and therefore incorrect. Cognitive Level: Applying. Client Need: Physiological Integrity/Pharmacological Therapies. Nursing Process: Implementation.
9. Answers: 2 and 3. Core Concept: 11.3. Rationale: In addition to being used to treat depression, duloxetine (Cymbalta), an SNRI, is also approved for the treatment of GAD and neuropathic pain. Duloxetin is not used for the treatment of phobias (option 1), seizures (option 4), or schizophrenia (option 5). Cognitive Level: Applying. Client Need: Physiological Integrity/Pharmacological Therapies. Nursing Process: Implementation.
10. Answer: 3. Core Concept: 11.3. Rationale: Depending on the medication, antidepressants improve mood by increasing levels of the neurotransmitters: norepinephrine, serotonin, or dopamine. Increasing levels of epinephrine (option 1) or GABA (option 4) have not shown to improve mood in patients suffering from depression. The reticular formation (option 2) is the area within the brain stem that is responsible for regulating the sleep–wake cycle and filtering stimuli received by the brain. Cognitive Level: Applying. Client Need: Physiological Integrity/Pharmacological Therapies. Nursing Process: Implementation.

Case Study Answers

1. Answer: 4. Core Concept: 11.5. Rationale: The primary use of mood stabilizers is to treat patients with severe mood swings (shifts between mania to depression), such as those diagnosed with bipolar disorder. Since Mrs. Coxilean does not exhibit these symptoms, the use of mood stabilizers would not be appropriate or helpful (option 1), and concerns about toxicity would not have been considered (option 2). Mrs. Coxilean did not state that she felt her condition was normal (option 3). Cognitive Level: Understanding. Client Need: Physiological Integrity/Pharmacological Therapies. Nursing Process: Planning.
2. Answer: 2. Core Concept: 11.3. Rationale: If Mrs. Coxilean were to take phenelzine (Nardil), an MAOI, the nurse would need to inform her that she should avoid eating foods containing tyramine such as chocolate. A reduction of sodium has not been shown to increase excretion of the drug (option 1). Some herbal supplements (option 3), for example, ginseng, should not be taken with MAOIs. Taken together, the patient may experience headache, tremors, mania, insomnia, irritability, and visual hallucinations. In addition, OTC medications for sleep (option 4) should also not be taken along with MAOIs because of possible drug interactions. Cognitive Level: Understanding. Client Need: Physiological Integrity/Pharmacological Therapies. Nursing Process: Planning.
3. Answer: 3. Core Concept: 11.3. Rationale: The drug of choice for Mrs. Coxilean would be sertraline (Zoloft), an SSRI. The therapeutic actions of this drug include the enhancement of mood and improvement of affect with maximum effects after several weeks. It also has been shown to have a greater safety profile than other antidepressants such as doxepin (option 1), a TCA, and tranylcypromine (option 2), an MAOI. Bupropion (option 4), an atypical antidepressant, would not be appropriate for Mrs. Coxilean because it is primarily used for changing moods, schizoaffective disorders, and quitting smoking. Cognitive Level: Understanding. Client Need: Physiological Integrity/Pharmacological Therapies. Nursing Process: Planning.
4. Answers: 1 and 3. Core Concept: 11.3. Rationale: Unfortunately, if Mrs. Coxilean were to start on an SSRI, such as Zoloft, she still may experience some of the adverse effects associated with this class of medication. Adverse effects may include sexual dysfunction, weight gain, nausea, headache, and insomnia. Loss of appetite (option 2) and problems with staying focused (option 4) are not adverse effects of SSRIs. Cognitive Level: Understanding. Client Need: Physiological Integrity/Pharmacological Therapies. Nursing Process: Evaluating.

Chapter 12

Review Answers

1. Answer: 2. Core Concept: 12.3. Rationale: Adverse effects, such severe muscle twitching or loss of sexual function, often diminish compliance with the medication regimen. Antipsychotic drugs cannot cure mental illness; they only provide symptom control (option 1). There is need to maintain a therapeutic level of medication in the blood to be effective; therefore, antipsychotics must be taken every day whether a person is symptomatic or not (option 3). It may take up to 8 weeks to see the full therapeutic effects of some antipsychotics (option 4). Cognitive Level: Understanding. Client Need: Physiological Integrity/Pharmacological Therapies. Nursing Process: Planning.
2. Answers: 1, 2, 3, and 4. Core Concept: 12.4. Rationale: Possible adverse effects of taking phenothiazines include sedation and muscle spasms early in therapy and tardive dyskinesia with long-term use. There are medications, such as Cogentin, that can help minimize or prevent some adverse effects. Phenothiazines are not known to cause hypertension (option 5). Cognitive Level: Applying. Client Need: Physiological Integrity/Pharmacological Therapies. Nursing Process: Implementation.

3. Answer: 3. Core Concept: 12.4. Rationale: Anticholinergic effects of chlorpromazine include dry mouth, tachycardia, and blurred vision. Hallucination, illusions, and paranoia are usually associated with the disease process of schizophrenia (option 1). Chlorpromazine does not cause hypertension, polyuria, or increased salivation (option 2). Although it can cause a high fever if the patient starts to exhibit signs of NMS, chlorpromazine does not cause confusion or muscle rigidity (option 4). Cognitive Level: Understanding. Client Need: Physiological Integrity/Pharmacological Therapies. Nursing Process: Evaluation.
4. Answer: 3. Core Concept: 12.4. Rationale: Phenothiazines, such as Mellaril, can cause EPS. These symptoms can include acute dystonia (severe spasms and muscle twitching), akathisia (uncontrolled, repetitive activity), secondary parkinsonism (shuffling gait), and tardive dyskinesia. Any or all of the adverse effects can cause difficulty sleeping. Anticholinergic effects of phenothiazines include dry mouth, tachycardia, and blurred vision (option 1). Cholinergic responses (option 2) and serotonin syndrome (option 4) are not associated with adverse effects of phenothiazines. Cognitive Level: Applying. Client Need: Physiological Integrity/Pharmacological Therapies. Nursing Process: Evaluation.
5. Answer: 4. Core Concept: 12.3. Rationale: Symptoms of psychosis remain in remission only as long as the patient takes the drug. If a patient chooses not to take the medication, symptoms of pretreatment illness quickly return. Hypertensive crisis does not occur upon withdrawal (option 1). Muscle twitching, a sign of EPS, may occur as a result of the dosage of medication and the length of therapy (option 2). Noncomplicance does not cause secondary parkinsonism, an adverse effect of some antipsychotics (option 3). Cognitive Level: Applying. Client Need: Physiological Integrity/Pharmacological Therapies. Nursing Process: Implementation.
6. Answer: 1. Core Concept: 12.4. Rationale: NMS is most likely to occur with phenothiazines, such as chlorpromazine. Aripiprazole (option 2), Risperidone (option 3), and Clozapine (option 4) are atypical antipsychotic drugs, which are not known to cause NMS. Cognitive Level: Understanding. Client Need: Physiological Integrity/Pharmacological Therapies. Nursing Process: Evaluation.
7. Answer: 2. Core Concept: 12.4. Rationale: Haloperidol (Haldol), a nonphenothiazine, is used for unprovoked aggressiveness and explosive hyperexcitability, often seen in those with severe behavior problems or psychotic disturbances. Seizures (option 1), severe mental depression (option 3), and alcoholism (option 4) are not indications for the use of haloperidol. Cognitive Level: Understanding. Client Need: Physiological Integrity/Pharmacological Therapies. Nursing Process: Planning.
8. Answer: 3. Core Concept: 12.5. Rationale: Some atypical antipsychotic drugs alter glucose metabolism, which can lead to type 2 diabetes. Phenothiazines (option 1) and nonphenothiazines (option 2) are not known to cause diabetes, so all antipsychotics (option 4) cannot be a correct answer. Cognitive Level: Understanding. Client Need: Physiological Integrity/Pharmacological Therapies. Nursing Process: Evaluation.
9. Answer: 2. Core Concept: 12.4. Rationale: The use of St. John's wort, sometimes used for depression, may increase the risk and severity of dystonia when used with conventional antipsychotic medications. Echinacea (option 1), black cohosh (option 3), and saw palmetto (option 4) have not been associated with the use of antipsychotic medications. Cognitive Level: Applying. Client Need: Physiological Integrity/Pharmacological Therapies. Nursing Process: Implementation.
10. Answer: 3. Core Concept: 12.5. Rationale: Aripiprazole (Abilify) controls both the positive symptoms of schizophrenia, such as delusional thinking and hallucinations, and negative symptoms. Aripiprazole does not directly increase mood or coping skills (option 1). It does not cause orthostatic hypotension or sedation (option 2). In addition, aripiprazole does not directly improve sleep or dietary habits (option 4). Cognitive Level: Applying. Client Need: Physiological Integrity/Pharmacological Therapies. Nursing Process: Evaluation.

Case Study Answers

1. Answer: 3. Core Concept: 12.2 and 12.3. Rationale: Mr. Wayne's symptoms of seeing people who are not there, talking about government agents who are trying to kill him, and communicating with "double agents" are considered positive symptoms (symptoms that add to normal behavior). Negative symptoms subtract from normal behavior, for example, lack of interest, motivation, lack of response, or pleasure (options 2 and 4). Regarding medications, atypical antipsychotics are more frequently prescribed because they produce significantly fewer adverse effects than conventional antipsychotic medications seen in options 1 and 2. Cognitive Level: Understanding. Client Need: Physiological Integrity/Pharmacological Therapies. Nursing Process: Planning.
2. Answers: 1, 2, 3, and 4. Core Concept: 12.5. Rationale: Risperidone may cause hyperactivity, shaking of the head and neck, fatigue, and fever. Risperidone may cause weight gain, not weight loss (option 5). Cognitive Level: Applying. Client Need: Physiological Integrity/Pharmacological Therapies. Nursing Process: Evaluation.
3. Answer: 2. Core Concept: 12.4. Rationale: Benztropine (Cogentin) is the preferred drug to help reduce dystonia caused by the antipsychotic Mr. Wayne is taking. Levodopa (option 1) is to be avoided because of its ability to increase dopamine functions, which enhances adverse effects. Thioridazine (option 3) and trifluoperazine (option 4) are conventional (phenothiazine) antipsychotic medications and are not given for adverse side effects. Cognitive Level: Applying. Client Need: Physiological Integrity/Pharmacological Therapies. Nursing Process: Implementation.
4. Answer: 3. Core Concept: N/A. Rationale: 15 mg (the order) ÷ 25 mg × 1 mL (amt. supplied) = 0.6 mL. Options 1, 2, and 4 are a result of miscalculations and therefore incorrect. Cognitive Level: Applying. Client Need: Physiological Integrity/Pharmacological Therapies. Nursing Process: Implementation.

Chapter 13

Review Answers

1. Answer: 4. Core Concept: 13.3. Rationale: Foods high in protein use the same pathways as levodopa for absorption into the bloodstream or brain and therefore compete for absorption. The effectiveness of the medication will be reduced. Vitamin C (option 1), carbohydrates (option 2), and folic acid (option 3) do not have the same effects on levodopa as protein. Cognitive Level: Applying. Client Need: Physiological Integrity/Pharmacological Therapies. Nursing Process: Implementation.
2. Answer: 2, 3, and 5. Core Concept: 13.5. Rationale: Nausea, diarrhea, and darkened urine are common adverse effects associated with donepezil. Donepezil has not been shown to cause sleepiness (option 1) or tinnitus (option 4). Cognitive Level: Applying. Client Need: Physiological Integrity/Pharmacological Therapies. Nursing Process: Implementation.
3. Answer: 3. Core Concept: 13.2. Rationale: Antiparkinson drugs are given to restore the balance of dopamine and ACh within the brain by either increasing accessibility of dopamine or by reducing the availability of ACh. Levodopa, a dopaminergic drug, helps to increase the synthesis of dopamine thus increasing the amount accessible for use. Increasing cholinergic stimulation in the brain (option 1), restoring ACh (option 2), and blocking or destroying dopamine (option 4) will cause an increase in Parkinson symptoms. Cognitive Level: Applying. Client Need: Physiological Integrity/Pharmacological Therapies. Nursing Process: Implementation.
4. Answer: 3. Core Concept: 13.3. Rationale: Benztropine (Cogentin) is used for relief of secondary parkinsonism and for the treatment of EPS brought on by antipsychotic pharmacotherapy such as Haldol. Levodopa–carbidopa, a dopaminergic drug (option 1);

risperidone, an antipsychotic drug (option 2); and cyclobenzaprine, a muscle relaxant (option 4), are not used to treat EPS. Cognitive Level: Applying. Client Need: Physiological Integrity/Pharmacological Therapies. Nursing Process: Implementation.

5. Answer: 2. Core Concept: 13.5. Rationale: One of the common adverse effects of rivastigmine (Exelon) is weight loss. Rivastigmine is not known to cause liver toxicity (option 1), renal failure (option 3), or EPS (option 4). Cognitive Level: Applying. Client Need: Physiological Integrity/Pharmacological Therapies. Nursing Process: Implementation.
6. Answer: 2. Core Concept: 13.13. Rationale: It is common for patients to complain of muscle pain when succinylcholine is used during surgery. Succinylcholine can also cause hyperthermia and hyperkalemia; therefore, hypothermia (option 1) and hypokalemia (option 4) are incorrect. In addition, succinylcholine is not associated with causing hypernatremia (option 3). Cognitive Level: Applying. Client Need: Physiological Integrity/Pharmacological Therapies. Nursing Process: Implementation.
7. Answer: 3. Core Concept N/A. Rationale: 350 mg × 3 (times a day) = 1050 mg/daily. Options 1, 2, and 4 are results of miscalculations and therefore incorrect. Cognitive Level: Applying. Client Need: Physiological Integrity/Pharmacological Therapies. Nursing Process: Implementation.
8. Answer: 1. Core Concept: 13.7. Rationale: Interferon drugs have unfavorable adverse effects such as flu-like symptoms (headaches, fever, chills, and muscle aches). Patients should be taught to report these symptoms to their healthcare provider. Interferon drugs are not known to cause orange colored urine (option 2) or diarrhea (option 3). Interferons should not require more than 6 months before the patient sees improvements (option 4). Cognitive Level: Applying. Client Need: Physiological Integrity/Pharmacological Therapies. Nursing Process: Implementation.
9. Answers: 1, 2, 3, and 5. Core Concept: 13.10. Rationale: Cyclobenzaprine (Flexeril) is a skeletal muscle relaxant that works on the CNS to relax muscles and reduce spasms. Adverse effects are drowsiness and blurred vision. Taking it with alcohol will increase drowsiness. In addition, patients need to know that this drug is only intended to be used for a short period of time (usually 2–3 weeks). Cyclobenzaprine is not known to cause headaches (option 4). Cognitive Level: Applying. Client Need: Physiological Integrity/Pharmacological Therapies. Nursing Process: Implementation.
10. Answer: 3. Core Concept: 13.12. Rationale: Dantrolene, a peripheral-acting skeletal muscle relaxant, helps control spasticity in patients with head, neck, or spinal cord injuries. An adverse effect of this drug is muscle weakness. It also can cause dry mouth and urinary retention; therefore, excessive salivation (option 1) and excessive urination (option 2) are incorrect. In addition, dantrolene does not cause insomnia (option 4). Cognitive Level: Applying. Client Need: Physiological Integrity/Pharmacological Therapies. Nursing Process: Implementation.

Case Study Answers

1. Answer: 2. Core Concept: 13.7. Rationale: The nurse will likely give interferon beta-1b (Betaseron), the immune system modulator. Amantadine (option 1) is an antiviral drug used for the treatment of PD, memantine (option 3) reduces the abnormally high levels of glutamate in patients with AD, and gabapentin (option 4) is an antiseizure drug used to treat anxiety in patients with MS. Cognitive Level: Applying. Client Need: Physiological Integrity/Pharmacological Therapies. Nursing Process: Implementation.
2. Answers: 1 and 4. Core Concept: 13.7. Rationale: Immune system modulators slow down the destruction of neurons caused by MS, thus reducing the number of relapses. These drugs do have a number of adverse effects such as flu-like symptoms (fever, chills, and muscle aches); therefore, option 2 is incorrect. Because of the possibility of toxicity, caution should be used in patients with preexisting liver problems (option 3). Serum levels

of the drug along with a CBC should be done periodically. Cognitive Level: Applying. Client Need: Physiological Integrity/Pharmacological Therapies. Nursing Process: Implementation.

3. Answer: 2. Core Concept: 13.7. Rationale: There is no cure for MS. Immune system modulators slow down the progression but usually only last for a short period of time. This class of drug does not provide long-term relief (option 1), nor does it make symptoms worse (option 3) or cause sedation (option 4). Cognitive Level: Applying. Client Need: Physiological Integrity/Pharmacological Therapies. Nursing Process: Implementation.
4. Answer: 3. Core Concept: 13.7. Rationale: Mitoxantrone (Novantrone), primarily a chemotherapeutic drug, is FDA-approved for patients with MS who have not responded to interferon or glatiramer therapy. Selegiline is used in the treatment of PD (option 1), gabapentin is an antiseizure drug used to treat anxiety pain related to MS (option 2), and donepezil is an AChE inhibitor used to treat AD (option 4). Cognitive Level: Applying. Client Need: Physiological Integrity/Pharmacological Therapies. Nursing Process: Implementation.

Chapter 14

Review Answers

1. Answer: 4. Core Concept: 14.2. Rationale: Most antiseizure medications are safety category D, which means that they may cause harm to the fetus but may provide benefit to the mother in a life-threatening situation. Category A (option 1) medications are lowest risk to the woman and fetus. Category B (option 2) medications have not shown a confirmed risk to fetus or woman. Category C (option 3) medications have shown a risk to fetus, but no studies have been performed in women. Cognitive Level: Understanding. Client Need: Physiological Integrity/Pharmacological Therapies. Nursing Process: Planning.
2. Answer: 3. Core Concept: 14.7. Rationale: Levels of antiseizure medications in the blood are analyzed to ensure that therapeutic levels are achieved or maintained (getting enough but not too much), helping healthcare providers to determine correct dosages for their patients. In addition, knowing levels allows the healthcare provider to monitor the effects that other medications, or even foods, have on the amount of medication available or utilized by the patient. Although hydantoin anticonvulsants should be administered cautiously in patients with preexisting blood dyscrasias or bone marrow depression, dilantin does not cause problems with the blood's plasma (option 1). The patient could ask the doctor, but the nurse should be able to understand and respond to this question (option 2). The primary way to determine the presence of adverse effects is usually by the patient's report and a physical assessment. Various diagnostic tests, such as drug levels, allow the healthcare provider to determine the patient's risk for developing some adverse effects (option 4). Cognitive Level: Applying. Client Need: Physiological Integrity/Pharmacological Therapies. Nursing Process: Implementation.
3. Answer: 4. Core Concept: 14.5. Rationale: Antiseizure medications are used to control seizure activity. Antiseizure medications are not used for curative purposes; therefore, the nurse cannot guarantee patients that they will be seizure-free within any specific time frame or that they can be cured (options 1–3). Cognitive Level: Applying. Client Need: Physiological Integrity/Pharmacological Therapies. Nursing Process: Implementation.
4. Answer: 1. Core Concept: 14.6. Rationale: Diazepam (Valium), a benzodiazepine, helps to terminate status epilepticus when given via the parenteral route. Its effects occur within minutes and can last for about 20 minutes. Clorazepate (option 3) and clonazepam (option 4), also benzodiazepines, are used to treat partial seizures and absence seizures. Gabapentin (option 2) is typically used to treat partial seizures. Cognitive Level: Understanding. Client Need: Physiological Integrity/Pharmacological Therapies. Nursing Process: Planning.

5. Answer: 2. Core Concept: 14.3. Rationale: Alternating contractions and relaxation of the muscles occur during the clonic phase of a generalized, tonic-clonic seizure. "Absence" (option 1) refers to a type of seizure that lasts only a few seconds with the patient appearing as if he or she is daydreaming. "Febrile" (option 3) refers to a type of seizure that usually lasts no more than a couple of minutes and occurs with a rapid rise of temperature during an illness. "Myoclonic" (option 4) refers to a type of seizure that is characterized by large, jerking body movements. Cognitive Level: Knowing. Client Need: Physiological Integrity/Pharmacological Therapies. Nursing Process: Data Collection.
6. Answer: 3. Core Concept: 14.7. Rationale: One of the most common adverse effects of hydantoin-related, antiseizure drugs is drowsiness. Other adverse effects include dizziness and blurred vision. The hydantoin-related drugs are not known to cause GI upset (option 1), spasms (option 2), or dry mouth (option 4). Cognitive Level: Applying. Client Need: Physiological Integrity/Pharmacological Therapies. Nursing Process: Implementation.
7. Answers: 1, 2, and 4. Core Concept: 14.6. Rationale: Taking more phenobarbital than prescribed can cause severe respiratory depression, coma, and death. Confusion and tachycardia (options 3 and 5) are not adverse effects of phenobarbital. Cognitive Level: Applying. Client Need: Physiological Integrity/Pharmacological Therapies. Nursing Process: Implementation.
8. Answer: 4. Core Concept: 14.8. Rationale: Taking ethosuximide (Zarontin) may cause depression. Urinary dysfunction (option 1), gingival hyperplasia (option 2), and tremors (option 3) are not typically associated with ethosuximide. Cognitive Level: Understanding. Client Need: Physiological Integrity/Pharmacological Therapies. Nursing Process: Evaluation.
9. Answer: 3. Core Concept: 14.7. Rationale: Phenytoin (Dilantin) can cause gingival hyperplasia. Valproic acid (option 1), carbamazepine (option 2), and primidone (option 4) are not associated with gingival hyperplasia. Cognitive Level: Understanding. Client Need: Physiological Integrity/Pharmacological Therapies. Nursing Process: Evaluation.
10. Answer: 1. Core Concept: 14.8. Rationale: Taking ethosuximide with phenytoin may cause an elevation in serum levels of phenytoin, causing phenytoin toxicity. An elevation in serum levels of phenytoin will not occur if taken with the barbiturate phenobarbital (option 2). Usually, phenytoin-like drugs such as carbamazepine (option 3) and valproic acid (option 4) would not be given with phenytoin because their actions are similar. Cognitive Level: Understanding. Client Need: Physiological Integrity/Pharmacological Therapies. Nursing Process: Evaluation.

Case Study Answers

1. Answer: 3. Core Concept N/A. Rationale: 66 pounds ÷ 2.2 kg/lb = 30 kg. The order is 20 mg/kg/day × 30 kg = 600 mg/day. Options 1, 2, and 4 are a result of miscalculations and are therefore incorrect. Cognitive Level: Applying. Client Need: Physiological Integrity/Pharmacological Therapies. Nursing Process: Implementation.
2. Answer: 3. Core Concept: 14.8. Rationale: Ethosuximide (Zarontin), a succinimide, controls seizures by delaying the entry of calcium into nerves, keeping them from firing too quickly. Enhancing the release or reception of GABA, a neurotransmitter (options 1 and 4), describes the action of some barbiturates, benzodiazepines, and newer GABA-related drugs. Delaying the amount of sodium going into the nerves, which decreases the ability of nerve impulses to travel (option 2), describes the action of hydantoin and hydantoin-like drugs. Cognitive Level: Applying. Client Need: Physiological Integrity/Pharmacological Therapies. Nursing Process: Implementation.
3. Answer: 3. Core Concept: 14.8. Rationale: Patients vary significantly in their ability to metabolize phenytoin; therefore, dosages are highly individualized. Because of the very narrow range between therapeutic dose and toxic dose, the patient's serum levels must be carefully monitored. Ethosuximide does not cause dependency (option 1) or anemia

(option 2) and is not known for a low margin of safety (option 4). Cognitive Level: Applying. Client Need: Physiological Integrity/Pharmacological Therapies. Nursing Process: Implementation.

4. Answer: 4. Core Concept: 14.8. Rationale: Taking ethosuximide with valproic acid, a hydantoin-like drug, may cause a fluctuation in serum ethosuximide levels. Taking ethosuximide with phenobarbital (option 1), diazepam (option 2), or pregabalin (option 3) should not cause a fluctuation in serum ethosuximide levels but may cause other adverse effects so the patient would still need to be monitored closely. Cognitive Level: Understanding. Client Need: Physiological Integrity/Pharmacological Therapies. Nursing Process: Evaluation.

Chapter 15

Review Answers

1. Answer: 4. Core Concept: 15.6. Rationale: Meloxicam is an NSAID used for both the pain and inflammation of osteoarthritis. Sumatripan (option 1) is used for migraines. Acetaminophen (option 2) is used for pain and fever but does not have the anti-inflammatory properties typically needed for conditions such as osteoarthritis. Fentanyl (option 3) is used both to control moderate to severe chronic pain and in surgical procedures. Cognitive Level: Understanding. Client Need: Physiological Integrity/Pharmacological Therapies. Nursing Process: Planning.
2. Answer: 1. Core Concept: 15.7. Rationale: Because of its vasoconstricting action, sumatriptan may cause chest pressure or pain. It should be used cautiously in patients with a recent MI or history of angina. Sumatriptan is not known to cause GI upset (option 2), bleeding (option 3), or lethargy (option 4). Cognitive Level: Understanding. Client Need: Physiological Integrity/Pharmacological Therapies. Nursing Process: Planning.
3. Answer: 1. Core Concept: 15.6. Rationale: NSAIDs are known to irritate the lining of the GI tract, resulting in GI upset and bleeding. NSAIDs are not known to cause urinary retention (option 2), blurred vision (option 3), or anorexia (option 4). Cognitive Level: Applying. Client Need: Physiological Integrity/Pharmacological Therapies. Nursing Process: Evaluation.
4. Answer: 4. Core Concept: 15.5. Rationale: Methadone is typically used to treat opioid dependency. Oxycodone (option 1), tramadol (option 2), and hydromorphone (option 3), all opioid agonists, are not used for the treatment of opioid dependency. Cognitive Level: Remembering. Client Need: Physiological Integrity/Pharmacological Therapies. Nursing Process: Planning.
5. Answer: 3. Core Concept: 15.2. Rationale: The sensation of pain begins at the nociceptors, free nerve endings located throughout the body. Once nociceptors are stimulated, the transmission travels to the spinal cord (option 1). Once in the spinal cord, a neurotransmitter called substance P (option 4) is thought to be responsible for the continuation of the transmission to the brain. The viscera (option 2) refers to the body's deeper, internal organs and the sensations associated with them. Cognitive Level: Understanding. Client Need: Physiological Integrity/Pharmacological Therapies. Nursing Process: Planning.
6. Answers: 2, 4, and 5. Core Concept: 15.1. Rationale: Prior to administering pain medication, the nurse must collect information about the location and severity of the patient's pain. The nurse should also ask the patient to describe their pain. Although the patient's medical diagnosis (option 1) and the last time a meal was eaten (option 3) are important, they are not specifically part of data collection. Cognitive Level: Applying. Client Need: Physiological Integrity/Pharmacological Therapies. Nursing Process: Data Collection.
7. Answer: 3. Core Concept: 15.5. Rationale: Because of the patient's LOC and shallow respirations, the nurse anticipates the opioid antagonist, naloxone (Narcan), would be ordered to reverse those and other adverse effects caused by opioids. Butorphanol

(option 1), hydrocodone (option 2), and oxycodone (option 4) are opioids. Cognitive Level: Understanding. Client Need: Physiological Integrity/Pharmacological Therapies. Nursing Process: Planning.

8. Answer: 1. Core Concept: 15.6. Rationale: Since the patient is allergic to aspirin (an NSAID), the nurse can administer acetaminophen, a centrally acting drug, for mild pain. Morphine (option 2) and fentanyl (option 4) are both opioids and are used for moderate to severe pain. Etodolac (option 3) is an NSAID and should not be used as an alternative to aspirin. Cognitive Level: Applying. Client Need: Physiological Integrity/Pharmacological Therapies. Nursing Process: Implementation.
9. Answers: 1, 2, 4, and 5. Core Concept: 15.7. Rationale: A patient using ergotamine (Ergostate), a medication used for migraines, should be monitored for tachycardia, nausea, vomiting, peripheral constriction, and signs of physical dependence. It does not cause peripheral dilation (option 3). Cognitive Level: Applying. Client Need: Physiological Integrity/Pharmacological Therapies. Nursing Process: Evaluation.
10. Answer: 4. Core Concept: N/A. Rationale: 400 mg (the order) ÷ 200 mg × 5 mL (amount supplied) = 10 mL. Options 1–3 are a result of miscalculations and therefore incorrect. Cognitive Level: Applying. Client Need: Physiological Integrity/Pharmacological Therapies. Nursing Process: Implementation.

Case Study Answers

1. Answers: 1, 2, and 4. Core Concepts: 15.2 and 15.6. Rationale: NSAIDs inhibit pain mediators at the body's nociceptors by preventing cyclooxygenase (COX), an enzyme responsible for the formation of prostaglandins. When COX is inhibited, inflammation and pain are reduced. NSAIDs do not work within the CNS (option 3). Cognitive Level: Understanding. Client Need: Physiological Integrity/Pharmacological Therapies. Nursing Process: Evaluation.
2. Answer: 1. Core Concept: 15.5. Rationale: The nurse would expect to give Percocet. It is an opioid combined with acetaminophen. Talwin (option 2), Dilaudid (option 3), and Demerol (option 4) are all opioids that are not available in a combination form with acetaminophen. Cognitive Level: Understanding. Client Need: Physiological Integrity/Pharmacological Therapies. Nursing Process: Planning.
3. Answers: 1–3. Core Concept: 15.5. Rationale: The combination of oxycodone and acetaminophen works well together to reduce pain. When combined, lower doses of the two drugs can be used to achieve therapeutic results and help to minimize the adverse effects. Combining the two medications does not ensure a lower cost (option 4). Cognitive Level: Applying. Client Need: Physiological Integrity/Pharmacological Therapies. Nursing Process: Implementation.
4. Answer: 3. Core Concept: 15.5. Rationale: Patients should report sedation to their healthcare provider. The goal is to prescribe enough medication to provide pain relief while minimizing adverse effects and enabling the patient to engage in ADLs. A dose that is too high or an overuse of narcotics can lead to sedation. Narcotics are not usually known to cause diarrhea (option 1), hallucinations (option 2), or insomnia (option 4). Cognitive Level: Applying. Client Need: Physiological Integrity/Pharmacological Therapies. Nursing Process: Implementation.

Chapter 16

Review Answers

1. Answer: 4. Core Concept: 16.5. Rationale: St. John's wort may intensify or prolong the effects of some opioids and anesthetics and should be discontinued 2 to 3 weeks prior to administration due to the possible risk of hypotension. Kava kava (option 1) is used to

treat anxiety, stress, and sleep problems. Oil of clove (option 2) is used for its antiseptic effect and ability to relieve tooth pain. Anise (option 3) is an herb used primarily in cooking. Cognitive Level: Applying. Client Need: Physiological Integrity/Pharmacological Therapies. Nursing Process: Implementation.

2. Answers: 1, 2, and 4. Core Concept: 16.3. Rationale: Lidocaine can cause excitement, irritability, and confusion. Lidocaine is not known to cause tachypnea (option 3) or hypotension (option 5). Cognitive Level: Applying. Client Need: Physiological Integrity/ Pharmacological Therapies. Nursing Process: Evaluation.

3. Answer: 2. Core Concept: 16.1. Rationale: The patient will have the anesthetic medication injected into the epidural space (area between the vertebrae and the spinal cord). For women in labor, it is common that a tube (catheter) is placed within this space so that multiple doses of the medication can be given during labor. An anesthetic drug injected into the affected area is known as infiltration (field block) anesthesia (option 1). An injection of anesthetic medication directly into the spinal cord is called spinal anesthesia (option 3). The application of anesthetic cream onto the skin is known as topical (surface) anesthesia (option 4). Cognitive Level: Applying. Client Need: Physiological Integrity/ Pharmacological Therapies. Nursing Process: Implementation.

4. Answer: 3. Core Concept: 16.5. Rationale: Patients with allergies to egg or soybean products should not be given propofol. Propofol is not contraindicated for those with allergies to peanuts (option 1), shellfish (option 2), or milk (option 4). Cognitive Level: Applying. Client Need: Physiological Integrity/Pharmacological Therapies. Nursing Process: Data Collection.

5. Answer: 1. Core Concept: 16.5. Rationale: A patient receiving nitrous oxide should be monitored for restlessness. Nitrous oxide has not been known to cause dysrhythmia (option 2), hypertension (option 3), or mania (option 4). Cognitive Level: Understanding. Client Need: Physiological Integrity/Pharmacological Therapies. Nursing Process: Planning.

6. Answer: 2. Core Concept: 16.6. Rationale: The nurse should explain that opioids, such as morphine, can provide some pain relief before surgery, and that atropine is used to decrease secretions. Patients have a right to know what medication they are receiving. The nurse should be prepared to educate the patient about their medication. Options 1 and 4 avoid the patient's question, which should not be done when administering medications. Option 3 is incorrect because morphine and atropine are nonanesthetic drugs used as adjuncts and do not help the anesthetic medications work more effectively. Cognitive Level: Applying. Client Need: Physiological Integrity/Pharmacological Therapies. Nursing Process: Implementation.

7. Answer: 1. Core Concept: 16.3. Rationale: Epinephrine constricts blood vessels, which may increase pressure within the vessels. As a result, adding epinephrine with anesthetics can cause tachycardia and hypertension in patients with a history of cardiovascular disease. Epinephrine is not known to cause bradycardia (options 2 and 4) or hypotension (option 3). Cognitive Level: Understanding. Client Need: Physiological Integrity/ Pharmacological Therapies. Nursing Process: Data Collection.

8. Answer: 2. Core Concept: 16.5. Rationale: Using both propofol (IV anesthetic) and nitrous oxide (gas anesthetic) together allows the dose of the inhaled agent to be reduced, thus lowering the potential for serious side effects. Together, these drugs can provide greater analgesia and greater muscle relaxation, not a decrease in muscle relaxation (option 1). Depending on the surgical procedure, both propofol and nitrous oxide can be used alone (options 3 and 4). Cognitive Level: Applying. Client Need: Physiological Integrity/ Pharmacological Therapies. Nursing Process: Implementation.

9. Answer: 4. Core Concept: N/A. Rationale: 1 mg (the order) $\div$ 0.8 mg/mL $\times$ 1 mL (amt. supplied) = 1.25 mL. Options 1–3 are a result of miscalculations and are therefore incorrect. Cognitive Level: Applying. Client Need: Physiological Integrity/Pharmacological Therapies. Nursing Process: Implementation.

10. Answer: 3. Core Concept: 16.6. Rationale: The nurse would expect that ondansetron would be ordered. Meperidine, an opioid, is used for anxiety and pain relief (option 1). Bethanechol is used to relieve constipation and urinary retention (option 2). Succinylcholine, a neuromuscular blocking agent, is used during surgery to ease intubation (option 4). Cognitive level: Understanding. Client Need: Physiological Integrity/Pharmacological Therapies. Nursing Process: Planning.

Case Study Answers

1. Answer: 2. Core Concept: 16.1. Rationale: The type of anesthesia used for stitches is infiltration (field block) anesthesia. It diffuses into the tissue to block a specific group of nerves in a small area very close to the area to be operated on. Option 1 describes topical (surface) anesthesia. Option 3 describes nerve block anesthesia, and option 4 describes epidural anesthesia. Cognitive Level: Applying. Client Need: Physiological Integrity/ Pharmacological Therapies. Nursing Process: Implementation.
2. Answer: 3. Core Concept: 16.3. Rationale: By constricting vessels, the addition of epinephrine to lidocaine increases the duration of the lidocaine. It is not added to prevent infection (option 1), prevent an allergic reaction (option 2), or decrease pain (option 4). Cognitive Level: Understanding. Client Need: Physiological Integrity/Pharmacological Therapies. Nursing Process: Planning.
3. Answer: 2. Core Concept: 16.3. Rationale: After administering lidocaine, the nurse monitors the patient for anxiety, one of several adverse effects. Unless the patient has an allergy to lidocaine, there should not be a constriction of airways (option 1). In addition, lidocaine is not known to cause tachycardia (option 3) or unresponsiveness (option 4). Cognitive Level: Applying. Client Need: Physiological Integrity/Pharmacological Therapies. Nursing Process: Evaluation.
4. Answer: 4. Core Concept: 16.3. Rationale: Even though it would have a calming effect, it would not be advisable to give a barbiturate to a patient if lidocaine is also being used. The barbiturate might decrease the effectiveness of the lidocaine. Barbiturates do not cause lidocaine toxicity (option 1), or increase the effectiveness of lidocaine (option 2). If a barbiturate were given, it would decrease the effectiveness of the lidocaine, but it would not be the cause of the patient becoming more irritable (option 3). Cognitive Level: Understanding. Client Need: Physiological Integrity/Pharmacological Therapies. Nursing Process: Planning.

Chapter 17

Review Answers

1. Answer: 3. Core Concept: 17.2. Rationale: HDL picks up cholesterol in the blood and other tissues and returns it to the liver, where it is used to make bile and used for the digestion of lipids. LDL (option 1) is made in the liver and released into the blood to be transported to the tissue, where it is used to make plasma membranes, synthesize steroids, or be stored. VLDL (option 2) is made in the liver and is the primary carrier of triglycerides (option 4). Cognitive Level: Remembering. Client Need: N/A. Nursing Process: N/A.
2. Answer: 3. Core Concept: 17.4. Lovastatin (Mevacor) is the only statin that needs to be taken with meals. Atorvastatin (option 1), simvastatin (option 2), and rosuvastatin (option 4) can be taken with or without food. Rationale: Cognitive Level: Understanding. Client Need: Physiological Integrity/Pharmacological Therapies. Nursing Process: Planning.
3. Answer: 2. Core Concept: 17.4. Rationale: Because the liver makes more cholesterol at night, it is best to take statin drugs in the evening before bedtime. Even though there are a couple of drugs in this class that can be taken anytime (option 1), it is more effective to take them in the evening. Taking statins with or without other medications (option 3) or

on an empty stomach (option 4) does not increase effectiveness. Cognitive Level: Applying. Client Need: Physiological Integrity/Pharmacological Therapies. Nursing Process: Implementation.

4. Answer: 3. Core Concept: N/A. Rationale: 20 mg (the order) ÷ 10 mg × 1 tablet (amount supplied) = 2 tablets. Options 1, 2, and 4 are a result of miscalculations and are therefore incorrect. Cognitive Level: Applying. Client Need: Physiological Integrity/Pharmacological Therapies. Nursing Process: Implementation.

5. Answer: 1. Core Concept: 17.5. Rationale: Bile acid resins are limited to the GI tract, so patients may experience adverse effects such as constipation, nausea, bloating, and indigestion. Because this drug class is not absorbed into the general circulation, symptoms such as headaches (option 2), anxiety (option 3), and double vision (option 4) are not associated with its use. Cognitive Level: Understanding. Client Need: Physiological Integrity/Pharmacological Therapies. Nursing Process: Evaluation.

6. Answer: 1. Core Concept: 17.5 Rationale: Colestipol (Colestid) is a bile acid resin that may cause adverse effects in the GI tract. Taking this medication along with a large amount of fluid can minimize these effects. Taking this drug on an empty stomach such as taking it 1 hour prior to meals (option 2), 4 hours after meals (option 3), or at bedtime (option 4) will increase the potential for adverse effects. Cognitive Level: Applying. Client Need: Physiological Integrity/Pharmacological Therapies. Nursing Process: Implementation.

7. Answers: 1, 2, and 4. Core Concept: 17.6. Rationale: Possible adverse effects of taking niacin include flushing, excess gas, and diarrhea. Niacin has not been shown to cause constipation (option 3) or headaches (option 5). Cognitive Level: Applying. Client Need: Physiological Integrity/Pharmacological Therapies. Nursing Process: Implementation.

8. Answer: 2. Core Concept: 17.3. Rationale: A total cholesterol value of 326 mg/dL places the patient at high risk for cardiovascular disease; therefore, drug therapy should be initiated. An exercise program should also be initiated (option 1) but not without including drug therapy because the laboratory values were so high. OTC supplements (option 3) may not be effective in reducing cholesterol, and an antihypertensive medication (option 4) may or may not be indicated at this time since because the blood pressure values are determined to be in prehypertensive stage. Cognitive Level: Understanding. Client Need: Physiological Integrity/Pharmacological Therapies. Nursing Process: Planning.

9. Answer: 3. Core Concept: 17.7. Rationale: Fibric acid agents such as gemfibrozil (Lopid) may cause gallstones to develop and affect liver function. These are not typical adverse effects of bile acid resins such as cholestyramine (option 1), niacin (option 2), or statins such as lovastatin (option 4). Cognitive Level: Understanding. Client Need: Physiological Integrity/Pharmacological Therapies. Nursing Process: Data Collection.

10. Answers: 1–3. Core Concept: 17.8. Rationale: Omega-3 acids, the beneficial component in fish oil (option 3), can cause minor adverse effects such as dyspepsia (indigestion) (option 1). In addition, some people who are allergic to seafood may not be able to take fish oil (option 2). Only very high doses of omega-3 fatty acids can cause a decrease in blood clotting (option 4), and it is not known to cause constipation (option 5). Cognitive Level: Applying. Client Need: Physiological Integrity/Pharmacological Therapies. Nursing Process: Implementation.

Case Study Answers

1. Answer: 2. Core Concepts: 17.5. Rationale: Cholestryamine, a bile acid binding drug, binds to cholesterol within bile acids in the intestines thus increasing cholesterol excretion in the feces. Cholestryamine does not inhibit enzymes that make cholesterol (option 1), increase the breakdown of cholesterol in the liver (option 3), or make more bile acids, which bind cholesterol (option 4). Cognitive Level: Applying. Client Need: Physiological Integrity/Pharmacological Therapies. Nursing Process: Implementation.

2. Answer: 1. Core Concept: 17.4. Rationale: Lovastatin, a statin drug, acts by inhibiting the enzyme HMG-CoA reductase that makes cholesterol and therefore reduces the amount of cholesterol made by the liver. The previous medication worked by binding bile acids in the intestine, which increases cholesterol excretion (option 2), so this answer is incorrect. Lovastatin does not increase the breakdown of cholesterol in the liver (option 3) or make more bile acids, which bind cholesterol (option 4). Cognitive Level: Applying. Client Need: Physiological Integrity/Pharmacological Therapies. Nursing Process: Implementation.
3. Answer: 3. Core Concept: 17.4. Rationale: Statin drugs can cause excessive muscle weakness and pain. Diarrhea (option 1), confusion (option 2), and indigestion (option 4) are not common serious adverse effects. Cognitive Level: Understanding. Client Need: Physiological Integrity/Pharmacological Therapies. Nursing Process: Evaluation.
4. Answer: 4. Core Concept: 17.4. Rationale: Statin drugs should increase HDL good cholesterol laboratory values rather than decrease them (option 3) or increase LDL (option 1) or VLDL (option 2) levels. Cognitive Level: Understanding. Client Need: Physiological Integrity/Pharmacological Therapies. Nursing Process: Data Collection.

Chapter 18

Review Answers

1. Answer: 3. Core Concepts: 18.1, 18.2, and 18.3. Rationale: The kidneys are not involved in the production of white blood cells (WBCs) but are involved in helping to maintain acid-base balance (option 1), the secretion of renin (option 2), and the production of calcitriol (option 4). Cognitive Level: Knowing. Client Need: N/A. Nursing Process: N/A.
2. Answer: 4. Core Concept: 18.5. Rationale: Dehydration is caused by not having enough fluid in the body. It can cause hypotension, headache, and dry mouth. Dehydration causes a decrease in urinary output, not an increase (option 1). Weight gain, edema (option 2), and HTN (option 3) can be signs of too much fluid in the body. Cognitive Level: Understanding. Client Need: Physiological Integrity/Pharmacological Therapies. Nursing Process: Data Collection.
3. Answer: 2. Core Concept: 18.6. Rationale: The most frequently used diuretics for HTN are thiazides such as hydrochlorothiazide. Ethacrynic acid (option 1) is a loop diuretic, spironolactone (option 3) is a potassium-sparing diuretic, and mannitol (option 4) is an osmotic diuretic. Cognitive Level: Applying. Client Need: Physiological Integrity/Pharmacological Therapies. Nursing Process: Implementation.
4. Answer: 2. Core Concept: 18.6. Rationale: Because diuretics can cause excess fluid loss, signs of hypotension can occur, such as dizziness when moving from a recumbent or sitting to a standing position. Patients are advised not to take their diuretics at night because they cause frequent urination (option 1). Patients should not increase sodium intake because it may cause fluid retention (option 3) or decrease fluid intake because it can cause dehydration (option 4). Cognitive Level: Applying. Client Need: Physiological Integrity/Pharmacological Therapies. Nursing Process: Implementation.
5. Answer: 3. Core Concept: 18.10. Rationale: The patient is receiving treatment to correct a problem with pH; therefore, the nurse will monitor pH status. Liver function tests (option 1), WBC count (option 2), and glucose levels (option 4) are not monitored for this reason. Cognitive Level: Understanding. Client Need: Physiological Integrity/Pharmacological Therapies. Nursing Process: Evaluation.
6. Answer: 2. Core Concept: 18.9. Rationale: KCl irritates the mucosa of the GI tract; therefore, nausea and vomiting may occur. Drowsiness (option 1), hypoglycemia (option 3), and muscle weakness (option 4) are not adverse effects of this medication. Cognitive Level: Understanding. Client Need: Health Promotion and Maintenance. Nursing Process: Evaluation.

7. Answer: 2. Core Concept: 18.7. Rationale: Patients taking potassium-sparing diuretics do not lose potassium in diuresis and therefore should not take potassium supplements or increase potassium-rich foods like patients taking loop or thiazide diuretics do (options 1 and 3). Magnesium levels (option 4) are not affected unless they are taken with loop or thiazide diuretics. Cognitive Level: Applying. Client Need: Health Promotion and Maintenance. Nursing Process: Implementation.
8. Answers: 2 and 3. Core Concept: 18.9. Rationale: Hyponatremia is caused by a decrease in serum sodium levels. This can occur through severe diarrhea, vomiting, prolonged fever, and sweating. Constipation (option 1), hemorrhage (option 4), and mild skin burns (option 5) do not contribute directly to this condition. Cognitive Level: Understanding. Client Need: Health Promotion and Maintenance. Nursing Process: Data Collection.
9. Answer: 4. Core Concept: 18.5. Rationale: Patients taking a diuretic should avoid or limit their intake of caffeine because of its ability to also cause increased urination. There is no need to avoid foods such as dark green, leafy vegetables (option 1), fruits (option 3), and nuts (option 2). Cognitive Level: Applying. Client Need: Health Promotion and Maintenance. Nursing Process: Implementation.
10. Answer: 2. Core Concept: N/A. Rationale: 1000 mL (total volume) ÷ 8 (total infusion hours) = 125 mL in 1 hour. Options 1, 3, and 4 are a result of miscalculations and are therefore incorrect. Cognitive Level: Applying. Client Need: Physiological Integrity/Pharmacological Therapies. Nursing Process: Implementation.

Case Study Answers

1. Answer: 3. Core Concept: 18.9. Rationale: Microzide is a thiazide diuretic, and potassium supplements should be taken, but combining supplements and a diet rich in potassium can cause hyperkalemia, a serious condition. Patients should limit the amount of food high in potassium when taking supplements or taking potassium-sparing diuretics (options 1, 2, and 4). Cognitive Level: Understanding. Client Need: Health Promotion and Maintenance. Nursing Process: Evaluation.
2. Answer: 1. Core Concept: 18.9. Rationale: The probable cause of Mr. Grant's symptoms is hyperkalemia (too much potassium). Hyperkalemia causes slow heart rate and weakness related to the cardiac symptoms. Hypokalemia (option 2) can cause similar symptoms, but his diet contraindicates this condition. Hyper- and hyponatremia (options 3 and 4) do not directly cause cardiac symptoms. Cognitive Level: Understanding. Client Need: Health Promotion and Maintenance. Nursing Process: Data Collection.
3. Answer: 4. Core Concept: 18.9. Rationale: Kayexalate is given to decrease high potassium levels. It is not used to affect fluid levels (options 1 and 2) or increase K^+ levels (option 3). Cognitive Level: Applying. Client Need: Health Promotion and Maintenance. Nursing Process: Implementation.
4. Answer: 3. Core Concept: 18.5. Rationale: Mr. Grant is now taking a loop diuretic. The same general principles concerning thiazide diuretics apply to loop diuretics (see case study question 1). Cognitive Level: Understanding. Client Need: Health Promotion and Maintenance. Nursing Process: Planning.

Chapter 19

Review Answers

1. Answer: 3. Core Concept: 19.6. Rationale: Adrenergic blockers are a second-line class of antihypertensive medications. ACE inhibitors (option 1), CCBs (option 2), and thiazide diuretics (option 4) are all first-line classes of medications used for hypertension. Cognitive Level: Knowledge. Client Need: Physiological Integrity/Pharmacological Therapies. Nursing Process: N/A.

2. Answer: 1. Core Concept: 19.9. Rationale: Cardizem, a CCB, regulates calcium flow into the muscle cells by blocking channels in the plasma membrane. This causes arteriole vasodilation and reduced peripheral resistance, which reduces the workload of the heart (slowing the heart rate). Because this drug affects heart rate and rhythm, baseline ECG and heart rate must be established. Micardis (option 2) is an ARB, Diruil (option 3) is a diuretic, and Nitropress (option 4) is a vasodilator. Cognitive Level: Understanding. Client Need: Physiological Integrity/Pharmacological Therapies. Nursing Process: Data Collection.
3. Answer: 3. Core Concept: 19.6. Rationale: Using a multidrug approach to treatment allows for smaller doses of each drug to be used. Using more than one medication does not necessarily mean that BP will decrease faster (option 1), that adverse effects are fewer (option 3), or that taking the two drugs together will treat other medical conditions (option 4). Cognitive Level: Understanding. Client Need: Physiological Integrity/Pharmacological Therapies. Nursing Process: Planning.
4. Answer: 2. Core Concept: 19.7. Rationale: A major adverse effect of furosemide (Lasix), a loop diuretic, is loss of potassium. The nurse must carefully monitor laboratory tests and instruct the patient to take potassium supplements. Hyperkalemia (option 1) is not usually a problem with this type of diuretic. Sodium and calcium levels (options 3 and 4) should be monitored, but they are not usually associated with significant side effects of this drug. Cognitive Level: Understanding. Client Need: Physiological Integrity/Pharmacological Therapies. Nursing Process: Evaluation.
5. Answer: 4. Core Concept: 19.8 Rationale: ARBs, such as losartan (Cozaar), are typically combined with loop diuretics, such as hydrochlorothiazide, for a more effective approach to BP management. Felodipine (option 1) is a CCB, methyldopa (option 2) is an alpha-adrenergic agent, and atenolol (option 3) is a beta-blocker. Cognitive Level: Understanding. Client Need: Physiological Integrity/Pharmacological Therapies. Nursing Process: Evaluation.
6. Answer: 3. Core Concepts: 19.8, 19.9, and 19.10. Rationale: When starting on an antihypertensive medication, the patient should be monitored for dizziness, a sign of low blood pressure, which can be caused by too much medication or is an adverse effect of some drug classes. Nausea, not including vomiting (option 1), can occur with vasodilators but is not associated with other types of antihypertensive medications. Diarrhea (option 2) and tetany (option 4) are not usually associated with antihypertensive drugs. Cognitive Level: Applying. Client Need: Health Promotion and Maintenance. Nursing Process: Evaluation.
7. Answer: 2. Core Concept: N/A. Rationale: 60 mg (the order) ÷ 120 mg × 1 tablet (amount supplied) = ½ tablet, twice a day, in the morning and again in the evening. Options 1, 3, and 4 are a result of miscalculations and are therefore incorrect. Cognitive Level: Applying. Client Need: Physiological Integrity/Pharmacological Therapies. Nursing Process: Implementation.
8. Answer: 3. Core Concept: 19.8. Rationale: ACE inhibitors block the effects of angiotensin II, which then decreases BP by dilating arteries and decreasing blood volume. CCBs (option 1) affect the flow of calcium, adrenergic blockers (option 2) act on receptors associated with the sympathetic nervous system, and direct-acting vasodilators (option 4) act directly on smooth muscle to allow dilation. Cognitive Level: Understanding. Client Need: Physiological Integrity/Pharmacological Therapies. Nursing Process: Planning.
9. Answer: 4. Core Concept: 19.11. Rationale: Vasodilators relax smooth muscles in the blood vessels to decrease peripheral resistance, which reduces BP. Option 1 is describing CCBs, option 2 is describing central-acting adrenergic blockers, and option 3 is describing ACE inhibitors. Cognitive Level: Understanding. Client Need: Physiological Integrity/Pharmacological Therapies. Nursing Process: Planning.

10. Answer: 2. Core Concept: 19.8. Rationale: Patients taking ACE inhibitors should be monitored for increased potassium levels. This can occur due to decreased aldosterone levels. Hypokalemia (option 1), hypernatremia (a high sodium level) (option 3), and hyperglycemia (a high glucose level) (option 4) are not associated with this medication. Cognitive Level: Applying. Client Need: Physiological Integrity/Pharmacological Therapies. Nursing Process: Evaluation.

Case Study Answers

1. Answer: 3. Core Concept: 19.11. Rationale: Mr. Rodriguez's blood pressure was extremely high and needed immediate attention. Direct-acting vasodilators are preferred because they act faster than any other antihypertensive drug. Nitroprusside is not typically used in most cases of HTN because of its adverse effects (option 1), and it does not have a long duration of action (option 2). The case study scenario does not mention allergies (option 4). Cognitive Level: Understanding. Client Need: Physiological Integrity/Pharmacological Therapies. Nursing Process: Planning.
2. Answer: 1. Core Concept: 19.8. Rationale: Thiazide and an ARB are combined in Hyzaar. Options 2, 3, and 4 do not contain this combination of medications. Cognitive Level: Remembering. Client Need: Physiological Integrity/Pharmacological Therapies. Nursing Process: Planning.
3. Answer: 1. Core Concept: 19.8. Rationale: Because Hyzaar is composed of two types of drugs used to reduce blood pressure, Mr. Rodriguez should have been taught to always rise slowly and avoid sudden changes in posture. Even though Hyzaar contains a thiazide, it is at a low dose and does not require a supplement as long as the patient eats a healthy diet with foods that contain potassium (option 2). It is not necessary to increase calcium (option 3), and exercise is a positive lifestyle routine that should be encouraged (option 4). Cognitive Level: Applying. Client Need: Physiological Integrity/Pharmacological Therapies. Nursing Process: Implementation.
4. Answer: 4. Core Concept: 19.9. Rationale: Reflex tachycardia and dizziness are adverse effects of fast-acting nifedipine. For those taking this medication, these symptoms are not caused by electrolyte imbalances (option 1), not taking enough of the medication (option 2), or excessive vasodilation of the arteries (option 3). Cognitive Level: Applying. Client Need: Physiological Integrity/Pharmacological Therapies. Nursing Process: Implementation.

Chapter 20

Review Answers

1. Answer: 2. Core Concept: 20.2. Rationale: Failure of the left side of the heart to pump effectively leads to congestion in the pulmonary system; signs include cough and shortness of breath. Ineffective pumping on the right side of the heart (option 1) leads to congestion (a back-up of blood) throughout the body, causing liver engorgement (option 3) and peripheral edema (option 4). Cognitive Level: Understanding. Client Need: Health Promotion and Maintenance. Nursing Process: Data Collection.
2. Answer: 4. Core Concept: 20.7. Rationale: Because digoxin is often used along with a diuretic in the treatment of HF, the patient must be carefully monitored for low potassium levels. Hypokalemia predisposes a patient to digoxin toxicity, a serious adverse effect. Levels of phosphate (option 1), amylase (option 2), and sodium (option 3) should be monitored periodically but do not have the same relationship with digoxin as potassium. Cognitive Level: Applying. Client Need: Physiological Integrity/Pharmacological Therapies. Nursing Process: Implementation.
3. Answer: 4. Core Concept: 20.8. Rationale: Because the mechanisms of actions are different, beta-blockers and ACE inhibitors work well together in the treatment of HF. ACE inhibitors

exhibit few serious adverse effects. Cardiac glycosides (option 1) and phosphodiesterase inhibitors (option 3) can cause serious adverse effects such as cardiac dysrhythmias so are not preferred drugs to work with beta-blockers. Diuretics (option 2) are sometimes used with other drugs, but patients also need to be monitored closely for hypokalemia and associated cardiac dysrhythmias. Cognitive Level: Applying. Client Need: Physiological Integrity/Pharmacological Therapies. Nursing Process: Implementation.

4. Answer: 1. Core Concept: 20.9. Rationale: Direct-acting vasodilators hydralazine and isosorbide dinitrate cause the vessels to relax, or open, by acting directly on the smooth muscle. Hydralazine works on the arterioles while isosorbide dinitrate works on the veins. This action decreases blood pressure and increases blood flow so that cardiac tissue can receive more oxygen, decreasing anginal pain. Carvedilol, a beta-blocker (option 2); chlorothiazide, a diuretic (option 3); and milrinone (Primacor), a phosphodiesterase inhibitor (option 4), are not combined with hydralazine to help relieve the pain of angina. Cognitive Level: Applying. Client Need: Physiological Integrity/Pharmacological Therapies. Nursing Process: Implementation.

5. Answer: 2. Core Concept: 20.10. Rationale: The most serious adverse effects of milrinone (Primacor), a phosphodiesterase inhibitor, are dysrhythmias. Milrinone (Primacor) can cause headaches (option 1), but it is a minor effect. Confusion (option 3) and drowsiness (option 4) are not usually associated with milrinone (Primacor). Cognitive Level: Applying. Client Need: Physiological Integrity/Pharmacological Therapies. Nursing Process: Implementation.

6. Answers: 1, 2, and 4. Core Concept: 20.5. Rationale: The pamphlet should include information that lisinopril may take several weeks to return blood pressure to normal range (option 1), and that potassium should be monitored from time to time because this drug may cause high potassium levels (option 2). In addition, taking lisinopril along with NSAIDs may cause a decrease in its antihypertensive effect (option 4). Lisinopril does not affect vision (option 3). Unless the patient starts to exhibit cardiac symptoms such as dysrhythmias or chest pain, there is no need to have an ECG done on a regular basis (option 5). Cognitive Level: Applying. Client Need: Physiological Integrity/Pharmacological Therapies. Nursing Process: Implementation.

7. Answer: 1. Core Concept: 20.8. Rationale: Beta-blockers lower heart rate and blood pressure. They do not increase heart rate and afterload (option 2). They do not produce systemic vasoconstriction (option 3) or increase the force of myocardial contractions (option 4). Cognitive Level: Applying. Client Need: Physiological Integrity/Pharmacological Therapies. Nursing Process: Implementation.

8. Answer: 1. Core Concept: 20.7. Rationale: The antidote for digoxin toxicity is digoxin immune fab, which should be ordered and available whenever digoxin is given. Milrinone (option 2) and inamrinone (option 3) are both phosphodiesterase inhibitors, which are not used along with digoxin. Flecainide, an antiarrhythmic (option 4), is not to be used with this drug because it increases digoxin levels, increasing the risk of toxicity. Cognitive Level: Applying. Client Need: Physiological Integrity/Pharmacological Therapies. Nursing Process: Implementation.

9. Answer: 1. Core Concept: 20.6. Rationale: Since the patient is taking furosemide (Lasix) (a loop diuretic), potassium is excreted in the urine and hypokalemia can occur. Potassium levels need to be monitored. Creatinine (option 2), sodium (option 3), and calcium (option 4) are not usually affected by furosemide or digoxin. Cognitive Level: Applying. Client Need: Physiological Integrity/Pharmacological Therapies. Nursing Process: Implementation.

10. Answer: 3. Core Concept: N/A. Rationale: 0.5 mg (the order) $\div$ 0.25 mg $\times$ 1 tablet (amount supplied) = 2 tablets. Options 1, 2, and 4 are a result of miscalculations and therefore incorrect. Cognitive Level: Applying. Client Need: Physiological Integrity/Pharmacological Therapies. Nursing Process: Implementation.

Case Study Answers

1. Answer: 2. Core Concept: 20.5. Rationale: ACE inhibitors, such as enalapril (Vascotec), are first-line drugs used for mild or moderate HF because of their limited adverse effects. Isosorbide dinitrate, a vasodilator (option 1), and milrinone, a phosphodiesterase inhibitor (option 3), are "second-line drugs" usually used for acute HF. Digoxin, a cardiac glycoside (option 4), may still be considered a first-line drug but has the potential to cause serious side effects and so is not the preferred drug when ACE inhibitors and diuretics are available. Cognitive Level: Applying. Client Need: Physiological Integrity/Pharmacological Therapies. Nursing Process: Implementation.
2. Answer: 2. Core Concept: 20.5. Rationale: An increase in cardiac output (without an increase in stress on the heart muscle) is a desired effect of drug therapy. An increase in heart rate (option 1), arterial blood pressure (option 3), and blood volume (option 4) causes the heart to work harder and weakens the heart muscle, eventually leading to HF. Cognitive Level: Applying. Client Need: Physiological Integrity/Pharmacological Therapies. Nursing Process: Implementation.
3. Answer: 1. Core Concept: 20.10. Rationale: Mr. Chen needs a drug such as inamrinone (Inocor) (a phosphodiesterase inhibitor) that is used for short-term support of severe or acute HF. Captopril, an ACE inhibitor (option 2); Carvedilol, a beta-blocker (option 3); and spironolactone, a potassium-sparing diuretic (option 4), are drugs used for HF but not for immediate use in severe or acute HF. Cognitive Level: Applying. Client Need: Physiological Integrity/Pharmacological Therapies. Nursing Process: Implementation.
4. Answer: 3. Core Concept: 20.6. Rationale: Furosemide (a loop diuretic) can cause cardiac dysrhythmias because it causes the loss of potassium (potassium is needed for proper cardiac conduction). Digoxin can also cause dysrhythmias, so the combination of the two drugs can be potentially dangerous and needs close monitoring. Furosemide does not cause hypotension (option 1), bradycardia (option 2), or hyperkalemia (option 4). Cognitive Level: Applying. Client Need: Physiological Integrity/Pharmacological Therapies. Nursing Process: Implementation.

Chapter 21

Review Answers

1. Answer: 2. Core Concept: 21.5. Rationale: Patients should be taught that Nitrostat tablets are to be given using the sublingual route, one tablet at a time, up to three tablets, one every 5 minutes. These tablets are not to be swallowed (option 1), nor should more than one tablet be taken at a time (option 4). If the healthcare provider is called prior to taking the tablets (option 3), the patient will be instructed the same way they were taught when initially given the medication. In addition, the time that the medication could have been working to aid the patient will have been lost. Cognitive Level: Applying. Client Need: Physiological Integrity/Pharmacological Therapies. Nursing Process: Implementation.
2. Answer: 1. Core Concept: 21.5. Rationale: The most common adverse effect of nitroglycerin is headache because it causes vasodilation, increasing blood flow to the brain. Nitroglycerin does not cause hypertension (option 2), diuresis (option 3), or bradycardia (option 4). Cognitive Level: Applying. Client Need: Physiological Integrity/Pharmacological Therapies. Nursing Process: Implementation.
3. Answer: 2. Core Concept: 21.6. Rationale: Beta-blockers block the beta receptors within the nervous system, decreasing heart rate, contractility, and blood pressure and thus reducing the oxygen needs of the heart and allowing healing. ACE inhibitors (option 1) prevent the formation of angiotensin, lowering blood pressure and reducing blood volume. Vasodilators (option 3) dilate blood vessels increasing blood flow. Diuretics (option 4) allow for excretion of excess fluid through the renal system. Cognitive Level: Applying. Client Need: Physiological Integrity/Pharmacological Therapies. Nursing Process: Implementation.

4. Answer: 2. Core Concept: 21.9. Rationale: The use of reteplase can cause bleeding because it interferes with the clotting process. It is not known to cause dehydration (option 1), confusion (option 3), or increased clotting time (option 4). Cognitive Level: Applying. Client Need: Physiological Integrity/Pharmacological Therapies. Nursing Process: Implementation.
5. Answer: 3. Core Concept: 21.9. Rationale: Because reteplase can cause an increase in bleeding (a serious adverse effect), the nurse must be vigilant to assess for abnormal bleeding during its infusion. Reteplase does not cause an increase in blood pressure (option 1), vomiting, or diarrhea (option 4). An increase in heart rate is not directly attributed to reteplase but can be seen with increased bleeding (option 2). Cognitive Level: Applying. Client Need: Physiological Integrity/Pharmacological Therapies. Nursing Process: Implementation.
6. Answers: 2. Core Concept: 21.11. Rationale: Hemorrhagic strokes are caused by the rupture of blood vessels in the brain, usually as a result of high blood pressure or weakening of the vessel wall (aneurysm). Therefore, thrombolytics are the exception among the options provided. They must never be used for a patient with a hemorrhagic stroke because they will prevent clotting and increase bleeding. Anticonvulsants (option 1) can be used to prevent convulsions, antihypertensives (option 3) are used to decrease blood pressure, and an osmotic diuretic (option 4) is used to reduce swelling in the brain. Cognitive Level: Understanding. Client Need: Physiological Integrity/Pharmacological Therapies. Nursing Process: Planning.
7. Answer: 4. Core Concept: N/A. Rationale: Ordered infusion 150 mL ÷ 60 minutes (1 hr) × 15 drops/mL = 37.5 (38 drops/min). Options 1–3 are a result of miscalculations and are therefore incorrect. Cognitive Level: Applying. Client Need: Physiological Integrity/Pharmacological Therapies. Nursing Process: Implementation.
8. Answer: 1. Core Concept: 21.6. Rationale: Beta adrenergics block norepinephrine and epinephrine from binding to beta receptors, slowing heart rate and decreasing contractility of the heart, thus reducing the workload of the heart. Beta blockers do not directly relax arterial and venous smooth muscle (option 2), cause increased contractility and heart rate (option 3), or decrease peripheral resistance (option 4). Cognitive Level: Applying. Client Need: Physiological Integrity/Pharmacological Therapies. Nursing Process: Implementation.
9. Answer: 3. Core Concept: 21.7. Rationale: Taking digoxin with CCBs enhances the effect of digoxin, possibly causing toxicity. Acetaminophen (option 1), ibuprofen (option 2), and ranitidine (option 4) are not contraindicated when taking CCBs. Cognitive Level: Applying. Client Need: Physiological Integrity/Pharmacological Therapies. Nursing Process: Implementation.
10. Answers: 1, 2, 3, and 4. Core Concept: 21.10. Rationale: Aspirin is given to prevent further clotting; beta-blockers are given to reduce the workload of the heart; and thrombolytics are given to dissolve existing clots when a person is diagnosed with a heart attack. In addition, an ACE inhibitor is usually given just after thrombolytic therapy is completed to aid in heart repair. Potassium-sparing diuretics (option 5) are not given to patients experiencing an MI. Cognitive Level: Applying. Client Need: Physiological Integrity/Pharmacological Therapies. Nursing Process: Implementation.

Case Study Answers

1. Answer: 2. Core Concept: 21.5. Rationale: Nitroglycerin is given to end an angina attack in progress. It relaxes and dilates the smooth muscle of vessels, allowing increased blood flow to the heart tissue. Nitroglycerin does not prevent future angina attacks (option 1), prevent MI or stroke (option 3), or relieve epigastric pain (option 4). Cognitive Level: Applying. Client Need: Physiological Integrity/Pharmacological Therapies. Nursing Process: Implementation.

2. Answer: 2. Core Concept: 21.5. Rationale: Ms. Bush should be instructed to take sublingual nitroglycerin at the first indication of chest pain. It is used for acute pain and not recommended to take for exercising (option 1) or throughout the day (options 3 and 4). Cognitive Level: Applying. Client Need: Physiological Integrity/Pharmacological Therapies. Nursing Process: Implementation.
3. Answer: 1. Core Concept: 21.6. Rationale: Ms. Bush has been prescribed metoprolol, a beta blocker, to help prevent acute angina attacks by reducing the workload of the heart. It is not used to end an angina attack (option 2) or prevent MI or stroke (option 3). It does lower blood pressure but it is not given to Ms. Bush for this reason at this time (option 4). Cognitive Level: Applying. Client Need: Physiological Integrity/Pharmacological Therapies. Nursing Process: Implementation.
4. Answer: 1. Core Concept: 21.9. Rationale: The nurse lets Ms. Bush know that reteplase is used in acute situations like hers and is dissolving any existing clots that are impeding blood flow to the brain. This drug is not used to prevent clot formation (option 2), stabilize blood pressure (option 3), or reduce the workload on the heart (option 4). Cognitive Level: Applying. Client Need: Physiological Integrity/Pharmacological Therapies. Nursing Process: Implementation.

Chapter 22

Review Answers

1. Answer: 2. Core Concept: 22.1. Rationale: Patients with severe burns lose fluid through the burns, resulting in loss of blood volume and possible hypovolemic (decreased blood volume) shock. Cardiogenic shock (option 1) is a result of the heart's inability to function properly. Septic shock (option 3) is caused by a systemic infection, and anaphylactic shock (option 4) is a severe response from an allergy. Cognitive Level: Understanding. Client Need: Physiological Integrity/Pharmacological Therapies. Nursing Process: Assessment.
2. Answer: 4. Core Concept: 22.2. Rationale: While it is important to monitor all of the vital signs (options 1–3), a drop in blood pressure is the most indicative of shock and its increase during treatment is considered an important parameter in determining effectiveness. Cognitive Level: Understanding. Client Need: Physiological Integrity/Pharmacological Therapies. Nursing Process: Assessment.
3. Answer: 2. Core Concept: 22.3. Rationale: As a colloid, normal serum albumin draws water from the body's cells and tissues into the blood vessels, thus increasing the blood volume. The 0.45% NS (option 1), 0.33% NS (option 3), and, once in the body, D5W (option 4) are all hypotonic solutions and would cause the fluid to shift from the intravascular space (within the blood vessels) to the intracellular and interstitial (tissue) spaces. Cognitive Level: Applying. Client Need: Physiological Integrity/Pharmacological Therapies. Nursing Process: Implementation.
4. Answers: 1, 2, and 3. Core Concept: 22.4. Rationale: Dopamine can cause an increase in blood flow to the kidneys at low doses, and at high doses it can increase cardiac output. Dopamine also causes vasoconstriction, which increases blood pressure. It is not used to treat anaphylaxis (options 4 and 5). Cognitive Level: Applying. Client Need: Physiological Integrity/Pharmacological Therapies. Nursing Process: Implementation.
5. Answer: 1. Core Concept: 22.6. Rationale: Epinephrine stimulates the sympathetic nervous system. Specifically, it stimulates the alpha-receptors, increasing blood pressure, and activates beta-receptors, opening the smooth muscles of the airways to relieve bronchospasms. Dobutamine (option 2) stimulates the beta-adrenergic receptors to increase cardiac output and maintain blood flow; digoxin (option 3) increases myocardial contractility, and dopamine (option 4) stimulates alpha-adrenergic receptors, causing vasoconstriction and raising blood pressure. Cognitive Level: Understanding. Client Need: Physiological Integrity/Pharmacological Therapies. Nursing Process: Planning.

6. Answer: 4. Core Concept: 22.6. Rationale: Vasodilators are not used to treat anaphylaxis. Common drugs used include antihistamines to prevent the release of histamines (option 1), corticosteroids to lessen the inflammatory response (option 2), and bronchodilators to relax smooth muscle in order to open airways (option 3). Cognitive Level: Understanding. Client Need: Physiological Integrity/Pharmacological Therapies. Nursing Process: Planning.
7. Answer: 2. Core Concept: 22.5. Rationale: Inotropic drugs can reverse the symptoms of shock by increasing the force of myocardial contractions, thus increasing cardiac output. These drugs do not cause a decrease in cardiac output (option 1), slow the heart rate (option 3), or increase afterload (option 4). Cognitive Level: Applying. Client Need: Physiological Integrity/Pharmacological Therapies. Nursing Process: Evaluation.
8. Answer: 3. Core Concept: 22.4. Rationale: Norepinephrine, a powerful vasoconstrictor, acts on the alpha-adrenergic receptors in the smooth muscle wall of the blood vessels, immediately raising blood pressure. Hypertension is a serious adverse effect that must be monitored continuously during administration. Norepinephrine does not cause bradycardia (option 1), hypotension (option 2), or liver failure (option 4). Cognitive Level: Applying. Client Need: Physiological Integrity/Pharmacological Therapies. Nursing Process: Evaluation.
9. Answer: 2. Core Concept: 22.4. Rationale: One advantage of using dobutamine is that it increases myocardial contractility, increasing cardiac output without significantly increasing heart rate. It is especially used for those in septic shock, cardiogenic shock, or with history of heart failure. Dobutamine does not increase heart rate (option 1) or decrease cardiac output (option 3). Its actions do not include vasoconstriction (option 4). Cognitive Level: Remembering. Client Need: Physiological Integrity/Pharmacological Therapies. Nursing Process: Planning.
10. Answer: 2. Core Concept: N/A. Rationale: Ordered infusion 1000 mL ÷ 5 hr = 200 mL/hr. 200 mL/hr ÷ 60 min/hr. × 15 drops/mL = 50 drops/min. Options 1, 3, and 4 are a result of miscalculations and are therefore incorrect. Cognitive Level: Applying. Client Need: Physiological Integrity/Pharmacological Therapies. Nursing Process: Implementation.

Case Study Answers

1. Answer: 4. Core Concept: 22.6. Rationale: Epinephrine activates beta-receptors, opening the smooth muscles of the airways to relieve bronchospasms. D5W (option 1) in an IV solution is given to supply dextrose to the body cells and to shift fluid out the intravascular space. Dobutamine (option 2) increases myocardial contractility, and hydrocortisone (option 3) lessens the inflammatory response of the immune system. Cognitive Level: Applying. Client Need: Physiological Integrity/Pharmacological Therapies. Nursing Process: Implementation.
2. Answer: 1. Core Concept: 22.3. Rationale: Because isotonic solutions such as 0.9% sodium chloride (normal saline) have the same concentration of solutes as plasma, they do not move into cells. They remain outside the cells within the intravascular space (blood/plasma), thus increasing blood volume and replacing lost fluids. The medications dobutamine (option 2), hydrocortisone (option 3), and epinephrine (option 4) do not directly impact blood volume. Cognitive Level: Applying. Client Need: Physiological Integrity/Pharmacological Therapies. Nursing Process: Implementation.
3. Answer: 4. Core Concept: 22.6. Rationale: Epinephrine stimulates the alpha-receptors of the nervous system, causing vasoconstriction and increasing blood pressure. 0.9% sodium chloride increases blood volume, which would eventually increase blood pressure but not in 2 minutes (option 1). Dobutamine (option 2) increases myocardial contractility, and hydrocortisone (option 3) lessens the inflammatory response of the

immune system; therefore, these do not have any direct impact on raising blood pressure. Cognitive Level: Understanding. Client Need: Physiological Integrity/Pharmacological Therapies. Nursing Process: Evaluation.

4. Answer: 4. Core Concept: 22.6. Rationale: Albuterol (Ventolin), a bronchodilator, relaxes muscles in the airways, increases air flow, and relieves shortness of breath. Diphenhydramine (Benadryl) (option 1) is used to prevent the release of histamines; hydrocortisone (option 2) is used to lessen inflammation; and phenylephrine, Neo-Synephrine (option 3), is a vasoconstrictor commonly used to maintain blood pressure and as a decongestant. Cognitive Level: Applying. Client Need: Physiological Integrity/Pharmacological Therapies. Nursing Process: Implementation.

Chapter 23

Review Answers

1. Answer: 3. Core Concept: 23.4. Rationale: Sodium is responsible for generating spontaneous contractions of the heart (action potential). The action (potential) of the heart occurs when sodium channels open, allowing sodium (and calcium) to rush into the cell, causing depolarization (contraction). Potassium (option 1) moves out of the cell because of the movement of sodium through potassium ion channels but returns after cardiac contraction (repolarization). Magnesium (option 2) and chloride (option 4) help to ensure proper levels of sodium, calcium, and potassium. Cognitive Level: Understanding. Client Need: Physiological Integrity/Pharmacological Therapies. Nursing Process: Data Collection
2. Answer: 2. Core Concept: 23.6. Rationale: Because of the role of sodium in cardiac conduction, sodium channel blockers slow the flow of sodium into the cell, thus slowing the impulse and cardiac contraction. This type of drug does not increase automaticity (option 1), prolong the refractory period (option 3), or increase impulse conduction (option 4). Cognitive Level: Applying. Client Need: Physiological Integrity/Pharmacological Therapies. Nursing Process: Implementation.
3. Answer: 2. Core Concept: N/A. Rationale: Ordered 15 mg, three times a day. 15 mg (ordered) ÷ 30 mg (available) × 1 tablet = ½ tablet per dose. In addition, the patient will receive a total of 45 mg per day (15 mg × 3 times/day). Options 1, 3, and 4 are a result of miscalculations and are therefore incorrect. Cognitive Level: Applying. Client Need: Physiological Integrity/Pharmacological Therapies. Nursing Process: Implementation.
4. Answer: 3. Core Concept: 23.8. Rationale: The use of amiodarone (Cararone) along with digoxin can cause an increase of digoxin in the blood. This increase can lead to digoxin toxicity. Therefore, if taken together, the dosage of digoxin must be decreased. When taken with amiodarone, digoxin does not have to be discontinued (option 1) but should never be increased or doubled (options 2 and 4). Cognitive Level: Understanding. Client Need: Physiological Integrity/Pharmacological Therapies. Nursing Process: Planning.
5. Answer: 1. Core Concept: Nursing Process Focus. Rationale: Because one of the effects of antidysrhythmic drugs is the slowing of cardiac conduction, a slower heart rate is expected. These drugs do not cause an increase in heart rate (option 2), renal insufficiency (option 3), or hepatic insufficiency (option 4). Cognitive Level: Applying. Client Need: Physiological Integrity/Pharmacological Therapies. Nursing Process: Evaluation.
6. Answer: 2. Core Concept: Nursing Process Focus. Rationale: Since antidysrhythmic drugs decrease heart rate, the patient should be instructed to notify the healthcare provider if their heart rate drops out of normal range (under 60 beats per minute). Constipation (option 1) is not normally related to this class of drugs. Antidysrhythmic drugs do not increase heart rate, so heart rate should not exceed 90 beats per minute (option 3).

The patient is taking an antidysrhythmic drug to correct a dysrhythmia: therefore, decreasing blood pressure may not be a goal and the patient would not have to notify their provider (option 4). Cognitive Level: Applying. Client Need: Physiological Integrity/Pharmacological Therapies. Nursing Process: Implementation.

7. Answers: 1, 2, and 3. Core Concept: Nursing Process Focus. Rationale: Patients should be instructed that common adverse effects of antidysrhythmic drugs include dizziness, hypotension, and weakness because of decreased cardiac output, heart rate, and blood pressure. Anorexia (option 4) and insomnia (option 5) are not adverse effects common to this class of drugs. Cognitive Level: Applying. Client Need: Physiological Integrity/Pharmacological Therapies. Nursing Process: Implementation.
8. Answer: 2. Core Concept: Nursing Process Focus. Rationale: Since antidysrhythmic drugs decrease heart rate, the patient should be instructed to take their pulse prior to taking the medication. The patient would not be taught to take medication only when feeling excessively tired (option 1). Being excessively tired may be a sign of decreased cardiac output so patients should notify their healthcare provider. Never drinking alcohol (option 3) or increasing sodium and potassium intake (option 4) would not be included in a teaching plan. Cognitive Level: Understanding. Client Need: Physiological Integrity/Pharmacological Therapies. Nursing Process: Planning.
9. Answer: 2. Core Concept: 23.9. Rationale: Verapamil (Calan), a CCB, is also used to treat angina because it causes vasodilation of the coronary arteries, allowing more oxygen to reach the myocardium. Digoxin, a cardiac glycoside (option 1); adenosine, a purine nucleoside (option 3); and quinidine sulfate, a class I antiarrhythmic agent (option 4), are not used to treat angina. Cognitive Level: Applying. Client Need: Physiological Integrity/Pharmacological Therapies. Nursing Process: Implementation.
10. Answer: 1. Core Concept: 23.9. Rationale: Diltiazem (Cardizem), a CCB, is the drug being administered. In addition to stabilizing dysrhythmias, it also decreases blood pressure and dilates the coronary arteries, reducing cardiac pain. Digoxin (option 2), adenosine (option 3), and quinidine sulfate (option 4) are not used for blood pressure control or angina. Cognitive Level: Applying. Client Need: Physiological Integrity/Pharmacological Therapies. Nursing Process: Implementation.

Case Study Answers

1. Answer: 4. Core Concept: 23.6. Rationale: Lidocaine, a sodium channel blocker, slows the speed of electrical conduction across the heart muscle by blocking the influx of sodium into the cells. Lidocaine does not increase heart rate (option 1); it slows the heart rate by affecting the conduction system. It does not lower blood pressure (option 2) or increase the strength of heart contractions (option 3). Cognitive Level: Client Need: Applying. Physiological Integrity/Pharmacological Therapies. Nursing Process: Implementation.
2. Answer: 2. Core Concept: 23.7. Rationale: In addition to being an antidysrhythmic, propranolol (a beta blocker) will also decrease Mrs. Duncan's blood pressure. Beta blockers should not increase blood pressure (option 1), have no effect on blood pressure (option 3), or increase and then decrease blood pressure (option 4). Cognitive Level: Client Need: Physiological Integrity/Pharmacological Therapies. Nursing Process: Planning.
3. Answer: 3. Core Concept: 23.8. Rationale: Both propranolol and amiodarone can affect the lungs. Propranolol may cause bronchospasm and amiodarone can cause a flu-like syndrome. Taking both of these drugs together increases the risk of developing problems, decreasing the amount of oxygen the patient receives and producing the adverse effects of dizziness, fainting, and fatigue. The symptoms Mrs. Duncan is experiencing are not related to her diet (option 1). These two drugs may cause bradycardia but would not cause HTN (option 2), nor would they cause her blood pressure to get out of control (option 4). Cognitive Level: Client Need: Physiological Integrity/Pharmacological Therapies. Nursing Process: Planning.

4. Answer: 1. Core Concept: Nursing Process Focus. Rationale: Mrs. Duncan will be instructed to take her pulse rate and blood pressure prior to taking her medication daily because these medications affect both. At this time, it is not necessary for Mrs. Duncan to keep a log of weight loss or gain (option 2), eat plenty of foods containing potassium (option 3), or avoid taking aspirin (option 4). Cognitive Level: Client Need: Physiological Integrity/Pharmacological Therapies. Nursing Process: Planning.

Chapter 24

Review Answers

1. Answer: 1, 2, 4, and 5. Core Concept: 24.5. Rationale: The adverse effects of clopidogrel (Plavix) include headache, diarrhea, bruising, and skin rash. Clopidogrel has not been known to cause constipation (option 3). Cognitive Level: Applying. Client Need: Physiological Integrity/Pharmacological Therapies. Nursing Process: Evaluation.
2. Answer: 2. Core Concept: 24.4. Rationale: Warfarin (Coumadin) is an anticoagulant. This class of drug prevents clot formation or prevents the further development of a clot. The use of an anticoagulant such as warfarin will not break down clots (options 1, 3, and 4). Cognitive Level: Applying. Client Need: Physiological Integrity/Pharmacological Therapies. Nursing Process: Implementation.
3. Answer: 1. Core Concept: 24.8. Rationale: The patient starting on oprelvekin (Neumega) should see an increase in platelets within 5–9 days, unlike option 2, which states that the results should be immediate. Oprelvekin helps create new platelets, not white blood cells (options 3 and 4). Cognitive Level: Applying. Client Need: Physiological Integrity/ Pharmacological Therapies. Nursing Process: Implementation.
4. Answer: 2. Core Concept: 24.4. Rationale: A common adverse effect of LMWHs, like enoxaparin (Lovenox), is bleeding because they decrease clotting time. The patient must be monitored for any signs of bruising and bleeding. LMWHs do not cause gingival hyperplasia (option 1) or increased pain (option 4). This class of drug would actually decrease the ability of clotting at an incision (option 3). Cognitive Level: Applying. Client Need: Physiological Integrity/Pharmacological Therapies. Nursing Process: Implementation.
5. Answers: 1, 2, 4, and 5. Core Concept: 24.5. Rationale: Coumadin (anticoagulant), ibuprofen (NSAID), aspirin (antiplatelet), and tissue plasminogen activators (thrombolytic) should not be used with clopidogrel unless the healthcare provider is consulted because all of them have the ability to increase the risk for bleeding, an adverse effect already associated with clopidogrel (Plavix). Taking diltiazem is not contraindicated while taking colpidogrel (option 3). Cognitive Level: Applying. Client Need: Physiological Integrity/Pharmacological Therapies. Nursing Process: Implementation.
6. Answers: 3 and 4. Core Concept: 24.8. Rationale: Because of their medical condition, a decrease in RBCs, patients should avoid excessive fatigue by taking frequent rest periods until RBC and iron levels return to normal. In addition, patients should monitor their blood pressure and pulse because one of the serious adverse effects of epoetin alfa is HTN. Patients do not need to stop eating raw vegetables (option 1) or avoid direct sunlight (option 2). Even though it is wise to protect the eyes from bright light by wearing sunglasses, the use of epoetin is not the reason for protecting the eyes (option 5). Cognitive Level: Understanding. Client Need: Physiological Integrity/Pharmacological Therapies. Nursing Process: Evaluation.
7. Answer: 1. Core Concept: 24.7. Rationale: Aminocaproic acid (Amicar) is the preferred drug to control postoperative bleeding. Aspirin (option 2) is an antiplatelet that reduces clotting time. Trombin (Evithrom), a hemostatic drug, is used to prevent blood loss following cardiopulmonary bypass surgery (option 3).Tranexamic acid, Cyklokapron, (option 4), another hemostatic drug, is used in dental surgery for patients with

hemophilia and for women with heavy menstrual bleeding. Cognitive Level: Understanding. Client Need: Physiological Integrity/Pharmacological Therapies. Nursing Process: Planning.

8. Answer: 1. Core Concept: 24.4. Rationale: Protamine sulfate reverses the anticoagulant effects of heparin. Anytime heparin is ordered, protamine sulfate should be available and used when a patient has elevated aPTT levels and abnormal bleeding is noted. Vitamin K (option 2) is the antidote for warfarin, Trental (option 3) improves blood flow through peripheral blood vessels, and ardeparin (option 4) is used to treat thrombosis. Cognitive Level: Understanding. Client Need: Physiological Integrity/Pharmacological Therapies. Nursing Process: Planning.
9. Answer: 4. Core Concept: N/A. Rationale: 35,000 units (ordered) ÷ 10,000 units (available) × 1 mL = 3.5 mL daily. Options 1–3 are a result of miscalculations and are therefore incorrect. Cognitive Level: Applying. Client Need: Physiological Integrity/Pharmacological Therapies. Nursing Process: Implementation.
10. Answer: 2. Core Concept: 24.6. Rationale: The nurse must monitor for the most common adverse effect of alteplase (activase): bleeding as seen in bruising and epistaxis. Alteplase is not known to cause an elevated temperature (option 1), skin rash, urticaria (option 3), or wheezing (option 4). Cognitive Level: Applying. Client Need: Physiological Integrity/Pharmacological Therapies. Nursing Process: Evaluation.

Case Study Answers

1. Answer: 4. Core Concept: 24.4. Rationale: The goal of anticoagulant therapy, such as heparin, is to prevent thrombi from forming. Anticoagulants do not dissolve pulmonary emboli (option 1), prevent excessive bleeding (option 2), or reduce blood viscosity (option 3). Cognitive Level: Understanding. Client Need: Physiological Integrity/Pharmacological Therapies. Nursing Process: Planning.
2. Answer: 3. Core Concept: 24.4. Rationale: The most common adverse effect of heparin is bleeding (anticoagulant properties). Common adverse effects of heparin do not include nausea or vomiting (option 1). Heparin also does not cause MI (option 2) or sedation (option 4). Cognitive Level: Applying. Client Need: Physiological Integrity/Pharmacological Therapies. Nursing Process: Implementation.
3. Answer: 2. Core Concept: 24.4. Rationale: Warfarin, an oral anticoagulant, is more convenient to take than heparin, which is given either IV or subcutaneously. Mr. Hawkins was not switched because warfarin is more effective (option 1), causes less risk for hemorrhage (option 3), or is less expensive (option 4). Cognitive Level: Applying. Client Need: Physiological Integrity/Pharmacological Therapies. Nursing Process: Implementation.
4. Answer: 1. Core Concept: 24.4. Rationale: Mr. Hawkins will need to have his PT/INR values tested during the 2 weeks after his release from the hospital to determine warfarin levels and effectiveness. CBCs (option 2), aPTT (option 3), and white blood cell counts (option 4) are not needed to monitor warfarin effectiveness. Cognitive Level: Applying. Client Need: Physiological Integrity/Pharmacological Therapies. Nursing Process: Implementation.

Chapter 25

Review Answers

1. Answer: 3. Core Concept: 25.4. Rationale: Acetaminophen does not have anti-inflammatory properties; therefore, it is not classified as an NSAID. Aspirin (option 1), ibuprofen (option 2), and Motrin, a trade name of ibuprofen (option 4), are all NSAIDs and are used for inflammation. Cognitive Level: Applying. Client Need: Physiological Integrity/Pharmacological Therapies. Nursing Process: Implementation.

2. Answer: 3. Core Concept: 25.4. Rationale: Tinnitus (ringing in the ears) and dizziness are two of the adverse effects that can be experienced when taking aspirin (ASA); therefore, the patient should not take ASA before consulting the healthcare provider. Sinus infections may cause dizziness if the eustachian tubes are blocked but do not usually cause tinnitus (option 1). The nurse should determine whether the patient is taking other medications that contain aspirin, but most OTC medications include acetaminophen, not aspirin (option 2). Taking aspirin with food or milk may help relieve gastric adverse effects but it will not prevent tinnitus or dizziness (option 4). Cognitive Level: Applying. Client Need: Physiological Integrity/Pharmacological Therapies. Nursing Process: Evaluation.
3. Answer: 3. Core Concept: 25.4. Rationale: The most common adverse effect of NSAIDs is GI irritation. NSAIDs are also known to cause edema (option 1), rashes (option 2), and bleeding (option 4). In addition, NSAIDs have a black box warning about the risk of MI or stroke (option 5). Cognitive Level: Applying. Client Need: Physiological Integrity/Pharmacological Therapies. Nursing Process: Implementation.
4. Answer: 4. Core Concept: 25.5. Rationale: Corticosteroids suppress the actions of chemical mediators of inflammation, such as histamine and prostaglandins. In addition, they inhibit the immune system by suppressing certain functions of phagocytes and lymphocytes. Therefore, a patient taking this class of medications should be monitored for the possibility of infections. Corticosteroids are not known to cause bleeding (option 1), respiratory distress (option 2), or dehydration (option 3). Cognitive Level: Applying. Client Need: Physiological Integrity/Pharmacological Therapies. Nursing Process: Implementation.
5. Answer: 2. Core Concept: 25.5. Rationale: When used for long-term therapy, Cushing syndrome can occur. This condition causes an elevation of blood glucose levels, and patients with diabetes must adjust their insulin doses. Without an evaluation of the patient's diet, the nurse cannot assume that the diet is not being followed (option 1). There is no evidence that the patient is developing an illness (option 3), or that their diabetes is getting worse (option 4). Cognitive Level: Understanding. Client Need: Physiological Integrity/Pharmacological Therapies. Nursing Process: Evaluation.
6. Answer: 4. Core Concept: N/A. Rationale: Convert grains to milligrams 65 mg/1 gr × 10 gr/1 = 650 mg. 650 mg (the order) ÷ 325 mg × 1 tablet (amt. supplied) = 2 tablets. Options 1–3 are a result of miscalculations and are therefore incorrect. Cognitive Level: Applying. Client Need: Physiological Integrity/Pharmacological Therapies. Nursing Process: Implementation.
7. Answers: 1, 2, 4, and 5. Core Concept: 25.6. Rationale: The effects of acetaminophen that should be reported include lethargy and anorexia, which are the results of acetaminophen poisoning. Acetaminophen can also cause severe allergic reactions such as difficulty breathing, angioedema, itching, and rash, which should also be reported. Acetaminophen is not known to cause tearing of the eyes (option 3). Cognitive Level: Applying. Client Need: Physiological Integrity/Pharmacological Therapies. Nursing Process: Implementation.
8. Answer: 4. Core Concept: 25.5. Rationale: A moon-shaped face, bruising, and shoulder hump are results of Cushing syndrome, a condition (adverse effect) that can result from the long-term use of prednisone. These signs or symptoms are not considered normal findings (option 1), birth defects (option 2), or the symptoms of myasthenia gravis (option 3). Cognitive Level: Applying. Client Need: Physiological Integrity/Pharmacological Therapies. Nursing Process: Evaluation.
9. Answer: 1. Core Concept: 25.6. Rationale: Because excessive use of both acetaminophen and alcohol can cause liver damage, combining these two drugs is not recommended due to the possibility of liver failure from hepatic necrosis. Combining alcohol and acetaminophen has not been known to cause renal damage (option 2), pulmonary damage (option 4), or a thrombosis (option 3). Cognitive Level: Applying. Client Need: Physiological Integrity/Pharmacological Therapies. Nursing Process: Implementation.

10. Answer: 2. Core Concept: 25.5. Rationale: Using the topical method of drug administration may prevent the serious adverse effects of corticosteroids. Topical corticosteroids are not prescribed because they are cheaper or easier to take than oral versions (options 1 and 4). Option 3 is incorrect because topical steroids should not be applied to a rash when an infection is present. Level: Applying. Client Need: Physiological Integrity/Pharmacological Therapies. Nursing Process: Implementation.

Case Study Answers

1. Answer: 2. Core Concept: 25.4. Rationale: The nurse should monitor the patient for the most common NSAID adverse effect: gastric irritation and upset. NSAIDs are not known to cause drowsiness (option 1), excessive dryness or stinging sensations of the nose (option 3), or rashes or dryness of the skin (option 4). Cognitive Level: Understanding. Client Need: Physiological Integrity/Pharmacological Therapies. Nursing Process: Planning.
2. Answer: 1. Core Concept: 25.4. Rationale: Taking NSAIDs with food will decrease stomach irritation. Because NSAIDs can cause gastric irritation, it is not advised to take them on an empty stomach (option 2). Taking two types of NSAIDs at the same time increases the risk of gastric irritation (option 3). NSAIDs can also cause dizziness and drowsiness (option 4). Cognitive Level: Applying. Client Need: Physiological Integrity/Pharmacological Therapies. Nursing Process: Implementation.
3. Answer: 3. Core Concept: 25.5. Rationale: The nurse would expect that a short-term, systemic corticosteroid would be used for a flare. This class of medication suppresses the inflammatory response seen in patients with arthritis. Biologic response modifiers (option 1), such as interferon and monoclonal antibodies, are substances that arouse the body's response to infection and are used to treat disorders like cancer. Sympathomimetics (option 4) are primarily used to treat heart and obstructive airway conditions. Intranasal corticosteroids (option 2) are used primarily for inflammation within the nasal cavity. Cognitive Level: Understanding. Client Need: Physiological Integrity/Pharmacological Therapies. Nursing Process: Planning.
4. Answer: 2. Core Concept: 25.5. Rationale: Prednisone, used for short periods of time, markedly reduces inflammation and pain. The healthcare provider had good reason to prescribe another stronger, anti-inflammatory drug to help the patient (option 1). Prednisone is used for its anti-inflammatory properties (option 3). Prednisone has severe adverse effects such as gastric irritation, and in long-term use, Cushing syndrome (option 4). Cognitive Level: Applying. Client Need: Physiological Integrity/Pharmacological Therapies. Nursing Process: Implementation.

Chapter 26

Review Answers

1. Answers: 1, 2, and 4. Core Concept: 26.4. Rationale: Adverse effects of interferon alfa-2b (Intron A) include thoughts of suicide, depression, and hepatotoxicity. This drug is not known to cause hypotension (option 3). Cognitive Level: Applying. Client Need: Physiological Integrity/Pharmacological Therapies. Nursing Process: Evaluation.
2. Answers: 1, 2, and 5. Core Concept: 26.4. Rationale: The nurse would question the use of aldesleukin (Proleukin) for liver disease, metastatic lung cancer, or colon cancer. Aldesleukin (Proleukin) is an interleukin 2 drug used in the treatment of metastatic renal cancer (option 3) and metastatic melanoma (option 4). Cognitive Level: Understanding. Client Need: Physiological Integrity/Pharmacological Therapies. Nursing Process: Planning.
3. Answer: 4. Core Concept: 26.4. Rationale: Oprelvekin (Neumega), an interleukin-11 drug, is used to stimulate platelet production in patients with weakened immune

systems to help fight infections. Oprelvekin does not suppress the immune system (option 1), reduce the inflammatory response of the body (option 2), or act as an antiviral (option 3). Cognitive Level: Applying. Client Need: Physiological Integrity/Pharmacological Therapies. Nursing Process: Implementation.

4. Answer: 1. Core Concept: 26.4. Rationale: A biologic response modifier, filgrastim (Neupogen) promotes the production of WBCs. These drugs are used to shorten the length of neutropenia (reduced leukocyte count) in patients with cancer and in those who have had a bone marrow transplant. Therefore, patients taking this medication should be evaluated for the therapeutic outcome of increased WBCs. This drug does not increase the production of platelets (option 2). It also does not increase (option 3) or decrease (option 4) the production of RBCs. Cognitive Level: Understanding. Client Need: Physiological Integrity/Pharmacological Therapies. Nursing Process: Evaluation.

5. Answer: 3. Core Concept: 26.3. Rationale: The recommended schedule for the administration of the DTaP vaccine is at 2 months, 4 months, 6 months, 15–18 months, and 4–6 years of age. The other options are incorrect: The vaccination schedule recommends that the first injection be given at 2 months instead of 1 month of age (option 1). It also recommends a series of five injections instead of four (options 2 and 4). Cognitive Level: Applying. Client Need: Physiological Integrity/Pharmacological Therapies. Nursing Process: Data Collection.

6. Answer: 3. Core Concept: 26.3 Rationale: In addition to the hepatitis B vaccine series, the HBIG vaccine is also given to those who have been exposed to the hepatitis B virus. It provides preformed antibodies (temporary, passive immunity), allowing the body time to build its own antibodies to the virus. It does not provide active immunity (option 4), and does not have an effect on the hepatitis B (Engerix-B) series of vaccines (options 1 and 2). Hepatitis B (Engerix-B) series is used to provide prophylaxis against exposure. Cognitive Level: Applying. Client Need: Physiological Integrity/Pharmacological Therapies. Nursing Process: Implementation.

7. Answer: 2. Core Concept: 26.5. Rationale: Because immunosuppressants cause a decrease in the body's ability to fight infection (suppression of the immune system), patient needs to be evaluated for any symptoms of infection. Immunosuppressants are not usually associated with hypotension (option 1), hypoglycemia (option 3), or bleeding (option 4). Cognitive Level: Applying. Client Need: Physiological Integrity/Pharmacological Therapies. Nursing Process: Evaluation.

8. Answer: 4. Core Concept: N/A. Rationale: Convert pounds to kilograms 100 pounds ÷ 2.2 kg = 45.45 kg. Order: 0.15 milligrams × 45.45 kg = 6.8175 mg (6.82 mg) per day ÷ 2 = 3.41 mg per dose. Options 1–3 are a result of miscalculations and are therefore incorrect. Cognitive Level: Applying. Client Need: Physiological Integrity/Pharmacological Therapies. Nursing Process: Implementation.

9. Answer: 4. Core Concept: 26.5. Rationale: Cyclosporine should not be taken with grapefruit juice because it increases blood levels of the drug. Options 1–3 are correct responses by the patient: Those taking cyclosporine should report a reduction of urine output (option 1), frequently wash their hands (option 2), and take their blood pressure every day (option 3). Cognitive Level: Understanding. Client Need: Physiological Integrity/Pharmacological Therapies. Nursing Process: Planning.

10. Answer: 2. Core Concept: 26.5. Rationale: The primary, major adverse effect of cyclosporine is a decrease in urinary output. Therefore, renal function tests should be done. This includes the laboratory tests measuring BUN and creatinine. Although CBC (option 1), liver enzymes (option 3), and electrolytes (option 4) should be monitored, they are not the primary adverse effects. Cognitive Level: Understanding. Client Need: Physiological Integrity/Pharmacological Therapies. Nursing Process: Evaluation.

Case Study Answers

1. Answer: 4. Core Concept: 26.3. Rationale: The hepatitis B vaccine works by stimulating the body to form antibodies to attack the virus and by generating memory cells to recognize the entry of the hepatitis B virus. This type of immunity is called active immunity. The hepatitis B vaccine series does not provide passive immunity (option 1). The hepatitis B vaccine is developed by using recombinant technology not an attenuated (option 2) or live virus (option 3). Cognitive Level: Applying. Client Need: Physiological Integrity/Pharmacological Therapies. Nursing Process: Implementation.
2. Answer: 1. Core Concept: 26.3. Rationale: The hepatitis B vaccine is typically given as a series of three injections: the first injection, the second injection a month after the first, and the last injection 6 months after the first injection. The other options are incorrect; it is not usually given as a series of either two (option 2) or four (option 4) injections. In addition, the third injection is given 6 months after the first one, not the second (option 3). Cognitive Level: Applying. Client Need: Physiological Integrity/Pharmacological Therapies. Nursing Process: Implementation.
3. Answer: 3. Core Concept: 26.3. Rationale: Patients allergic to yeast or yeast products should not receive the hepatitis B vaccines unless approved by their healthcare provider. Smoking cigarettes (option 1) or drinking alcohol (option 4) will not prevent a patient from receiving the vaccine. A fear of needles and injections may inhibit a person from receiving the vaccine but it is not a reason that they should not be able to receive it (option 2). Cognitive Level: Understanding. Client Need: Physiological Integrity/Pharmacological Therapies. Nursing Process: Data Collection.
4. Answers: 1, 3, and 4. Core Concept: 26.3. Rationale: Hepatitis B vaccines may cause pain or inflammation at the injection site, fatigue, and fever. It is not known to cause nausea (option 2). Cognitive Level: Applying. Client Need: Physiological Integrity/Pharmacological Therapies. Nursing Process: Implementation.

Chapter 27

Review Answers

1. Answer: 4. Core Concept: 27.4. Rationale: More teaching is needed when the patient states, "I will take my medication until I feel better." All antibiotics should be taken as prescribed, even if the patient is feeling better, to prevent development of resistant bacteria. Patient understanding is demonstrated through the statements made about taking the medication until it is gone (option 1), calling the doctor if a rash or fever develops (option 2), and not taking the amoxicillin with orange juice (option 3). Cognitive Level: Applying. Client Need: Physiological Integrity/Pharmacological Therapies. Nursing Process: Evaluation.
2. Answer: 2. Core Concept: 27.7. Rationale: Although cephalosporins, such as cefazolin, offer a reasonable alternative for most patients unable to take penicillins, some patients who are allergic to penicillin will also be allergic to cephalosporins. In this case, cephalosporins are contraindicated if the patient has previously experienced a *severe* allergic reaction to penicillin. There is no known relationship between cefazolin (Ancef) and yeast (option 1), sulfonamides (option 3), or macrolides (option 4). Cognitive Level: Applying. Client Need: Physiological Integrity/Pharmacological Therapies. Nursing Process: Data Collection.
3. Answer: 3. Core Concept: 27.8. Rationale: The nurse should include that tetracyclines should be taken 1 to 2 hours before or after eating or drinking dairy or calcium products. Tetracyclines bind ions such as calcium and iron, thereby decreasing the drug's absorption by as much as 50%. Tetracyclines are not taken with food (option 1). Pregnant patients and those who are breastfeeding should not take tetracyclines because they are pregnancy category D medications (option 2). Tetracyclines cause few adverse

effects; gastric upset and photosensitivity are most common (option 4). Cognitive Level: Understanding. Client Need: Physiological Integrity/Pharmacological Therapies. Nursing Process: Planning.

4. Answer: 1. Core Concept: 27.10. Rationale: The patient taking aminoglycosides should be monitored for nephrotoxicity. Aminoglycosides are not known to cause hepatic failure (option 2), superinfections (option 3), or hypertension and rash (option 4). Cognitive Level: Applying. Client Need: Physiological Integrity/Pharmacological Therapies. Nursing Process: Evaluation.
5. Answer: 2. Core Concept: 27.11. Rationale: If ciprofloxin, a fluoroquinolone, is taken with antacids, absorption is decreased. As previously stated, taking ciprofloxin with antacids does affect absorption (option 3) but does not increase (option 1) or delay (option 4) absorption. Cognitive Level: Applying. Client Need: Physiological Integrity/Pharmacological Therapies. Nursing Process: Implementation.
6. Answer: 1. Core Concept: 27.13. Rationale: The patient taking vancomycin should be told that this medication can cause flushing. Other adverse effects are frequent (option 2) and include hypotension, not hypertension (option 4), and rash on upper body called red man syndrome (option 3). Cognitive Level: Understanding. Client Need: Physiological Integrity/Pharmacological Therapies. Nursing Process: Planning.
7. Answer: 4. Core Concept: 27.14. Rationale: Although rare, hepatotoxicity (liver toxicity) is a serious and sometimes fatal adverse effect of INH; thus, the patient should be monitored carefully for jaundice, fatigue, elevated hepatic enzymes, or loss of appetite. Liver enzyme tests are usually performed monthly during therapy. INH is not known to be associated with the laboratory testing of PT/PTT (option 1) or BUN (option 3). CBC (option 2) is a standard laboratory test done with most conditions, not specific to those taking INH. Cognitive Level: Understanding. Client Need: Physiological Integrity/Pharmacological Therapies. Nursing Process: Evaluation.
8. Answers: 1, 2, 3, and 4. Core Concept: 27.6. Rationale: Common adverse effects of penicillin G include diarrhea, nausea, vomiting, pain at the injection site, and rashes. Penicillin G is not known to cause constipation (option 5). Cognitive Level: Applying. Client Need: Physiological Integrity/Pharmacological Therapies. Nursing Process: Implementation.
9. Answer: 4. Core Concept: 27.9. Rationale: Lovastatin should not be taken with erythromycin because it may increase the risk of muscle toxicity. Erythromycin is not known to interact with lisinopril (option 1), ibuprofen (option 2), or Lasix (option 3). Cognitive Level: Applying. Client Need: Physiological Integrity/Pharmacological Therapies. Nursing Process: Data Collection.
10. Answer: 4. Core Concept: N/A. Rationale: Order 500 mg ÷ 250 mg/tablet = 2 tablets × 4 times a day = 8 tablets a day (24 hours). Options 1–3 are a result of miscalculations and are therefore incorrect. Cognitive Level: Applying. Client Need: Physiological Integrity/Pharmacological Therapies. Nursing Process: Implementation.

Case Study Answers

1. Answer: 1. Core Concept: 27.10. Rationale: Because gentamicin may cause nephrotoxicity, Ms. Jackson's intake and output should be monitored. Monitoring liver enzymes (option 2), visual acuity (option 3), and fasting blood glucose levels (option 4) are not usually associated with gentamicin. Cognitive Level: Applying. Client Need: Physiological Integrity/Pharmacological Therapies. Nursing Process: Evaluation.
2. Answer: 2. Core Concept: 27.10. Rationale: Ms. Jackson should be taught that gentamicin may cause ototoxicity with symptoms that include persistent headaches, dizziness, and ringing in the ears. Gentamicin is not known to cause anemia (option 1), nausea and vomiting (option 3), or liver failure (option 4). Cognitive Level: Applying. Client Need: Physiological Integrity/Pharmacological Therapies. Nursing Process: Implementation.

3. Answer: 3. Core Concept: 27.12. Rationale: The nurse anticipates that the new medication for Ms. Jackson's kidney infection would be trimethoprim–sulfamethoxazole (Septra). The combination of sulfamethoxazole (SMZ), a sulfonamide, with the anti-infective trimethoprim (TMP) is most frequently used in the pharmacotherapy of UTIs. Sulfacetamide (option 1) is used for treatment of acne and seborrheic dermatitis, silver sulfadiazine (option 2) is used for burns, and vancomycin (option 4) is an antibiotic usually reserved for severe infections from gram-positive organisms such as MRSA. Cognitive Level: Understanding. Client Need: Physiological Integrity/Pharmacological Therapies. Nursing Process: Planning.
4. Answers: 1 and 3. Core Concept: 27.12. Rationale: The adverse effects of sulfonamides are increased sensitivity of skin to sunlight and nausea and vomiting. Liver failure (option 2) and hypotension (option 4) are not usually associated with sulfonamides. Cognitive Level: Applying. Client Need: Physiological Integrity/Pharmacological Therapies. Nursing Process: Implementation.

Chapter 28

Review Answers

1. Answer: 3. Core Concept: 28.2. Rationale: The patient taking amphotericin B should be monitored for nephrotoxicity, a common adverse effect of the medication. Kidney function tests are usually performed. Amphotericin B is not known to cause ototoxicity (option 1), hepatic toxicity (option 2), or anoxia (option 4). Cognitive Level: Understanding. Client Need: Physiological Integrity/Pharmacological Therapies. Nursing Process: Evaluation.
2. Answer: 4. Core Concept: 28.2. Rationale: The nurse would expect a patient with oral candidiasis to be prescribed nystatin (Mycostatin), an antifungal medication that can be used systemically or topically. Terbinafine (option 1) is used for skin and nail mycoses; clotrimazole (option 2) is used topically for vaginal and skin mycoses; and ketoconazole (option 3) is used for severe systemic mycoses. Cognitive Level: Understanding. Client Need: Physiological Integrity/Pharmacological Therapies. Nursing Process: Planning.
3. Answer: 3. Core Concept: 28.3. Rationale: Treatment of nail mycoses may require several months of therapy. Treatment of nail mycosis requires more than one tablet (option 1) or 3 days (option 2). The nurse should know enough about the medication regimen to be able to answer the patient's question (option 4). Cognitive Level: Applying. Client Need: Physiological Integrity/Pharmacological Therapies. Nursing Process: Implementation.
4. Answer: 3. Core Concept: 28.6. Rationale: Immunity from the flu vaccine begins about two weeks after vaccination. Immunity does not occur within a couple of days (option 1) or within a week of vaccination (option 2). However, it does not take as long as 3 to 4 weeks after vaccination to achieve immunity (option 4). Cognitive Level: Applying. Client Need: Physiological Integrity/Pharmacological Therapies. Nursing Process: Implementation.
5. Answers: 1 and 3. Core Concept: 28.6. Rationale: The use of acyclovir (Zovirax) can reduce the frequency, duration, and severity of herpes. Acyclovir cannot cure herpes (option 2) and is not used to treat viral influenza (option 4) or HIV (option 5). Cognitive Level: Applying. Client Need: Physiological Integrity/Pharmacological Therapies. Nursing Process: Implementation.
6. Answer: 4. Core Concept: 28.6. Rationale: The nurse would expect a neuroamidase inhibitor to be ordered. These drugs are used to treat active influenza virus infections. If given within 48 hours of the onset of symptoms, oseltamivir (Tamiflu) and zanamivir (Relenza) are reported to shorten the duration of symptoms. Protease inhibitors

(option 1), nonnucleoside (option 2), and nucleoside (option 3) reverse transcriptase inhibitors are antiretroviral medications used in the treatment of HIV. Cognitive Level: Understanding. Client Need: Physiological Integrity/Pharmacological Therapies. Nursing Process: Planning.

7. Answers: 2–4. Core Concept: 28.7. Rationale: The patient taking metronidazole (Flagyl) should be monitored for anorexia, headaches, a metallic taste, and dry mouth. Metronidazole is not known to cause constipation (option 1). Cognitive Level: Understanding. Client Need: Physiological Integrity/Pharmacological Therapies. Nursing Process: Evaluation.
8. Answer: 2. Core Concept: 28.3. Rationale: A patient taking topical antifungals should be taught that gloves should be worn when applying medication in order to prevent the spread of infection. Other antifungals can be taken as ordered by the healthcare provider (option 1). In some cases, antifungals can be applied to open skin areas (option 3), and unless the patient has other medical conditions, there is no need to take vital signs prior to the application of topical antifungals (option 4). Cognitive Level: Understanding. Client Need: Physiological Integrity/Pharmacological Therapies. Nursing Process: Planning.
9. Answers: 1, 3, and 4. Core Concept: 28.3. Rationale: Burning, itching, and irritation are all possible adverse effects of clotrimazole. An increase in discharge (option 2), or the development of ulcers (option 5), are not known to be associated with clotrimazole. Cognitive Level: Applying. Client Need: Physiological Integrity/Pharmacological Therapies. Nursing Process: Implementation.
10. Answer: 1. Core Concept: 28.7. Rationale: Caregivers must be taught that good hand hygiene practices are very important in preventing the spread of pinworms and roundworms. Worms can be deposited on the toys then ingested by children when they put their hands into their mouths (option 2). Wearing shoes while outside can help prevent the transmission of worms (option 3). Reinfection can occur if proper hygiene is not practiced (option 4). Cognitive Level: Applying. Client Need: Physiological Integrity/Pharmacological Therapies. Nursing Process: Implementation.

Case Study Answers

1. Answer: 4. Core Concept: 28.5. Rationale: Current medication regimens for HIV/AIDS help patients to live symptom free, for a longer period of time. At this time, no medication can cure someone with HIV (option 1), drugs have not been developed for multiple resistant HIV strains (option 2), and antiretroviral medications are not used for the treatment of the flu (option 3). Cognitive Level: Understanding. Client Need: Physiological Integrity/Pharmacological Therapies. Nursing Process: N/A.
2. Answer: 3. Core Concept: 28.5. Rationale: Antiretroviral medications act by blocking the replication process of the HIV. These medications do not strengthen the immune system (option 1), interfere with the ability of the virus to enter a cell (option 2), or bind to proteins found on the viral surface (option 4). Cognitive Level: Understanding. Client Need: Physiological Integrity/Pharmacological Therapies. Nursing Process: Implementation.
3. Answers: 1, 3, and 4. Core Concept: 28.5. Rationale: It is very important that patients with HIV understand that they will be taking antiretrovirals for the rest of their lives, and for the treatment to be fully effective, the medications must be taken according to the prescribed schedule. In addition, patients need to be instructed to notify their healthcare provider if adverse effects make taking the drugs difficult and to keep all laboratory appointments so that health status can be properly monitored. Patients should never just stop taking their medications because this may result in a rapid rebound of HIV replication (option 2). Cognitive Level: Understanding. Client Need: Physiological Integrity/Pharmacological Therapies. Nursing Process: Planning.

4. Answer: 4. Core Concept: 28.5. Rationale: Anemia in patients with HIV may be caused by drug toxicity. This severe adverse effect is associated with antiretroviral medications that cause a decrease in red blood cell production. Abuse does not usually cause anemia (option 1). Anemia is not considered a minor adverse effect of medications (option 2). Not taking the HIV medications does not cause anemia (option 3). Cognitive Level: Understanding. Client Need: Physiological Integrity/Pharmacological Therapies. Nursing Process: Evaluation.

Chapter 29

Review Answers

1. Answer: 3. Core Concept: 29.6 and Nursing Process Focus: Patients Receiving Antineoplastic Therapy. Rationale: Most antineoplastic drugs cause nausea and vomiting; therefore, antiemetic drugs should be given just prior to their administration to prevent these adverse effects. In addition, patients may be given an antiemetic to take after each round of chemotherapy in case they need it. Waiting to administer antiemetic drugs until after the patient vomits allows unwarranted suffering (option 1). Waiting until after the treatment regimen is complete will not prevent the onset of nausea and vomiting (option 2). The patient should not have to request the antiemetic drug (option 4). Cognitive Level: Applying. Client Need: Physiological Integrity/Pharmacological Therapies. Nursing Process: Implementation.
2. Answer: 2. Core Concept: 29.7. Rationale: Monitor any patient taking cisplatin, an alkylating drug, for bone marrow suppression—specifically looking for a decrease in RBCs, WBCs, and platelets. Cisplatin is not known to cause irreversible heart failure (option 1), cardiac toxicity (option 3), or peripheral neuropathy (option 4). Cognitive Level: Understanding. Client Need: Physiological Integrity/Pharmacological Therapies. Nursing Process: Planning.
3. Answers: 1, 4, and 5. Core Concept: 29.8. Rationale: Patients receiving methotrexate, an antimetabolite, should not use NSAIDs, including aspirin, because they interfere with the excretion of methotrexate, causing increased blood levels and toxicity. In addition, live oral vaccines should not be given during the use of methotrexate because it may decrease antibody response and increase adverse reactions to the vaccine. Methotrexate is not known to interact with iron supplements (option 2) or acetaminophen (option 3). Cognitive Level: Understanding. Client Need: Physiological Integrity/Pharmacological Therapies. Nursing Process: Data Collection.
4. Answer: 2. Core Concept: 29.9. Rationale: Severe local necrosis may occur if extravasation (leaking) occurs when administering doxorubicin (Adriamycin) intravenously. Leaking of this powerful drug out of the vessel and into the interstitial tissue causes pain. Extravasation of the medication or pain at the IV site does not indicate an allergic reaction (option 1), loss of neural reflexes (option 3), or the development of a blood clot (option 4). Cognitive Level: Understanding. Client Need: Physiological Integrity/Pharmacological Therapies. Nursing Process: Evaluation.
5. Answer: 2. Core Concept: N/A. Rationale: Order: 20 mg daily ÷ 10 mg/tablet available = 2 tablets daily. 2 tablets per day × 7 days (one week) = 14 tablets per week. Options 1, 3, and 4 are a result of miscalculations and are, therefore, incorrect. Cognitive Level: Applying. Client Need: Physiological Integrity/Pharmacological Therapies. Nursing Process: Implementation.
6. Answer: 4. Core Concept: 29.7. Rationale: Nausea, vomiting, and diarrhea are common adverse effects of most antineoplastic drugs, including cyclophosphamide (Cytoxan), a cytotoxic antibiotic drug. In most cases, alopecia caused by chemotherapy drugs is reversible (option 1). Since cyclophosphamide does not cause neurotoxicity or renal toxicity, it is not necessary to teach patients the signs and symptoms of these effects (options 2 and 3). Cognitive Level: Applying. Client Need: Physiological Integrity/Pharmacological Therapies. Nursing Process: Implementation.

7. Answers: 2 and 4. Core Concept: 29.8. Rationale: The patient receiving methotrexate should be monitored for adverse effects such as bruising (due to low platelet counts), diarrhea, and nausea. Methotrexate has not been known to cause cardiac dysthymias (option 1) or a decrease in urinary output (option 3). Cognitive Level: Applying. Client Need: Physiological Integrity/Pharmacological Therapies. Nursing Process: Evaluation.

8. Answer: 2. Core Concept: 29.12. Rationale: Rituximab (Rituxan), a type of monoclonal antibody, works by binding to surface proteins present on cancer cells and destroying (shattering) them. Alkylating drugs change the structure of the cancer cell's DNA, preventing them from replicating (option 1). Antimetabolites block a specific step in cancer cell metabolism (option 3). Cytotoxic antibiotics attach to the DNA of cancer cells, inhibiting their growth (option 4). Cognitive Level: Applying. Client Need: Physiological Integrity/Pharmacological Therapies. Nursing Process: Implementation.

9. Answer: 3. Core Concept 29.6 and Nursing Process Focus: Patients Receiving Antineoplastic Therapy. Rationale: Patients with decreased WBC counts, specifically neutrophils (neutropenia), have compromised immune systems and should not handle or eat raw food due to an increased risk of acquiring an infection from the surface of the foods. Patients should be taught to have others prepare and thoroughly cook raw foods to reduce bacteria levels. Alcohol-based mouthwashes should not be used (option 1). Increasing fluid intake is acceptable but it does not help prevent infection due to a weakened immune system (option 2). Megace is used to stimulate appetite (option 4). Cognitive Level: Applying. Client Need: Physiological Integrity/Pharmacological Therapies. Nursing Process: Implementation.

10. Answer: 2. Core Concept: 29.11. Rationale: The most serious problem associated with tamoxifen use is the increased risk of endometrial (uterine) cancer. Therefore, any patient taking this hormone agent should be closely monitored. Tamoxifen is not usually known to cause flu-like symptoms (option 1), alopecia (option 3), or thrombocytopenia (option 4). Cognitive Level: Understanding. Client Need: Physiological Integrity/Pharmacological Therapies. Nursing Process: Planning.

Case Study Answers

1. Answer: 3. Core Concept: 29.13. Rationale: Ms. Novak is taking filgrastim (Neupogen), an immune stimulant, to boost her immune system. Vincristine, a natural product antineoplastic that destroys cancer cells, adversely causes immunosuppression (option 1). Epoetin alfa is given to prevent anemia by stimulating RBCs (option 2). Tamoxifen is being given to inhibit tumor growth (option 4). Cognitive Level: Applying. Client Need: Physiological Integrity/Pharmacological Therapies. Nursing Process: Implementation.

2. Answer: 2. Core Concept: 29.13. Rationale: Epoetin is given to stimulate the production of RBCs, thus preventing anemia. Epoetin does not stimulate the WBCs needed to boost the immune system (option 1), reduce neurotoxicity (option 3), or kill cancer cells (option 4). Cognitive Level: Applying. Client Need: Physiological Integrity/Pharmacological Therapies. Nursing Process: Implementation.

3. Answer: 2. Core Concept: 29.10. Rationale: The nurse should monitor patients taking vincristine for signs of peripheral neuropathy. Symptoms include numbness and tingling in the limbs, muscular weakness, loss of neural reflexes, and pain. Vincristine is not usually known to cause issues related to blood glucose levels (option 1) or ototoxicity (option 3). Although CNS effects of vincristine may include seizures, depression, and hallucinations, it does not cause confusion (option 4). Cognitive Level: Applying. Client Need: Physiological Integrity/Pharmacological Therapies. Nursing Process: Evaluation.

4. Answer: 1. Core Concept: 29.13. Rationale: Usually, pain management proceeds up a ladder, starting with NSAIDs, to the weak opioid analgesics, and eventually to the strongest opioids. However, in cases like Ms. Novak's, drug combinations (an anti-inflammatory and opioid) may be used to achieve optimal pain control. NSAIDs (option 2) are not strong enough to reduce neuropathy pain caused by vincristine. A weak opioid (option 3) also may not be enough to manage her pain, and strong opioids produce undesirable effects (option 4). Cognitive Level: Understanding. Client Need: Physiological Integrity/Pharmacological Therapies. Nursing Process: Planning.

Chapter 30

Review Answers

1. Answer: 1. Core Concept: 30.9. Rationale: For an acute asthma attack, albuterol (Proventil HFA), a SABA drug, would be given. This class of drugs stimulates the sympathetic nervous system, relaxing the smooth muscle of the bronchial tubes and allowing more airflow and oxygen to the alveoli. Budesonide (option 2) and Fluticasone (option 3) are corticosteroids used to treat asthma and allergic rhinitis. Zafirlukast (option 4) is a leukotriene modifier used to treat allergic rhinitis and as a prophylactic drug for chronic asthma. Cognitive Level: Understanding. Client Need: Physiological Integrity/Pharmacological Therapies. Nursing Process: Data Collection.
2. Answer: 2. Core Concept: 30.9. Rationale: The patient taking salmeterol (Serevent), a LABA drug, must understand that this drug is used to prevent asthma attacks and must be taken every day to be effective. Salmeterol has not been known to cause nausea and vomiting (option 1). The patient should be taught that long-term use of salmeterol may cause tremors (option 3) and that caffeinated food and beverages should be avoided (option 4). The goal of therapy is the prevention of attacks, so ensuring that the patient follows the medication schedule is of the highest priority. Cognitive Level: Understanding. Client Need: Physiological Integrity/Pharmacological Therapies. Nursing Process: Planning.
3. Answers: 1, 2, 3 and 5. Core Concept: 30.4. Rationale: The nurse will monitor the patient taking Benadryl (an H_1-receptor blocker/antihistamine) for drowsiness, dry mouth, and tachycardia. This medication can also cause mild hypotension. Benadryl has not been known to cause nausea (option 4). Cognitive Level: Understanding. Client Need: Physiological Integrity/Pharmacological Therapies. Nursing Process: Evaluating.
4. Answer: 2. Core Concept: 30.11. Rationale: Montelukast (Singulair) is a leukotriene modifier, approved for the prophylaxis of chronic asthma. Taken orally it can take as long as a week to provide therapeutic benefit. Leukotrienes are ineffective at relieving acute bronchospasm (option 3). Their onset of action is not rapid (option 1) but it does not take as long as several weeks to provide therapeutic benefits (option 4). Cognitive Level: Applying. Client Need: Physiological Integrity/Pharmacological Therapies. Nursing Process: Implementation.
5. Answer: 2. Core Concept: 30.7. Rationale: The nurse informs the patient that *antitussives* suppress cough, while *mucolytics* loosen bronchial secretions. These terms are not interchangeable (option 3), nor do both types of drugs loosen and remove secretions (options 1 and 4). The drugs that stimulate the removal of secretions are known as *expectorants*. Cognitive Level: Applying. Client Need: Physiological Integrity/Pharmacological Therapies. Nursing Process: Implementation.
6. Answer: 2. Core Concept: 30.10. Rationale: Corticosteroids, such as budesonide, are the most effective drugs for the *prevention* of acute asthmatic episodes; so the nurse informs the patient that budesonide should be taken on a regular basis to work. The approved dose is one to two inhalations daily; four inhalations would cause an overdose of the

medication (option 1). Corticosteroids used for asthma are only available in inhalation form (option 3), so the patient cannot get the medication in a tablet form. It is not necessary to clear the nose prior to using the medication (option 4). Cognitive Level: Applying. Client Need: Physiological Integrity/Pharmacological Therapies. Nursing Process: Implementation.

7. Answer: 1. Core Concept: 30.7. Rationale: Benzonatate (Tessalon), an antitussive, has a local anesthetic-like effect on stretch receptors in the lung, which interrupts the cough message. Patients taking this drug must be instructed to swallow, not chew, the soft capsules, because chewing will cause numbness of the throat and tongue. The patient should not stop taking the medication (option 3), nor should the dosage be decreased (option 2). Once the patient stops chewing the medication, the numbness will go away (option 4). Cognitive Level: Applying. Client Need: Physiological Integrity/Pharmacological Therapies. Nursing Process: Implementation.
8. Answer: 3. Core Concept: N/A. Rationale: Ordered 4 mg ÷ 2 mg × 5 mL (available) = 10 mL. Options 1, 2, and 4 are a result of a miscalculation and are therefore incorrect. Cognitive Level: Applying. Client Need: Physiological Integrity/Pharmacological Therapies. Nursing Process: Implementation.
9. Answer: 2. Core Concept: 30.5. Rationale: Patients taking intranasal corticosteroids may experience an intense burning sensation. Intranasal corticosteroids are not known to cause rebound congestion (option 1), drowsiness (option 3), or nervousness (option 4). Cognitive Level: Applying. Client Need: Physiological Integrity/Pharmacological Therapies. Nursing Process: Implementation.
10. Answer: 1. Core Concept: 30.6. Rationale: Afrin, a sympathomimetic decongestant, may cause rebound congestion and should not be used for longer than 3 to 5 days. Afrin is administered in an intranasal form and is not known to affect blood pressure (option 2) or cause anxiety (option 3). No clinically significant drug interactions have been found (option 4). Cognitive Level: Understanding. Client Need: Physiological Integrity/Pharmacological Therapies. Nursing Process: Planning.

Case Study Answers

1. Answer: 4. Core Concept: 30.9. Rationale: Ipratropium, an anticholinergic drug, will help resolve his dyspnea by relaxing the smooth muscle of the bronchi, rapidly relieving bronchospasms to allow more air flow and available oxygen. Hydrocodone (option 1), an opioid, is given for its antitussive properties. Acetaminophen is being given for fever and discomfort (option 2). Guaifenesin is an expectorant (option 3). Cognitive Level: Applying. Client Need: Physiological Integrity/Pharmacological Therapies. Nursing Process: Implementation.
2. Answer: 3. Core Concept: 30.7. Rationale: Guaifenesin, an expectorant, is given to reduce the thickness or viscosity of bronchial secretions, thus aiding in its removal from the respiratory tract. Hydrocodone (option 1), an opioid, is given for its antitussive properties. Acetaminophen is being given for fever and discomfort (option 2). Ipratropium is being given for its bronchodilation effects (option 4). Cognitive Level: Applying. Client Need: Physiological Integrity/Pharmacological Therapies. Nursing Process: Implementation.
3. Answer: 1. Core Concept: 30.7. Rationale: Hydrocodone, an opioid-antitussive, acts by raising the cough threshold in the cough center, thereby decreasing both the frequency and intensity of coughs. Even though doses are low, patients not used to taking this type of drug may experience the effect of most opioids, drowsiness. Acetaminophen (option 2), guaifenesin (option 3), and ipratropium (option 4) are not known to cause drowsiness. Cognitive Level: Understanding. Client Need: Physiological Integrity/Pharmacological Therapies. Nursing Process: Evaluation.

4. Answer: 3. Core Concept: 30.12. Rationale: For continued treatment, the nurse expects Mr. Thomas to receive a prescription for budesonide, an inhaled corticosteroid used to reduce inflammation within the airways. Salmeterol (option 1), a LABA drug, is used to prevent asthma attacks. Tiotropium (option 2), an anticholinergic bronchodilator, is already being given in the drug ipratropium. Olopatadine (option 4) is an antihistamine used for minor allergies. Cognitive Level: Understanding. Client Need: Physiological Integrity/Pharmacological Therapies. Nursing Process: Planning.

Chapter 31

Review Answers

1. Answer: 3. Core Concept: 31.2. Rationale: The primary cause of peptic ulcers is the bacteria *H. pylori.* Although lifestyle factors such as stress (option 1) and smoking (option 2) are associated with ulcers, they do not cause them. Family history (option 4) has not been shown to be a determining factor in the formation of ulcers. Cognitive Level: Applying. Client Need: Physiological Integrity/Pharmacological Therapies. Nursing Process: Implementation.
2. Answers: 1, 4 and 5. Core Concept: 31.5. Rationale: The patient should know that drug therapy using ranitidine (Zantac) will extend over a period of several weeks to several months. Taking antacids at the same time as H_2-receptor antagonists will lessen absorption: Therefore, antacids should not be given within 1 hour of taking H_2-receptor antagonists. Although rare, ranitidine can cause a decrease in RBC, WBCs, and platelets, so a CBC should be done periodically. Although some H_2-receptor blockers, such as cimetidine (Tagamet), may cause CNS depression (option 2), ranitidine does not cross the blood–brain barrier. Drug therapy will last longer than a few days (option 3). Cognitive Level: Understanding. Client Need: Physiological Integrity/Pharmacological Therapies. Nursing Process: Planning.
3. Answer: 1. Core Concept: N/A. Rationale: 10 mL/dose of Lomotil (order) ÷ 5 mL × 2.5 mg (available) = 5 mg/dose × 4 times a day = 20 mg/day. Options 2–4 are a result of a miscalculation and are incorrect. Cognitive Level: Applying. Client Need: Physiological Integrity/Pharmacological Therapies. Nursing Process: Implementation.
4. Answer: 2. Core Concept: 31.4. Rationale: The teaching plan should include that omeprazole (Prilosec) is not taken for a prolonged period of time because it can interfere with calcium absorption and result in fractures due to weakened bones. It is not safe for long-term use (option 1). Therapeutic levels can take 2 hours (option 3). Omeprazole can be taken with antacids and is available in oral form combined with antacid sodium bicarbonate; however, it does not have to be taken with an antacid to be effective (option 4). Cognitive Level: Understanding. Client Need: Physiological Integrity/Pharmacological Therapies. Nursing Process: Planning.
5. Answer: 1. Core Concept: 31.6. Rationale: For the patient taking magnesium hydroxide (Mylanta), the nurse should monitor for diarrhea, a possible adverse effect. Magnesium hydroxide is not known to cause peripheral disease (option 2), neuropathy (option 3), or respiratory disorders (option 4). Cognitive Level: Applying. Client Need: Physiological Integrity/Pharmacological Therapies. Nursing Process: Evaluating.
6. Answer: 2. Core Concept: 31.9. Rationale: Patients should be advised not to overuse laxatives because the smooth muscle in the colon can lose its tone and cause chronic constipation. Patients should not use laxatives daily because it can lead to overuse (option 1). A decrease of either fluids (option 3) or food (option 4) intake is not advised because some laxatives may cause a depletion of fluids and electrolytes. Cognitive Level: Applying. Client Need: Physiological Integrity/Pharmacological Therapies. Nursing Process: Implementation.
7. Answer: 2. Core Concept: 31.11. Rationale: In order to prevent chemotherapy-induced nausea and vomiting, ondansetron is started at least 30 minutes prior to chemotherapy and continued for several days after. Because chemotherapy-induced nausea and

vomiting are more difficult to control or stop once they have started, medication administration should not be dependent on the patient complaining of nausea (option 3) or actually vomiting (option 4). In addition, patients may complain of nausea more frequently than is possible to give the medication (option 1). Cognitive Level: Applying. Client Need: Physiological Integrity/Pharmacological Therapies. Nursing Process: Implementation.

8. Answer: 1. Core Concept: 31.3. Rationale: It is not advisable for patients with PUD to take aspirin and other NSAIDs because they can cause irritation to the gastric mucosa and contribute to the formation of ulcers. It is not contraindicated to eat raw vegetables (option 2) or take antiemetics (option 4) while taking medications for PUD. In addition, patients being treated for PUD should avoid the use of alcohol (option 3). Cognitive Level: Applying. Client Need: Physiological Integrity/Pharmacological Therapies. Nursing Process: Evaluating.
9. Answers: 1. Core Concept: 31.8. Rationale: Patients taking sucralfate (Carafate), a medication used for the treatment of PUD, should be monitored for the adverse effect of constipation. Sucralfate is not known to cause dizziness (option 2), muscle pain (option 3), or diarrhea (option 4). Cognitive Level: Understanding. Client Need: Physiological Integrity/Pharmacological Therapies. Nursing Process: Evaluating.
10. Answer: 1. Core Concept: 31.12. Rationale: Taking pancrelipase (Cotazym) with meals ensures that the enzymes contained within pancrelipase are available when food reaches the duodenum. Pancrelipase should not be taken on an empty stomach (option 2). Pancrelipase contains enzymes used to digest fats, carbohydrates, and proteins; therefore, taking this medication only with carbohydrates minimizes its effectiveness and availability when other types of foods are eaten (option 3). A decrease (not increase) in dosage may be needed if the patient exhibits symptoms of overuse such as nausea, vomiting, or diarrhea (option 4). Cognitive Level: Analyzing. Client Need: Physiological Integrity/Pharmacological Therapies. Nursing Process: Evaluating.

Case Study Answers

1. Answer: 1. Core Concept: 31.4. Rationale: PPIs, such as omeprazole, act by blocking the enzyme responsible for secreting hydrochloric acid in the stomach. Antacids are used to neutralize stomach acid (option 2). Clarithromycin and amoxicillin are antibiotics used to eliminate *H. pylori* (options 3 and 4). Cognitive Level: Applying. Client Need: Physiological Integrity/Pharmacological Therapies. Nursing Process: Implementation.
2. Answers: 2 and 3. Core Concept: 31.7. Rationale: Clarithromycin and amoxicillin are antibiotics commonly used to help eliminate *H. pylori*. Omeprazole (Prilosec) blocks the secretion of stomach acid (option 1), and antacids neutralize stomach acid (option 4). Cognitive Level: Applying. Client Need: Physiological Integrity/Pharmacological Therapies. Nursing Process: Implementation.
3. Answers: 1 and 2. Core Concept: 31.7. Rationale: Using two or more antibiotics increases the effectiveness of therapy and lowers the potential for bacterial resistance. Even though studies have shown that a combination of PPIs and two antibiotics has been successful in eradicating *H. pylori*, total destruction of the bacteria cannot be *guaranteed* because some strains are resistant to specific antibiotics (option 3). The current use of antibiotics does not affect the cost of future drug therapy (option 4). Cognitive Level: Applying. Client Need: Physiological Integrity/Pharmacological Therapies. Nursing Process: Implementation.
4. Answer: 1. Core Concept: 31.9. Rationale: Mr. Han can take methylcellulose (Citrucel), a bulk-forming laxative, to help relieve constipation. Famotidine (option 2), an H2 receptor blocker, is used to treat PUD and GERD. Omeprazole (option 3) is a PPI used for PUD that blocks the secretion of acid. Bismuth salts are an antidiarrheal medication (option 4). Cognitive Level: Analyzing. Client Need: Physiological Integrity/Pharmacological Therapies. Nursing Process: Planning.

Chapter 32

Review Answers

1. Answer: 3. Core Concept: 32.4. Rationale: Vitamin B_{12} is given to patients who have pernicious anemia. Patients with this condition cannot absorb enough vitamin B_{12} from food because they lack the intrinsic factor, a protein made in the stomach. Vitamin B_{12} is usually administered via injections. Vitamin B_{12} is not specifically indicated for those with liver disease (option 1), chronic inflammatory disease (option 2), or inadequate exposure to sunlight (option 4). Cognitive Level: Understanding. Client Need: Physiological Integrity/Pharmacological Therapies. Nursing Process: Planning.
2. Answer: 4. Core Concept: 32.4. Rationale: If a patient has an *overdose* of warfarin (a drug that slows the clotting process given to prevent the formation of clots), the nurse would administer the antidote, vitamin K, which is normally used by the body to promote blood clotting. Vitamins A (option 1), D (option 2), and E (option 3) do not affect warfarin. Cognitive Level: Applying. Client Need: Physiological Integrity/Pharmacological Therapies. Nursing Process: Implementation.
3. Answer: 1. Core Concept: 32.5. Rationale: Patients taking ferrous sulfate need to know not to take it with antacids. Antacids decrease the absorption of iron. Ferrous sulfate is not known to cause severe diarrhea (option 2) or affect blood pressure (option 4). Although taking iron with meals will lessen GI upset, food can decrease the absorption of iron by as much as 70% (option 3). It is recommended that iron preparations be administered 1 hour before or 2 hours after a meal. Cognitive Level: Applying. Client Need: Physiological Integrity/Pharmacological Therapies. Nursing Process: Implementation.
4. Answer: 2. Core Concept: 32.4. Rationale: The nurse will monitor the patient with a history of alcohol abuse for thiamine deficiency. Alcohol inhibits the absorption of thiamine and folic acid. It is the most common cause of thiamine deficiency in the United States. Alcohol is not known to directly affect biotin (option 1), niacin (option 3), or riboflavin (option 4). Cognitive Level: Understanding. Client Need: Physiological Integrity/Pharmacological Therapies. Nursing Process: Evaluation.
5. Answer: 3. Core Concept: 32.5. Rationale: Loop or thiazide diuretics can cause significant potassium loss through urination; therefore, the nurse should monitor the patient for symptom of hypokalemia. These diuretics are not known to directly impact selenium (option 1), calcium (option 2), or magnesium (option 4). Cognitive Level: Applying. Client Need: Physiological Integrity/Pharmacological Therapies. Nursing Process: Evaluation.
6. Answer: 4. Core Concept: 32.5 and Nursing Process Focus: Patients Receiving Iron Supplements. Rationale: Because liquid iron supplements are known to stain teeth, the nurse would teach patients to rinse their mouth with water after swallowing the medication. Swishing the iron will stain the teeth (option 1). Absorption of iron decreases when taken with food (option 2). Iron is given as a supplement for specific conditions, such as iron-deficiency anemia, so avoidance of foods high in iron content is not necessary (option 3). Cognitive Level: Applying. Client Need: Physiological Integrity/Pharmacological Therapies. Nursing Process: Implementation.
7. Answer: 2. Core Concept: 32.5. Rationale: Weakness, hypertension, and dysrhythmias are all symptoms of a lack of magnesium. In addition to recognizing the symptoms of hypomagnesemia, the nurse should monitor the laboratory reports for electrolyte levels. Altered calcium levels can cause muscle weakness and cardiac dysrhythmias but do not directly cause hypertension (option 1). Altered aluminum (option 3) or chromium (option 4) levels do not cause weakness, hypertension, or dysrhythmias. Cognitive Level: Understanding. Client Need: Physiological Integrity/Pharmacological Therapies. Nursing Process: Planning.

8. Answers: 1, 2 and 5. Core Concept: 32.7. Rationale: Patients taking topiramate (Qysmia), an appetite suppressant, must be monitored for possible adverse effects such as constipation, dizziness, and dry mouth. Qysmia is not known to cause hypertension (option 3) or diarrhea (option 4). Cognitive Level: Understanding. Client Need: Physiological Integrity/Pharmacological Therapies. Nursing Process: Evaluation.
9. Answer: 3. Core Concept: 32.6. Rationale: Because the patient's GI tract is not functioning (swallowing and movement within the intestinal tract), and the metabolic needs of the patient cannot be met through enteral nutrition, the patient will need to have TPN. TPN is nutrition provided IV through a peripheral vein. If a patient's GI tract is nonfunctioning, the patient cannot receive adequate nutrition via the oral route (option 1), through any of the enteral routes (option 2), or directly into the GI tract (option 4). Cognitive Level: Understanding. Client Need: Physiological Integrity/Pharmacological Therapies. Nursing Process: Planning.
10. Answer: 3. Core Concept: N/A. Rationale: 250 mL to be infused over 4 hours (the order). 250 mL ÷ 4 hours = 62.5 mL/hour. Options 1, 2, and 4 are a result of miscalculations and are therefore incorrect. Cognitive Level: Applying. Client Need: Physiological Integrity/Pharmacological Therapies. Nursing Process: Implementation.

Case Study Answers

1. Answer: 2. Core Concept: 32.2. Rationale: The nurse explains that B complex vitamins are water soluble because of their ability to dissolve easily in water. Vitamins A (option 1), D (option 3), and E (option 4) are all fat-soluble vitamins. Cognitive Level: Understanding. Client Need: Physiological Integrity/Pharmacological Therapies. Nursing Process: Evaluation.
2. Answer: 4. Core Concept: 32.3. Rationale: The RDA establishes the *minimum* amount of nutrient needed to prevent a deficiency in healthy adults. The RDA is not the amount of nutrient required by *all* people (option 1), the *maximum* amount of nutrient needed to prevent deficiency (option 2), or the amount of nutrient needed by an *average* person (option 3). Cognitive Level: Understanding. Client Need: Physiological Integrity/Pharmacological Therapies. Nursing Process: Evaluation.
3. Answers: 1, 2, 3, and 4. Core Concepts: 32.4 and 32.6. Rationale: The nurse should collect information about Ms. Chin's diet, the presence of any chronic diseases, and her use of alcohol. All three of these factors can influence not only if she should take a multivitamin supplement but what type she should take. Although weight may not be an indicator of an inadequate diet, it should be taken to help determine nutritional and caloric recommendations. Cognitive Level: Applying. Client Need: Physiological Integrity/Pharmacological Therapies. Nursing Process: Data Collection.
4. Answer: 3. Core Concept: 32.3. Rationale: The nurse should inform Ms. Chin not to take more than the recommended dose until she speaks to the healthcare provider about the problems associated with her diet. Based on Ms. Chin's problems, diet analysis, a physical exam, and laboratory results, only the healthcare provider should speak with her regarding any changes to the supplements outside the recommended dosages (options 1, 2, and 4). Cognitive Level: Applying. Client Need: Physiological Integrity/Pharmacological Therapies. Nursing Process: Implementation.

Chapter 33

Review Answers

1. Answer: 1. Core Concept: 33.8. Rationale: High doses of corticosteroids, taken over a long period of time, can cause symptoms like those seen in Cushing disease. These symptoms can include changes in behavior and vision, osteoporosis, HTN, delayed

wound healing, and peptic ulcers. Graves disease (option 2) is a form of hyperthyroidism. Patients with this disorder may exhibit tachycardia, anxiety, insomnia, weight loss, and heat intolerance. Diabetes insipidus (option 3) is caused by a deficiency of ADH, which results in large volumes of very dilute urine and increased thirst. Diabetes mellitus (option 4) is a metabolic disorder that causes a state of hyperglycemia (increased glucose in the blood) as the result of a deficiency in insulin or a decrease in the sensitivity of insulin receptors on target cells. Cognitive Level: Applying. Client Need: Physiological Integrity/Pharmacological Therapies. Nursing Process: Implementation.

2. Answer: 4. Core Concept: 33.8. Rationale: Patients taking hydrocortisone (Cortef) and fludrocortisones (Florinef) need to understand that it is a lifelong therapy, taken every day, and that precautions should be taken to ensure that the patient has enough medication when going away in case there is a delay returning home. The patient does not need to take his or her blood pressure more than two to three times a week (option 1), avoid indoor crowds (option 2), or have his or her vision checked before leaving on a trip (option 3). Cognitive Level: Understanding. Client Need: Physiological Integrity/Pharmacological Therapies. Nursing Process: Planning.
3. Answer: 3. Core Concept: 33.6. Rationale: The nurse will inform the patient that PTU may decrease white blood cell production, therefore increasing the risk of infection. The patient should report signs of infection such as sore throat, chills, and low-grade fever. PTU has not been known to cause tinnitus, altered taste, thickened saliva (option 1); insomnia, nightmares, night sweats (option 2); or dry eyes, decreased blinking, or reddened conjunctiva (option 4). Cognitive Level: Understanding. Client Need: Physiological Integrity/Pharmacological Therapies. Nursing Process: Planning.
4. Answer: 2. Core Concept: N/A. Rationale: Ordered 5 units ÷ 20 units × 1 mL (available) = 0.25 mL. Options 1, 3, and 4 are a result of miscalculations and are therefore incorrect. Cognitive Level: Applying. Client Need: Physiological Integrity/Pharmacological Therapies. Nursing Process: Implementation.
5. Answer: 2. Core Concept: 33.8. Rationale: It is extremely important that the patient taking methylprednisolone (Medrol) understand that he or she must not stop taking this medication abruptly. The adrenal glands will not be able to secrete sufficient corticosteroids, and symptoms of adrenocortical insufficiency will appear. Weight gain (option 1), sleeplessness (option 3), and restlessness (option 4) are usually not associated with methylprednisolone (Medrol). Cognitive Level: Analyzing. Client Need: Physiological Integrity/Pharmacological Therapies. Nursing Process: Evaluation.
6. Answers: 1 and 2. Core Concept: 33.8. Rationale: An adverse effect of dexamethasone is osteoporosis. In order to reduce this risk, the nurse informs the patient to perform weight-bearing exercises three to four times a week and to increase dietary intake of calcium and vitamin D. Remaining sedentary (option 3) and increasing fluid intake, for example, with carbonated sodas (option 4), will actually increase the risk of osteoporosis. Participating in highly strenuous activities may cause injury and is not necessary for bone health. Cognitive Level: Applying. Client Need: Physiological Integrity/Pharmacological Therapies. Nursing Process: Implementation.
7. Answer: 3. Core Concept: 33.4. Rationale: Desmopressin (DDAVP) is an ADH replacement that causes the body to retain fluid by acting on the kidneys. Adverse effects include edema and weight gain; therefore, patients are advised to take and record their weight every day. Patients are not encouraged to drink plenty of fluids (option 1). It is not necessary that patients taking DDAVP avoid close contact with children or pregnant women (option 2) or wear a mask (option 4). Cognitive Level: Understanding. Client Need: Physiological Integrity/Pharmacological Therapies. Nursing Process: Planning.
8. Answer: 4. Core Concept: 33.4. Rationale: DI is caused by a deficiency in ADH, which causes an increase in urinary output. DDAVP is given to replace the ADH; therefore, the patient taking this medication should see a decrease in urinary output. An increase

in urinary output would be evidence that the medication was not effective (option 1). DDAVP should not cause blood pressure to fall below the normal range, nor should it affect blood sugar (options 2 and 3). Cognitive Level: Understanding. Client Need: Physiological Integrity/Pharmacological Therapies. Nursing Process: Evaluation.

9. Answer: 1. Core Concept: 33.4. Rationale: The nurse should plan to inform the parents that somatropin (Humatrope) will need to be given by subcutaneous injection several times a week during periods of active growth and may continue until adulthood. It is not given to prevent mental deficiencies (option 2). The medication is usually effective during a patient's normal growth period; 6 to 8 inches in late adolescence is usually seen (option 3). Daily laboratory monitoring is not required during the first weeks of therapy (option 4). Cognitive Level: Understanding. Client Need: Physiological Integrity/Pharmacological Therapies. Nursing Process: Planning.
10. Answers: 2, 3, and 5. Core Concept: 33.8. Rationale: Methylprednisolone can cause edema, visual changes, and mood changes. Methylprednisolone is not known to cause tinnitus (option 1) or lower abdominal pain (option 4). Cognitive Level: Applying. Client Need: Physiological Integrity/Pharmacological Therapies. Nursing Process: Planning.

Case Study Answers

1. Answers: 3 and 4. Core Concept: 33.6. Rationale: Adverse effects of levothyroxine include tachycardia and insomnia. This medication may also cause anxiety, weight loss, and heat intolerance. Levothyroxine is not known to cause constipation (option 1) or weight gain (option 2). Cognitive Level: Applying. Client Need: Physiological Integrity/Pharmacological Therapies. Nursing Process: Implementation.
2. Answer: 3. Core Concept: 33.6. Rationale: To closely reflect the body's own hormone levels, Mrs. Brookfield should take levothyroxine in the morning, at the same time every day. Taking levothyroxine with food or meals containing high fiber may affect the absorption of the drug (option 1). Many fruits and vegetables inhibit thyroid secretion, reducing the effectiveness of levothyroxine (option 2). If diarrhea occurs, the patient should notify the healthcare provider to determine the need to take or skip the dose (option 4). Cognitive Level: Applying. Client Need: Physiological Integrity/Pharmacological Therapies. Nursing Process: Implementation.
3. Answer: 3. Core Concept: 33.6. Rationale: A sign of hypothyroidism is a low pulse rate (Mrs. Brookfield's pulse was 58). An increase in the patient's pulse would indicate medication effectiveness. Sleeping more hours a day (option 1), increasing weight (option 2), and complaints of being tired (option 4) are all signs of continuing hypothyroidism, thus indicating that the medication dose is ineffective and may need to be increased. Cognitive Level: Understanding. Client Need: Physiological Integrity/Pharmacological Therapies. Nursing Process: Evaluation.
4. Answer: 4. Core Concept: 33.6. Rationale: Nervousness, palpitations, and tremors are all signs of hyperthyroidism, an adverse effect of levothyroxine. These signs indicate that the dosage of the drug needs to be decreased. Nervousness, palpitations, and tremors are not symptoms of hypothyroidism (option 1), do not indicate that the thyroid is functioning normally (option 2), and do not indicate that diabetes has developed (option 3). Cognitive Level: Understanding. Client Need: Physiological Integrity/Pharmacological Therapies. Nursing Process: Evaluation.

Chapter 34

Review Answers

1. Answers: 1, 2, 3, and 5. Core Concept: 34.2. Rationale: Polyuria (excessive urination), polyphagia (increased hunger), and polydipsia (increased thirst) are all primary symptoms of type 1 diabetes mellitus, and can sometimes be seen in type 2 diabetes. Another

sign of type 1 DM is weight loss (option 5). This occurs when glucose is unable to enter cells so lipids are used as the primary energy source. Weight gain (option 4) is not a symptom of type 1 DM. Cognitive Level: Applying. Client Need: Physiological Integrity/Pharmacological Therapies. Nursing Process: Data Collection.

2. Answer: 3. Core Concept: 34.3. Rationale: The subcutaneous route is the most common route of administration for insulin, although insulin can be administered through the IV route in emergencies. Insulin is not administered via the oral (option 1), intradermal (option 2), or intramuscular (option 4) routes. Level: Knowing. Client Need: Physiological Integrity/Pharmacological Therapies. Nursing Process: Planning.
3. Answer: 2. Core Concept: 34.5. Rationale: Incretin enhancers, an oral hypoglycemic drug class, stimulate the release of insulin from the pancreas and suppress the production of glucagon. Incretin enhancers do not decrease the uptake of glucose by the cells (option 1) or increase (option 3) or decrease (option 4) insulin production. Cognitive Level: Applying. Client Need: Physiological Integrity/Pharmacological Therapies. Nursing Process: Implementation.
4. Answer: 4. Core Concept: 34.3. Rationale: It is important that the nurse evaluate the patient's awareness of when hypoglycemia, an adverse effect of insulin administration, may occur. Normally, blood glucose levels are at their lowest when insulin levels are at their peak. Exercise can also decrease blood glucose. To decrease the risk of a hypoglycemic reaction, the patient should not plan to exercise during peak times (option 3). The patient does not need to give insulin around the previous insulin's peak time (options 1 and 2). Cognitive Level: Applying. Client Need: Physiological Integrity/Pharmacological Therapies. Nursing Process: Evaluation.
5. Answer: 3. Core Concept: 34.3. Rationale: The patient statement "I must draw the NPH insulin first if I am mixing it with regular insulin" shows a lack of understanding. When mixing two types of insulin, the rapid or short-acting insulin is always drawn into the syringe first; then the intermediate insulin is drawn into the syringe. This is done to prevent contamination of the faster acting insulin vials. Options 1, 2, and 4 are correct statements: If experiencing a hypoglycemic reaction, the patient should drink something with sugar in it (option 1). Illness puts stress on the body and causes an increase in glucose, so an increase in insulin may be necessary (option 2). If blood glucose levels remain above 140 mg/dL, the patient should notify the healthcare provider in case an adjustment to insulin amounts is needed (option 4). Cognitive Level: Applying. Client Need: Physiological Integrity/Pharmacological Therapies. Nursing Process: Evaluation.
6. Answer: 1. Core Concept: N/A. Rationale: The healthcare provider orders 500 mg ÷ 1,000 mg × 1 tablet = ½ tablet per dose × two times a day = 1 tablet for the day. The tablet is scored, which means it can be broken in half, one half to be given in the morning and the other half given in the evening. Options 2–4 are a result of miscalculation and are therefore incorrect. Cognitive Level: Applying. Client Need: Physiological Integrity/Pharmacological Therapies. Nursing Process: Implementation.
7. Answer: 2. Core Concept: 34.3. Rationale: During exercise, cellular demand for glucose (energy) is increased, which causes decreasing levels of glucose in the blood. Shortly after exercise there is a risk of a hypoglycemic reaction. During this time, the patient does not need more insulin, but instead may need to eat a carbohydrate snack in order to prevent hypoglycemia. Options 1, 3, and 4 are incorrect. There is not an increase of blood glucose during exercise but blood glucose levels are affected. And even though there is a decrease in blood glucose during exercise, more insulin should not be given because it will cause a further drop in blood glucose. Cognitive Level: Understanding. Client Need: Physiological Integrity/Pharmacological Therapies. Nursing Process: Evaluation.
8. Answers: 1, 2, 3, and 5. Core Concepts: 34.2 and 34.3. Rationale: Factors that can influence the amount of insulin needed by a patient include exercise (lowers blood glucose, decreasing insulin need at the time), diet (depending on what is eaten, insulin need may

increase or decrease), and illness (stress on the body raises blood glucose levels which may mean an increase in insulin). Changes in weight can also influence the amount of insulin needed (option 5). Insulin needs during sleep are determined when the normal insulin regimens are set up for each patient (option 4). Cognitive Level: Applying. Client Need: Physiological Integrity/Pharmacological Therapies. Nursing Process: Implementation.

9. Answer: 4. Core Concept: 34.5. Rationale: The nurse should administer glipizide (Glucotrol) just before breakfast so that its onset begins with the first meal and lasts through the day. This oral antidiabetic drug should not be administered subcutaneously (option 1), after meals (option 2), or at bedtime (option 3). Cognitive Level: Applying. Client Need: Physiological Integrity/Pharmacological Therapies. Nursing Process: Implementation.
10. Answer: 4. Core Concept: 34.3. Rationale: Glargine (Lantus), a long-acting insulin, may be given any time of day as long as it is given the same time every day. Bedtime is usually the most convenient time for most patients. Lantus does not have to be given before meals (option 1), with meals (option 2), or only at bedtime (option 3). Cognitive Level: Applying. Client Need: Physiological Integrity/Pharmacological Therapies. Nursing Process: Implementation.

Case Study Answers

1. Answers: 1 and 2. Core Concepts: 34.2 and 34.4. Rationale: Factors that contributed to his laboratory results include his diet and level of stress. Smoking (option 3) and hypertension (option 4) do not directly cause hyperglycemia but will contribute to any long-term complications associated with this condition. Cognitive Level: Applying. Client Need: Physiological Integrity/Pharmacological Therapies. Nursing Process: Data Collection.
2. Answers: 1, 2, and 4. Core Concepts: 34.2 and 34.4. Rationale: Regular exercise, oral antidiabetic medication, and learning how to cope with stress will all help Mr. Jones control his blood glucose levels. Since he is overweight, maintaining his current weight will not aid him in better glucose control (option 3). His healthcare provider will help him form a weight loss plan. Cognitive Level: Applying. Client Need: Physiological Integrity/Pharmacological Therapies. Nursing Process: Implementation.
3. Answers: 2–4. Core Concept: 34.5. Rationale: The adverse effects of metformin include diarrhea, abdominal discomfort, and headaches. It can also cause nausea, vomiting, a metallic taste, anorexia, dizziness, agitation, and fatigue. Metformin is not known to cause constipation (option 1). Cognitive Level: Applying. Client Need: Physiological Integrity/Pharmacological Therapies. Nursing Process: Implementation.
4. Answer: 1. Core Concept: 34.5. Rationale: The nurse understands there is an increased risk of hypoglycemia if Mr. Jones takes both metformin for diabetes and either captopril, furosemide, or nifedipine for his high blood pressure. The combination of medications used for high blood pressure and metformin are not known to cause a decrease in renal excretion (option 2), an increase in renal excretion (option 3), or a decreased risk for hypoglycemia (option 4). Cognitive Level: Understanding. Client Need: Physiological Integrity/Pharmacological Therapies. Nursing Process: Planning.

Chapter 35

Review Answers

1. Answer: 2. Core Concept: 35.2. Rationale: The type of birth control where the estrogen level remains constant throughout the treatment cycle but the progestin level increases toward the end of the menstrual cycle is called biphasic. Monophasic OCs (option 1) deliver a constant dose of estrogen and progestin throughout the treatment cycle. With triphasic OCs (option 3), the amounts of both estrogen and progestin vary in three distinct phases during the treatment cycle. The quadriphasic OC called Natazia (option 4)

contains a synthetic estrogen called estradiol valerate and a progestin called dienogest; it is supposed to more closely replicate normal monthly hormone levels than other types. Cognitive Level: Applying. Client Need: Physiological Integrity/Pharmacological Therapies. Nursing Process: Implementation.

2. Answer: 1. Core Concept: 35.7. Rationale: Before taking sildenafil (Viagra), the patient should be evaluated for any cardiovascular problems such as angina. Patients with a history of angina usually take a nitrate drug (nitroglycerine). Both sildenafil and nitroglycerine dilate blood vessels, and taking both together markedly increases the effect, which causes a drop in blood pressure and decreased blood flow to the heart, possibly causing a heart attack. Having diabetes (option 2), having allergies to dairy products (option 3), or being treated for migraines (option 4) does not inhibit the patient from taking sildenafil. Cognitive Level: Applying. Client Need: Physiological Integrity/Pharmacological Therapies. Nursing Process: Data Collection.

3. Answer: 3. Core Concepts: 35.3 and 35.4. Rationale: Estrogen–Progesterone OCs, such as medroxyprogesterone (Prempro), may cause thrombosis and would be contraindicated for a 40-year-old woman with a history of deep vein thrombosis. A woman with dysfunctional uterine bleeding (option 1) may benefit from OC therapy. This drug may also be one of the drugs used in the treatment of uterine cancer (option 2). In addition, a 21-year-old healthy woman may use an estrogen–progesterone OC for birth control (option 4). Cognitive Level: Understanding. Client Need: Physiological Integrity/Pharmacological Therapies. Nursing Process: Planning.

4. Answer: 2. Core Concept: 35.2. Rationale: One of the drugs used for emergency contraception is levonorgestrel, otherwise known as "Plan B." It is approved for purchase OTC and involves taking 0.75 mg of levonorgestrel in two doses, 12 hours apart. Oxytocin (option 1) is a natural hormone, which is used to induce labor and control postpartum bleeding. Medroxyprogesterone (option 3), a synthetic progestin, is used primarily to treat dysfunctional uterine bleeding. Magnesium sulfate (option 4) is used to inhibit uterine contractions in pregnant women at risk for preterm labor. Cognitive Level: Understanding. Client Need: Physiological Integrity/Pharmacological Therapies. Nursing Process: Planning.

5. Answers: 1, 2, 3, and 5. Core Concept: 35.5. Rationale: The nurse monitors a patient on oxytocin (Pitocin) for possible adverse effects such as uterine rupture, seizures, and fetal dysrhythmias. Oxytocin may also cause hypertension (option 5), not hypotension (option 4). Cognitive Level: Applying. Client Need: Physiological Integrity/Pharmacological Therapies. Nursing Process: Evaluation.

6. Answer: 2. Core Concept: 35.6. Rationale: A complication of testosterone therapy is hepatic (liver) failure. Testosterone therapy is not known to cause renal failure (option 1) or decrease cholesterol (option 3). Maturation of the male sex organs is caused by naturally occurring testosterone in pubescent boys. (option 4). Cognitive Level: Applying. Client Need: Physiological Integrity/Pharmacological Therapies. Nursing Process: Implementation.

7. Answer: 3. Core Concept: 35.2 and Nursing Process Focus: Patients Receiving Oral Contraception. Rationale: A patient who has not taken her OC for the last 2 days should use additional birth control until her regular schedule is reestablished. She can take the missed two pills on the day remembered and the next two pills on the following day (option 1). She should follow the remaining schedule just after the second day of taking the two pills (option 2). It is too early to obtain and use a home pregnancy kit (option 4). Cognitive Level: Applying. Client Need: Physiological Integrity/Pharmacological Therapies. Nursing Process: Implementation.

8. Answer: 4. Core Concept: N/A. Rationale: Ordered 50 mg (every 2 weeks) ÷ 100 mg/mL = 0.5 mL x 4 (2 weeks ÷ 8 weeks) = 200 mg. Options 1–3 are a result of a miscalculation and therefore are incorrect. Cognitive Level: Applying. Client Need: Physiological Integrity/Pharmacological Therapies. Nursing Process: Implementation.

9. Answer: 4. Core Concept: 35.3. Rationale: The best response is to inform the patient to discuss risks versus benefits of HRT with her healthcare provider. HRT has adverse effects, but is commonly prescribed to relieve menopausal symptoms (options 1 and 2). It is not within the nurse's scope of practice to make the decision of whether or not a patient should be started on HRT (option 3). Cognitive Level: Applying. Client Need: Physiological Integrity/Pharmacological Therapies. Nursing Process: Implementation.
10. Answer: 4. Core Concept: 35.8. Rationale: The patient with BPH may be treated with finasteride (Proscar). Finasteride (Proscar) shrinks enlarged prostates and helps restore urinary function. Propecia is used to treat hair loss (option 1). Sildenafil is used to treat erectile dysfunction (option 2), and estrogen is used to treat uterine dysfunction and as an OC (option 3). Cognitive Level: Understanding. Client Need: Physiological Integrity/Pharmacological Therapies. Nursing Process: Planning.

Case Study Answers

1. Answer: 3. Core Concept: 35.3. Rationale: Dysfunctional uterine bleeding may be treated by the use of OCs (estrogen/progesterone). The use of condoms will not affect uterine bleeding (option 1). A patient with dysfunctional uterine bleeding should not wait until the pain gets really bad to see a healthcare provider (option 2). Screening of sexual partners does not treat dysfunctional uterine bleeding (option 4). Cognitive Level: Understanding. Client Need: Physiological Integrity/Pharmacological Therapies. Nursing Process: Planning.
2. Answer: 4. Core Concept: 35.4. Rationale: In order to determine if Ms. Philips is a good candidate for Depo-Provera (a synthetic progestin also used as birth control), the nurse needs to ask her if she has any plans of becoming pregnant. Having diabetes (option 1), losing weight (option 2), or having a diet high in protein (option 3) does not inhibit the use of Depo-Provera. Cognitive Level: Applying. Client Need: Physiological Integrity/Pharmacological Therapies. Nursing Process: Data Collection.
3. Answers: 1 and 3. Core Concept: 35.4. Rationale: The nurse should inform the patient that smoking increases the risk of serious cardiovascular adverse effects and to notify the healthcare provider if she misses two or more consecutive periods. Depo-Provera should be taken daily at the same time each day (option 2). Caffeine is not beneficial (option 4). Cognitive Level: Applying. Client Need: Physiological Integrity/Pharmacological Therapies. Nursing Process: Implementation.
4. Answers: 2 and 4. Core Concept: 35.4. Rationale: The nurse tells Ms. Philips that possible adverse effects of Depo-Provera include breast tenderness and breakthrough bleeding. Depo-Provera is not known to cause weight loss (option 1) or loss of appetite (option 3). Cognitive Level: Applying. Client Need: Physiological Integrity/Pharmacological Therapies. Nursing Process: Implementation.

Chapter 36

Review Answers

1. Answer: 2. Core Concept: 36.4. Rationale: The trade name of a medication that lowers serum alkaline phosphatase is Fosamax, a bisphosphonate used to treat osteoporosis. Azulfidine (option 1) is a DMARD used to treat RA. Colchicine (option 3) and Benemid (option 4) are uric acid-inhibiting drugs used to treat gout. Cognitive Level: Applying. Client Need: Physiological Integrity/Pharmacological Therapies. Nursing Process: Implementation.
2. Answer: 4. Core Concept: 36.4. Rationale: Since one of the adverse effects of raloxifene is the risk of venous thromboembolism, a patient taking this drug along with warfarin should have a PT/INR test to determine baselines. Even though it is beneficial to monitor a patient's platelet (option 1), WBC (option 2), and sodium (option 3) levels, they are not necessary when the patient begins to take warfarin. Cognitive Level: Applying. Client Need: Physiological Integrity/Pharmacological Therapies. Nursing Process: Planning.

3. Answer: 1. Core Concept: 36.1. Rationale: Calcitriol is the active form of vitamin D and its primary function is to increase calcium absorption. A patient taking calcitriol should be monitored for dysrhythmias because calcium ions influence the excitability of all neurons including the electrical impulses within the heart muscle. It is not necessary to monitor for hypercalcemia (option 2), fluid overload (option 3), or flu-like symptoms (option 4). Cognitive Level: Understanding. Client Need: Physiological Integrity/Pharmacological Therapies. Nursing Process: Planning.
4. Answer: 3. Core Concept: 36.8. Rationale: The patient with gout would take allopurinol. Calcitriol (option 1) is used for osteoporosis, osteomalacia, and rickets. Azathioprine (option 2) is a DMARD used for RA. Raloxifene (option 4), a SERM, is used to treat osteoporosis. Cognitive Level: Understanding. Client Need: Physiological Integrity/Pharmacological Therapies. Nursing Process: Planning.
5. Answer: 3. Core Concept: 36.4. Rationale: Alendronate (Fosamax), a bisphosphonate used to treat osteoporosis, must be taken on an empty stomach and the patient needs to remain in an upright position for 30 minutes after taking it. Allopurinol (option 1), a drug used to treat gout; calcitonin (option 2), a hormone that stimulates bone building; and raloxifene (option 4), a SERM used to treat osteoporosis, do not require the patient to remain upright after administration. Cognitive Level: Applying. Client Need: Physiological Integrity/Pharmacological Therapies. Nursing Process: Implementation.
6. Answer: 1. Core Concept: 36.4. Rationale: Calcitonin, a hormone that stimulates the building of bones by adding calcium, is available as a nasal spray. One of its adverse effects is nasal irritation. Calcitonin is not known to cause headaches (option 2), watery eyes (option 3), or sinus infections (option 4). Cognitive Level: Applying. Client Need: Physiological Integrity/Pharmacological Therapies. Nursing Process: Implementation.
7. Answer: 3. Core Concept: 36.7. Rationale: Hydroxychloroquine (Plaquenil), a DMARD, is used to treat RA. One of its adverse effects is blurred vision. It can also cause GI disturbances, hair loss, headaches, and mood changes. Hydroxychloroquine is not known to cause cardiac dysrhythmias (option 1), joint stiffness (option 2), or decreased muscle strength (option 4). Cognitive Level: Understanding. Client Need: Physiological Integrity/Pharmacological Therapies. Nursing Process: Evaluation.
8. Answer: 3. Core Concept: 36.3. Rationale: Calcium phosphate has the highest potency at 19.3 mEq/g. Calcium chloride (option 1) has 13.6 mEq/g, calcium citrate (option 2) has 12 mEq/g, and calcium gluconate (option 4) has 4.5 mEq/g. Cognitive Level: Applying. Client Need: Physiological Integrity/Pharmacological Therapies. Nursing Process: Evaluation.
9. Answers: 1, 2, and 4. Core Concepts: 36.4 and 36.5. Rationale: The nurse would include calcitonin in the plan of care for patients who have Paget disease, hypercalcemia, and osteoporosis. Calcitonin is not commonly used to treat hypocalcemia (option 3) or osteoarthritis (option 5). Cognitive Level: Understanding. Client Need: Physiological Integrity/Pharmacological Therapies. Nursing Process: Planning.
10. Answer: 4. Core Concept: N/A. Rationale: The patient will receive 62.5 mL/hour (250 mL÷4 hours = 62.5 mL/hour). Options 1–3 are a result of a miscalculation and are therefore incorrect. Cognitive Level: Applying. Client Need: Physiological Integrity/Pharmacological Therapies. Nursing Process: Implementation.

Case Study Answers

1. Answer: 4. Core Concept: 36.8. Rationale: Allopurinol works by reducing the production of uric acid. Allopurinol does not work by directly decreasing deposits of uric acid in the joint spaces (option 1) or reducing pain associated with joint inflammation (option 2), although these effects usually result when uric acid levels are reduced. Allopurinol does not increase renal excretion of uric acid (option 3). Cognitive Level: Applying. Client Need: Physiological Integrity/Pharmacological Therapies. Nursing Process: Implementation.

2. Answers: 1–4. Core Concept: 36.8. Rationale: Allopurinol can cause headaches, vertigo, toxic epidermal necrolysis, and skin rash. Cognitive Level: Applying. Client Need: Physiological Integrity/Pharmacological Therapies. Nursing Process: Implementation.
3. Answer: 3. Core Concept: 36.8. Rationale: Alcohol may inhibit the renal excretion of uric acid, thus raising the uric acid levels in the blood. Alcohol does not significantly increase allopurinol levels (option 1), interfere with the absorption of antigout medications (option 2), or cause the urine to become more alkaline (option 4). Cognitive Level: Applying. Client Need: Physiological Integrity/Pharmacological Therapies. Nursing Process: Implementation.
4. Answer: 4. Core Concept: 36.8. Rationale: Since aspirin has been known to cause gout, Mr. Hurtt shows that he needs additional instructions when he says that he will continue taking aspirin. Options 1–3 are correct statements about allopurinol. He should take his medications as prescribed (option 1), stop drinking alcohol (option 2), and avoid high purine foods (option 3). Cognitive Level: Understanding. Client Need: Physiological Integrity/Pharmacological Therapies. Nursing Process: Evaluation.

Chapter 37

Review Answers

1. Answer: 2. Core Concept: 37.4. Rationale: Benzocaine, an OTC medication used for minor skin irritation such as sunburn, pruritus, minor wounds, and insect bites, should *not* be used on open lesions or sores; therefore, option 4 is incorrect. Benzocaine can be used on minor sunburns (option 1). It is not known to cause blisters (option 3). Cognitive Level: Applying. Client Need: Physiological Integrity/Pharmacological Therapies. Nursing Process: Implementation.
2. Answer: 4. Core Concept: 37.6. Rationale: In a plan of care for patients taking Topicort, the possible adverse effect of skin irritation and redness should be included. Topicort is not known to cause localized pruritus and hives (option 1), hair loss in the application area (option 2), or a worsening of acne (option 3). Cognitive Level: Applying. Client Need: Physiological Integrity/Pharmacological Therapies. Nursing Process: Planning.
3. Answer: 4. Core Concept: 37.3. Rationale: The medication used for lice that is applied to the body and rinsed out after 10 minutes is permethrin. Lindane (option 1) is also used for the treatment of lice but is only prescribed after other drugs have failed because it can cause serious nervous system toxicity. Crotamiton (option 2), another pediculicide, is prescribed as a 10% cream. Cortizone (option 3) is a topical corticosteroid used to treat the inflammation of dermatitis. Cognitive Level: Applying. Client Need: Physiological Integrity/Pharmacological Therapies. Nursing Process: Implementation.
4. Answer: 1. Core Concept: 37.4. Rationale: The nurse would include the use of Benzocaine (Solarcaine) in the plan of care for someone with minor sunburn. Cortizone (option 2) is a topical corticosteroid used to treat the inflammation of dermatitis. Benzoyl peroxide (option 3) is an OTC medication used for minor skin irritation such as acne. Doxycycline (option 4) is an antibiotic used in combination with other medications such as benzoyl peroxide to treat acne. Cognitive Level: Understanding. Client Need: Physiological Integrity/Pharmacological Therapies. Nursing Process: Planning.
5. Answer: 2. Core Concept: 37.5. Rationale: Tretinoin, a retinoid medication used for acne, is not recommended for use during pregnancy. Hydrocortisone (option 1) is a corticosteroid used to decrease the inflammation associated with minor skin irritations. Benzoyl peroxide (option 3), an OTC medication, is used for minor skin irritation such as acne. At low percentages, pregnant women can use it. Benzocaine (option 4), an OTC medication, is used for minor skin irritation such as sunburn, pruritus, minor wounds, and insect bites. Cognitive Level: Applying. Client Need: Physiological Integrity/Pharmacological Therapies. Nursing Process: Implementation.

6. Answers: 1, 2, and 4. Core Concept: 37.6. Rationale: The systemic adverse effects that can be caused by the use of topical corticosteroids are mood changes, bone defects, and adrenal insufficiency. Liver toxicity (option 3) is not usually an adverse effect of topical corticosteroid use. Whereas topical corticosteroids can cause skin irritation, this adverse effect is not a result of the systemic absorption of the drug (option 5). Cognitive Level: Understanding. Client Need: Physiological Integrity/Pharmacological Therapies. Nursing Process: Evaluation.
7. Answer: 2. Core Concept: 37.5. Rationale: One of the most effective treatments for rosacea is topical metronidazole (Metrogel). Calcipotriene (option 1), Acitretin (option 3), and Cyclosporine (option 4) are all drugs used to treat psoriasis. Cognitive Level: Understanding. Client Need: Physiological Integrity/Pharmacological Therapies. Nursing Process: Planning.
8. Answer: 2. Core Concept: 37.5. Rationale: Medications that promote the shedding of skin, like some of the drugs used to treat acne, are called keratolytic agents. Pediculicides (option 1) are used to treat lice infestations. Retinoids (option 3) are vitamin A–like compounds used to treat acne. Corticosteroids (option 4) are used to treat the inflammation of dermatitis, eczema, and psoriasis. Cognitive Level: Remembering. Client Need: Physiological Integrity/Pharmacological Therapies. Nursing Process: Planning.
9. Answer: 1. Core Concept: 37.7. Rationale: Betamethasone is one of the topical corticosteroids used in the initial treatment of psoriasis. It has a reputation for being effective, safe, and inexpensive. Doxycycline (option 2) is an antibiotic used alone or in combination with other medications such as benzoyl peroxide for the treatment of acne. Cyclosporine (option 3) is a drug used to treat psoriasis. Benzocaine (option 4), an OTC medication, is used for minor skin irritation such as sunburn, pruritus, minor wounds, and insect bites. Cognitive Level: Understanding. Client Need: Physiological Integrity/Pharmacological Therapies. Nursing Process: Planning.
10. Answer: 3. Core Concept: N/A. Rationale: Order: infliximab 5 mg/kg. Convert pounds to kilograms and multiply by 5 mg. 198 pounds ÷ 2.2 kg/pound = 90 kg × 5 mg/kg = 450 mg. Options 1, 2, and 4 are a result of a miscalculation and are therefore incorrect. Cognitive Level: Applying. Client Need: Physiological Integrity/Pharmacological Therapies. Nursing Process: Implementation.

Case Study Answers

1. Answer: 2. Core Concept: 37.5. Rationale: Benzoyl peroxide is an OTC medication used to treat acne. Improvements begin in the first week but the full effects may take several weeks to a month or longer. Benzoyl peroxide takes longer than a week to be fully effective (option 1). With benzoyl peroxide, improvements should be evident within a few weeks (option 3). Burt has not taken the medication long enough for it to become effective, although his skin condition may justify the addition of an antibiotic (option 4). Cognitive Level: Applying. Client Need: Physiological Integrity/Pharmacological Therapies. Nursing Process: Implementation.
2. Answer: 4. Core Concept: 37.5. Rationale: Because of the severity of Burt's acne, the healthcare provider may prescribe an antibiotic to inhibit bacterial growth, thus lessening the redness and inflammation associated with his disorder. Metronidazole (option 1) is a medication effective against certain bacteria and is used for psoriasis. Benzocaine (option 2), an OTC medication, is used for minor skin irritation such as sunburn, pruritus, minor wounds, and insect bites. Corticosteroids (option 3) are used to treat the inflammation in disorders such as dermatitis, eczema, and psoriasis. Cognitive Level: Understanding. Client Need: Physiological Integrity/Pharmacological Therapies. Nursing Process: Planning.
3. Answer: 2. Core Concept: 37.5. Rationale: Tretinoin, a retinoid, is a vitamin A–like compound that decreases oil production by reducing the size and number of oil glands. It

does not act by shedding the outer layer of skin like keratolytic agents (option 1). In addition, it does not inhibit bacterial growth like antibiotics (option 3) or reduce inflammation like corticosteroids (option 4). Cognitive Level: Applying. Client Need: Physiological Integrity/Pharmacological Therapies. Nursing Process: Implementation.

4. Answers: 2–4. Core Concept: 37.5. Rationale: Tretinoin may cause dry mouth and nose, photosensitivity, and skin irritation such as burning and redness. Tretinoin is not known to cause swelling around the mouth (option 1). Cognitive Level: Applying. Client Need: Physiological Integrity/Pharmacological Therapies. Nursing Process: Implementation.

Chapter 38

Review Answers

1. Answer: 2. Core Concept: 38.6. Rationale: The patient having her eyes examined will need to have mydriatic drops put into her eyes to dilate the pupil so the healthcare provider can see the retina. Eyedrops that constrict the pupil, such as miotics and others (options 1 and 3), cannot be used in an eye examination. Corticosteroid drops (option 4) are used to reduce inflammation. Cognitive Level: Applying. Client Need: Physiological Integrity/Pharmacological Therapies. Nursing Process: Implementation.
2. Answer: 3. Core Concept: 38.4. Rationale: In order to relieve pressure within the eye by increasing the outflow of aqueous humor, the patient would need to receive a miotic drug, such as pilocarpine (Ocusert). Timolol (option 1) and betaxolol (option 2) are beta blockers that decrease pressure within the eye by decreasing the formation of aqueous humor. Ciprofloxacin (option 4) is an antibiotic used to treat infections. Cognitive Level: Applying. Client Need: Physiological Integrity/Pharmacological Therapies. Nursing Process: Planning.
3. Answer: 1. Core Concept: 38.5. Rationale: In order to relieve pressure within the eye by decreasing the production of aqueous humor, the patient would need to receive a beta-blocker like timolol (Timoptic). Atropine sulfate (option 2), a cycloplegic drug, is used to relax ciliary muscles during eye examinations. Pilocarpine (option 3), a miotic, is used to decrease pressure within the eye by increasing the flow of aqueous humor. Ciprofloxacin (option 4) is an antibiotic used to treat infections. Cognitive Level: Applying. Client Need: Physiological Integrity/Pharmacological Therapies. Nursing Process: Implementation.
4. Answer: 4. Core Concept: N/A. Rationale: Ordered 250 mg × four (4) times in 24 hours = 1000 mg per day. This includes the initial dose of 250 mg. Options 1, 2, and 3 are a result of a miscalculation and are therefore incorrect. Cognitive Level: Applying. Client Need: Physiological Integrity/Pharmacological Therapies. Nursing Process: Implementation.
5. Answer: 1. Core Concept: 38.7. Rationale: A patient with inflammation would be given an anti-inflammatory drug such as a corticosteroid. For ear infections, corticosteroids are combined with antibiotics, for example, ciprofloxacin and hydrocortisone (Cipro HC). Aluminum sulfate and calcium acetate (Domeboro) (option 2) are used for the relief of minor skin irritations. Osmotic diuretics (option 3) and carbonic-anhydrase inhibitors (option 4) are used to treat glaucoma. They work by lowering pressure within the eye by decreasing the formation of aqueous humor. Cognitive Level: Understanding. Client Need: Physiological Integrity/Pharmacological Therapies. Nursing Process: Planning.
6. Answer: 3. Core Concept: 38.7. Rationale: The nurse should inform the patient that the instillation of eardrops would cause a decrease in hearing for a few minutes, just until the drops can be absorbed. The solution will stay within the ear canal until it is absorbed (options 1 and 2) and, depending on the medication, may take between an hour to a few days to become effective (option 4). Cognitive Level: Understanding. Client Need: Physiological Integrity/Pharmacological Therapies. Nursing Process: Planning.

7. Answers: 1, 2, 3, and 5. Core Concept: 38.7. Rationale: Ciprofloxacin can cause rashes, white patches in the mouth, and ear pain. In females, it can also cause vaginal itching and discharge. Ciprofloxacin has not been known to cause a total loss of hearing (option 4). Cognitive Level: Applying. Client Need: Physiological Integrity/Pharmacological Therapies. Nursing Process: Implementation.
8. Answer: 1. Core Concept: 38.3. Rationale: The rationale for giving antiglaucoma medication is to reduce the pressure within the eye by either decreasing the production of aqueous humor or increasing the flow of aqueous humor out of the eye. Increasing the production of aqueous humor would increase the pressure within the eye (options 2 and 4). Decreasing the outflow of aqueous humor would also increase the pressure within the eye (options 2 and 3). Cognitive Level: Understanding. Client Need: Physiological Integrity/Pharmacological Therapies. Nursing Process: Implementation.
9. Answer: 3. Core Concept: 38.4. Rationale: The patient taking travoprost (Travatan), a prostaglandin, should be instructed that the medication might darken the pigmentation of the iris. This medication is not administered *only* in the morning (option 1). Travoprost works by increasing the outflow of aqueous humor to treat glaucoma. It does not constrict or dilate the pupils (options 2 and 4). Cognitive Level: Applying. Client Need: Physiological Integrity/Pharmacological Therapies. Nursing Process: Implementation.
10. Answer: 1. Core Concept: 38.5. Rationale: Methazolamide (Neptazane) is a sulfonamide carbonic-anhydrase inhibitor. Sulfonamides are drugs known to cause allergic reactions; therefore, patients allergic to sulfonamides should not take methazolamide. Betaxolol and carteolol (options 2 and 3) are specific beta blockers (option 4), which are also used to treat glaucoma. Cognitive Level: Understanding. Client Need: Physiological Integrity/Pharmacological Therapies. Nursing Process: Planning.

Case Study Answers

1. Answer: 3. Core Concept: 38.2. Rationale: If left untreated, glaucoma can lead to blindness. Glaucoma is not known to cause options 1, 2, and 4. Mydriasis (option 1) refers to drugs that cause dilation of the pupils. Cycloplegia (option 2) is the paralysis of the ciliary muscle of the eye. Vertigo (option 4) refers to dizziness. Cognitive Level: Applying. Client Need: Physiological Integrity/Pharmacological Therapies. Nursing Process: Implementation.
2. Answer: 1. Core Concept: 38.5. Rationale: The most common adverse effect of timolol is local burning and stinging. Timolol is not known to cause sinus irritation (option 2) or edema around the eyes (option 4). If applied correctly, timolol should not be significantly absorbed into the blood stream, but if absorption does occur, it may cause bronchoconstriction (option 3). Cognitive Level: Applying. Client Need: Physiological Integrity/Pharmacological Therapies. Nursing Process: Implementation.
3. Answers: 1 and 3. Core Concept: 38.5. Rationale: It is not advisable to take epinephrine or nitrates with timolol. Taking epinephrine can lead to HTN; nitrates can lead to hypotension and bradycardia. Ciprofloxacin (option 2), an antibiotic, and the anti-inflammatory corticosteroids (option 4) are not known to interact with timolol. Cognitive Level: Applying. Client Need: Physiological Integrity/Pharmacological Therapies. Nursing Process: Implementation.
4. Answer: 3. Core Concept: 38.5. Rationale: It may require 2 to 4 weeks of treatment before the maximum therapeutic effect is realized. It will take more than a week or two (options 1 and 2) before Ms. Saunders can tell any difference in her vision but it should not take as long as 2 months (option 4). Cognitive Level: Applying. Client Need: Physiological Integrity/Pharmacological Therapies. Nursing Process: Implementation.

Appendix B

Calculating Dosages

I. Calculating Dosage Using Ratios and Proportions

A. A *ratio* is used to express a relationship between two or more quantities. Ratios may be written using the following notations.

1:10 means 1 part of drug A to 10 parts of solution/solvent.

In drug calculations, ratios are usually expressed as a fraction:

$$\frac{\text{1 part drug A}}{\text{10 part solution}} = \frac{1}{10}$$

A *proportion* shows the relationship between two ratios. It is a simple and effective means for calculating certain types of doses.

$$\frac{\text{Dose on hand}}{\text{Quantity on hand}} = \frac{\text{Desired dose}}{\text{Quantity desired } (X)}$$

Using cross-multiplication, we can write the same formula as follows:

$$\text{Quantity desired } (X) = \frac{\text{Desired dose} \times \text{Quantity on hand}}{\text{Dose on hand}}$$

Example 1: The healthcare provider orders erythromycin 500 mg. It is supplied in a liquid form containing 250 mg in 5 mL. How much drug should the nurse administer?

To calculate the dosage, use the formula:

$$\frac{\text{Dose on hand (250 mg)}}{\text{Quantity on hand (5 mL)}} = \frac{\text{Desired dose (500 mg)}}{\text{Quantity desired } (X)}$$

Then, cross-multiply:

$$250 \cancel{\text{mg}} \times X = 5\text{mL} \times 500 \cancel{\text{mg}}$$

Therefore, the dose to be administered is 10 mL.

B. The same proportion method can be used to solve solid dosage calculations.

Example 2: The healthcare provider orders methotrexate 20 mg/day. The methotrexate is available in 2.5-mg tablets. How many tablets should the nurse administer each day?

$$\frac{\text{Dose on hand (2.5 mg)}}{\text{1 tablet}} = \frac{\text{Desired dose (20 mg)}}{\text{Quantity desired } (X \text{ tablets})}$$

Cross-multiplication gives:

$$2.5 \text{ mg } X = 20 \text{ mg} \times 1 \text{ tablet}$$

Therefore, the nurse should administer 8 tablets daily.

II. Calculating Dosage by Weight

Doses for pediatric patients are often calculated by using body weight. The nurse must use caution to convert between pounds and kilograms, as necessary (see Table 3.2 in Chapter 3, page 25). Use the formula:

$$\text{Body weight (kg)} \times \text{amount mg/kg} = X \text{ mg of drug}$$

Example 3: The healthcare provider orders 10 mg/kg of methsuximide for a client who weighs 90 kg. How much should be administered?

The patient should receive 900 mg of methsuximide.

Example 4: The healthcare provider orders 5 mg/kg/day of amiodarone. The patient weighs 110 pounds. How much of the drug should be administered daily?

Step 1: Convert pounds to kilograms.

$$110 \text{ Ib} \times 1 \text{ kg}/2.2 \text{ Ib} = 50 \text{ kg}$$

Step 2: Perform the drug calculation.

$$50 \cancel{\text{kg}} \text{ (body weight)} \times 5 \text{ mg}/\cancel{\text{kg}} = 250 \text{ mg}$$

The patient should receive 250 mg of amiodarone per day.

III. Calculating Dosage by Body Surface Area

Many antineoplastic drugs and most pediatric doses are calculated using body surface area (BSA).

The formula for BSA in metric units is:

$$\text{BSA} = \sqrt{\frac{\text{weight (kg)} \times \text{height (cm)}}{3600}}$$

The formula for BSA in household units is

$$\text{BSA} = \sqrt{\frac{\text{weight (Ib)} \times \text{height (inches)}}{3131}}$$

Example 5: The healthcare provider orders 10 mg/m2 of an antibiotic for a child who is 2 feet tall and weighs 30 lb. How many milligrams should be administered?

Step 1: Calculate the BSA of the child.

$$\text{BSA} = \sqrt{\frac{30 \times 24}{3131}}$$

$$\text{BSA} = \sqrt{\frac{720}{3131}}$$

$$\text{BSA} = \sqrt{0.230} = 0.48 \text{ m}^2$$

Step 2: Calculate the drug amount.

$$10 \text{ mg/m}^2 \times 0.48 \text{ m}^2$$

The nurse should administer 4.8 mg of the antibiotic to the child.

IV. Calculating IV Infusion Rates

Intravenous fluids are administered over time in units of mL/min or gtt/min (gtt = drops). The basic equation for IV drug calculations is as follows:

$$\frac{\text{mL of solution} \times \text{gtt/mL}}{\text{h of administration} \times 60 \text{ min/h}} = \frac{\text{gtt}}{\text{min}}$$

Example 6: The healthcare provider orders 1,000 mL of 5% normal saline to infuse over 6 hours. What is the flow rate?

$$\frac{1{,}000 \cancel{\text{mL}} \times 10 \text{ gtt}/\cancel{\text{mL}}}{6 \cancel{\text{h}} \times 60 \text{ min}/\cancel{\text{h}}} = \frac{28 \text{ gtt}}{\text{min}}$$

Other IV conversion formulas you may use include the following:

$$\text{mcg/kg/h} \rightarrow \text{mL/h}$$

$$\cancel{\text{kg}} \times \frac{\cancel{\text{mcg}}/\cancel{\text{kg}}}{\text{h}} \times \frac{\cancel{\text{mg}}}{1{,}000\ \cancel{\text{mcg}}} \times \frac{\text{mL}}{\cancel{\text{mg}}} = \frac{\text{mL}}{\text{h}}$$

$$\text{mcg/m}^2\text{/h} \rightarrow \text{mL/h}$$

$$\cancel{\text{m}^2} \times \frac{\cancel{\text{mcg}}/\cancel{\text{m}^2}}{\text{h}} \times \frac{\cancel{\text{mg}}}{1{,}000\ \cancel{\text{mcg}}} \times \frac{\text{mL}}{\cancel{\text{mg}}} = \frac{\text{mL}}{\text{h}}$$

$$\text{mcg/kg/ min} \rightarrow \text{gtt/ min}$$

$$\text{kg} \times \frac{\cancel{\text{mcg}}/\cancel{\text{kg}}}{\text{min}} \times \frac{\cancel{\text{mg}}}{1{,}000\ \cancel{\text{mcg}}} \times \frac{\text{mL}}{\cancel{\text{mg}}} \times \frac{10\ \text{gtt}}{\cancel{\text{mL}}} = \frac{\text{gtt}}{\text{min}}$$

Guide to Special Features

CAM Therapy

Fast Facts

Lifespan and Diversity

New Drug Focus

Nursing Process Focus

Patients Need to Know

Prototype Drug

Safety Alert

Glossary

Aδ fibers nerves that transmit sensations of sharp pain *(15) / page 223*

absorption (ab-SORP-shun) the process of moving a drug across body membranes *(4) / page 45*

acetylcholine (ACh) (ah-SEET-ul-KOH-leen) primary neurotransmitter of the parasympathetic nervous system; also present at somatic neuromuscular junctions and at parasympathetic and sympathetic preganglionic nerves *(9) / page 104*

acetylcholinesterase (AChE) (AS-ee-til-KOH-lin-ES-ter-ays) an enzyme that degrades acetylcholine within the synapse, enhancing the effects of the neurotransmitter *(13) / page 186*

acidosis (ah-sid-OH-sis) condition of having too much acid; plasma pH below 7.35 *(18) / page 286*

acquired resistance when a microbe is no longer affected by a drug following treatment with anti-infectives *(27) / page 424*

acromegaly (AKROW-megah-lee) excess secretion of growth hormone in adults *(33) / page 556*

action potential (poh-TEN-shial) an electrical signal of a single cell (muscle or nerve) generated by the opening and closing of special ion channels located on the cell's membrane *(14) / page 212*

activated partial thromboplastin time (aPTT) (throm-bow-PLAS-tin) blood test used to determine how long it takes clots to form to regulate heparin dosage *(24) / page 380*

active immunity stimulating the body to produce antibodies through the administration of a vaccine *(26) / page 411*

acute gouty arthritis (ah-CUTE GOW-ty are-THRYE-tis) condition where uric acid crystals quickly accumulate in the joints of the big toes, heels, ankles, wrists, fingers, knees, or elbows, resulting in red, swollen, or inflamed tissue *(36) / page 617*

adaptive body defenses a second line of immune defenses that are specific to particular threats *(26) / page 408*

addiction (ah-DIK-shun) the continued use of a substance despite its negative health and social consequences *(8) / page 84*

Addison disease (ADD-iss-un) hyposecretion of glucocorticoids and aldosterone by the adrenal cortex *(33) / page 562*

adenoma (AH-den-OH-mah) benign tumor of glandular tissue *(29) / page 468*

adjuvant analgesics (ADD-jeh-vent an-ul-JEE-ziks) additional pain killers provided when another is not providing sufficient relief *(15) / page 225*

adjuvant chemotherapy (AD-ju-vent) technique in which antineoplastics are administered *after* surgery or radiation to effect a cure *(29) / page 470*

adrenal atrophy (AT-troh-fee) shrinkage of the adrenal glands *(33) / page 562*

adrenergic (add-rah-NUR-jik) a term relating to nerves that release norepinephrine or epinephrine *(9) / page 104*

adrenergic blockers drugs that block the actions of the sympathetic nervous system, as in marijuana *(9) / page 105*

adrenergic drugs autonomic drugs that work by activating the sympathetic nervous system *(9) / page 105*

adrenocorticotropic hormone (ACTH) (uh-dreen-oh-kor-tik-o-TRO-pik) hormone secreted by the pituitary that stimulates the release of glucocorticoids by the adrenal cortex *(33) / page 561*

adverse drug effect adverse event resulting from drug administration; often called an *adverse drug reaction (3) / page 25*

adverse event any undesirable experience associated with the use of a medical product in a patient *(3) / page 25*

aerosol (AIR-oh-sol) suspension of small liquid droplets of drug, usually to cause bronchodilation *(30) / page 493*

afterload pressure that must be overcome for the ventricles to eject blood from the heart *(20) / page 316*

agonists (AG-on-ists) drugs that are capable of binding with receptors in order to cause a cellular response *(4) / page 50*

akathisia (ACK-ah-THEE-shea) uncontrolled limb and body movements *(12) / page 167*

alcohol intoxication (AL-ku-hol in-tak-su-KA-shun) a condition of altered mental and physical function resulting from drinking more alcoholic beverages within a time frame than the body can tolerate *(8) / page 89*

aldosterone (al-DOH-stair-own) hormone secreted by the adrenal cortex that increases sodium reabsorption in the distal tubule of the kidney *(18) / pages 281*

alimentary canal (AL-uh-MEN-tare-ee) the hollow tube in the digestive system that starts in the mouth and includes the esophagus, stomach, small intestine, and large intestine *(31) / page 516*

alkalosis (al-kah-LOH-sis) condition of having too much base; plasma pH above 7.45 *(18) / page 286*

alkylation (AL-kill-AYE-shun) process by which certain chemicals attach to DNA and change its structure and function *(29) / page 473*

allergic reaction a hyper-response of body tissues to a foreign substance (allergen), in which patients experience uncomfortable and potentially serious symptoms, including difficulty breathing, pain, swelling, skin rash, and other unfavorable signs *(3) / page 25*

allergic rhinitis (rye-NYE-tis) syndrome of sneezing, itchy throat, watery eyes, and nasal congestion resulting from exposure to antigens; also known as *hay fever (30) / page 494*

alopecia (AL-oh-PEESH-ee-uh) hair loss *(29) / page 472*

alpha (α) receptor type of subreceptor found in the sympathetic nervous system *(9) / page 105*

alternate-day therapy taking a drug every other day in order to minimize adverse effects *(25) / page 401*

alveoli (al-VEE-oh-lie) dilated sacs at the end of the bronchial tree where gas exchange occurs *(30) / page 492*

Alzheimer disease (AD) (ALLZ-heye-mer) most common dementia, characterized by loss of memory, confusion, disorientation, and loss of judgment; hallucinations and delusions may also occur *(13) / page 185*

amenorrhea (ah-men-oh-REE-ah) lack of normal menstrual periods *(35) / page 592*

amides (AM-ides) type of chemical linkage found in some local anesthetics involving carbon, nitrogen, and oxygen (—NH—CO—) *(16) / page 243*

analgesics (an-ul-JEE-ziks) drugs used to reduce or eliminate pain *(8, 15) / pages 83, 225*

anaphylactic (ann-ah-fuh-LAK-tick) shock acute, life-threatening type of shock characterized by a history of allergy with a sudden onset of symptoms following food or drug intake *(22) / page 347*

anaphylaxis (ANN-a-fah-LAX-iss) an acute allergic response to an antigen that results in severe hypotension and may cause death if untreated *(3, 25) / pages 25, 346*

androgens (AN-droh-jens) steroid sex hormones that promote the appearance of masculine characteristics *(35) / page 595*

anesthesia (ANN-ess-THEE-zee-uh) medical procedure involving drugs that block the transmission of nerve impulses and cause loss of sensation and/or consciousness *(16) / page 243*

angina pectoris (an-JEYE-nuh PEK-tore-us) acute pain in the chest on physical or emotional exertion due to inadequate oxygen supply to the myocardium *(21) / page 330*

angiotensin II (AN-geo-TEN-sin) chemical released in response to falling blood pressure that causes vasoconstriction and release of aldosterone *(19) / page 300*

angiotensin-converting enzyme (ACE) (angeo-TEN-sin) enzyme responsible for converting angiotensin I to angiotensin II *(19) / page 300*

anorexia (AN-oh-REX-ee-uh) loss of appetite *(31) / page 518*

anorexiants (AN-oh-REX-ee-ants) drugs used to suppress appetite *(32) / page 543*

antacid (an-TASS-id) drug that neutralizes stomach acid *(31) / page 523*

antagonism type of drug interaction in which one drug inhibits the effectiveness of another *(27) / page 426*

antagonists (an-TAG-oh-nists) drugs that block the response of another drug *(4) / page 50*

anterior pituitary an area of the pituitary gland also known as *adenohypophysis (33) / page 552*

antibiotic (ann-tie-bye-OT-ik) substance produced by a microorganism that inhibits or kills other microorganisms *(27) / page 424*

antibodies (ANN-tee-BOD-ees) proteins produced by the body in response to an antigen; used interchangeably with the term *immunoglobulin (26) / page 408*

anticholinergics drugs that inhibit the action of acetylcholine at its receptor *(9) / page 105*

anticoagulants (ANT-eye-co-AG-you-lent) agents that inhibit the formation of blood clots *(24) / page 377*

antidepressants (AN-tee-dee-PRESS-ahnts) drugs used for the treatment of depression and a range of anxiety disorders, including panic, obsessive-compulsive, social phobia, and post-traumatic stress disorders *(10, 11) / pages 126, 142*

antidiuretic hormone (ADH) (ANT-eye-deye-your-ET-ik) hormone produced by the hypothalamus that stimulates the kidneys to conserve water *(19, 33) / pages 296, 555*

antiemetic (AN-tie-ee-MET-ik) drug that prevents vomiting *(31) / page 528*

antiflatulents (an-tie-FLAT-u-lentz) drugs that reduce gas formation in the GI tract *(31) / page 523*

antigen (ANN-tih-jenz) a foreign organism or substance that induces the formation of antibodies *(22, 26) / pages 353, 407*

anti-infective (ann-tie-in-FEK-tive) general term for any medication effective against pathogens *(27) / page 424*

antiplatelet drugs (ant-eye-PLAY-tuh-let) medications that decrease the coagulation function of platelets *(24) / page 377*

antipsychotic drugs class of drugs used to treat psychosis and other mental and emotional conditions *(11) / page 153*

antipyretics drugs used to treat fever *(25) / page 401*

antiretrovirals (an-tie-RET-roh-veye-ral) drugs effective against retroviruses *(28) / page 452*

antitussives (anti-TUSS-ive) drugs used to suppress cough *(30) / page 501*

anxiety state of apprehension or dread due to a perceive threat or danger *(10) / page 121*

anxiolytics (ANG-zee-oh-LIT-iks) drugs that relieve anxiety agents for mood stabilization *(10) / page 124*

apothecary system (ah-POTH-eh-kare-ee) former system of weights and measures used by healthcare providers and pharmacists; replaced by the metric system *(3) / page 29*

assessment phase appraisal of a patient's condition that involves gathering and interpreting data *(5) / page 56*

asthma (AZ-muh) chronic inflammatory disease of the airways *(30) / page 502*

astringent effect (ah-STRIN-jent) the shrinkage of swollen membranes or binding together of body surface material *(3) / page 35*

atherosclerosis (ath-ur-oh-skler-OH-sis) a buildup of fatty substances and loss of elasticity of the arterial walls *(17, 21) / pages 259, 330*

atrioventricular (AV) node (ay-tree-oh-ven-TRIK-you-lur noad) small area of specialized fibers that lies in the wall separating the two atria *(23) / page 361*

atrioventricular bundle (ay-tree-oh-ven-TRIK-you-lur BUN-dul) specialized cardiac tissue that receives electrical impulses from the AV node and sends them to the bundle branches; also known as the *bundle of His (23) / page 361*

attention-deficit/hyperactivity disorder (ADHD) a disorder typically diagnosed in childhood and adolescence characterized by hyperactivity as well as attention, organization, and behavior control issues *(8, 11) / pages 92, 154*

auras (AUR-uhs) sensory cues such as bright lights, smells, or tastes that precede a migraine *(15) / page 235*

autoantibodies (AW-tow-ANN-tee-BAH-dees) proteins called rheumatoid factors released by B lymphocytes; these tear down the body's own tissue *(36) / page 615*

automaticity (aw-toh-muh-TISS-uh-tee) ability of certain myocardial cells to spontaneously generate an action potential *(23) / page 361*

B cell type of lymphocyte that is essential for the humoral immune response *(26) / page 408*

bactericidal (bak-teer-ih-SY-dall) substance that has ability to kill bacteria *(27) / page 424*

bacteriostatic (bak-teer-ee-oh-STAT-ik) substance that can inhibit the growth of bacteria *(27) / page 424*

balanced anesthesia use of multiple medications to induce unconsciousness, cause muscle relaxation, and maintain deep anesthesia *(16) / page 248*

barbiturates (bar-bi-CHUR-ates) class of drugs derived from barbituric acid; they act as CNS depressants and are used for their sedative and antiseizure effects *(10) / page 131*

baroreceptors (BARE-oh-ree-sep-tours) nerves located in the walls of the atria, aortic arch, vena cava, and carotid sinus that sense changes in blood pressure *(19) / page 295*

benign (bee-NINE) neither life threatening nor fatal *(29) / page 468*

benign prostatic hypertrophy (BPH) (bee-NINE pros-TAT-ik hy-PURR-tro-fee) nonmalignant enlargement of the prostate gland *(35) / page 597*

benzodiazepines (ben-zo-di-AZ-eh-peenz) class of drugs used to treat anxiety and insomnia *(10) / page 129*

beta-lactam ring (bay-tuh LAK-tam) chemical structure found in most penicillins and some cephalosporins *(27) / page 427*

beta-lactamase/penicillinase (bay-tuh-LAK-tam-ace/pen-uh-SILL-in-ace) enzyme present in certain bacteria that is able to inactivate many penicillins and some cephalosporins *(27) / page 427*

beta (β)-receptor type of subreceptor found in the sympathetic nervous system *(9) / page 105*

bile acids (BEYE-ul) chemicals secreted in bile that aid in the digestion of fats *(17) / page 265*

bioavailability (BEYE-oh-ah-VALE-ah-BILL-ih-TEE) the ability of a drug to reach its target cells and produce its effect *(2) / page 18*

bioequivalence (BEYE-oh-ee-KWIV-oh-LENZ) the property wherein two drugs with identical active ingredients or two different dosage forms of the same drug possess similar bioavailability and produce the same effect at the site of physiological activity *(2) / page 18*

biologic response modifiers natural substances that are able to enhance or stimulate the immune system *(26) / page 412*

biologics (beye-oh-LOJ-iks) chemical agents that produce biological responses within the body; they are synthesized by cells of the human body, animal cells, or microorganisms *(1) / page 4*

biologic response modifiers (BEYE-oh-LAH- jick) biologic agents that block steps in the inflammatory cascade, reduce joint inflammation, and slow the progression of joint damage *(36) / page 616*

bioterrorism (beye-o-TEH-or-izm) the intentional use of infectious biologic agents, chemical substances, or radiation to cause widespread harm or illness *(1) / page 11*

biotransformation (BEYE-oh-trans-for-MAY-shun) the chemical conversion of drugs from one form to another that may result in increased or decreased activity *(4) / page 46*

bipolar disorder (bi-PO-ler) a disorder characterized by extreme and opposite feelings, such as euphoria and depression or calmness and rage; also called *manic depression (11) / page 152*

bisphosphonates (bis-FOSS-foh-nayts) family of drugs that block bone resorption by inhibiting osteoclast activity *(36) / page 611*

black box warning warning label surrounded by a black border and issued by the FDA to emphasize the important and serious life-threatening risks associated with use of the drug *(1, 10) / pages 7*

bone deposition the opposite of bone resorption; the process of depositing mineral components into bone *(36) / page 605*

bone resorption (ree-SORP-shun) process of bone demineralization or the breaking down of bone into mineral components *(36) / page 605*

boosters additional doses of a vaccine given months or years after the initial dose to increase the effectiveness of the vaccine *(26) / page 409*

bradycardia (bray-dee-KAR-DEE-ah) a condition of slow heartbeat *(19) / page 308*

bradykinin (bray-dee-KYE-nin) chemical mediator of pain released following tissue damage *(15) / page 233*

breakthrough bleeding bleeding at abnormal times during the menstrual cycle *(35) / page 592*

broad-spectrum antibiotic anti-infective that is effective against many different gram-positive and gram-negative organisms *(27) / page 426*

bronchi (BRON-ky) primary passageways of the bronchial tree that contain smooth muscle *(30) / page 492*

bronchioles (BRON-key-oles) very small bronchi that contain a considerable amount of smooth muscle that can make breathing easier by dilating, or more difficult by constricting *(30) / page 492*

bronchoconstriction (BRON-koh-kun-STRIK-shun) decrease in diameter of the airway due to contraction of bronchial smooth muscle *(30) / page 502*

bronchodilation (BRON-koh-dye-LAY-shun) increase in diameter of the airway due to relaxation of bronchial smooth muscle *(30) / page 504*

bronchospasm (bron-koh-SPAZ-um) rapid constriction of the airways *(30) / page 502*

buccal route (BUCK-ahl) the administration of medications by the cheek or mouth *(3) / page 32*

bundle branches (BUN-dul BRAN-chez) electrical conduction pathways in the heart leading from the AV bundle and through the wall between the ventricles *(23) / page 361*

C fibers nerves that transmit dull, poorly localized pain *(15) / page 223*

calcifediol (kal-SIF-eh-DYE-ol) intermediate form of vitamin D *(36) / page 605*

calcitonin (kal-sih-TOH-nin) treatment typically administered to women who cannot take estrogen or bisphosphonate therapy or for clients with Paget disease *(36) / page 605*

calcitriol (kal-si-TRY-ol) substance that is transformed in the kidneys during the second step of the conversion of vitamin D to its active form *(36) / page 605*

calcium channel blockers (CCBs) drugs that block the flow of calcium ions into myocardial cells *(19) / page 304*

calcium ion channels (KAL-see-um) pathways in a plasma membrane that allows calcium ions to enter the cell during an action potential *(23) / page 362*

cancer (KAN-sir) malignant disease characterized by rapidly growing, invasive cells that spread to other regions of the body and eventually kill the host *(29) / page 468*

capsid (CAP-sid) protein coat that surrounds a virus *(28) / page 452*

carbonic anhydrase (kar-BON-ik an-HY-drase) enzyme that forms carbonic acid by combining carbon dioxide and water *(18) / page 282*

carcinogens (kar-SIN-oh-jenz) any physical, chemical, or biological factors that cause or promote cancer *(29) / page 469*

cardiac output amount of blood pumped by each ventricle in 1 minute *(19) / page 295*

cardiogenic shock (kar-dee-oh-JEN-ik) type of shock caused when the heart is diseased such that it cannot maintain circulation to the tissues *(22) / page 347*

cathartic (kah-THAR-tik) drug that causes complete evacuation of the bowel *(31) / page 525*

chemical name strict chemical nomenclature used for naming drugs established by the International Union of Pure and Applied Chemistry (IUPAC) *(2) / page 16*

chemoprophylaxis (kee-moh-pro-fill-AX-is) use of a drug to prevent an infection *(27) / page 426*

chemotherapy drug treatment of cancer *(29) / page 469*

cholecalciferol (KOH-lee-kal-SIF-er-ol) inactive form of vitamin D *(36) / page 605*

cholinergic (kol-in-UR-jik) a term relating to nerves that release acetylcholine *(9) / page 104*

cholinergic blockers drugs that block the actions of the parasympathetic nervous system *(9) / page 105*

cholinergic drugs another name for parasympathomimetic drugs *(9) / page 105*

chronic bronchitis (KRON-ik bron-KEYE-tis) chronic disease of the lungs characterized by excess mucus production and inflammation *(30) / page 509*

clinical depression a major depressive disorder comprising a depressed affect plus at least five of the common symptoms lasting for a minimum of 2 weeks *(11) / page 141*

clinical pharmacology an area of medicine devoted to the evaluation of drugs used for human therapeutic benefit *(1) / page 9*

closed-angle glaucoma (glaw-KOH-mah) called acute glaucoma, this type of glaucoma is caused by the iris blocking trabecular meshwork, hindering outflow of aqueous fluid *(38) / page 642*

closed comedones (KOME-eh-dones) commonly called whiteheads, this type of acne develops just beneath the surface of the skin *(37) / page 630*

clotting factors substances contributing to the process of blood clotting *(24) / page 376*

club drugs substances taken at dance clubs, all-night parties, and raves *(8) / page 83*

CNS depressants (dee-PRESS-ahnts) drugs that lower neuronal activity within the CNS *(10) / page 126*

coagulation (co-ag-you-LAY-shun) the process of blood clotting *(24) / page 376*

coagulation cascade (cass-KADE) a complex series of steps by which blood flow stops *(24) / page 376*

cognitive symptoms cognitive symptoms of schizophrenic patients include poor ability to pay attention, make decisions, and understand information; and problems applying information once learning has occurred *(12) / page 163*

colloids (KO-loyds) type of IV fluid replacement solution consisting of large protein molecules that are unable to cross membranes *(22) / page 350*

combination drugs drug products with more than one active generic ingredient *(2) / page 17*

complementary and alternative medicine (CAM) therapies an extremely diverse set of therapies and healing systems that are considered to be outside of mainstream healthcare *(1, 7) / pages 4, 72*

compliance (kom-PLY-ans) taking a medication in the way it was prescribed by the practitioner; in the case of OTC drugs, following the instructions found on the label *(3) / page 26*

constipation (kon-stah-PAY-shun) infrequent passage of abnormally hard and dry stools *(31) / page 524*

contractility (kon-trak-TILL-eh-tee) the strength by which the myocardial fibers contract *(20) / page 316*

contraindications (CON-trah-EN-deh-KAY-shuns) situations under which drugs should not be used *(3) / page 24*

controlled substance in the United States, a drug restricted by the Comprehensive Drug Abuse Prevention and Control Act *(2) / page 20*

convulsions (kon-VULL-shuns) uncontrolled muscle contractions or spasms that occur in the face, torso, arms, or legs *(14) / page 204*

coronary arteries (KOR-un-air-ee AR-tur-ees) vessels that bring oxygen and nutrients to the myocardium *(21) / page 329*

corpora cavernosa (KORP-us kav-ver-NOH-sum) tissues in the penis that fill with blood during an erection *(35) / page 596*

corpus luteum (KORP-us LUTE-ee-uhm) temporary hormone-secreting gland in women that is formed when a follicle releases its oocyte *(35) / page 585*

corticosteroids (KORT-ik-ko-STARE-oyds) class of hormones secreted by the outer cortex of the adrenal glands *(33) / page 560*

cretinism (KREE-ten-izm) dwarfism and mental retardation caused by lack of thyroid hormone during infancy *(33) / page 556*

Crohn disease (KROHN) chronic inflammatory bowel disease affecting the ileum and sometimes the colon *(31) / page 519*

cross-tolerance (krause TOL-er-ans) the process of adapting to a new drug as a result of having already been exposed to a related drug *(8) / page 87*

crystalloids (KRIS-tuh-loyds) type of IV fluid replacement solution that resembles blood plasma and is capable of crossing membranes *(22) / page 350*

culture and sensitivity (C&S) testing laboratory test used to identify bacteria and to determine which antibiotic is most effective *(27) / page 426*

Cushing syndrome (KUSH-ing) condition caused by excessive corticosteroid secretion by the adrenal glands or by overdosage with corticosteroid medication *(25, 33) / pages 401, 562*

cyclooxygenase (COX) (sye-klo-OK-sah-jen-ays) key enzyme in the prostaglandin metabolic pathway that is blocked by aspirin and other NSAIDs *(15, 25) / pages 233, 397*

cycloplegia (sy-kloh-PLEE-jee-ah) blurred vision *(38) / page 643*

cycloplegic drugs (sy-kloh-PLEE-jik) drugs that relax or temporarily paralyze ciliary muscles *(38) / page 647*

cytokines (SYE-toh-kines) chemicals produced by white blood cells, such as interleukins, leukotrienes, interferon, and tumor necrosis factor, that guide the immune response *(26) / page 408*

cytotoxic T cell type of lymphocyte that directly attacks and destroys antigens *(26) / page 409*

data collection the systematic collection, organization, validation, and documentation of patient data *(5) / page 56*

deep vein thrombosis (DVT) a condition in which thrombi in the venous system form in the veins of the legs due to sluggish blood flow *(24) / page 377*

defecation (def-ah-KAY-shun) evacuation of the colon; bowel movement *(31) / page 525*

delirium (dee-LEAR-ee-um) erratic behavior involving hallucinations *(12) / page 165*

delta 9-tetrahydrocannabinol (THC) (TEH-trah-HEYE-droh-cah-NAB-in-ol) the active chemical in marijuana *(8) / page 90*

dementia (dee-MEN-she-ah) degenerative disorder characterized by progressive memory loss, confusion, and the inability to think or communicate effectively *(12) / page 165*

depolarization (dee-po-lur-eye-ZAY-shun) condition in which the plasma membrane charge is changed such that the inside is made less negative *(23) / page 362*

depression (dee-PRESS-shun) an emotional disorder characterized by many symptoms, including changes in sleeping, eating, and daily activities, and persistent mood changes such as feeling constant sadness, shame, and, guilt *(11) / page 140*

dermatitis (dur-mah-TIE-tiss) inflammatory condition of the skin characterized by itching and scaling *(37) / page 140*

designer drugs (de-ZEYE-ner drugs) drugs that are produced in a laboratory and are intended to mimic the effects of other psychoactive controlled substances *(8) / page 83*

diabetes insipidus (die-uh-BEE-tees in-SIP-uh-dus) excessive urination due to lack of secretion of antidiuretic hormone *(33) / page 555*

diabetic ketoacidosis (DKA) potentially life-threatening condition of patients with diabetes mellitus caused by acidosis and the uncontrolled accumulation of ketones bodies *(34) / page 572*

diarrhea abnormal frequency and liquidity of bowel movements *(31) / page 527*

diastolic pressure (DEYE-ah-stall-ik) blood pressure during the relaxation phase of heart activity *(19) / page 293*

dietary fiber substance neither digested nor absorbed that contributes to the fecal mass *(31) / page 525*

Dietary Supplement and Nonprescription Drug Consumer Protection Act law that requires companies that market herbal and dietary supplements to include their address and phone number on the product labels so consumers can report adverse events *(7) / page 79*

Dietary Supplement Health and Education Act (DSHEA) of 1994 primary law in the United States regulating herb and dietary supplements *(7) / page 78*

dietary supplements nondrug substances regulated by the DSHEA *(7) / page 72*

digestion (dye-JES-chun) process by which the body breaks down ingested food into small molecules that can be absorbed *(31) / page 516*

directly observed therapy (DOT) treatment protocol by which a healthcare worker or other trained individual administers the medications and watches the patient swallow the dose to ensure that the medication is taken exactly as prescribed to decrease the risk for relapse, the spread of the infection in the community, and the development of drug resistance that could result from erratic or partial treatment *(27) / page 442*

disease-modifying antirheumatic (ANTY-roo-MATIK) drugs (DMARDs) drugs that reduce destruction of the joints and progression of rheumatoid arthritis *(36) / page 615*

disruptive mood dysregulation disorder (dis-REG-you-lay-shun) characterized in children by severe and recurrent temper tantrums that exceed conditions warranted by the situation *(11) / page 141*

distribution (dis-tree-BU-shun) the process of transporting drugs through the body *(4) / page 45*

diuretic (deye-your-ET-ik) drug that increases urine flow *(18) / page 277*

drug abuse the recurrent use of legal or illegal drugs, or the improper use of prescription or over-the-counter drugs with negative consequences *(8) / page 83*

drug misuse the use of a drug for purposes for which it was not intended or using a drug in excessive quantities *(8) / page 83*

dry powder inhaler (DPI) device used to convert a solid drug to a fine powder for the purpose of inhalation *(30) / page 493*

duration of drug action the amount of time it takes for a drug to maintain its desired effect *(4) / page 49*

dwarfism below normal height caused by a deficiency in thyroid hormone or growth hormone *(33) / page 555*

dysentery (DISS-en-tare-ee) severe diarrhea that may include bleeding *(28) / page 460*

dysfunctional uterine bleeding hemorrhage that occurs at abnormal times or in abnormal quantities during the menstrual cycle *(35) / page 592*

dyslipidemia (dys-lip-i-DEEM-ee-uh) an abnormal amount of lipid in the blood *(17) / page 259*

dyspnea shortness of breath *(30) / page 503*

dysrhythmias (diss-RITH-mee-uhz) abnormalities in cardiac rhythm *(23) / page 359*

dysthymic disorder (dis-THEYE-mick) a chronic condition persisting for at least 2 years that is characterized by moderate depressive symptoms of an unknown origin that prevents a person from feeling happiness or functioning normally *(11) / page 141*

dystonia (diss-TONE-ee-ah) muscle spasm characterized by rigidity and abnormal, occasionally painful, movements or postures *(13) / page 194*

eclampsia (ee-KLAMP-see-uh) condition in which seizures and/or a coma develop in a patient with preeclampsia *(14) / page 209*

ectopic foci/pacemakers (ek-TOP-ik FO-si) cardiac tissue outside the normal cardiac conduction pathway that generates action potentials *(23) / page 361*

eczema (ECK-zih-mah) also called *atopic* dermatitis, a skin disorder with unexplained symptoms of inflammation, itching, and scaling *(37) / page 632*

efficacy (EFF-ik-ah-see) the effectiveness of a drug in producing a more intense response as its concentration is increased *(4) / page 51*

electrocardiogram (ECG) (e-lek-tro-KAR-dee-oh-gram) device that records the electrical activity of the heart *(23) / page 361*

electrolytes (ee-LEK-troh-lites) charged substances in the blood, such as sodium, potassium, calcium, chloride, and phosphate *(18) / page 284*

embolus (EM-boh-luss) a blood clot carried in the bloodstream *(24) / page 377*

emesis (EM-eh-sis) vomiting *(31) / page 528*

emetics (ee-MET-ikz) drugs used to induce vomiting *(31) / page 529*

emollients drugs employed to soothe psoriasis symptoms *(37) / page 634*

emphysema (em-fuss-EE-muh) terminal lung disease characterized by dilation of the alveoli *(30) / page 509*

endogenous opioids (en-DAHJ-en-nuss O-pee-oyds) chemicals produced naturally within the body that decrease or eliminate pain; they closely resemble the actions of morphine *(15) / page 224*

endometrial carcinoma (en-doh-MEE-tree-ahl CAR-sin-OH-mah) cancer of the endometrium *(35) / page 592*

endometriosis (en-doh-MEE-tree-oh-sis) abnormal location of endometrial tissues *(35) / page 592*

end-stage renal disease (ESRD) when the kidneys are no longer able to function at a level necessary for day-to-day living, and dialysis and kidney transplantation become treatment alternatives *(18) / page 277*

enteral nutrition treatment of undernutrition by the oral route or through a feeding tube *(32) / page 543*

enteral route (EN-tur-ul) the major route by which drugs enter the body through the digestive tract *(3) / page 31*

enteric-coated (in-TARE-ik) hard, waxy coating that enables drugs to resist the acidity of the stomach; enables drugs to dissolve in the small intestine *(3) / page 31*

enterohepatic recirculation (EN-ter-oh-HEE-pah-tik) recycling of drugs and other substances by the circulation of bile through the intestine and liver *(4) / page 48*

epilepsy (EPP-ih-lepp-see) condition characterized by two or more recurrent seizures that have not been provoked by specific events such as trauma, infection, fever, or chemical change *(14) / page 204*

epinephrine (EH-pin-NEF-rin) neurotransmitter or medication that activates the sympathetic nervous system *(9) / page 104*

erythema (ear-ih-THEE-mah) redness associated with skin irritation *(37) / page 625*

erythropoietin (ee-rith-ro-po-EE-tin) hormone secreted by the kidney that stimulates red blood cell production *(18) / page 277*

esters (ES-turs) type of chemical linkage found in some local anesthetics involving carbon and oxygen (—CO—O—) *(16) / page 245*

estrogen (ES-troh-jen) class of steroid sex hormones produced by the ovary *(35) / page 586*

etiologies (e-tee-OL-o-gees) causes of the patient's disease or condition *(5) / page 57*

evaluation criteria objective assessment of the effectiveness and impact of interventions *(5) / page 58*

evaluation phase part of the nursing process that provides an objective assessment of the effectiveness of the interventions *(5) / page 61*

excretion (eks-KREE-shun) the process of removing substances from the body *(4) / page 47*

expectorants (eks-PEK-tor-ent) drugs used to increase bronchial secretions *(30) / page 502*

external otitis (oh-TYE-tiss) commonly called swimmer's ear, this is inflammation of the outer ear *(38) / page 648*

extrapyramidal symptoms (EPS) (peh-RAM-ed-el) symptoms where muscles become very rigid because of overmedication with antipsychotics or by lack of dopamine function in the corpus striatum *(12) / page 167*

false neurotransmitter (NYUR-oh-TRANS-mitt-ur) chemical that simulates a natural neurotransmitter but does not produce the same physiologic effect *(19) / page 308*

febrile seizures abnormal states of neuronal discharge resulting from high fever *(14) / page 205*

fibrillation (fi-bruh-LAY-shun) type of dysrhythmia in which the chambers beat in a highly disorganized manner *(23) / page 359*

fibrin (FEYE-brin) an insoluble protein formed from fibrinogen by the action of thrombin in the blood-clotting process *(24) / page 376*

fibrinogen (feye-BRIN-oh-jen) blood protein converted to fibrin by the action of thrombin in the blood-clotting process *(24) / page 376*

fibrinolysis (feye-brin-OL-oh-sis) removal of a blood clot *(24) / page 377*

filtrate (FIL-trate) fluid in the nephron that is filtered at Bowman's capsule *(18) / page 274*

first-pass effect a mechanism whereby drugs are absorbed across the intestinal wall and enter into blood vessels, known as the hepatic portal circulation, which carries blood directly to the liver *(4) / page 47*

folic acid (foh-lik) B vitamin that is a coenzyme in protein and nucleic acid metabolism; also known as *folate (29) / page 475*

follicle-stimulating hormone (FSH) hormone secreted by the pituitary gland that regulates sperm or egg production *(35) / page 585*

follicular cells (fo-LIK-yu-lur) cells in the thyroid gland that secrete thyroid hormone *(33) / page 556*

formularies (FOR-mew-LEH-reez) lists of drugs and drug recipes commonly used by pharmacists *(1) / page 5*

fungi (FUN-jeye) kingdom of organisms that includes mushrooms, yeasts, and molds *(28) / page 447*

ganglia (GANG-lee-ah) collections of neuron cell bodies located outside the CNS *(9) / page 104*

gastroesophageal reflux disease (GERD) (GAS-troh-ee-SOF-ah-JEEL REE-flux) the regurgitation of stomach contents into the esophagus *(31) / page 518*

general anesthesia medical procedure that causes gradual loss of consciousness accompanied by loss of sensation to the entire body *(16) / page 243*

generalized anxiety disorder (GAD) difficult-to-control, excessive anxiety that lasts 6 months or more *(10) / page 122*

generalized seizures seizures that travel throughout the entire brain on both sides *(14) / page 206*

generic name (je-NARE-ik) nonproprietary name of a drug assigned by the government *(2) / page 16*

glaucoma (glaw-CO-muh) an eye disease that is characterized by gradual changes in peripheral vision, possibly advancing to blindness *(38) / page 641*

gliomas (glee-OH-muhz) malignant tumors of the brain *(29) / page 468*

glucagon (GLUE-kah-gon) pancreatic hormone that increases blood sugar *(34) / page 570*

glucocorticoids (glu-ko-KORT-ik-oydz) type of hormone secreted by the outer portion of the adrenal gland that includes cortisol *(33) / page 561*

glycoprotein IIb/IIIa (GLEYE-koh-proh-teen) enzyme responsible for platelet aggregation *(24) / page 384*

goal an objective that the patient or nurse seeks to attain or achieve *(5) / page 58*

gonadocorticoids (go-NAD-oh-KORT-ikoyds) hormones secreted by the adrenal cortex; they are mostly androgens (male sex hormones), though small amounts of estrogens (female sex hormones) are produced *(33) / page 562*

gonadotropin releasing hormone (GnRH) (go-NAD-oh-TROPE-en) hormone secreted by the hypothalamus that travels to the pituitary gland to stimulate the secretion of follicle-stimulating hormone *(35) / page 585*

gout (GOWT) metabolic disorder characterized by the accumulation of uric acid in the bloodstream or joint cavities *(36) / page 617*

Graves disease syndrome caused by hypersecretion of thyroid hormone *(33) / page 557*

H^+, K^+-ATPase enzyme responsible for pumping acid onto the mucosal surface of the stomach *(31) / page 519*

H_1-receptor blocker drug that blocks the effects of histamine in smooth muscle in the bronchial tree *(30) / page 496*

H_2-receptor blocker drug that inhibits the effects of histamine at its receptors in the GI tract *(31) / page 521*

half-life ($t_{1/2}$) the length of time required for a drug to decrease its concentration in the plasma by one-half of the original amount *(4) / page 49*

healthcare-associated infections (HAIs) infections acquired in a healthcare setting such as a hospital, physician's office, or nursing home *(27) / page 425*

heart failure (HF) disease in which the heart muscle cannot contract with sufficient force to meet the body's metabolic needs *(20) / page 315*

***Helicobacter pylori* (hee-lick-oh-BAK-tur py-LOR-eye)** bacterium associated with a large percentage of peptic ulcer disease *(31) / page 518*

helminths (HELL-minth) type of flat, round, or segmented worms *(28) / page 460*

helper T cell type of lymphocyte that coordinates both the humoral and cell-mediated immune responses and that is the target of the human immunodeficiency virus *(26) / page 409*

hematopoiesis (hee-mato-po-EE-sis) the process of blood cell production *(24) / page 387*

hemorrhagic stroke (hee-moh-RAJ-ik) type of stroke caused by bleeding from a blood vessel in the brain *(21) / page 341*

hemostasis (hee-moh-STAY-sis) the slowing or stopping of blood flow *(24) / page 375*

hemostatics (hee-moh-STAT-iks) drugs used to prevent and treat excessive bleeding from surgical sites *(24) / page 378*

herb a plant with a soft stem that is used in healing or as a seasoning *(7) / page 73*

high-density lipoprotein (HDL) lipid-carrying particle in the blood that contains high amounts of protein and lower amounts of cholesterol; considered to be "good" cholesterol *(17) / page 260*

highly active antiretroviral therapy (HAART) type of drug therapy for HIV infection that includes high doses of multiple medications that are given together *(28) / page 454*

histamine (HISS-tuh-meen) chemical released by mast cells in response to an antigen; causes dilation of blood vessels, smooth muscle constriction, tissue swelling, and itching *(25) / page 396*

HMG-CoA reductase (ree-DUCK-tase) primary enzyme in the biochemical pathway for the synthesis of cholesterol *(17) / page 262*

hormone replacement therapy (HRT) treatment for menopausal symptoms and to prevent long-term consequences of estrogen loss that provides doses of estrogen, sometimes combined with a progestin *(35) / page 591*

hormones chemicals secreted by endocrine glands that act as chemical messengers to affect homeostasis *(33) / page 551*

host an organism that is being infected by a microbe *(28) / page 452*

host flora (host FLOR-uh) normal microorganisms found in or on a patient *(27) / page 426*

household system older system of measurement involving teaspoons, tablespoons, cups, drops, pounds, etc. *(3) / page 29*

humoral immunity (HYOU-mor-ul eh-MEWN-uh-tee) a specific body defense mechanism involving the production and release of antibodies *(26) / page 408*

hypercholesterolemia (HEYE-purr-koh-LESS-tur-ol-EEM-ee-uh) high levels of cholesterol in the blood *(17) / page 260*

hyperglycemic effect (hi-pur-gli-SEEM-ik) describes the action of lowering blood sugar *(34) / page 571*

hyperkalemia (heye-purr-kah-LEE-mee-ah) dangerously high potassium levels in the blood *(18) / page 281*

hyperlipidemia (HEYE-purr-LIP-id-EEM-ee-uh) excess amounts of lipids in the blood *(17) / page 259*

hypernatremia high sodium level in the blood *(18) / page 284*

hypertension (HTN) (heye-purr-TEN-shun) high blood pressure *(19) / page 292*

hypertriglyceridemia (HEYE-purr-tri-gliss-ur-i-DEEM-ee-uh) elevated triglycerides *(17) / page 260*

hypervitaminosis excess intake of vitamins *(32) / page 538*

hypoglycemic effect (hi-po-gli-SEEM-ik) describes the action of increasing blood sugar *(34) / page 570*

hypogonadism (hi-poh-GO-nad-izm) below normal secretion of the steroid sex hormones *(35) / page 595*

hypokalemia (hi-poh-kah-LEE-mee-ah) low potassium levels in the blood *(18) / page 279*

hyponatremia (hi-po-nay-TREE-mee-uh) low levels of sodium in the blood *(18) / page 285*

hypothalamus (hi-po-THAL-ih-mus) region of the brain that triggers unconscious responses to extreme stress, such as increased blood pressure, elevated breathing rate, and dilated pupils *(10, 33) / pages 124, 551*

hypovolemic shock (hi-poh-voh-LEEM-ik) type of shock caused by loss of fluids such as that which occurs during hemorrhaging, extensive burns, or severe vomiting or diarrhea *(22) / page 347*

immune response adaptive response to defend the body against a particular threat *(26) / page 408*

immunization (IH-mewn-ize-AYE-shun) the process of introducing a foreign substance (a vaccine) into the body to trigger immune activation *before* the patient is exposed to the real pathogen *(26) / page 409*

immunoglobulin (Ig) (ih-MEW-noh-GLOB-you-lin) protein produced by the body in response to an antigen; used interchangeably with the term *antibody (26) / page 408*

immunomodulator (ih-mew-no-MOF-you-layter) a general term referring to any drug that affects body defenses *(26) / page 407*

immunosuppressants (ih-MEW-noh-suh-PRESS-ents) any drug, chemical, or physical agent that lowers the natural immune defense mechanisms of the body *(26) / page 413*

implementation phase part of the nursing process during which the nurse carries out activities that assist in accomplishing established goals *(5) / page 60*

impotence (IM-poh-tense) inability to obtain or sustain an erection; also called erectile dysfunction *(35) / page 596*

incretin enhancers (in KREE tin) the dipeptidyl peptidase-4 (DPP-4) inhibitors that prevent the breakdown of natural incretins, allowing the hormone levels to rise and produce a greater response *(34) / page 578*

incretin mimetics injectable drugs that mimic the effects of incretins *(34) / page 577*

incretins hormones secreted by the intestines in response to a meal when blood glucose is elevated *(34) / page 577*

inflammation (IN-flah-MAY-shun) nonspecific body defense that occurs in response to an injury or antigen *(25) / page 395*

inflammatory bowel disease (IBD) diseases with ulceration of the intestine, including Crohn disease and ulcerative colitis, characterized by abdominal cramping, diarrhea, and weight loss *(31) / page 519*

influenza (in-flew-EN-zah) common viral infection of the respiratory system; often called *flu (28) / page 459*

innate body defenses first line of protection from pathogens that serve as general barriers to microbes or environmental hazards *(26) / page 407*

inotropic drug (eye-noh-TROW-pik) medication that changes the force of contraction of the heart *(22) / page 407*

inotropic effect (in-oh-TRO-pik) change in the strength or contractility of the heart *(20) / page 317*

insomnia (in-SOM-nee-uh) the inability to fall asleep or stay asleep *(10) / page 125*

insulin (IN-sule-in) pancreatic hormone that decreases blood sugar levels *(34) / page 570*

insulin analogs (ANNAH-logs) recombinant human DNA insulins that have been modified to have rapid or prolonged durations *(34) / page 572*

insulin resistance phenomena in which target tissues have become unresponsive to insulin *(34) / page 576*

integrative healthcare applying both conventional and complementary approaches to healing the patient *(7) / page 72*

international normalized ratio (INR) laboratory value used to monitor the degree of blood anticoagulation during warfarin therapy *(24) / page 381*

interventions actions that produce an effect or that is intended to alter the course of a disease or condition *(5) / page 57*

intracellular parasites infectious microbes that live inside host cells *(28) / page 452*

intradermal (ID) route (IN-trah-DERM-ul) method of parenteral drug delivery in which drugs are injected into the dermis of the skin *(3) / page 37*

intramuscular (IM) route (IN-trah-musk-u-lar) method of parenteral drug delivery in which drugs are injected into layers of muscle beneath the skin *(3) / page 39*

intravenous (IV) route (IN-trah-VEE-nus) method of parenteral drug delivery in which drugs are injected into the venous circulation *(3) / page 40*

intrinsic factor chemical secreted by the stomach that is required for absorption of vitamin B_{12} *(32) / page 538*

islets of Langerhans (EYE-lits of LANG-gur-hans) clusters of cells in the pancreas responsible for the secretion of insulin and glucagon; also called the pancreatic islets *(34) / page 570*

keratinization (keh-RAT-en-eye-zay-shun) development of the stratum corneum or horny layer of epithelial tissue *(37) / page 630*

keratolytic agents (keh-RAT-oh-lih-tik) drugs used to promote shedding of old skin *(37) / page 631*

ketoacids (KEY-to-ass-ids) waste products of fat metabolism that lower the pH of the blood *(34) / page 572*

leukemia (lew-KEE-mee-ah) cancer of the blood characterized by overproduction of white blood cells *(29) / page 468*

libido (lih-BEE-do) interest in sexual activity *(35) / page 595*

limbic system (LIM-bik) area in the brain responsible for emotion, learning, memory, motivation, and mood *(10) / page 123*

lipomas (lip-OH-mahs) benign tumors of fat tissue *(29) / page 468*

lipoproteins (LIP-oh-PROH-teenz) substances carrying lipids in the bloodstream *(17) / page 260*

liposomes (LIP-oh-sohms) small sacs of lipids designed to carry drugs inside them *(29) / page 477*

local anesthesia loss of sensation to a relatively small part of the body without loss of consciousness *(16) / page 243*

low-density lipoprotein (LDL) lipid-carrying particle that contains lower amounts of protein and high amounts of cholesterol; considered to be "bad" cholesterol *(17) / page 260*

low molecular weight heparins (LMWHs) heparin-like drugs that inhibit blood clotting *(24) / page 379*

lumen (LOO-men) the cavity or channel of a hollow tube such as a blood vessel *(19) / page 295*

luteinizing hormone (LH) (LEW-ten-iz-ing) hormone secreted by the pituitary gland that triggers ovulation in the female and stimulates sperm production in the male *(35) / page 585*

lymphomas (lim-FOH-mahz) cancer of lymphatic tissue *(29) / page 468*

macrominerals (major minerals) inorganic compounds needed by the body in amounts of 100 mg or more daily *(32) / page 539*

major depressive disorder a disorder characterized by at least five symptoms of depression *(11) / page 141*

malaria (mah-LARE-ee-ah) tropical disease characterized by severe fever and chills; caused by the protozoan *Plasmodium* *(28) / page 460*

malignant (mah-LIG-nent) life threatening or fatal *(29) / page 468*

mast cells connective tissue cells located in tissue spaces that release histamine following injury *(25) / page 396*

mastoiditis (mass-toy-DYE-tuss) inflammation of the mastoid sinus *(38) / page 468*

mechanism of action how a drug exerts its effects *(2) / page 15*

medication error any preventable event that may cause or lead to inappropriate medication use or patient harm while the medication is in the control of the healthcare professional, patient, or consumer *(6) / page 64*

medication error index places medication errors into nine categories based on the extent of the harm an error can cause *(6) / page 65*

medications substances designed to prevent or treat diseases *(1) / page 4*

megaloblastic anemia condition caused by a deficiency of vitamin B_{12} *(32) / page 538*

menopause (MEN-oh-paws) time when females stop secreting estrogen and menstrual cycles cease *(35) / page 591*

menorrhagia (men-oh-RAGE-ee-uh) prolonged or excessive menstruation *(35) / page 592*

metabolic bone disorders (meh-tuh-BAHL-ik) skeletal disorders such as osteomalacia, osteoporosis, and Paget disease *(36) / page 605*

metabolism (meh-TAHB-oh-liz-ehm) the sum total of all chemical reactions in the body or an organ (e.g., the liver) *(4) / page 46*

metastasis (mah-TAS-tah-sis) travel of cancer cells from their original site to a distant tissue *(29) / page 468*

metered-dose inhalers (MDIs) devices used to deliver a precise amount of drug to the respiratory system *(30) / page 493*

metric system the most common system of measurement; involves kilograms (kg), grams (g), milligrams (mg), micrograms (mcg), and so on *(3) / page 28*

microminerals (trace minerals) inorganic compounds needed by the body in amounts of 20 mg or less daily *(32) / page 539*

migraine (MYE-grayne) severe headache preceded by auras that may include nausea and vomiting *(15) / page 235*

mineralocorticoid (min-ur-al-oh-KORT-ik-oyd) hormone involved in the regulation of fluid and electrolytes by its effects in the kidney *(33) / page 561*

minimum effective concentration the amount of drug required to produce a therapeutic effect *(4) / page 49*

miosis (my-OH-sis) constriction of the pupil *(38) / page 642*

monoamine oxidase inhibitors (MAOIs) (mon-oh-AHM een OK-se-daze) drugs inhibiting monoamine oxidase, an enzyme that terminates the actions of neurotransmitters such as dopamine, norepinephrine, epinephrine, and serotonin *(11) / page 148*

mood stabilizers drugs that level mood to treat bipolar disorder and mania *(11) / page 152*

mucolytics drugs used to loosen thick mucus *(30) / page 502*

multiple sclerosis (MS) (skle-ROH-sis) autoimmune disorder of the central nervous system; a condition in which antibodies slowly destroy tissues in the brain and spinal cord *(13) / page 188*

muscarinic (MUS-kah-RIN-ik) type of cholinergic receptor found in smooth muscle, cardiac muscle, and glands *(9) / page 104*

mutations (myou-TAY-shuns) permanent, inheritable changes to DNA *(27) / page 424*

mycoses (my-KOH-sees) diseases caused by fungi *(28) / page 447*

mydriasis (mih-DRY-uh-siss) dilation of the pupil *(38) / page 642*

mydriatic drugs (mih-DRY-atik) drugs that dilate the pupils *(38) / page 647*

myocardial infarction (MI) (meye-oh-KAR-dee-ul in-FARK-shun) medical emergency in which a blood clot blocks a portion of a coronary artery *(21) / page 337*

myocardial ischemia (meye-oh-KAR-dee-ul ik-SKEE-mee-uh) condition in which there is a lack of blood supply to the myocardium due to a constriction or obstruction of a blood vessel *(21) / page 330*

myxedema (mix-uh-DEEM-uh) condition caused by insufficient secretion of thyroid hormone *(33) / page 557*

narcolepsy (NAR-koh-lep-see) condition characterized by uncontrolled daytime sleepiness *(8) / page 92*

narcotic (nar-KOT-ik) natural or synthetic drug related to morphine; may be used as a broader legal term referring to hallucinogens (LSD), CNS stimulants, marijuana, and other illegal drugs *(15) / page 225*

narrow-spectrum antibiotic anti-infective that is effective against only one or a small number of organisms *(27) / page 426*

natriuretic peptide (hBNP) (na-tree-ur-ET-ik) hormone that increases the urinary excretion of sodium and dilates blood vessels *(20) / page 323*

natural alternative therapies herbs, natural extracts, vitamins, minerals, or dietary supplements *(1) / page 4*

nebulizers (NEB-you-lyes-urz) devices used to convert liquid drugs into a fine mist for the purpose of inhalation *(30) / page 493*

negative feedback a common feature of endocrine gland homeostasis in which the last hormone or action in the pathway prevents the production and release of the first hormone *(33) / page 551*

negative symptoms symptoms that *subtract from* normal behavior; signs that are used to assist with the diagnosis of schizophrenia *(12) / page 163*

neoplasm (NEE-oh-PLAZ-um) same as *tumor*; an abnormal swelling or mass *(29) / page 468*

nephrons (NEF-ronz) functional units of the kidney *(18) / page 274*

nephrotoxicity (NEF-row-toks-ISS-ih-tee) an adverse effect on the kidneys *(27) / page 433*

neurogenic shock (nyoor-oh-JEN-ik) type of shock resulting from brain or spinal cord injury *(22) / page 347*

neuroleptanalgesia (new-row-lept-an-ul-JEE-zee-ah) a state produced by combining the opioid fentanyl (Sublimaze) with the antipsychotic agent droperidol (Inapsine) in which patients are conscious though insensitive to pain and unconnected with surroundings *(16) / page 249*

neuroleptic malignant syndrome (NMS) (noo-roh-LEP-tik) a potentially fatal condition caused by some antipsychotic medications; symptoms include an extremely high body temperature, drowsiness, changing blood pressure, irregular heartbeat, and muscle rigidity *(12) / page 166*

neuroleptics (noo-roh-LEP-ticks) drugs used to treat "nervous-type" conditions such as psychoses *(12) / page 165*

neuromuscular blockers anesthetics that cause paralysis without loss of consciousness *(16) / page 252*

neuromuscular blocking drugs (NEWR-oh-musc-you-lahr) drugs that bind to acetylcholine receptors, preventing contraction of skeletal muscle *(13) / page 197*

nicotinic (NIK-oh-TIN-ik) type of cholinergic receptor found in ganglia of both the sympathetic and parasympathetic nervous systems *(9) / page 104*

nitrogen mustards class of chemicals that are alkylating agents *(29) / page 473*

nociceptor (no-si-SEPP-ter) receptor connected with nerves that receive and transmit pain signals to the spinal cord and brain *(15) / page 223*

norepinephrine (nor-EH-pin-NEF-rin) primary neurotransmitter in the sympathetic nervous system *(9) / page 104*

nursing diagnosis clinically based judgment about the patient and his or her response to health and illness *(5) / page 57*

nursing process five-part decision-making system that includes assessment, nursing diagnosis, planning, implementation, and evaluation *(5) / page 56*

obsessive-compulsive disorder (OCD) anxiety characterized by recurrent, intrusive thoughts or repetitive behaviors that interfere with normal activities or relationships *(10) / page 122*

off-label use when a drug is being prescribed for a condition for which it is not FDA-approved *(1) / page 10*

oligomenorrhea (ol-ego-men-oh-REE-uh) infrequent menstruation *(35) / page 592*

onset of drug action the amount of time it takes to produce a therapeutic effect after drug administration *(4) / page 49*

open-angle glaucoma (glaw-KOH-mah) also called chronic simple glaucoma, this type of glaucoma is caused by congestion in trabecular meshwork, hindering outflow of aqueous fluid *(38) / page 642*

open comedones type of acne in which sebum has plugged the oil gland; commonly called blackheads *(37) / page 630*

opiates (OH-pee-ahts) natural substances extracted from the poppy plant *(15) / page 225*

opioid (OH-pee-oyd) natural or synthetic morphine-like substance obtained from the unripe seeds of the poppy plant *(8, 15) / pages 85, 225*

orally disintegrating tablets (ODTs) drug formulations that allow for quick dissolving and absorption of medications *(3) / page 31*

orthostatic hypotension (or-tho-STAT-ik) fall in blood pressure that occurs when someone changes position from recumbent to upright *(19) / page 146*

osteoarthritis (OA) (OSS-tee-oh-are-THRYE-tis) disorder characterized by degeneration of joints such as the fingers, spine, hips, and knees *(36) / page 614*

osteomalacia (OSS-tee-oh-muh-LAY-shee-uh) rickets in children; disease characterized by softening of the bones without alteration of basic bone structure *(36) / page 607*

osteoporosis (OSS-tee-oh-poh-ROH-sis) condition in which bones become brittle and susceptible to fracture *(36) / page 609*

otitis media (oh-TYE-tuss MEE-dee-ah) inflammation of the middle ear *(38) / page 648*

ototoxicity (OH-toh-toks-ISS-ih-tee) an adverse effect on hearing *(27) / page 433*

outcome objective measures of goals *(5) / page 58*

ovulation (ov-you-LAY-shun) release of an egg by the ovary *(35) / page 585*

oxytocics (ox-ee-TOH-sicz) drugs that *stimulate* uterine contractions to promote the induction of labor *(35) / page 594*

oxytocin (ox-ee-TOH-sin) hormone secreted by the pituitary gland that stimulates uterine contractions and milk ejection *(35) / page 594*

Paget disease (PAH-jets) disorder characterized by weak, enlarged, and abnormal bones *(36) / page 614*

palliation (PAL-ee-AYE-shun) form of chemotherapy intended to alleviate symptoms rather than cure the disease *(29) / page 470*

pancreatic insufficiency condition in which the pancreas is not secreting sufficient amounts of digestive enzymes, resulting in malabsorption syndromes *(31) / page 530*

pandemic (pan-DIM-ik) events or diseases of epidemic proportion that spread across human populations *(1) / page 11*

panic disorder anxiety characterized by intense feelings of immediate apprehension, fearfulness, terror, or impending doom *(10) / page 122*

papules (PAP-yools) inflammatory bumps without pus that swell, thicken, and become painful *(37) / page 631*

parafollicular cells (par-uh-fo-LIK-u-lur) cells in the thyroid gland that secrete calcitonin *(33) / page 556*

parasympathetic nervous system (PAIR-ah-SIM-pah THET-ik) portion of the autonomic system that is active during periods of rest and digestion *(9) / page 101*

parasympathomimetics (PAIR-ah-SIM-path-oh-mah-MET-iks) drugs that mimic the actions of the parasympathetic nervous system *(9) / page 105*

parenteral route (pah-REN-tur-ul) the major route by which drugs enter the body other than the enteral or topical route *(3) / page 36*

parkinsonism degenerative disorder of the nervous system caused by a deficiency of the brain neurotransmitter dopamine; this deficiency results in disturbances of muscle movement *(13) / page 180*

partial (focal) seizures seizures that start on one side of the brain and travel a short distance before stopping *(14) / page 206*

passive immunity administration of antibodies; provides short-term immunity *(26) / page 411*

pathogen (PATH-oh-jen) organism that is capable of causing disease *(27) / page 422*

pathogenicity (path-oh-jen-ISS-ih-tee) ability of an organism to cause disease in humans *(27) / page 423*

pathophysiology (PATH-oh-fiz-ee-OL-oh-jee) the study of diseases and the functional changes occurring in the body as a result of diseases *(1) / page 3*

patient-controlled analgesia (PCA) (an-ul-JEE-ziah) use of an infusion pump to deliver a prescribed amount of pain relief medication over a designated time *(15) / page 228*

peak plasma level when the medication has reached its highest concentration in the bloodstream *(4) / page 49*

pediculicides (puh-DIK-you-lih-sides) medications that kill lice *(37) / page 628*

peptic ulcer erosion of the mucosa in the alimentary canal, most commonly in the stomach and duodenum *(31) / page 517*

percutaneous coronary intervention (PCI) (per-cue-TAIN-ee-us) procedure in which a severely narrowed coronary artery is opened during cardiac catheterization *(21) / page 331*

perfusion (purr-FEW-shun) blood flow through a tissue or organ *(30) / page 492*

peripheral edema (purr-IF-ur-ul eh-DEE-mah) swelling in the limbs, particularly the feet and ankles, due to an accumulation of interstitial fluid *(20) / page 316*

peripheral resistance (per-IF-ur-ul) the amount of friction encountered by blood as it travels through the vessels *(19) / page 295*

peristalsis (pair-ih-STAL-sis) involuntary wavelike contraction that occurs in the alimentary canal *(31) / page 517*

pernicious anemia (pur-NISH-us ah-NEE-mee-ah) type of anemia usually caused by lack of secretion of intrinsic factor *(32) / page 538*

pH a measure of the acidity or alkalinity of a solution *(18) / page 286*

pharmaceutics (far-mah-SOO-tiks) the science of preparing and dispensing drugs *(1) / page 5*

pharmacodynamics (FAR-mah-koh-deye-NAM-iks) the study of how the body responds to drugs and natural substances *(4) / page 50*

pharmacokinetics (FAR-mah-koh-kee-NET) the study of what the body does to drugs *(4) / page 45*

pharmacologic classification (FAR-mah-koh-LOJ-ik) method for organizing drugs on the basis of their mechanism of action (how they work pharmacologically) *(2) / page 15*

pharmacology (far-mah-KOL-oh-jee) the study of medicines; the discipline pertaining to how drugs improve the health of the human body *(1) / page 3*

pharmacopoeia (far-mah-KOH-pee-ah) medical reference summary indicating standards of drug purity, strength, and directions for synthesis *(1) / page 6*

pharmacotherapeutics (far-mah-koh-THER-ah-PEW-tiks) treatment of diseases by the use of drugs *(1) / page 4*

pharmacy the preparation and dispensing of drugs *(1) / page 5*

phobias (FO-bee-ahs) fearful feelings attached to situations or objects *(10) / page 122*

phosphodiesterase (fos-fo-die-ES-tur-ase) enzyme in muscle cells that cleaves phosphodiester bonds; its inhibition increases myocardial contractility *(20) / page 324*

photosensitivity condition that occurs when the skin is very sensitive to sunlight *(27) / page 431*

physical dependence (FI-zi-kul dee-PEN-dens) the condition of experiencing unpleasant withdrawal symptoms when a substance is discontinued *(8) / page 85*

pituitary gland (pit-TOO-it-air-ee) endocrine gland in the brain responsible for controlling many other endocrine glands *(33) / page 551*

planning phase stage of the nursing process that links strategies or interventions to established goals and outcomes *(5) / page 58*

plaque (PLAK) fatty material that builds up in the lining of blood vessels and may lead to hypertension, stroke, myocardial infarction, or angina *(17, 21) / pages 259, 330*

plasma cells type of cells derived from B cells that produce antibodies *(26) / page 408*

plasmids (PLAZ-midz) small pieces of circular DNA found in some bacteria that are able to transfer resistance from one bacterium to another *(27) / page 424*

plasmin (PLAZ-min) enzyme formed from plasminogen that dissolves blood clots *(24) / page 377*

plasminogen (plaz-MIN-oh-jen) protein that prevents fibrin clot formation *(24) / page 377*

polarized (POLE-uh-rized) condition in which the inside of a cell is more negatively charged than the outside of the cell *(23) / page 362*

positive symptoms symptoms that *add on to* normal behavior; signs that are used to assist with the diagnosis of schizophrenia *(12) / page 163*

posterior pituitary area of the pituitary gland, also known as *neurohypophysis* *(33) / page 552*

postmenopausal bleeding (POST-men-oh-pause-ahl) hemorrhage following menopause *(35) / page 592*

postpartum depression depression experienced by a woman during the first several weeks after the birth of her baby *(11) / page 141*

post-traumatic stress disorder (PTSD) anxiety characterized by a sense of helplessness and the reexperiencing of a traumatic event, for example, war, physical or sexual abuse, natural disaster, or murder *(10) / page 123*

potassium ion channel (po-TASS-ee-um) pathway in a plasma membrane that allows potassium to leave the cell during an action potential *(23) / page 362*

potency (POH-ten-see) the power or strength of a drug at a specified concentration or dose *(4) / page 51*

preeclampsia (pree-ee-KLAMP-see-uh) condition in which hypertension develops because of pregnancy or recent pregnancy. Hypertension is accompanied by proteinuria and/or edema *(14) / page 209*

preload degree of stretch of the cardiac muscle fibers just before they contract *(20) / page 316*

premenstrual dysphoric disorder (dis-FOR-ick) a condition in which women express signs of irritability and tension before menstruation *(11) / page 141*

premenstrual syndrome (PMS) (PREE-men-stroo-ahl) symptoms develop during the luteal phase of the menstrual cycle *(35) / page 592*

prn order Latin *pro re nata*; physician's order; means "to administer as required by the patient's condition" *(3) / page 27*

prodrugs drugs that become more active after they are metabolized *(4) / page 47*

progesterone (pro-JESS-ter-own) hormone responsible for building up the uterine lining in the second half of the menstrual cycle and during pregnancy *(35) / page 586*

prolactin (pro-LAK-tin) hormone secreted by the pituitary gland that stimulates milk production in the mammary glands *(35) / page 594*

prostaglandins (pros-tah-GLAN-dins) chemicals released after tissue damage, leading to pain, inflammation, and other body reactions *(15, 35) / pages 233, 594*

prothrombin (PRO-throm-bin) blood protein converted to thrombin in the blood-clotting process *(24) / page 376*

prothrombin time (PT) blood test used to determine the time needed for plasma to clot, used to regulate warfarin dosage *(24) / page 381*

proton-pump inhibitors (PPIs) drugs that inhibit the enzyme H^+, K^+-ATPase *(31) / page 519*

prototype drug (PRO-toh-type) an original, well-understood drug model from which other drugs in a pharmacologic class have been developed *(2) / page 16*

protozoans (PRO-toh-ZOH-en) single-celled microorganisms *(28) / page 460*

provitamins inactive chemicals that are converted to a vitamin in the body *(32) / page 536*

pruritus (proo-RYE-tus) itching associated with dry, scaly skin *(37) / page 625*

pseudoseizures (SU-do-SEE-zhurrs) paroxysmal (sharp recurrent) episodes that resemble and are often misdiagnosed as epileptic seizures; also called psychogenic nonepileptic seizures (PNES) *(14) / page 205*

psoralens (SOR-uh-lenz) drugs used along with phototherapy for the treatment of psoriasis and other severe skin disorders *(37) / page 634*

psoriasis chronic, noninfectious inflammatory skin disorder that is characterized by red patches of skin covered with flaky, silver-colored scales called *plaques (37) / page 634*

psychedelics (seye-keh-DEL-iks) substances that alter perception and reality *(8) / page 91*

psychological dependence (seye-koh-LOJ-i-kul dee-PEN-dens) an unpleasant, intense craving for a drug after it has been withdrawn *(8) / page 85*

psychotic depression condition characterized by the expression of mood shifts and unusual behaviors. Intense behaviors include hallucinations, combativeness, and disorganized speech patterns *(11) / page 141*

purines (PYUR-eenz) building blocks of DNA and RNA, either adenine or guanine *(29) / page 476*

Purkinje fibers (purr-KEN-gee FI-burrs) electrical conduction pathway leading from the bundle branches to all portions of the ventricles *(23) / page 361*

pustules (PUSS-chools) inflammatory bumps with pus *(37) / page 631*

pyrimidines (peer-IM-uh-deen) building blocks of DNA and RNA, either thymine or cytosine in DNA, and cytosine and uracil in RNA *(29) / page 476*

reabsorption movement of substances from the kidney tubule back into the blood *(18) / page 276*

rebound congestion a condition of hypersecretion of mucus following use of intranasal sympathomimetics *(30) / page 500*

rebound insomnia increased sleeplessness that occurs when long-term antianxiety or hypnotic medication is discontinued *(10) / page 125*

receptor (ree-SEP-tor) the structural component of a cell to which a drug binds in a dose-related manner to produce a response *(4) / page 50*

receptor theory a cellular mechanism by which most drugs produce their effects *(4) / page 50*

recommended dietary allowance (RDA) amount of vitamin or mineral needed daily to avoid a deficiency in a healthy adult *(32) / page 537*

red man syndrome flushing, hypotension, itching, and rash on the upper body caused by certain anti-infectives *(27) / page 436*

reflex tachycardia (ta-kee-CAR-dee-ah) temporary speeding up of heart rate that occurs when blood pressure falls *(19) / page 296*

refractory period (ree-FRAK-tor-ee) time during which the myocardial cells rest and are not able to contract *(23) / page 363*

releasing hormones hormones secreted by the hypothalamus that travel via blood vessels a short distance to tell the pituitary which hormone to release *(33) / page 551*

renal failure decrease in the kidneys' ability to maintain electrolyte and fluid balance and excrete waste products *(18) / page 276*

renin-angiotensin-aldosterone system (RAAS) (REN-in–an-geo-TEN-sin-al-DOS-ter-own) series of enzymatic steps by which the body raises blood pressure *(19) / page 300*

respiration (res-purr-AY-shun) exchange of oxygen and carbon dioxide *(30) / page 492*

reticular activating system (RAS) the brain structure that projects from the brainstem and thalamus to the cerebral cortex; responsible for sleeping and wakefulness and performs an alerting function *(10) / page 124*

reticular formation (re-TIK-u-lurr) a network of neurons found along the entire length of the brainstem connected with the reticular activating system *(10) / page 124*

retinoids (RETT-ih-noydz) vitamin A-like compounds used in the treatment of severe acne and psoriasis *(37) / page 631*

retinol (RETT-in-nall) chemical name for vitamin A *(37) / page 632*

reverse transcriptase (ree-VERS trans-CRIP-tace) viral enzyme that converts RNA to DNA *(28) / page 454*

rheumatoid arthritis (RA) (ROO-mah-toyd are-THRYE-tis) systemic autoimmune disorder characterized by inflammation of multiple joints *(36) / page 615*

rosacea (roh-ZAY-shee-uh) skin disorder characterized by clusters of papules *(37) / page 631*

routine orders orders not written as single, STAT, or prn *(3) / page 27*

salicylism (sal-IH-sill-izm) poisoning due to aspirin and aspirin-like drugs *(25) / page 398*

scabicides (SKAY-bih-sides) drugs that kill scabies and mites *(37) / page 628*

scabies (SKAY-beez) skin disorder caused by the female mite burrowing into the skin and laying eggs *(37) / page 627*

scheduled drugs in the United States, a term describing a drug placed into one of five categories (I through V) based on its potential for misuse or abuse *(2) / page 19*

schizoaffective disorder (SKIT-soh-ah-FEK-tiv) disorder with symptoms similar to schizophrenia and mood disorders *(12) / page 163*

schizophrenia (SKIT-soh-FREN-ee-uh) type of psychosis characterized by abnormal thoughts and thought processes, withdrawal from other people and the outside environment, and apparent preoccupation with one's own mental state *(12) / page 162*

seasonal affective disorder (SAD) depression experienced during the winter months; associated with a reduced release of the brain neurohormone melatonin *(11) / page 141*

seborrhea (seb-oh-REE-ah) condition characterized by overactivity of oil glands *(37) / page 630*

secondary parkinsonism results from abnormal neuronal activity in areas of the corpus striatum and substantia nigra mainly due to medications, such as those used to treat psychosis, major psychiatric disorders, or nausea *(12) / page 167*

secretion movement of substances from the blood into the kidney tubule after filtration has occurred *(18) / page 276*

sedative-hypnotic (SED-ah-tiv hip-NOT-ik) drug that produces a calming effect when given in lower doses, and produces sleep when given in higher doses *(10) / page 126*

sedatives (SED-ah-tivs) drugs that relax or calm the patient *(10) / page 126*

seizure (SEE-zhurr) symptom of epilepsy characterized by abnormal neuronal discharges within the brain *(14) / page 204*

selective estrogen-receptor modulators (SERMs) drugs that directly produce an action similar to estrogen in body tissues; used for the treatment of osteoporosis in postmenopausal women *(36) / page 610*

selective serotonin-reuptake inhibitors (SSRIs) (sir-eh-TO-nin) drugs that selectively inhibit the reuptake of serotonin into nerve terminals *(11) / page 144*

sentinel event one that results in an unexpected, serious, or fatal injury following the administration (or lack of administration) of a medication *(6) / page 67*

septic shock (SEP-tik) type of shock caused by severe infection in the bloodstream *(22) / page 347*

serotonin-norepinephrine reuptake inhibitors (SNRIs) drugs that block the recycling of two neurotransmitters, serotonin and norepinephrine *(11) / page 146*

serotonin syndrome (SES) a set of signs and symptoms associated with overmedication with antidepressants *(11) / page 145*

shock condition in which there is inadequate blood flow to meet the body's needs *(22) / page 347*

side effects nontherapeutic reactions to a drug *(3) / page 25*

single order a physician's order for a drug that is to be given only once and at a specific time; an example is a preoperative order *(3) / page 27*

sinoatrial (SA) node (si-no-AYE-tree-ul noad) center of autorhythmicity, the ability of excitable cells to rhythmically generate their own action potentials in the heart *(23) / page 361*

situational depression short-term depression resulting from circumstances in a person's life *(11) / page 141*

six rights of drug administration practical guidelines for nurses to use during drug preparation, delivery, and administration of drugs *(3) / page 25*

social anxiety disorder social phobia, a kind of anxiety disorder characterized by excessive and unreasonable fear of social situations *(10) / page 122*

sodium ion channels (SO-dee-um) pathways in the plasma membrane that allow sodium ions to enter the cell during an action potential *(23) / page 362*

somatotropin (so-mat-oh-TROH-pin) another name for growth hormone *(33) / page 555*

spasticity (spas-TISS-ih-tee) condition in which certain muscle groups remain in a continuous contracted state *(13) / page 193*

specialty supplements dietary products intended to enhance (or complement) a specific body function, such as supporting joint health or immune function *(7) / page 77*

stable angina type of angina that occurs in a predictable pattern, usually relieved by rest *(21) / page 330*

standing order a physician's order written in advance of a situation, which is to be carried out under specific circumstances *(3) / page 27*

STAT order comes from *statim*, the Latin word meaning "immediately"; the time frame between writing the STAT order and administering the drug may be five minutes or less, depending on facility rules *(3) / page 27*

status asthmaticus (STAT-us az-MAT-ik-us) acute form of asthma requiring immediate medical attention *(30) / page 503*

status epilepticus (ep-ih-LEP-tih-kus) condition characterized by repeated seizures *(14) / page 207*

stroke a major cause of permanent disability caused by blockage of blood to the brain or rupture of a blood vessel in the brain *(21) / page 341*

subcutaneous route (sub-kew-TAY-nee-us) method of parenteral drug delivery in which drugs are injected into the hypodermis of the skin *(3) / page 37*

sublingual (SL) route (sub-LIN-gwal) method of enteral drug delivery in which drugs are placed under the tongue *(3) / page 32*

substance abuse the self-administration of a drug in a way that one's culture or society views as abnormal and unacceptable *(8) / page 83*

substance dependence when a person has an overwhelming desire to take a drug and cannot stop *(8) / page 83*

substance P neurotransmitter within the spinal cord involved in the neural transmission of pain *(15) / page 224*

superficial mycoses fungal diseases of the hair, skin, nails, and mucous membranes *(28) / page 447*

superinfection condition caused when a microorganism grows rapidly as a result of having less competition in its environment *(27) / page 426*

sustained-release tablets or capsules that are designed to dissolve very slowly *(3) / page 31*

sympathetic nervous system (SIM-pah-THET-ik) portion of the autonomic system that is active during periods of stress and which produces the fight-or-flight response *(9) / page 101*

sympatholytics (SIM-path-oh-LIT-iks) drugs that block the actions of the sympathetic nervous system *(9) / page 105*

sympathomimetics (sim-path-oh-mih-MET-iks) drugs that mimic the actions of the sympathetic nervous system *(9) / page 105*

systemic mycoses fungal diseases affecting internal organs *(28) / page 448*

systolic pressure (SIS-tol-ik) blood pressure during the contraction phase of heart activity *(19) / page 293*

T cell type of lymphocyte that is essential for the cell-mediated immune response *(26) / page 408*

tardive dyskinesia (TAR-div dis-ki-NEE-zee-uh) involuntary movements of facial muscles and the tongue that occur due to long-term antipsychotic therapy *(12) / page 167*

targeted therapies antineoplastic drugs that target specific aspects of cancer cell physiology *(29) / page 480*

taxanes (TAKS-anez) natural antineoplastics isolated from the Pacific yew *(29) / page 477*

tension headache common type of head pain caused by stress and relieved by nonnarcotic analgesics *(15) / page 235*

teratogen any substance that will harm a developing fetus or embryo *(2) / page 20*

termination of drug action when the drug effect stops *(4) / page 49*

testosterone (test-AHST-erh-own) the primary male sex hormone responsible for male secondary sex characteristics *(35) / page 586*

therapeutic classification (ther-ah-PEW-tik) method for organizing drugs on the basis of their *therapeutic usefulness (2) / page 15*

therapeutic (therah-PEW-tick) range the plasma drug concentration *between* the minimum effective concentration and the toxic concentration *(4) / page 49*

therapeutic interchange exchange of medicines within the same therapeutic or pharmacologic class that may be authorized for distribution to patients through an interdisciplinary approach *(2) / page 19*

therapeutic lifestyle changes nondrug changes that, when implemented, can reduce blood cholesterol levels *(17) / page 261*

therapeutics (ther-ah-PEW-tiks) the branch of medicine concerned with the treatment of disease and suffering *(1) / page 4*

three checks of drug administration checks used by nurses together with the six rights to help ensure patient safety and drug effectiveness *(3) / page 26*

thrombin (THROM-bin) enzyme formed in coagulating blood from prothrombin; it converts fibrinogen to fibrin, which forms the basis of a blood clot *(24) / page 376*

thromboembolic disorder (THROM-bow-EM-bow-lik) disease associated with the formation of blood clots *(24) / page 377*

thrombolytics (throm-bow-LIT-iks) drugs used to dissolve existing blood clots *(24) / page 378*

thrombotic stroke (throm-BOT-ik) type of stroke caused by a blood clot blocking an artery in the brain *(21) / page 341*

thrombus (THROM-bus) blood clot *(24) / page 377*

tissue plasminogen activator (tPA) natural enzyme and a drug that dissolves blood clots *(24) / page 377*

titer (TIE-ter) measurement of the amount of a substance in the blood *(26) / page 409*

tocolytics (toh-koh-LIT-iks) drugs used to inhibit uterine contractions *(35) / page 594*

tolerance (TOL-er-ans) the process of adapting to a drug over time and requiring higher doses to achieve the same effect *(8) / page 86*

tonometry (toh-NAHM-uh-tree) technique for measuring eye tension and pressure *(38) / page 642*

topical route (TOP-ik-ul) the route by which drugs are placed directly onto the skin and associated membranes *(3) / page 33*

topoisomerase (TOH-poh-eye-SOM-er-ase) enzyme that assists in the repair of DNA damage *(29) / page 477*

total parenteral nutrition (TPN) treatment of undernutrition through the parenteral infusion of dextrose, amino acids, emulsified fats, vitamins, and minerals *(32) / page 543*

toxic concentration the level of drug that will result in serious adverse effects *(4) / page 49*

toxins (TOX-inz) chemicals produced by a microorganism that are able to cause injury to its host *(27) / page 423*

toxoid vaccines (TOX-oid vaks-EENs) vaccines containing bacterial toxins that have been chemically modified to be incapable of causing disease *(26) / page 410*

trade name proprietary name of a drug assigned by the manufacturer; also called the *brand name* or *product name* *(2) / page 17*

transdermal (trans-DER-mul) method of drug delivery, usually by a patch, in which drugs are absorbed across the layers of the skin for the purpose of entering the bloodstream *(3) / page 33*

transmucosal (trans-mew-KOH-sul) method of topical drug delivery in which drugs are applied directly to mucosal membranes, including the nasal and respiratory pathways and vagina *(3) / page 35*

transplant rejection when the immune system recognizes a transplanted tissue as being foreign and attacks it *(26) / page 413*

tricyclic antidepressants (TCAs) (treye-SICK-lick) drugs with a three-ring chemical structure that inhibit the reuptake of norepinephrine and serotonin into nerve terminals *(11) / page 146*

triglycerides (tri-GLISS-ur-ide) types of lipid that contain three fatty acids and a chemical backbone of glycerol *(17) / page 259*

triple therapy common therapy for the management of PUD consisting of a combination of a proton pump inhibitor plus two antibiotics *(31) / page 519*

tubercles (TOO-burr-kyouls) cavity-like lesions in the lung characteristic of infection by *Mycobacterium tuberculosis* *(27) / page 439*

tumor (TOO-more) abnormal swelling or mass *(29) / page 468*

tumor suppressor genes genes that inhibit the transformation of normal cells into cancer cells *(29) / page 468*

type 1 diabetes mellitus (die-uh-BEE-tees MEL-uh-tiss) disease characterized by lack of secretion of insulin by the pancreas that usually begins in the early teens *(34) / page 572*

type 2 diabetes mellitus disease characterized by insufficient secretion of insulin by the pancreas or by lack of sensitivity of insulin receptors that usually begins in middle age, though increasingly diagnosed in younger people *(34) / page 575*

ulcerative colitis (UL-sir-ah-tiv koh-LIE-tuss) inflammatory bowel disease of the colon *(31) / page 519*

undernutrition taking in or absorbing fewer nutrients than required for normal body growth and maintenance *(32) / page 542*

unstable angina type of angina that occurs frequently with severe symptoms and that is not relieved by rest *(21) / page 330*

uricosurics (YOUR-ik-cose-youriks) drugs that increase the excretion of uric acid by blocking its reabsorption in the kidney *(36) / page 617*

urinary antiseptics drugs given by the PO route for their antibacterial action in the urinary tract *(27) / page 436*

urticaria (EHR-tik-air-ee-ah) raised, red, itchy bumps, commonly referred to as hives *(37) / page 625*

vaccination (VAK-sin-AYE-shun) the process of introducing a foreign substance (a vaccine) into the body to trigger immune activation *before* the patient is exposed to the real pathogen *(26) / page 409*

vaccines (vaks-EEN)s preparations of microorganism particles that are injected into a patient to stimulate the immune system with the intention of preventing disease *(26) / page 407*

vasomotor center (VAZO-mo-tor) area of the medulla that controls baseline blood pressure *(19) / page 295*

vasopressin (vaz-oh-PRESS-in) another name for antidiuretic hormone *(33) / page 555*

vasospastic (Prinzmetal's) angina type of angina in which decreased myocardial blood flow is caused by *spasms* of the coronary arteries *(21) / page 330*

ventilation (ven-tah-LAY-shun) process by which air is moved into and out of the lungs *(30) / page 492*

very low-density lipoprotein (VLDL) lipid-carrying particle that is converted to LDL in the liver *(17) / page 260*

vinca alkaloids (VIN-ka AL-kah-loids) chemicals obtained from the periwinkle plant *(29) / page 477*

virulence (VEER-you-lens) the severity of disease that an organism is able to cause *(27) / page 423*

virulization (veer-you-lih-ZAY-shun) appearance of masculine secondary sex characteristics *(35) / page 595*

viruses nonliving particles containing RNA or DNA that are able to cause disease *(28) / page 452*

vitamins organic compounds required by the body in small amounts *(32) / page 536*

withdrawal syndrome (with-DRAW-ul SIN-drom) unpleasant symptoms experienced when a physically dependent client discontinues the use of an abused drug *(8) / page 85*

yeasts (YEESTz) type of fungus that is unicellular and divides by budding *(28) / page 447*

Zollinger–Ellison syndrome (ZOLL-in-jer ELL-ih-sun) disorder of having excess acid secretion in the stomach *(31) / page 520*

Index

Indexing style: Prototype drugs appear in **bold face**. Information in tables is denoted with a "*t*" after the page number. Information in figures is denoted with an "*f*" after the page number.

D

H

I

J

K

L

M

P

Q

R

T

U

V

W

X

Y

Z

Credits

Photo Credits

Cover: ESB Professional/Shutterstock

Chapter 1: Page 1 (middle right): LaCameraChiara/Shutterstock; Pages 1 (top), 2, 12: Nomad Soul/Shutterstock; Page 1 (middle left): Real Deal Photo/Shutterstock; Page 1 (bottom): Sheff/Shutterstock

Chapter 2: Pages 14, 21: Dirk Ecken/Shutterstock

Chapter 3: Pages 23, 42: Sheff/Shutterstock

Chapter 4: Pages 44, 53: Alexander Raths/Shutterstock

Chapter 5: Pages 55, 62: Real Deal Photo/Shutterstock

Chapter 6: Pages 64, 69: Svetamart/Fotolia

Chapter 7: Pages 71, 80: Olga Miltsova

Chapter 8: Pages 82, 97: LaCameraChiara/Shutterstock

Chapter 9: Page 99 (middle right): Bikeriderlondon/Shutterstock; Page 99 (middle left): DALSTOK/Shutterstock; Page 99 (bottom): Michael Spring/Fotolia; Pages 99 (top), 100, 118: Vbaleha/Fotolia.

Chapter 10: Pages 120, 137: ChameleonsEye/Shutterstock

Chapter 11: Pages 139, 159: Picture Factory/Fotolia

Chapter 12: Pages 161, 176: DALSTOK/Shutterstock

Chapter 13: Pages 178, 201: Jenny Sturm/Shutterstock

Chapter 14: Pages 203, 219: Bikeriderlondon/Shutterstock

Chapter 15: Pages 221, 240: Michael Spring/Fotolia

Chapter 16: Pages 242, 255: pzRomashka/Shutterstock

Chapter 17: Page 257 (top): PT Images/Shutterstock; Page 257 (middle left): Larry Mulvehill/Science Source; Page 257 (middle right): Monkey Business Images/Shutterstock; Page 257 (bottom): Jack Cronkhite/Shutterstock; Pages 258, 271: Upthebanner/Shutterstock

Chapter 18: Pages 273, 289: PT Images/Shutterstock

Chapter 19: Pages 291, 312: Gstockstudio/Fotolia

Chapter 20: Pages 314, 327: Hunta/Fotolia

Chapter 22: Pages 346, 357: Larry Mulvehill/Science Source

Chapter 23: Pages 358, 372: Jack Cronkhite/Shutterstock

Chapter 24: Pages 374, 390: Monkey Business Images/Shutterstock

Chapter 25: Page 393 (middle Left): Felix Mizioznikov/Shutterstock; Page 393 (middle right): Lisa F. Young/Shutterstock; Pages 393 (top), 394, 404: Amble Design/Shutterstock; Page 393 (bottom): Poznyakov/Shutterstock

Chapter 26: Pages 406, 418: Felix Mizioznikov/Shutterstock

Chapter 27: Pages 420, 445: Poznyakov/Shutterstock

Chapter 28: Pages 446, 464: Focus Pocus LTD/Fotolia

Chapter 29: Pages 466, 487: Lisa F. Young/Shutterstock

Chapter 30: Page 489 (bottom left): Happymay/Shutterstock; Pages 489 (top), 490, 512: Stephen Orsillo/Shutterstock; Page 489 (bottom right): Svyatoslav Lypynskyy/Fotolia

Chapter 31: Pages 514, 533: Happymay/Shutterstock

Chapter 32: Pages 535, 546: Svyatoslav Lypynskyy/Fotolia

Chapter 33: Page 549 (bottom left): Flashon Studio/Shutterstock; Page 549 (bottom right): Pathdoc/Fotolia

Chapter 34: Pages 569, 582: Flashon Studio/Shutterstock

Chapter 35: Pages 584, 601: pathdoc/Fotolia

Chapter 36: Page 603 (bottom right): Jeffrey B. Banke/Shutterstock; Page 603 (bottom left): Jorg Hackemann/Shutterstock; Pages 603 (top), 604, 621: T-Design/Shutterstock

Chapter 37: Pages 623, 637: Jorg Hackemann/Shutterstock

Chapter 38: Pages 639, 651: Jeffrey B. Banke/Shutterstock